THE PHYSICIAN'S GUIDE TO DIVING MEDICINE

THE PHYSICIAN'S GUIDE TO DIVING MEDICINE

Edited by
Charles W. Shilling
Catherine B. Carlston
and
Rosemary A. Mathias

Undersea Medical Society
Bethesda, Maryland

PLENUM PRESS • NEW YORK AND LONDON

Library of Congress Cataloging in Publication Data

Main entry under title:

The Physician's guide to diving medicine.

Includes bibliographies and index.

1. Submarine medicine. 2. Diving, Submarine—Physiological aspects. I. Shilling, Charles W. (Charles Wesley) II. Carlston, Catherine B. III. Mathias, Rosemary A. IV. Undersea Medical Society. [DNLM: 1. Diving. 2. Submarine Medicine. WD 650 P577]
RC1005.P49   1984   616.9'8022   84-14817
ISBN 0-306-41428-7

©1984 Plenum Press, New York
A Division of Plenum Publishing Corporation
233 Spring Street, New York, N.Y. 10013

All rights reserved

No part of this book may be reproduced, stored in a retrieval system, or transmitted in any form or by any means, electronic, mechanical, photocopying, microfilming, recording, or otherwise, without written permission from the Publisher

Printed in the United States of America

Contributors

The contributors who authored this book are listed alphabetically below. Their names also appear in the text following contributed chapters or sections.

N. R. Anthonisen, M.D., Ph.D.
Professor of Medicine
University of Manitoba
Winnipeg, Manitoba, Canada

Arthur J. Bachrach, Ph.D.
Director, Environmental Stress Program
Naval Medical Research Institute
Bethesda, Maryland

C. Gresham Bayne, M.D.
Assistant Adjunct Professor of Medicine
University of California, San Diego

Albert R. Behnke, Jr., M.D.
Adjunct Professor of Exercise Science
University of Massachusetts, Amherst

Peter B. Bennett, Ph.D.
Director, F. G. Hall Laboratory
Duke University Medical Center
Durham, North Carolina

Walter R. Bergman
Special Assistant for Diving
Naval Sea Systems Command
Washington, District of Columbia

Robert J. Biersner, Ph.D.
Naval Medical Research and Development Command
Bethesda, Maryland

Mark E. Bradley, M.D.
Naval Medical Research Institute
Bethesda, Maryland

Carl Edmonds, M.B., B.S. — Diving Medical Centre, Cremorne, New South Wales, Australia

Delbert E. Evans, Ph.D. — Naval Medical Research Institute, Bethesda, Maryland

Morris D. Faiman, Ph.D. — Department of Pharmacology and Toxicology, University of Kansas, Lawrence

Joseph C. Farmer, Jr., M.D. — Division of Otolaryngology, Duke University Medical Center, Durham, North Carolina

William P. Fife, Ph.D. — Professor of Physiology, Texas A & M University, Bryan

Harold M. Ginzburg, M.D. — National Institute on Drug Abuse, Bethesda, Maryland

Robert F. Goad, M.D. — U.S. Navy Medical Corps, Duke University Medical Center, Durham, North Carolina

John M. Hallenbeck, M.D. — Naval Medical Research Institute, Bethesda, Maryland

R. W. Hamilton, Ph.D. — Hamilton Research, Ltd., Tarrytown, New York

George B. Hart, M.D. — Director, Baromedical Department, Memorial Hospital Medical Center, Long Beach, California

H. V. Hempleman, Ph.D. — Superintendent, Admiralty Marine Technology Establishment, Alverstoke, United Kingdom

Donald D. Hickey, M.D. — Hyperbaric Research Laboratory, Department of Physiology, State University of New York at Buffalo

Suk Ki Hong, M.D., Ph.D. — Department of Physiology, State University of New York at Buffalo

Eric P. Kindwall, M.D. — Director, Department of Hyperbaric Medicine
St. Luke's Hospital
Milwaukee, Wisconsin

Jo Ann S. Kinney, Ph.D. — Naval Submarine Medical Research Laboratory
Groton, Connecticut

Kenneth W. Kizer, M.D., M.P.H. — Division of Occupational Medicine
University of California, San Francisco

David R. Leitch, M.B., Ch.B., Ph.D., M.F.O.M. — Institute of Naval Medicine, Royal Navy
Gosport, United Kingdom

Paul G. Linaweaver, Jr., M.D. — Santa Barbara Medical Foundation Clinic
Santa Barbara, California

Claes E. G. Lundgren, M.D., Ph.D. — Hyperbaric Research Laboratory
Department of Physiology
State University of New York at Buffalo

H. F. Nicodemus, M.D. — Chairman, Department of Anesthesia
Naval Hospital, Bethesda, Maryland

Arvid Påsche, M.Sc. — Research Scientist
Norwegian Underwater Technology Center
Bergen, Norway

R. R. Pearson, M.D., M.F.O.M. — Institute of Naval Medicine
Alverstoke, United Kingdom

David H. Peterson, B.S. — National Oceanic and Atmospheric Administration
Rockville, Maryland

Paul J. Sheffield, Ph.D. — Hyperbaric Medicine Division
USAF School of Aerospace Medicine
Brooks Air Force Base, Texas

Charles W. Shilling, M.D. — Executive Secretary
Undersea Medical Society, Inc.
Bethesda, Maryland

Joel Kevin Sims, M.D. — Chief, Emergency Medical Services Systems Branch
Department of Health, Hawaii
Honolulu, Hawaii

Charles J. Stahl, M.D.   Professor of Pathology
                               Quillen-Disner College of Medicine
                               East Tennessee State University, Johnson City

Barbara B. Tabeling, M.D.   Department of Anesthesiology
                               Mercy Hospital, Urbana, Illinois

D. N. Walder, M.D.   Department of Surgery
                               University of Newcastle-upon-Tyne
                               United Kingdom

J. Michael Walsh, Ph.D.   National Institute on Drug Abuse
                               Bethesda, Maryland

Reviewers

An expert reviewer was selected for each chapter. Their voluntary effort is greatly appreciated. They are listed alphabetically.

E. E. P. Barnard, M.B., B.S., D.Phil.	Operational Medical Services, Royal Navy Institute of Naval Medicine Alverstoke, United Kingdom
C. Gresham Bayne, M.D.	Assistant Adjunct Professor of Medicine University of California, San Diego
Alfred A. Bove, M.D., Ph.D.	Mayo Medical School and Mayo Clinic Rochester, Minnesota
John M. Hallenbeck, M.D.	Naval Medical Research Institute Bethesda, Maryland
R. deG. Hanson, M.D., Ph.D.	Consultant in Occupational Medicine Royal Navy, United Kingdom
William L. Hunter, Jr., M.D.	Naval Regional Medical Center Jacksonville, Florida
Paul G. Linaweaver, Jr., M.D.	Santa Barbara Medical Foundation Santa Barbara, California
Norman K. I. McIver, M.B., B.S.	North Sea Medical Center Great Yarmouth, United Kingdom
John Naquin, M.A.	Naval Medical Research Institute Bethesda, Maryland

Reviewers

Lawrence W. Raymond, M.D.	Assistant Medical Director Exxon Corporation, New York Associate Professor, Cornell University Medical College, New York, New York
Albert J. Smith	U.S. Navy
Edward D. Thalmann, M.D.	U.S. Navy Experimental Diving Unit Panama City, Florida
O. E. VanDerAue, M.D.	U.S. Navy (Retired) Washington, District of Columbia
James Vorosmarti, Jr., M.D.	Commanding Officer Naval Medical Research Institute Bethesda, Maryland
S. A. Warner, D.Sc.	Department of Energy United Kingdom

Advisory Committee

James Vorosmarti, Jr., M.D.　　　Commanding Officer
　　　　　　　　　　　　　　　　Naval Medical Research Institute
　　　　　　　　　　　　　　　　Bethesda, Maryland

Robert C. Bornmann, M.D.　　　　Medical Corps, U.S. Navy

Claes E. G. Lundgren, M.D., Ph.D.　Hyperbaric Research Laboratory
　　　　　　　　　　　　　　　　Department of Physiology
　　　　　　　　　　　　　　　　State University of New York at Buffalo

Preface

This book is designed to be a physician's guide for those interested in diving and hyperbaric environments. It is not a detailed document for the erudite researcher; rather, it is a source of information for the scuba-diving physician who is searching for answers put to him by his fellow nonmedical divers.

Following the publication of *The Underwater Handbook: A Guide to Physiology and Performance for the Engineer* there were frequent requests for a companion volume for the physician. This book is designed to fill the void. Production of the book has been supported by the Office of Naval Research and by the Bureau of Medicine and Surgery, Research and Development Command, under Navy Contract No. N000014-78-C-0604.

Our heartfelt thanks go to the many authors without whose contributions the book could not have been produced. These articles are signed by the responsible authors, and the names are also listed alphabetically in these preliminary pages.

Every chapter was officially reviewed by at least one expert in the field covered and these reviewers are also listed on these pages. Our thanks go to them for their valuable assistance.

We are grateful to Marthe Beckett Kent for editing Chapter III. Our thanks also go to Mrs. Carolyn Paddon for typing and retyping the manuscripts, and to Mrs. Catherine Coppola, who so expertly handled the many fiscal affairs.

The Advisory Committee—Drs. Vorosmarti, Lundgren, and Bornmann—along with the three of us have deliberated on every section of the text several times. We believe it covers the field adequately. The context, however, does not necessarily reflect the position of the Navy or the Government, and no official endorsement should be inferred.

CHARLES W. SHILLING
CATHERINE B. CARLSTON
ROSEMARY A. MATHIAS

Foreword

Submarine Medicine Practice (NAVMED P-5054) was a Navy classic. Published initially in 1956, it was a beautifully written training text and reference for the Navy submarine and diving medical officer. Very popular inside and outside the Navy, within the U.S.A. and overseas, its appearance was also timely as deep diving and underwater swimming began the tremendous development and expansion which they experienced in the 1960s and 1970s. Physicians and medical scientists were taxed to make these longer and deeper dives possible, useful, and safe. The subsequent explosion of new information and new applications eventually outstripped the descriptions of "Submed Practice." But no second edition, revision, or new volume was published by the Navy. It would be a daunting task—outside the single ability of any one man, no matter how brilliant, inspired, or hard working. However, with the establishment of the Undersea Medical Society as an active force in the continuing education of the diving medical community, and especially after the assumption of the job of Executive Secretary by Charles W. Shilling, there was an organization with an energetic leader/editor to whom the Navy could turn to put the necessary book together.

This volume is truly a community effort. The roll of authors, reviewers, and editors spans the professional membership of the Undersea Medical Society. It is an afghan of varied-size pieces that have been interwoven and stitched together by the Editor into a final pattern of his design. For the three of us in the Management Committee it has been a rewarding and stimulating task to work with Chuck Shilling in the production of this, his latest book.

ROBERT C. BORNMANN
CLAES E. G. LUNDGREN
JAMES VOROSMARTI, JR.

Contents

I
The Diving Environment

A.	Introduction .... Charles W. Shilling	1
B.	Types of Diving .... Charles W. Shilling	1
	1. General	1
	2. Breath-Hold Diving	2
	3. Scuba Diving	3
	4. Surface-Supplied Diving	4
	5. Bounce Diving	4
	6. Saturation Diving	4
	7. Excursion Diving	6
C.	Natural Diving Environments .... Charles W. Shilling	6
	1. General	6
	2. Oceans	6
	3. Lakes	7
	4. Rivers	7
	5. Harbors	7
	6. Cave Diving	8
	7. Diving in Kelp	8
	8. Diving in Polluted Water	9
	9. Diving in Wrecks	9
	10. Diving in Cold Water	10
	11. Diving under Ice	10
References		12
D.	Man-Made Diving Environments .... R. W. Hamilton	12
	1. Introduction	12
	2. Caissons and Tunnels	12
	3. Deck Decompression Chambers	14
	4. Diving Systems	16
	5. System Characteristics	21

6. Hyperbaric Facilities 26
7. Rescue Chambers 28
8. Undersea Habitats and Underwater Welding Chambers 30
References 32

II
Physics of Diving and Physical Effects on Divers

Charles W. Shilling and Morris D. Faiman

A. Introduction 35
B. Pressure 35
   1. Units of Pressure 36
   2. Pressure Nomenclature 36
C. Pathophysiology of Gases Associated With Diving 37
   1. Air 38
   2. Oxygen 38
      a. Description 38
      b. Partial Pressure 39
      c. Toxicity 39
      d. Use of High Pressure Oxygen (HBO) 41
   3. Nitrogen 41
      a. Description 41
      b. Physiological Effects 42
   4. Helium 42
   5. Hydrogen 43
   6. Neon 43
   7. Carbon Dioxide 43
      a. Description 43
      b. Human Production 44
      c. Control of Breathing 44
      d. Transport 45
      e. Symptoms and Signs of Carbon Dioxide Retention 45
      f. Diving Implications 46
      g. Causes of Carbon Dioxide Excess 46
      h. Remedial Measures and Prevention 47
   8. Carbon Monoxide 47
      a. Description 47
      b. Causes of Carbon Monoxide Poisoning in Diving 47
      c. Symptoms 48
      d. Treatment 49
D. Gas Laws 49
   1. Boyle's Law 49
   2. Charles' Law 51
   3. General Gas Law 51
   4. Dalton's Law 52
   5. Henry's Law 54

E.	Characteristics of Gas		54
	1. Diffusion		54
	2. Moisture		55
	3. Density		55
	4. Viscosity		55
F.	Buoyancy		56
G.	Energy in Diving		57
	1. Light		57
	2. Sound		58
	3. Heat		58
	4. Temperature		59
	5. Specific Heat		59
	6. Conduction		59
	7. Convection		60
	8. Radiation, Evaporation		60
H.	Effects of Changing Pressure on the Diver		60
	1. Aural Barotrauma		60
	2. Blowup		61
	3. Gastrointestinal Barotrauma		66
	4. Pulmonary Barotrauma		66
	5. Sinus Barotrauma		67
	6. Squeeze		67
	7. Toothache or Aerodontalgia		68
	8. Vertigo		68
I.	Summary		68
References			68

III
Physiology of Diving

A.	Respiration	N. R. Anthonisen	71
	1. Lung Volumes: Effects of Gas Compression and Expansion		71
	a. Dynamics of Gas Flow in the Lungs		74
	2. Gas Density, Ventilation Distribution, Gas Exchange		80
	a. Control of Ventilation and Carbon Dioxide Retention		81
References			84
B.	Immersion Effects	Claes E. G. Lundgren and A. J. Påsche	86
	1. Respiratory Function		87
	2. Circulatory Function		91
	a. Significance		92
	3. Renal Effects		94
	a. Significance		95
	4. Gastrointestinal System Effects		95
	a. Significance		96
	5. Buoyancy Effects		97
References			98
C.	Cardiovascular Effects	Delbert E. Evans	99
	1. Hyperbaric Bradycardia		100
	a. Early Studies		100

		b.	Effects of Increased Partial Pressure of Oxygen	100

		b.	Effects of Increased Partial Pressure of Oxygen	100
		c.	Effects of Increased Gas Density	101
		d.	Effects of Increased Hydrostatic Pressure	102
		e.	Effects of Increased Gas Tensions of Helium and Nitrogen	104
		f.	Autonomic Mediation of Hyperbaric Bradycardia	105
	2.	Cardiovascular Effects of Saturation Exposure		106
	3.	Summary		107
References				107
D.	High Pressure Nervous Syndrome .... Peter B. Bennett			109
	1.	Signs and Symptoms in Man		109
	2.	Strategies for Amelioration of HPNS		117
		a.	Variation in Susceptibility and Personnel Selection	117
		b.	Choice of Compression Rate	117
		c.	Use of Excursions	118
		d.	Adaptation	120
		e.	Use of Narcotic Agents	120
References				126
E.	Inert Gas Narcosis .... Albert R. Behnke, Jr.			128
	1.	Nitrogen Narcosis		128
	2.	Other Gases and Narcosis		130
		a.	Argon	130
		b.	Xenon	130
		c.	Helium	130
		d.	Neon	131
		e.	Hydrogen	131
	3.	Quantification of Narcotic Effects		131
		a.	Rapid Compression Effects	132
		b.	Carbon Dioxide Effects	132
		c.	Individual Differences in Narcotic Response	132
	4.	Mechanisms of Action Underlying Inert Gas Narcosis		132
	5.	Inert Gas Effects		133
		a.	Model Surface Membrane Effects	133
		b.	Inert Gas Protection against the High Pressure Nervous Syndrome	133
		c.	Opposing Physiological Effects of Pressure and Inert Gases	134
		d.	Clinical Use of Nitrogen Narcosis as a Benign Stress	134
References				135
F.	Women and Diving .... William P. Fife			136
	1.	History		136
	2.	Physical Performance and Adaptability		136
	3.	Decompression Sickness		137
		a.	Extra Fat Burden	137
		b.	Oral Contraceptives	138
		c.	Intrauterine Devices	138
		d.	Premenstrual Fluid Retention and Menstruation	138
		e.	Summary	139

	4.	Pregnancy and Diving	140
	5.	Questions Frequently Asked	143
References			143
G.	Monitoring of Vital Signs; Doppler Monitoring ....C. Gresham Bayne		144
	1.	Voice Communication	146
	2.	Cardiovascular Monitors	146
	3.	Pulmonary Monitoring	147
	4.	Temperature Monitoring	148
	5.	Bubble Detection	149
		a. Ultrasound Research and Methods	150
		b. Clinical Significance	151
References			152
H.	Thermal Considerations ....Suk Ki Hong		153
	1.	Heat Exchanges in Air at One Atmosphere	153
	2.	Thermal Balance in Water at One Atmosphere Absolute	156
		a. Heat Transfer Coefficient of Water and Critical Water Temperature	156
		b. Quantity of Heat Loss	157
		c. Protection by Wet Suits	159
		d. Regional Heat Loss	162
		e. Effects of Exercise	163
		f. Symptoms of Severe and Prolonged Cold Exposure	165
		g. Treatment of Immersion Hypothermia	166
		h. Effects of Alcohol and Marijuana	167
		i. Cold Acclimatization	168
	3.	Thermal Balance in Dry Hyperbaric Environments	169
		a. Heat Transfer Properties	169
		b. Heat Exchange	172
	4.	Thermal Balance in Wet Hyperbaric Environments	175
References			177
I.	Metabolism and Dietary Effects ....Suk Ki Hong		178
	1.	Energy Metabolism in Divers	181
		a. Energy Metabolism in the Ama	181
		b. Energy Metabolism in Saturation Divers	183
	2.	Electrolyte Metabolism in Divers	186
	3.	Dietary Effects	187
References			188
J.	Hyperbaric Arthralgia ....Mark E. Bradley		190
References			192
K.	Vestibular and Auditory Function ....Joseph C. Farmer, Jr.		192
	1.	Auditory Function	193
	2.	Vestibular Function	195
References			198
L.	Vision ....Jo Ann S. Kinney		199
	1.	Physical Factors in Underwater Seeing	199
		a. Vision without a Face Mask	199

		b.	Effects of Refraction	199
		c.	Effects of Absorption and Scatter	201
	2.	Physiological Factors in Underwater Vision		203
		a.	Effect of Hyperbaric Oxygen	203
		b.	Effects of Nitrogen	204
		c.	Effect of Pressure	204
References				205
M.	Breath-Hold Diving .... Donald D. Hickey and Claes E. G. Lundgren			206
	1.	Physiology		206
		a.	Mammalian Dive Reflex	206
		b.	Limits of Breath Holding	207
		c.	Depth Limits of Breath-Hold Diving	214
		d.	Acclimatization to Breath-Hold Diving in Man	216
	2.	Medical Considerations		217
		a.	Drowning and Near-Drowning	217
		b.	Cardiological Considerations	217
		c.	Barotrauma	218
		d.	Decompression Sickness	219
		e.	Vertigo and Disorientation	219
References				220

IV
Decompression Theory H. V. Hempleman

A.	Introduction	223
B.	Defining the Problem	226
C.	The Haldane Concepts	229
D.	Using the Haldane Concepts	232
E.	Post-Haldane Difficulties	237
F.	U.S. Navy Initiative	242
G.	Diffusion vs. Perfusion	248
H.	Data From Tunnel Workers	254
I.	Bubble Generation and Growth	258
J.	Diving Tables Today	264
K.	General Observations	266
References		269

V
Immediate Medical Evaluation of the Diving Casualty Eric P. Kindwall

A.	Introduction		273
B.	Emergency Care		274
	1.	General Statement	274
	2.	Divers Alert Network	274
	3.	Diving Medics	274
	4.	Immediate Action	275

C.	Diagnosis		275
	1. Background		275
	2. Air Embolism		276
		a. General Statement	276
		b. Signs and Symptoms	276
		c. Emergency Treatment	276
	3. Decompression Sickness		277
		a. General Statement	277
		b. Symptoms	277
		c. Treatment	278
	4. Determining the Cause of the Accident		280
References			280

VI
Diagnosis and Treatment of Decompression Sickness

A.	General Survey .... Robert F. Goad		283
	1. History		283
	2. Symptoms and Signs		287
		a. Cutaneous and Lymphatic Symptoms	288
		b. Musculoskeletal Symptoms	289
		c. Central Neurological Symptoms	290
		d. Peripheral Neurological Symptoms	290
		e. Audiovestibular Symptoms	290
		f. Respiratory and Cardiovascular Symptoms	291
		g. Shock and Other Manifestations	291
		h. Aseptic Bone Necrosis	291
	3. Diagnosis		292
	4. Therapy		295
	5. New Ideas		309
References			310
B.	Inner Ear Decompression Sickness .... Joseph C. Farmer, Jr.		312
	1. Introduction		312
		a. Recent Human Studies	313
		b. Recent Animal Studies	314
	2. Management of Inner Ear Decompression Sickness		314
References			316
C.	Neurological Forms of Decompression Sickness David R. Leitch and John M. Hallenbeck		316
	1. Overview and Introduction		316
	2. Clinical Presentation		318
		a. Onset	318
		b. Signs and Symptoms	318
		c. Diagnosis	320
	3. Mechanisms of Neurological Decompression Sickness		321
	4. Prognosis		324

5. Concepts of Treatment 325
    a. Philosophy 325
    b. Initial Treatment 325
    c. Adjuvant Therapy 325
    d. Clinical Management 326
References 326
D. Delay After Decompression Sickness before Diving Again ....
.... R. W. Hamilton   328

VII
Diagnosis and Treatment of Gas Embolism   R. R. Pearson

A. Pulmonary Barotrauma and Arterial Gas Embolism 333
B. Pulmonary Barotrauma 333
  1. Introduction and Definitions 333
  2. Intravascular Gaseous Emboli 336
    a. Effect on Pulmonary Circulation 339
    b. Cerebral Arterial Gas Embolism 340
  3. Etiology of Pulmonary Barotrauma 344
  4. Presentation and Diagnosis 347
C. Arterial Gas Embolism 349
  1. Presentation 349
  2. Diagnosis 352
  3. Therapy 354
    a. Pressure 355
    b. Oxygen 357
    c. Adjuvant Therapy 358
  4. Relapse after Initial Response to Therapy 360
  5. Other Considerations 361
References 361

VIII
Near-Drowning   Barbara B. Tabeling

A. Definitions 369
B. Modifying Factors 370
C. History 370
D. Physiological Changes 372
  1. Oxygenation and Acid-Base Balance 372
  2. Anatomical Pulmonary Changes 373
  3. Blood Volume and Electrolyte Concentrations 374
  4. Cardiovascular System 375
  5. Hematology 376
  6. Renal Function 376
  7. Central Nervous System 376
  8. Infection 377
E. Treatment 378
  1. Immediate First Aid 378
  2. Emergency Transportation 379

	3.	Emergency Room Care	380
	4.	Respiratory Care	380
	5.	In-Hospital Monitoring and Therapy	382
	6.	Brain Resuscitation	383
	7.	Corticosteroids and Antibiotics	383
	8.	Hyperbaric Oxygen Therapy	384
	9.	Summary	384

Case Histories 385
    1   Case No. 1: DD, 1972 385
    2   Case No. 2: VYW, 1979 386
    3   Case No. 3: CV, 1980 387
References 387

IX
Diagnosis and Treatment of Other Diving-Related Conditions

A. The Unconscious Diver .... R. W. Hamilton 391
    1. Factors Leading to Loss of Consciousness 391
        a. Relevant Physiology 391
        b. Predisposing Conditions 392
        c. Environmental Factors 392
        d. Physiological Factors 394
    2. Recovering an Unconscious Diver 395
        a. Unconscious Diver in the Water 395
        b. Unconscious Bell or Habitat Diver 396
    3. Resuscitation 396
        a. Check Vital Signs 396
        b. Insert Airway 396
        c. Mouth-to-Mouth Resuscitation 396
        d. Cardiac Resuscitation 396
        e. Treat Significant Bleeding 397
        f. Transfer Injured Diver 397
        g. Report the Incident 397
References 397
B. Osteonecrosis .... D. N. Walder 397
    1. Introduction 397
    2. Diagnosis by Radiology 398
        a. Juxta-articular Lesions 399
        b. Head, Neck, and Shaft Lesions 400
    3. Other Methods of Diagnosis 400
    4. Clinical Management and Treatment 401
    5. Underlying Pathological Changes 402
    6. Etiology 402
Appendix 403
References 405

C. Microbes and the Diver .... Carl Edmonds and Charles W. Shilling 406
   1. Introduction 406
   2. Cross-Infections 406
   3. Diving with an Infection 406
   4. Local Infections Associated with Diving 407
      a. Sinusitis 407
      b. Skin Infection 407
      c. Infections from Wounds, Bites, Stings 408
   5. Systemic Infections 408
      a. Disease From Polluted Water 408
      b. Leptospirosis 408
      c. Pharyngoconjunctival Fever 408
      d. Near-Drowning 408
   References 409
D. Ear and Sinuses .... Joseph C. Farmer, Jr. 409
   1. Otologic Barotrauma 409
      a. Middle Ear Barotrauma 409
      b. External Ear Canal Barotrauma 414
      c. Inner Ear Barotrauma 414
   2. Otitis Externa 416
   3. Inner Ear Injuries at Stable Deep Depths 417
   4. Inner Ear Injuries and High Background Noise during Diving 418
   5. Paranasal Sinus Barotrauma 418
   References 420
E. Blast .... Charles W. Shilling 421
   1. Physical Aspects 422
   2. Clinical Aspects and Pathology 423
   3. Treatment 425
   4. Prevention and Protective Measures 425
   References 426
F. Dangerous Marine Life .... Joel Kevin Sims 427
   1. Infections from Marine Microorganisms............................. 427
      a. Infections Associated with Near-Drowning 427
      b. Tetanus 428
      c. Gas Gangrene 428
      d. *Mycobacterium marinum* Infections 429
      e. Erysipelothrix Infections 429
      f. Marine Vibrio Infections 429
      g. Coral Trauma Infections 429
      h. Marine Wounds 430
      i. Marine Fungal Infections 430
      j. Schistosome Cercarial Dermatitis 430
      k. Marine Viral Infections 430
   2. Poisonous and Venomous Marine Organisms 431
      a. Blue-Green Algae 431
      b. *Gymnodinium breve* (Red Tide) 431

		c.	Dogger Bank Itch	431
		d.	Green Algae (Phylum Chlorophyta)	431
		e.	Brown Algae (Phylum Phaeophyta)	432
		f.	Sponges	432
		g.	Nematocyst Envenomizations	432
		h.	Spine Puncture Envenomizations	433
		i.	Venomous Octopus Bites	434
		j.	Sea Snake Envenomizations	434
	3.	Human Toxic Ingestions		435
		a.	Scombroid Poisoning	435
		b.	Ciguatera Poisoning	435
		c.	Puffer Poisoning	436
	4.	Marine Trauma		436
	5.	Conclusion		437
References				437
G.	Spontaneous Pneumothorax .... Kenneth W. Kizer			441
References				443

X
Emergency Treatment While under Pressure

A.	Use of Drugs and Related Substances under Diving Conditions J. Michael Walsh and Harold M. Ginzburg			445
	1.	Physiological Background		446
		a.	Direct Effects of Pressure	446
		b.	Interactions of Pressure and Gas	447
		c.	Physical and Emotional State of Diver	447
		d.	Known Interactions of Drugs with Environment	448
	2.	Clinical Applications		449
		a.	Drugs Acting on Central Nervous System	449
		b.	Cardiovascular Agents	452
		c.	Respiratory Agents	452
		d.	Otorhinolaryngeal Agents	452
		e.	Antiallergenic Agents	455
		f.	Antibiotics	455
		g.	Abused Psychoactive Agents	458
	3.	Conclusions		458
References				459
B.	Anesthesia for Emergency Surgery under High Pressure Honorato F. Nicodemus			460
	1.	Protection of the Airway		461
		a.	Direct Visual Tracheal Intubation	464
		b.	Blind Nasotracheal Intubation	466
	2.	Regional Anesthesia		466

		a.	Toxicity of Local Anesthetics	467
		b.	Techniques	468
	3.	General Anesthesia		475
		a.	Inhalation Agents	476
		b.	Intravenous Anesthesia	476
		c.	Suggested Course of Action for General Anesthesia under High Pressure	483
References				485

XI
Physical and Psychological Examination for Diving

A.	Physical Standards for Diving ....Paul G. Linaweaver	489
	1. Background	489
	a. Military Diving	490
	b. Commercial Diving	490
	c. Scientific and Technical Diving	491
	d. Semiprofessional Diving	491
	e. Recreational Diving	491
	2. Physical Evaluation of Divers	492
	a. Age	494
	b. Sex	494
	c. Body Build	494
	d. Nervous System	494
	e. Ear, Nose, Throat	495
	f. Eyes	497
	g. Respiratory System	498
	h. Cardiovascular System	502
	i. Alimentary System	503
	j. Musculoskeletal System	504
	k. Skin	505
	l. Metabolic Disorders	506
	m. Genitourinary Disorders	506
	3. Special Studies Required for Divers	506
	4. Physical Fitness to Dive	506
Appendix A		508
Appendix B		510
Appendix C		513
Appendix D		515
Appendix E		517
References		519
B.	Psychological Standards for Diving .... Robert J. Biersner	520
	1. Recent Selection and Evaluation Research	521
	a. Mechanical and Arithmetic Aptitudes	521
	b. Age	523

		c.	Demographic Factors, Medical History, Social Adjustment	523
	2.		Summary and Conclusions	528

References 530

XII
Stress Physiology and Behavior Underwater
Arthur J. Bachrach

- A. Introduction 531
- B. Concept of Stress 531
- C. Stress in Diving 534
  - 1. Training to Alleviate Stress 534
    - a. Organized Training Programs 534
    - b. Physician's Role in Training 535
  - 2. Diver Motivation—A Stress Factor? 536
  - 3. Physical and Physiological Stress Factors 537
    - a. Fatigue 537
    - b. Cold 538
    - c. Cardiovascular Disorders and Sudden Death 543
  - 4. Cardiovascular Effects of Stress: Emotional Factors 544
- D. Diving Accidents 546
  - 1. Hazards and Accidents 547
  - 2. Diving Hazards and Accidents 549
- E. Diver Panic 553
  - 1. Helplessness and Anxiety 555
    - a. Behavioral Reactions 555
  - 2. Physiological Events in Panic 558
    - a. Hyperventilation 558
    - b. Hypoventilation 560
- F. Concluding Remarks 560

References 561

XIII
Safety Considerations
Charles W. Shilling

- A. Introduction 567
- B. The Diver 568
  - 1. Selection of the Diver 569
    - a. Physical Examination 569
    - b. Pyschological Evaluation 569
    - c. Diving History Evaluation 569
  - 2. Training 570
  - 3. Predive Condition 570
    - a. Age 570
    - b. Drugs 570
    - c. Alcohol 571
    - d. Cigarettes 571
    - e. Diet 572
    - f. Obesity 572
    - g. Fatigue 572
    - h. Physical Condition 575

xxx Contents

		i.	Emotional Stability	576
		j.	Infections	577
		k.	Previous Diving History	577
C.	The Dive			578
	1.	Organization and Planning		578
	2.	General Safety Precautions		578
	3.	Personnel: Qualified, Trained, Ready to Dive		579
	4.	Natural Hazards: Environmental Conditions		579
	5.	On-Site Hazards		581
		a.	Traffic	581
		b.	Sonar	581
		c.	Radioactive Contamination	581
	6.	Object Hazards		581
		a.	Fouling	582
		b.	Pollution	582
	7.	Special Situations		583
	8.	Recompression Chamber		583
	9.	Equipment, Regular and Emergency		584
	10.	Orientation		584
	11.	Diving Operations		584
		a.	Diving Platform	584
		b.	Warning Signals	584
		c.	Line Signals	586
		d.	Hand Signals	587
		e.	Descent	587
		f.	Fouling	587
		g.	Explosives	587
		h.	Electric Power	587
		i.	Shark Defense	589
		j.	Decompression	589
D.	Diving at Altitudes above Sea Level			589
E.	Flying after Diving			590
F.	Fire Safety			592
G.	Electrical Safety			592
H.	Blast			592
I.	Drowning			593
J.	Hazards of Marine Life			593
K.	Escape and Rescue			594
	1.	Submarines		594
		a.	Escape	594
		b.	Rescue	595
	2.	Submersibles and Habitats		595
L.	Ice Diving			596
References				597

XIV
Equipment and Procedures

A.	Treatment Chambers		601
	1.	Multiplace Chambers .... Paul J. Sheffield	601
		a. Introduction	601
		b. Contributions of Caisson Work	602
		c. Contributions of Diving	603

		d.	Contributions of Aviation	607
		e.	Contributions of Clinical Chambers	608
		f.	Development of Safety Codes	609
		g.	Principles of Safe Treatment Chamber Operations	610
		h.	Summary	618
References				619
	2.	Monoplace Chambers .... George B. Hart		621
		a.	Introduction	621
		b.	Optimal Monoplace Chamber System	622
		c.	Application of the Monoplace Chamber	624
		d.	Maintenance and Safety	624
		e.	Conclusion	625
References				625
B.	Scuba Diving .... David H. Peterson			625
	1.	Introduction		625
	2.	Development of Modern Scuba		626
	3.	The Scuba Diving Community		626
	4.	Scuba Procedures		627
	5.	Basic Scuba Diving Equipment		629
		a.	Cylinder Group	630
		b.	Regulator Group	633
		c.	Masks, Fins, Snorkels	636
		d.	Buoyancy Control Group	638
		e.	Protective Clothing Group	640
		f.	Instrument Group	642
	6.	Conclusion		643
References				644
C.	Surface-Supplied Diving .... Walt Bergman			645
	1.	Air Diving		645
	2.	Mixed-Gas Diving		651
D.	Deep Diving and Saturation Systems .... R. W. Hamilton			654
	1.	Diving With a Deep Diving System: Deep Bounce Diving		655
	2.	Saturation and Saturation-Excursion Diving		657
	3.	Habitat Diving		660
References				660

XV
Diving Accident Investigation
Charles J. Stahl

A.	Accident Reporting	661
B.	Objectives of Diving Accident Investigation	662
	1. Human Factors	663
	2. Environmental Factors	663
	3. Equipment Factors	663
	4. Other Factors Bearing on the Accident	663
C.	Authority for Investigation and Autopsy	664
D.	The Autopsy in Diving Accident Investigations	666
E.	Medical Investigation of Fatal Diving Accidents	667

	1.	Identification of Victim	667
	2.	Examination of Equipment	669
	3.	Total Body Radiography of Victim	669
	4.	Photographic Record of Investigation	669
	5.	Postmortem Examination	670
		a. External Examination and Search for Evidence of Injury	670
		b. Internal Examination and Search for Evidence of Injury	671
		c. Microscopic Examination	673
		d. Chemical and Toxicological Examinations	673
		e. Microbiological and Serological Examinations	676
F.	Summary		677
Appendix			677
References			681

Appendixes

Appendix A: Glossary	687
Appendix B: Abbreviations and Acronyms	717
Appendix C: Pressure Conversion Table	721
Author Index	723
Subject Index	725

The Diving Environment

A. Introduction

Homo sapiens is a terrestrial being, and moving into and under water requires special knowledge and special equipment. It is possible to descend into the water either as an individual diver exposed to the ambient pressure of the depth to which he goes, or to descend into the "deep" as the occupant of a submarine or other type submersible, where the occupant remains at atmospheric pressure, protected by a shield of unyielding armor. An individual may also be exposed to increased pressure in a hyperbaric dry chamber or wet pot ashore or in a lockout submersible under the water. Whenever or wherever exposed to the hyperbaric or underwater environment, the diver must be prepared to cope with the physical effects of pressure, which are described in Chapter II, "Physics of Diving."

The material in this chapter is divided into three sections: B. *Types of Diving*, C. *Natural Diving Environments*, and D. *Man-Made Diving Environments*. The aim is to cover the material in order to acquaint the reader with the possibilities without exhaustive detail.

B. Types of Diving

1. General

In discussing diving the ordinary person is thinking of a "plunge into water executed in a prescribed manner," as defined by Webster. That it is well for the physician to remember this is illustrated by an incident seen by this writer in the early days at the U.S. Navy Experimental Diving Unit. The emergency call came for the doctor to report to the Unit at once. Upon his arrival at the Unit it was determined that the injured diver was en route from Annapolis, Maryland, to the Unit at the Washington Navy Yard. When the diver arrived, instead of being rushed into the chamber, as everyone expected, a few questions elicited the information that he had taken a dare to dive from the superstructure of his yacht and that when he hit the surface, "something popped" in his back; he was paralyzed from the waist down. Now, the ideal treatment for a fractured back is not to be bounced around in the back seat of a touring car for 34 miles! Without asking any questions, the local doctor had responded to a call about a paralyzed diver by referring him to the nearest pressure chamber.

Before discussing the various types of diving it is well to present some definitions that will help in understanding the following presentation; see also the Glossary at the end of this book.

Air diving: Compressed air is the most commonly used breathing medium because it is so readily available. The medical and decompression aspects of air diving are generally well understood.

Bottom time: The time spent at maximum pressure.

Decompression dive: The commonly used term to indicate a dive in which the ascent or decompression is deliberately slowed compared to no-decompression dives. This slowing of the decompression may be in stages or it may be continuous, and the most time is taken at shallower depths. It is observed to allow inert gas to be eliminated from the body.

Decompression stop: The designated depth and time at which a diver must stop and wait during ascent from a decompression dive; the depth and time are specified by the decompression schedule used.

Decompression table: Decompression schedules in tabular presentation.

Mixed-gas diving: A mixture of inert gases with oxygen may be used as a breathing medium in a dive. Such gases may be: nitrogen-oxygen, helium-oxygen, hydrogen-oxygen, or other mixtures. Often the ratio of the diluent gas to oxygen is changed to keep the partial pressure of oxygen at or near the normal atmospheric (normoxic) level.

No-decompression dive: Commonly called "no-D" dive. It is a misnomer in that any ascent or movement toward the surface from a depth in the water allows some decompression. It refers to a dive of such duration or depth that the diver can safely return to the surface without decompression stops or deliberate slowing. Synonym: no-stop diving.

Other types of diving are presented in more detail in the following material.

2. Breath-Hold Diving

Breath-hold diving is the oldest type of diving and is performed without breathing equipment by simply holding the breath while under water. It is also called "free diving" and "skin diving."

Greek mythology is filled with references to the underwater world and with stories of breath-hold diving exploits. Herodotus tells of a diver, Scyllias, who was hired by Xerxes to dive for treasure on sunken Persian vessels. He was not allowed to leave when his mission was complete, but during a storm he dived into the sea, cut the moorings of Xerxes' galleys, causing great havoc, and escaped by swimming underwater.

The ama of Japan and Korea and the pearl and sponge divers the world over have for centuries used the breath-hold technique in their trades. Most of them wear goggles or masks and dive as deep as 145 ft (44 m, or to 5.4 ATA). In 1969, Bob Croft, a U.S. Navy diver, made a world's record breath-hold dive to 247 ft (75 m, or to 8.4 ATA).

The advantage of breath-hold diving is the complete freedom of the diver, but the obvious disadvantage is the time limitation, since the diver takes down with him only the air he filled his lungs with at the surface. Another advantage is that breath-hold diving practically eliminates the danger of air embolism or decompression sickness. A very recent case is interesting from the standpoint of Boyle's law. A scuba diver was working at 100 ft (30 m) and his buddy on the surface decided to breath-hold dive down and see how he was doing. Upon return to the surface the breath-hold buddy developed a typical case of air embolism. How could this happen? While under recompression treatment he admitted to breathing from the octopus rig of the scuba diver buddy, thus filling his lungs with compressed air; he then forgot to exhale on the way up.

The most dangerous aspect of breath-hold diving is the practice of hyperventilation prior to the dive. It is physiologically correct to assume that the increase in rate or volume of respiration above normal, or both, will reduce alveolar carbon dioxide tension and slightly increase alveolar oxygen tension and thus prolong the time before the breaking point. (The breaking point is defined as the termination of breath holding in response to the development of a net ventilatory stimulus too strong to be further resisted by voluntary effort.) Swimming pool blackouts are examples of this; the swimmer runs out of oxygen before the carbon dioxide buildup signals the breaking point. For a comprehensive presentation see Chapter III M, *Breath-Hold Diving*.

In breath-hold diving there is the additional factor that, although the partial pressure of oxygen (P_{O_2}) may be sufficient to maintain consciousness at depth, the move toward the surface with the decrease in hydrostatic pressure and the associated reduction in the partial pressure of oxygen may lead to unconsciousness. An experience that came close to tragedy will dramatically illustrate this point. At the Submarine Escape Training Tank at New London, Connecticut (illustrated in Chapter XIV, "Equipment and Procedures), it was the custom to put on a "show" for visiting dignitaries. This was done at night, so that no light would be reflected from the surface; with the lights on at the bottom of the 100-ft (30-m) tower every move could be clearly seen. After the preliminary training demonstration with the submarine escape apparatus (Momsen lung), one of the instructors would dive into the water and swim down to about 18 feet (5.5 m), where he became negatively buoyant, and then would just drop to the bottom. On one particular evening, with both the station Admiral and a visiting British Admiral in attendance, the men were putting on a particularly good show. When the diver reached the bottom he sat down on the submarine escape hatch, took off his shoe, and pretended to take out a stone. He was obviously staying too long, but at that time there was no means of communicating with him (a condition that was corrected the next day!). All the spectators were relieved when he went over to the ascending line and started coming up hand over hand. But at about the 15-ft level his head dropped back, bubbles began coming out of his mouth, he lost his grip on the line, and the submarine medical officer yelled, "Get him." The diving chief dove into the tank, swam down, and carried the diver into the open door of the 18-ft lock. The time interval until the chief's arm came out signaling that all was well was the longest ever experienced by the doctor in charge—he could see the court-martial table in front of him and the newspaper headlines: "Navy doctor loses diver in show for Admiral." But when the show was over, best of all was the reaction of the Admirals: the station Admiral said, "Well done, Doctor!" and the British Admiral said, "That was the most realistic drill I have ever seen."

3. Scuba Diving

Scuba is an acronym derived from Self-Contained Underwater Breathing Apparatus. It is commonly used to describe apparatus in which the inspired gas is delivered by demand regulator and exhaled into the surrounding water (open-circuit scuba) and the gas supply is carried on the diver's back. The closed-circuit scuba is a self-contained underwater breathing apparatus in which the breathing gas is recirculated through purifying and oxygen-replenishing systems; newer forms of scuba are controlled by oxygen sensors, and no exhaled gas is lost into the surrounding water. There are also semiclosed-circuit systems, in which a portion of the exhaled gas is lost into the surrounding water.

The equipment and procedures for scuba diving are presented in Chapter XIV, "Equipment and Procedures." Here it is important to note that with the advent of scuba the diver was freed from the air hose to the surface and became mobile and free for lateral movement. For this reason and because of the simplicity of the open-circuit scuba, it is universally used for diving and even is used in some situations in commercial diving.

4. Surface-Supplied Diving

Surface-supplied diving is a form of diving in which the breathing gas is supplied from a compressor or one or more cylinders at the surface—a dock, boat, platform, or rig. As the name implies, the diver is connected to this gas supply by a length of air hose, and thus his movements are severely limited. The many types of helmets and suits worn with this type of diving are well described in Chapter XIV, "Equipment and Procedures." The suits and helmets may be lightweight or heavy, and they usually carry communication cables along with the air hose. And, of course, the breathing mixture supplied can be air or any mixture of nitrogen-oxygen, helium-oxygen, hydrogen-oxygen, or other inert gas with oxygen.

For many years U.S. Navy diving was almost entirely surface supplied, and today most commercial diving, especially deep diving, is surface supplied.

5. Bounce Diving

Bounce diving is described as a short non-saturation dive beginning and ending at the surface; it is also called an intervention dive. It is obvious that this type of dive, which was the only type of diving prior to the saturation mode, can be made with any type of equipment and any mixture of breathing gases. The decompression time depends on depth and time of exposure.

6. Saturation Diving

As both scientific and commercial interest in the oceans increase it becomes apparent that facilities must be provided so that the research or working diver can remain at depth for long periods of time.

The problem is that in diving to greater depths and in tackling time-consuming jobs the most serious limiting factor is the need for prolonged decompression, since decompression time lengthens markedly as time increases at any given depth. Eventually, however, and probably within 24 to 36 hr, the body becomes saturated with nitrogen or other inert gas at the pressure of depth. Once the diver's tissue gases have reached equilibrium with the pressure environment, the time required for decompression at the end of the dive for a given depth does not increase with additional time spent at that depth.

In 1957, U.S. Navy medical officers R. D. Workman, G. F. Bond, and W. F. Mazzone (Workman et al. 1962) reported on the concept of saturation diving. They reasoned that after a period of time at a fixed pressure the diver will absorb into his tissues all of the inert gas he is capable of absorbing.

Of course, this saturated diver must decompress with a much longer schedule than dives to the same depth but of shorter duration (see Chapter IV, "Decompression Theory"), but he decompresses only once instead of the many times required in bounce diving, thus minimizing the physical risks of decompression and reducing dramatically the time of decompression for long periods of working time under standard diving conditions. In 1966, Captain George Bond (Bond 1966) reported on experimental work that gave confirmation to this principle. Both laboratory and field research in using this saturation technique led to the U.S. Navy "undersea habitat" idea put into practice in the SeaLab projects.

Two basic approaches are commonly used in saturation diving:

(i) Habitat/Ocean Floor Laboratory. A habitat may be defined as a seafloor structure that is usually maintained at ambient pressure and that provides a base of operation for the saturated diver and his equipment. Gas pressure inside the habitat prevents flooding by seawater and makes it possible for the diver to enter and exit through an opening in the floor.

(ii) Deep-Dive Saturation System. The deep-dive saturation system is used almost exclusively by commercial diving organizations and consists of two elements: (1) a deck decompression chamber (DDC), which is located on a surface support platform, is really the living quarters for the divers during the long periods at pressure, and (2) a pressurized personnel transfer capsule (PTC) in which the divers commute to and from the work site. The PTC may be a diving bell or a lock-out submersible that will carry more than one diver. Both are maintained at the working depth pressure so that the divers may be brought to the surface, the PTC married to the DDC, and the divers transferred to the DDC without any change in pressure.

The most crucial point to remember is that the saturated diver must not be decompressed quickly and thus must not go shallower than a prescribed depth above his saturated depth without undergoing a decompression schedule that will bring him safely to this lesser pressure and, ultimately, to atmospheric pressure. Thus the saturated diver should not wear a flotation device that could become inflated and carry him to the surface, nor should he wear a quick-release weight belt. And he must be properly trained, must become familiarized with the habitat or bell, and must conduct his working dives so that he can return to the pressurized (ambient) chamber easily. For the saturated diver to go directly to the surface, even from a depth of only 100 ft, would be hazardous.

One of the life support problems is that of supplying a proper gas mixture. It is obvious that oxygen should be maintained at an adequate level. Carbon dioxide must be elminated to prevent buildups in habitats, bells, or PTCs; this is done by venting or a scrubbing system that contains a chemical absorbent such as barium hydroxide, soda lime, or lithium hydroxide. The length of time these absorbents will remain active is directly related to the number of divers and to the temperature and humidity in the support equipment.

Emergency situations (treated in detail in Chapter XIII, "Safety Considerations") are particularly difficult when the divers are saturated, for removal and rapid decompression are impossible. Great precautions must therefore be taken against a number of potentially hazardous situations. Fire, for example, is probably the greatest hazard of the hyperbaric environment, and its possibility must be guarded against. Loss of power to operate the life-support systems and loss of communication with the surface are mechanical problems that can be dealt with by the inclusion of backup systems. And the obvious possibility that a diver could be lost or experience blowup becomes a grave danger to the saturated diver.

7. Excursion Diving

An excursion is the movement of the diver either upward from the saturation depth or downward from the saturation depth; the permissible safe distance and lapsed time of the excursion dive depend on the saturation depth. In this activity a saturation diver may be compared to a diver at the surface who is saturated at 1 atm, whereas the habitat or bell diver is saturated at pressures greater than 1 atm. The surface diver can make dives (excursions) to depth and return directly to the surface provided he has not absorbed more gas during the excursion than the body can safely release (no-decompression dive). In the same way, habitat divers can make prescribed excursions either to greater depths (downward) or to lesser depths (upward) in the water by following the depth and time limitations of the no-decompression excursion tables. General rules cannot be given, since factors such as cold, work loads, types of equipment used, or experience must be considered in any excursion or decompression from saturation.

C. Natural Diving Environments

1. General

Environmental characteristics such as temperature, visibility, marine life, tides, currents, and type of bottom may vary signficantly from place to place. The only variable that approaches stability is the relationship between depth of water and hydrostatic pressure, and that varies according to the density (salinity) of the water. One atmosphere is generally accepted as being equal to 33 ft (10 m) of seawater, or 34 ft (10.2 m) of fresh water.

Because diving conditions can vary greatly within a chosen locality, it is important to obtain as much information as possible about local conditions from divers who are familiar with the diving areas. A checkout dive with a diver from the area is a good idea.

2. Oceans

Such factors as density, temperature, and salinity of water; atmospheric conditions (barometric pressure, air temperature, humidity, winds); tides and currents; water clarity; bottom topography; and marine organisms make the ocean a challenging environment for the diver. In fact the diver's effectiveness is severely limited by ocean environmental factors, e.g., high hydrostatic pressure, dynamic forces from waves and currents, limited visibility, and low temperature. For a detailed coverage of the ocean environment as it affects diving, three references are recommended: Adolfson and Berghage (1974), Miller (1979), and Shilling et al. (1976).

3. Lakes

Lake diving has many of the same variables as ocean diving with one significant difference: the change in ambient pressure due to the altitude of the lake above sea level. Thus, in mountain lake diving, the decompression schedules normally used by sport and professional divers at sea level must be adjusted to compensate for lowered atmospheric pressure. This means that for the same depth and the same bottom time a longer decompression time is necessary. Details of this problem are presented in Chapter XIII, "Safety Considerations."

Another factor to consider in lake diving is that in some localities lakes have become the dumping ground for the area and may contain everything from broken bottles to old cars. Man-made lakes often cover old houses and barns that were not cleared away before the flooding, so a careful checkout is most important.

4. Rivers

Most of the problems of ocean and lake diving are also found in river diving, but one major problem is not shared to the same extent with the ocean and lakes—the current. For example, the Colorado River downstream from the Hoover Dam runs at from 6 to 8 knots (about 11–15 km/hr); there a diver who grabs something so as to stop and look around will find that the current is swift enough to tear off his face mask unless he can hold it with one hand. A diver wearing standard deep-sea gear, with a life line and heavy weights, can usually work in currents up to 1.5 knots (about 2.8 km/hr) without major difficulty. If supplied with an additional weighted belt, he should be able to accomplish useful work in currents as fast as 2.5 knots (about 4.6 km/hr). A scuba diver, who is essentially floating in the moving water, is severely handicapped by currents of greater than one knot, or a little less than 2 km/hr.

Another problem in diving in rivers is visibility, which may be practically zero if the river carries large amounts of sediment, either normally or as the result of recent rainfall. Bubbles also block the light, so that in or under white water it may be almost dark. Diving with underwater lights is not much help, because the light is attenuated by the suspended particulate matter.

5. Harbors

Diving in a bay or harbor presents the diver with most of the difficulties faced in ocean or lake diving, with the added factor of the tide and its associated current. Tidal current, the periodic horizontal flow of water accompanying the rise and fall of the tide, is of considerable significance to the diver who must work in such restricted areas as bay mouths or channels. Essentially, tides are long-period waves, the period lasting 12 hr, 25 min, and the wave length being equal to one-half the circumference of the earth. The tidal cycle is 24 hr, 50 min. Offshore, where the direction of flow is not restricted by any barriers, the tidal current flows continuously, the direction changing through all points of the compass during the tidal periods. When restricted to certain channels, such as harbors, bays, rivers, or straits, the current reverses with the rise and fall of the tides. Tidal current movement toward shore or upstream is the *flood*; movement away from shore or downstream is the *ebb*. At each reversal of current a short period of little or no current exists that is called *slack water*. The speed of the current varies with the width of the channel, and it may be so swift that diving should be restricted to the period of slack water.

6. *Cave Diving*

Cave diving, although not very common, is intriguing to the sport diver and offers a new area of research for the scientist. But the natural hazards, which include an overhead ceiling, darkness, low visibility, current, and the physical characteristics of the cave, are such that only experienced and specially trained and equipped divers should undertake cave diving.[1]

Thus it is important to determine the physical and psychological limits of the least experienced person of the team, to assemble the appropriate equipment, and to develop safe contingency plans for emergency situations. This last is imperative, for more than once all participants have perished inside a cave. In a recent tragedy four young people were found entangled in the fish line they had intended to use to find their way out. Temporary lines should consist of a suitable safety reel, a line guide, a drum with a buoyancy chamber, and should carry at least 400 ft of $1/16$-in., 100-lb test line (125 m, 1.5 mm, 45 kg, respectively).

Special consideration must be given to lighting and to buoyancy control, but of paramount importance is a large enough supply of air.

7. *Diving in Kelp*

Various types of kelp grow in the waters along the west coast of the United States; in fact, the growth extends from Mexico to the Aleutians. They grow in water depths of 10 to 60 ft (3–18 m) or more, depending on the clarity of the water. When mature they reach the surface, where their foliage may form a dense, almost impenetrable mat. This dense canopy, however, often has thin spots or holes through which a diver can enter or

---

[1] A helpful monthly newsletter is published by the National Association for Cave Diving (P.O. Box 14492, Gainesville, FL 32604). This professional organization promotes training, safety, education, conservation, and service for cave divers.

exit. A diver swimming through the kelp on the surface can become entangled in the kelp. He must remain calm as he attempts to free himself. The diver who must swim on the surface should seek open paths or attempt to pass over the kelp if it cannot be parted. Swimming under the surface canopy is easier, provided a sufficiency of breathing air remains.

From a boat, water entry with feet first and legs together is preferable to the head-first roll or back entry, because of the likelihood of entanglement in the kelp. Once through the surface canopy the divers will find themselves in a forestlike area that may be quite dark. It is important to realize that any irregular surface, even a knife strapped to the outside of the leg, is likely to catch kelp; thus all equipment should be streamlined. When approaching the surface the diver should raise the arms over the head so as to move the fronds aside to provide an opening. The diver should stay in the upright position and not thrash around, or entanglement may result. As in many diving situations, panic is the enemy in this type of diving.

8. *Diving in Polluted Water*

There is a generally accepted notion that running water soon purifies itself, and that salt water does not harbor microorganisms. Neither of these concepts is true, for the water abounds with microorganisms, most of which are fortunately not pathogenic for man, and many rivers have raw sewage discharged into them along the way and are little better than open sewers. A number of superficial or systemic infections that are due to specific, or in some cases nonspecific, organisms are presented in Chapter IX.

It is well to remember that there may be gross chemical pollution that may also be hazardous to the diver. If it is necessary to dive near a sewage outflow or in known polluted water it is important to wear a standard dry suit with helmet so as to protect the body from contact with the water, to rinse down with fresh water before removing any equipment, and to bathe carefully afterward.

9. *Diving in Wrecks*

Since a number of inherent dangers are associated with diving in or around a wreck, it follows that extra care must be taken both in planning and in carrying out the dive. Of prime importance is the route to the surface, especially if there are a number of deck levels, passageways, and small entrances. It is well to remember that the only known way out is the way in!

If the diver is surface-supplied there may be a problem with the air hose, and the *U.S. Navy Diving Manual* (1978) recommends that a tender be at the entrance to each level (it is obvious that all underwater tenders must be divers); this type of maneuver requires careful planning and execution. In scuba diving a line must be carried into the wreck so as to mark the safe exit route.

For either type of diving there are a number of special considerations (Miller 1979). For obvious reasons visibility will be markedly reduced and a flashlight must be carried.

Passage through an opening that is too small should never be forced, for the return may be even more difficult. The diver should go feet first into any space, remembering that decayed wood and corroded metal can collapse. The diver must always be on the lookout for sharp objects that may be hidden by algae, sea polyps, or other marine growth, and because underwater enclosures are havens for all types of sea life, hazardous marine life should be considered at all times. (See Chapter IX-F on *Dangerous Marine Life*.) As in cave diving, it is imperative that an adequate air supply be available, for one never knows how long it may be necessary to stay inside a wreck. If warranted because of depth and dive duration, a spare air supply and regulator should be placed outside the entrance to the wreck as a safety measure.

10. *Diving in Cold Water*

Diving in cold water presents many problems, the most important of which is keeping the diver warm and maintaining his core temperature. This is necessary not only for comfort but because temperature changes can drastically affect a diver's performance, his ability to concentrate, and his working efficiency. The temperature zone of highest efficiency and comfort is rather narrow (see Figure I-1), for between 60°F and 70°F (15°C and 21°C) body heat loss to the water can soon bring on chilling and excessive fatigue, whereas water temperature higher than 86°F (30°C) may lead to overheating and may cause exhaustion. Details of physiological effects are found in Chapter III under the topic *Thermal Considerations*.

Three general types of exposure suits are available that are designed to help keep the diver's body warm (Miller 1979). In moderately cold water the standard ¼- to ⅜-in. foam neoprene wet suit with a hooded neoprene vest usually is satisfactory for dives as long as 60 min, provided the diver is actively working. It is possible to double the time under water by using a variable-volume dry suit. For very cold water the hot water wet suit affords thermal protection but tethers the diver to the water supply.

Diving in cold water also presents several equipment problems that need to be considered. Single-hose regulators are especially susceptible to freezing, although some new models are built to resist this. Standard double-hose regulators are more resistant to freezing malfunction and are preferable for diving in extreme cold. Also, the diver's mask may show an increased tendency to fog or freeze in cold water; partially flooding the mask and flushing seawater over the faceplate temporarily relieves the condition.

Hands should be protected with gloves or mittens—the loss of manual dexterity is overridden by the added warmth provided. Wearing a knitted watch cap under the hood of the dry suit is especially effective in conserving body heat. Heavy insulating socks under the boots in either a wet or dry suit will help keep the feet warm.

11. *Diving under Ice*

Precautions additional to the problems discussed in connection with cold-water diving must be taken when diving under ice.

Most ice diving is done in lakes, where the ice forms a relatively flat platform that

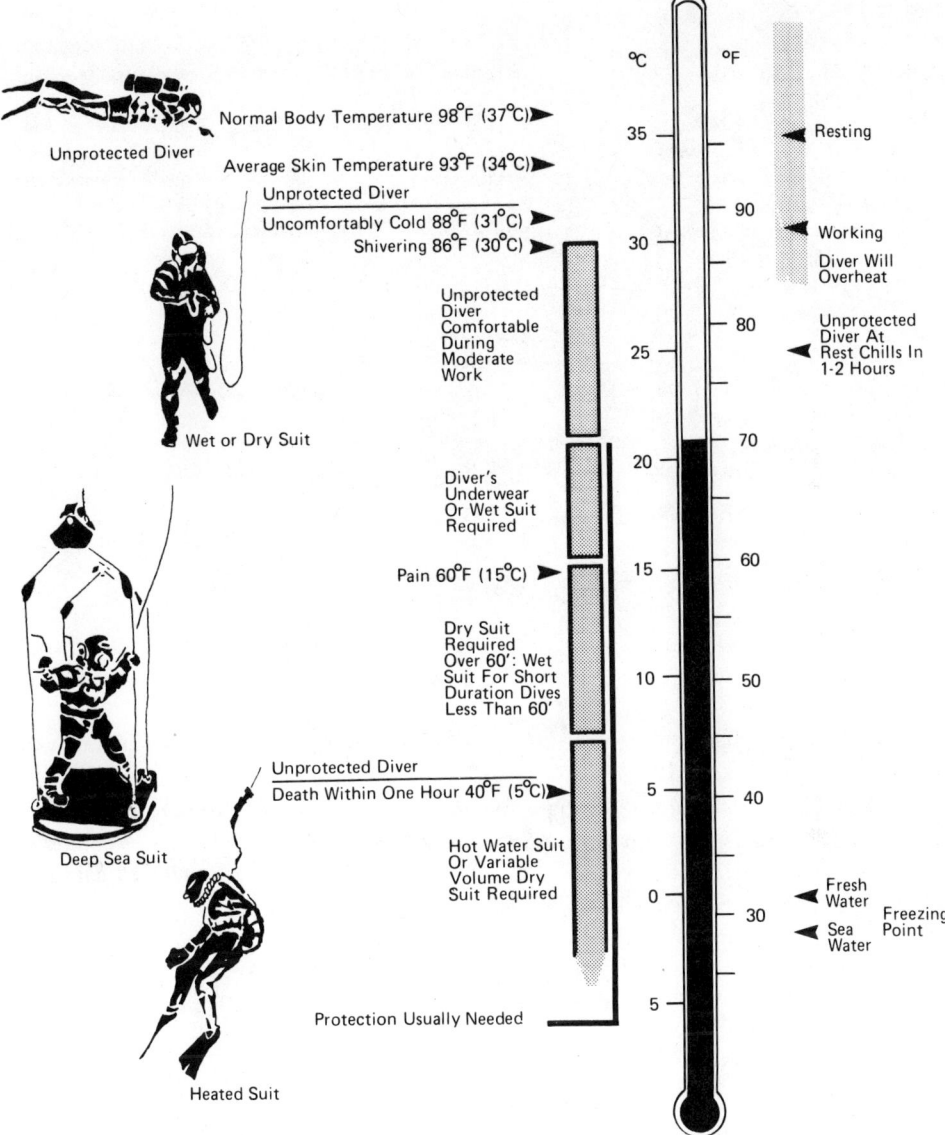

Figure I-1. Water temperature protection chart. [From U.S. Navy (1978).]

is firmly frozen to the shore. Diving from drifting ice or in the midst of broken free ice is dangerous and should be done only if absolutely necessary.

Diving is done in the Arctic, but the ice cover, darkness, cold, and currents combine to make polar waters the most hostile of all underwater environments.

The safety measures for ice diving are treated in Chapter XIII, "Safety Considerations."

CHARLES W. SHILLING

References

ADOLFSON, J. A., AND T. E. BERGHAGE 1974. *Perception and Performance under Water*. New York: John Wiley and Sons.
BENNETT, P. B., AND D. H. ELLIOTT (editors) 1975. *The Physiology and Medicine of Diving and Compressed Air Work* (2nd ed.). Baltimore: Williams and Wilkins.
BOND, G. F. 1966. Effects of new and artificial environments on human physiology. *Arch. Environ. Health* 12: 85–90.
COUNCIL FOR NATIONAL COOPERATION IN AQUATICS 1974. *The New Science of Skin and Scuba Diving* (4th ed.). New York: Association Press.
MILLER, J. W. (editor). 1979. *The NOAA Diving Manual* (2nd ed.). Washington, DC: National Oceanic and Atmospheric Administration, U.S. Dept. Commerce.
SHILLING, C. W., M. F. WERTS, AND N. R. SCHANDELMEIER (editors) 1976. *The Underwater Handbook: A Guide to Physiology and Performance for the Engineer*. New York: Plenum Press.
U.S. NAVY 1978. *U.S. Navy Diving Manual (Change 2). Air Diving*. Washington, DC: U.S. Navy Dept., Vol. 1. (NAVSHIPS 0994-001-9010.)
WORKMAN, R. D., G. F. BOND, AND W. F. MAZZONE 1962. Prolonged exposure of animals to pressurized normal and synthetic atmospheres. Res. Rep. 26, No. 5. New London, CT: U.S. Navy Med. Res. Lab., p. 1–19.

D. Man-Made Diving Environments

1. Introduction

This section describes various types of facilities by means of which humans may be exposed to hyperbaric pressures. Its intent is not to impart engineering or operational details but to acquaint the reader with the overall scope of hyperbaric systems and devices by which the human being may be subjected to pressure. These include deck decompression chambers, deep diving systems and diving bells, submersibles, undersea habitats, and the chambers associated with tunnel and caisson work. In addition to these operational facilities there are various types of treatment and rescue systems. Some of the important general characteristics and subsystems common to the different systems are discussed. The classic decompression chamber is the basic model of a man-made pressure environment.

Hyperbaric facilities have a few characteristics in common. For one thing, they are all in one way or another pressure vessels. Most chambers have some type of entry lock or pass-through lock large enough for people to be transferred into and out of the chamber while it is at pressure. The chambers generally have viewports and interior lighting and some type of communication system. Needed are a source of suitable gas or air for compression, a piping system for carrying it to and from the chamber, and suitable gauges and valves for control. Most other elements are functions of the specific application.

2. Caissons and Tunnels

Until 20 years or so ago the greatest source of hyperbaric exposure for commercial workers was in caisson and tunnel work. When underground construction work has to be carried out below the level of the water table, the contractor has the problem of keeping water out of the working area. This problem is commonly encountered in building bridge abutments and deep foundations, where caissons must be sunk, and in tunneling for roads and railroads beneath rivers and lakes. Compressed air is used to keep the water out of the head of the tunnel or the bottom of the caisson.

In 1841 M. Triger (described in Bert 1878) exploited the innovation of using compressed air to keep water out of subterranean excavations. He constructed the first caisson from sections of iron cylinders sunk to a depth of 66 ft (20 m). By means of a pump at the surface the air in the caisson was compressed to a pressure corresponding to the pressure head of the surrounding water. At the top a lock was provided through which the excavated material could be hoisted and through which the workers could pass.

In caissons and tunnels the physiological problems are the same, but there are differences from the construction point of view. In both, large air compressors are used to pressurize the working area—at the bottom of the caisson or at the face of the tunnel. The nonworking end of the caisson or of the tunnel is sealed off by a large lock through which elevators or railway cars may pass; such a lock in a tunnel is called the *mud lock* and is used for locking materials and supplies in and excavated material out. Generally workers are locked in and out of the pressure area through another lock, a *man lock* or *long lock*. A separate chamber, called a *medical lock*, is usually located nearby and used for treatment of any casualties. The medical lock is equipped with oxygen-breathing equipment, a first aid kit, and appropriate medical supplies. There is also a *pass-through lock* for obtaining additional supplies as needed.

The first reported cases of caisson disease, now called decompression sickness (DCS), occurred during the Triger caisson work in 1841. Two laborers, after working for seven hours in the caisson, experienced severe pains—in the left arm of one worker, in the knees of the other—one-half hour after emerging into open air.

In construction of the St. Louis Eads Bridge over the Mississippi River in 1869 the highest pressure was 4.45 ATA. There was 352 workers, and among these were 30 serious cases of decompression sickness and 12 deaths (Jarcho 1968).

In the construction of the East River tunnels in New York City for the Pennsylvania Railroad in 1909 there were 20 deaths, although the incidence of reported decompression sickness arising from a total of 557,000 man-decompressions was low, an incidence of 0.7% (Keays 1909). (A detailed presentation of decompression sickness is presented in Chapter VI, "Diagnosis and Treatment of Decompression Sickness.")

The first compressed air work regulations for New York State were compiled in 1912; progressively from that time hours of work were shortened and the interval between shifts lengthened. Nevertheless, despite curtailed hours of work and somewhat longer intervals in air at normal pressure, there were still occurrences of serious disability. Among 300 cases of DCS reported by Thorne (1941) in connection with the Queens Midtown Tunnel, New York City, in 1938 there were 25 cases of paralysis, 15 cases characterized by cardiopulmonary symptomatology (chokes), and 30 cases of vertigo (staggers).

These New York tables were revised by U.S. Navy Medical Officers O. E. VanDerAue, G. Duffner, and A. R. Behnke, Jr, at the request of the New York Authority. Not only were maximal hours of work in compressed air reduced, but decompression time was extended in accordance with Navy experience.

Use of these revised tables in New York in the construction of the third tube of the Lincoln Tunnel in 1955–57 resulted in a remarkable record of only 44 cases of Type I (mild) decompression sickness and no deaths—out of 138,034 man-decompressions (Kooperstein and Schuman 1957).

One of the problems not solved for either the caisson and tunnel worker or for the deep sea diver, however, is development of aseptic bone necrosis (dysbaric osteonecrosis), which may be sequential to compressed air work. For a presentation of this problem, see that section in Chapter IX.

Because of the many problems associated with the use of compressed air, the contractor usually tries to avoid its use and resorts to such techniques as pumping down the water table, trenching, or pumping a slurry ahead of the boring machine. Union and insurance rules have often become more decisive than engineering problems or physiology in deciding whether to use compressed air.

3. Deck Decompression Chambers

By far the most common manned hyperbaric facility is the classic deck decompression chamber (DDC). This chamber has two main uses. First, it is used at locations where bounce diving is being conducted, for the purpose of treating decompression sickness in the event it occurs following a dive. A second and actually more frequent application is for surface decompression. In this technique, which is discussed in more detail in Chapter IV, "Decompression Theory," the diver is brought to the surface before his schedule of decompression (decompression obligation) is complete and is recompressed to an intermediate depth, generally 40 feet of seawater (fsw), or 12 meters of seawater (msw), and the decompression is completed in the chamber; this often involves the breathing of oxygen. The safety and operational advantages of surface decompression are substantial; for most air diving operations deeper than about 30 fsw (9 msw) a chamber is an economic necessity if a substantial amount of diving is to be done (U.S. Navy 1978; Zinkowski 1971).

The inside of a DDC is all too familiar to most experienced diving doctors. This is the type of facility that is available for a large percentage of the treatments of decompression sickness. Shore-based treatment facilities are often quite similar in both structure and function and in many cases are nothing more than permanently mounted deck chambers.

The most common deck decompression chamber in commercial use is about 54 in. (1.4 m) in diameter and about 12 ft (4 m) long (Figure I-2). It has an inner lock about 7 ft (2 m) long, and an outer or entry lock takes up the remainder of its length. The control plumbing is mounted in a box on the side of the chamber, usually with a cover that forms a shelter when opened. Many U.S. Navy deck chambers are a bit larger, about 5 ft (1.5 m) in diameter, and they may be equipped with bunks, whereas often the commercial chambers have only a mattress or merely the deck plates. All have at least a built-in breathing system (BIBS) for breathing oxygen and then disposing of exhaled oxygen, some type of lighting, and a loudspeaker-type intercom system. [The deck decompression chamber is illustrated and described in some detail in the *U.S. Navy Diving Manual* (1978), p. 8-35.]

The Diving Environment   15

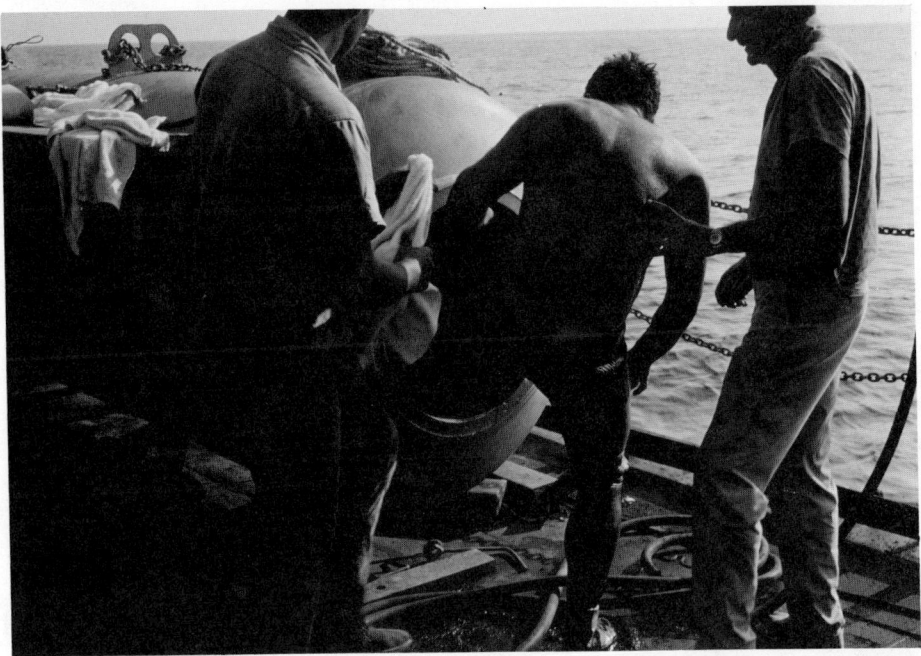

Figure I-2. Diver entering typical deck decompression chamber. He is entering the outer lock; the inner lock is already at a pressure of 40 fsw (12 msw). He will be pressurized to that depth for a period of oxygen breathing as the "surface" portion of his surface decompression procedure. (Photo, R. W. Hamilton.)

In a normal surface decompression operation, the chamber inner lock is taken to the proper pressure depth, generally 40 fsw (12 msw), and the diver after surfacing enters the outer lock, which is then pressurized. He may or may not be accompanied by a tender, depending on whether he can doff without help the particular type of gear he is wearing, but he usually decompresses alone. The total elapsed time for this transfer must not exceed 5 min, so the procedure is simplified as much as possible and is directed toward getting the diver back to appropriate pressure as quickly as possible.

The DDC normally relies on purging or ventilation with air to reduce the CO_2 generated by the occupants and to maintain a safe oxygen environment in the event that the built-in breathing system does not contain an overboard dump mechanism for the expired oxygen when oxygen is being breathed. Criteria are given in the *U.S. Navy Diving Manual* (1978) (p. 8-38 to 8-41) for ventilation; it is done by opening both the pressurization and the exhaust valves at the same time.

Operation of these chambers is simple and straightforward and can be easily learned by studying the plumbing, which is generally exposed. Most chambers have the capability for both pressurization and exhaust control to be handled from inside, with an external override. Thus, the physician when he is locking in (being pressurized) to treat a patient who is already at pressure may have the option of controlling his own pressurization. (If this is not the case, it is advisable to make sure the communication system is dependable during the high noise accompanying pressurization and that arrangement is made for some other signaling system in the event of an ear block.)

4. Diving Systems

Diving systems include the most exciting and expensive hyperbaric equipment, from the simple systems with a small bell and deck decompression chamber to the sophisticated saturation "spreads," and they include as well the lockout submersibles and 1-atm systems (Brown and Stott 1980; Gilman 1974a; Usquin and Wide 1974; Wilson 1974, Haux 1982).

A discussion of the various dive modes might aid in describing the systems. Diving systems were first used commercially in support of the exploration phase of petroleum production, where the job was to make occasional dives from 10 to 40 min long, on short notice, and generally in some remote part of the world. As the oil fields went through the transition from exploration to production, this "rig" diving gave way to construction diving, where many hours of continuous work were required, and this led to the extensive commercial exploitation of saturation diving techniques. The diving systems reflected the application—some were designed to be small and efficient, others for steady work.

A deep diving system has a minimum of two primary components: a deck decompression chamber, and a diving bell that can be mated to it (Figure I-3). Also required

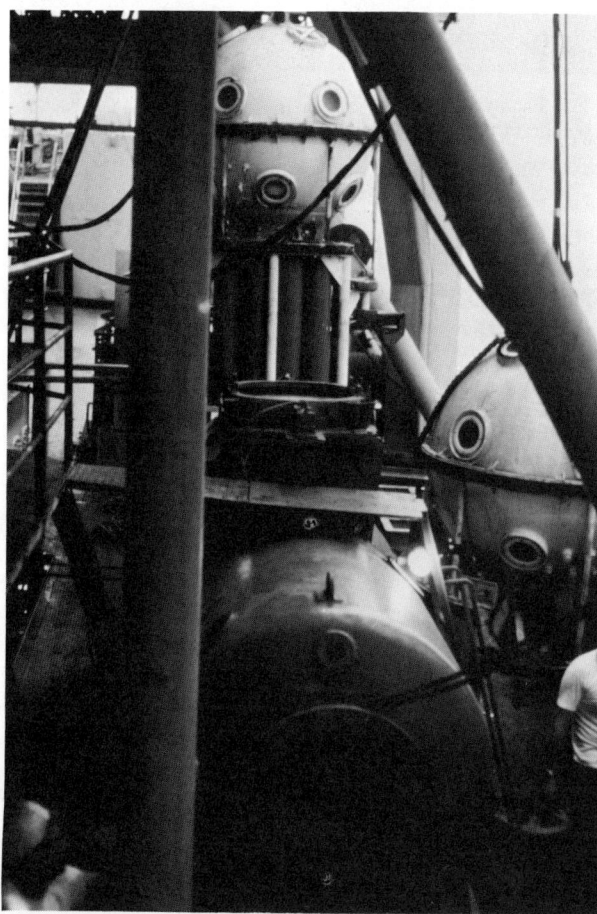

Figure I-3. A small deep diving system tucked on board a drill ship. This system has two bells but is too small for extended saturation diving. (Photo, Claude Harvey.)

is some type of handling system for putting the bell in and out of the water and for mating it to the deck chamber; in rare cases the ship's crane is used. These units normally have a pressure rating somewhere between 400 and 600 fsw (120 and 185 msw).

The bell is generally a sphere 5–6 ft (1.5–1.8 m) in diameter and may mate with the deck chamber in several ways (Figure I-4). In the smaller systems probably the most common bell has a single hatch at the bottom; the bell must be rotated 90° in mating so

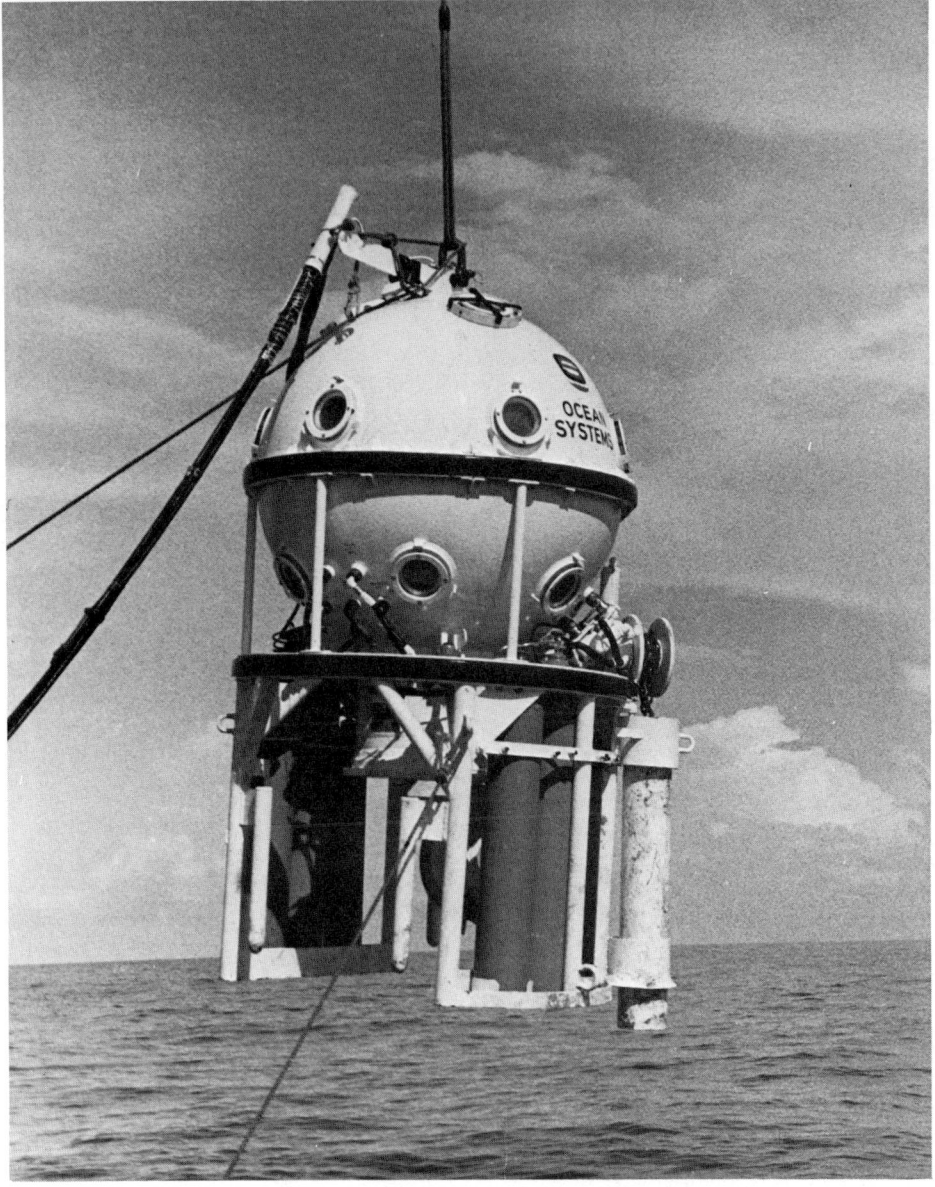

Figure I-4. Commercial diving bell, ADS-4, being lowered over the side. To the lower right of the bell is the drop weight connected to its hydraulically operated winch. (Courtesy of Ocean Systems, Inc.)

that this hatch can then be joined to a horizontal one on the deck chamber. Or the bell may be lifted and mated vertically on top of the deck chamber's transfer lock (this mode is used by the early ADS-4 and Mark I systems). In some cases a bell may have a mating capability on the side, but this makes it more expensive and heavier because it will still have the bottom hatch.

Typically the chamber system is mounted near the side of the vessel. The bell is transferred over the side by a handling system that often consists of a framework in the shape of an inverted U and a winch, all mounted on the same skid as the chamber. The bell may also be lowered directly through the bottom of the vessel, via an opening called a *moon pool*.

Bells are attached to a conventional steel cable to be used as a lifting wire and to a separate bundle of hoses that serves as an umbilical to carry gases, power, and communication; or there may be an integrated strength, power, and communications cable (SPCC). On deck the umbilical may be wound on a separate winch or be coiled into a large basket by hand. Most umbilicals are bundled by taping every few feet with duct tape, but some are preformed with a molded vinyl covering. An auxiliary cable member is normally bundled into the umbilical so that the bell can be brought to the surface by the umbilical if the lifting wire fails.

A bell may or may not be positively buoyant, and a good case can be made for each condition. Some will float and are made sinkable by the addition of a *drop weight* or *clump* that can be released if free ascent is desired.

In a typical dive the divers lock themselves into the bell at sea level atmospheric pressure and are lowered to the work site with the bell still pressurized at atmospheric pressure. When they are ready to go to work, they pressurize the bell—usually with a premixed helium-oxygen mixture—until the bell is at the same pressure as ambient water pressure and the hatches can be opened; a working diver, the lockout diver, can then exit the bell and perform his work. At least one, maybe two, divers remain in the bell to tend the lockout diver and act as his standby.

Breathing is normally by demand apparatus of a premixed lockout mix of gases supplied from the surface through the umbilical. A few *push-pull* systems (see Glossary) have the capability of recovering the diver's expired gas and returning it to either the bell or the surface for scrubbing and reuse.

For short dives under moderately cold conditions, the diver's thermal protection may be a dry suit, but in deeper and longer dives hot water is circulated through a hot water (diving) suit. The bell may have a heat exchanger so that its interior can be heated by the same hot water supply, and it may be insulated.

In addition to controls for the diver's breathing gas and for hot water supplied from the surface, a bell should also carry an auxiliary or emergency supply of breathing gas (Figure I-5). The bell is normally equipped with interior and exterior lighting and with communications from the bell and the diver to the surface vessel, but it is quite common for the man in the bell (bellman) to be unable to talk directly with the diver. Most bells have several viewports.

The bell contains at least one oxygen analyzer covering the range likely to be encountered, but colorimetric tubes are adequate for any CO_2 analysis that may be required. At least one cylinder of oxygen is normally available and piped so that it can be metered in as a replacement for oxygen consumed in metabolism. A bell also contains a CO_2 scrubber, possibly portable.

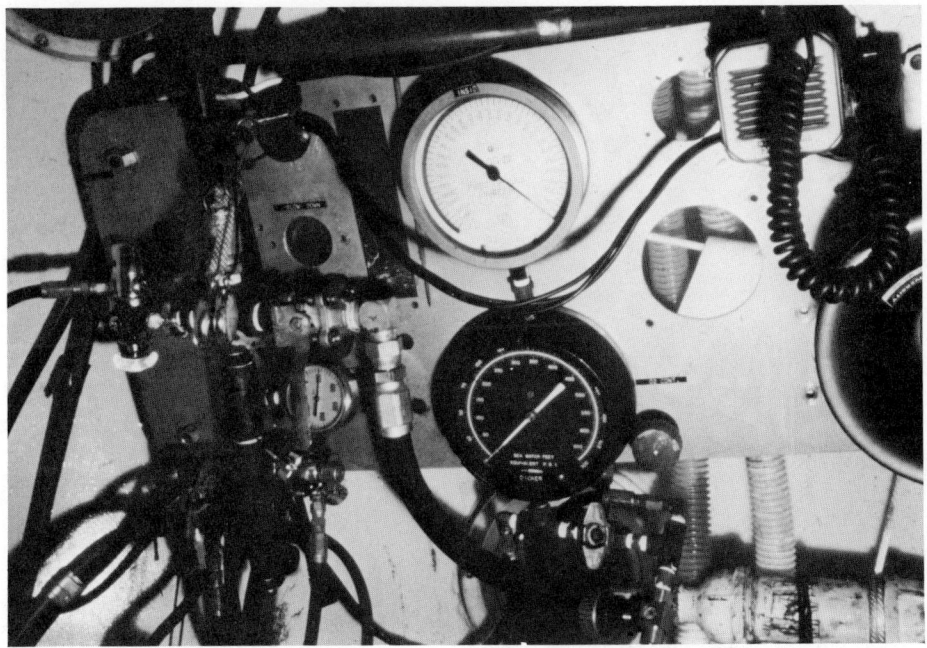

Figure I-5. Inside of typical diving bell; pressure gauges are in the center and gas supply controls on the left. (Photo, J. MacInnis.)

A bell may contain a number of items for use in aiding an injured or disabled diver. There should be a pulley, or a small block and tackle arrangement, in the top so that an unconscious diver can be hoisted into the bell by the bellman. Some bells are equipped with a flooding valve to permit the bell to be partially filled with water. This enables the bellman to float the disabled diver into the bell. The bell first aid kit should contain, as a minimum, an airway, wound dressings, a tourniquet, and scissors. There also may be survival equipment for use in case the umbilical is accidentally cut; these supplies should include thermal protection garments and respiratory gas warmers, some type of lung-powered or hand-powered CO_2 scrubber, through-water wireless communications, and an acoustical pinger, or beacon.

Most bells can be used for observation only, whereby divers (or even nondivers) are lowered at 1 atm for the purpose of making observations or controlling work carried out by the vessel crew, but some saturation bells can not take external pressure. Some bells are equipped with manipulator arms that permit a certain amount of work to be done without a diver in the water.

The term bell is in general use for all types of diving. A bell used for short dives in which decompression begins while divers are still in it is properly called a submersible decompression chamber (SDC), and one used for transferring divers in saturation might be called a personnel transfer capsule (PTC).

The deck chamber portion of the deep diving system (Figure I-6) has at least two compartments, one of which is the transfer lock through which the bell is mated. This lock and the main lock serve essentially the same functions as those in a deck decompression chamber but are equipped for longer occupation. The main lock contains

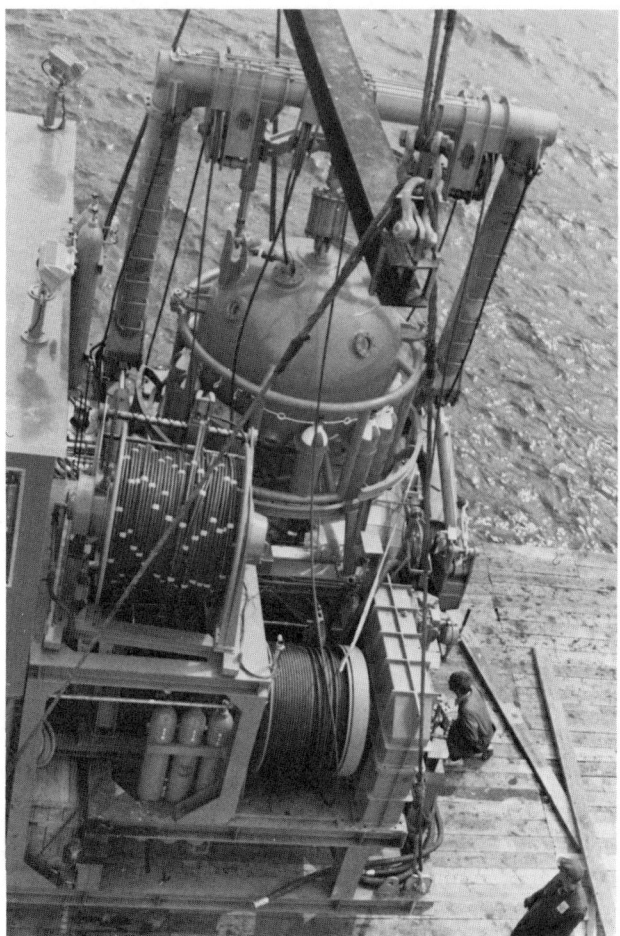

Figure I-6. Deep diving/saturation system; handling system and winches for lifting bell and spooling the umbilical. Bell is mated on top of the entry lock and main living chamber. (Photo, Mark Freitag.)

bunks and some type of environmental control capability, which may be a portable CO_2 scrubber in the simplest cases or a complete environmental control system in the more sophisticated ones. For deep helium diving a heater is desirable.

Deep diving systems may be controlled by valves and gauges mounted on the side of the chamber in much the same way as the basic DDCs (Figure I-6), but the more sophisticated systems have a control van or shack so that operator and instruments can be kept out of the weather.

Saturation systems differ from deep diving systems primarily in matters of degree. Saturation systems are usually much larger, have complete living facilities, and are equipped with environmental conditioning capability that makes continuous habitation not only feasible but reasonably comfortable (Figure I-7). A large saturation spread incorporates several chambers so that different crew schedules can be followed and some divers can be decompressed while others are carrying out the regular diving work schedule. Both temperature and humidity control are essential for a long-term habitation.

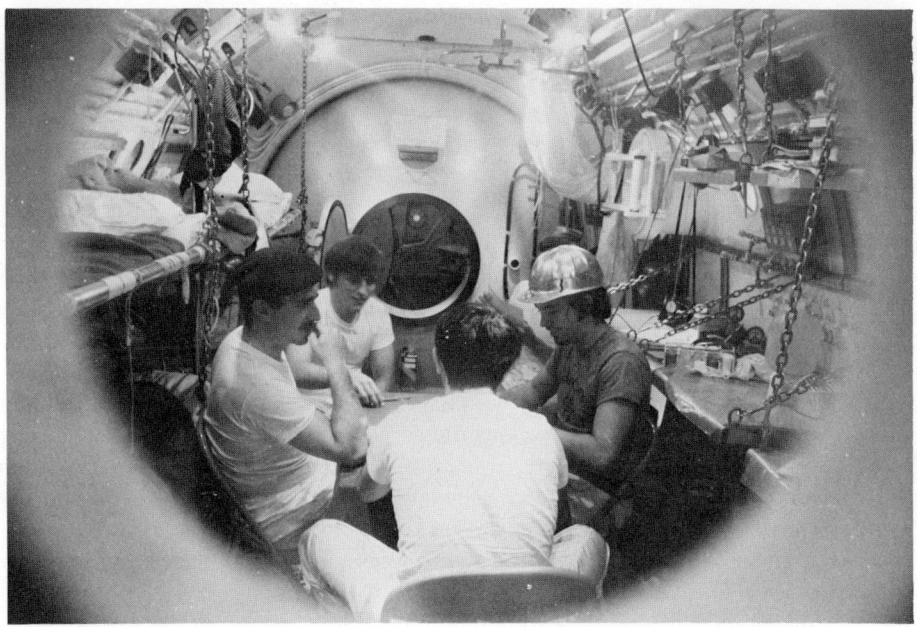
Figure I-7. Divers decompressing in saturation. (Photo, R. W. Hamilton.)

Lockout submersibles are small submarines that have a pressure hull for the pilots and a separate one for the divers. This latter chamber is essentially the same as a diving bell, is used in the same way, and has many of the same features. One important difference, however, is that an untethered submersible has no umbilical and consequently is severely limited in gas stores and power. Conventional open-circuit hot water heating can not be used. The divers are usually transferred to the submersible in saturation at the working depth, so pressurization gas need not be carried; lockout breathing gas is limited also, unless a rebreather or push-pull is used. These and other limitations, plus the high operating expense, tend to restrict the use of lockout submersibles.

Another category of equipment that does not impose increased pressure but is part of the diving operation is that of one-atmosphere systems. These may be submersibles, observation bells (e.g., ARMS, MOB 1001), subsea wellhead capsules (SEAL, Lockheed), and anthropomorphic diving suits (one type is called a JIM). They usually have some type of manipulator as well as capability for viewing of the operation from the surface. Avoiding pressure eliminates many of the familiar diving medical problems, but atmosphere control and thermal protection and protection against other hazards remain; a need for survival and rescue is always a possibility (Hopkins 1974; Morrison et al. 1976).

5. *System Characteristics*

The prime environmental variable associated with diving systems is pressure. Pressure is increased by the valved release of gas into the chamber from a high pressure source, such as a bank of high pressure cylinders, and is reduced by venting gas overboard, i.e., into the ambient environment. Chamber pressure is measured by a conventional pressure gauge; it is usually read to a degree of accuracy far more exacting than is required physiologically. Electronic pressure transducers may be used with digital readouts and for pressure recording, but they are not so reliable that the conventional pressure gauge can be dispensed with (see Figure I-8).

Important to any pressure system is the structure that contains or holds the pressure (the "pressure boundary"). A diving system is predominantly one or more steel pressure vessels, but it is also equipped with viewports, hatches, and a variety of penetrations to the hull itself. Pressure vessels, pipes, and other equipment follow a rule familiar to physicians—Laplace's law, which states that the tension in the wall is proportional to its radius of curvature, and which is the phenomenon that makes an aneurism grow once it has started. Thus the larger a system is, the heavier its wall must be. A ⅛-in. (3-mm) gas sampling line may stand the same pressure as the ½-in. (13-mm) hull of the chamber itself. These principles are, of course, critical to the initial design of the system but are also important to users who are rigging such auxiliary equipment as sampling lines and may be required to make ad hoc arrangements on an emergency basis.

This is perhaps the place to touch on a very important aspect of the use and operation of pressure vessels, that of certification. For many years in the United States the only standard for the construction of a hyperbaric chamber was the code of the American Society of Mechanical Engineers (ASME) for unfired pressure vessels—that is, pressure vessels not used as boilers. These standards dealt adequately with the construction of the

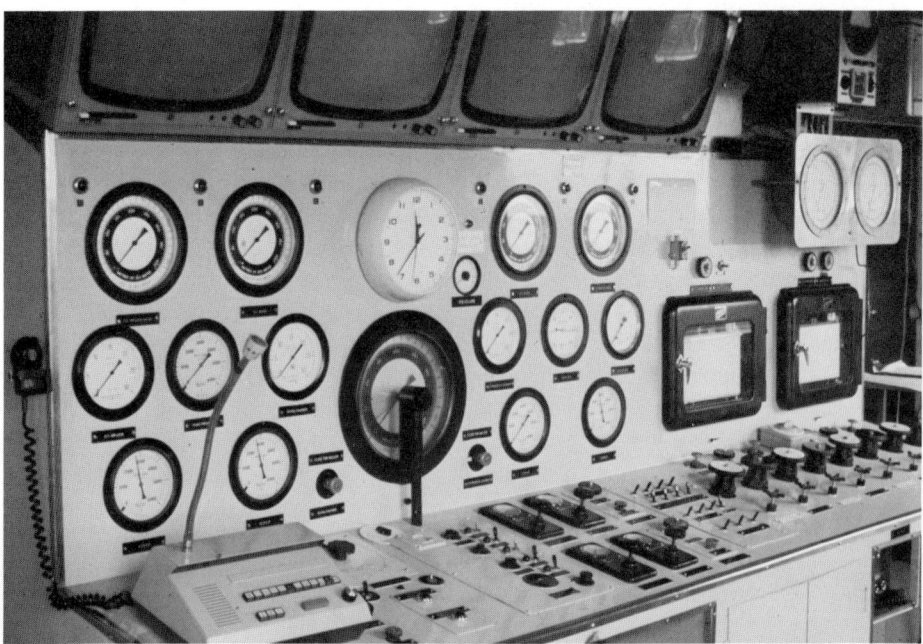

Figure I-8. Control console for deep diving-saturation system. (Photo, Mark Freitag.)

pressure chamber itself but were concerned entirely with the safety of those outside a pressure vessel and did not consider the possibility that someone might be inside. In recent years certification has matured and there are now a variety of agencies involved in these specifications. The ASME now has rules for pressure vessels for human occupancy (PVHO), and diving systems are also certified in the United States by the U.S. Coast Guard and the American Bureau of Shipping. Each country has its own standards (see Det Norske Veritas, 1982).

Most diving systems being built today meet requirements of many if not all of these agencies. An additional and substantially more complex certification is that of the U.S. Navy, which deals with virtually all aspects of a hyperbaric facility; it has been applied to all Navy installations and to all major contract research facilities. But all in all, no amount of certification can substitute for competence and good judgment in the use of such facilities.

Gas storage is a major problem for most diving operations; the needs are met by having on board many high pressure tanks. These may be individual cylinders, or *quads* (a quad is a cluster of from 4 to as many as 28 standard cylinders with a common manifold; see Figure I-9), or a *tube skid* of several large cylinders; sometimes gas semitrailers are used. These tanks may contain various mixtures, or pure gases. The number of gas mixes can be kept to a minimum by having a gas blender (e.g., Mixmaker) on board. Various methods are used for reclaiming and reusing diving gas mixtures; these range from simple recapture and recompression to sophisticated refining devices using cryogenic or molecular sieve technology. Systems are now practical enough to be in regular use commercially.

Air-filled chambers may be pressurized directly from a compressor (high volume,

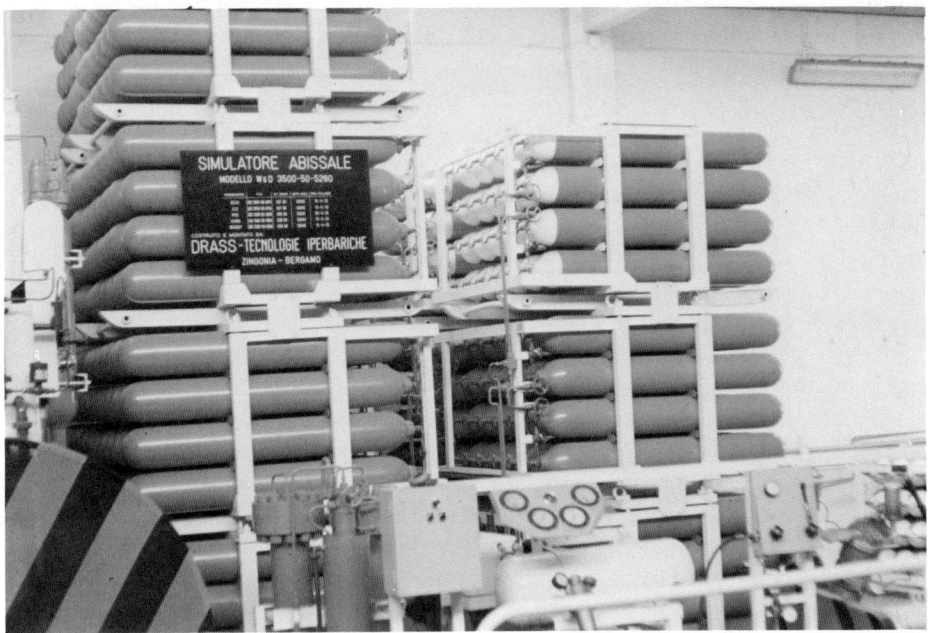

Figure I-9. Stores of breathing gas in "quads" as used for deep diving. (Photo, R. W. Hamilton.)

low pressure), possibly mediated with a small volume tank, or "receiver," kept filled by the compressor. An important consideration in the use of a compressor for chamber pressurization is the oil used as a compressor lubricant. To maintain adequate fire safety in the chamber it is essential that the compressor either be nonlubricated or lubricated with water, or that the compressor output be filtered adequately to remove oil vapor before the air goes into the chamber.

The critical life-support variable in a diving system is oxygen; control of oxygen involves both analysis and makeup. Some type of gas analysis is essential for any type of hyperbaric system that is filled with any mixtures other than just air. Oxygen can be analyzed by several physicochemical methods, and the analyzer may operate by having a sensor or detector unit within the chamber or by reducing the sample gas to atmospheric pressure for analysis. In the first case the analyzer can be read directly for partial pressure, but in the second case a compensation for the reduction of pressure needs to be made. The proper level of oxygen to be maintained in the chamber is a function of the duration of the exposure, and it may range between a low of around 0.21 atm partial pressure to as great as 1.6 or 1.7 atm.

Oxygen makeup or "metabolic O_2" is managed by bleeding oxygen (or a mixture richer in oxygen than the chamber atmosphere) into the chamber at a rate equal to the consumption of the occupants, or at a higher rate if the oxygen partial pressure in the chamber is to be raised. Oxygen is metered into the chamber by means of a flowmeter, but the pressure drop in a cylinder of predetermined volume can also be used to estimate the correct amount. In the case of an air-filled chamber purging or ventilating with air normally maintains an adequate oxygen level.

Carbon dioxide is removed from the basic deck decompression chamber by purging with air. In other systems some type of scrubber is used. For a diving bell and the smaller systems for deep diving a portable electrically powered scrubber is adequate. This uses a blower to force chamber gas through a canister containing a granulated CO_2 absorbing agent (such as Baralyme or Sodasorb). For the larger systems and saturation spreads, CO_2 is normally removed in an external environmental control system (ECS) loop that is serviced by surface personnel. Although more sophisticated regenerative scrubbers have been developed for military submarines, and although there are numerous other chemical reactions that can remove CO_2 economically, no such systems have proved suitable for use in diving. Carbon dioxide is routinely analyzed in most systems and is kept below a partial pressure of 3–4 mmHg (U.S. Navy 1978).

Humidity is controlled in one of two ways. The first is by cooling the gas being conditioned to a temperature low enough to reduce the water vapor content by condensation to achieve the appropriate relative humidity. This method is limited by the available temperature range and the necessity of rewarming the cooled gas before returning it to the chamber. Nevertheless, this system is the most practical for most installations, since it uses traditional refrigeration technology and can be used in an external loop or by means of a dehumidifier element (followed by a reheater) with a blower contained within the chamber. A thermostatically controlled heater in this circuit is the normal means of temperature control. The other approach is to use a regenerable moisture absorbent such as silica gel. This is used in a scrubber system entirely equivalent to those used for removal of CO_2 and often may be contained in the same canister. It takes a rather large amount of silica gel to remove the moisture generated by diving activity, but this method is feasible and is quite practical to use for reducing humidity in the event of a special need or an equipment failure. Desirable relative humidity is in the range 50% to 75%, and temperature is set to the comfort of the divers. This ranges between 26°C and 32°C in a helium atmosphere and increases with depth.

Saturation systems usually contain shower and toilet facilities, generally located in the entry lock. These are straightforward in use but involve considerable engineering. Shower water may be provided by means of a pump or a pressurized holding tank (one each for hot and cold water). Waste is collected in a holding tank by gravity or suction. Toilets are designed so as to prevent suction injury, using interlocks or relief valves.

Transfer locks are used to pass both people and supplies into and out of pressure vessels. They operate with exactly the same principle as a lock in a canal. The small lock for passing in supplies and food was originally called the medical lock, a term that dates back to the day when the only use of a pressure chamber was for treatment. (Note that the term *medical lock* in the jargon of tunnel and caisson workers is the lock for decompressing the workers on their way out.) In a well-managed diving operation these locks need be used only rarely for medical supplies and therefore terms like *lunch lock* or *food lock* are more appropriate. Generally, these locks have an interlock mechanism that makes it impossible to open the hatch unless pressures have been equalized. It is important when using a lock to be sure that the things being passed through can undergo the pressure change safely and without damage.

Fires in hyperbaric chambers have cost a number of lives. Fire safety is a function of both design and operating procedures, and a comprehensive coverage is beyond the scope of this chapter. The fundamental requirements for a fire are the same in a chamber as anywhere—an oxidizer, a fuel, and a source of ignition. All three of these are dealt with in Chapter XIII, "Safety Considerations." (See also Shilling et al. 1976.) If the oxygen in the atmosphere can be kept below about 6%, fire is impossible. The use of materials not flammable in enriched oxygen is also helpful. Necessary wiring is insulated with Teflon or mineral insulation and enclosed in metal conduit; instrument housings are purged with inert gas. Some installations also limit the voltage allowed inside the chamber to an arbitrary value, but the benefit of this voltage limitation is doubtful and may lead to a false sense of security. In addition to provision for fire prevention each chamber should have some means of extinguishing a fire should it start, and there should always be a breathable mix on the BIB system and a mask for every occupant. Whenever possible the chamber hatches should be arranged to permit escape to another compartment should a fire occur.

The principles of hyperbaric chamber fire safety play an important role in hyperbaric medicine and should be thoroughly understood by a hyperbaric physician. It may be as important to know what is *not* a hazard as what is.

One subsystem not yet mentioned is that of communication. The basic deck chamber has a two-way speaker and possibly has sound-powered phones as a backup. More sophisticated systems usually have these plus a headphone system that works with both dry headsets and diving helmets. Closed-circuit television may show the dive supervisor what is going on both inside and outside of the bell, and views of the insides of the chambers are normally available to the surface crew controlling a saturation complex. As part of the communication apparatus for a deep diving system there should be a helium voice unscrambler. (See Figure I-7, which shows divers decompressing in saturation.)

6. *Hyperbaric Facilities*

Ground based hyperbaric facilities are of two general types: those dedicated exclusively to hyperbaric oxygen therapy or treatment of decompression sickness, and those equipped for research in diving. Many facilities combine both applications (NAS/NRC 1966; Sheffield et al. 1977).

Hyperbaric medical facilities are located in most major cities; they are equipped in the same general way as deck decompression chambers but are much larger and have more sophisticated capabilities. They are pressurized with air and, as has been discussed previously, may use high-volume, low-pressure compressors ("low" meaning about 125 psi) or banks of air stored at high (2000–3000 psi) pressure. Many systems have both.

Hyperbaric medical facilities are generally large enough to have "walk-in" doors; very often these chambers have capability for automatic pressure control and venting. They may be equipped for surgery or for the treatment of many patients at a time, have provision for mask breathing, and have tents to use in supplying oxygen exposure to wounds. The pressure rating of most such facilities is adequate for treatment of decompression sickness and embolism. Some chambers are equipped with such sophisticated instrumentation as defibrillators and blood gas analyzers. Because the environment can not be kept in the zone of no combustion ($<6\% \; O_2$), instruments must either be purged with nitrogen or be of special design. They must also be capable of withstanding the pressurization. Most hyperbaric treatment chambers are equipped with water-deluge type of fire extinguishing systems, but all chambers should include a hand-controlled water spray as well.

Monoplace or one-man chambers may also be used for medical treatment (Figure I-10). These chambers are generally made of acrylic plastic and are capable of only 20 or

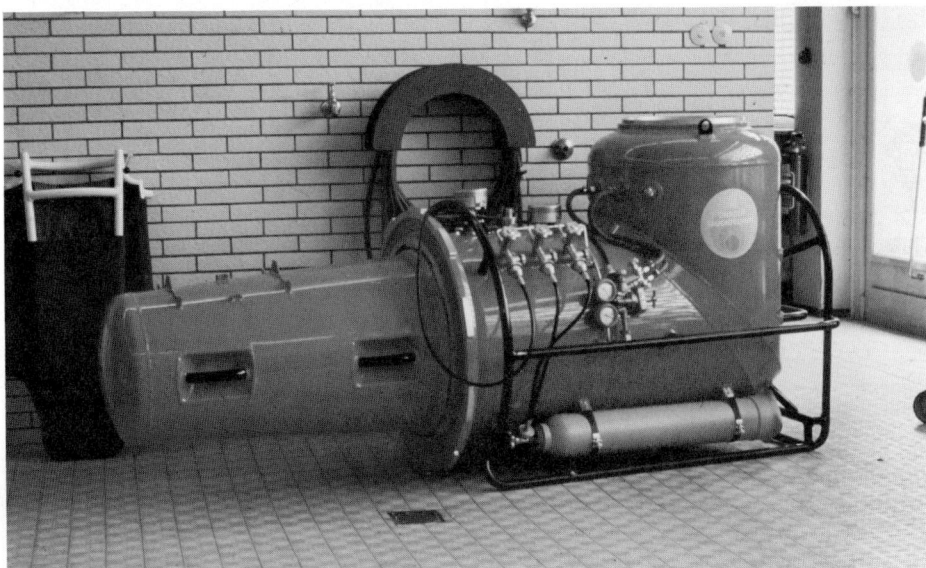

Figure I-10. Chamber for transporting an injured diver; there is adequate space in chamber for attendent. (Photo, R. W. Hamilton.)

30 psi pressure, but this is adequate for hyperbaric oxygen therapy. Use of the monoplace chamber is preferred in the treatment of burns covering large portions of the body; for smaller areas an oxygen tent covering the wound area can be used in the conventional chamber. The monoplace chambers are not acceptable where a great deal of hands-on treatment or care is required, but they are effective in many circumstances. In view of the rather good safety record in the use of this type of chamber the strong prejudice of some experts against monoplace chambers is possibly unwarranted (Hart and Kindwall 1977).

There are a dozen or so major facilities worldwide (Figures I-11–I-13) dedicated to the study of the human being in high pressures, the equipment necessary to support him, and the training of people for work in that environment. These generally have pressure capability of at least several hundred feet and have the ability to use various gas mixtures both for the chamber atmosphere and for the breathing gas; many facilities also have the capability for hyperbaric experimental work under water. These facilities are generally equipped in much the same way as a deep diving system and, in fact, in some cases can be used both ashore and at sea. They are generally larger and have more compartments and much more instrumentation and equipment for communication.

Two different methods are used for providing a wet environment for research and training. The first is a vertically oriented cylinder, the bottom portion of which is filled with water. It may be entered through a hatch right into the water or it may have an igloo space above the water. This is usually the chamber with the highest pressure in the complex, and the dimensions may vary between space enough for several divers to swim around to that of merely exposing a single diver to the wet environment. The other type

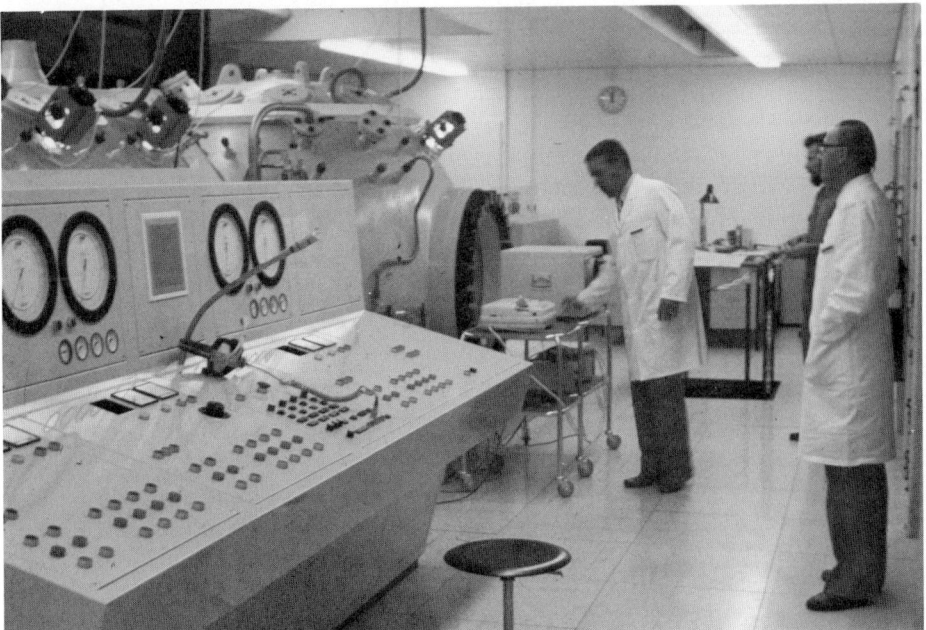

Figure I-11. Laboratory at Kantonspital, University of Zurich, Switzerland. Chambers have a depth rating of 3050 fsw (1000 msw), wet and dry. (Photo, R. W. Hamilton.)

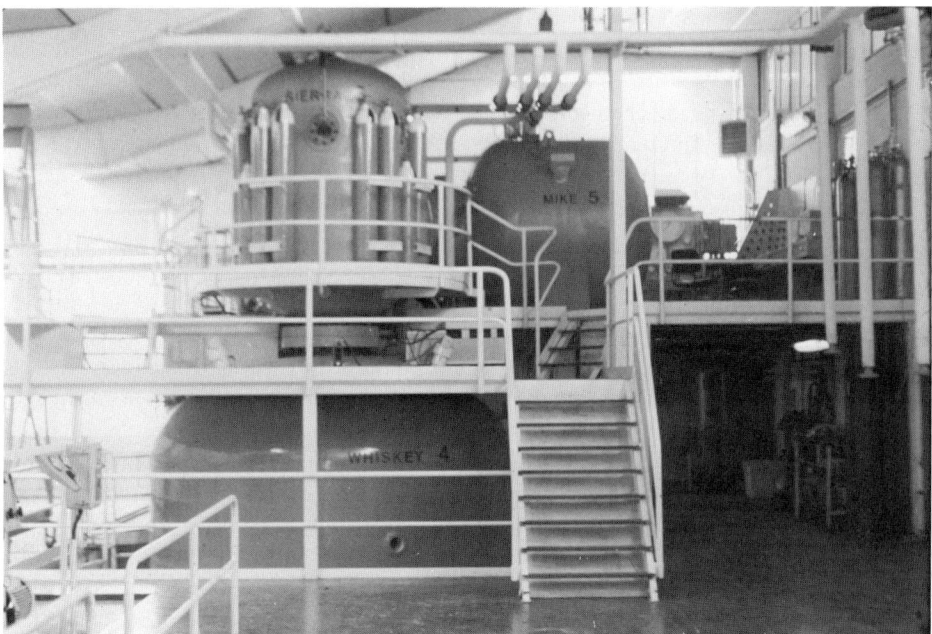

Figure I-12. Training and research facility of SubSea Oil Services, Zingonia, Italy. A bell is shown locked on to a wet pot, simulating the actual lockout environment at sea, to a depth of 500 msw. (Photo, R. W. Hamilton.)

is a horizontally oriented cylinder with a baffle arrangement (a Lanphier–Morin baffle) whereby one end of the chamber is filled with water and accessible to the dry area through a surface located between the baffles. Water is held up in the wet portion by a counterbalancing Torricellian vacuum. Both methods have advantages and disadvantages, and both are effective (Fullerton 1978).

Maintaining the water in a hyperbaric facility requires at least the filtration equipment of a swimming pool and generally also involves temperature control. Some facilities are capable of cooling the water to as low as the freezing point. Fresh water is most often used, or a calcium chloride solution if the additional density is important; seawater is rarely used, because of its corrosive nature. Special-purpose chambers have been built that allow the simulation of exit from a diving bell into the water, simulation of escape from a submarine, or full-opening doors for admitting large items of equipment into the chamber for testing.

7. Rescue Chambers

The category of rescue chambers comprises a wide variety of chambers and is a field that is subject to rapid change in its technology. In the Norwegian sector of the North Sea a diving system is required to have a chamber that can be used to transfer divers in saturation from a vessel that has to be abandoned. These rescue chambers consist of a diving bell that can be cut loose, a portion of the diving system that is skid-mounted and separable, or a complete life boat in which a pressure chamber has been installed

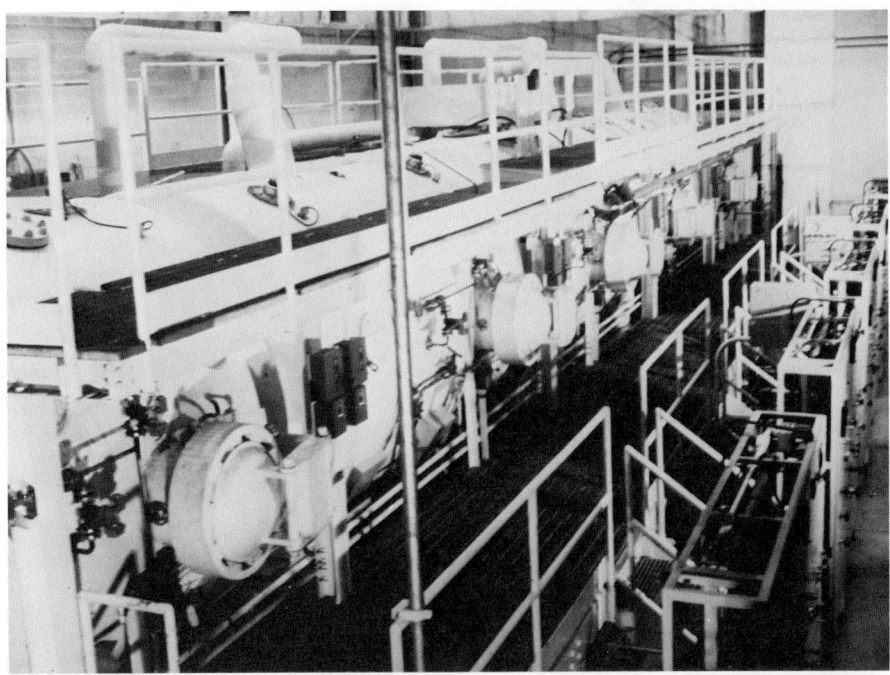

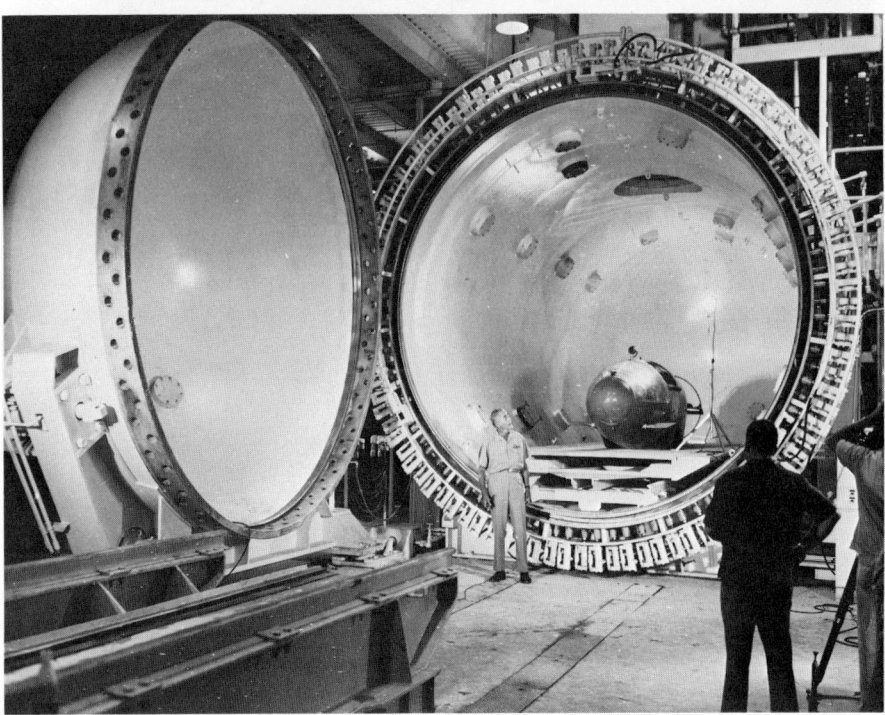

Figure I-13. Navy Ocean-Pressure Simulation Facility at Navy Experimental Diving Unit, Panama City, FL. *Top*: view of exterior of dry chamber. *Bottom*: wet pot for simulation of ocean environments to a depth of 2250 fsw (685 msw). (Photos, U.S. Navy.)

and to which the divers can transfer (under pressure) by tunnel. All are supposed to have autonomous life-support capability, which definitely must include temperature control. The efficacy of the concept of a rescue chamber is controversial, but the chambers are legally required and are available for use.

Another rescue chamber concept is the helicopter-transportable titanium chamber operated by a medical services firm in Aberdeen, Scotland. Two titanium chambers constitute the system. The first is a one-man chamber capable of being carried by several men and occupied by one or possibly two divers. It is intended to transfer the divers from the diving system to a larger eight-man rescue chamber that can be carried by helicopter and has autonomous life-support capabilities good for several hours. The performance of this system has been demonstrated. It can be mated to many of the diving systems currently in use in the North Sea. Pressure capability is great enough to make a transfer at 750 fsw (230 msw). (See Galerne 1978.)

Several other one-man chambers are in use. One of these, built by a civilian contracting agency, has been tested by the U.S. Navy and found to be acceptable for a transfer period of a few hours (Riegel 1974).

Another available system has room for an injured diver and an attendant and is still small enough to be manhandled. This permits a patient to be moved under pressure without isolating him; it is of European manufacture.

8. Undersea Habitats and Underwater Welding Chambers

There are a number of undersea habitats that allow divers or scientists, or both, to live and work on the bottom of the sea at ambient pressure (Figure I-14). The habitats may be either filled with air, if in the proper depth range (less than 50–60 fsw or 15–18 msw), or with a mixture of nitrogen-oxygen or helium-oxygen. There are about as many different types of life support for these systems as there are systems. These may involve purge of the chambers by a large volume of air from the shore, or a buoy that floats above the habitat and with its own diesel-powered compressor conditions the chamber gas, or some more or less self-contained or autonomous systems. The functions that the life support systems perform are essentially the same as those of a diving system or decompression chamber; it is essential that anyone providing medical support to such a facility understand thoroughly its capabilities and limitations.

Decompression from habitats has been carried out in a variety of ways. The Hydrolab, for example, was depressurized to atmospheric pressure and divers then exited and swam to the surface. In another operation (FLARE) the divers locked out, swam to the surface, and were properly decompressed in a surface chamber. In many systems (e.g., Aegir) the entire habitat is recovered and decompression is carried out at the surface under surface control.

As offshore oil fields continue to be developed the advantages of welding the pipelines under the sea are stimulating the development of a variety of underwater, ambient pressure, welding chambers (Figure I-15). These fit down over a pipeline joint and provide a gas-filled space in which welders can make a dry weld using more or less conventional surface techniques. These chambers are often called *habitats* by analogy with the undersea habitat, but they are not used for living (Gilman 1974b). Their use imposes a substantial atmospheric toxicity problem that has been dealt with in a variety of ways ranging from absolute

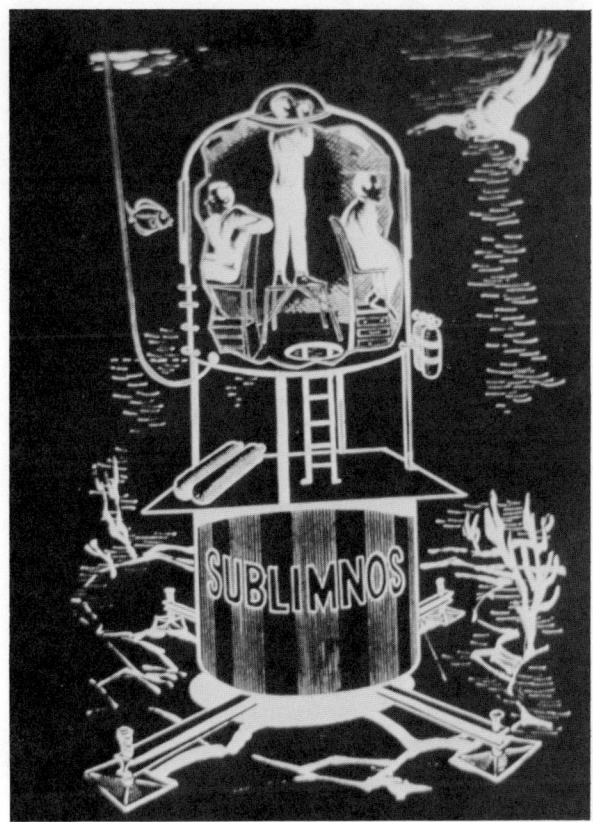

Figure I-14. Sketch of Sublimnos habitat. Facility consists of a living chamber ballasted by a lower compartment full of ballast. This habitat was operated in Lake Huron.

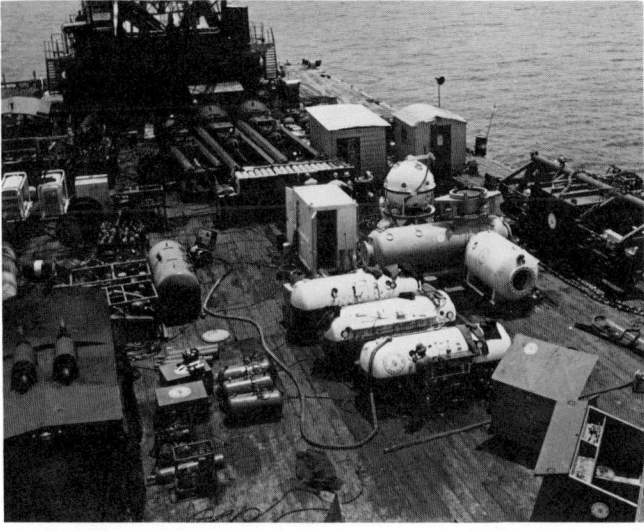

Figure I-15. Equipment "spread" for an active diving operation on board a work barge. Base of crane is in background; underwater welding chamber is at right. In foreground are three deck decompression chambers, while another, smaller one is at left. Behind them is a deep diving system with a bell and control shack. (Photo, Ocean Systems, Inc.)

prohibition of breathing the chamber atmosphere once welding has begun to shirt-sleeve welding with an appropriate scrubbing system. The important gases are carbon monoxide, oxides of nitrogen, and ozone. Carbon monoxide may also be given off by the process of preheating the pipe prior to the commencement of welding, and dangerous levels of carbon monoxide have been detected. Most welding is done deep enough for maintenance of a fire-safe atmosphere and for the oxygen level still to be within normal physiological limits (Jones 1975). Electrical safety is another consideration in underwater welding and is discussed in Chapter XIII, "Safety Considerations."

R. W. HAMILTON

References

BERT, P. 1878. *Barometric Pressure* (transl. by M. A. and F. A. Hitchcock). Columbus, OH: College Book Co., 1943. Republ. Bethesda, MD: Undersea Medical Society, 1978, p. 355–410; 890–895.

BROWN, E., AND M. STOTT 1980. Apache/"Cachalot" 1500 ft saturation system. In: *International Diving Symposium '80*. Gretna, LA: Assoc. of Diving Contractors; p. 27–38. (Tenth Annual International Diving Symposium, New Orleans, Feb. 1980.)

DET NORSKE VERITAS 1982. *Rules for Certification of Diving Systems*. Oslo: Det Norske Veritas.

FULLERTON, D. J. 1978. Canada's new hyperbaric research facility. In: *The Working Diver 1978*. Washington, DC: Marine Technol. Soc., p. 87–107. (Sixth Biennial Working Divers Symposium, Columbus, OH, Mar. 1978.)

GALERNE, A. 1978. North Sea hyperbaric center. In: *The Working Diver 1978*. Washington, DC: Marine Technol. Soc., p. 67–73. (Sixth Biennial Working Divers Symposium, Columbus, OH, Mar. 1978.)

GILMAN, B. C. 1974a. Design, fabrication and installation of commercial diving systems. In: *The Working Diver—1974*. Washington, DC: Marine Technol. Soc., p. 99–123. (Fourth Annual Diving Safety Symposium, Morgan City, LA, Jan. 1974.)

GILMAN, B. C. 1974b. Industry's move into deeper water creates new diving systems demand. *Offshore* 34: 74–78.

HART, G. B., AND E. P. KINDWALL 1977. Hyperbaric chamber clinical support: Monoplace. In: *Hyperbaric Oxygen Therapy*, edited by J. C. Davis and T. K. Hunt. Bethesda, MD: Undersea Medical Society, p. 41–46. (Undersea Med. Soc. Workshop, San Francisco, 1975.)

HAUX, G. 1982. *Subsea Manned Engineering*. Carson, CA: Best Publishing.

HOPKINS, J. W. 1974. The development of the Lockheed subsea oil and gas well production system. In: *National Needs and Ocean Solutions*. Washington, DC: Marine Technol. Soc., p. 557–567. (Proceedings Tenth Annual Conference.)

JARCHO, S. 1968. Alphonse Jaminet on caisson disease (1871). *Am. J. Cardiol.* 21: 258–260.

JONES,, J. J. 1975. Underwater, hyperbaric, dry environment welding. In: *Proceedings, Fifth Annual International Diving Symposium, Morgan City, LA, Jan. 1975*. Gretna, LA: Assoc. Diving Contractors, p. 36–43.

KEAYS, F. L. 1909. Compressed-air illness with a report of 3,692 cases. *Cornell Univ. Med. Coll. Publ. Res. Dept. Med.* 2: 1–55.

KOOPERSTEIN, S. I., AND B. J. SCHUMAN 1957. Acute decompression sickness—a report of forty-four cases. *Ind. Med. Surg.* 26: 492–496.

MORRISON, J. B., A. B. GISBORNE, W. S. BUTT, AND J. T. FLORIO 1976. Biomechanical evaluation of a one atmosphere diving suit. In: *The Working Diver 1976*. Washington, DC: Marine Technol. Soc. p. 38–54. (The Working Diver Syposium, Columbus, OH, Mar. 1976.)

NAS/NRC COMMITTEE ON HYPERBARIC OXYGENATION 1966. *Fundamentals of Hyperbaric Medicine*. Washington, DC: Natl. Acad. Sci./Natl. Res. Council. (Publ. 1298.)

RIEGEL, P. S. 1974. One-man portable recompression chamber. In: *The Working Diver—1974*. Washington, DC: Marine Technol. Soc. p. 219–235. (Fourth Annual Diving Safety Symposium, Morgan City, LA, Jan. 1974.)

SHEFFIELD, P. J., J. C. DAVIS, G. C. BELL, AND T. J. GALLAGHER 1977. Hyperbaric chamber clinical support: Multiplace: In: *Hyperbaric Oxygen Therapy*, edited by J. C. Davis and T. K. Hunt. Bethesda, MD: Undersea Medical Society, 1977, p. 25–39. (Undersea Med. Soc. Workshop, San Francisco, 1975.)

SHILLING, C. W., M. F. WERTS, AND N. R. SCHANDELMEIER (editors) 1976. *The Underwater Handbook: A Guide to Physiology and Performance for the Engineer*. New York: Plenum Press.

THORNE, I. J. 1941. Caisson disease: Observations and report of 300 cases at the Queen's Midtown Tunnel Project. *JAMA* 117: 585–588.

U.S. NAVY 1978. *U.S. Navy Diving Manual (Change 2). Air Diving*. Washington, DC: U.S. Navy Dept., vol. 1. (NAVSEA 0994-LP-001-9010.)

USQUIN, B., AND P. WIDE 1974. A 2200 feet modular D.D.S. In: *The Working Diver—1974*. Washington, DC: Marine Technol. Soc. p. 83–98. (Fourth Annual Diving Safety Symposium, Morgan City, LA, Jan. 1974.)

WILSON, H. D. 1974. Commercial saturation diving operations. In: *The Working Diver—1974*. Washington, DC: Marine Technol. Soc. p. 29–39. (Fourth Annual Diving Safety Symposium, Morgan City, LA, Jan. 1974.)

ZINKOWSKI, N. B. 1971. *Commercial Oilfield Diving*. Centreville, MD: Cornell Maritime Press.

Physics of Diving and Physical Effects on Divers

A. *Introduction*

Everyone on earth is continuously exposed, under normal circumstances, to the pressure of the earth's atmosphere, which at sea level amounts to 14.7 pounds per square inch (psi) of body surface. Most of the time people do not think about air pressure or the air they breathe. They become aware, however, of a change in pressure when they fly in an unpressurized airplane or when they climb a mountain, because in these situations atmospheric pressure is reduced, as is the partial pressure of oxygen, which causes shortness of breath.

When the body moves away from sea level or rises above the earth, pressure on it decreases, but no matter how far above the earth a body moves, the atmospheric pressure never decreases by more than one atmosphere (1 atm). For divers, however, the pressure increases by 1 atm with every additional 33 ft of seawater depth. This increase in pressure complicates medical problems associated with work underwater or in a chamber that is under pressure.

Before the effects of pressure on the human body are considered, we must first understand the physics of pressure. These principles of physics provide the keystone in understanding the reasons for employing various diving techniques and procedures, and the operation of associated equipment. They also assume particular significance in studying the effects of the underwater environment upon the human body (U.S. Navy 1973) and, it should be added, to sound clinical judgment of pressure-related injuries and illnesses.

B. *Pressure*

Pressure is force acting on a unit area; expressed mathematically,

$$\text{Pressure} = \frac{\text{force}}{\text{area}} \quad \text{or} \quad P = \frac{F}{A}$$

Thus, as you sit reading this there is a force acting on your body equal to approximately 42,336 lb, or more than 20 tons, since the body skin surface of an average male equals 20 ft^2, and the sea level pressure is 14.7 psi. You are completely unaware of this enormous pressure, because of equalization of the pressure within and outside the body.

1. Units of Pressure

Pressure units in this field are too numerous to remember: feet or meters of salt or fresh water; inches of mercury (in. Hg); millimeters of mercury (mmHg); pounds per square inch (psi); grams or kilograms per square centimeter (g/cm^2 or kg/cm^2); bars or millibars (bar or mbar); pascal (Pa); torricelli (torr); and standard physical atmosphere (atm). The more common units are expressed at sea level as follows:

$$\begin{aligned}
1 \text{ atm} &= 29.9 \text{ inches of mercury (in. Hg)} \\
&= 760 \text{ millimeters of mercury (mmHg)} \\
&= 101.3 \text{ kilopascals (kPa)} \\
&= 33 \text{ feet of seawater (fsw)} \\
&= 34 \text{ feet of fresh water} \\
&= 14.7 \text{ pounds per square inch (lb/in.}^2\text{; psi)} \\
&= 1033 \text{ grams per square centimeter (g/cm}^2\text{)} \\
&\quad \text{(seen only in the old literature)} \\
&= 10.08 \text{ meters of seawater (msw)} \\
&= 1013.3 \text{ millibars (mbar)}
\end{aligned}$$

2. Pressure Nomenclature

Definition of a number of types of pressure is appropriate here.

(i) Absolute Pressure. Absolute pressure is the sum of all pressures acting on an object; in diving, the sum of the atmospheric pressure and the hydrostatic pressure acting on a submerged object.

(ii) Ambient Pressure. Ambient pressure is the absolute pressure surrounding an object.

(iii) Atmospheric Pressure. Atmospheric pressure is the pressure exerted by the earth's atmosphere, which varies with altitude above sea level; at sea level atmospheric pressure is equal to 14.7 psi.

(iv) Design Pressure. Design pressure is a pressure rating of a component established by physical characteristics and stress analysis.

(v) Gauge Pressure. Since gauges are normally calibrated to read zero at sea level, it follows that gauge pressure is the increase above atmospheric pressure in the pressure being measured; thus, gauge pressure is the difference between absolute pressure and atmospheric pressure (syn.: overpressure).

(vi) Hydrostatic Pressure. Hydrostatic pressure in open water is the weight of the column of water above, and acting on, a body immersed in the water. The pressure is equal in all directions at a specific depth, and pressure exerted at any point is the same if the fluid

is at rest. But the most important consideration for diving is that water in its liquid form is virtually incompressible; i.e., it is a liquid that, in general, does not change significantly in volume or other characteristics because of changes in either temperature or pressure. Any outside pressure exerted on a confined body of water will spread throughout the liquid—equally and in all directions. Since water is incompressible, it follows that "liquid man" can work comfortably at a depth of 500 feet of seawater (fsw) where the pressure is 237 psi of body surface or about 339 tons. (For the time being we will not consider the air-filled parts of the body, such as the lungs, middle ear, sinuses, and the gas in the gastrointestinal tract.)

A young woman said that she had a "hole" in her head the size of an egg following an operation for a benign growth, and only the scalp had been used to cover the opening. She had been told that if she went underwater, the pressure would squeeze her brain and kill her. Because the brain is largely water and subject to hydrostatic laws, she could be assured that the pressure change was not a problem. On the other hand it was not wise for her to dive: the possible irritable focus resulting from surgical penetration of the dura increased the risk of a seizure, and a seizure while underwater could easily lead to drowning.

(vii) Partial Pressure. In a mixture of gases, the proportion of the total pressure contributed by a single gas in the mixture is called the partial pressure of that gas. A mixture of gases rather than a single pure gas is usually used for diving or for working in a pressure chamber. Thus, partial pressure computations are necessary for mixed-gas diving and are useful in understanding diving physiology. The principles of these computations are presented with Dalton's law, later in this chapter.

Accounts of two accidents illustrate how partial pressure affects the diver who is breathing under pressure. A scuba diver picked up his compressed air tanks that had been in the basement for the winter and was glad to see that the pressure was still up for his first dive of the season. Just as he went under the water he lost consciousness and sank to the bottom. Fortunately he had obeyed the first rule of diving and had a buddy, who pulled him out and resuscitated him. Examination of the air in his tank revealed that it contained only 2% oxygen by volume, which is only 15.2 mmHg partial pressure (at the surface)—far below the level required to maintain life. During the winter, the oxygen had reacted with the moisture and the iron of the tank to form iron oxide, thus using up the oxygen.

In deep commercial diving it is the usual practice to use gas mixtures with the oxygen partial pressure held so that at the working depth it will be normal—a normoxic mixture. Two men were working at 300 ft, or at a pressure of about 10 atm. For such a mixture at that depth the oxygen percentage should be 2%. But the mixing equipment failed and the men were breathing 100% oxygen at that depth, or a partial pressure of 7600 mmHg, which caused convulsions and death in moments.

C. *Pathophysiology of Gases Associated with Diving*

In all underwater activity the individual must continue to breathe; thus for survival there must be available some oxygen-containing gas mixture. The breathing mixture may be supplied through an umbilical from the surface to the diver, or the diver may carry his gas in a cylinder on his back, as in scuba diving. Air is the most common diving gas, but since other combinations are used, it is important to be familiar with the diving gases and the properties and behavior of these most elusive and intangible of substances.

Gases such as oxygen (O_2), carbon monoxide (CO), carbon dioxide (CO_2), and nitrogen (N_2) play an important role in underwater activity and hyperbaric exposure. Each gas alone, or the interaction between the gases, has an effect on physiological function and may have a deleterious effect on the organism.

For the purpose of this presentation we are assuming that as physicans you know the physiology of respiration, particularly the alveolar blood-gas exchange, the blood transport of the gases to the tissues, and metabolism. It might be well, however, to review the gas laws, which are defined in this chapter and the Glossary. For a review of the pathology of the above gases as they are affected by increased pressure experienced in diving and other hyperbaric activity, the following reading is suggested: Bennett and Elliott (1975); Shilling et al. (1976); Miller (1979); Miles and Mackey (1976).

While each gas is discussed separately in this chapter, the gases themselves are almost always used in some mixture. Air is a naturally occurring mixture of many of them. In certain types of diving special mixtures may be blended, using one or more of the inert gases with oxygen. Further details of the gases can be found in U.S. Navy (1978), Miller (1979), Shilling (1964).

1. Air

Compressed air is the most commonly used breathing gas for diving operations. Normal air is a mixture of gases and vapors; the composition of dry air is shown in Table II-1.

2. Oxygen

a. Description

Oxygen. Symbol O; atomic number 8; atomic weight 16.000; molecular weight 31.9998. Used as the standard of comparison for the atomic weight of each of the other elements. A colorless, odorless, tasteless gas. Nontoxic at atmospheric pressure but becomes highly toxic under increased partial pressure. Discovered by Priestley in 1774 and independently by Scheele the same year. Named from the Greek, for *acid*, to mean *acid-forming*. The most abundant of all elements on earth; is found free in the atmosphere, 23.15% by weight in dry air and 20.98% by volume, and is the most abundant element (85.8%) in the ocean. Occurs in combination with silicon, aluminum, iron, and other metals in all rocks, making up, in fact, an average 46.7% of the solid crust of the earth. A constituent of practically all plant and animal substances, except the hydrocarbons. The best general text on the subject of oxygen is probably the one by Gilbert (1981).

Three radioactive isotopes have been identified: ^{19}O, with a radioactive half-life of 29.4 sec; ^{14}O, half-life 76.5 sec; and ^{15}O, half-life 118.0 sec.

Oxygen is essential in the process of respiration of all animals. In the air we breathe it is the oxygen—and only the oxygen—that is actually used by the body. The burning of

Table II-1
Composition of Dry Air

Component	Percent by volume
Nitrogen	78.084
Argon	0.934
Oxygen	20.946
Carbon dioxide	0.033
Rare gases	0.003
Neon	
Helium	
Krypton	
Hydrogen	
Xenon	
Carbon monoxide	

fuels is a process of combination with free oxygen, and oxygen is used as a propellant for rockets. Oxygen is capable of reacting chemically with all other elements except the inert gases and fluorine.

b. Partial Pressure

The duality of oxygen depends on its partial pressure and it may be life sustaining, therapeutic, or lethal as the partial pressure increases. (See Dalton's law in the next section.) The partial pressure of oxygen considered normoxic and to which man is adapted is 0.21 ATA. However, a healthy person can maintain proper blood oxygenation with inspired oxygen pressures down to about 0.16 ATA. Below this level performance is impaired, and unconsciousness occurs when the level gets lower than about 0.1 ATA. Levels much below this may cause brain damage or death if maintained for more than 3 or 4 min. Oxygen poisoning of the individual depends, of course, on the partial pressure of oxygen but also on the length of exposure, the level of activity in work, and the temperature.

In diving it is important to know the oxygen dose to the individual and to keep it as near the normoxic level as possible. The problem is handled by mixing gases rather than using air at the deeper depths (over 300 ft). For example a mixture of nitrogen and oxygen (nitrox) for use at 10 atm absolute would have only 2% oxygen, for at depth the diver would be breathing 20%, or a normoxic level. Mixtures of helium and oxygen (heliox) are also used in deep diving.

c. Toxicity

Prolonged exposure to increased partial pressure of oxygen can result in toxic effects which become progressively more severe as the inspired partial pressure or duration of exposure is increased. The most dramatic of the effects are on the respiratory system (the Lorrain Smith effect) and on the central nervous system (the Paul Bert effect). There are other physiological effects but they are not generally of pathological importance and not of immediate trouble for the diver.

(i) Measurement and Limits. In the interest of prevention it is important to know the partial pressure limits for oxygen. The accompanying table (U.S. Navy Diving Manual 1973) gives the oxygen partial pressure limits for oxygen in mixed-gas mixtures during working dives. They are deliberately conservative.

Exposure time, min	Maximum oxygen partial pressure, ATA
30	1.6
40	1.5
50	1.4
60	1.3
80	1.2
120	1.1
240	1.0

For calculating the individual total oxygen exposure incurred during all phases of a dive, including decompression, the Institute for Environmental Medicine of the University of Pennsylvania developed a measure called the Unit Pulmonary Toxicity Dose (UPTD).

(ii) Pulmonary Toxicity. The harmful effects of breathing increased partial pressure of oxygen have been amply demonstrated on lung membranes and on lung function. The damage is the result of chemical actions related to the inspired partial pressure of oxygen and to the physical consequences of excluding the inert carrier gas from the pulmonary passage; Clark and Lambertson (1971) point out that the rate of development and degree of chemical damage to the respiratory passages are proportional to both the amount of oxygen and the duration of exposure.

Pulmonary edema is one of the most common pathological manifestations of pulmonary oxygen toxicity; it first appears as a widening of interstitial spaces and progresses, in most cases, to form massive pleural effusions. Atelectasis is another finding that may be related to chemical action on alveolar surfactant. Associated with the atelectasis, edema, congestion, asymmetric narrowing of the airways, and decrease in alveolar surfactant is a loss of elastic properties of the pulmonary tissue. This leads to an early demonstrable reduction in vital capacity.

(iii) Central Nervous System Damage. Whereas the respiratory system is affected by long-term (i.e., hours of) continuous exposure to partial pressure not exceeding 2.0 atm, the exposure to oxygen partial pressures of several atmospheres rapidly affects the central nervous system first and can culminate in convulsions, paralysis, and possible death.

Early warning signs usually precede the onset of convulsions: Localized muscular twitching, especially around the face; incoordination of diaphragm in respiration; nausea; paresthesis (pins and needles); dizziness, incoordination; light-headedness; euphoria; dyspnea (subjective distress or difficulty); confusion; visual symptoms; dilated pupils; bradycardia. These early warning signs may be barely noticeable and the convulsion may come on almost immediately. The latency or "safe latent period" decreases sharply with increasing partial pressure. There is also a marked individual difference in tolerance.

The latent period for oxygen poisoning is shortened by administration of a low concentration of carbon dioxide, and it is decreased by exercise; hypothermia should delay convulsions.

d. Use of High Pressure Oxygen (HBO)

(i) Surface Decompression. "Sur-D" is a technique for discharging all or a portion of the diver's decompression obligation in a decompression chamber on the surface rather than in the water. It is recommended that oxygen be breathed in the recompression chamber to significantly reduce the decompression time.

(ii) Omitted Decompression. Certain emergencies may interrupt or prevent a diver from taking the regular specified decompression stops. Blowup, exhausted air supply, or bodily injury may constitute such emergencies. Even if the diver shows no symptoms or ill effects the omitted decompression must be made up at once to avoid later difficulty. An appropriate way is to use the oxygen surface decompression tables.

(iii) Treatment Tables. The standard treatment tables allow for oxygen breathing at the 30-, 20-, and 10-ft stops. This has proved to be an excellent treatment regime.

(iv) Hyperbaric Oxygen Therapy. Oxygen is used in the treatment of both decompression sickness and air embolism. It is also used as hyperbaric oxygen (100% breathed under increased pressure) for the treatment of a number of nondiving disease conditions: carbon monoxide poisoning; anemia, exceptional blood loss; cyanide poisoning; gas gangrene; compromised skin grafts; smoke inhalation; Meleney's ulcer; and many other diseases and conditions (Davis and Hunt 1977 and *Hyperbaric Oxygen Therapy: A Committee Report* 1981).

3. Nitrogen

a. Description

Nitrogen. Symbol N; atomic number 7; atomic weight 14.008; molecular weight 28,0134. A colorless, odorless, tasteless, nontoxic, chemically inert gas. Discovered by Rutherford in 1772. Named from the Latin words for *niter-forming*. Found in great abundance in our atmosphere (78.03% nitrogen by weight) to an estimated amount of more than four trillion tons. Natural abundance furnished by two stable isotopes: ^{14}N, 99.635%, and ^{15}N, 0.365%. Although chemically and biologically inert, there are important active compounds: the nitrates in fertilizers as plant nutrition; nitroglycerine as an explosive, nitrous oxide as an anesthetic (laughing gas); and in the form of protein as a food for man and animals.

In diving, since nitrogen in the air or in a nitrogen-oxygen mixture (nitrox) is inert in the free state, it is essentially a carrier for the oxygen and may be considered to dilute the oxygen. Because of the anesthetic properties of nitrogen breathed under pressure (increased partial pressure), a condition known as nitrogen narcosis may develop, which can result in a loss of orientation, performance, and judgment by the diver. (See Chapter III-E, *Inert Gas Narcosis*). Nitrogen is also incriminated in bubble formation during too-rapid decompression and thus the development of decompression sickness.

b. Physiological Effects

Since the air we breathe contains about 80% nitrogen, it follows that the blood and all of the tissues of living and breathing men and animals are saturated with nitrogen at a tension (partial pressure) equal to the partial pressure of nitrogen in the atmosphere. Let us assume that in the average person with normal lungs, the alveoli contain air equal to the pressure of the atmosphere, and thus the partial pressure of nitrogen to the alveoli will be about 570 mmHg. If such a person is exposed to a breathing medium other than air or is taken to a depth or to an altitude, the change will alter the partial pressure of nitrogen in the alveoli, and the blood and tissues must either lose or take up nitrogen in order to reach equilibrium with the changed alveolar nitrogen pressure.

(i) Absorption and Elimination. The process of taking up more nitrogen is called *absorption, saturation,* or *nitrogenation*. The process of giving up nitrogen is correspondingly called *elimination, desaturation,* or *denitrogenation*. In diving both processes are important: saturation is critical when the diver is exposed to an increased partial pressure of nitrogen at depth and desaturation is important when the diver returns to the surface. The sequence of events involved in saturation can be illustrated by the changes that occur in the body of a diver taken rapidly from the surface to a depth of 100 fsw. The process can briefly be described as follows: Let us say that the tension of nitrogen in a diver's blood upon leaving the surface is roughly eight-tenths (0.8) of 1 atm; when the diver reaches 100 fsw, the alveolar pressure of nitrogen will be about 0.8 of 4 atm (or 3.2 atm), while the nitrogen tension in the blood and tissues will remain temporarily at 0.8 atm. The partial pressure difference or gradient between the alveolar air and the blood and tissues is thus $3.2 - 0.8 = 2.4$ atm. This is the force that makes molecules of nitrogen move from the alveolar air to the alveolar capillaries and from the bloodstream to the tissues. This process of reaching a new equilibrium is of course influenced by the amount of the blood supplied to each particular tissue, e.g., bone and cartilage with a meager supply and liver with a generous supply. It is also dependent on the saturation efficiency of the tissue, nitrogen being about five times as soluble in fat as in water. Time at a given depth is most important in determining the degree of saturation.

(ii) Implications for Decompression. If the diver were to come to the surface without any stops for decompression there would be a gradient of 2.4 atm tending to force the nitrogen in his blood out of solution. Forgoing decompression is, of course, not permitted, since time must be allowed for slow desaturation on the way to the surface. (The principles of decompression are presented in detail in Chapter IV, "Decompression Theory.") If sufficient time is not allowed during decompression, bubbles may form. These bubbles are the basis of decompression sickness, which is described in detail in Chapter VI.

4. *Helium*

Helium. Symbol He; atomic number 2; atomic weight 4.003. A colorless, odorless, nontoxic gas. Discovered in 1868 by English astronomers Lockyer and Frankland in the gas surrounding the sun and therefore named from Greek work for *sun*. Discovered in 1895 by the Scottish chemist Ramsay in the mineral clevite. Also occurs with some natural gases, four wells in Texas having produced 55 million ft^3 of helium; has also been found in wells in Canada, Poland, and the USSR. Almost totally inert, does not even combine with itself. No biological, medical, or agricultural usefulness. Two stable isotopes, ^{3}He and ^{4}He, account for its natural abundance, ^{4}He furnishing almost 100%.

Since helium is seven times lighter than air, its primary use in the early twentieth century was for inflation of balloons and dirigibles. Because of its low density it is also used extensively for deep diving, since it does not have the narcotic effect of nitrogen. It does, however, have some disadvantages: breathing helium-oxygen mixtures causes speech distortion (Donald Duck effect), which hinders communication; its high thermal conductivity results in rapid loss of body heat.

5. Hydrogen

Hydrogen. Symbol H; atomic number 1; atomic weight 1.0080. A colorless, odorless, tasteless, nontoxic gas. First recognized as a distinct element by the English physicist Cavendish in 1766. Named by Lavoisier to mean *water-forming*. Occurs chiefly combined with oxygen in water, with carbon in hydrocarbons, with other elements in acids and bases, and with carbon, oxygen, and nitrogen in a vast variety of organic substances. Occurs throughout living material. Natural abundance furnished by two stable isotopes: ^{1}H, 99.9849%, and ^{2}H, 0.0151%.

For years hydrogen was used in balloons and dirigibles because it is the lightest of all elements, but it is violently explosive when mixed with air in proportions such that more than 5.3% oxygen is present. The flaming crash of the German dirigible airship *Hindenburg* in 1937 at the Naval Air Station in Lakehurst, New Jersey, put an effective end to the general use of hydrogen for lighter-than-air ships.

Hydrogen is used in diving in some parts of the world where helium is difficult to get, and it can be used safely for very deep diving, where the percentage of oxygen would be well below the explosive range.

6. Neon

Neon. Symbol Ne; atomic number 10; atomic weight 20.183. An inert, monatomic, colorless, odorless, tasteless gas. Found in ordinary air, 1 part neon to about 65,000 parts air. Discovered by the Scottish chemists Ramsay and Travers in 1898 and named from the Greek word for *new*. Natural abundance from three stable isotopes: ^{20}Ne, 90.92%; ^{21}Ne, 0.26%; and ^{22}Ne, 8.82%.

Since neon has superior thermal insulating properties, and since it does not exhibit the narcotic properties of nitrogen and does not cause speech distortion, neon has been the subject of some diving research. It is not commonly used, however, as a diving gas.

7. Carbon Dioxide

a. Description

Carbon dioxide. Symbol CO_2; molecular weight 44.0103. Occurs in the atmosphere as approximately 0.03% of the total and at that concentration is colorless, odorless, tasteless, and nontoxic. However, in greater concentration it has an acid taste and odor and can be extremely toxic.

Carbon dioxide is produced by the natural processes of animal metabolism, combustion, and fermentation. In man it is the result of the production of energy from the oxidation of carbon, and it is constantly eliminated through the process of respiration.

Carbon dioxide is also produced in the burning of fossil fuels (particularly coal), and as its atmospheric levels increase in the United States it may, in time, become a serious public health problem. Production of carbon dioxide in the process of fermentation holds no threat to the general public, and the level must only be controlled in the brewery itself.

b. Human Production

The production of carbon dioxide (CO_2) in the human diver is closely related to the consumption of oxygen: for every liter of oxygen consumed, almost a liter of carbon dioxide is produced. As with other gases, the volume of a given quantity of gas varies with depth, but the actual number of molecules involved does not so vary. However, CO_2 production does vary with type of diet and changes markedly with exercise or various levels of work.

The relationship between the amount of carbon dioxide produced and the amount of oxygen consumed can be expressed as a ratio, the respiratory quotient:

$$\text{Respiratory quotient} = \frac{CO_2 \text{ produced}}{O_2 \text{ consumed}}$$

This ratio can range from 0.7 to 1.0, depending on the diet and the rate of exercise or work; the average ratio for a working diver is 0.85.

According to the *U.S. Navy Diving Manual* (1973), the process of respiration includes six phases that are important to the life of the cells and thus to the entire body: (1) breathing or ventilation of the lungs; (2) exchange of gases between the blood and air in the lungs; (3) transport of gases carried by the blood; (4) exchange of gases between blood and body tissues; (5) exchange of gases between the tissue fluids and cells; and (6) use and production of gases by the cells. These phases are discussed below in relation to CO_2 metabolism.

c. Control of Breathing

The respiratory center of the brain, sensitive to the level of carbon dioxide and acid in the blood, controls the rate and volume of breathing. When the level of CO_2 becomes too high, the center triggers an increase in breathing so as to move more air through the lungs to achieve a normal CO_2 level. The peripheral chemoreceptors monitor the level of oxygen and carbon dioxide in the blood leaving the lungs. When the oxygen partial pressure falls, these chemoreceptors send impulses to the respiratory center, signaling the need for an increase in breathing. However, a low oxygen level, by itself, may not increase the breathing rate until a dangerously low oxygen partial pressure has been reached.

The volume of breathing is closely related to oxygen consumption and carbon dioxide production, since it is through ventilation (breathing) that the body maintains normal levels of these gases. Increased atmospheric pressure will not increase the alveolar carbon dioxide tension because CO_2 is formed in the body, and if the tidal volume of air being breathed is unchanged, CO_2 is expired as it is formed. In fact, the body strives not so much to get rid of carbon dioxide as to maintain the proper tension of that gas in the arterial blood and throughout the system. Either too much CO_2 (hypercapnia) or too little (hypocapnia) may have deleterious effects.

d. Transport

Blood can take up a much greater quantity of oxygen and of carbon dioxide than can be carried in simple solution. Hemoglobin, which is the principal constituent in red blood cells, has the chemical property of combining with oxygen and with carbon dioxide. The blood's normal hemoglobin content increases the blood's oxygen- and carbon-dioxide–carrying capacity by a factor of 50%. Also, although a small amount of carbon dioxide is carried in the blood in simple solution, a much larger amount is found in chemical combinations such as carbonic acid or bicarbonate. The transport of respiratory gases is enhanced by the fact that the taking up of oxygen by hemoglobin in the lung capillaries actually favors the unloading of carbon dioxide at the same time that the absorption of carbon dioxide into the blood in the tissues favors the release of oxygen. In the tissues, oxygen, which is continuously being used, is at a lower partial pressure than it is in the blood. Carbon dioxide is produced inside the tissue cells, which increases its concentration relative to that of the blood reaching the tissues. Therefore, blood supplied by the arteries gives up oxygen and receives carbon dioxide during its transit through the tissue capillaries.

The *U.S. Navy Diving Manual* (1973) describes the relationship of air volume to carbon dioxide elimination so well that we quote:

> Under normal conditions at the surface and, more particularly, under usual diving conditions where the partial pressure of oxygen is increased by compression of more molecules into the same volume of air, a man breathes mainly to eliminate excess carbon dioxide. If he succeeds in eliminating this excess, an ample supply of oxygen is generally assured. The actual *volume* of air required to eliminate carbon dioxide and keep the body's carbon dioxide tensions at a certain level does not change noticeably with depth. A man who is doing the same amount of work and holding the same arterial carbon dioxide tension will, therefore, have almost exactly the same RMV [respiratory minute volume]—in terms of volume as measured at his depth—regardless of the depth to which he goes. Because of the compression of gas, this means that the volume of molecules of air (and the volume as measured at the surface) increases in proportion to the absolute pressure. This is why a demand apparatus cylinder which suffices for an hour at a certain work rate at the surface may last only 30 minutes at a depth of 33 feet or 15 minutes at a depth of 99 feet. If a man's actual lung ventilation does decrease at a depth, this means that he either has reduced his carbon dioxide production by slackening his work rate or has allowed his carbon dioxide tension to rise.

e. Symptoms and Signs of Carbon Dioxide Retention

When carbon dioxide retention is associated with and contributes to hypoxia, there may be no signs and symptoms. However, the usual symptoms include labored breathing, air hunger, headache, dizziness, weakness, unusual perspiration, nausea, and mental changes, and confusion may also occur. The signs of carbon dioxide retention may include slowing of responses, clumsiness, and foolish actions; loss of consciousness is obviously the most dangerous sign.

Carbon dioxide retention has been blamed for a number of fatal and near-fatal accidents. Schaefer (1974) noted: "Carbon dioxide plays a major role in the physiology of the high-pressure environment, since the increased breathing resistance easily leads to carbon dioxide retention. The latter has been observed frequently in scuba and helmet diving." He also pointed out that carbon dioxide retention is often associated with deep diving and the performance of heavy, exhausting work. However, even in air excursions from a shallow dive in the nitrogen-oxygen saturation mode, carbon dioxide retention has been observed.

Loss of consciousness underwater is fatal unless rescue is prompt, so any light that can be thrown on the cause of the unconsciousness is important to divers. Results of a recent workshop (Thomas and Shilling 1980) state that one of the major causes of loss of consciousness in divers is carbon dioxide retention. Some physicians feel so strongly about this factor that they recommend that any diver showing any of the signs or symptoms of CO_2 retention be carefully examined to determine if he or she is a CO_2 retainer, and be prohibited from diving if found to have this tendency. Carbon dioxide retention also potentiates both nitrogen narcosis and oxygen poisoning.

f. Diving Implications

For the diver carbon dioxide is a serious problem both in the control of the amount of this gas in the breathing medium supplied, and particularly in the removal of the respiratory carbon dioxide. Removal in semiclosed- and closed-circuit breathing systems is accomplished by forcing the expired air through an absorbent (e.g., lithium hydroxide, Baralyme, or Sodasorb). Removal of CO_2 from closed living spaces is essential for submarines, submersibles, and habitats and is accomplished by the use of carbon dioxide scrubbers.

If the absorbent fails to function, the diver or person in the closed space will be in a hazardous situation. The function of the absorbent is slowed by cold temperature, and death has occurred as a result of failure of the system to properly absorb the carbon dioxide in a cold environment.

It is important to remember that effects of carbon dioxide, as well as any other gas, depend on the partial pressure of the gas. (See *Dalton's Law* in this chapter.) For example, breathing 1% carbon dioxide at 132 ft (5 ATA) would have the same effect on a diver as if he were breathing 5% carbon dioxide at the surface (1 ATA). This is true because the partial pressure of carbon dioxide is the same in both cases.

g. Causes of Carbon Dioxide Excess

The most frequent cause of CO_2 problems in diving is failure of the diver's supply of carbon dioxide absorbent, caused by a poorly designed absorbent canister, too little or improperly packed absorbent, water leakage into the canister, or exhaustion of the canister's supply. Deaths have occurred simply because of the failure to fill the canister.

Other causes of CO_2-related problems in diving are: increased breathing resistance, overexertion, excessive attempts to control breathing, and carbon dioxide retention.

h. Remedial Measures and Prevention

The first preventive measure is self-evident: proper care of the carbon dioxide absorbent and its canister. In addition, divers should rest when breathing becomes labored and discontinue the dive if breathing difficulty continues to be excessive or if mental changes are noted. Finally, if an individual is proved to be a carbon dioxide retainer, further diving is contraindicated.

8. *Carbon Monoxide*

a. Description

Carbon monoxide. Symbol CO; molecular weight 28.0106. A colorless, odorless, tasteless gas and thus difficult to detect. A poisonous gas that, when breathed for even short periods, may be lethal. Produced by the incomplete combustion of fuels and found most commonly in the exhaust of internal combustion engines. A level of 10 ppm should not be exceeded in a pressurized breathing system.

It is interesting to note that human metabolic processes produce 0.3 to 1.0 ml/hr of CO, a sufficient amount to be a consideration in planning for groups living in enclosed spaces. Vorosmarti and his co-workers (1970), reporting on helium-oxygen saturation dives, said: "The volume percent of CO increased throughout the dives, which indicates that in long deep exposures CO may reach dangerous levels unless a method of CO removal is provided."

b. Causes of Carbon Monoxide Poisoning in Diving

A typical problem for divers is contamination of the air supply or the air in the tanks from improperly placing the compressor engine exhaust where the CO can be blown into the air intake of the pump, sucked up, and sent to the diver under pressure and thus under increased partial pressure of CO.

As mentioned above, carbon monoxide is produced by internal combustion engines. This means that great care must be exercised not to draw engine exhaust into the air compressor that supplies a diver's breathing air. A case history presented by Edmonds and his colleagues (1981) clearly illustrates this danger: "An experienced diver planned a dive in an area subject to tidal currents. He planned to dive at slack water and anchored his boat a short time before low tide. The hookah compressor was correctly arranged with the inlet upwind of the exhaust and the dive commenced. After an hour at ten metres the diver felt dizzy and lost consciousness but was fortunately pulled aboard by his attendant and revived." The diagnosis was carbon monoxide poisoning confirmed by blood analysis. The explanation was straightforward. As the tide turned, so did the boat. This put the compressor inlet downwind of the motor exhaust and carbon monoxide from the exhaust was breathed under pressure by the diver.

According to the prevailing air purity standards, the maximum carbon monoxide allowable in the workplace is 0.002% by volume, or 20 ppm. If carbon monoxide is considered a small part of the "other" gases in the atmosphere and the same rules are applied, the partial pressure of CO at 1 atm is 0.00002%, while at 137 ATA (4500 fsw) there is a highly significant increase in the partial pressure to 0.003%. These implications of Dalton's law are significant, and should be understood by the diver and by his physician.

Smoking is another factor directly affecting the oxygen-carrying capacity of the blood (Miller 1979). The smoke from a typical American cigarette contains about 4% carbon monoxide (20,000 ppm). The average concentration inhaled is 400–500 ppm, which produces from 3.8 to 7.0% carboxyhemoglobin (HbCO) in the blood. This compares with 0.5% HbCO in the nonsmoker. Erickson (1976) discusses a study by Goldsmith (1963) that relates smoking habits to percent HbCO. Results of this work are summarized in the following table:

Smoking habits	Median HbCO level, %	Expired CO, ppm
Light smoker (less than ½ pack/day)	3.8	17.1
Moderate smoker (more than ½ pack/day and less than 2)	5.9	27.5
Heavy smoker (2 packs/day or more)	6.9	32.4

Since the maximum level of carbon monoxide allowed in the breathing air for U.S. Navy divers is 20 ppm, the *expired* air of even a moderate smoker exceeds U.S. Navy air purity standards. Since the carboxyhemoglobin level of a nonsmoker in a smoke-filled environment can rise to a level of 5%, smoking should be prohibited in long-term habitat or diving bell exposures.

Furthermore, considering that it takes a heavy smoker approximately 8 hr to eliminate 75% of the CO inhaled, and that smoking has such deleterious effects on the cardiorespiratory system, the *NOAA Diving Manual* (Miller 1979) says: ". . . divers are well advised not to smoke. If the habit cannot be 'kicked,' smoking should be avoided for several hours before diving."

c. Symptoms

When breathed, this toxic gas reacts with hemoglobin to form carboxyhemoglobin—the affinity of hemoglobin for carbon monoxide, according to Rodkey and his colleagues (1969), "being 218 times that for oxygen at 37°[C]." Thus the hemoglobin is prevented from carrying oxygen to the tissues and the subject develops hypoxia. Hypoxia is aggravated by a shift of the oxygen-hemoglobin curve to the left. In addition, carbon monoxide has a toxic effect at the cellular level that may be significant clinically.

Early symptoms of CO toxicity are headache, dizziness, and breathlessness upon exertion. These symptoms occur when divers breathe air contaminated with 800 parts per million (ppm) of carbon monoxide for an hour. At 1600 ppm, confusion occurs, followed by collapse, and, at 3200 ppm, unconsciousness. At higher levels there is profound coma and death. However, diagnosis may be difficult. Furgang (1972) describes a case of carbon monoxide intoxication that presented as an air embolism. The *U.S. Navy Diving Manual* (1978) states that "a particularly treacherous factor in carbon monoxide poisoning is that conspicuous symptoms may be delayed until the diver begins to surface. This is because, while at depth, the greater partial pressure of oxygen in the breathing supply will force more oxygen into solution in the blood plasma. Some of this additional oxygen will reach the cells, and some of it may forcibly displace carbon monoxide from the hemoglobin. During ascent, as the partial pressure of oxygen diminishes, the full effect of the carbon monoxide will be felt."

d. Treatment

The Undersea Medical Society's Committee on Hyperbaric Oxygenation (1981) lists carbon monoxide as a Category 1 condition (a disorder for which hyperbaric oxygen is the primary mode of treatment) and says: "There is ample evidence from animal experiments and clinical experience that hyperbaric oxygen is a primary mode of therapy in acute carbon monoxide poisoning. It is assumed that other adjunctive measures such as control of electrolyte imbalance and adequate supportive care are used in conjunction with hyperbaric oxygenation. Medical opinion now holds that more than one [hyperbaric] treatment is often indicated in the hours or days immediately following acute poisoning."

D. Gas Laws

Gases are subject to three closely interrelated factors—temperature, pressure, and volume. As the kinetic theory of gases points out, a change in one of these factors, such as an increase in temperature, must result in some measurable change in the other factors. Basic gas laws have been established to help predict the changes that will be reflected in temperature, pressure, or volume as the conditions of the operating environment are changed. These laws are: Boyle's law, Charles' law, the general gas law, Dalton's law and Henry's law.

It is important to note that in working with the gas laws, all pressure is absolute pressure, all temperature is absolute temperature, and all units used in the equations should be in only one system of units, i.e., either English or metric.

1. Boyle's Law

At a constant temperature the volume of a perfect gas varies inversely as the pressure to which the gas is subjected, and the pressure varies inversely as the volume. That is, the higher the pressure, the smaller the volume, and vice versa. It follows that the density will vary directly with the absolute pressure. Boyle's law (stated above in italics) is of fundamental importance to underwater physiology, since it means that if the pressure on a given confined gas is doubled, it must be compressed to half its volume, and an enclosed volume of a gas cannot be subjected to increased pressure unless it occupies a smaller space. This is illustrated in the schematic sketch of a submarine escape training tank (Figure II-1). It will be noted that the open-bottom bell is filled with air at the surface, but as it is lowered into the water the air is compressed to one-half its original volume

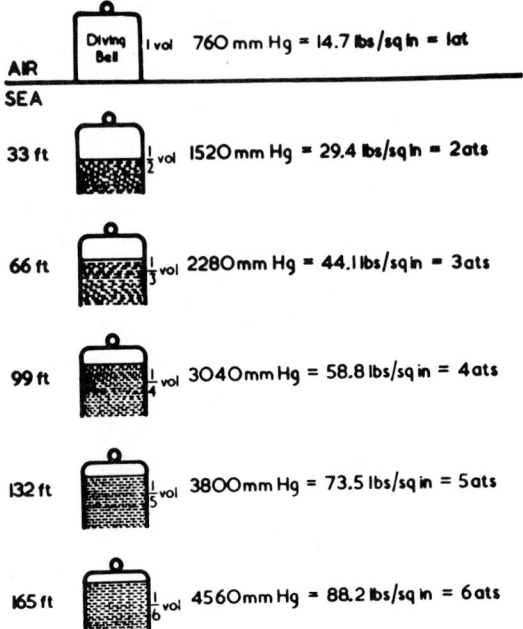

Figure II-1. Boyle's law and diving. $PV = K$. [Reprinted from Miles (1969) by permission of the author and Staples Press.]

at a depth of 33 ft (10 m), to one-third at 66 ft (20 m), and to one-fourth its original volume at 99 ft (30 m).

The reverse is also true: if the bell is filled with compressed air at 99 ft, this air will expand as the bell goes to the surface and will bubble out the bottom until three volumes are discharged. From the standpoint of the diver this is vitally important, for air in the lungs will act in the same manner. An example is a case that occurred during a 50-lb pressure test in the tank at the Submarine Base, New London, Connecticut. During the early stages of decompression, which was rapid and continuous, one of the men signaled he was in distress. Upon examination of the lungs it became obvious at once that he had a collapsed left lung (pneumothorax), and as the pressure on the outside was being lowered, the compressed air in his left chest was expanding and pressing on the mediastinum, embarrassing the heart and causing pain. The other men were put in the outer lock and their decompression was completed; a surgeon and a large trocar were called for, and the air in the chest was released while the decompression was proceeding for the subject with the collapsed lung. Within a few days after decompression the lung had expanded and there were no aftereffects—except that the patient was turned down for submarine duty and warned not to take up diving.

One of the difficult concepts to understand is how a diver can breath-hold dive and go to a depth of several hundred feet and return to the surface with no problem, yet a scuba diver at equalized pressure (equilibrium) at a very shallow depth who comes to the surface holding his breath may develop an air embolism and die. To illustrate this let us assume that a breath-hold diver is going from the surface down to 99 ft. During descent the gas in his lungs will be compressed, until at 99 ft it will be reduced to one-fourth the original volume. As he turns around and comes directly to the surface the original volume will expand, and once again the lungs will be full.

Now let us assume that as part of a training exercise a diver is to make a free ascent from a depth of 66 ft (20 m). On the bottom he is breathing in his scuba gear, and he is in pressure balance with his environment. He takes one last deep breath and ditches the scuba and heads for the surface. The inexperienced diver has a natural tendency to hold his breath so as to be sure there is air enough to reach the surface. By the time he reaches 33 ft, according to Boyle's law, the air in his lungs will have increased in volume to match the reduction in absolute pressure. His lungs will now be stretched and uncomfortable. This contributes to panic, and the rest of the ascent from 33 ft to the surface may well prove fatal, for the lungs cannot accommodate to the doubling in size necessary for halving the pressure. The alveoli will rupture, and air will be driven into the circulation, resulting in massive air embolism.

Failure to understand and practice this elimination of pressurized air or gas is probably the cause of more scuba deaths than any other single factor. Under conditions of extreme stress it is possible to hold the glottis closed so that no air can escape from the lungs, and surfacing under this condition from only 6 ft underwater may be fatal. Even when the diver exhales correctly, lung abnormality may cause local retention or trapping of gas, and when the stretched alveoli rupture, air will flow into the circulation. Air embolism due to pulmonary barotrauma is usually fatal if treatment by immediate recompression is not instituted. This problem is treated fully in Chapter VII, "Diagnosis and Treatment of Gas Embolism."

2. Charles' Law

For any gas at a constant pressure, the volume of the gas varies directly with the absolute temperature. For any gas at a constant volume, the pressure of the gas varies directly with the absolute temperature; i.e., change in either volume or pressure is directly related to the change in the absolute temperature. A French scientist, Jacques Charles, found that if the pressure was kept constant—as in some sort of freely expanding container—the volume of gas would increase as the temperature increased. Conversely, if the volume was restrained in a rigid container, the pressure would increase with the temperature. This is all in accordance with the kinetic theory of gases—higher temperature, higher molecular speeds.

3. General Gas Law

As noted above, Boyle and Charles demonstrated that with any gas the factors of temperature, volume, and pressure were so interrelated that a change in any of the three factors must be balanced by a corresponding change in one or both of the others. The general gas law (also known as the Boyle-Charles law and the ideal gas law) is a convenient combination of these two laws in predicting the behavior of a given quantity of gas when changes may be expected in any or all of the variables. Since

$$\frac{P_1 V_1}{T_1} = K \quad \text{and} \quad \frac{P_2 V_2}{T_2} = K$$

the formula for the general gas law is

$$\frac{P_1 V_1}{T_1} = \frac{P_2 V_2}{T_2}$$

where P_1 = initial pressure (absolute), V_1 = initial volume, T_1 = initial temperature (absolute), P_2 = final pressure (absolute), V_2 = final volume, T_2 = final temperature (absolute), and K = a constant.

In working with this formula, a few simple rules must be kept in mind: there can be only one unknown; if it is established that a value remains unchanged (such as the volume of an air tank), or that the change in one of the variables will be of little consequence, simplify the computation by canceling out the value on both sides of the equation.

If a diver used only one gas for all underwater work, the general gas law would suffice for most of the necessary calculations. Since the only life-supporting gas that could be used is oxygen, and since it is toxic when breathed for extended periods at increased pressure, it follows that a mixture is required. The common mixture is air (21% oxygen, 78% nitrogen, 1% other gases) or one of the inert gases serving as a carrier for oxygen. The human body has a wide range of reactions to various gases under different pressure conditions, and thus another gas law is required to help compute the differences between breathing at the surface and breathing under pressure.

4. Dalton's Law

Dalton's law—named for the English scientist who discovered the principle involved—states: *The total pressure exerted by a mixture of gases is equal to the sum of the pressure of each of the different gases making up the mixture, each gas acting as if it alone were present and occupying the total volume.* In other words, the whole is equal to the sum of the parts, and each part is not affected by any of the other parts. The pressure contributed by any gas in the mixture is proportional to the number of molecules of that gas in the total volume, and the pressure of that gas is called its partial pressure, meaning its part of the whole. Thus Dalton's law is sometimes referred to as the "law of partial pressure."

The partial pressure contributed by a single gas is in direct proportion to its percentage of the total volume (V) of the mixture. Stated in another way, the total pressure (P) exerted by a mixture of gases is equal to the sum of the pressures of each of the different gases in the mixture (x, y, z)—each gas acting as if it alone were present and occupied the total volume.

Stated algebraically,

$$P_{total} = P_x + P_y + P_z$$

and

$$P_x = P_{total} \times V_x/100$$

Let us consider the diver breathing air at the surface just before he goes underwater. For the purpose of this illustration (disregarding the presence of water vapor), air is 21% oxygen, 79% nitrogen and other inert gases, and 0.03% carbon dioxide (see Figure II-1). Using the above formula and the conventional notation of respiratory physiologists, the partial pressure of oxygen at the surface would be:

$$P_{O_2} = 21\% \times 760 \text{ mmHg} = 160 \text{ mmHg}$$

the inert gas pressure would be:

$$P_{inert} = 79\% \times 760 \text{ mmHg} = 600 \text{ mmHg}$$

and the carbon dioxide pressure would be

$$P_{CO_2} = 0.03\% \times 760 \text{ mmHg} = 0.23 \text{ mmHg}$$

Now let us consider the man in the training tank bell who is about to escape to the surface. He is breathing air that is pressurized to 3040 mmHg (760 mmHg × 4 ATA). The composition of the air is not changed, but the quantity is four times as great and the partial pressure of each gas is increased:

$$P_{O_2} = 21\% \times 3040 \text{ mmHg} = 638 \text{ mmHg}$$
$$P_{inert} = 79\% \text{ (approx)} \times 3040 \text{ mmHg} = 2402 \text{ mmHg}$$
$$P_{CO_2} = 0.03\% \times 3040 \text{ mmHg} - 0.912 \text{ mmHg}$$

An easily understood example is that of a container at atmospheric pressure (14.7 psi). If the container were filled with oxygen alone, the partial pressure of the oxygen would be 1 atm. If the same container at 14.7 psi (1 atm) were filled with dry air, the partial pressure of all the constituent gases would contribute to the total pressure, as shown in the following tabulation:

Percentage of Component × Total Pressure (Absolute) = Partial Pressure

Gas	Percentage of component	Atmospheres partial pressure
N_2	78.08	0.7808
O_2	20.95	0.2095
CO_2	0.03	0.003
Other	0.94	0.0094
Total	100.00	1.000

If the same container, for example a scuba cylinder, were filled with air to 2000 psi (137 ATA), the partial pressures of the various components would reflect the increased pressure in the same proportion as their percentage of the gas, as illustrated in the following tabulation:

Gas	Percentage of component	Atmospheres partial pressure
N_2	78.08	106.97
O_2	20.95	28.70
CO_2	0.03	0.04
Other	0.94	1.29
Total	100.00	137.00

5. Henry's Law

Whenever a gas is in contact with a liquid, a portion of the gas molecules will enter into solution with the liquid; they are said to be dissolved in the liquid. This factor of solubility is of vital importance in diving, since significant amounts of gases are dissolved in body tissues at the gas pressures encountered.

Apart from the individual characteristics of the various gases and liquids, two physical conditions have an effect on the quantity of gas that will be absorbed: temperature and pressure. Since a diver is always operating under unusual conditions of pressure, an understanding of gas laws is particularly important.

Thus, Henry's law states: *The amount of any given gas that will dissolve in a liquid at a given temperature is a function of the partial pressure of that gas in contact with the liquid* (and of the solubility coefficient of the gas in the particular liquid). Since a large percentage of the human body is water, the law simply says that as one dives deeper and deeper, more gas will dissolve in the body tissues. It follows that during ascent, the dissolved gas must be released.

Some gases are more soluble than others, and some liquids are better solvents than other liquids. For example, nitrogen is five times more soluble (on a weight-for-weight basis) in fat than in water. These facts and the differences in blood supply have led to the postulate of tissues with different saturation times (5-min tissues, 10-min tissues, 20-, 40-, 75-, etc.), the basis on which decompression tables are calculated.

The significance of this phenomenon coupled with the comparatively slow rates of solution in and release of gas from body tissues is developed fully in Chapter IV, "Decompression Theory."

E. Characteristics of Gas

1. Diffusion

Gas diffusion is the process of intermingling or mixing of gas molecules. If two gases are placed together in a container, they will eventually mix completely, even though one gas may be heavier than the other. The mixing occurs as a result of constant molecular action.

Gas will also pass through a permeable membrane (a solid that permits molecular transmission) until pressure is equalized (equilibrium). The direction of movement depends on the partial pressure: the gas molecules will move from the higher pressure side to the lower pressure side until the partial pressure is equalized. Numerous body tissues act as permeable membranes.

2. Moisture

The amount of water vapor in a gaseous atmosphere is referred to as humidity. Absolute humidity is the mass of water vapor per unit volume of a gas mixture. Relative humidity is the ratio, expressed in percent, of the amount of water actually in a gas mixture to the amount of water vapor that could be present if the mixture were saturated at the same temperature.

Breathing gas must have sufficient moisture for comfort, as too little can cause an uncomfortable sensation of dehydration of the diver's mouth, throat, nasal passages, and sinus cavities; but too much moisture in the system can increase breathing resistance and produce congestion.

Expired gas contains moisture that may condense in the breathing tubes or mask. This water is easily blown out through the exhaust valve and, in general, causes no problems. In very cold weather, however, freezing can occur, and if this happens the dive should be aborted.

Condensation of expired moisture or evaporation from the skin may cause fogging of the glass of the face mask. Moistening the glass with saliva, liquid soap, or commercially available antifog compounds will reduce or prevent this difficulty (Miller 1979).

3. Density

Gas density is related to absolute pressure as an almost linear function. As a diver's depth increases, the density of the breathing gas increases. High gas densities act to limit the diver's ability to ventilate his lungs and to increase the respiratory work required; this effect acts on both the diver and his equipment. In an experimental situation men have been able to accomplish tasks with a gas density 18 times normal, although work ability was drastically restricted.

4. Viscosity

The property of a gas to resist internal flow, or viscosity, does not change appreciably with increase in depth. For practical applications the diver should note that as resistance is increased due to density, and to a lesser extent due to viscosity, the flow is reduced in direct proportion. Therefore, if the length of the air hose is doubled, the pressure must be doubled in order to maintain the same flow (Miller 1979).

Both density and viscosity must be considered in the engineering design of respiratory equipment. Relevant to this it is worth noting that equipment must be designed to provide maximum desired *peak flow* during a breathing cycle, rather than just the average minute volume.

Practically, breathing-gas density is not a limiting problem in the use of air or nitrogen-oxygen mixtures, since narcosis becomes a problem before density becomes limiting.

F. *Buoyancy*

The buoyant effect of liquids is expressed by Archimedes' principle, which may be stated: Any object wholly or partially immersed in a liquid is buoyed up by a force equal to the weight of the liquid displaced. The laws of flotation based on Archimedes' principle can be summarized as follows (U.S. Navy 1978):

1. A body sinks in a fluid if the weight of fluid it displaces is less than the weight of the body. This is called negative buoyancy, which connotes a tendency to sink.
2. A submerged body remains in equilibrium, neither rising nor sinking, if the weight of the fluid it displaces is exactly equal to its own weight. This condition is called neutral buoyancy and reflects a condition of balance wherein an object will tend to neither rise nor sink but will remain suspended.
3. If a submerged body weighs less than the volume of the liquid it displaces, it will rise and float with part of its volume above the surface; it will be considered to have positive buoyancy, indicating a tendency to float.

The buoyant force of the fluid depends on its density (weight per unit volume). Salt water, with a density of 64 lb/ft^3 (1.025 g/cm^3) has a slightly greater buoyant force than fresh water, which has a density of 62.4 lb/ft^3 (1.0 g/cm^3). This is why it is noticeably easier for a swimmer to float in the ocean than in a lake, a greater percentage of his body remaining out of the water.

The tendency of a substance to float (or not to float) is also indicated by its specific gravity. For a solid this is a number assigned on the basis of the ratio of the density of the substance to the density of fresh water. Water is given a specific gravity of 1.0. Cork, which has one-fourth the density of water (15 lb/ft^3 or 0.24 g/cm^3) has a specific gravity of 0.24.

The average human body has a specific gravity of approximately 1.0. This varies slightly, the fat man floating more easily and the thin person having more difficulty. After a deep breath most individuals are positively buoyant; i.e., they remain on the surface. In fresh water about 10% will sink, but in seawater only 2% are negatively buoyant. Buoyancy can be regulated by inflation of the standard hard-hat diving outfit. The Archimedes principle as it applies in this case is illustrated in Figure II-2.

> The diver, with his helmet and dress, weighs 384 pounds. If he inflates his dress so that he displaces 6.5 cubic feet of water, he will be buoyed up by a force equal to the weight of 6.5 cubic feet of water. Because sea water weighs 64 pounds per cubic foot, the buoyant force acting on this diver would be 6.5 × 64 = 416 pounds. This force is 32 (416 − 384) pounds more than his total weight. Such an excess of buoyancy force is called positive buoyancy. In this example, the diver would actually float with half a cubic foot of his volume out of water. The

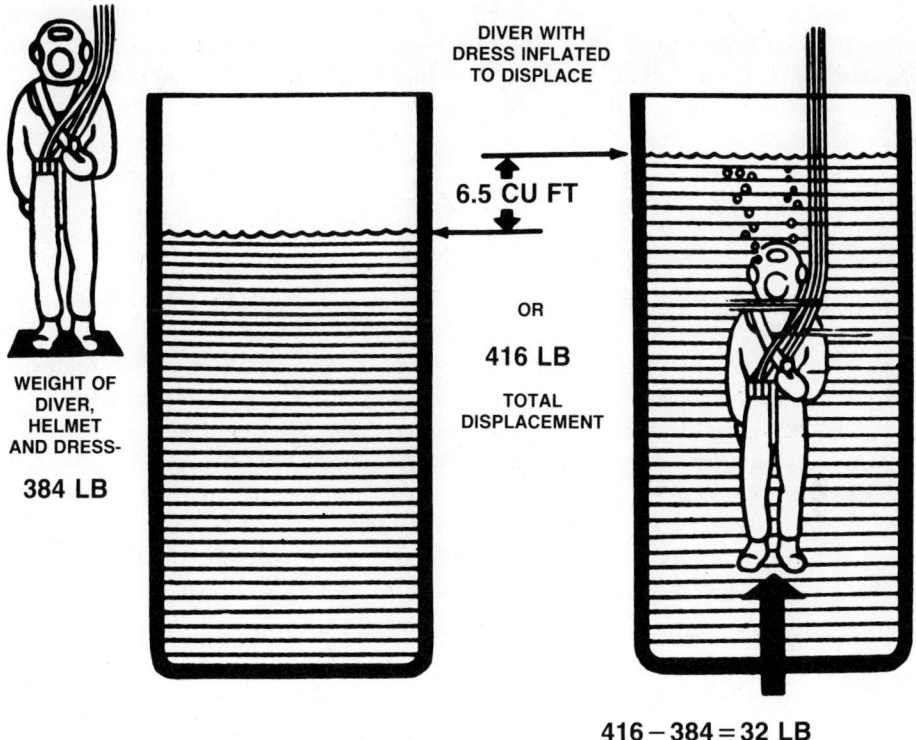

Figure II-2. Buoyancy—the Archimedes principle (U.S. Navy 1970).

volume of water displaced would then be 6 cubic feet, the weight of which (6 × 64 = 384 pounds) would equal his own weight. To give himself neutral buoyancy, with which he would neither rise nor sink in the water, the diver could either exhaust one-half of a cubic foot of air from his dress or wear an additional 32 pounds of weight. If he required negative buoyancy (the state of being heavy in the water), he would have to add still more weight or let out more air. (U.S. Navy 1970).

G. Energy in Diving

Energy is the capacity to do work. Six basic forms of energy exist: mechanical, heat, light, chemical, electrical, and nuclear. All forms of energy except nuclear energy are commonly found in diving activity, but only those forms that have unusual effects underwater are discussed in this section—light, sound, and heat.

1. Light

The human eye needs light in order to see, because what it sees is actually an image created by the reflection of light from various surfaces, objects, or particles in the air.

A diver underwater has to deal with a number of factors not usually encountered in air on the surface, and these directly influence what he sees. Among these factors are *diffusion*, which scatters the light; *turbidity*, which blocks the light; *absorption*, which alters the color and intensity of the light; and *refraction*, which "bends" the light. For further details of this problem see *Vision* in Chapter III.

2. Sound

Sound is produced by the vibration of an object, which sets up a pattern of waves of moving molecules in the air, water, or other medium. These waves in turn cause a sympathetic vibration in a detector such as an eardrum or the diaphragm of a microphone. Sound travels best in a dense medium, since the more closely packed the molecules, the more efficient the transmission of the sound waves. Sound will not travel in a vacuum. Sound travels about four times as fast in water as in air.

Although most acoustic energy loss results from geometric spreading, loss by absorption is also appreciable. Other problems are related to dispersion, scattering, and reflection. Underwater hearing is thus affected by several conditions not encountered in the atmosphere. These include (Miller 1979)

1. Reverberations of sound resulting from reflections from the bottom.
2. Gradients and discontinuities in the water resulting from thermal and salinity conditions and microorganisms.
3. Noises caused by water movement and passing ships and marine life.
4. Type of head covering.

In the air sound travels at the rate of about 1100 ft/sec. The slight time lapse from the time sound hits one ear and then the other allows localization of the sound source. Since sound travels at the rate of about 4900 ft/sec in water, localization is much more difficult but is possible, especially for the low-frequency or broad-band signals (less than 6000 Hz).

Further detail relating the ear and diving will be found in Chapter IX. High-intensity sound is transmitted by high-intensity waves, which may damage the ear. (See Chapter IX, under *Blast*.)

3. Heat

Heat, or the absence of it, is crucial to man's enviromental balance. As the physician well knows the human body functions only within a very narrow range of internal temperature, and it contains delicate control mechanisms. Consideration of heat is a many-faceted subject and is treated in several sections of this guide. Water temperature is a major consideration for the diver and is treated in Chapter I, "The Diving Environment." The problem of the diver as an individual in this environment is handled in Chapter III, "Physiology of Diving," under *Thermal Considerations*. And the relationship of hypothermia to near-drowning is presented in Chapter VIII. In this chapter we consider only the physical aspects. It is well to remember that of all of man's natural enemies, none is more awesome than cold. And in no place is cold more relentless a foe than in the oceans, where in many places the temperature is too low at depth for a diver to survive unprotected for more than a short time. Thus there is a definite need for the diver to have adequate life-support systems for cold-water diving.

Heat is energy that causes an increase in the temperature of matter to which it is added and a decrease in the temperature of matter from which it is removed, provided that the matter does not change state during the process. Heat is a form of energy associated with and is proportional to the molecular motion of a substance. Defined in another way, heat is energy possessed by a substance as a result of the motion of its molecules. Heat added to a substance results in increased molecular speed and an associated rise in its temperature. The most common example of heat energy is the boiling of water over an open flame.

Heat is generated in many different ways—for example, by friction and by electricity.

Quantities of heat are measured in British Thermal Units (Btu), calories (cal), or kilogram calories (kcal), and more recently the joule (J). One Btu is the amount of heat required to raise the temperature of one pound of water one degree Fahrenheit. A calorie is the amount of heat required to raise the temperature of a gram of water one degree Celsius, and a kilogram calorie (frequently kilocalorie, or large calorie) is the corresponding amount for a kilogram of water.

4. Temperature

Temperature and heat are closely related but must be distinguished because different substances do not necessarily contain the same heat energy even though their temperatures are the same. Temperature is the degree of hotness or coldness measured on a definite scale. It may be measured as degrees centigrade or Celsius, degrees Fahrenheit, Kelvin, or degrees Rankine.

5. Specific Heat

Specific heat is the ratio between the amount of transferred heat that can raise a unit mass of a substance one degree and that required for raising a unit mass of water one degree. Specific heat, like specific gravity, is a ratio that uses water as the base, with a value of 1.0. The specific heat of air is 0.24, which means that 0.24 calorie will raise the temperature of a gram of air by 1°C. If one converts air from a weight to a volume basis and compares it with water, it will be found that a volume of water will absorb 3600 times as much heat as a volume of air for the same rise in temperature (Miller 1979).

6. Conduction

Heat is transmitted from one place to another in three ways: by conduction, convection, and radiation.

Conduction is the transmission of heat by direct material contact, as in the heating of the cooking-pot handle. Of the three, conduction is of most significance to divers. Some substances are excellent conductors of heat—for example, iron, helium, and water.

Some, like air, are very poor conductors. Thus, since water is a much better conductor of heat than air, an unprotected diver can lose a great deal of body heat to the surrounding water by direct conduction.

7. Convection

The transmission of heat by the movement of heated fluids is a form of convection. As pointed out by the *U.S. Navy Diving Manual* (1978): "A diver, seated on the bottom of a tank of water in a cold room, can lose heat not only by direct conduction to the water, but also by convection currents in the water. The warmed water next to his body will rise and be replaced by colder water in the tank. The warmed water passing along the walls of the tank, or reaching the surface, will lose heat to the cooler surroundings. Once cooled the water will sink only to be warmed again as part of a continuing cycle."

8. Radiation, Evaporation

Radiation is the transmission of heat by electromagnetic waves of energy. Heat from the sun, from electric heaters, and from fireplaces is primarily radiant heat. This type of heat transmission is, in general, not of great importance to the diver. Heat is also lost through evaporation of moisture on the body surface when it is in a gaseous environment.

H. Effects of Changing Pressure on the Diver

In the underwater environment the diver is always experiencing changes in pressure as well as the associated changes in volume of the air or gas being breathed. The effect of these changes in pressure and gas volume on the diver may induce *barotrauma*. In this chapter we consider the physical effects, describing only enough physiological response to illustrate the problem.

"Gas cavities of the body must adjust to large and rapid changes in pressure during diving. It is worthwhile to think of the gas volume system of the body as divided into the right and the collapsible chambers, as illustrated in [Figure II-3]. Since the rigid chambers cannot collapse to accommodate pressure changes, air must be able to flow into them or there will be congestion and bleeding to accommodate the relative vacuum situation" (Shilling et al. 1976).

The conditions and situations that result from these pressure and volume changes are discussed below in alphabetical order. They vary greatly in severity and frequency of occurrence and thus in importance to diving, but they are included because they are due to physical factors related to changes in pressure.

1. Aural Barotrauma

Remembering that the middle ear is an air-filled cavity sealed on the outer side by the eardrum and open to the throat through the eustachian tube, it is not hard to understand

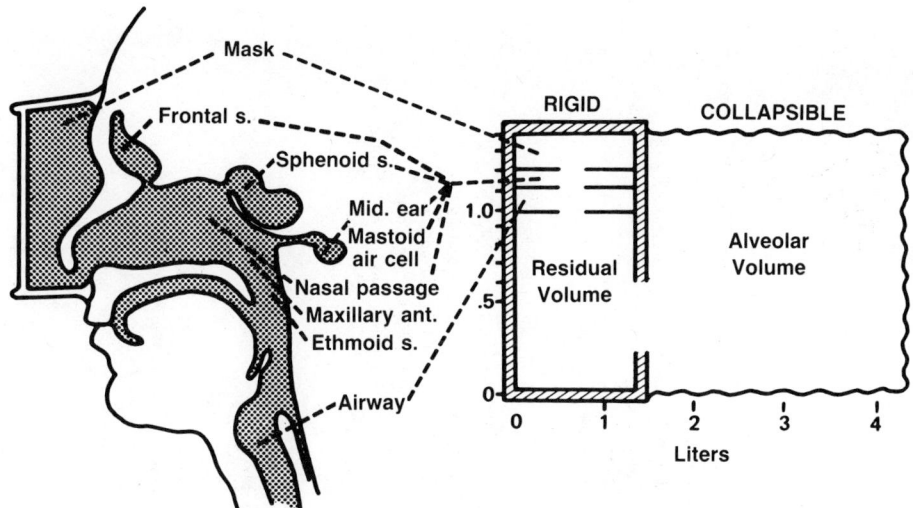

Figure II-3. Schematic presentation of the various rigid chambers in the human being that must be properly pressure-compensated during a dive. The figures for a typical ama give relative proportions. [Reprinted from Rahn and Yokoyama (1965), National Academy of Sciences–National Research Council, Washington, D.C.]

that the most common complaint of anyone experiencing changes in air pressure is difficulty in "clearing" or "popping" the ears. Normally, equalization of air pressure in the middle ear is accomplished during the act of swallowing, and there is no trauma either to the eardrum or to the middle ear. Chronically in some individuals, however, and in the presence of an upper respiratory infection in most individuals, the eustachian tube does not open freely. Difficulty may thus ensue with the dramatic pressure changes encountered by hyperbaric activity. It is important to remember that "it is the difference between the pressure in the middle ear and the ambient pressure, not the absolute value of either pressure, that calls forth the series of tissue changes known collectively as aerotitis media" (Shilling et al. 1946). This condition (aerotitis media) is most frequently referred to incorrectly in the literature as otitis media, but is also known as aero-otitis, aerotitis, aural barotrauma, otitic barotrauma, and aerosalpingotympanitis; among divers it is known as *ear squeeze*, and among aviators, simply as *aviators' ear*.

Aural barotrauma may be classified as due to ascent or descent, and also as to the part of the ear affected. Problems with the ears as they relate to pressure changes are discussed in *Vestibular and Auditory Function* in Chapter III, *Inner Ear Decompression Sickness* in Chapter VI, and *Ear and Sinuses* in Chapter IX.

2. Blowup

Blowup is one of the uncommon but serious accidents that may occur when diving in a suit and helmet. When a diver moves toward the surface, water pressure decreases and air inside the suit expands, creating positive buoyancy. Control may be lost and the diver propelled to the surface, the excess pressure in the suit causing maximum inflation to the extent that the suit may become so rigid that the diver cannot move but is spread-eagled on the surface. See Table II-2 for further details. Holding the breath on the way

Table II-2
Factors Relating to Changes in Pressure

Conditions	Causes	Symptoms and signs	Treatment	Prevention
Aural barotrauma Aural barotrauma of ascent	Expansion of gas trapped in the middle ear as ambient pressure decreases	Sensation of pressure or pain; dizziness (alternobaric vertigo)	Usually none is needed	Do not dive with a head cold or infection that blocks eustachian tubes; slow ascent when symptoms occur
Aural barotrauma of descent (middle-ear squeeze)	Diving with blocked eustachian tube; failure to "pop" ears on descent	Symptoms: pain in ear during descent; sudden relief of pain if eardrum ruptures Signs (dependent on extent of damage): redness and swelling of eardrum; bleeding into eardrum or middle-ear space; rupture of eardrum with bleeding; spitting up of blood; bleeding to outside if eardrum is ruptured May result in otitis media	Report to medical officer Mild case without rupture: avoid pressure until damage heals and ears can be readily cleared Ruptured eardrum: no diving until healed (usually about two weeks); keep water and all objects and materials (including medications) out of ear; keep hands away from ears Return to medical officer at once if pain increases or if drainage appears (these signs may indicate infection requiring antibiotic treatment)	Do not accept men who cannot pass pressure test "Pop" ears properly during descent—swallow or yawn; move jaw; blow gently against closed nostrils Do not dive with a head cold or infection that blocks eustachian tubes Use nose drops, spray, or inhaler for mild difficulty
External-ear barotrauma (external-ear squeeze)	Suit squeeze; hood sealing over external ear; use of ear plugs	Symptoms: pain on descent even though able to "pop" ears; feels almost same as middle-ear squeeze; pain stops if eardrum ruptures Signs: drum may have same appearance as in middle-ear squeeze; often see	Same as in middle-ear squeeze (keep hands away from ears); report any signs of infection	If using closed rubber swimsuit be sure to admit air for equalization during descent (pinch face seal at junction with mask to make a channel) Line hood (ear aura) with flannel or porous rubber to prevent sealing

Physics and Physical Effects of Diving 63

		blood blisters on or around eardrum or in canal; eardrum may be ruptured, but bleeding to outside *does not* necessarily mean rupture May result in otitis media	Never use ear plugs
Blowup	In deep-sea or helium-oxygen rig: any mishap or error that causes overinflation of dress, poor adjustment of air-control and exhaust valves, or plugging of exhaust openings; loss of shoe or weights; allowing legs to be higher than body (if legs are not properly laced or shoes are too light); too strong or rapid a pull by tenders, suddenly breaking free from being stuck in mud; strong tide causing diver to lose hold on bottom or descending line, thus sweeping him to surface In self-contained diving: unintentional dropping of weights; accidental overinflation of breathing bag; excess air in closed dry suit as result of efforts to equalize suit squeeze; failure of vent valves on suit during ascent; unintentional inflation of lifejackets	Air embolism: if breath is held during blowup even from extremely shallow depth (i.e., 7 ft above diver's head) Decompression sickness: If diver required decompression stops or was close to nondecompression limits (the rapid ascent of blowup may cause trouble even in a dive not requiring stops) Mechanical injury resulting from striking bottom of boat or other object at surface Squeeze may result from falling back into deeper water after reaching surface and exhausting air from diving dress Drowning not unlikely to occur if suit ruptures at surface	Diagnose all the mishaps that may have occurred during blowup and act accordingly If diver is unconscious, recompress immediately (probable air embolism) If dive did not require decompression and diver appears all right, watch him closely and keep him near recompression chamber; if symptoms of decompression sickness develop, treat according to treatment tables in Chapter VI If dive did require decompression, follow procedure described in Chapter VI Apply first aid and other measures as required for injuries if any	First, guard against the cause with careful safety procedures Prohibit use of controlled blowup as a means of ascent *Exhale* continously if blowup occurs Tenders: take in at once all slack in diver's line when diver reaches surface after blowing up Diver: exhaust only enough air to prevent rupture of suit and retain positive buoyancy until tender has taken in slack

(Continued)

Table II-2—Cont.

Conditions	Causes	Symptoms and signs	Treatment	Prevention
Gastrointestinal barotrauma	Gas trapped in the gastrointestinal tract during ascent	Abdominal discomfort; collicky pains; rarely severe	Belching or flatus Slowing the rate of ascent or stopping for a time—in severe cases, descending again	Avoid carbonated beverages and heavy meals before diving
Pulmonary barotrauma	Imbalance between pressures in physiological gas spaces and body tissues On descent may occur in breath-hold diving by descending too deep On ascent (more common), internal air trapping; inadequate exhalation caused by faulty apparatus; panic, water inhalation In scuba diving, throwing off the mask and coming to the surface holding the breath	Symptoms: pulmonary tissue damage; emphysema; pneumothorax; air embolism Signs: difficult breathing; cough; bloody sputum	Adequate respiration with 100% oxygen; drug support for the cardiovascular system; if severe, immediate recompression For pneumothorax: *at surface*: bed rest and supportive treatment and, when necessary, suction to withdraw air and fluid *during decompression*: it may be necessary to put a trocar through the chest wall to release trapped gas For air embolism: immediate recompression	All care should be taken to condition divers to react rationally and with patience when breathing problems occur Equipment should be kept in perfect condition and should never be used without prior checking Do not descend further than 99 ft during breath-hold diving In scuba diving, divers should be trained never to remove their masks to come to the surface holding the breath; in an emergency it seems to be very hard to remember to exhale during ascent
Sinus barotrauma	Blocking of the passage from the sinus to the nose	Symptoms: congestion of the lining of the sinus; hemorrhage into the sinus cavity Signs: blood and mucus may be expelled		Medical screening for abnormal nasal passage or polyps; do not dive when you have a cold or nasal congestion

Squeeze	Face Squeeze: when wearing a face mask, failure to equalize internal and external pressure Body squeeze: falling through the water	Tissues will swell and may even bleed In a hard-hat rig, if a diver falls he may be slammed into his helmet and severely injured or killed	Blowing air into the diver's mask to equalize pressure Emergency rescue operations to achieve medical aid as soon as possible	Same as treatment Use self-contained systems whenever possible; take safety precautions against accidents, especially falling off platform
Vertigo*	Vestibular problems; middle-ear barotrauma of descent; overforceful Valsalva maneuvers; unilateral caloric stimulation; vestibular decompression sickness	Dizziness; disorientation nausea	Recompress immediately Stop ascent, descent, compression, or decompression—whichever is in effect when dizziness occurs—until dizziness passes When there is topside communication, reassurance can sometimes prevent panic; if not, a diving companion may prevent a serious accident by helping the diver cope with his confusion	Medical selection to rule out abnormalities of the ear and vestibular system, and routine predive examination for ear, nose, and throat infections "Buddy system"

Data from Riu et al. 1969. U.S Navy 1970. Reuter 1971. Williams and Cohen 1972. Edmonds et al. 1973. *See also Chapter III, *Vestibular and Auditory Function*. [Table adapted from Shilling et al. (1976).]

up may lead to air embolism, and inadequate decompression may lead to decompression sickness.

3. Gastrointestinal Barotrauma

There is ordinarily as much as a liter or more of gas trapped in the gastrointestinal tract. Since this is a soft tissue organ, there is normally compression and reexpansion of this gas with no special problem. But if, as is fairly common with the neophyte scuba diver, air is swallowed while under pressure, or if gas from a previously ingested heavy meal accumulates, there may be sufficient expansion of gas to cause discomfort or even colicky pains, and if severe it may cause difficulty in breathing.

4. Pulmonary Barotrauma

Tissue damage and its sequelae may result from an imbalance between pressure in physiological gas spaces and body tissue in the lungs as well as the ears and sinuses.

Pulmonary barotrauma of descent is not very common but may possibly occur in breath-hold diving. According to Boyle's law, as the diver descends in the water the lung volume decreases with increasing pressure, so that 6 liters of gas of the normal lung will be compressed to 1.5 liters at 99 ft (30 m). This is approximately the normal residual volume, and further descent may cause pulmonary congestion, edema, and hemorrhage, but this is a very rare condition.

Pulmonary barotrauma associated with ascent is a much more common and serious occurrence. Lanphier (1957) believes it to be second only to drowning as a cause of death among scuba divers. We must remember that the diver is in equilibrium with the pressure at depth. Thus at 99 ft he will have his lungs filled with air (or other mixture of breathing gas) under a pressure of 60 psi. His body will also be exposed to a pressure of 60 psi. As he moves toward the surface he will have no problem if he continues to breathe normally. But if through panic he holds his breath or inhales water, inducing laryngospasm, there will be an internal pressure of about 60 psi and an external pressure of 15 psi when he reaches the surface. In a situation like this, rupture of the thin-stretched walls of the alveoli will occur and either air embolism, pneumothorax, or emphysema will be the end result. This can occur from very shallow depths, for according to Edmonds and Thomas (1972), "pressure gradients necessary to cause pulmonary barotrauma are approximately 80 mmHg near the surface. Hence barotrauma may supervene when the ambient water pressure falls to 80 mmHg or more below the intrapulmonary pressure—i.e., with an ascent of four feet to the surface."

A fatal case occurred with an experienced diver who ascended to the surface on a line anchored to a habitat on the bottom. He had a valuable camera in his hand and upon surfacing found a heavy sea running, and he held on to the buoy while 8-ft waves rolled over him. In what was surmised to be greater concern for his camera than for his own safety, he obviously breathed at the wrong time and had a lung full of air as the external pressure was suddenly lowered. Air embolism was the result.

Air or gas embolism; pneumothorax; and emphysema, whether mediastinal or subcutaneous, are treated in detail in Chapter VII, "Diagnosis and Treatment of Gas Embolism," but they are mentioned here because they are part of the physical pressure effects on divers.

Gas embolism is the most serious result of pulmonary overpressurization resulting in rupture of the alveoli. The gas is dispersed into the pulmonary venous system and is carried to the heart and then into the systemic circulation, resulting in gas emboli in the coronary, cerebral, and other systemic arterioles. And the gas bubbles continue to expand with further decreases in pressure, increasing the damage.

Pneumothorax may result from distended alveoli rupturing through the visceral pleural lining of the lung and allowing air into the pleural cavity. Trapped interpleural gas will expand with decrease of pressure on the diver, and a collapsed lung may result.

Mediastinal emphysema, or the presence of air in the mediastinal tissues, is the result of rupture of lung tissue that allows air to dissect along the plane of the trachea and the large vessels.

Subcutaneous emphysema, which may be associated with mediastinal emphysema, is the result of air being forced into the tissues of the neck (in diving). It is frightening to the individual, as demonstrated by the near-hysteria of a young submarine candidate who had worked so hard trying to "clear his ears" with the Valsalva maneuver that he had ruptured an alveolus, allowing air to escape into the mediastinum and to dissect up into the neck. The swelling and crepitus and mild pain frightened the neophyte diver, but breathing oxygen for a short period cleared up the situation with no residual effects.

5. *Sinus Barotrauma*

Sinus barotrauma, if it occurs during descent, is often referred to as sinus squeeze and results from blocking of the air passages from the nose to the sinuses. Congestion of the lining of the sinus and hemorrhage into the cavity compensate for the contraction of the air within the sinus cavity, and during ascent blood and mucus may be expelled.

Sinus barotrauma of ascent may occur as a result of occlusion of the sinus openings by folds of tissue or by polyps, preventing escape of the expanding gases, and hemorrhage may follow.

6. *Squeeze*

Squeeze can occur when the diver is unable to equalize the pressure differential during ascent or descent. It is most common in the ears and sinuses and occurs most seriously during descent. Squeeze may occur associated with the face mask and the diving suit.

Face mask squeeze results from wearing a tight face mask and not equalizing pressure by blowing air into the mask during descent. The relative vacuum caused by the increased external pressure must be satisfied, or the facial tissues will swell and even bleed as they are forced into the space between the rigid mask and the face. Wearing goggles while breath-hold diving can also result in conjunctival hemorrhage.

Body squeeze is caused by falling through the water without adequate air pressure to fill the relative vacuum between the suit and the diver. In a hard-hat outfit, unless extra gas is added during descent to compensate for the volume changes, the diver may be forced up into the helmet and subjected to a bizarre injury. The scuba set is dangerous only if it fails and the diver falls through the water. The depth of the diver at the time of the fall is most important. If he falls from the surface to 33 feet, the pressure change will be such as to decrease the air volume to one-half the original volume; whereas, if the diver were to fall from 132 to 165 feet (the same number of feet) the volume changes would be only 16.7%.

7. Toothache or Aerodontalgia

Although not very common, pain in a tooth can be caused by pressure changes and can be operationally important. If this happens, the diver should consult a dentist.

8. Vertigo

Vertigo may result from overpressurization of the middle ear during ascent (alternobaric vertigo), from middle-ear barotrauma of descent, from overforceful Valsalva maneuvers (see Glossary), or unilateral caloric stimulation (cold water entering through a perforated eardrum), but it is more commonly the result of other situations and conditions. (See Chapter III section on *Vestibular and Auditory Function*.)

Vertigo is a common problem among divers and is related to the problem of disorientation, which may have serious consequences. In the presence of vertigo, it is wise for the diver to "freeze" on the line until the dizziness passes, usually for only a few minutes.

I. Summary

As pointed out in the *Introduction* to this chapter, understanding of the physics of diving is essential to the safe and effective performance of the diver, and it is thus important for the physician to master the material. For easy reference Table II-2 presents a thumbnail sketch of the various conditions and their causes, symptoms and signs, treatment, and prevention.

CHARLES W. SHILLING
MORRIS D. FAIMAN

References

ARMSTRONG, H. G., AND J. W. HEIM 1937. The effect of flight on the middle ear. *JAMA* 109: 417–421.
BENNETT, P. B., AND D. H. ELLIOTT 1975. *The Physiology and Medicine of Diving and Compressed Air Work* (2nd ed.). Baltimore: Williams and Wilkins.
CLARK, J. M., AND C. J. LAMBERTSEN 1971. Pulmonary oxygen toxicity: A review. *Pharmacol. Rev.* 23: 37–133.

COLES, R. R. A. 1964. Eustachian tube function. *J. R. Nav. Med. Serv.* 50: 23–29.

DAVIS, J. C., AND T. K. HUNT (editors) 1977. *Hyperbaric Oxygen Therapy*. Bethesda, MD: Undersea Medical Society.

EDMONDS, C., AND R. L. THOMAS 1972. Medical aspects of diving. Part 3. *Med. J. Aust.* 2: 1300–1304.

EDMONDS, C., P. FREEMAN, R. THOMAS, J. TONKIN, AND F. A. BLACKWOOD 1973. *Otological Aspects of Diving*. Glebe, N.S.W., Australia: Australasian Med. Publ. Co.

EDMONDS, C., C. LOWRY, AND J. PENNEFATHER 1981. *Diving and Subaquatic Medicine* (2nd ed.). Mosman, Australia: Diving Medical Centre.

ERICKSON, P. R. 1976. The toxicity of carbon monoxide under pressure and consideration for standards setting. In: *Proceedings of the 1976 Diver's Gas Purity Symposium*. Columbus, OH: Batelle Laboratories.

FLISBERG, K., S. INGELSTEDT, AND D. ORTEGREN 1963. The valve and "locking" mechanisms of the eustachian tube. *Acta Oto-Laryngol. Suppl.* 182: 57–68.

FURGANG, F. A. 1972. Carbon monoxide intoxication presenting as air embolism in a diver. A case report. *Aerosp. Med.* 43: 785–786.

GILBERT, D. L. 1981. *Oxygen and Living Processes*. New York: Springer-Verlag.

GOLDSMITH, J. R., AND S. A. LANDAW. 1968. Carbon monoxide and human health. *Science* 162: 1352–1359.

Hyperbaric Oxygen Therapy: A Committee Report 1981. Bethesda, MD: Undersea Medical Society.

KELLER, A. P. 1958. A study of the relationship of air pressure to myringorupture. *Laryngoscope* 68: 2015–2028.

LANPHIER, E. H. 1957. Diving medicine. *N. Engl. J. Med.* 256: 120–131.

MILES, S. 1969. *Underwater Medicine* (3rd ed.). Philadelphia: J. B. Lippincott Co.

MILES, S., AND MACKAY, D. E. 1976. *Underwater Medicine*. Philadelphia: J. B. Lippincott.

MILLER, J. W. (editor) 1979. *The NOAA Diving Manual* (2nd ed.). Washington, DC: National Oceanic and Atmospheric Administration, U.S. Dept. of Commerce.

PERLMAN, H. B. 1943. The effect of explosions on the acoustic apparatus. *Trans. Am. Acad. Ophthalmol. Otolaryngol.* 47: 442–453.

RAHN, H., AND T. YOKOYAMA (editors) 1965. *Physiology of Breath-Hold Diving and the Ama of Japan*. Washington, DC: Natl. Acad. Sci./Natl. Res. Council.

REUTER, S. H. 1971. 95% of divers' ear problems start in the eustacian tube. *Clin. Trends* 10: 8.

RIU, R., L. HOTTES, R. GUILLERM, R. BADRE, AND R. LEDEN 1969. La trompe d'eustache dans la plonge. *Rev. Physiol. Subaquatique Med. Hyperbare* 1: 194–198.

RODKEY, F. L., J.D. O'NEAL, AND H. A. COLLISON 1969. Oxygen and carbon monoxide equilibria of human adult hemoglobin at atmospheric and elevated pressure. *Blood* 33: 57–65.

SCHAEFER, K. 1974. Carbon dioxide effects under conditions of raised environmental pressure. Rep. 804. Groton, CT: U.S. Navy Submarine Medical Research Laboratory.

SHILLING, C. W. 1964. *Atomic Energy Encyclopedia in the Life Sciences*. Philadelphia: W. B. Saunders.

SHILLING, C. W., M. F. WERTS, AND N. R. SCHANDELMEIER (editors) 1976. *The Underwater Handbook. A Guide to Physiology and Performance for the Engineer*. New York: Plenum Press.

THOMAS, S. C., AND C. W. SHILLING (editors) 1980. *Carbon Dioxide Effects on Mammalian Tissue*. Bethesda, MD: Undersea Medical Society.

U.S. NAVY 1970. *US Navy Diving Manual*. Washington, DC: Department of the Navy. (NAVSHIPS 0994-001-9010.)

U.S. NAVY 1973. *Diving Manual*, Vol. I, Change 2. Washington, DC: U.S. Department of the Navy. (NAVSHIPS 0994-001-9010.)

U.S. NAVY 1978. *U.S. Navy Diving Manual*. Washington, DC: Department of the Navy. (NAVSEA 0994-LP-001-9010.)

WILLIAMS, D. H., AND E. COHEN 1972. Human thresholds for perceiving sudden changes in atmospheric pressure. *Percept. Mot. Skills* 35: 437–438.

VAIL, H. H. 1929. Traumatic conditions of the ear in workers in an atmosphere of compressed air. *Arch. Otolaryngol.* 10: 113–126.

VOROSMARTI, J., JR., M. E. BRADLEY, P. G. LINAWEAVER, J. C. KLECKNER, AND W. F. ARMSTRONG 1970. Helium-oxygen saturation diving. I. Hematologic, lactic acid dehydrogenase and carbon monoxide-carboxyhemoglobin studies. *Aerosp. Med.* 41: 1347–1353.

III

Physiology of Diving

A. Respiration

1. Lung Volumes: Effects of Gas Compression and Expansion

The significant subdivisions of lung or respiratory system volume are functional residual capacity, residual volume, and total lung capacity; these are shown in Figure III-1. Functional residual capacity (FRC) is the volume of gas in the respiratory system at the end of a normal expiration. Residual volume (RV) is the gas volume in the system at maximal expiration, and total lung capacity (TLC) is the gas volume at maximal inspiration. Vital capacity (VC), the maximum amount of gas an individual can move, is the difference between TLC and RV. The determinants of these subdivisions of lung volume are shown for a young man in Figure III-2, which plots the passive pressure-volume characteristics of the lung, the chest wall, and the total respiratory system.

The curves of Figure III-2 were obtained by measuring the pressure differences across the lungs, chest wall, and total system in a relaxed subject with airway occluded at lung volumes ranging from TLC to RV. The pressure difference across each of these structures defines its elastic recoil. The elastic recoil of the lung was measured as the difference between alveolar pressure, which during breath hold equals pressure at the mouth, and pleural pressure, usually estimated by measuring pressure in the thoracic esophagus. The pressure difference across the chest wall or the elastic recoil of the chest wall is the difference between esophageal pressure and pressure at the body surface. The elastic recoil of the total system is the difference between alveolar and body surface pressures, which is the sum of the recoils of the lung and chest wall. At FRC all respiratory muscles are relaxed, and alveolar pressure equals body surface pressure; the recoil of the chest wall is equal and opposite to that of the lung. At TLC, the recoil of the lung far exceeds that of the chest wall; this is the maximal lung volume because the lung is so stiff that the inspiratory muscles are unable to overcome lung recoil. At RV, the respiratory system has a very negative recoil: during relaxation at RV, pressure in the occluded airway and alveolar pressure are much less than body surface pressures. This is almost entirely caused by the stiffness of the chest

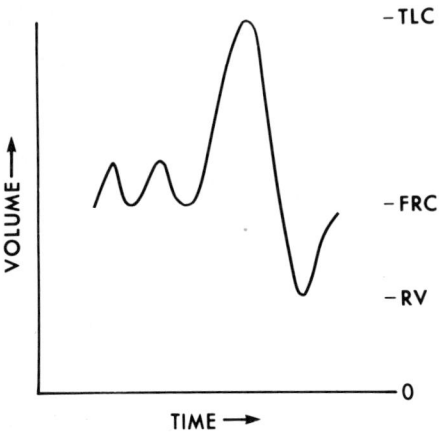

Figure III-1. Lung volumes illustrated by a spirogram. *Ordinate*, lung volume; *abscissa*, time. After period of normal breathing, subject took a maximum inspiration to total lung capacity (TLC), followed by a maximum expiration to residual volume (RV).

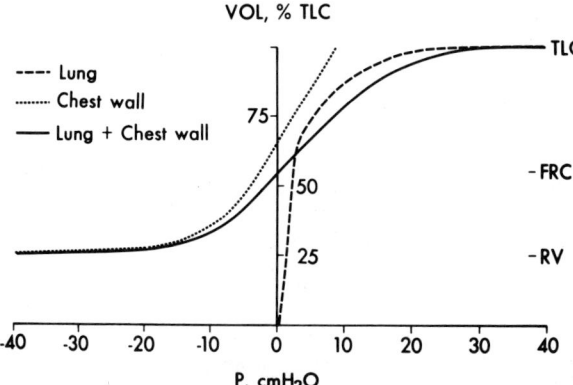

Figure III-2. Static pressure volume curves of lungs, chest wall, and total respiratory system. *Ordinate*, lung volume; *abscissa*, pressure across each structure. In the lungs, this pressure is the alveolar-pleural pressure difference; in the chest wall, it is the pleural-body surface pressure difference; in the total system, it is the alveolar-body surface pressure difference.

wall at low volumes. Residual volume is the minimum volume because the expiratory muscles cannot compress the chest wall further. To summarize, at both volume extremes the respiratory system is very stiff; that is, there is little volume change in response to large changes of pressure. At TLC this stiffness occurs in the lung, while at RV it resides in the chest wall.

In diving as in few other situations, pressures larger than those achieved by the respiratory muscles (shown in Figure III-2) may be imposed across the respiratory system, often with disastrous results. The case of the breath-hold diver is illustrative. As the diver descends, gas in the lungs is compressed; at 33 feet of seawater (fsw) the volume of the respiratory system is half what it was at the surface. If the diver descends far enough for lung volume to shrink to RV, the alveolar pressure will be some 40 cmH$_2$O less than body surface pressure and the chest wall will be very stiff. Because of this stiffness, further descent will not compress the chest and decrease lung volume but will greatly increase the difference between alveolar and body surface pressure. Blood is shifted toward the low alveolar pressure, engorges the pulmonary vessels, and ruptures them. The resulting alveolar hemorrhage and edema, called *lung squeeze*, limit the depth attainable by breath-hold divers (Strauss and Wright 1971). Lung squeeze also occurs in surface-supplied divers when the supply pressure fails or when the diver falls from one pressure level to another faster than the surface supply pressure can be increased.

Since RV is normally 20% to 25% of TLC, one would predict that if breath-hold divers take a maximal inspiration before submerging, they would be able to descend to a depth equivalent to 4–5 ATA, that is, 99–132 fsw. In fact, breath-hold divers have descended to depths of 250 fsw. Part of this discrepancy may be caused by these individuals having unusually small values of RV/TLC, but a better explanation is that blood shifts into the chest allow decreases of gas volume below the RV measured at the surface (Schaefer et al. 1972; Strauss and Wright 1971). Such shifts have been demonstrated at more modest depths, and at 250 fsw gas volume is about half of RV, while the remainder is blood.

Some diving mammals regularly descend to depths greater than 1000 fsw; this can be achieved only with respiratory system mechanics different from those in man. Diving mammals have very flexible chest walls, and potentially large intrathoracic blood storage spaces (Anderson 1967; Harrison and Tomlison 1960). Further, in at least some of these animals, small airways have cartilage in their walls (Denison et al. 1971). At low lung volumes, these airways resist collapse better than do the alveoli. Thus at great depths, the alveoli may collapse completely and express their remaining gas volume into the airways. By contrast, in most terrestrial mammals small airways close at low lung volumes before the alveoli collapse, so that at great depths gas remains in the alveoli. At depth, having gas-filled alveoli is a disadvantage. Alveoli contain an enormous number of thin-walled capillaries that can leak and rupture because alveolar gas pressure is lower than body surface pressure; when the alveoli are airless this pressure difference does not exist. Further, the relatively large alveolar blood flow is very efficient at taking up inert gas, and human decompression sickness has been reported after repeated breath-hold dives (Paulev 1965). The airway blood supply is much more meager than that of the alveoli, so that alveolar collapse may protect diving mammals against both decompression sickness and lung squeeze.

Figure III-2 also shows the genesis of pulmonary barotrauma. If divers take breaths of compressed air and ascend while holding their breath, lung volume will increase as the gas expands. If a diver is ascending from 33 fsw, the lung volume will double by the time the diver surfaces. If the diver began breath holding at a lung volume greater than 50% of TLC, at the surface the lung gas will have expanded to a volume greater than 100% of TLC. At large volumes the lungs are so stiff that they will not accommodate volume increments without large increases in transpulmonary pressure, and when transpulmonary pressure reaches 60–80 cmH$_2$O, the lungs rupture and gas escapes into either the pleural space or the lung interstitium (Lanphier 1965). In the former case the result is pneumothorax; if the gas escapes into the interstitium, it may dissect along interstitial planes to the mediastinum or it may enter the pulmonary veins to cause air embolism. The probability of pulmonary barotrauma therefore depends upon the depth and lung volume at which breath hold begins. If divers hold their breath near TLC, very short ascents (from 3 to 6 ft) can produce lung rupture. Obviously, the way to avoid lung rupture is to expire continuously during ascent, without allowing the lung volume to increase. However, U.S. Navy case records contain well-documented instances of air emboli during ascents in which the subject expired continuously. Though the explanation remains speculative, it seems likely that the individuals so affected had airway closure within their lungs, which caused the alveoli served by these closed airways to overexpand and rupture (Liebow et al. 1959). Indeed, radiological signs of extra-alveolar gas have been detected in individuals who have completed asymptomatic ascents (James 1969).

a. Dynamics of Gas Flow in the Lungs

As gas is compressed, its density increases. To breathe at depth is therefore to breathe gas of increased density. To understand the physiological significance of this, it is necessary to review the rules governing gas flow in branching tubes (Anthonisen et al. 1971; Wood and Bryan 1971), such as the human airways, and to review briefly the mechanics of breathing.

The laws governing gas flow depend on the velocities of the gas and the geometry of the system considered. At relatively low velocities, flow is laminar. Laminar flow, as illustrated in Figure III-3 *top*, is characterized by an orderly motion of gas; the gas in the center of the tube moves more rapidly than that at the periphery. In laminar flow:

$$\dot{V} = \Delta P K \eta^{-1} \tag{1}$$

where $\dot{V}$ = flow, ΔP is the pressure drop driving flow, K is a constant describing airway geometry, and η is gas viscosity.

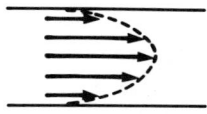

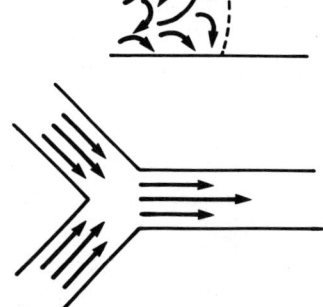

Figure III-3. Schematic of flow regimes in the lung; arrows represent relative gas velocities. *Top*: laminar flow: flow is orderly in that gas at the center has higher velocities than gas adjacent to the airway wall, which may approximate zero. Velocity increases from edge to center of airway in a smooth parabolic fashion. *Middle*: tubulent flow: motion of individual gas molecules is haphazard and disorderly and the flow advances down the airway in a relatively square front. *Bottom*: flow undergoes convective acceleration as two airways join to become one. Because flow in the single airway must equal that in its two tributaries, which have a greater cross-sectional area, gas velocity in the single airway must be increased.

When gas velocities are greater, the orderly patterns of gas motion are disrupted and flow becomes turbulent, as illustrated in Figure III-3 *middle*. Turbulent flow may be approximately characterized as

$$\dot{V} = \frac{\sqrt{\Delta P}}{\sqrt{\rho}} K' \tag{2}$$

where V is flow, P is the pressure driving flow, K' is a constant describing airway geometry, and ρ is gas density.

Finally, during expiration gas in the lung flows from peripheral airways to central ones, and the cross-sectional area of the central airways is less than that of the peripheral ones. Therefore, to maintain equal flow in center and periphery, gas velocities must be relatively high in the central airways; that is, the gas must be speeded up as it moves centrally (Figure III-3 *bottom*). This process is called convective acceleration, and it imposes pressure losses; there is a flow resistance associated with convective acceleration. In flow with convective acceleration:

$$\dot{V} = \frac{\sqrt{\Delta P}}{\sqrt{\rho}} K'' \qquad (3)$$

where $\dot{V}$ is flow, P is the pressure driving flow, K'' is a constant describing geometry, and ρ is gas density.

These equations indicate that when velocities are low enough for flow to be laminar (Eq. 1), density does not affect flow resistance, but that when flow is turbulent or undergoes convective acceleration, the flow achieved for a given pressure drop is decreased by increasing density. In flow that is turbulent or undergoing convective acceleration, flow and resistance are density dependent.

The act of breathing may be regarded as being carried out by applying forces to the lungs that cause them cyclically to inflate and deflate, and the forces necessary to achieve this depend on the mechanical characteristics of the lungs. A static pressure-volume curve of the lung was illustrated in Figure III-2, and a more detailed example is shown in Figure III-4. This curve was generated by inflating and deflating the lung in a series of steps and measuring transpulmonary pressure—the pressure difference between alveoli and pleural surface—in the intervals between the steps. At all lung volumes the lung exhibits positive elastic recoil; the transpulmonary pressure is positive, that is, alveolar pressure is greater than pleural pressure. This means that if left to itself, the lung's elastic recoil is such that it always tends to deflate. It is also evident that to increase volume, transpulmonary pressure must be increased, and that for a given change in lung volume there must be a greater

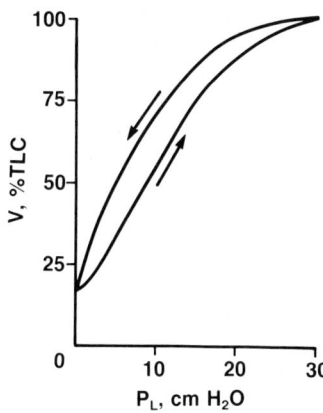

Figure III-4. Static pressure volume curve of the mammalian lung. *Ordinate*, lung volume; *abscissa*, transpulmonary pressure (alveolar-pleural pressure difference).

change in transpulmonary pressure at high lung volumes than at low. Further, lung inflation necessitates greater changes in transpulmonary pressures than does lung deflation. This behavior is termed hysteresis: the pressure-volume path followed during inflation differs from that followed during deflation.

Part of the static pressure-volume behavior of the lung is caused by the mechanical characteristics of the lung tissue, but a larger part is related to the fact that the lung represents an air-liquid interphase (Radford 1964). Such interphases tend to contract by virtue of the surface tension of the liquid, and most of the elastic recoil of the lung is related to its surface tension. Indeed, the normal lung contains a phospholipid (surfactant) that lowers the surface tension of the fluid at the alveolar surface. Without this material, lungs undergo massive atelectasis. In addition, surfactant is responsible for most of the pressure-volume hysteresis of the lung.

The lung pressure-volume curves of Figure III-2 and Figure III-4 show the pressure necessary to inflate the lung and hold it at a volume in the absence of gas flow. Breathing, however, is not a static maneuver: there is gas flow in and out of the lungs. Equations 1 to 3 indicate that whatever the type of flow, its maintenance demands a driving pressure, and the amount of driving pressure per unit of flow ($\Delta P/\dot{V}$) in turn defines airways resistance.

A model of the respiratory system is presented in Figure III-5, which allows more detailed consideration of the physiological factors governing airways resistance and gas flow in the lungs. The thorax is depicted as a rigid box, and the respiratory muscles as driving a piston. The lung is a balloon within the box, connected to the outside world via an airway. The space between the box and the balloon is therefore analogous to the pleural space, and the piston, or respiratory muscles, change balloon or lung volume by changing the pressure in this space, which in turn changes the pressure within the lung alveoli. The relationship of alveolar to pleural pressure is defined by the pressure-volume curve of the lung. Now consider the airways. Part of the airways are within the lung, part are inside the thorax but outside the lung, and part are outside the thorax. All airways are nonrigid, which is to say they are to some extent collapsible. The total cross-sectional area of the airways increases sharply as one moves from the mouth to the periphery (Weibel 1964); though individual peripheral airways are small, the sum of their cross-sectional areas is large.

Inspiration is induced by the inspiratory muscles, which expand the thorax and lower pleural pressure. Alveolar pressure is also lowered and gas flows into the lung. During normal tidal breathing, expiration is passive; that is, the inspiratory muscles relax and the elastic recoil of the lung forces the gas out and restores the lung and thorax to their original volumes (FRC). Most of the pleural pressure applied to the lung during such breathing is used to overcome the static elastic recoil of the lung: differences between mouth and alveo-

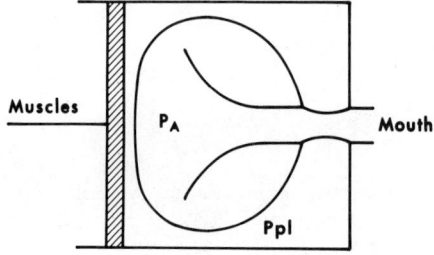

Figure III-5. Model for examining dynamics of the respiratory system. Box represents chest wall, and the piston is powered by the respiratory muscles. Lung is a balloon within the box and communicates with the mouth via the airways. P_A is alveolar pressure, Ppl is pleural pressure.

lar pressure are relatively small. However, during increased breathing efforts, such as those that occur with exercise, gas flows increase greatly, and ever greater fractions of the applied pressure are needed to overcome airways resistance. Further, expiratory muscles are used to increase pleural and alveolar pressures: expiration is no longer passive.

The maximum ventilation achievable is limited by expiratory flow rate. Gas flow during inspiration is, for a given airways resistance, determined by inspiratory effort. The more forceful the inspiratory muscle contraction, the greater the decrease in pleural and alveolar pressures, the greater the pressure difference between alveolar and mouth pressures, and the higher the inspiratory flow. Similar events do not occur during expiration. During forced expiration, contraction of the expiratory muscles increases pleural and alveolar pressures, and expiratory flow commences. However, if the airways resistance is such that the pressure drop in the intrapulmonary airways is equal to the elastic recoil of the lung (P_A − Ppl, Figure III-5), the pressure within the airways leaving the lungs is equal to Ppl. Immediately downstream (mouthward) from this point, pressure in the airway is less than Ppl; the pressure inside the airway is less than the pressure outside it. The nonrigid airway undergoes dynamic compression and becomes flow limiting; greater expiratory efforts, though they increase P_A and Ppl, also serve to compress further the extrapulmonary intrathoracic airways and do not increase expiratory flow (Pride et al. 1967). In the presence of dynamic compression of central airways, expiratory flow is independent of expiratory effort, once a certain expiratory effort has been achieved. Thus, expiratory flow limits the maximal ventilation an individual can achieve because expiratory flow attains a maximum at submaximal efforts, while inspiratory flow increases continuously with inspiratory effort. Thus tests that assess maximum expiratory flow are commonly and successfully used to predict maximum voluntary ventilation (MVV).

If maximum expiratory flow is independent of effort, what are its determinants? A useful illustrative analysis of forced expiration has been presented by Macklem and Mead (1968). They defined the point in the airway where airway pressure equaled pleural pressure as the equal pressure point and divided the airway into segments upstream and downstream from this point. Flow through both segments is equal. Flow in the upstream segment is dependent on the resistance of the airways of that segment and on the pressure drop in the segment. This pressure drop is by definition P_A − Ppl, which is the elastic recoil of the lung. Maximal expiratory flow is therefore determined by the resistance of the upstream segment and the elastic recoil of the lung. Thus, maximum expiratory flow decreases as lung volume decreases, because as volume decreases so does elastic recoil; at the same time, airway resistance increases.

Given the preceding primer of fluid dynamics and lung mechanics, several general predictions may be made about the effect of breathing dense gases on pulmonary dynamics. First, at depth as at the surface, maximum expiratory flow determines maximum voluntary ventilation. Second, flow in peripheral airways is probably laminar and unaffected by gas density (Eq. 1) because the total cross-sectional area of peripheral airways is so large that gas velocities must be very low. Third, because the total cross-sectional area of the central airways is small, velocities are relatively high and flow is likely to be turbulent and density dependent. Fourth, irrespective of turbulence, flow in central airways is almost certainly density dependent because airway geometry is such that flow must undergo considerable convective acceleration. Fifth, at high lung volumes when expiratory flow and gas velocities are high, flow and resistance should be more density dependent than at low lung volumes when flow and velocities are relatively low. Finally, because of the large cross-sectional area of peripheral airways, peripheral airways resistance is low in relation to central airways resistance, and the latter is the chief determinant of the total airways resistance.

These predictions are borne out by the data. Figure III-6 plots maximum expiratory flow against gas density at a number of lung volumes. This kind of plot is particularly appropriate because at a given lung volume the elastic recoil of the lung, which is the pressure driving flow, is fixed and independent of effort, flow, and gas density. Flow and gas density are linearly related on the log-log plot of Figure III-6. At high lung volumes (50% of VC), the slope of the line is such that

$$\dot{V} = K\rho^{-0.5} = K/\sqrt{\rho} \tag{4}$$

indicating that flow is either turbulent or dominated by convective acceleration (Eqs. 2 and 3). At low lung volumes, flow is less dependent on density, indicating that a significant portion is laminar.

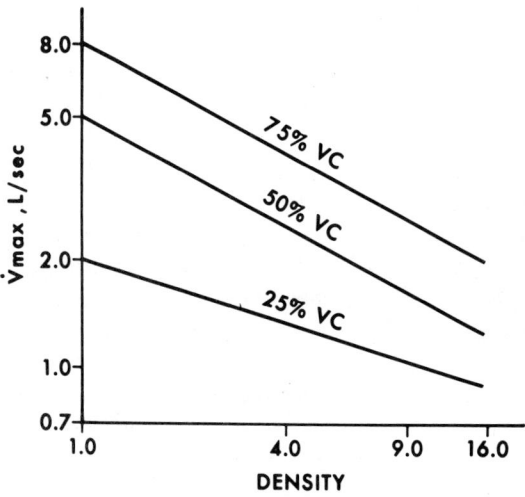

Figure III-6. Maximum expiratory flow as a function of gas density. *Ordinate*, maximum flow in liters/sec. *Abscissa*, gas density relative to that of air, which is assigned a density of 1.0. Both ordinate and abscissa are logarithmic. Data measured as three lung volumes (75% VC, 50% VC, and 25% VC) are shown.

For reasons discussed above, maximum voluntary ventilation (MVV) is dependent on maximum expiratory flow and should relate to gas density in similar fashion. Figure III-7 shows MVV as a function of absolute pressure. The MVV is halved in an air-breathing diver at 100 fsw (4 ATA). At greater depths, helium-oxygen mixtures are often substituted for air because of the nonnarcotic properties of helium (He). This practice is advantageous from the respiratory point of view because helium is much less dense than air. Figure III-7 also shows MVV for a subject breathing 80% helium (He) and 20% oxygen (O_2); at a given depth the MVV is considerably greater on the helium mixture than on air. Actually, the oxygen-helium data of Figure III-7 underestimate MVV in real life because as depth increases the fractional concentration of O_2 decreases and that of He increases. Thus a diver working at 60 ATA (nearly 2000 fsw) is likely to be breathing

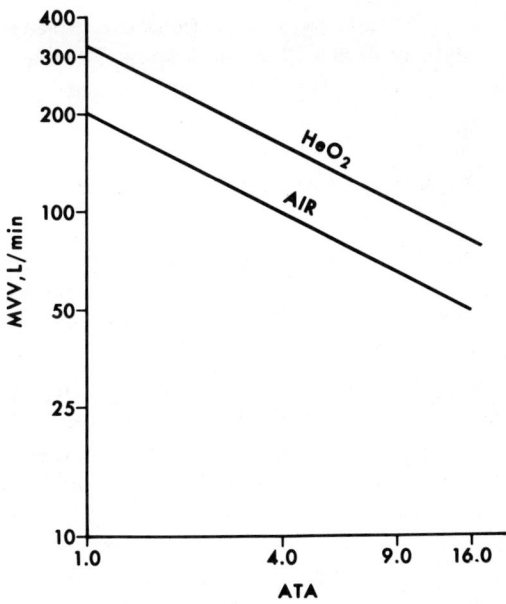

Figure III-7. MVV as a function of depth, breathing air and 20% O_2, 80% He. *Ordinate*, MVV is liters/min on a logarithmic scale. *Abscissa*, depth in ATA, also on a logarithmic scale.

a mixture of 0.5 ATA O_2 and 59.5 ATA He; the density of this mixture is roughly 16 times that of air. Maximum expiratory flow and therefore MVV would (Eqs. 2 and 3) be roughly one-fourth of that attained breathing air on the surface.

In normal individuals, the maximal ventilation attained during exercise (MVE) is 50%–60% of the MVV. According to Figure III-7, MVE remains less than MVV until a depth of 4 ATA is reached during air breathing and a depth of 9 ATA during oxygen-helium breathing. At greater depths MVE cannot be kept constant because it exceeds the MVV. At these depths MVE should appoximate the MVV, a prediction that accords with some results (Anthonisen et al. 1976; Wood and Bryan 1971) but not with others (Dwyer et al. 1977; Thalmann and Lundgren 1978). In any event, when the normal MVE exceeds the MVV, ventilatory ability limits exercise capacity; subjects cannot sustain exercise that at 1 ATA is associated with ventilation greater than the MVV. This exercise limitation increases as the MVV decreases with depth. However, even at 2000 fsw (60 ATA) breathing 0.5 ATA O_2 and the balance helium, a diver should be able to achieve ventilations of 40–50 liters per minute (liters/min) (25% of surface MVV), enough to allow useful work. However, several groups have reported the onset of severe, "choking" dyspnea during exercise at depths that required levels of ventilation approximating MVV (Anthonisen et al. 1976; Wood and Bryan 1971). This dyspnea was qualitatively different from that observed during maximal exercise at 1 ATA and may have been caused by dynamic compression of the airways. Because MVE is always less than MVV at 1 ATA, dynamic airway compression does not occur.

Finally, this discussion has considered only the intrapulmonary limitations of gas flow. The working scuba diver has to cope not only with the mechanics of lungs and airways but also with the additional mechanical loads on the respiratory system imposed by mouthpieces, hoses, and valves. The size of these loads varies with the design of the equipment. Modern single-hose scuba gear does not impose a very large load. Further, because maximum ventilation is limited by dynamic collapse of the intrathoracic airways, substantial external static and resistive loads may be added to the respiratory system without decreasing ventilatory performance.

2. Gas Density, Ventilation Distribution, Gas Exchange

At rest, a normal individual inhales about 0.5 liter with each breath. This tidal volume is relatively small compared to the FRC, which in an average man is about 3.0 liters. To maintain adequate gas exchange with pulmonary capillary blood, the fresh air in the inspirate must mix with the gas in the FRC. This is accomplished at least in part by diffusion; the oxygen from the inspirate diffuses toward the alveolar wall and the carbon dioxide released from the capillaries diffuses in the opposite direction (Figure III-8). The speed of these diffusive processes is dependent on the number and size of inert gas molecules in the system. Thus gas in gas diffusion is slowed in the lungs of individuals at depth. If this slowing were critical, pulmonary gas exchange would be compromised, and the effect would be the same as increasing the respiratory dead space by making the subject breathe through a large tube. This problem has been investigated theoretically by several workers using lung models, and, not surprisingly, results have varied with the model chosen (Cumming et al. 1966; Paiva 1973). Some results have indicated that diffusive mixing of gas within alveoli, alveolar ducts, and respiratory bronchioles is completed in the time allowed by the respiratory cycle, while others have suggested that this mixing is incomplete. If the latter were the case at 1 ATA, one would expect failure of diffusive mixing to be accentuated at depth, especially if inspired oxygen were maintained at 0.2 ATA. Indeed, pulmonary gas exchange, as assessed by comparing arterial to inspired O_2, might be compromised. Such is not the case. In fact, there is persistent evidence that at least in dogs, alveolocapillary oxygen exchange is actually improved by breathing dense gas (Martin et al. 1972; Worth et al. 1976). The mechanism responsible

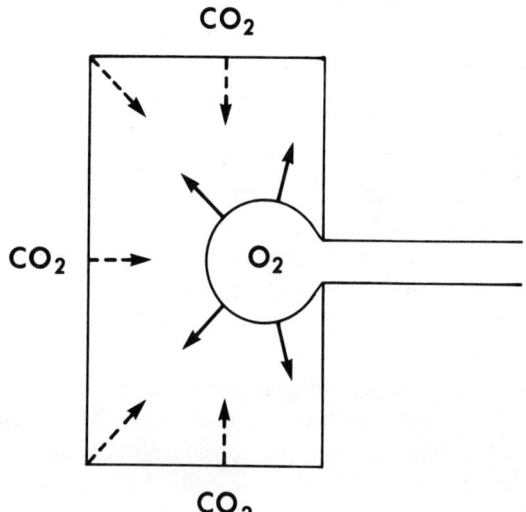

Figure III-8. Schematic showing importance of diffusion mixing in the lung. A 500-ml breath is inhaled through a 250-ml dead space (the airway) into a 3000-ml gas volume—the FRC. Oxygen must diffuse from the inspirate throughout the FRC, while CO_2 must do the reverse. (Though drawn to scale, this diagram neglects gas mixing during inspiration and does not indicate the finely divided structure of the lung, which shortens diffusing distances.)

for this improvement is obscure, but these experiments do show that pulmonary gas exchange is unlikely to be compromised by delayed gas in gas diffusion at depth. This may be caused in part by the close contact between the lungs and the heart; changes in cardiac volume and position caused by the heart beat tend to "shake" the lungs and improve gas mixing within them (Engel et al. 1973).

a. Control of Ventilation and Carbon Dioxide Retention

It has been observed repeatedly that divers at depth tend to ventilate less at rest and exercise than they do at the surface (Lanphier 1975). Indeed, early reports indicated that working divers could show striking increases in end-tidal carbon dioxide (CO_2) (Lanphier 1963). In people with normal lungs, end-tidal CO_2 equals alveolar CO_2 ($P_{A_{CO_2}}$), which in turn equals arterial CO_2 (Pa_{CO_2}). At a given level of metabolism, Pa_{CO_2} is inversely proportional to alveolar ventilation ($\dot{V}_A$): Pa_{CO_2} multiplied by $\dot{V}_A$ is proportional to the metabolic output of CO_2. Increases in alveolar CO_2 therefore indicate alveolar hypoventilation. The partial pressure of CO_2 in arterial blood is normally 40 mmHg and does not change with exercise. In the early studies cited, $P_{A_{CO_2}}$ averaged 66 mmHg and in some cases rose to 70 mmHg. These figures suggest that $\dot{V}_A$ was reduced by 25%–45% below the normal figure. Since the experiments were conducted at 4 ATA and involved only moderate exercise, the observed carbon dioxide retention did not occur because the ventilation demanded by the exercise exceeded the divers' MVV: at 4 ATA during maximal exercise, ventilation approximates the MVV. These divers therefore hypoventilated because they chose to hypoventilate, and this choice implied that under the circumstances of the study these individuals' control of ventilation differed from the normal.

Classically, the ventilatory control system has been considered a system concerned with error detection and minimization. The signals are the partial pressures of carbon dioxide and oxygen in the arterial blood: when Pa_{CO_2} rises or Pa_{O_2} falls, an error is detected and ventilation is increased in an effort to restore the signal to its original values. Arterial oxygen is sensed in the carotid bodies; these organs also sense Pa_{CO_2}, but most of the ventilatory responses to CO_2 can be attributed to the sensing of Pa_{CO_2} by receptors located in the medulla oblongata. Carbon dioxide response is commonly assessed by having people inhale CO_2 while keeping Pa_{O_2} constant and measuring the ventilation elicited by a given (increased) level of alveolar or arterial CO_2. The response to hypoxia is evaluated by lowering alveolar and arterial Po_2 while measuring ventilation and keeping Pa_{CO_2} constant. The results of this kind of testing are shown in Figure III-9, which illustrates features of the human ventilatory control system. The response to carbon dioxide is much more vigorous than the response to hypoxia: a 20-mmHg increase in Pa_{CO_2} results in a tenfold increase in ventilation, while a change in Pa_{O_2} of 60 mmHg produces a smaller increase in ventilation. The ventilatory response to carbon dioxide is linear, and small elevations produce detectable changes of ventilation. The response to hypoxia is, on the other hand, hyperbolic. Arterial oxygen may be lowered from 100 mmHg to 60 mmHg with little ventilatory response, but further decreases in Pa_{O_2} are attended by a vigorous ventilatory response. When both hypoxia and hypercapnia are present, responses to increases in Pa_{CO_2} or decreases in Pa_{O_2} are greatly magnified. Indeed, summing the response to pure hypercapnia and pure hypoxia results in a lower level of ventilation than when comparable levels of hypoxia and hypercapnia are present simultaneously.

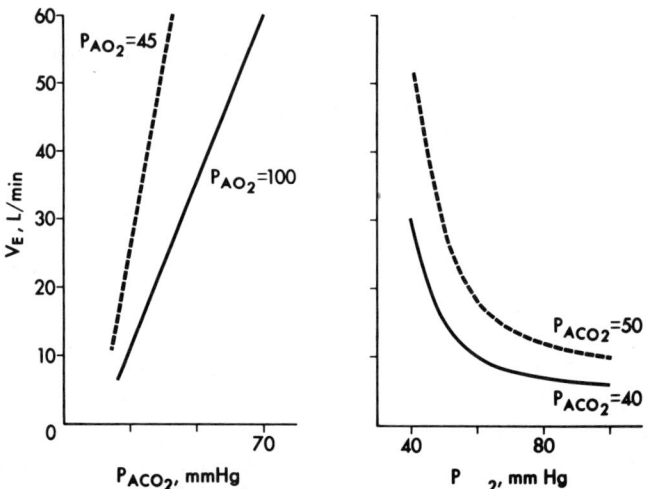

Figure III-9. Hypercapnic and hypoxic ventilatory responses. *Left*, ventilatory response to CO_2 at two levels of oxygenation. Ventilation is plotted against alveolar CO_2. *Right*, ventilatory response to hypoxia at two levels of CO_2. Ventilation is on *ordinate*, alveolar Po_2 on *abscissa*.

It has long been known that the control of ventilation is influenced by factors other than Pa_{O_2} and Pa_{CO_2}. For example, when normal people exercise, ventilation increases but Pa_{O_2} and Pa_{CO_2} change little. Neural input from the chest wall, lungs, and exercising limbs may all influence ventilation. Also, breathing may be voluntarily controlled as it is in speaking, singing, and playing wind instruments. One such nonchemical control important in this discussion is the response to respiratory loads. When normal humans are forced to breathe through external resistances or when they are subjected to acute bronchospasm, ventilation does not decrease and Pa_{O_2} and Pa_{CO_2} remain normal (Mann et al. 1978). The added load is sensed, probably by the chest wall or lungs, and respiratory efforts are increased enough to maintain ventilation and blood gases. These load-compensating reflexes have been shown to operate whenever normal breathing is impeded.

Given the characteristics of normal ventilatory control outlined above, let us see how they apply to the diving situation. Hypoxia is uncommon in diving situations; the inspired partial pressure of oxygen is usually greater than that in air at 1 ATA. Hypoxic ventilatory response should therefore not be important to divers. However, we have seen that elevations of Pa_{CO_2} may occur in divers; carbon dioxide responses must therefore be considered. Divers breathe through resistive equipment, and because of gas density their airway resistance is increased. Divers are frequently subjected to inert gas narcosis that could depress central ventilatory control. Finally, divers are frequently taught, or spontaneously learn, atypical breathing patterns that they use at depth, and divers represent a selected subpopulation of humans who may have atypical ventilatory control.

Though load-compensating reflexes are adequate for maintaining normal resting ventilation in the face of most respiratory loads, this is not necessarily true when breathing is stimulated. The ventilatory response to carbon dioxide is depressed by increased gas density (Figure III-10) (Doell et al. 1973; Linnarsson and Hesser 1978), and may be more depressed by external resistance (Milic-Emili and Tyler 1963). Although there is evidence of load compensation (Linnarsson and Hesser 1978), the compensation is not entirely effective, and ventilation at a given carbon dioxide level is less with an added load than without it. On the other hand, load compensation during exercise appears to be better. Although breathing at 4 ATA depresses the carbon dioxide response, exercise at 4 ATA is not accompanied by decreased ventilation until near maximum levels are reached, at least in normal nondivers (Anthonisen et al. 1976).

At depth it is difficult to separate the effects of gas density from those of inert gas narcosis. However, breathing 30%–50% nitrous oxide at the surface induces a state very similar to fairly severe narcosis. Under these circumstances hypoxic response is depressed but carbon dioxide and load-compensating responses are not (Yacoub et al. 1976).

Divers tend to ventilate less during exertion than nondivers (Lally et al. 1974). It is not known whether this is a learned response or whether divers are different because of preselection. Divers are reported to have smaller ventilatory responses to carbon dioxide than nondivers (Lanphier 1963), which might influence exercise ventilation. Divers tend to use low breathing frequencies and large tidal volumes to attain a given level of ventilation; this is particularly true at depth. Again, it is not clear whether this breathing pattern is innate or learned. Divers are sometimes trained to "skip breathe," which involves a pattern of very low frequencies, very large tidal volumes, and end-inspiratory breath-holds. It can be shown that this pattern is very efficient in terms of pulmonary

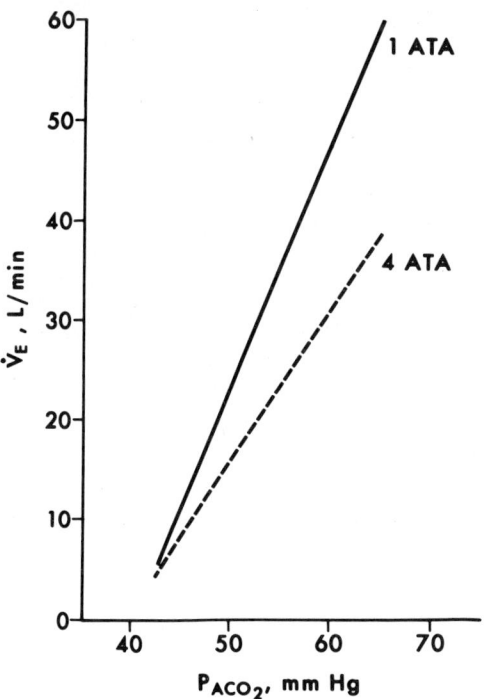

Figure III-10. Ventilatory responses to CO_2 at 1 and 4 ATA. *Ordinate*: ventilation in liters/min; *abscissa*: alveolar P_{CO_2}.

gas exchange (Nye 1970). On the other hand, voluntary limitation of breathing frequency sharply diminishes carbon dioxide response.

To summarize, increased resistance both inside and outside the lungs, combined with the tendency to breathe slowly and deeply, may account for carbon dioxide retention in divers who at the surface tend to ventilate less than nondivers in response to both carbon dioxide and exercise. Nondivers retain carbon dioxide only in trivial amounts during very heavy exercise at depth. Whether the difference between nondivers and divers is innate or acquired is an interesting and unanswered question. It should be noted that carbon dioxide retention at depth may not be a useful adaptation. Hypoventilation conserves both gas supply and breathing effort, but acute carbon dioxide retention decreases mental acuity and probably potentiates both inert gas narcosis and oxygen toxicity.

Some workers have noted mild elevations of resting $P_{A_{CO_2}}$ at depth when divers breathed oxyhelium (Saltzman et al. 1971). Because similar elevations of $P_{A_{CO_2}}$ were not noted when the same subjects breathed air at depths with inspired gas densities similar to those of the oxyhelium mixtures, it was concluded that the increases in $P_{A_{CO_2}}$ were due to the greater hydrostatic pressures of the oxyhelium experiments. Although this interpretation is intriguing, it is not apparent why it is true, and recent work has not confirmed the original findings (Clark et al. 1978).

N. R. ANTHONISEN

References

ANDERSON, H. T. 1967. Cardiovascular adaptations in diving mammals. *Am. Heart J.* 74:255.
ANTHONISEN, N. R., M. E. BRADLEY, J. VOROSMARTI, AND P. G. LINAWEAVER 1971. Mechanics of breathing with helium-oxygen and near-oxygen mixtures in deep saturation diving. In: *Underwater Physiology IV. Proceedings of the Fourth Symposium on Underwater Physiology*, edited by C. J. Lambertsen. New York: Academic Press, p. 339–346.
ANTHONISEN, N. R., G. UTZ, M. H. KRYGER, AND J. S. URBANETTI 1976. Exercise tolerance at 4 and 6 ATA. *Undersea Biomed. Res.* 3:95–102.
CLARK, J. M., R. GELFAND, C. D. PUGLIA, AND C. J. LAMBERTSEN 1978. Work capability and physiological effects in He-O₂ excursions to pressures of 400-800-1200 and 1600 feet of sea water. Philadelphia: Univ. of Pennsylvania Medical Center, Institute for Environmental Medicine, p. E14-1–E14-34.
CUMMING, G., J. CRANK, K. HORSFIELD, AND I. PARKER 1966. Gaseous diffusion in the airways of the human lung. *Respirat. Physiol.* 1:58–74.
DENISON, D. M., D. A. WARREN, AND J. B. WEST 1971. Airway structure and alveolar emptying in the lungs of sea lions and dogs. *Respirat. Physiol.* 13:253–260.
DOELL, D., M. ZUTTER, AND N. R. ANTHONISEN 1973. Ventilatory responses to hypercapnia and hypoxia at 1 and 4 ATA. *Respirat. Physiol.* 18:338–346.
DWYER, J., H. A. SALTZMAN, AND R. O'BRYAN 1977. Maximal physical work capacity of man at 43.4 ATA. *Undersea Biomed. Res.* 4:359–473.
ENGEL, L. A., L. D. H. WOOD, G. UTZ, AND P. T. MACKLEM 1973. Gas mixing during inspiration. *J. Appl. Physiol.* 35:18–24.
HARRISON, R. J., AND J. D. W. TOMLISON 1960. Normal and experimental diving in the common seal (*Phoca vitulina*). *Mammalia* 24: 386.

JAMES, J. E. 1969. Extra alveolar air resulting from submarine escape training. Rep. 550 Groton, CT: U.S. Navy Submarine Medical Center.

LALLY, D. A., F. W. ZECHMAN, AND R. A. TRACY 1974. Ventilatory responses to exercise in divers and nondivers. *Respirat. Physiol.* 20:117–129.

LANPHIER, E. H. 1963. Influence of increased ambient pressure upon alveolar ventilation. In: *Underwater Physiology II. Proceedings of the Second Symposium on Underwater Physiology*, edited by C. J. Lambertsen and L. J. Greenbaum. Washington, DC: Natl. Acad. Sci./Natl. Res. Council, p. 124–133. Publication 1181.

LANPHIER, E. H. 1965. Underwater physiology. E. Overinflation of lungs. In: *Handbook of Physiology. Respiration*, edited by W. O. Fenn and H. Rahn. Washington, DC: American Physiological Society, Sect. 3, Vol. II, p. 1189–1230.

LANPHIER, E. H. 1975. Pulmonary function. In: *The Physiology and Medicine of Diving and Compressed Air Work* (2nd ed.), edited by P. B. Bennett and D. H. Elliott. Baltimore: Williams & Wilkins, p. 102–154.

LIEBOW, A. A., J. E. STARK, J. VOGEL, AND K. E. SCHAFER 1959. Intrapulmonary trapping in submarine escape training casualties. *U.S. Armed Forces Med. J.* 10:265.

LINNARSSON, D., AND C. M. HESSER 1978. Dissociated ventilatory and central nervous responses to CO_2 at raised N_2 pressure. *J. Appl. Physiol.: Respir. Environ. Exercise Physiol.* 45: 756–761.

MACKLEM, P. T., AND J. MEAD 1968. Factors determining expiratory flow in dogs. *J. Appl. Physiol.* 25:159–169.

MANN, J., C. A. BRADLEY, AND N. R. ANTHONISEN 1978. Occlusion pressure in acute bronchospasm induced by methylcholine. *Respirat. Physiol.* 33:339–347.

MARTIN, R. R., M. ZUTTER, AND N. R. ANTHONISEN 1972. Pulmonary gas exchange in dogs breathing SF_6 at 4 ATA. *J. Appl. Physiol.* 33:86–92.

MILIC-EMILI, J., AND J. M. TYLER 1963. Relation between worker output of respiratory muscles and CO_2 tension. *J. Appl. Physiol.* 18:497–504.

NYE, R. E. 1970. Influence of the cyclical pattern of ventilatory flow on pulmonary gas exchange. *Respirat. Physiol.* 10:321–337.

PAIVA, M. 1973. Gas transport in the human lung. *J. Appl. Physiol.* 35:401–410.

PAULEV, P. E. 1965. Decompression sickness following repeated breath-hold dives. *J. Appl. Physiol.* 20:1028–1031.

PRIDE, N. B., S. PERMUTT, R. L. RILEY, AND B. BRAMBERGER-BARNEA 1967. Determinants of maximum expiratory flow from the lungs. *J. Appl. Physiol.* 23:646–662.

RADFORD, E. P. 1964. Static mechanical properties of mammalian lungs. In: *Handbook of Physiology. Respiration*, edited by W. O. Fenn and H. Rahn. Washington, DC: American Physiological Society, Sect., 3, Vol. I, p. 429–450.

SALTZMAN, H. A., J. U. SALZANO, G. D. BLENKARN, AND J. A. KYLSTRA 1971. Effects of pressure on ventilation and gas exchange in man. *J. Appl. Physiol.* 30:443–449.

SCHAFER, K. E., R. D. ALLISON, C. R. CAREY, AND R. STRAUSS 1972. The effects of simulated breath-hold dives in dry and wet chambers on blood shifts into the thorax. Rep. 729. Groton, CT: U.S. Navy Submarine Research Laboratory.

SCHAFER, K. E., R. D. ALLISON, J. H. DOUGHERTY, JR., C. R. CAREY, R. WALKER, F. YOSTRAND, AND D. PARKER 1968. Pulmonary and circulatory adjustments determining the limits of breath-hold diving. Rep. 531. Groton, CT: U.S. Navy Submarine Research Laboratory.

STRAUSS, M. C., AND P. W. WRIGHT 1971. Thoracic squeeze diving casualty. *Aerosp. Med.* 46:673–675.

THALMANN, E. D., AND C. E. G. LUNDGREN 1978. The effect of static lung loading on $\dot{V}O_2$max, V_E and MVV at depth. *Undersea Biomed. Res. Suppl.* 5:11–12.

WEIBEL, E. 1964. Morphometrics of the lung. In: *Handbook of Physiology. Respiration*, edited by W. O. Fenn and H. Rahn. Washington, DC: American Physiological Society, Sect. 3, Vol. I, p. 285–305.

WOOD, L. D. H., AND A. C. BRYAN 1971. Mechanical limits of exercise ventilation at increased ambient pressure. In: *Underwater Physiology, IV. Proceedings of the Fourth Symposium on Underwater Physiology*, edited by C. J. Lambertsen. New York: Academic Press, p. 307–316.

WORTH, H., H. TAKAHASHI, H. WILLMER, AND J. PIIPER 1976. Pulmonary gas exchange in dogs ventilated with mixtures of oxygen with various inert gases. *Respirat. Physiol.* 28:1–15.

YACOUB, O., D. DOELL, M. H. KRYGER, AND N. R. ANTHONISEN 1976. Depression of hypoxic ventilatory response by nitrous oxide. *Anesthesiology* 45:385–389.

B. *Immersion Effects*

One aspect of immersion that most divers and swimmers have personally experienced is the drastic change in thermal environment that frequently accompanies immersion. A diver may encounter a thermoregulatory problem not only when immersed but also in the pressure chamber, as discussed in Chapter IV, "Decompression Theory." Another aspect of immersion is that water may carry pathogenic organisms and induce changes in the skin that enhance penetration by various microorganisms and parasites. (Chapter IX presents various immersion-related aspects of dermatological and infectious diseases.)

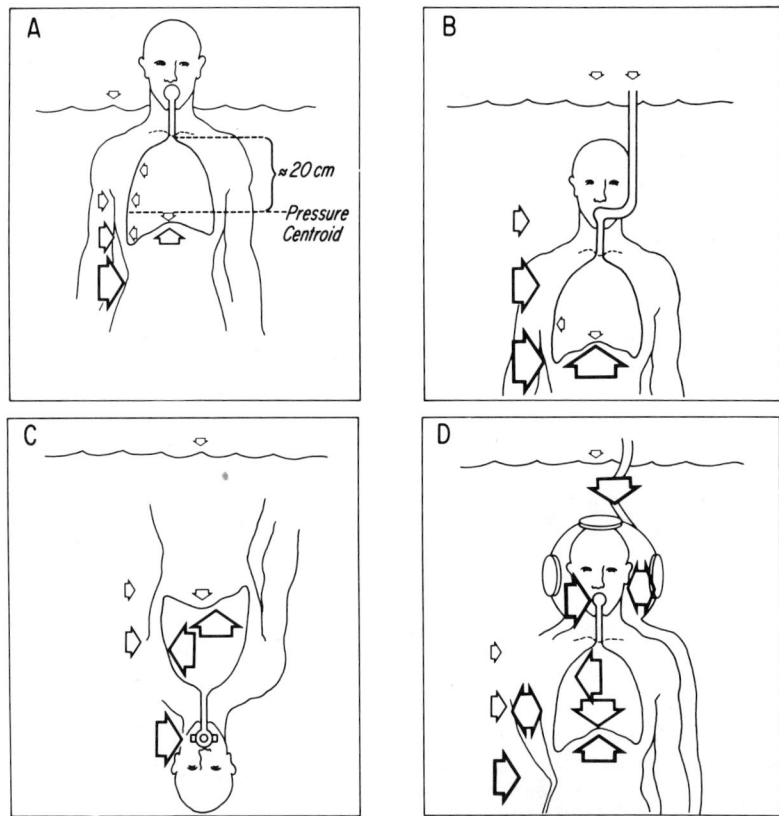

Figure III-11. Pressure forces acting on and exerted by thorax and lungs. Widths of *arrows* symbolize relative magnitude of forces. A: During head-out immersion in upright posture, lower portions of chest are exposed to increasingly higher hydrostatic pressures (according to depth). Mean effect of this corresponds to pressure 8 inches (20 cm) below jugular notch. Alveolar pressure is equal to 1.0 atm (on outside of the chest it is 1.0 atm plus water pressure). In this situation pressure on inside of chest is lower than mean pressure on the outside. B: Snorkel breathing while submersed (note risks) corresponds to situation in Figure III-11A except that in this situation the external pressure is even greater. C: Breathing from scuba regulator at mouth level in head-down posture. Regulator supplies air to alveolar space at pressure determined by depth of regulator. Pressure on outside of chest is less than on inside. D: Hard hat diver in suit that is air-filled to waist level. Air pressures in suit, helmet, and alveoli equal water pressure at waist level. Pressures on outside and inside of chest are equal.

One important effect of immersion is to alter the influence of gravity upon the body. This change, which is caused by the density of the water, occurs immediately beneath the water surface and is therefore in essence independent of depth. However, it is influenced by type of breathing gear and body posture under water. To illustrate these statements, for the simplest case, Figure III-11A shows a person immersed with his head above the water. In this situation gravitational effects on blood distribution are counterbalanced and tend to redistribute blood from the dependent regions into the thorax. In addition, there is a tendency toward chest compression so that breathing is performed at a smaller average lung volume.

Examples of different immersion effects are offered by the snorkel diver, the hard hat diver, and the scuba diver who assumes a head-down position. Although the snorkel diver (Figure III-11B) is subjected to an overpressure on the outside of the chest, the scuba diver is breathing against an overpressure inside the chest (Figure III-11C). If the suit of a hard hat diver contains little air, he may be in a situation similar to that of the snorkel diver. By contrast, if his suit is well inflated (Figure III-11D), he may be more like the nonimmersed person against whose body no significant outside overpressure is exerted.

It follows that for a discussion of immersion effects on the body, it is necessary to define the interplay of hydrostatic forces and opposing forces, i.e., to state whether the subject is in an upright position, at what relative pressure breathing gas is provided, and so forth.

1. Respiratory Function

The influence of immersion on the respiratory system can be traced to direct pressure effects as well as to indirect effects caused by blood distribution changes. Alterations in the respiratory system during immersion are reflected in many different variables. A brief overview of these alterations is given below, followed by a more detailed discussion of possible mechanisms and their significance.

The vast majority of studies to date have employed subjects immersed to the neck and in an upright position. Comparisons with the nonimmersed condition have usually shown that during immersion:

(1) Vital capacity (VC) is reduced;
(2) Functional residual capacity (FRC) is reduced, primarily as a result of lowered expiratory reserve volume (ERV);
(3) Closing volume (CV) and volume of trapped air are increased;
(4) Lung compliance (C_L) is reduced;
(5) Diffusing capacity of the lungs is increased;
(6) Distribution of ventilation is shifted toward more ventilation in apical regions and less in basal regions of the lungs;
(7) Flow resistance is increased;
(8) Strenuous exercise at depth may be associated with increased dyspnea.

The effects of immersion on VC have been addressed in more than 20 publications over the years (for a review, see Dahlbäck 1978). The reported changes in VC range from 0% to −15%, and the average change that can be computed from these studies is −6%.

Dahlbäck et al. (1978) showed that if the blood redistribution that normally occurs during immersion was prevented there was no change in VC. Blood redistribution was prevented by a technical device allowing immersion of the thoracoabdominal part of the subject while leaving the legs out of the water. The hydrostatic forces acting on the chest, although restricting maximal inspiratory excursions somewhat, aided in expiration so as to allow for an unchanged VC (relative to the nonimmersed condition). The importance of immersion-induced blood redistribution for VC changes is further borne out by our observation that when arterial occlusion was applied on arms and legs before immersion there was almost no reduction in VC as the subjects were lowered into the water (Kurss et al. 1980). In the same study it was shown that water temperature markedly modifies immersion effects on VC. Thus, in thermoneutral water (35°C) the VC reduction was, on the average, 5%, while in cool water (20°C) the decrease was 10%, reflecting peripheral vasoconstriction forcing blood into the thorax, and in warm water (40°C) there was no significant change in VC, indicating that a considerable amount of peripheral blood pooling persisted.

The intrathoracic blood volume apparently competes with air for space. Furthermore, as explained below in more detail, engorgement of pulmonary capillaries may make the lungs stiffer and limit VC. To describe immersion effects on the FRC, it is useful to employ the pressure centroid of the chest and the eupneic pressure concepts.

Because of the high density of water, immersion creates sizable pressure differences between locations of the body that are at different depths. Thus, the lower parts of the chest are subject to higher pressure than the upper parts. The net effect of these pressure loads on the outside that are opposed by the outward recoil of the chest and the intra-alveolar pressure (equal to gas pressure at mouth level) is to make the system settle at a new lower volume at which the outward recoil balances the mean water pressure on the chest (Figures III-12A and III-12B).

As will be evident later, breathing at a reduced FRC may entail certain "physiological disadvantages." If one is to be able to evaluate immersion effects quantitatively, information about the hydrostatic forces acting on the chest is required. If the alveolar pressure increased to equal the mean water pressure, the chest wall and lungs would be brought back out so as to restore nonimmersed FRC. One way to find this balancing pressure is to connect an immersed subject to a diver's breathing regulator and gradually move the regulator deeper in the water until the subject's FRC has been restored. The level of the chest at which the membrane of the regulator is then located defines the vertical position of the pressure centroid of the chest.

The bulk of evidence indicates that the reduction in FRC that occurs in the absence of the above-mentioned balancing pressure usually is caused by a diminution of the ERV, while no firm conclusion can be drawn about RV changes. The mean reduction in ERV that may be calculated from a review of the results of 14 articles (Dahlbäck 1978) amounts to 66%. Jarrett (1965) determined the pressure required to restore FRC and found that during immersion to the sternal notch the pressure centroid was 7.5 in. (19 cm) below the sternal angle in the upright posture and 2.8 in. (7 cm) behind it in the horizontal

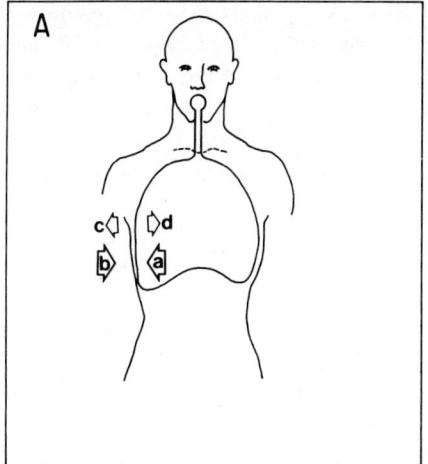 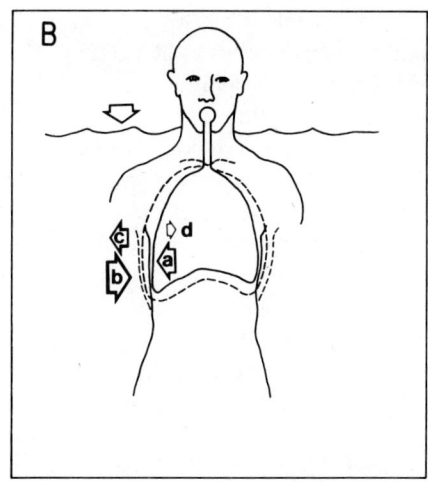

Figure III-12. Pressure forces acting on and exerted by thorax and lungs. Widths of *arrows* symbolize relative magnitude of forces. *A*: Nonimmersion. Gas pressure (a and b) on inside and outside of thorax-lung complex equal atmospheric pressure. Outward recoil force of thoracic wall (c) is balanced by equally large inward recoil force exerted by lungs (d) at functional residual capacity level (i.e., a + c = b + d). *B*: Head-out immersion. Inside pressure (a) equals atmospheric pressure, outside pressure (b) is sum of atmospheric and average water pressure. Outward recoil force of thoracic wall (c) is enlarged due to chest compression and inward recoil force of lungs (d) slightly reduced. New balance of forces (a + c = b + d) is reached at a reduced functional residual capacity level. *Dashed contours* correspond to nonimmersed condition.

posture. It is tempting to suggest that a diver's breathing gear should be designed to provide breathing gas at the pressure prevailing at his or her pressure centroid. As early as 1947, Paton and Sand (1947) determined the respiratory gas pressure subjectively most acceptable (eupneic pressure) to diver-subjects. Remarkably, they found the eupneic pressure point to be at a much shallower location than the "isovolume" centroid determined by Jarrett (1965). Thus, the eupneic point at rest was 6–8 in. (15–20 cm) above the sternal angle in the erect position. It was lowered to 4–6 in. (10–15 cm) above the sternal angle when there was hyperpnea from any cause (distances from external auditory meatus recalculated). These differences between Paton and Sand's (1947) and Jarrett's (1965) results were ascribed by the latter to differences in experimental techniques. In the earlier work a mouthpiece had been used and the subjects had to bite on it to keep it from popping out at high mouth pressures, while Jarrett used an oronasal mask that allowed the subjects to relax fully.

In the search for guidelines for choosing suitable intrapulmonary pressures for divers, experiments have recently been carried out in submersed exercising subjects at depth (Thalmann et al. 1979). The divers wore full-face masks and assumed the prone position. Intrapulmonary pressures were varied within a range of -23 cmH$_2$O to $+17$ cmH$_2$O relative to the sternal angle. Although these pressure extremes had no appreciable influence on respiratory gas exchange and end-tidal carbon dioxide tensions, an intrapulmonary pressure of about $+7$ cmH$_2$O relative to the pressure centroid was clearly subjectively preferable. At this pressure the dyspnea experienced when doing heavy exercise at depth was less pronounced than at more negative intrapulmonary pressures.

One notable effect of immersion is that it changes the distribution of pulmonary ventilation (Arborelius et al. 1972b). The apical regions that are distended (at FRC) and underventilated in nonimmersion become less distended due to compression during immersion and therefore amenable to larger volume changes with each breath. By contrast, ventilation in basal regions is reduced, presumably mostly because of airway closure. This airway closure can be demonstrated by measurement of trapped air volume (Dahlbäck and Lundgren 1972) or closing volume (Bondi et al. 1976).

There are presumably several mechanisms behind the airway closure during immersion. With increased blood content the lungs are likely to be heavier, and therefore they tend to compress airways in dependent regions. Furthermore, an erectile effect on the alveolar walls by blood-engorged capillaries may reduce the recoil of the lungs. This will increase pleural pressure and therefore pressure on the outside of the airways, increasing the tendency for them to close. The fact that breathing is performed at a lower FRC also reduces the recoil force of the lungs, adding to the closing mechanism just described. Measurements of closing volume (CV) (or closing capacity) during head-out immersion have given somewhat conflicting results (presumably for technical reasons). However, the bulk of the evidence indicates a tendency for increased CV during immersion (Bondi et al. 1976; Prefaut et al. 1978; Prefaut et al. 1979). Clearly, when the FRC is low, as in immersion, and CV is increased, there is a greater possibility that some airway closure will occur within the span of the tidal volume (toward the end of the expiration).

A possible consequence of this is disturbances in the arterialization of the blood going through the lungs. Indeed, Prefaut and his colleagues (1978) have demonstrated that the more an individual's tidal volume (V_T) is within the CV envelope, the higher the alveolar-arterial oxygen tension difference will be. Furthermore, they showed that the older or more overweight the individual is, the more overlap between the breathing range (ERV + V_T) and CV there will be during immersion. In subjects whose CV's were below end-expiratory levels, there was even a reduction in the alveolar-arterial oxygen tension difference (from about 12 mmHg nonimmersed to 8 mmHg immersed), while for those breathing completely within the CV envelope, that difference increased markedly (from about 13 to 24 mmHg). The improvement in the former group was ascribed to improved perfusion conditions.

One aspect of the erectile effects on the lungs caused by vascular engorgement during immersion is that the lungs become stiffer, i.e., their compliance is reduced. A 30% reduction in static compliance (Dahlbäck et al. 1978) and 37% in dynamic compliance (Dahlbäck et al. 1979) have been recorded.

As explained earlier, the reduced FRC during immersion tends to decrease airway diameter, and this has been given as the explanation for an observed increase of about 30% in average pulmonary gas flow resistance during tidal breathing (Dahlbäck et al. 1979). The increased flow resistance is reflected in a 15% decrease in maximum voluntary ventilation, as demonstrated by Flynn et al. (1975). They also concluded that the inertia of the water on the chest was of no consequence.

The increase in lung stiffness, gas flow resistance during immersion, and hydrostatic pressure on the chest will increase respiratory work. Direct measurements of total respiratory work during transition from immersion to the xiphoid to immersion to the neck have shown an increase in the work of respiration from about 6000 gram-centimeters (g-cm) to 10,000 g-cm per 1-liter breath (Hong et al. 1969). Although this is a 65% increase, the respiratory work performed is still very small and presumably of little practical significance. This information pertains to resting conditions at 1 ATA, however, and information about respiratory work during immersion in combination with exercise and inspiration of high-density gas mixtures is still lacking.

2. Circulatory Function

It is well known that man's circulation during terrestrial life is influenced considerably by gravitational force. If this influence is offset by immersion, a marked increase in cardiac output (CO) may occur. Thus, head-out immersion in thermoneutral (35°C) water resulted in a 32% increase in CO that was caused entirely by enlarged stroke volume (SV), as determined by the dye-dilution technique (Arborelius et al. 1972a). Even larger increases (about 66% in CO and 80% in SV) have been recorded with a CO_2 rebreathing technique (Farhi and Linnarsson 1977). This study also showed that the increase in cardiac output was gradual as immersion progressed to the hip, to the xiphoid, and to the chin. Immersion to the neck redistributes about 0.7 liter of blood from the periphery into the thorax (Arborelius et al. 1972a), and the diastolic filling of the heart is enhanced, as illustrated by roentgen cinematography (Risch et al. 1978). Thus, increases of 130 ml have been recorded in the diastolic volume of the heart during immersion of the standing subject to the diaphragm and of an additional 120 ml upon further immersion to the neck (Risch et al. 1978). This distension evokes the Starling mechanism and increases SV. Peripheral vasodilation may cause the arterial blood pressure to remain essentially unchanged (Arborelius et al. 1972a). Increased peripheral perfusion during immersion has been demonstrated in muscle tissue by the radioactive tracer technique (Balldin et al. 1971b) and also as an increase in the rate of whole-body nitrogen elimination during oxygen breathing (Balldin and Lundgren 1972). It appears that the immersion effect on the circulation diminishes as the water temperature decreases. Rennie and his colleagues (1971) found cardiac output values obtained during rest and in water below 34°C somewhat lower than those taken during nonimmersion. During exercise, however, the cardiac output approached the levels achieved under "dry" conditions. There is presently a lack of information about circulatory adjustment to exercise in response to immersion, presumably because it is difficult to design experiments in which exactly the same exercise is performed under both wet and dry conditions.

The increase in central blood volume is accommodated to 25% by the large intrathoracic vessels (Risch et al. 1978), and also by the heart and the pulmonary capillaries. The extra blood accumulation in the latter, estimated by Farhi and Linnarsson (1977) to be about 170 ml (i.e., another 25%) accounts for an increase in diffusing capacity of about 45%–60% (Begin et al. 1976). However, another analysis showed that while young individuals had an increase in diffusing capacity, older subjects showed a decrease, presumably because of airway closure (Prefaut et al. 1978). These observations, together with the fact that members of the former group tended to breathe above their CV while in the water while members of the latter breathed below it, was given as the reason why immersion reduced the alveolar-arterial oxygen tension difference in young people and increased it in older people. Although experimental data are lacking, it is conceivable that the deeper inspiration caused by physical exercise might decrease the difference between these two groups. Another rather dramatic effect of immersion, presumably elicited by distension of the heart, is the appearance of extrasystoles during the first minutes of immersion (Arborelius et al. 1972a).

Immersion has been used to simulate the weightless state in space travel. After several hours of immersion, a state of cardiovascular deconditioning may be demonstrated, and, surprisingly, it has been shown that the concomitant reduction in orthostatic tolerance on a tilt table is more marked in physically trained than in untrained subjects (Stegman et al. 1969). In a later study it was found that intermittent exercise during a 6-hr immersion period offered considerable protection against the orthostatic instability (Stegman et al. 1975). These authors suggested that this might be related to a reduction in immersion diuresis caused by exercise and thought to conserve plasma volume. Nonetheless, the untrained subjects in this study exhibited a higher diuresis during immersion than the athletes, whether resting or active. The athletes' overall greater orthostatic impairment after immersion was hypothesized to be caused by a considerably reduced effectiveness of the blood pressure control system (Stegman et al. 1975).

a. Significance

The standard immersion situation is one in which the subject assumes an upright posture and the alveolar gas pressure is the same as the pressure at the subject's mouth level, while pressure on the chest is higher by about 20–30 cmH$_2$O. Although this posture causes changes in pulmonary mechanics and blood perfusion, there is as yet little evidence that these changes seriously jeopardize respiratory function. However, subjects performing heavy exercise at depth and breathing against a hydrostatic load on the chest become dyspneic; adjusting the pulmonary pressure to a slight overpressure eased this dyspnea. Consequently, breathing apparatus for divers should be designed to minimize intrapulmonary negative pressure.

Under special conditions the changes in cardiorespiratory function may be of consequence. It may be theorized that the large alveolar-arterial oxygen tension difference (amounting to about 24 mmHg) seen by Prefaut et al. (1978) in some subjects could increase the risk if $P_{A_{O_2}}$ is already low, perhaps because of a marginally functioning piece of diving gear. In connection with oxygen breathing, such as may be done to enhance inert gas elimination during decompression, airway closure may pose special problems. Thus, Balldin et al. (1971a) observed reductions in VC of more than 22% when oxygen was inhaled for 2 hr during head-out immersion. This phenomenon could be ascribed to total absorption of the oxygen and atelectasis formation in the closed-off regions. Deep inhalations, although painful, restored VC. Atelectasis formation could also be prevented by taking a deep inspiration every 5 min during the oxygen-breathing period. As an alternative remedy, an admixture of moderate amounts of inert gas to the oxygen would prevent the collapse of closed-off lung regions.

It has been hypothesized that air trapping during diving may introduce the danger of local overdistension of the lung, lung rupture, and air embolism (Dahlbäck and Lundgren 1972). During ascent the air in a closed-off region expands. If the pressure required to reopen the closed airway is higher than the pressure the walls of the expanding lung section can withstand, rupture will result. Although no quantitative information about these pressures is available, it seems prudent to suggest that ascent or decompression should not be performed while divers retain a low lung volume for any length of time.

Behnke and Austin (1974) have reported a case of fatal embolism in connection with submarine escape training; they stated that the case was best explained by expansion of trapped air as a result presumably of "overdeflation" during the initial phase of ascent. In this case the trainee, starting a free ascent from 100 fsw (3 ATA), was seen to exhale on his way to the surface. At 50 fsw (1.5 ATA), his ascent slowed (possibly from loss of buoyancy due to excess exhalation), and he was given a boost upward by his instructor. When the trainee reached 40 fsw (1.2 ATA), he released a large amount of air and shortly afterward lost consciousnes. The trainee died during the subsequent recompression treatment aimed at resolving gas emboli.

The distension exerted on the heart by immersion might cause frequent extrasystoles even in the healthy young individual. This observation clearly dictates caution in allowing persons who may have heart pathology to swim or dive.

A special case of greatly accentuated immersion effects may occur in snorkel swimming if the snorkel is erroneously used to get down below the surface. In this case, although the intra-alveolar pressure is still atmospheric, the water depth allowed by the snorkel is added to the hydrostatic load on the chest. One obvious effect of this is that inspiration will eventually become impossible: the maximum pressure the inspiratory muscles can overcome is about 130 cmH$_2$O (Ringqvist 1966). There is an early account of Stigler (1911) of systematic experiments attempting to determine the maximum depth at which "snorkelbreathing" can be performed. The primary goal of those experiments, which also dramatically illuminated the dangers of deep-immersion snorkel breathing, was actually to measure the maximum force of the inspiratory muscles. In one experiment Stigler was rapidly lowered into the water in an erect position while breathing through tubes supplying air at atmospheric pressure. He remained at depth, his nipples 2 m under the surface, for 18 sec, during which time he made forceful but fruitless attempts to inspire. Immediately after the experiment he had an irregular and weak pulse and a heart rate of 200 beats per minute. Physicians determined, by means of percussion, that Stigler had developed a two-finger-wide lateral displacement of the heart borders. They diagnosed his condition as heart dilatation. He remained bedridden for 7 weeks. Even months after the episode, Stigler believed that his heart could not cope with the level of athletic activities he had engaged in earlier. Stigler (1911) discussed the mechanism of heart dilatation in terms that have since gained support from results of the earlier-mentioned measurements in catheterized immersed subjects, i.e., he assumed that the heart dilatation was due to an accumulation of blood in the heart caused by much higher pressure on the outside of the body relative to the interior of the thorax.

However, cardiac output and peripheral circulation may be enhanced when the immersion depth is moderate, i.e., during immersion to the neck. This change in circulation may influence the rate of inert gas exchange. It is reasonable to expect that if immersion acts to make circulation hyperkinetic while a diver is at depth, his uptake of inert gas may be enhanced. Similarly, Balldin and Lundgren (1972) have demonstrated that nitrogen elimination during oxygen breathing is considerably enhanced if the subject is immersed to the neck. Balldin (1973) went on to demonstrate that if the immersion effect was used to enhance nitrogen elimination, the incidence of decompression sickness was significantly reduced in experimental decompressions in volunteer subjects.

Theoretically, the reduced orthostatic tolerance after extended immersion may be of some practical consequence. Especially in physically well-trained persons, who apparently are particularly sensitive to the deconditioning effect on blood pressure regulation, it is conceivable that imposing a sudden orthostatic load after several hours of immersion could cause fainting. We have observed a diver who complained of severe faintness after having climbed out of the water after several long-lasting dives. When he was forced to stand on the ladder for a while, there was clearly a risk that he might faint and fall back into the water.

3. Renal Effects

Immersion influences renal function through a multitude of hormonal and other mechanisms that are still insufficiently understood. Epstein (1978) published an excellent review of the renal effect of immersion. The following discussion of these effects is largely based on his review.

Head-out immersion causes both a water diuresis and a natriuresis, which are apparently controlled by different mechanisms. Although the increase in diuresis is usually manifest by the first or second hour, the natriuresis usually peaks by the fourth or fifth hour.

The diuretic response is determined by the state of hydration. In well-hydrated subjects the response is prompt, and diuresis, dominated by an increased free-water clearance, may reach about three times the level achieved during preimmersion periods. In the hydropenic state, the increase in diuresis is smaller and caused solely by increased osmolar clearance peaking in the fourth hour of immersion.

The dominating factor behind the immersion diuresis is a suppression in the release of antidiuretic hormone (ADH). This suppression appears to be brought about as a reflex response to distension of left atrial or pulmonary vein mechanoreceptors; the distension is caused by the previously described increase in central blood volume. As mentioned in Epstein's (1978) review, there is also a possibility that this mechanoreceptor stimulation may cause reduced renal sympathetic activity, which increases diuresis by altering intrarenal perfusion, and by direct tubular effects. There are also observations indicating that immersion enhances renal prostaglandin E excretion, which could enhance diuresis via several mechanisms.

Immersion causes increased natriuresis, but this increase is strongly correlated to salt intake and also varies among individuals. The sodium excreted may amount to 200%–300% of preimmersion levels. The lack of dependence of this phenomenon on diuresis is evident from the fact that even if ADH is administered to prevent diuresis, natriuresis may still increase in response to immersion.

The mechanism triggering natriuresis appears to be the same as that responsible for immersion diuresis, i.e., a stimulation of intrathoracic circulatory mechanoreceptors. The effector site is located in the tubules where increased sodium rejection is induced; this rejection is in turn mediated by diverse hormonal and neural mechanisms. Immersion causes a decrease in plasma aldosterone levels, apparently as a secondary effect of the suppression of renin-angiotensin levels. However, even when this effect is counteracted by administering an exogenous mineralocorticoid, the natriuresis persists, although it is blunted. This led Epstein and his co-workers (1978) to postulate the presence of a natriuretic hormonal factor. However, Epstein (1978) has also considered other mechanisms, such as alteration in intrarenal blood flow distribution and direct changes in tubular function caused by reduced sympathetic tone and increased release of renal prostaglandin.

Although the natriuresis of immersion is accompanied by kaliuresis, there is a lack of consensus about the reproducibility of this effect. Bicarbonate excretion is increased during immersion and is associated with an increase in urinary P_{CO_2} and a marked increase in urinary pH. The titratable acid, urinary ammonium, and net acid excretion are suppressed in immersion, effects that are not related to any systematic acid-base balance changes.

a. Significance

One practical aspect of immersion diuresis, which may reach a level of about 350 ml/hr, is the necessity to urinate frequently. For a diver wearing a suit this is not a small problem. Although the problem of increased thirst apparently has not been studied directly, it is probably one of the immersion effects, since the subject is gradually becoming dehydrated.

It is known that dehydration reduces a subject's work time because of exhaustion and also interferes with his ability to dissipate heat (Costill 1972). However, this latter circumstance would rarely cause problems for a diver. As discussed in a review by Cook (1951) there appears to be a relationship between individual differences in water balance and morbidity in altitude decompression sickness. The possibility that immersion-related disturbances in fluid-electrolyte balance may cause circulatory or other changes that could influence individual susceptibility to decompression sickness should therefore be considered.

4. Gastrointestinal System Effects

During head-out immersion in the upright position the abdomen, being at greater depth, is subjected to a proportionately higher water pressure than the thorax. This pressure is transmitted to the abdominal content. The pressures on each side of the diaphragm, which are equal (and negative) in the nonimmersed state, change so that the pressure on the abdominal side becomes positive and considerably higher than on the thoracic side (by about 15 cmH_2O) (Agostoni et al. 1966).

The diaphragm is displaced in the cranial direction and the compression of the lungs generates an increase in pleural pressure and therefore in esophageal pressure. Johnson et al. (1975) have shown that although the pressure increased by about 5 mmHg, the esophageal pressure went up by about 5 mmHg (cf. Figure III-13). This creates a marked pressure difference that would tend to push the gastric contents into the esophagus, were it not for the distal esophageal sphincter, whose pressure during immersion also increases and remains up to 15 mmHg higher than gastric pressure. However, the authors made the point that in the case of faulty sphincter function the increased gastroesophageal pressure gradient may predispose to gastric reflux (Johnson et al. 1975).

When a diver swims head-down toward the bottom, the vertical pressure differences on his body are reversed in comparison to the head-up posture. Thus, the diver's mouth and breathing regulator are at a greater depth than the lungs, and especially the stomach. This reversal of the esophageal pressure profile compared to the head-up posture is shown in Figure III-13 (Lundgren 1975). The high air pressure in the oral cavity relative to the esophagus may lead to considerable air ingestion (Brattström et al. 1975). Change in

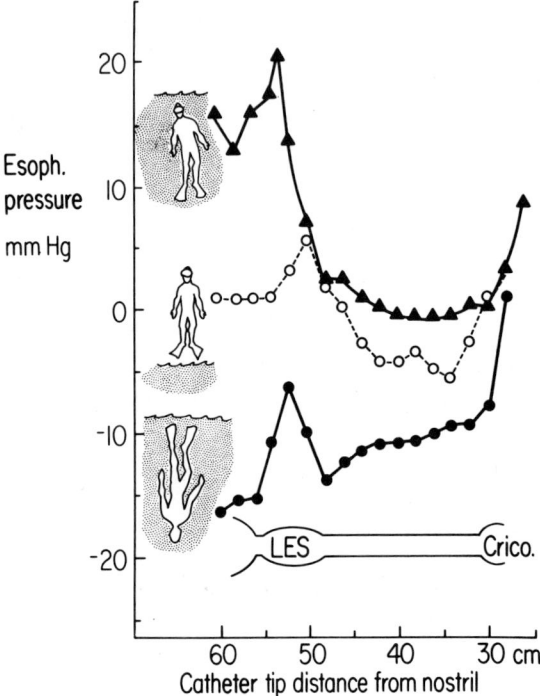

Figure III-13. Esophageal pressure profiles (end-expiratory measured relative to mouth pressure in one subject) during erect immersion, nonimmersion and head-down immersion. Schematic figure of esophagus with lower esophageal sphincter (LES) and cricopharyngeus is shown for orientation. [From Lundgren (1976).]

body buoyancy, determined by underwater weighing, was taken as a measure of aerophagia during diving. It was demonstrated that, although descending feet-first to 30 m (96 fsw) caused a mean weight reduction equivalent to that caused by ingesting about 0.17 qt (0.16 liter) of air (1 atm equivalent), descending head-first caused 0.31 qt (0.29 liter) of air to be swallowed. In one dive the subject was exposed to seven cycles of pressure changes between 25 and 30 m while simulating swimming along an uneven bottom contour. In this case the subject surfaced with 1.42 qt (1.34 liters) of air in the stomach, which caused considerable distension and pain. The same study demonstrated that only negligible amounts of air entered the stomach when the ears were cleared by blowing against the clamped nose.

a. Significance

The high gastric pressure relative to esophageal pressure during head-out immersion or when assuming an upright posture under water is probably conducive to gastric reflux only when the sphincter pressure is deficient. Although this may be a relatively rare condition, vomiting while under water is very dangerous. It is conceivable that if the diver is near vomiting for other reasons, such as seasickness, high gastric pressure might precipitate reflux that would otherwise be avoided. The golden rule not to go swimming (or diving) on a full stomach may indeed be rationally based. Also, as pointed out by Johnson and colleagues (1975), drugs that might lower distal esophageal sphincter pressure should not be taken by swimmers and divers.

Gastrointestinal distension by gas may be more of a problem in diving than is usually recognized. Thus an epidemiologic study of more than 2000 sport divers showed that at one time or another 5.4% had experienced gastric pain, nausea, and vomiting apparently caused by gastrointestinal overdistention (Lundgren and Örnhagen 1975). Notably, these causes were frequently connected to steep head-first descents or difficulties in ear clearing that may have promoted aerophagia. The potential seriousness of aerophagia during diving is further borne out by a recent case report describing an incidence of gastric rupture during decompression (Wolkiewicz et al. 1979). This occurred in a diver after she had swallowed seawater mixed with air when trying to cope with a leaking breathing regulator.

From the practical point of view it seems prudent to warn divers against excessive swallowing (for instance for the purpose of ear clearing), especially in the head-down posture. If a diver experiences a sensation of fullness or pain in the stomach during ascent, he or she should descend until the sensation goes away and then, before continuing the ascent, should try to expel the excess gas by belching while in the upright position.

5. Buoyancy Effects

One striking effect of immersion is the apparent weightlessness of the body. Although this situation may be modified by attaching various pieces of equipment to the body, the distribution of weight and abnormal buoyancy of the body is still a common problem. The easily achieved state of neutral buoyancy is enjoyable, since it allows a diver freedom to move in the vertical plane. However, lack of sufficient body weight is a great disadvantage when stationary work is to be performed under water. For instance, when using a saw the diver may have to hold himself to the object being sawed with one hand to avoid moving back and forth while the other hand tries to move the saw. This calls for an expenditure of considerable additional energy in the form of static work. An interesting example of the importance of weight-buoyancy distribution in the water has been offered by Pendergast and co-workers (1977). They found that female swimmers were more proficient than male swimmers in relation to their power output. This was explained by the fact that the female swimmers have a better weight-buoyancy distribution, which allows them to assume a more horizontal position (with less drag) in the water than males.

The amount of energy expended to move in water is quite large because of the viscous resistance of water. The mechanical efficiency of the front crawl stroke has been rated at about 3% to 7.5% (Pendergast et al. 1977), and the efficiency of underwater fin swimming at roughly twice this level (Rennie et al. 1971). By comparison, running and bicycling are performed at 20% to 25% efficiency. The viscous resistance of water dampens rapid movements and makes the use of a club or hammer more difficult.

Having the normal sensation of weight eliminated or disturbed deprives the diver of important proprioceptive clues for orientation. The situation is further aggravated when vision is limited by murky water or by equipment. The diver then has to rely primarily on his vestibular function, and this frequently turns out to be inadequate. Experienced divers have aborted dives and shown signs of severe anxiety in response to the sensory deprivation accompanying a dive with neutrally buoyant gear in very turbid water.

This section was written with partial support of the Office of Naval Research and the Naval Medical Research and Development Command through Office of Naval Research Contract N00014-78-C-0205, and with partial support from a Fellowship Grant for A. J. Påsche under the auspices of the Norwegian Underwater Institute and granted by the Royal Norwegian Council for Scientific and Industrial Research, Grant No. KS1850.7552.

CLAES E. G. LUNDGREN
A. J. PÅSCHE

References

AGOSTONI, E., G. GURTNER, G. TORRI, AND H. RAHN 1966. Respiratory mechanics during submersion and negative-pressure breathing. *J. Appl. Physiol.* 21: 251–258.
ARBORELIUS, M., JR., U. I. BALLDIN, B. LILJA, AND C. E. G. LUNDGREN 1972a. Hemodynamic changes in man during immersion with the head above water. *Aerosp. Med.* 43:592–598.
ARBORELIUS, M., JR., U. I. BALLDIN, B. LILJA, AND C. E. G. LUNDGREN 1972b. Regional lung functions in man during immersion with the head above water. *Aerosp. Med.* 43:701–707.
BALLDIN, U. I. 1973. The preventive effect of denitrogenation during warm water immersion on decompression sickness in man. *Försvarsmedicin* 9:239–243.
BALLDIN, U. I., AND C. E. G. LUNDGREN 1972. Effects of immersion with the head above water on tissue nitrogen elimination in man. *Aerosp. Med.* 43:1101–1108.
BALLDIN, U. I., G. O. DAHLBÄCK, AND C. E. G. LUNDGREN 1971a. Changes in vital capacity produced by oxygen-breathing during immersion with the head above water. *Aerosp. Med.* 42:384–387.
BALLDIN, U. I., C. E. G. LUNDGREN, J. LUNDVALL, AND S. MELLANDER 1971b. Changes in the elimination of ^{133}Xenon from the anterior tibial muscle in man induced by immersion in water and by shifts in body position. *Aerosp. Med.* 42:489–493.
BEGIN, R., M. EPSTEIN, M. A. SACKNER, R. LEVINSON, R. DOUGHERTY, AND D. DUNCAN 1976. Effects of water immersion to the neck on pulmonary circulation and tissue volume in man. *J. Appl. Physiol.* 40:293–299.
BEHNKE, A. R., AND L. F. AUSTIN 1974. Introduction to SCUBA diving. *J. Sports Med.* 11:276–290.
BONDI, K. R., J. M. YOUNG, R. M. BENNETT, AND M. E. BRADLEY 1976. Closing volumes in man immersed to neck in water. *J. Appl. Physiol.* 40:736–740.
BRATTSTRÖM, P., B. LINDVALL, C. E. G. LUNDGREN, AND H. ÖRNHAGEN 1975. Influence of body posture and ear clearing on body buoyancy during diving. *Undersea Biomed. Res.* 2:161–166.
COOK, S. F. 1951. Role of exercise, temperature, drugs and water balance in decompression sickness. Part II. In: *Decompression Sickness, Caisson Sickness, Diver's and Flier's Bends and Related Syndromes*, edited by J. F. Fulton. Philadelphia: Saunders Company, p. 223–241.
COSTILL, D. L. 1972. Water and electrolytes. In: *Ergogenic Acids and Muscular Performance*, edited by W. P. Morgan. New York: Academic Press, p. 293–318.
DAHLBÄCK, G. O. 1978. Lung mechanics during immersion in water—with special reference to pulmonary air trapping (unpublished thesis). University of Lund, Sweden: Laboratory of Aviation and Naval Physiology, Institute of Physiology and Biophysics.
DAHLBÄCK, G. O., AND C. E. G. LUNDGREN 1972. Pulmonary air trapping induced by water immersion. *Aerosp. Med.* 43:768–774.
DAHLBÄCK, G. O., B. JONSON, AND C. E. G. LUNDGREN 1979. Influence of hydrostatic thorax compression and intrathoracic blood pooling on dynamic lung mechanics during head-out immersion. *Undersea Biomed. Res. Suppl.* 6:23.
DAHLBÄCK, G. O., E. JÖNSSON, AND M. H. LINÉR 1978. Influence of hydrostatic compression of the chest and intrathoracic blood pooling on static lung mechanics during head-out immersion. *Undersea Biomed. Res.* 5:71–85.
EPSTEIN, M. 1978. Renal effects of head-out immersion in man. Implications for an understanding of volume homeostasis. *Physiol. Rev.* 58:529–581.
EPSTEIN, M., N. S. BRICKER, AND J. J. BOURGOIGNIE 1978. Presence of a natriuretic factor in urine of normal men undergoing water immersion. *Kidney Int.* 13:153–158.
FARHI, L. E., AND D. LINNARSSON 1977. Cardiopulmonary readjustments during graded immersion at 35°C. *Respir. Physiol.* 30:35–50.

FLYNN, E. T., JR., E. M. CAMPORESI, AND S. A. NUNNELEY 1975. Cardiopulmonary responses to pressure breathing during immersion in water. In: *Man, Water, Pressure*, edited by E. H. Lanphier and H. Rahn. Buffalo: State Univ. of New York at Buffalo, Dept. of Physiology, p. 79–94.

HONG, S. K., P. CERRETELLI, J. CRUZ, AND H. RAHN 1969. Mechanics of respiration during submersion in water. *J. Appl. Physiol.* 27:535–538.

JARRETT, A. S. 1965. Effect of immersion on intrapulmonary pressure. *J. Appl. Physiol.* 20:1261–1266.

JOHNSON, L. F., Y. C. LIN, AND S. K. HONG 1975. Gastroesophageal dynamics during immersion in water to the neck. *J. Appl. Physiol.* 38:449–454.

KURSS, D. I., C. E. G. LUNDGREN, AND A. J. PÅSCHE 1980. The effect of water temperature on vital capacity during head-out immersion. In: *Underwater Physiology VII. Proceedings of the Seventh Symposium on Underwater Physiology*, edited by A. J. Bachrach and M. M. Matzen. Bethesda, MD.: Undersea Medical Society.

LUNDGREN, C. E. G. 1975. Immersion effects on pulmonary, circulatory and gastrointestinal systems. In: *International Symposium on Man in the Sea*, edited by S. K. Hong. Bethesda, Md.: Undersea Medical Society.

LUNDGREN, C. E. G., AND H. ÖRNHAGEN 1975. Nausea and abdominal discomfort—possible relation to aerophagia during diving: an epidemiologic study. *Undersea Biomed. Res.* 2:155–160.

PATON, W. D. M., AND A. SAND 1947. The optimum intrapulmonary pressure in underwater respiration. *J. Physiol.* 106:119–138.

PENDERGAST, D. R., P. E. DIPRAMPERO, A. B. CRAIG, JR., D. R. WILSON, AND D. W. RENNIE 1977. Quantitative analysis of the front crawl in men and women. *J. Appl. Physiol.: Respir. Environ. Exercise Physiol.* 43:475–479.

PREFAUT, CH., F. DUBOIS, CH. ROUSSOS, R. AMARL-MARQUES, P. T. MACKLEM, AND F. RUFF 1979. Influence of immersion to the neck in water on airway closure and distribution of perfusion in man. *Respir. Physiol.* 37:313–323.

PREFAUT, CH., M. RAMONATXO, R. BOYER, AND G. CHARDON 1978. Human gas enchange during water immersion. *Respir. Physiol.* 34:307–317.

RENNIE, D. W., P. DIPRAMPERO, AND P. CERRETELLI 1971. Effects of water immersion on cardiac output, heart rate, and stroke volume of man at rest and during exercise. *Med. Sport* 24:223–228.

RINGQVIST, T. 1966. The ventilatory capacity in healthy subjects. *Scand. J. Clin. Lab. Invest. Suppl.* 88:18.

RISCH, W. D., H.-I. KOUBENEC, U. BECKMANN, S. LANGE, AND O. H. GAUER 1978. The effect of graded immersion on heart volume, central venous pressure, pulmonary blood distribution and heart rate in man. *Pfluegers Arch.* 374:115–118.

STEGMAN, J., H. D. FRAMING, AND M. SCHIEFELING 1969. Der Einfluss einer 6-stündigen Immersion in thermodifferentem Wasser auf die Regulation des Kreislaufes und des Leistungsfähigkeit bei Trainierten und Untrainierten. *Pfluegers Arch.* 312:129–138.

STEGMAN, J., U. MEIER, W. SKIPKA, W. HARTLIEB, B. HEMMER, AND U. TIBES 1975. Effects of a multi-hour immersion with intermittent exercise on urinary excretion and tilt table tolerance in athletes and non-athletes. *Aviat. Space Environ. Med.* 46(1):26–29.

STIGLER, R. 1911. Die Kraft unserer Inspirations Muskulatur. *Pfluegers Arch.* 139:234–254.

THALMANN, E. D., D. K. SPONHOLTZ, AND C. E. G. LUNDGREN 1979. Effects of immersion and static lung loading on submerged exercise at depth. *Undersea Biomed. Res.* 6:259–290.

WOLKIEWIEZ, J., A. VALICI, P. MAESTRACCI, AND M. MARCILLON 1979. L'association rupture gastrique et MD.D. problemes diagnostic et therapeutique. *Med. Aeronaut. Spat. Med. Subaquat. Hyperbare* 18(21):251–253.

C. Cardiovascular Effects

The cardiovascular effects of diving vary widely and depend to a large degree on the type of exposure. Hyperbaric exposure is associated with certain cardiovascular changes that may be affected in turn by other factors in the hyperbaric environment, such as immersion, thermal stress, breathing against increased external resistance, breath holding, and exercise. This section discusses primarily the effects of hyperbaric exposure per se on the cardiovascular system, without specific reference to other factors, such as immersion, that are covered elsewhere.

1. Hyperbaric Bradycardia

The most widely recognized effect of hyperbaric pressure on the cardiovascular system is a slowing of heart rate. This relative bradycardia has been observed in animals and man; it occurs in air and helium-oxygen exposures both at rest and during exercise.

a. Early Studies

In one of the first reports of this phenomenon, Heller, Mager, and von Schrötter (1897) described the results of studies made on caisson workers exposed to 1.5 and 2.6 atmospheres of air pressure (2.5 and 3.6 ATA). Resting heart rates were reduced by approximately 15 beats per minute (bpm) during exposure to either pressure. Heller and his colleagues also noted that the average increase in heart rate after work at increased pressure was "decidedly smaller than the average increase of pulse rate of workers under normal atmospheric conditions" (Heller et al. 1897).

The first systematic study of the effects of pressure on heart rate and blood pressure was performed at the U.S. Navy Experimental Diving Unit in 1935. Shilling, Hawkins, and Hansen (1936) measured the heart rate and blood pressure of subjects reclining, standing, and exercising during exposure to air at 2, 4, 6, 7, and 10 ATA (60, 120, 180, 220, and 330 fsw). Each exposure to increased pressure was preceded by control measurements taken in the pressure chamber at normal atmospheric pressure. Shilling and his colleagues (1936) found a consistent decrease in heart rate with exposure to pressure. The average decreases in heart rate for all pressures were 9.12 bpm while the subjects were reclining, 11.1 bpm while standing, and 12.1 bpm while exercising. A decrease in blood pressure also occurred during exposure to increased air pressure.

Since the work of Shilling and his associates (1936) a number of investigators have attempted to determine which physical factors of the hyperbaric environment are responsible for the slowing in heart rate. Among factors that have been investigated are increased partial pressure of oxygen, increased gas density, increased pressure per se, and increased gas tensions of nitrogen and of helium.

b. Effects of Increased Partial Pressure of Oxygen

As air is compressed, the partial pressure of oxygen increases proportionally. Knowledge of this fact led early workers to question whether the slowing in heart rate was caused by the increased partial pressure of oxygen (Po_2). Shilling and his co-workers (1936) discussed this possibility, citing the work of Dautrebande and Haldane (1921), who had observed that pure oxygen breathed at 1 and 2 ATA caused a slowing of the pulse rate. More recent studies by Fagraeus (1974) and by Hesser and Fagraeus and Linnarsson (1968, 1974) have demonstrated that the increased Po_2 is only partially responsible for the bradycardia induced by exposure to compressed air. These investigators measured heart rate and other physiological variables in exercising subjects exposed to either (1) 1 ATA air, (2) 1 ATA oxygen, or (3) 4.5 ATA air. Because the inspired P_{O_2} was approximately the same in exposures (2) and (3), the investigators could determine the degree to which increased oxygen tension contributed to the overall decrease in heart rate. Fagraeus and colleagues (1974) found that for each of four levels of oxygen consumption (induced by increasing the work load), heart rate was reduced by approximately 12–16 bpm during exposure to 4.5 ATA air. When the experiment was repeated with the subjects breathing oxygen at 1 ATA, there was a reduction in heart rate of approximately 4–7 bpm. Fagraeus and his associates (1974) concluded that only about one-third of the decrease in heart rate was caused by the increased P_{O_2} (oxygen dependent); the remaining decrease (non-oxygen dependent) was caused by some factor or factors related to the increased nitrogen pressure. Although most of the decrease in heart rate caused by exposure to compressed air is not oxygen dependent, Whalen and his associates (1965) have shown that breathing 100% oxygen at 3.04 ATA causes a further reduction in heart rate.

Other investigators have observed bradycardia with increased pressures of helium. For example, Matsuda and colleagues (1975) found a decrease in heart rate in exercising subjects exposed to 7 ATA (220 fsw) helium containing 0.3 ATA oxygen of approximately 20% compared to measurements made at 1.2 ATA air. This decrease was almost entirely non-oxygen dependent because the level of oxygen throughout the exposure was kept to approximately 0.3 ATA.

In summary, the bradycardia resulting from exposure to compressed air is partially caused by the increased P_{O_2} (oxygen dependent) but to a greater degree is caused by other non-oxygen-dependent factors related to the increased inert gas pressure.

c. Effects of Increased Gas Density

After the demonstration by Hesser and his associates (1968), and others, that a large part of hyperbaric bradycardia was not oxygen dependent, studies were begun in 1971 at the U.S. Navy Experimental Diving Unit to determine which physical factors in the hyperbaric environment were responsible for this phenomenon. These studies by Flynn and associates (1972) were carefully designed to separate and quantify the effects of increased gas density and increased ambient pressures on the bradycardia induced by hyperbaric exposure. Heart rate was measured in human subjects at rest and at three consecutive work levels of 30, 60, and 90 W. Subjects were exposed to gas mixtures of constant density at varying ambient pressures and to gas mixtures of different densities at constant ambient pressures. Flynn and colleagues (1972) used various mixtures of helium, nitrogen, and oxygen to provide a constant level of inspired oxygen of 147–150 mmHg at all pressures. The pressures, gas mixtures, and resulting densities are shown in Table III-1. From the table, it can be seen that gas mixtures at pressures of 1.0 to 5.45 ATA and gas densities ranging from 0.77 g/liter to 6.02 g/liter were used. The effects of these exposures on heart rate at rest and at three levels of work are shown in Figures III-14 and III-15. Figure III-14 shows that with a constant gas density increased pressure alone reduces heart rate at each level of work. Figure III-15 illustrates that at a constant pressure, increasing the density of the inspired gas caused a further reduction

Table III-1
Composition and Density of Gas Mixtures[a]

Depth, ATA	Gas mixture	Density, g/liter
1.0	21% O_2–38.7% He–40.3% N_2	0.77
	21% O_2–79.0% N_2	1.11
3.27	6.1% O_2–93.9% He	0.77
	6.1% O_2–82.6% He–11.3% N_2	1.11
	6.1% O_2–93.9% N_2	3.61
5.45	3.6% O_2–96.4% He	1.11
	3.6% O_2–96.4% N_2	6.02

[a]From Flynn et al. (1972).

in heart rate at each level of work. From these results, Flynn and colleagues (1972) concluded that both the increased density of the inspired gas and the increased pressure (or some factor relating to it) contribute to the development of non-oxygen-dependent hyperbaric bradycardia.

d. Effects of Increased Hydrostatic Pressure

The effects of increased pressure per se are, of course, difficult to study in man or any whole animal. Lundgren and Örnhagen (1976), however, were able to study the heart rate response to pressure alone in liquid-breathing mice. They employed a technique in which unanesthetized mice breathed a liquid fluorocarbon of high gas-dissolving capacity; use of this technique made it possible to increase hydrostatic pressure without increasing the inert gas tensions. These authors found that increasing the hydrostatic pressure to 2000 ATA (6600 fsw) caused a progressive decrease in heart rate, which first became evident at 25 ATA (825 fsw). At 175 ATA (5775 fsw), the average heart rate was 48% of the control value. This effect was not altered by treating the animals with autonomic blocking agents, which suggests that the bradycardia was caused by the direct action of pressure on cardiac pacemaker cells. This mechanism was confirmed by Örnhagen and Hogan (1977), who used sinus node preparations isolated from mouse, rat, guinea pig, rabbit, and dog hearts. Compression to 150 ATA (4950 fsw) caused an averaged 43% reduction in spontaneous beating frequency, which was unaltered by autonomic blocking agents. This slowing of heart rate may be the result of the slowed cardiac conduction and decreased excitability that Doubt and Hogan (1978) have found at 150 ATA.

These and other studies indicate that pressure alone may have an effect on heart rate. In evaluating the relevance of these studies to human diving, however, it is important to note the circumstances under which these effects have been found. In each of the above-mentioned studies, bradycardia occurred only at extreme pressures. For example, in liquid-breathing mice, no significant reduction in heart rate occurred until the pressure reached 90 ATA (approximately 3000 fsw). In the isolated sinus node preparations, only the effects of exposure to 150 ATA (approximately 5000 fsw) were studied. In contrast, Fagraeus (1971) found that neither the heart rate nor the contractile force of the isolated guinea pig heart was altered by exposure to 9 ATA (300 fsw). Thus, although there is evidence suggesting that pressure alone could cause a slowing of heart rate at great pressure, there is little evidence indicating that such an effect could account for the bradycardia seen in humans during hyperbaric exposure.

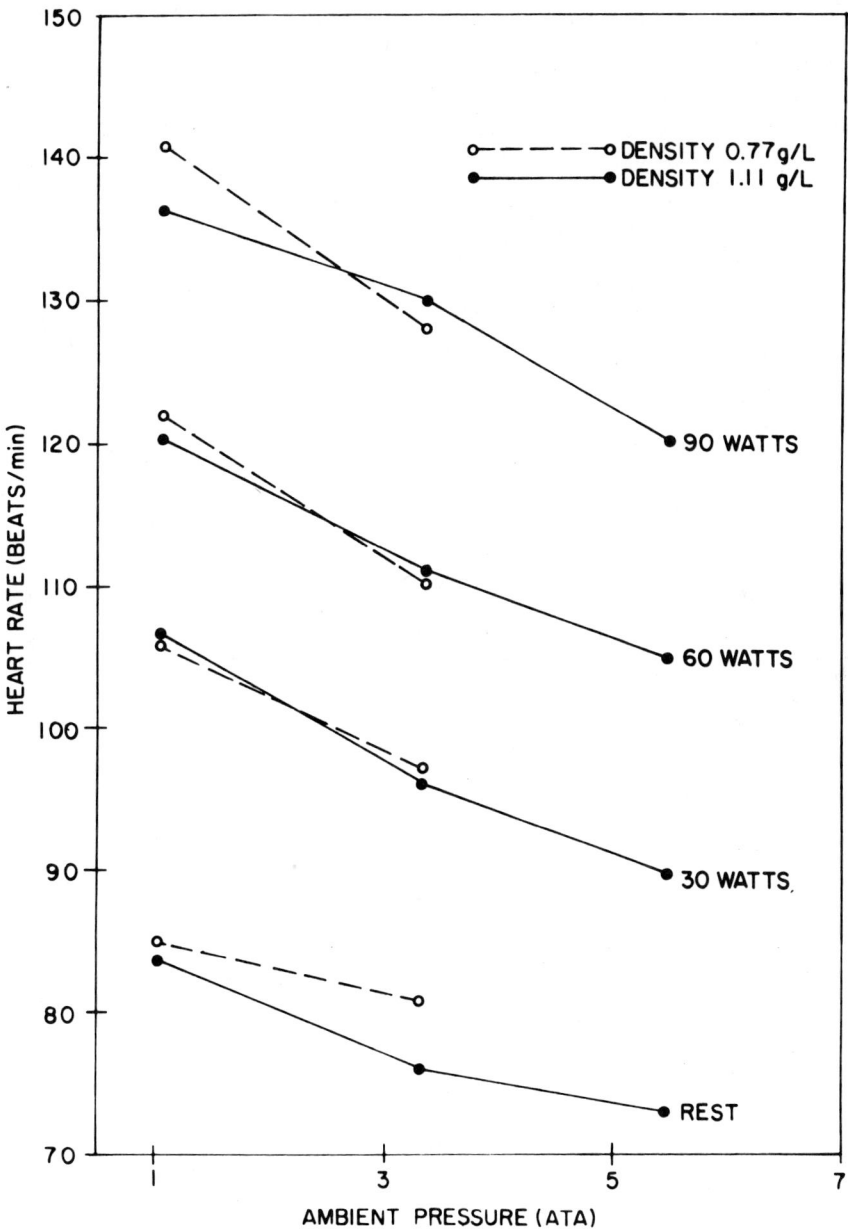

Figure III-14. Relationship between heart rate and ambient pressure at a constant inspired gas density of 0.77 and 1.11 g/liter. [From Flynn et al. (1972).]

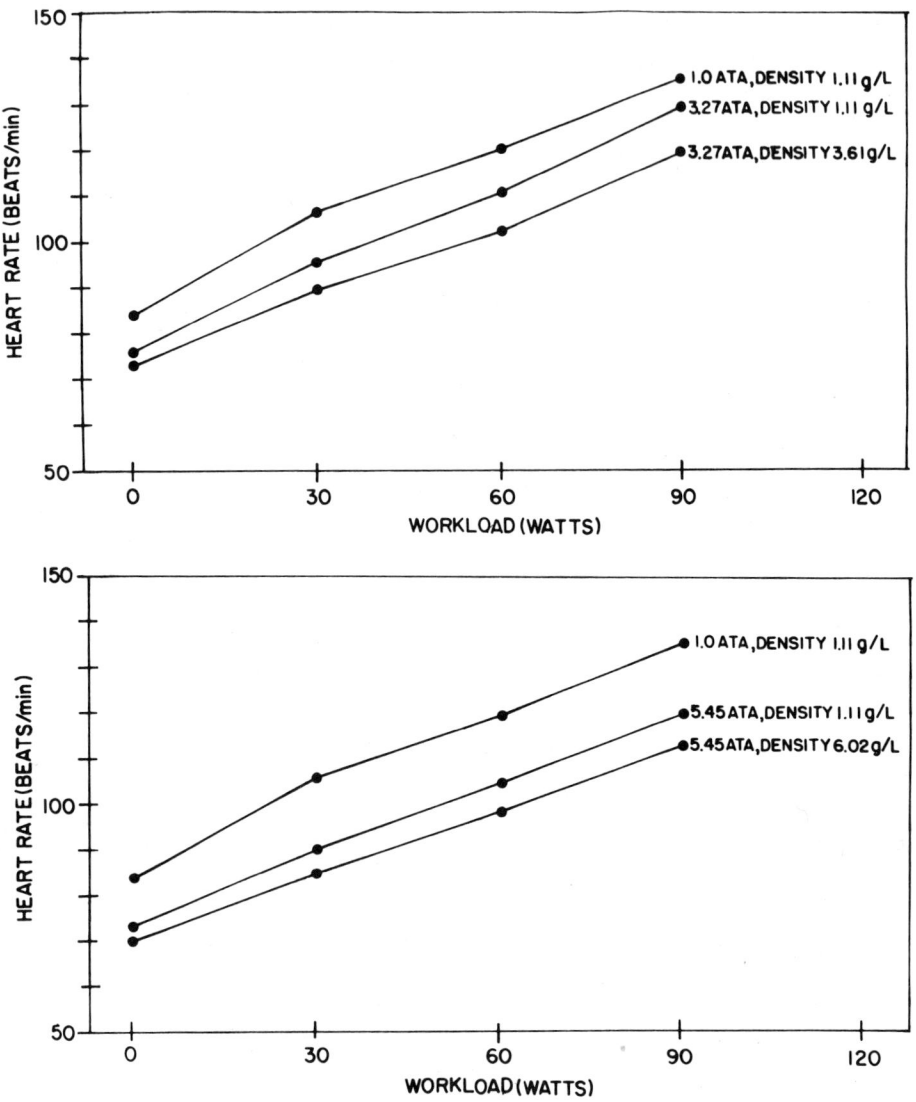

Figure III-15. Relationships between heart rate and work load as a function of ambient pressure and gas density. [From Flynn et al. (1972).]

e. Effects of Increased Gas Tensions of Helium and Nitrogen

Another possible factor in the development of hyperbaric bradycardia is a direct effect of increased tensions of nitrogen or helium. These effects are also difficult to study in isolation, but some consideration has been given to them. For example, Flynn and colleagues (1972) questioned whether the bradycardia they attributed to increased gas density might be related to the increased partial pressure of nitrogen, because under pressure this gas is known to have profound effects on the central nervous system. When

Flynn and associates (1972) compared their findings to those of Bradley and Dickinson (1976), in which a small decrease in heart rate was seen with subjects breathing 15% nitrous oxide (approximately equivalent in narcotic potency to breathing air at 150 fsw), they concluded that nitrogen itself was a small contributor to the bradycardia they had observed under pressure.

Whether helium itself might be partially responsible for a slowing in heart rate has also been considered. Although helium had long been considered physiologically inert, studies indicating that helium breathing at 1 ATA had an antiarrhythmic effect in animals after coronary ligation generated interest in its cardiovascular effects (Pifarre et al. 1968, 1969, 1970; Raymond et al. 1972). A reduction in heart rate was also observed in animals breathing helium. This reduction was associated with a reduction of sympathetic tone (Lin and Kato 1974) or a decrease in levels of circulating catecholamines (Raymond et al. 1972). Helium breathing has also been found to decrease circulating catecholamine levels in human subjects (Gledhill et al. 1975). Nevertheless, other studies involving a variety of animals have failed to demonstrate an antiarrhythmic effect of helium breathing (Evans et al. 1977; Holland et al. 1973; Nicholas et al. 1975) or an effect of helium on the autonomic nervous system (Hardenbergh et al. 1978; Nicholas et al. 1974). Moreover, Wade and associates (1979) have found no antiarrhythmic effect of helium breathing in humans with spontaneous premature ventricular beats.

Because of the conflicting results of previous studies and their questionable relevance to human diving, studies were recently begun at the Naval Medical Research Institute to determine the effects of breathing helium-oxygen at 1 ATA on the cardiovascular system (D. E. Evans, unpublished observations). Ten male subjects performed continuous bicycle exercise at approximately 50% of aerobic capacity for 30 min. Each subject breathed air during one experimental period and 80% helium–20% oxygen during another. Measurements of oxygen consumption, heart rate, and cardiac output failed to show any cardiovascular differences between helium-oxygen and air breathing. Similarly, no differences in plasma epinephrine or norepinephrine levels occurred in the helium-oxygen or air breathing conditions. These observations suggest that helium-oxygen breathing at 1 ATA in human subjects does not cause changes in the cardiovascular system or in plasma catecholamine levels during rest or exercise. Whether helium under pressure has physiological or pharmacological effects on the cardiovascular system is unknown.

f. Autonomic Mediation of Hyperbaric Bradycardia

From the previous discussion it is apparent that both oxygen-dependent and non-oxygen-dependent factors contribute to hyperbaric bradycardia. Several investigators have sought to determine the degree to which these effects are mediated by the autonomic nervous system (Daly and Bondurant 1961; Fagraeus 1974; Fagraeuus and Linnarsson 1973). In the most comprehensive of these studies, Fagraeus and Linnarsson (1973) used cholinergic and β-adrenergic blocking agents in human subjects in whom both oxygen-dependent and non-oxygen-dependent bradycardia were studied. Fagraeus and Linnarsson (1973) found during light exercise in air at 1 ATA, in oxygen at 1.3 ATA, and in air at 6.0 ATA that the oxygen-dependent bradycardia was caused primarily by a direct action on the heart, with a proportionally smaller effect mediated by the parasympathetic nervous system. In contrast, the non-oxygen-dependent bradycardia was caused primarily by a reduced β-adrenergic stimulation of the heart. Recent animal studies (D. E. Evans, unpublished observations) at the Naval Medical Research Institute have also revealed both direct cardiac effects and autonomic nervous mediation of bradycardia caused by helium-oxygen exposure to 16 ATA. How these changes in heart and autonomic nervous system effects affect humans during heavy exercise at greater depths is not known.

2. Cardiovascular Effects of Saturation Exposure

In recent years, several saturation exposures have been made in which human subjects were exposed to pressures of approximately 3 to 50 ATA (100 to 1650 fsw) for periods ranging from several days to several weeks. Saturation exposures to 200 fsw (6.0 ATA) have been made using nitrogen-oxygen; deeper exposures have involved helium-oxygen mixtures. During these exposures many physiological measurements have been made, including measurements of heart rate and other indexes of cardiovascular function. As might be expected from earlier work, bradycardia has been a frequent, although not totally consistent, finding in these exposures. For example, Wilson and co-workers (1977) studied cardiovascular responses to saturation exposures of nitrogen-oxygen at 50 and 200 fsw (1.5 to 6 ATA). The oxygen level in these exposures ranged from approximately 0.3 to 0.5 ATA. A consistent 20% to 30% decrease in heart rate was observed at saturation depth. During saturation exposures to 50 fsw (1.5 ATA) brief excursions to deeper depths (down to 250 fsw or 7.5 ATA) were accompanied by a further reduction in heart rate. Alterations in cardiac conduction and some cardiac arrhythmias were also observed (Wilson et al. 1977). Although various degrees of bradycardia have been seen in almost all deep saturation dives using helium-oxygen, the decrease in heart rate has not been found to be linear with depth. For example, in compression of human subjects to 850 fsw (25 ATA), Flynn and associates (1972) found a decrease in heart rate from 120 bpm at surface to 108 bpm at 300 fsw in subjects exercising at 60 W. From 300 fsw to 850 fsw (9 to 25 ATA) however, there was no further reduction in heart rate. In a 1500-fsw (45 ATA) saturation exposure, Morrison and colleagues (1976) observed bradycardia at rest and during exercise at 600 fsw but no further reduction in heart rate upon compression to 1500 fsw. Thus, deeper exposures appear to have little additional effect on heart rate.

Although heart rate has been measured in many saturation diving exposures, heart rate is only one factor in the complex regulation of cardiovascular performance. The more important question with regard to human diving is whether hyperbaric exposure causes a decrease in cardiac output and thus diminishes blood flow to the tissues. During several recent saturation exposures, indirect measurements of cardiac output have been made in an attempt to address this question. Smith and co-workers (1977) and Matsuda and associates (1978) have used impedance cardiography to measure stroke volume and cardiac output in human subjects exposed to 18.6 ATA (600 fsw) and 11 ATA (360 fsw), respectively. These investigations have shown that hyperbaric bradycardia is accompanied by an increase in stroke volume that maintains or increases cardiac output under pressure. Hempleman and colleagues (1978), using a carbon dioxide and nitrous oxide rebreathing technique, have found an overall decrease in cardiac output at 600 and 900 fsw (200 and 300 msw) even though the bradycardia was accompanied by some increase in stroke volume during rest and light exercise. During heavy work at these depths, stroke volume fell to below surface values, indicating a further decrease in cardiac output. Because of the limited number of studies available and the conflicting results obtained, the question of changes in stroke volume and cardiac output under hyperbaric exposure is unresolved.

3. Summary

The most consistent effect of hyperbaric exposure on the cardiovascular system is a slowing of heart rate. Hyperbaric bradycardia occurs at rest and during exercise, in hyperoxic and normoxic exposures of nitrogen-oxygen or helium-oxygen, from relatively shallow to deep depths, and during brief and saturation exposures. Factors that contribute to hyperbaric bradycardia include increased tensions of oxygen, increased gas density, increased hydrostatic pressure, and, possibly, increased tensions of nitrogen and of helium. The decrease in heart rate is mediated partially by the autonomic nervous system and partially by direct effects on the heart.

The significance for human diving of changes in heart rate is still relatively unknown. The effect of hyperbaric exposure on cardiac output in humans has been studied, but conflicting results preclude a definitive statement about the cause of this effect. Because changes in cardiac output or regional blood flow may limit diver performance and influence the uptake and elimination of inert gases, understanding these cardiovascular effects is important to diving safety and to the extension of man's diving capability.

The author wishes to express appreciation to Mr. David LeGrys and Mrs. Mary M. Matzen for their assistance in the preparation of this manuscript.

DELBERT E. EVANS

References

BRADLEY, M. E., AND J. G. DICKSON, JR. 1976. The effects of nitrous oxide narcosis on the physiological and psychologic performance of man at rest and during exercise. In: *Underwater Physiology V. Proceedings of the Fifth Symposium on Underwater Physiology*, edited by C. J. Lambertsen. Bethesda, MD: Fed. Am. Soc. Exp. Biol., p. 617–626.

DALY, W. J., AND S. BONDURANT 1961. Effects of oxygen breathing on the heart rate, blood pressure, and cardiac index of normal men—resting, with reactive hyperemia, and after atropine. *J. Clin. Invest.* 41: 126–132.

DAUTREBANDE, L., AND J. S. HALDANE 1921. The effects of respiration of oxygen breathing and circulation. *J. Physiol.* 55: 296–299.

DOUBT, T. J., AND P. M. HOGAN 1978. Effects of hydrostatic pressure on conduction and excitability in rabbit atria. *J. Appl. Physiol.: Respir. Environ. Exercise Physiol.* 45: 24–32.

EVANS, D. E., E. HARDENBERGH, L. W. RAYMOND, AND M. E. BRADLEY 1977. Effect of helium breathing on cardiac arrhythmias induced by coronary occlusion and digitalis in the cat. *Undersea Biomed. Res.* 4: 381–389.

FAGRAEUS, L. 1971. Performance of the isolated guinea-pig heart in the hyperbaric environment. Stockholm, Sweden: Karolinska Institutet, Laboratories of Aviation and Naval Medicine.

FAGRAEUS, L. 1974. Cardiorespiratory and metabolic functions during exercise in the hyperbaric environment. *Acta Physiol. Scand. Suppl.* 414: 1–40.

FAGRAEUS, L., C. M. HESSER, AND D. LINNARSSON 1974. Cardiorespiratory responses to graded exercise at increased ambient air pressure. *Acta Physiol. Scand.* 91: 259–274.

FAGRAEUS, L., AND D. LINNARSSON 1973. Heart rate in the hyperbaric environment after autonomic blockade. *Försvarsmedicin* 9: 260–264.

FLYNN, E. T., T. E. BERGHAGE, AND E. F. COIL 1972. Influence of Increased Ambient Pressure and Gas Density on Cardiac Rate in Man. Rep. 4-72. Panama City, FL: U.S. Navy Experimental Diving Unit.

GLEDHILL, N., A. K. CHIN, and A. C. BRYAN 1975. Plasma catecholamines in humans during helium breathing. *Physiologist* 18: 22.

HARDENBERGH, E., J. A. MILES, AND L. W. RAYMOND 1978. Lack of effect of helium breathing on catecholamine levels in the adrenal vein blood of the rabbit. *Aviat. Space Environ. Med.* 49: 573–575.

HELLER, R., W. MAGER, AND H. V. SCHRÖTTER 1897. On the physiological behavior of pulse with change of air pressure. *Z. Klin. Med.* 33(3):1–60. (NAVSHIPS Trans. No. 1349.)

HEMPLEMAN, H. V., B. ANDREWS, D. W. BURGESS, R. F. CARLYLE, AND S. A. COLLIS 1978. Observations on men at pressures of up to 300 msw (31 bar). Rep. 78401. Gosport, Hants, U.K.: Admiralty Marine Technology Establishment.

HESSER, C. M., L. FAGRAEUS, AND D. LINNARSSON 1968. Cardiorespiratory responses to exercise in the hyperbaric environment. Stockholm, Sweden: Karolinska Institutet, Laboratories of Aviation and Naval Medicine.

HOLLAND, J. A., W. G. WOLFE, AND J. A. KYLSTRA 1973. Helium: Absence of antiarrhythmic effect in anesthetized dogs. *J. Thorac. Cardiovasc. Surg.* 66: 478–480.

LIN, Y. C., AND E. N. KATO 1974. Effects of helium gas on heart rate and oxygen consumption in unanesthetized rats. *Undersea Biomed. Res.* 1: 281–289.

LUNDGREN, C. E. G., AND H. C. ÖRNHAGEN 1976. Heart rate and respiratory frequency in hydrostatically compressed, liquid-breathing mice. *Undersea Biomed. Res.* 3: 303–320.

MATSUDA, M., H. NAKAYAMA, H. ARITA, J. F. MORLOCK, J. CLAYBAUGH, R. M. SMITH, AND S. K. HONG 1978. Physiological responses to head-out immersion in water at 11 ATA. *Undersea Biomed. Res.* 5: 37–52.

MATSUDA, M., H. NAKAYAMA, A. ITOH, N. KIRIGAYA, F. K. KURATA, R. H. STRAUSS, AND S. K. HONG 1975. Physiology of man during a 10-day dry heliox saturation dive (SEATOPIA) to 7 ATA. I. Cardiovascular and thermoregulatory functions. *Undersea Biomed. Res.* 2: 101–117.

MORRISON, J. B., P. B. BENNETT, E. E. P. BARNARD, AND W. J. EATON 1976. Physiological studies during a deep, simulated oxygen-helium dive to 1500 feet. In: *Underwater Physiology V. Proceedings of the Fifth Symposium on Underwater Physiology*, edited by C. J. Lambertsen. Bethesda, MD: Fed. Am. Soc. Exp. Biol., p. 3–20.

NICHOLAS, T. E., J. L. HART, AND P. A. KIM 1974. Effect of breathing helium on sympathetic nervous and cardiovascular functions. *Undersea Biomed. Res.* 1: 271–280.

NICHOLAS, T. E., J. L. HART, AND, P. A. KIM 1975. Inability of helium to influence the occurrence of arrhythmias in cats, rats and mice. *Undersea Biomed. Res.* 2: 28–34.

ÖRNHAGEN, H. Ch., AND P. M. HOGAN 1977. Hydrostatic pressure and mammalian cardiac-pacemaker function. *Undersea Biomed. Res.* 4: 347–358.

PIFARRE, R., W. D. COX, M. JASUJA, AND W. E. NEVILLE 1969. Helium in the prevention of ventricular fibrillation. *Dis. Chest* 56: 135–138.

PIFARRE, R., T. K. RAGHUNATH, R. M. VANECKO, F. S. CHUA, J. U. BALIS, AND W. E. NEVILLE 1970. Effect of oxygen and helium mixtures on ventricular fibrillation. *J. Thorac. Cardiovasc. Surg.* 60: 648–652.

PIFARRE, R., S. M. WILSON, AND C. A. HUFNAGEL 1968. The influence of oxygen and helium upon ventricular fibrillation: a preliminary report. *J. Thorac. Cardiovasc. Surg.* 55: 535–537.

RAYMOND, L., R. B. WEISKOPF, AND M. J. HALSEY 1972. Possible mechanism for the antiarrhythmic effect of helium in anesthetized dogs. *Science* 176: 1250–1252.

SHILLING, C. W., J. A. HAWKINS, AND R. A. HANSEN 1936. The influence of increased barometric pressure on the pulse rate and arterial blood pressure. *US Nav. Med. Bull.* 34: 39–47.

SMITH, R. M., S. K. HONG, R. H. DRESSENDORFER, H. J. DWYER, E. HAYASHI, AND C. YELVERTON 1977. Hana Kai II: A 17-day dry saturation dive at 18.6 ATA. IV. Cardiopulmonary functions. *Undersea Biomed. Res.* 4: 267–281.

WADE, C. E., E. W. BANISTER, D. G. BAKER, AND Y. C. LIN 1979. Absence of antiarrhythmic effects of helium in patients with spontaneous premature ventricular beats at rest. *Undersea Biomed. Res.* 6: 313–318.

WHALEN, R. E., H. A. SALTZMAN, D. H. HOLLOWAY, JR., H. D. McINTOSH, H. O. SIEKER. AND I. W. BROWN, JR. 1965. Cardiovascular and blood gas responses to hyperbaric oxygenation. *Am. J. Cardiol.* 15: 638–646.

WILSON, J. M., P. D. KLIGFIELD, G. M. ADAMS, C. HARVEY. AND K. E. SCHAEFER 1977. Human ECG changes during prolonged hyperbaric exposures breathing N_2-O_2 mixtures. *J. Appl. Physiol.: Respir. Environ. Exercise Physiol.* 42: 614–623.

D. High Pressure Nervous Syndrome

When vertebrates, including men, are exposed to pressures greater than 500 feet of seawater (15 ATA) either in the dry hyperbaric environment of a pressure chamber or in actual submersion, signs and symptoms may appear; these include tremors of the extremities, severe myoclonic jerks, fatigue, and, ultimately, convulsions. In association with these symptoms, changes in the electrical activity of the brain and, at times, nausea, dizziness, and somnolence also occur. These may cause a decrement in the performance of divers working at deep depths, and although divers have not convulsed at the depths which have been attained to date, equivalent to 2250 feet of seawater (fsw) or 68 ATA (Bennett et al. 1982), such convulsions have been seen in other primates (monkeys). In the case of animals, death may ensue if pressures are increased still further.

In humans, the group of signs and symptoms associated with very deep diving is called the High Pressure Nervous Syndrome (HPNS); its development is affected by the rate of compression and the hydrostatic pressure attained. The faster the rate of compression and the higher the pressure, the more severe the signs and symptoms. Thus, the speed with which divers can be compressed and remain fit to work is limited. At depths greater than 1500 fsw (46 ATA), even with very long compressions of many days, slow compression rates, and stages (which have been effective in ameliorating signs and symptoms), HPNS may affect the performance, health, and safety of the deep diver.

Further, since the etiology of HPNS is unclear, whether frequent HPNS causes any permanent damage to the brain is not known. For these reasons, HPNS may well set limits on the conditions under which man may perform useful work in the ocean.

This section reviews the more important practical aspects of HPNS, including its signs, symptoms, and factors that potentiate or prevent the syndrome. More detailed reviews are available elsewhere (Bachrach and Bennett 1973; Bennett 1975, Bennett et al. 1976; Hunter and Bennett 1974).

1. Signs and Symptoms in Man

In 1965 the Royal Navy carried out a series of simulated oxygen-helium deep dives in the pressure chamber of the Royal Naval Physiological Laboratory (RNPL), with compression rates of 100 fsw/min, depths of 600 fsw (9 ATA) and 800 fsw (25 ATA), and durations at depth of 1 to 4 hr (Bennett 1965; Bennett and Dossett 1967). Helium was not expected to be narcotic at such depths. Surprisingly, however, new signs and symptoms were noted, including coarse tremors of the extremities, myoclonic jerking, dizziness, nausea, and vomiting, accompanied by a severe decrement in any task requiring manual dexterity, and some decrement in intellectual ability (Table III-2). Further, in

Table III-2

Change from Predive Values in
Performance at 600 and 800 fsw
Breathing Oxygen-Helium

Task	Decrease, %	
	600 fsw	800 fsw
Arithmetic multiplication ($98 \times 6 = \_\_$)		
(a) Number correct	18 (6)	42 (4)
(b) Number attempted	4 (6)	6 (4)
Fine manual dexterity		
(a) Ball bearing test	25 (6)	53 (4)

Numbers in parentheses = n. Data derived from Bennett (1965), Bennett and Dossett (1967).

contrast to compressed air intoxication, most of these signs and symptoms disappeared after about 90 min. Other experimental oxygen-helium dives conducted at about that time confirmed that this new syndrome occurred in divers exposed to these and deeper depths (Bennett 1967; Hamilton et al. 1967; Zaltsman 1968) and also showed that slowing the compression rate reduced the severity of the symptoms.

In 1968, however, a relatively slow 2-hr compression to 1190 fsw (37 ATA) by the French was aborted after 4 min at depth because a considerable amount of slow-wave theta activity (4–8 Hz) developed in the electroencephalogram (EEG), accompanied by tremors, somnolence, and fatigue. Similar EEG changes have also occurred immediately before mice under hyperbaric pressure convulsed (Brauer et al. 1968).

A few months later three Swiss diver-subjects were compressed at 16–17 fsw/min to 1000 fsw (31 ATA), in a joint Swiss–Royal Navy experiment. They remained at 1000 fsw for 3 days and made three excursions to 1150 fsw (36 ATA) for periods as long as 2 hr (Buehlmann et al. 1970). During the excursions the divers used semiclosed breathing apparatus and performed physical work without developing symptoms. Again in 1968, men were compressed at 40 fsw/hr to 1000 fsw in a Duke University–U.S. Navy experiment, without any signs or symptoms of HPNS (Summitt et al. 1969).

Efficiency during the Buehlmann dives to 1000 fsw (31 ATA) was impaired by tremors (Table III-3) in the first 1.5 hr, as revealed by performance in the ball bearing test, which involves picking up ball bearings with tweezers and placing them in a tube. Performance on less sensitive tests, however, showed little change, and there was no evidence of mental impairment. Some nausea and vertigo were also reported.

During excursions, performance efficiency did not deteriorate. The HPNS was therefore considered a compression syndrome, caused by the heat of compression, psychological stress, and the unexplained effect of an overfast change of pressure, combined with helium hyperventilation. Urine electrolyte measurements were made under these conditions, as were other measurements of blood morphology and biochemistry. The urine showed a reduction in sodium, calcium, magnesium, and chloride ions, and diuresis of phosphorus and potassium (Buehlmann et al. 1970).

Similar measurements were made in a dive to 800 fsw (25 ATA) at 3 to 5 fsw/min, with excursions at 27 and 28 fsw/min to 1050 (33 ATA) and 1100 fsw (34 ATA),

Table III-3
Performance Impairment in Deep Saturation Oxygen-Helium and Excursion Dives

Test	At surface	After compression	Time at 31 ATA (1000 fsw)						2-hr Excursions to 36 ATA
			1 hr	2 hr	3 hr	24 hr	48 hr	72 hr	
Ball bearing	12 ± 4	6 ± 5	10 ± 6	11 ± 4	12 ± 5	16 ± 6	18 ± 3	17 ± 4	19 ± 4
Dotting	69 ± 12	66 ± 9	63 ± 9	63 ± 7	62 ± 13	61 ± 6	67 ± 6	69 ± 8	63 ± 9
Dotting in squares	38 ± 4	32 ± 4	32 ± 4	34 ± 3	35 ± 5	39 ± 2	36 ± 3	41 ± 2	38 ± 3
Errors, %	2	6	3	0	3	6	5	10	9
Letter code	39 ± 6	33 ± 5	30 ± 6	32 ± 4	33 ± 6	38 ± 8	35 ± 4	41 ± 5	37 ± 3
Errors, %	0	7	7	2	0	0	0	2	0
Arithmetic correct	9 ± 1	—	11·5 ± 3	—	11 ± 3	14 ± 2	—	14 ± 2	12 ± 2
Arithmetic attempted	9·5 ± 1	—	13·5 ± 2	—	13 ± 3	15 ± 3	—	17 ± 2	14 ± 2

Values are mean number correct ± SD.   Data derived from Buehlmann et al. (1970).

conducted by International Underwater Contractors, Inc. (IUC), and a U.S. Navy team of scientists from the New London Submarine Medical Center (Proctor et al. 1972; Schaefer et al. 1970). Tremors were observed during the excursions and, as with many early dives to 1000 fsw (31 ATA) that had relatively rapid compressions, arthralgia and aching muscles occurred. Psychological performance was unimpaired.

Urinary pH, carbon dioxide, and bicarbonate increased significantly; in contrast to the Swiss/British dive to 1000 fsw (31 ATA), sodium, potassium, and phosphorus excretion increased, calcium was unchanged, and chloride decreased. The IUC-USN results are believed to have been caused by hyperventilation-induced respiratory alkalosis, a common finding in early deep oxygen-helium diving. That the Swiss divers had been trained not to hyperventilate at depth may account for the differences in urine electrolytes seen in the Swiss–RN experiments.

The excellent physical condition of the divers in these experiments made it seem unlikely that there was a "barrier" to deep diving at depths greater than 1200 fsw (37 ATA). An intensive scientific study of HPNS, which culminated in the exposure of two men to a simulated depth of 1500 fsw (46 ATA) for 10 hr (Bennett and Gray 1971; Bennett and Towse 1971a, 1971b) was therefore undertaken. Instead of continuous compression, compression was made in stages to permit research to be conducted. However, as later became apparent, these stages, coupled with a relatively slow rate of compression (16 to 17 fsw/min), permitted the divers to reach 1500 fsw able to function effectively despite some HPNS symptoms.

Initial compression was made to the first stage at 600 fsw (19 ATA), at which the two divers stayed 24 hr before compressing to 1000 fsw (31 ATA) for a further 24-hr stay (Figure III-16). During the remainder of the compression, 1-hr stages were made at 1100, 1200, and 1400 fsw (34, 37, and 43 ATA), and an additional 24 hr were spent at 1300 fsw (48 ATA). On arrival at both 600 fsw (19 ATA) and 1000 fsw (31 ATA), the subjects reported tremors, myoclonic jerks, dizziness, and slight nausea, which improved during the first hours at these depths. For the first time, on-line frequency analysis was made of the electroencephalograms. These showed a progressive increase in theta activity (4 to 6 Hz) and a reduction in electrical activity at the faster frequencies, which was most evident when the divers' eyes were open (Figure III-17). This increased theta activity occurred especially during each compression phase and continued to increase for 6 hr

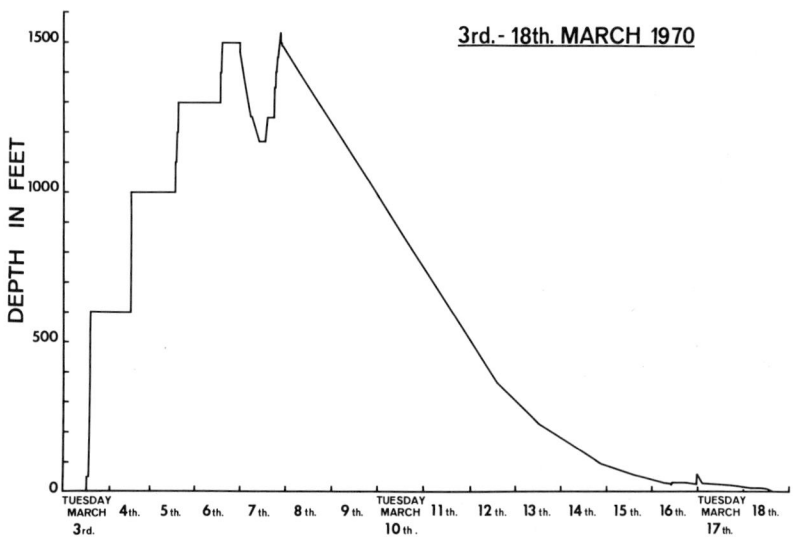

Figure III-16. Dive profile for first dive to 1500 fsw at RNPL, England. Recompression to 1535 fsw during decompression was caused by vestibular decompression illness. [From Bennett and Towse (1971a).]

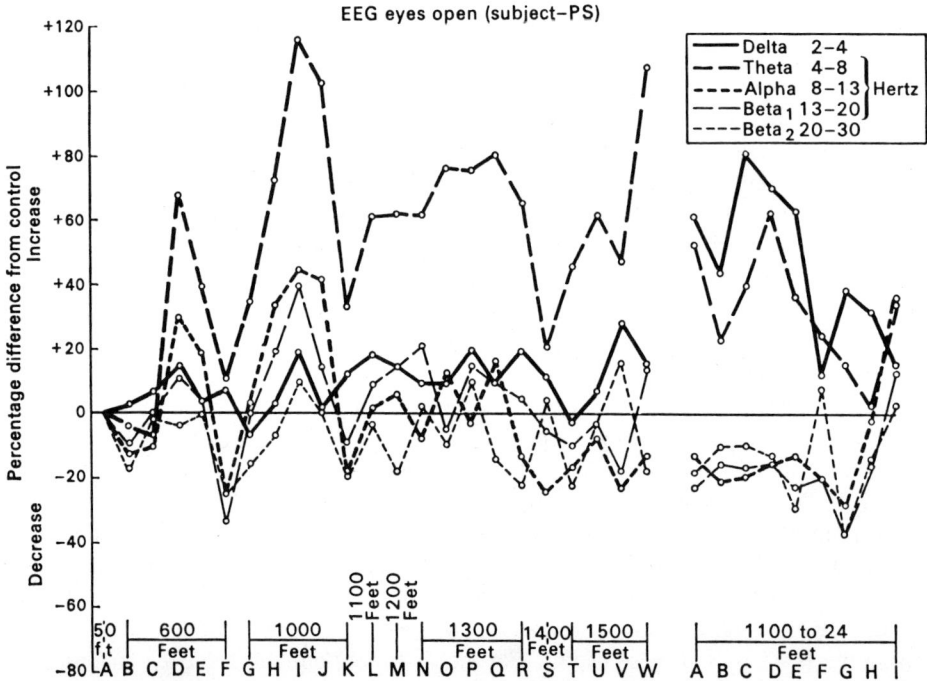

Figure III-17. Percentage change in frequencies of electrical activity of brain in a subject during a 1500 fsw oxygen-helium dive at RNPL, taken at various stable stages of the dive, compared to control values obtained at 50 fsw. Marked increase in theta activity (4–8 Hz) is initiated by each compression phase and continues for 6 hr even though compression has stopped. [From Bennett and Towse (1971b).]

after compression ceased. For an additional 12 hr, this 4- to 6-Hz activity slowly decreased. With increasing depth, however, there was a consistent rise in the basic theta activity, which seemed to be caused by hydrostatic pressure rather than the rate of compression.

Performance tests indicated no change in intellectual functions such as arithmetic multiplication, but psychomotor tasks, especially those involving fine neuromuscular coordination, such as the so-called ball bearing test, did show significant decreases from predive performance levels (Figure III-18). The effects of HPNS are therefore different from those of nitrogen narcosis, in which intellectual performance rather than psychomotor ability primarily is affected (Bennett 1975).

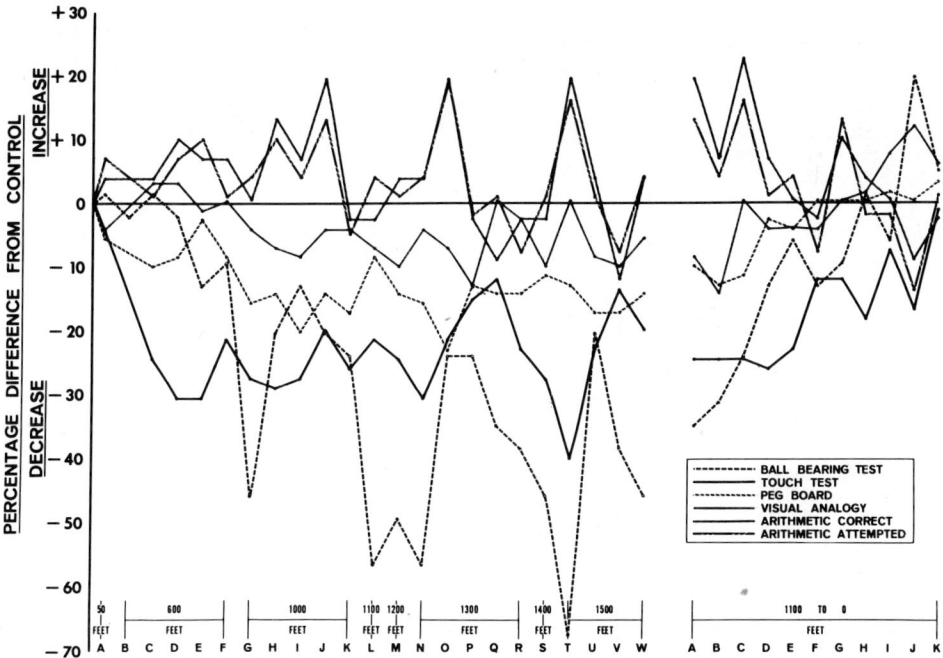

Figure III-18. Percentage change from predive control measurements of effects of exposure to oxygen-helium on performance during British 1500-fsw experimental dive shown in Figure III-16. Intellectual performance (arithmetic) is unaffected but tests of fine motor dexterity show a decrease due to tremors and myoclonic jerking. [From Bennett and Towse (1971a).]

Much of the psychomotor performance decrement was caused by tremors and myoclonic jerking. Accelerometer measurements of the tremor showed considerable individual variation, as did the other tests. One subject's resting postural tremor increased during each compression phase, and his base tremor also increased with greater depth (Figure III-19).

Despite decreases in performance, however, the subjects were able to function surprisingly well, especially considering that earlier exposures to 1190 fsw (37 ATA) had to be aborted after only 4 min. These studies supported the inference, based on lipid solubilities and other factors, that helium does not possess narcotic properties. However,

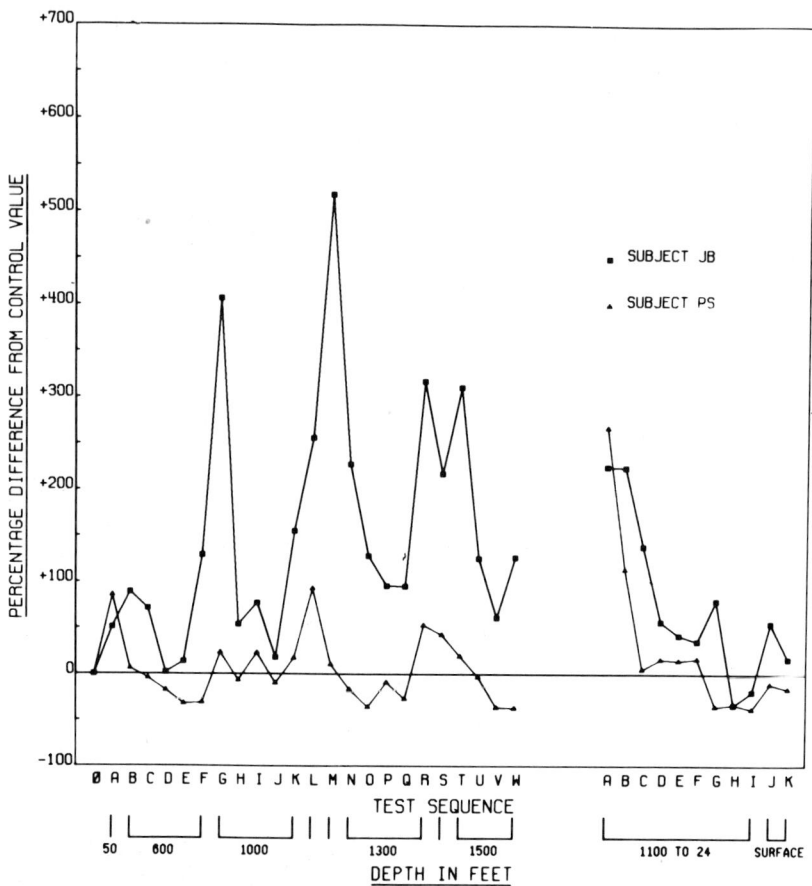

Figure III-19. Percentage change in degree of finger tremor measured by an accelerometer on the index finger in two subjects exposed to 1500 fsw during the RNPL dive in 1970. One subject shows an increase in tremor with each compression phase while the other is unaffected. In Subject JB, there is also a progressive increase in base-line tremor with increasing depth. [From Bennett and Towse (1971a).]

as the earlier Bennett studies of 1965 and 1967 showed, intellectual performance may be affected by nausea, fatigue, and somnolence if the compression rate is fast enough to cause severe HPNS.

In 1970, the French diving company COMEX, using similar staging techniques and an increasingly slow rate of compression, attained 1700 fsw (53 ATA) and observed similar increases in EEG theta activity and a reduction of fast alpha (8 to 13 Hz) and beta (14 to 22 Hz) frequencies during a dive called Physalie V (Fructus 1972). Tremor was present from 1000 fsw (31 ATA) and became much more apparent at 1600 fsw (50 ATA) and deeper. Performance tests also showed decrements, and in moments of relaxation the divers experienced a reduction in awareness that the French termed *microsleep*.

In June 1972, Physalie VI was carried out; this dive exposed two men to 2001 fsw (62.5 ATA) for the first time; this depth was at that time the limit of human deep oxygen-helium diving (Figure III-20). In this dive the slow rate of compression and long stages

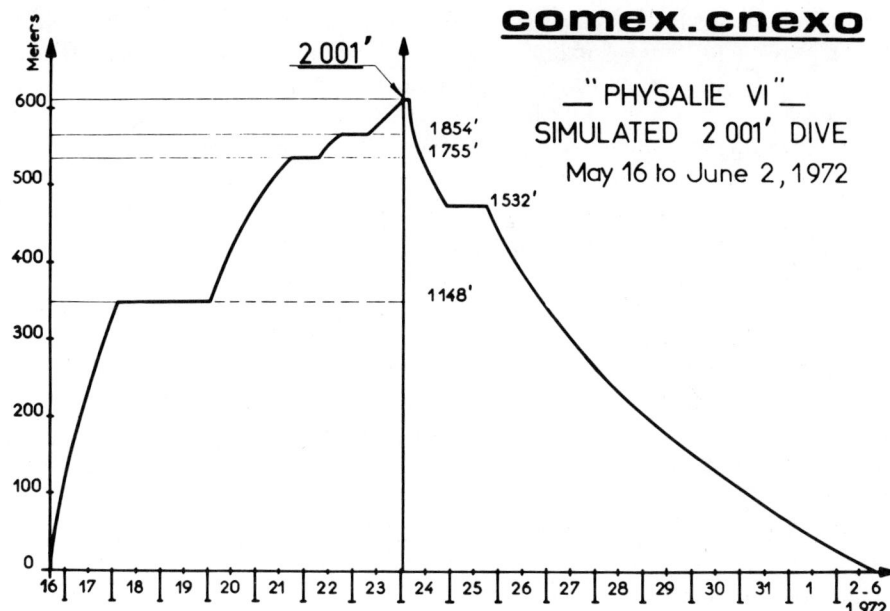

Figure III-20. Dive profile for deepest experimental dive made by COMEX. Note that the rate of compression decreased with depths and stages are used to permit adaptation to HPNS.

meant that 7 days were required to attain this depth. Although there was some decrement in performance, it was considered less than that seen in the earlier 1500-fsw British experiment.

Another dive made by the French laboratory was called Sagittaire IV and involved the divers attaining and staying at 2001 fsw (60.5 ATA) for 50 hr. Again, compression involved stages of 17 hr at 640 fsw (21 ATA), 45 hr at 1280 fsw (41 ATA), 46 hr at 1760 fsw (56 ATA) and 1850 fsw (59 ATA), and a slow exponential rate of compression to 1280 fsw (41 ATA) with a 9-fsw/hr rate from 1280 to 1760 fsw and a 30-fsw/hr rate between 1760 and 1950 fsw. Although the amount of tremor during this dive was less even than in the previous Physalie V dive, it did not decrease during the stages or at maximum depth, where it was very marked. This was believed to be caused by the more rapid rate of compression of 30 fsw/hr in the last phase, which probably caused a 40 to 50% decrement in intellectual performance but a 20% decrement in manual dexterity only.

The French group has characterized the clinical signs of HPNS as tremor, dysmetria, fasciculation, myoclonus, and drowsiness (microsleep). Major EEG modifications are augmentation of theta waves (slow activity), diminution of alpha waves (fast activity), and microsleep. There are also disturbances in the organization of sleep. The group did not notice any disorganization, nausea, or dizziness—symptoms that are probably dependent on compression rate (Naquet et al. 1975; Rostain and Naquet 1974).

They concluded also that the degree of tremor is a function of compression rate. For example, during Physalie V, using rapid compressions between 1120 and 1280 fsw (35 to 40 ATA) and 1500 and 1560 fsw (44 to 50 ATA), tremor reached a level 700%

above normal between 1500 and 1660 fsw (50 to 53 ATA) while during Physalie VI, with compression to 1950 fsw (62 ATA), tremor did not increase more than 250% above the normal level. Tremor persisted as long as the subjects stayed at constant depths, and remained notable even when 100 hr had been spent at 1560 fsw (51 ATA). Tremor disappeared during decompression, and more rapidly at bottom depth if it was not serious.

Classic neurological tests show that dysmetria occurs with the HPNS; it varies in intensity from subject to subject. It can appear at depths as shallow as 960 fsw (31 ATA) during rapid compression but is generally observed below 1280 fsw (41 ATA) and disappears during decompression. Fasciculations and myoclonia are superimposed on the tremor when it reaches high intensity. Fasciculations generally appear before myoclonia; both occur predominantly in the upper limbs, and sometimes, at high pressures, in the face and neck muscles. Onset of these symptoms occurs between 640 and 960 fsw (21 and 31 ATA) during rapid compressions, and below 1600 fsw (51 ATA) for slow compressions. These symptoms regress slightly during prolonged stays at constant depths and disappear during decompression at the same depths at which they appeared during compression.

Drowsiness appears in some subjects left at rest but does not appear consistently in every subject. It is less constant and affects fewer subjects during slow compressions with intermediate stages. Drowsiness persists during extended stays at depth, and usually disappears in the 640 fsw (21 ATA) decompression zone. Other symptoms observed by the French group were nasal congestion, which occurred below 1280 fsw (41 ATA) whether the humidity was above or below 70%, and light sleep, with vivid dreams or nightmares.

In the United States six U.S. Navy divers in 1973 (Spaur 1974) made a dive designed to document the divers' ability to perform useful work in the water using Navy breathing apparatus and procedures. Compression, using standard U.S. Navy compression rates of 40 fsw/hr between 400 and 1000 fsw (13 to 31 ATA), slowing to 30 fsw/hr from 1000 to 1300 fsw (31 to 40 ATA) and to 20 fsw/hr from 1300 to 1600 fsw (40 to 49 ATA), and several stages, required 6 days. The divers spent 7 days at 1600 fsw. They were able to perform light to moderate work at 1600 fsw in the water using the Mark 10 (Mod 4) closed-circuit underwater breathing apparatus. Tests indicated tremor below 1000 fsw (31 ATA). Statometer measurements revealed a marked loss in balancing ability with increasing depth, but vestibular function tests revealed no abnormalities.

The deepest open ocean dive was made in October 1977, when the COMEX group, in conjunction with the French Navy, exceeded the 1975 U.S. Navy depth of 1148 fsw (36 ATA) and conducted pipeline-connecting operations at 460 msw (46.5 ATA) from the dynamically positioned drillship *Petrel* off the southern coast of France. During the dive, called Janus IV, two French Navy divers and four COMEX divers were saturated in two teams of three men each. Compression to 430 msw (47.3 ATA), the saturation depth, took 30 hr, with an additional 30 min for compression to the excursion depth of 460 msw (46.5 ATA). Decompression required 7 days and 18 hr.

Working dives involving 10 hr at 1508 fsw (46.5 ATA) were made by the divers, each of whom performed two excursions to the working depth during the 3 days of saturation at 1410 fsw (47 ATA). On October 20, two 10-min dives were made to 1644 fsw (49 ATA). The experiment proved that men can work as capably at that great depth as at 700 or 1000 fsw (21 to 31 ATA).

The success of Janus IV was ensured by using several strategies that facilitate deep diving with a minimum of HPNS; these techniques range from personnel selection, choice of suitable compression rate, use of stages and excursions, addition of nitrogen (trimix or other narcotic) to the breathing gas, and diver adaptation.

2. Strategies for Amelioration of HPNS

a. Variation in Susceptibility and Personnel Selection

Individual susceptibility to HPNS varies widely. For example, during helium-nitrogen-oxygen research dives at the Duke Medical Center (Bennett et al. 1974) one of the subjects showed marked tremor during each compression phase, another showed no tremor, and one showed moderate tremor. This variability was reflected in their performance (Figure III-21). Subjective symptoms and reactions to such conditions as nausea and dizziness vary among divers.

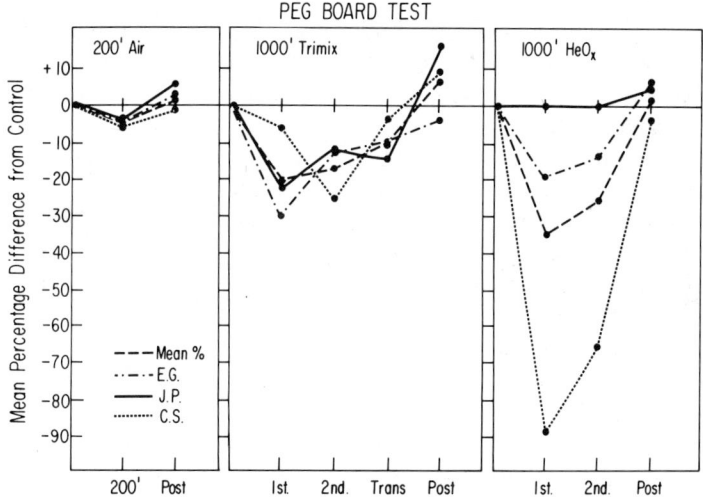

Figure III-21. Mean percentage difference in a psychomotor task from control values in three men exposed to either 200 fsw compressed air, compression to 1000 fsw helium-oxygen or 1000 fsw trimix (i.e., helium-oxygen with 18% nitrogen for 33 min—the same partial pressure of N_2 as in the 200-fsw air dive). Trimix suppresses tremors of HPNS that cause psychomotor decrement in heliox, but with trimix there is still some decrement due to nitrogen narcosis. [From Bennett et al. (1974).]

b. Choice of Compression Rate

The more rapid the rate of compression, the shallower the depth of onset and the more intense the signs and symptoms of HPNS. Slowing the rate of compression is therefore advantageous in reducing HPNS. Various attempts have been made to develop mathematical models to compute an effective compression profile. However, these models have been based on highly speculative hypotheses about the causes of HPNS; at present, it is best to rely on the simple rule that compression should follow a mainly exponential rate, with a slower and slower rate as depth increases. It is also necessary to use compression stages at various points to permit the divers to adapt to the effects of hydrostatic pressure (Figures III-16 and III-20). Compression to very great depths therefore requires a time-depth profile not unlike that of decompression. The optimum rate between given depths or the optimum staging depths or times are not known, but guidelines based on the 100–150 laboratory dives made in the United States, United Kingdom, and France to depths greater than 1000 fsw (31 ATA) can be obtained from the literature (Bennett et al. 1976).

c. Use of Excursions

As in decompression, where sizable excursions can be made from a saturation depth without decompression stops, excursions can be used to ameliorate the signs and symptoms of HPNS. In 1969, Buehlmann and his co-workers (1970) made a 3-day laboratory saturation dive to 1000 fsw (31 ATA) at the RNPL; this dive involved an initial linear compression rate of 16 to 17 fsw/min, and caused some HPNS, nausea, and vertigo with mild tremor, which resolved in 1–2 hr (Table III-3). Excursions of up to 2 hr were later made to 1150 fsw (36 ATA) at a rate of 16 to 17 fsw/min. During the excursion the divers swam underwater wearing semiclosed apparatus and were able to perform heavy work; tests revealed no HPNS symptoms.

During an experimental dive in New London by the U.S. Navy (Proctor et al. 1972; Schaefer et al. 1970), excursions were made from 800 to 1112 fsw (25 to 34 ATA) and 800 to 1050 fsw (25–33 ATA) at the faster rate of 27 and 28 fsw/min. This compression rate caused some weakness and the onset of tremors, but reducing the rate to 17 fsw/min the next day solved these problems. Yet after 24 hr at 1000 to 1100 fsw (31–34 ATA) and at 1300 to 1400 fsw (40–43 ATA), the same rate of compression to 1500 fsw did cause an increase in tremor (Figure III-19) and changes in brain electrical activity (Figure III-17). These differences in compression rate effects may merely have reflected individual variations in susceptibility.

During a collaborative experiment with Oceaneering International, Inc., at Duke University Medical Center (Bachrach and Bennett 1973), six men were compressed over a 2-day period to 870 fsw (27 ATA) using four stages and compression rates declining from 25 fsw/min to 2 fsw/min. During the 4 days at 870 fsw, three of the subjects together made excursions to 1000 fsw (31 ATA) on different days, using rates of 16.7 fsw/min, 50 fsw/min, and 100 fsw/min. During the 2 hr at maximum depth, tests of performance efficiency were made, and one of the divers carried out various tasks under water. No HPNS effects were seen as a result of either the saturation or the excursion (Table III-4).

The COMEX group has used excursion procedures adapted with considerable success from its Ludion experimental dive series and the Janus ocean series, which consisted of three dives (Figure III-22). In 1968 during Janus 1, two men lived for 5 days at 290 fsw (10 ATA) and made 10 dives to the wellhead at 500 fsw (16 ATA). A second team carried out 12 excursions. In February 1970, an additional series of dives was made with saturations at 656 fsw (21 ATA) and excursions to a wellhead at 840 fsw (26 ATA).

Table III-4

Performance Efficiency during Excursion from Saturation at 850 fsw to 1000 fsw at 100 fsw/min

Test	Predive	870 fsw	Time at depth Arrival at 1000 fsw	105 min at 1000 fsw
Ball bearing	15.67 ± 3.79	19.00 ± 2.08	18.33 ± 2.08	18.33 ± 2.08
Peg board	28.67 ± 3.26	32.67 ± 4.73	31.33 ± 4.51	30.00 ± 1.00
Visual analogy	47.00 ± 6.25	49.33 ± 5.51	51.00 ± 7.00	48.33 ± 2.31
Arithmetic	11.00 ± 5.57	8.00 ± 8.89	9.00 ± 7.81	13.33 ± 8.08

Values are number correct ± SD. Data derived from Bachrach and Bennett (1973).

This method permitted two men to work 34 hr in 1 week. The final experiment of the Janus series involved excursions from 1250 fsw (39 ATA) to 1350 fsw (42 ATA).

However, use of the excursion technique is limited by the risk of vestibular decompression sickness or incapacitating HPNS symptoms if too fast a compression is used in a very deep excursion. This risk was illustrated in a British dive to 1500 fsw (46 ATA) in 1970, when a therapeutic recompression was made from 1170 fsw (36 ATA) to 1535 fsw (47 ATA) with short compressions and stages totaling 8.5 hr, and during which the diver experienced confusion and a sense of impending loss of consciousness that required immediate decompression. Surprisingly, during experiments at the University of Pennsylvania in 1975, excursions of 400 fsw (13 ATA) in a period of 20 min were tolerated. The University of Pennsylvania results may possibly be explained by variability in diver susceptibility or differences in the type of depth-time profile used for the whole study, which involved compression to 800 fsw (25 ATA), followed by compression from 800 to 1200 fsw (25–37 ATA) in 50 min, and which produced fatigue, nausea, and vomiting.

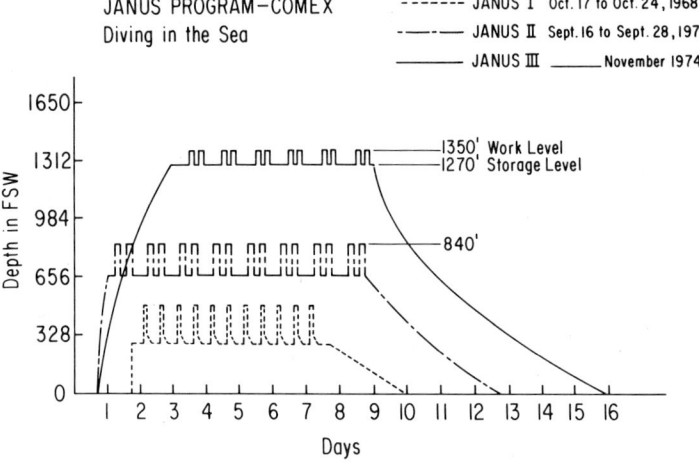

Figure III-22. COMEX excursion dive series in the open sea. The deeper the depth, the shorter the excursion from the saturation storage depth.

The success of excursions as inhibitors of HPNS is apparently related to the total time spent at depths greater than 1000 fsw (31 ATA) before the excursion is made. More work is required to establish the value of excursion diving in preventing HPNS and the relationship of diver adaptation to the success of deep excursion diving.

d. Adaptation

As early as 1965, when quantitative measurements of the performance decrement in divers compressed at 100 fsw/min with heliox to 600 fsw (19 ATA) and 800 fsw (25 ATA) were first made (Bennett 1965; Bennett and Dossett 1967), it was noted that, in contrast to the performance decrement caused by compressed air narcosis, divers developed considerable adaptation to HPNS after spending time at depth. Signs and symptoms of HPNS are at their worst either during compression or immediately upon reaching depth; within 1 to 1.5 hr they decrease markedly. However, this pattern is less noticeable at depths greater than 1500 fsw (46 ATA). For example, in the first dive to 1500 fsw (46 ATA) at the RNPL in 1970, tremors, nausea, and dizziness occurred after each phase of the 3-day compression, which was performed with three 24-hr stages and a compression rate of 16–17 fsw/min (Bennett and Towse 1971a, 1971b). However, the divers recovered rapidly, although it was 20 hr before the electrical activity of their brains returned to normal. Each subsequent compression phase again stimulated the marked rise of slow-wave theta activity (Figure III-17).

Rostain and his COMEX group colleagues noted, however, that during their Physalie VI dive to 2001 fsw (60.5 ATA) for 80 min in 1972, which involved a compression of 7.3 days and three stages [46 hr at 1150 fsw (40 ATA) and 14 hr each at 1765 fsw (54 ATA) and 1855 fsw (57 ATA)], the tremor did not decrease during the stages or the bottom stay. Similarly, during their Sagittaire IV dive in 1974 to 2001 fsw (60.5 ATA) for 50 hr after a compression with one stage of 17 hr at 658 fsw (20 ATA) and three stages each of 45 hr, and a slower compression rate than was used during Physalie VI, there was no appreciable adaptation to tremor. In fact, after 4 days at 1640 fsw (51 ATA), the tremor was still noticeable, disappearing only during decompression. In the Sagittaire IV dive, jerkiness did, however, show some adaptation. Fatigue and drowsiness persisted during the extended stays at depth, and sometimes even into the decompression period.

Thus, although adaptation may not occur for all signs and symptoms of HPNS at all depths, it is probably advantageous for divers involved in dives between 1000 fsw (31 ATA) and 1500 fsw (46 ATA) to rest in the personnel transfer capsule or deck decompression chamber for the first hour or more before entering the water to work. However, modifying the rate of compression may be equally effective in controlling or reducing symptoms.

e. Use of Narcotic Agents

In Russia in 1961, Zaltsman reported that helium (pressure) exerted a so-called antagonism on the narcotic effect of nitrogen (Zaltsman 1961). This effect was observed during dives to 527 fsw (16 ATA) using air-helium mixtures and a maximum nitrogen partial pressure of 4.5 ATA. Under these conditions, divers could perform heavy work $(221–580 \text{ kg} \cdot \text{m}^{-2} \cdot \text{min}^{-1})$ with few or no tremors or signs of HPNS and no thermal balance or voice distortion problems. What Zaltsman was in fact doing was reproducing in humans a study conducted by Johnson and Flagler (1950), which showed that tadpoles would fall to the bottom of a tank of water after ethyl alcohol was added to the water but that increasing the hydrostatic pressure nullified the effect of the alcohol and permitted the tadpoles to return to normal behavior.

Brauer and co-workers (1974) and Lever et al. (1971) also noted that in a variety of animals, adding anesthetic agents to the helium-oxygen atmosphere ameliorated or prevented HPNS.

The F. G. Hall Laboratory for Environmental Research at Duke University has studied the value of using trimix (O_2-He-N_2) as the breathing gas in ameliorating HPNS. In 1973, four divers from the Harbor Branch Foundation and Oceaneering International were compressed in 20 min to 720 fsw (22 ATA) on a breathing mixture of 25% N_2, 0.5 ATA O_2, and the remainder helium. The same divers were exposed also to 1000 fsw (31 ATA) in 33 min with 18% N_2 (i.e., in both cases 5.6 ATA of nitrogen), to 1000 fsw breathing only helium-oxygen, and to 200 fsw (6 ATA) breathing compressed air (equivalent to the same 5.6 ATA of N_2). These procedures allowed the effects of trimix and heliox on HPNS to be compared and also permitted any nitrogen narcosis to be observed (Bennett et al. 1974).

The diver-subjects took a battery of neurophysiological and performance tests. Two of the subjects were HPNS sensitive and preferred to have nitrogen in their mixtures. The 1000-fsw He-O_2 dive had to be aborted 10 min early because one of these subjects suffered severe HPNS. The other two subjects reported that nitrogen narcosis on the He-O_2-N_2 dive reduced their efficiency (Figure III-23). However, nitrogen did effectively prevent tremor and nausea (Figure III-24).

Additional studies were made during 1974 when five divers from Oceaneering International and Duke University were compressed to 1000 fsw (31 ATA) for 2 hr breathing 10% N_2 (3.2 ATA N_2) (Bennett et al. 1975). The 33-min compression profile was modified to provide an increasingly slower descent beginning with 60 fsw/min and

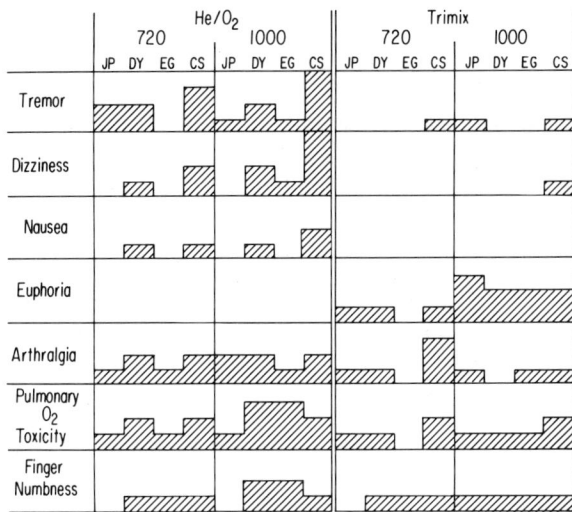

Figure III-23. Subjective sensations of four divers during exposure to helium-oxygen or trimix (He-N_2-O_2) at 720 fsw with trimix (N_2 was 25% at 720 fsw and 18% at 1000 fsw). Variation in susceptibility of divers to HPNS and efficacy of narcotic nitrogen in suppressing the signs and symptoms of HPNS are indicated. [From Bennett et al. (1974).]

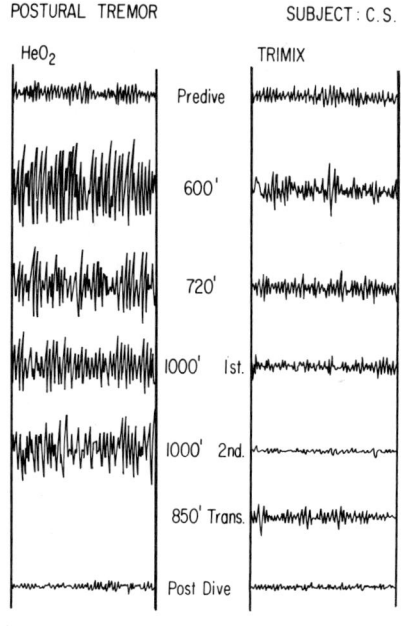

Figure III-24. Changes in finger tremor measurements of one diver exposed to helium-oxygen and another exposed to trimix (18% N_2) during 33-min compression to 1000 fsw. Nitrogen was added at 600 fsw when tremor was beginning to increase. Removing nitrogen at 850 fsw results in return of tremors. [From Bennett et al. (1974).]

from 700 to 1000 fsw (22–31 ATA) a rate of 20 fsw/min and three short stages were used. One of the divers worked at bolting two flanges together for 44 min in cold water (56°F). Performance tests indicated no narcosis and few or no signs of HPNS (Figure III-25). However, the "wet" diver did experience some euphoria. The COMEX group, which studied trimix in its experimental CORAZ dive series, also reported euphoria when a 9% N_2 mixture was used.

In 1976, K. D. Marine (A. Krasberg, personal communication) used a similar compression profile in a 35-min compression to 1000 fsw (31 ATA), using a breathing mixture of only 6.4% N_2 augmented by 1.5 ounces of 70-proof British scotch whiskey; the philosophy behind this technique was that as the alcohol is metabolized and its effect decreases the diver would be adapting to HPNS and would not need as much N_2. During a 44-min period performing a typical oilfield task, one of these subjects, who had apparently not consumed more than half the alcohol, did have mild tremors. However, although alcohol may be effective, it should be used with care because hangover effects could cause performance decrements and other problems.

In 1976, a team from the Harbor Branch Foundation, Oceaneering International, and Duke University's F. G. Hall Laboratory carried out a series of experiments in the chambers at the University and at RNPL to study trimix at depths greater than 1000 fsw (31 ATA). Two dives were made to 1000 fsw with 10% N_2 in the helium-oxygen mixture, primarily to test decompression procedure modifications involving the use of 0.6 ATA of O_2, which necessitated increasing the decompression period from 4 to 5 days.

The compression to 1312 fsw (48 ATA) made by two Oceaneering divers was accomplished in 100 min using only 6% N_2, 0.5 ATA O_2, and the remainder helium. Nitrogen was reduced to 6% to lessen the narcotic effects seen when 10% N_2 is used at this depth. The divers experienced some dizziness, lightheadedness, nausea, and HPNS

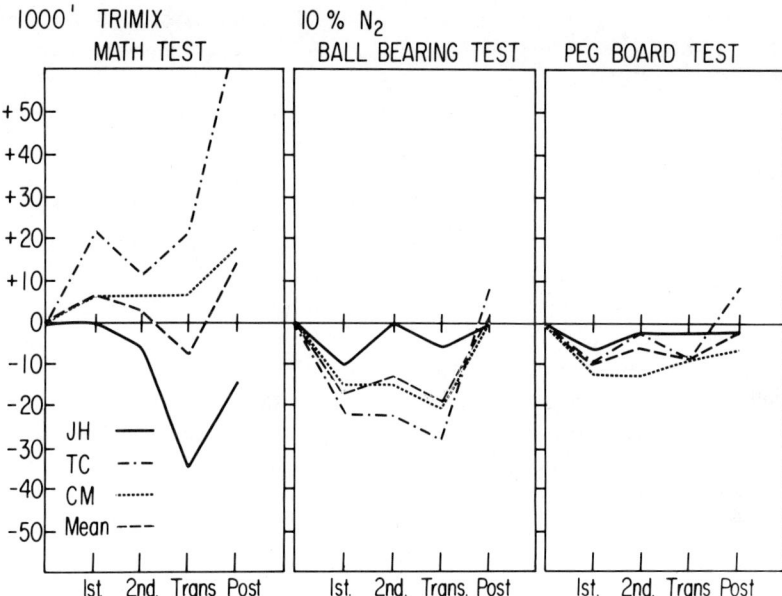

Figure III-25. Percentage change in test results of three subjects compressed to 1000 fsw in 33 min breathing trimix (10% N_2). First test period refers to arrival at 1000 fsw and second 100 min later. *Trans* means transfer to helium-oxygen only. [From Bennett et al. (1975).]

tremors, and appeared fatigued but reported that they could function and would have been able to work in the water if the dive had been in the open sea. However, it was clear that they would have been in better condition had a slower compression and a 10% nitrogen mixture been used. During compression to the 1600 fsw (49 ATA) depth a week after the successful 6-day decompression from 1312 fsw (41 ATA), a slower compression rate that took 150 min rather than 100 min was used. At the 30-min stage at 1312 fsw the divers were in better condition than on the previous dive, with only mild dizziness; the divers reported feeling fit and confident. Compression from the 1312 fsw (41 ATA) stage to 1600 fsw (49 ATA) was planned at 3 fsw/min, for a total travel time of 92 min. However, at 1521 fsw (46 ATA), the dive was aborted because of tremors, dizziness, nausea, sleepiness, and fatigue. Although these symptoms would have decreased with time, it was evident that the 5% to 6% N_2 and the slower rate, although more effective for exposures to 1312 fsw (41 ATA), were not sufficient to protect against HPNS at the deeper depth. It is possible that a mixture including 10% nitrogen would have suppressed many of these symptoms; whether nitrogen narcosis would have occurred, adding to the fatigue and sleepiness, was the subject of later research.

Thus in 1979 a series of dives were planned at Duke termed Atlantis which had two main objectives. One was to establish the relationship between the nitrogen percentage to be added to heliox and the rate of compression to control the HPNS. The second was to determine the effects of inspired gas density, hydrostatic pressure, and narcosis on various respiratory and circulatory parameters such as the often reported dyspnea. Only one factor, either the nitrogen percentage or the compression rate, was to be changed per dive—from either 5% or 10% nitrogen and 12 hr 20 min or 24 hr 40 min to 1509 fsw (46.6 ATA), respectively. Additional studies included reflexes, hematology, sleep, EEG, and clinical neuropsychological investigations.

The first two dives in 1979 and 1980 utilized the same compression rate of 12 hr 20 min to 1509 fsw (460 m), but with 5% trimix in Atlantis I and 10% trimix in Atlantis II and two of the subjects in the dives the same and one different (Bennett et al. 1981).

For Atlantis I the especially rapid compression (the previous fastest rate to this depth was three times slower) of 12 hr 20 min was expected to cause HPNS as was the case. One subject vomited during compression and another exhibited fatigue and lapses of consciousness (the French microsleep). However the three divers were able to function very well by the second day of the dive. This was in spite of decrements in the tests of performance ability; these results seemed mainly because the divers were working more slowly than previously, for all tests were completed satisfactorily, including the very complex pulmonary function measurements, arterial catheterization and blood gas sampling and analysis. Work-limiting dyspnea (a sense of air hunger or breathing through a straw) was present during moderate exercise, but the arterial blood gases were within normal limits. Indeed, the dyspnea seemed worse when the subjects were required to breathe helium-oxygen alone rather than trimix, suggesting it may be another part of HPNS mediated centrally.

Atlantis II in March 1980 was planned also to 1509 fsw (46.6 ATA) and utilized two of the same divers and one new one, but with 10% nitrogen rather than the 5% of Atlantis I. This proved very successful in controlling the debilitating effects of HPNS and after 6 days at 1509 fsw the dive was extended to 2132 fsw (65.5 ATA) by compression with helium producing a 7.8% nitrogen mixture at a depth deeper than man had ever been previously. In October 1980 the British Admiralty Marine Technology Establishment (AMTE) made a dive to 2165 fsw (66.5 ATA) with 10% trimix but with an especially rapid compression from 1378 fsw (42.6 ATA) that resulted in the two divers being incapacitated during 37 hr at 2165 fsw. This illustrated that even with trimix there is an optimal compression rate to prevent HPNS.

In Atlantis II, however, during the 24-hr stay at 2132 fsw the subjects between them clearly demonstrated that it is possible to lead a normal existence without nausea, dizziness, vomiting, somnolence, undue tremors, or myoclonic jerking, to carry out complicated tasks requiring fine manual dexterity such as venepunctures, and to do moderately heavy work on a bicycle ergometer without undue distress. However, the performance tests indicated the same decrement in efficiency as for Atlantis I and there was reason to believe from other French and British dives (described earlier) that much of this was due to the especially rapid compression.

Atlantis III therefore was planned and took place from January to March 1981 with direct compression of three divers over a period of 7 days to 2132 fsw (65.5 ATA) using a rate of compression twice as slow as for Atlantis II in 1980 (Bennett et al. 1982). Compression was with 10% nitrogen in helium-oxygen (10% Trimix) throughout and the duration at 2132 fsw was 4 days to permit, as at 1509 fsw (46.6 ATA) in Atlantis II, a full series of tests of psychological and neurophysiological performance and lung function and arterial blood gases in the resting and working diver. After the 4 days the divers were compressed further to 2250 fsw (69 ATA), where they spent 24 hr and carried out additional tests before beginning the long decompression (Figure III-26).

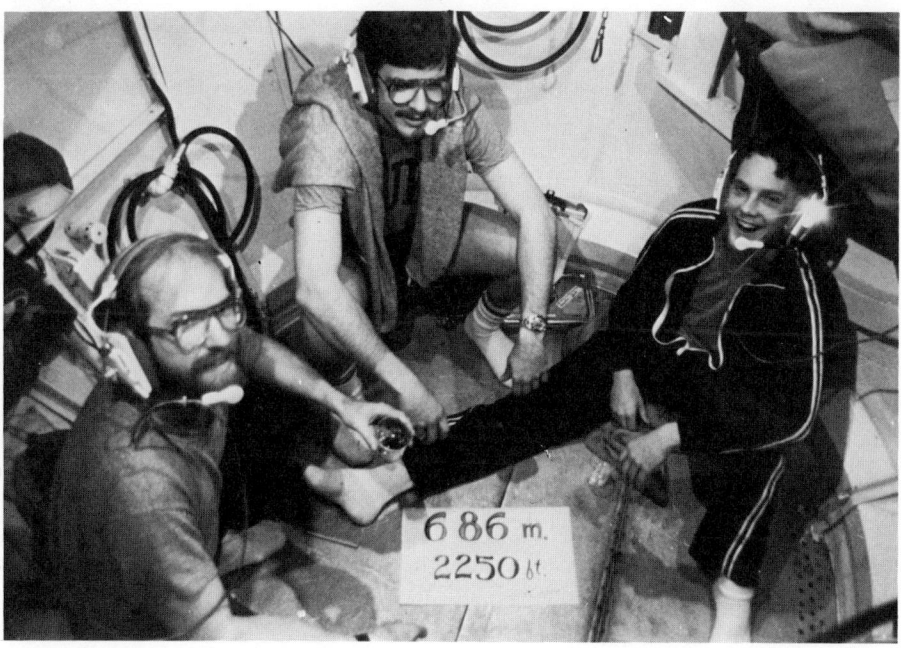

Figure III-26. The three divers of Atlantis III arrive at a depth of 2250 fsw in a fit and competent condition.

During Atlantis III the divers broke both depth and duration records and in fact were 11 days at depths greater than 2000 fsw (61.5 ATA), 7 days deeper than 2132 fsw (65.5 ATA), and 1 day at 2250 fsw (69 ATA) compared to the Atlantis II in which only 1 day was spent at 2132 fsw. The trimix, as with Atlantis II, was very effective in preventing the debilitating signs and symptoms of HPNS. Lung function studies showed that very hard work was possible at these pressures, one of the three divers carrying out 240 W of work on a bicycle ergometer for 5 min (classified as maximal hard work) and yet his arterial blood gases showed only 53 mmHg carbon dioxide, which is equivalent to that expected on the surface. The divers did not experience dyspnea or breathlessness (probably due to the 10% nitrogen rather than the 7.8% of Atlantis II) but stopped work at the higher work loads because of muscular irregularities.

One of the three divers appeared to get less control of HPNS by the nitrogen than the others, with some mild increase in hand tremors with depth and mild increase in the slow waves of the electrical activity of his brain. However, the deeper the dive the better he became. The larger performance decrements of 40%–50% on the first day at 1509 fsw (46.6 ATA) due to rapid compression seen in Atlantis I and II were not seen with the slower compression of Atlantis III, but the tests still showed much the same decrement in performance as for Atlantis I and II for a given depth, regardless of nitrogen percentage or rate of compression. This decrement for most tests was 15%–20% and was at its maximum at 1165 fsw (36 ATA) and encouragingly no worse at 2250 fsw (69 ATA). There did appear to be slight difficulty with concentration at 2250 fsw that was identified by a greater decrement in arithmetic ability than the other tests. This improved with time at maximum depth. That divers did not sleep as effectively as usual could also have added to the problem. In general, however, the divers were in a fit condition and able to perform satisfactorily all the many tasks and research operations required of them, and all of the planned scientific data were obtained. None of the adverse effects noted in the 1980 British dive were seen, which seems to confirm that these were due to too rapid a compression with trimix.

During the decompression two mild bends resulted, one at 1733 fsw (53.5 ATA) and one at 1690 fsw (52 ATA). These responded well to recompression and oxygen therapy; slow removal of the nitrogen from the trimix from this point to 5% at 1500 fsw (46 ATA) and 0% at 1000 fsw (31 ATA) resulted in no further problems.

Atlantis IV took place in October 1982 and utilized virtually the same compression profile as Atlantis III but with 5% rather than 10% nitrogen in heliox. The performance data in Atlantis III (Bennett et al. 1982) indicated that the decrements at depths greater than 1870 fsw (57.5 ATA) of 30% to 40% were because the nitrogen was too high. The results of Atlantis IV confirmed this and indicated that decrements of only some 10% were seen initially, which returned to control values at 1968 fsw (60.6 ATA) during the decompression. Dyspnea was seen during exercise at 2132 fsw (65.5 ATA) as was seen also in Atlantis I, again with 5% trimix. This was not seen to any similar extent when the nitrogen was 10%. This appears to confirm that the dyspnea is probably mediated centrally through the brain as another sign of the HPNS.

Other studies with trimix also were made in the early 1980s in Norway at 985 fsw (31 ATA) and 1642 fsw (50.6 ATA) (Peterson et al. 1982; Vaernes et al. 1982) and in France at 1511 fsw (46.7 ATA) (Rostain et al. 1982); these have clarified the value of adding nitrogen to heliox in controlling HPNS, but they emphasized also the importance of a slow compression rate and careful selection of the divers.

It is not possible to consider all the rapidly increasing amount of data concerning HPNS here but further information can be obtained elsewhere (Bennett 1982). In conclusion, although the mechanism of HPNS is not known, increased hydrostatic pressure does appear to be a primary factor. Despite the failure to understand the underlying mechanisms of HPNS, however, much has been learned through laboratory experiments that has enabled the depths to which man may be exposed to be extended steadily. In 1903, the limiting depth for deep diving was believed to be 200 fsw (6 ATA); 80 years later, it is more than ten times as great. There are people today, as in 1903, who maintain that we have now reached the limits of human diving. However, since these "limits" have been broken consistently in the past, there is no reason to believe that careful research will not continue to extend the depths attainable by human divers.

PETER B. BENNETT

References

BACHRACH, A. J., AND P. B. BENNETT 1973. Tremor in diving. *Aerosp. Med.* 44: 613–623.
BENNETT, P. B. 1965. Psychometric impairment in men breathing oxygen-helium at increased pressures. Underwater Physiology Rep. 251. U.K. Medical Research Council, Royal Naval Personnel Research Committee.

BENNETT, P. B. 1967. Performance impairment in deep diving due to nitrogen, helium, neon and oxygen. In: *Underwater Physiology III. Proceedings of the Third Symposium on Underwater Physiology*, edited by C. J. Lambertsen. Baltimore: Williams & Wilkins.
BENNETT, P. B. 1975. The high pressure nervous syndrome: man. In: *The Physiology and Medicine of Diving and Compressed Air Work*, edited by P. B. Bennett and D. H. Elliott. London: Baillière, Tyndall.
BENNETT, P. B. 1982. The high pressure nervous syndrome. In: *The Physiology and Medicine of Diving and Compressed Air Work* (3rd ed.) edited by P. B. Bennett and D. H. Elliott. London: Baillière Tyndall, p. 262–296.
BENNETT, P. B., AND A. N. DOSSETT 1967. Undesirable effects of oxygen-helium breathing at great depths. Underwater Physiology Sub-committee Rep. 260, U.K. Medical Research Council, Royal Naval Personnel Research Committee.
BENNETT, P. B., AND S. P. GRAY 1971. Changes in human urine and blood chemistry during a simulated oxygen-helium dive to 1500 ft. *Aerosp. Med.* 42: 868–874.
BENNETT, P. B., AND E. J. TOWSE 1971a. Performance efficiency of men breathing oxygen-helium at great depths between 100 ft and 1500 ft. *Aerosp. Med.* 42: 1147–1156.
BENNETT, P. B., AND E. J. TOWSE 1971b. The high pressure nervous syndrome during a simulated oxygen-helium dive to 1500 ft. *EEG Clin. Neurophysiol.* 31: 383–393.
BENNETT, P. B., A. BACHRACH, R. BRAUER, J. ROSTAIN, AND L. RAYMOND 1976. The high pressure nervous syndrome. In: *National Plan for the Safety and Health of Divers in Their Quest for Subsea Energy*, edited by M. W. Beckett. Bethesda, MD: Undersea Medical Society.
BENNETT, P. B., G. D. BLENKARN, J. ROBY, AND D. YOUNGBLOOD 1974. Suppression of the high pressure nervous syndrome in human deep dives by He-N_2-O_2. *Undersea Biomed. Res.* 1: 221–237.
BENNETT, P. B., R. COGGIN, AND M. MCLEOD 1982. Effect of compression rate on use of trimix to ameliorate HPNS in man to 686 m (2251 ft). *Undersea Biomed. Res.* 9: 335–351.
BENNETT, P. B., R. COGGIN, AND J. ROBY 1981. Control of HPNS in humans during rapid compression with trimix to 650 m (2132 ft). *Undersea Biomed. Res.* 8: 85–100.
BENNETT, P. B., J. ROBY, S. SIMON, AND D. YOUNGBLOOD 1975. Optimal use of nitrogen to suppress the high pressure nervous syndrome. *Aviat. Space Environ. Med.* 46: 37–40.
BRAUER, R. W., M. R. JORDAN, AND R. O. WAY 1968. Modification of the convulsive seizure phase of the high pressure excitability syndrome in mice. *Fed. Proc.* 27: 284.
BRAUER, R. W., S. M. GOLDMAN, R. W. BEAVER, AND M. E. SHEEHAN 1974. N_2, H_2 and N_2O antagonism of high pressure neurological syndrome in mice. *Undersea Biomed. Res.* 1: 59–72.
BUEHLMANN, A. A., H. MATTHYS, G. OVERRATH, P. B. BENNETT, D. H. ELLIOTT, AND S. P. GRAY 1970. Saturation exposures of 31 ATA in an oxygen-helium atmosphere with excursions to 36 ATA. *Aerosp. Med.* 41: 394–402.
FRUCTUS, X. R. 1972. Down below the great depths. In: *Proceedings of the Third International Conference on Hyperbaric and Underwater Physiology*. Paris: Doin.
HAMILTON, R. W., J. B. MACINNIS, A. D. NOBLE, AND H. R. SCHREINER 1967. Saturation diving at 650 feet. Tech. Memo. B1411. Tonawanda, NY: Ocean Systems, Inc.
HUNTER, W. L., AND P. B. BENNETT 1974. The causes, mechanisms and prevention of the high pressure nervous syndrome. *Undersea Biomed Res.* 1: 1–28.
JOHNSON, F. H., AND E. A. FLAGLER 1950. Hydrostatic pressure reversal of narcosis in tadpoles. *Science* 112: 91–92.
LEVER, M. J., K. W. MILLER, W. D. M. PATON, AND E. B. SMITH 1971. Pressure reversal in anaesthesia. *Nature* 231: 371–386.
NAQUET, R., J. C. ROSTAIN, AND X. FRUCTUS 1975. High pressure nervous syndrome: Clinical and electro-physiological studies in man. In: *Strategy for Future Diving to Depths Greater Than 1000 ft*. Bethesda, MD: Undersea Medical Society. (Workshop Rep. WS G-15-75.)
PETERSON, R. E., P. B. BENNETT, R. VAERNES, A. P. DICK, AND S. TONJUM 1982. Testing of compression strategies for diving to 500 msw. *Undersea Biomed. Res. Suppl.* 9: 21.
PROCTOR, L. D., C. R. CAREY, R. M. LEE, K. E. SCHAEFER, AND H. VAN DEN ENDE 1972. Electroencephalographic changes during saturation excursion dives to a simulated sea water depth of 1000 ft. *Aerosp. Med.* 43: 867–877.
ROSTAIN, J. C., AND R. NAQUET 1974. Le syndrome nerveux des hautes pressions: caracteristiques et evolution en fonction de divers modes de compression. *Rev. Electroencephalogr. Neurophysiol.* 4: 107–124.

ROSTAIN, J. C., C. LEMAIRE. AND R. NAQUET 1982. HPNS in man during a 12 day stay at 450 m in He-N$_2$-O$_2$ breathing mixture. *Undersea Biomed. Res. Suppl.* 9: 22.

SCHAEFER, K. E., C. R. CAREY, AND J. DOUGHERTY 1970. Pulmonary gas exchange and urinary electrolyte excretion during saturation-excursion diving to pressures equivalent to 800 and 1000 ft of seawater. *Aerosp. Med.* 41: 856–864.

SPAUR, W. H. 1974. 1600-ft Dive. In: *The Working Diver 1974*. Washington, DC: Marine Technology Society.

SUMMITT, J. K., J. S. KELLEY, J. M. HERRON, AND H. A. SALTZMAN 1969. Joint U.S. Navy-Duke University 1000 ft saturation dive. Rep. 3-69. Washington, DC: U.S. Navy Experimental Diving Unit.

VAERNES, R., P. B. BENNETT, D. HAMMERBORG, B. ELLERTSEN, R. E. PETERSON, AND S. TONJUM 1982. Central nervous system reactions during heliox and trimix dives to 31 ATA. *Undersea Biomed. Res.* 9: 1–14.

ZALTSMAN, G. L. 1961. Physiological principles of a sojourn of a human in conditions of raised pressures of the gaseous medium. (Eng. transl. Wright-Patterson AFB, OH, 1967.)

ZALTSMAN, G. L. 1968. *Hyperbaric Epilepsy and Narcosis (Neurophysiological Studies)*. Leningrad: Sechenov Institute of Evolutionary Physiology and Biochemistry, USSR Acad. Sci.

E. Inert Gas Narcosis

The inert gases include those gases that are believed to exert their biological effects without changing their own chemical structure or modifying the chemical structure of other substances. The general term includes such gases as nitrous oxide, ethylene, and cyclopropane, as well as nitrogen, helium, argon, neon, krypton, and xenon. Although several of these gases are not anesthetic at pressures of less than 1 atm, all except helium and neon have been shown to produce narcotic effects at elevated pressures (Featherstone and Muehlbaecher 1963). Interest has focused particularly on the effects of nitrogen in hyperbaric atmospheres because it both impairs the functioning of divers in diving operations and has potential clinical applications.

1. Nitrogen Narcosis

When men were first exposed to hyperbaric atmospheres, they did not expect the narcotic effects of nitrogen. For more than a century the origin of the impaired performance of workers in compressed air remained obscure, although the effects were manifest. In the older literature dealing with caisson (compressed air) operations, workmen were reported to sing spontaneously, and the prevailing mood in the compressed air atmosphere was described as euphoric. The expansive feeling experienced by scuba divers at pressure has been described euphemistically as "rapture of the depths."

During the course of arduous diving operations in 1927 to salvage gold from the *Laurentic*, which had been sunk to a depth of 132 fsw during World War I, Captain Damant, who was in charge of diving operations, reported the following observations: "One unexpected and rather awkward finding was that, though all of the divers were picked men and had been put through a specially searching medical examination, some of them became abnormal mentally (or emotionally as Sir Leonard Hill put it) whilst under this high pressure, and on their return to the surface could remember nothing of what they had been doing before they began to ascend. This effect might be attributed to the high partial pressure of oxygen in pure air when breathed at 130 lb, or to impurities in the air which was actually supplied to the divers, but Sir Leonard Hill has made tests on the same men which satisfy him that neither oxygen nor carbon dioxide is responsible. It seems to be an extreme case of the subtle change in character and behaviour which comes over some men at less high air pressures and is well known to experienced diving officers'' (Damant 1930).

In 1932, during the course of dives to depths in excess of 300 fsw, divers had difficulty in assimilating facts and in making quick decisions; their symptoms were summarized as "a slowing of the process of cerebration" (Hill and Phillips 1932). In addition to severe emotional disturbances, loss of consciousness was reported. The origin of the impairments was not discerned.

During the early 1930s, Behnke and co-workers (1935) conducted laboratory tests that required dexterity in the large, well-illuminated chamber at the Harvard School of Public Health. They found that compressed air at a pressure of 3 to 4 ATA was associated with euphoria, retardation of higher mental processes, and impaired neuromuscular coordination. Errors were made in recording data and making arithmetic calculations, and fine hand manipulative movements were impaired. Increased effort ("subjective re-enforcement") tended to counteract these aberrations, but at 10 ATA, the signs and symptoms amounted to incipient stupefaction that severely retarded task performance. The untoward effects were best described by the general term *narcosis*. Attention focused on the similarity between the molar concentration of nitrogen at pressures in excess of 10 ATA and the concentration of ethyl ether in the blood under conditions of light anesthesia. The relatively high solubility of nitrogen in lipids accorded with a tenet of the Meyer-Overton hypothesis, namely, that there is a parallel between the affinity of an aliphatic anesthetic for lipid and its narcotic potency. Table III-5 displays the relative solubilities and various effects of several of the inert gases.

In the course of rescue attempts made after the sinking of the *U.S.S. Squalus* in 1939, two experienced divers were incapacitated by the symptoms of nitrogen narcosis. These divers, who were breathing compressed air at a depth of 240 fsw, reported having difficulty thinking clearly, and one diver apparently lost consciousness (Behnke 1945).

Other symptoms of nitrogen narcosis resemble those of ethanol intoxication and include slurred speech, incoordination, and sagittal and lateral body sway. A recent article

Table III-5
Relative Solubilities of Inert Gases and Inert Gas Anesthetic Potencies

	Relative solubility*		Pressures in ATA, required to produce:		
Gas	In benzene, 25°C	In olive oil, 37°C	Loss of righting reflex,* in 50% of mice	Protection against electroshock,** in 50% of mice	Protection against radiosensitivity,† bean seedlings
Helium	1.0	1.0	190	163	55
Neon	1.41	1.29	110	—	—
Hydrogen	3.31	3.35	85	—	—
Nitrogen	5.67	4.47	35	18	12.5
Argon	11.24	8.82	24	12.6	2.0
Krypton	35.0	28.8	3.9	1.8	2.0
Nitrous oxide	172.0	94.1	1.5	0.58	—

*Data derived from Smith (1969). **From Carpenter (1954). †From Ebert et al. (1958).

(Jones et al. 1979) reported that the ingestion of ethanol potentiates the nitrogen-induced body sway observed in elevated air atmospheres. Physicians who have performed cardiac surgery in a hyperbaric chamber have reported that the narcotic effects of nitrogen may interfere with the surgeon's ability to make judgments, especially in situations involving surgical emergencies.

The narcotic effects of the nitrogen component of compressed air have had important consequences for the development of human diving, including the search, which continues today, for inert gases to serve as oxygen diluents in breathing gas mixtures at depths below 150–200 fsw.

2. Other Gases and Narcosis

a. Argon

Inhaling argon with a normal concentration of oxygen at 10 ATA (330 fsw) causes an even greater stupefaction than breathing compressed air at the same pressure (Behnke and Yarbrough 1939). Its narcotic properties and density make it inappropriate for use as a breathing gas. Argon is between two and four times as narcotic as nitrogen; for example, when divers are breathing an argon-oxygen mixture, their performance on visual tasks is severely impaired at pressures less than half as great as those causing an equivalent impairment during nitrogen breathing (Ackles and Fowler 1971).

b. Xenon

Xenon produces anesthesia in human beings at pressures as low as 1 ATA (33 fsw) (Cullen and Gross 1951). The history of xenon is unique in that much of the early work with this gas was performed on man (Featherstone and Muehlbaecher 1963). Xenon has much greater narcotic effects than nitrogen and has only been used in research on breathing mixtures.

c. Helium

Helium is colorless and odorless and is the lightest of the rare gases (molecular weight 4.002). It is monatomic and devoid of chemical activity except under the influence of electron bombardment, which causes it to combine with tungsten, iodine, and other substances. Helium is currently the diluent gas of choice for all breathing gas mixtures used to supply divers diving to depths deeper than 150 fsw (5 ATA). It does not produce narcosis, even at depths of 2000 fsw (61.6 ATA). Helium's only disadvantages as a breathing gas are that it distorts the speech of divers breathing it, and also causes rapid heat loss from their bodies (or overheating at temperatures higher than 33°C to 35°C (approximately 94°F) because of its conductivity, which is six times greater than that of nitrogen.

d. Neon

Studies comparing the usefulness of neon as a breathing gas diluent with nitrogen and helium have shown that neon can be breathed at 200 fsw (37 ATA) without narcotic effects (Hamilton and Kenyon 1976). Voice communication is less distorted by neon than by helium, and the amount of heat lost to the water is apparently less than that with helium. Neon's disadvantages as a breathing gas include high cost and increased breathing resistance at moderate or heavy work loads (Shilling et al. 1976).

e. Hydrogen

Hydrogen, although not one of the inert gases, was used as an experimental breathing gas as early as 1914, and systematic investigations were carried out in 1941 (Case and Haldane 1941). The explosiveness of hydrogen is its principal disadvantage, but it can be used as a breathing gas diluent if the oxygen concentration in the mixture is maintained below 4%. In addition, preliminary research sponsored by the Office of Naval Research and the Bureau of Medicine and Surgery (Projects Hydrox I and II) revealed that hydrogen can be used in the diving range from 400 to 1000 fsw (Edel 1976). The use of a hydrogen-oxygen breathing mixture (rather than helium-oxygen) for decompressions after saturation dives would apparently increase decompression times by about 33% (Edel 1976). However, hydrogen has two important advantages as a breathing gas: it is available without limit, and it produces less breathing resistance at depth than other gases (Edel 1976).

3. Quantification of Narcotic Effects

Shilling and Willgrube (1937) provided the first quantitative evidence of the narcotic properties of compressed air using psychometric tests on 46 men breathing air at pressures between 3.7 and 10 ATA. The results of the arithmetic and cancellation tests found by these investigators have been repeatedly confirmed. Kiessling and Maag (1962), using sophisticated techniques, showed that at the relatively low pressure of 4 ATA (132 fsw) there were performance decrements of 33% in reasoning ability, 21% in reaction time, and 8% in manual dexterity. The length of time spent at pressure did not significantly affect the degree of narcosis.

The statometer tests of Adolphson et al. (1972) are of special significance with reference to the importance of lateral and sagittal body sway in the evaluation of the narcotic effects of gases. In tests to 10 ATA (330 fsw) these investigators found a quadratic relationship between deterioration in balance and increasing depth. At 10 ATA (330 fsw) the amplitude of body sway was doubled. The elevated carbon dioxide tension in the lungs produced a synergistic effect with nitrogen.

In the wet environment, Adolphson (1967) reported that submersion made it more difficult for divers to perform tasks but did not affect the primary impairment induced by nitrogen at high pressures. "Although at 10 ATA the psychomotor functions were in most cases markedly reduced, only slight behavioural changes were observed. At 13 ATA the behavioural changes were strongly accentuated, however, and the majority of subjects showed a behavioural pattern entirely different from normal. In several cases, psychotic and alcoholic-like symptoms appeared" (Adolphson 1967). The parallel between the effects of nitrogen narcosis and alcoholic intoxication has been confirmed (Jones et al. 1979).

a. Rapid Compression Effects

Normally, rapid compression and carbon dioxide retention combine to potentiate nitrogen narcosis. However, if the time at depth is too short to permit the critical concentration of nitrogen to affect the brain, narcosis does not occur. Compressing divers to 13 ATA (400 fsw) and 16 ATA (500 fsw) in 20 sec, followed 40 sec later by decompression, caused only a 15% decrease in two-choice reaction times at 16 ATA and no significant decrement at 13 ATA (Bennett 1975).

b. Carbon Dioxide Effects

Although some investigators believe carbon dioxide to be the primary cause of narcosis, this hypothesis has been disproved. Nevertheless, carbon dioxide substantially augments the impairment caused by nitrogen at high pressures. The physiological cause of this synergism is the dilatation of cerebral blood vessels, accompanied by accelerated cerebral blood flow, in response to elevated pulmonary carbon dioxide tensions. The effect of any neuroactive gas in the lungs is markedly augmented by increasing carbon dioxide tensions.

c. Individual Differences in Narcotic Response

Studies of the narcotic action of inert gases have shown that there are large differences in the range of individual responses. It is therefore difficult to establish a regular pattern or sequence of symptoms and signs that will apply to a randomly selected group of individuals. Of greater significance, perhaps, is the fact that all of the neuromuscular and behavioral aberrations attributed to nitrogen narcosis are reversed when the pressure is reduced, and residual impairments have not been reported.

4. *Mechanisms of Action Underlying Inert Gas Narcosis*

At present, it is still only possible to develop hypotheses about the mechanisms of action responsible for producing inert gas narcosis, despite the number and importance of recent studies in anesthesia research. In general, the narcotic potency of inert gases correlates with various physical properties of the gases, such as their solubility in lipids or in proteins, or decreases in the surface tension of monomolecular layers, polarizability, or molecular volume, as reflected by van der Waal constants. Although the site of action of a narcotic gas does not correspond to any simple bulk phase such as lipid, fluid, or protein (Smith 1969), the following data are known:

Meyer and Hopff (1923) investigated the narcotic effects of gases under pressure on mice, frogs, and salamanders. They postulated that the threshold of narcosis was related to the solubility of the particular gas in lipid rather than to the partial pressure of the gas, and they reported that the narcotic threshold occurred when the anesthetic concentration reached approximately 0.06 mole per liter. Later studies by Lever and co-workers (1971) of anesthetic gas solubility in membrane lipids confirmed this earlier work by establishing that the critical anesthetic concentration in lipid was 0.05 mole per liter.

Such an anesthetic dose produces a lipid expansion of about 0.4%, and the hydrostatic pressure required to nullify an expansion of such magnitude would be about 100 ATA (3300 fsw), a value that agrees with experimental data. It would appear that the narcotic potency of inert gases is due to their effect on the "free volume" (or "empty volume"), perhaps in lipid in the cell membrane of nerve tissue (Stern and Frisch 1973). "Thus, the anesthetic potency of a gas depends upon its lipid solubility, thermal expansivity, and compressibility of the liquid phase, environmental temperature, and hydrostatic pressure, rather than only on the lipid solubility as in the Meyer-Overton hypothesis" (Bennett 1975).

5. *Inert Gas Effects*

a. Model Surface Membrane Effects

The interactions of inert gases are best observed in a model system consisting of monomolecular film made from stearic acid, cholesterol, lecithin, and lipoprotein extracted from beef lung; this film, which is spread on the surface of distilled water, has the gross characteristics of nerve membrane. Exposing the film to anesthetics lowers the film's surface tension, and anesthetic potency is measured by determining the affinity of the anesthetic for the surface film. Anesthetic potency is directly and linearly related to the anesthetic's affinity for the lipid film (Clements and Wilson 1962).

The relationship between the action of inert gases in this model system and in cell membranes was explained by Clements and Wilson as follows:

> Inert gases at partial pressures sufficient to bring about a standard effect in a biological system act on a lipoprotein-water interface to cause a standard decrease of 0.39 dyne/cm of interfacial tension . . . . Since the composition and structure of cellular membranes and of the experimental films are very similar, it would seem reasonable to think that these narcotic agents are also sorbed into the cellular interfaces, where they may change the effective dielectric constant and permeability . . . . Insofar as we understand the behavior of the model, it does not permit us to state whether the interactions occur primarily between lipid film and narcotic or between water and narcotic facilitated by the presence of lipid. In either interpretation our data suggest that lipid plays an essential role.

b. Inert Gas Protection against the High-Pressure Nervous Syndrome

Adding nitrogen to a helium-oxygen breathing mixture provides some protection against the effects, collectively called the High Pressure Nervous Syndrome (HPNS), of pressure per se. (For a detailed description of HPNS, see Section D of this chapter.) The most convincing evidence of the protective effect of additive nitrogen is the results of the classic mice experiments conducted by Rahn and associates (Rahn 1975; Rahn and Rokitka 1976). Mice were compressed at a rate of 0.25 ATA/min to 100 ATA (3300 fsw). The physical condition of the mice was assessed by measuring the distance run on an activity wheel during the dark part of the 24-hr cycle. Results were as follows:

1. If normoxic mixtures of helium were used, typical signs of HPNS were observed above 50 ATA.
2. When compressed with the addition of 10 or 20 ATA of nitrogen HPNS effects were not present.

Over a 48- to 72-hr period of observation, four colonies of mice ran an average of 0.3 km (0.2 mile) per day when the atmosphere contained no nitrogen and an average of 1.0 km (0.6 mile) per day when the atmosphere included 10 ATA of nitrogen. When the atmosphere contained 20 ATA of nitrogen, one colony ran an average of 5.0 km (3.1 miles) per day. The conclusion of these elegant tests of the responses of a whole, intact organism was that under the best conditions, overall running activity decreases to approximately one-half of the activity level at surface pressure.

c. Opposing Physiological Effects of Pressure and Inert Gases

Miller (1977) has analyzed the mechanisms of the opposing physiological effects of high pressure and inert gases. He states, "The use of anesthetic gases to ameliorate the effects of pressure re-introduces the problem of inert gas narcosis into deep diving. However, this problem is mitigated by the remarkable observation that pressure reverses the effects of anesthetics . . .. The pressure reversal of anesthesia suggests that the anesthetics not only dissolve in, but also expand and fluidize the lipid bilayer regions of biomembranes. Anesthetics have in fact been observed to fluidize membranes and this fluidization is reversed by pressures of the same magnitude as those observed physiologically." Miller's challenging conclusion is that anesthesia occurs when the volume of a hydrophobic region is caused to expand beyond a certain critical volume by absorption of an inert substance. Applying pressure opposes this expansion and reverses the anesthesia. Convulsions (in animals) occur when some hydrophobic region is compressed beyond a certain critical amount by the application of pressure. The absorption of an inert gas will compensate for such compression and raise the convulsion threshold pressure.

d. Clinical Use of Nitrogen Narcosis as a Benign Stress

Using pressure and inert gases to regulate the contraction and expansion of neural membranes has not been sufficiently developed to apply to specific instances of neurological dysfunction. However, increasing the atmospheric pressure has permitted physicians to detect and assess normally covert behavioral and neuromuscular deficits without residual effects (Behnke 1945; Adolphson 1967; Adolphson et al. 1972). Use of a pressurized nitrogen modality may thus become a routine procedure in the diagnosis of certain types of neurological impairments in the future.

ALBERT R. BEHNKE, JR.

References

ACKLES, K. N., AND B. FOWLER 1971. Cortical evoked response and inert gas narcosis in man. *Aerosp. Med.* 43: 1181–1184.

ADOLPHSON, J. 1967. Human performance and behaviour in hyperbaric environments. In: *Acta Psychologica Gothoburgensia*, edited by J. Elmgren. Stockholm: Almqvist and Wiksell.

ADOLPHSON, J., L. GOLDBERG, AND T. BERGHAGE 1972. Effects of increased ambient air pressures on standing steadiness in man. *Aerosp. Med.* 43: 520–524.

BEHNKE, A. R. 1945. Psychological and psychiatric reactions in diving and in submarine warfare. *Am. J. Psychiatry* 101: 720–725.

BEHNKE, A. R., R. M. THOMSON, AND E. P. MOTLEY 1935. The psychologic effects of breathing air at 4 atmospheres pressure. *Am. J. Physiol.* 112: 554–558.

BEHNKE, A. R., AND O. D. YARBROUGH 1939. Respiratory resistance, oil-water solubility and mental effects of argon compared with helium and nitrogen. *Am. J. Physiol.* 126: 409–415.

BENNETT, P. B. 1975. Inert gas narcosis. In: *The Physiology and Medicine of Diving and Compressed Air Work*, edited by P. B. Bennett and D. H. Elliott. London: Baillière, Tindall.

CASE, E. M., AND J. B. S. HALDANE 1941. Human physiology under high pressure. *J. Hyg. (Cambridge)* 41: 225–249.

CLEMENTS, J. A., AND K. M. WILSON 1962. The affinity of narcotic agents for interfacial films. *Proc. Natl. Acad. Sci.* 48: 1008–1014.

CULLEN, S. C., AND E. G. GROSS 1951. The anesthetic properties of xenon in animals and human being with additional observations on krypton. *Science* 113: 580–582.

DAMANT, G. C. C. 1930. Physiological effects of work in compressed air. *Nature (Lond.)* 126: 606–608.

EDEL, P. O. 1976. Use of other gases: hydrogen and neon. In: *Decompression Procedures for Depths in Excess of 400 Feet*, edited by R. W. Hamilton, Jr. Bethesda, MD: Undersea Medical Society.

FEATHERSTONE, R. M., AND C. A. MUEHLBAECHER 1963. The current role of inert gases in the search for anesthesia mechanisms. *Pharmacol. Rev.* 15: 97–121.

HAMILTON, R. W., JR., AND D. J. KENYON 1976. Decompression work at Tarrytown. In: *Decompression Procedures for Depths in Excess of 400 Feet*, edited by R. W. Hamilton, Jr. Bethesda, MD: Undersea Medical Society.

JONES, A. W., R. D. JENNINGS, J. ADOLPHSON, AND C. M. HESSER 1979. Combined effects of ethanol and hyperbaric air on body sway and heart rate in man. *Undersea Biomed. Res.* 6: 15–25.

KIESSLING, R. J., AND C. H. MAAG 1962. Performance impairment as a function of nitrogen narcosis. *J. Appl. Psychol.* 46: 91–95.

LEVER, M. J., K. W. MILLER, W. D. M. PATON, AND E. B. SMITH 1971. Pressure reversal of anaesthesia. *Nature (Lond.)* 231: 368–371.

MEYER, K. H., AND H. HOPFF 1923. Narcosis by inert gases under pressure. *Hoppe-Seyler's Z. Physiol. Chem.* 126: 288–298.

MILLER, K. W. 1977. The opposing physiological effects of high pressures and inert gases. *Fed. Proc.* 36: 1663–1667.

RAHN, H. 1975. Performance during mouse saturation dives to 100 ATA. In: *The Strategy for Future Diving to Depths Greater than 1000 ft.*, M. J. Halsey, W. Settle, and E. B. Smith, rapporteurs. Bethesda, MD: Undersea Medical Society.

RAHN, H., AND M. A. ROKITKA 1976. Narcotic potency of N_2, A, and N_2O evaluated by physical performance of mouse colonies. *Undersea Biomed. Res.* 3: 25–34.

SHILLING, C. W., M. F. WERTS, AND N. R. SCHANDELMEIER (editors) 1976. *The Underwater Handbook: A Guide to Physiology and Performance for the Engineer.* New York: Plenum Press, p. 193–205.

SHILLING, C. W., AND W. W. WILLGRUBE 1937. Quantitative study of mental and neuro-muscular reactions as influenced by increased air pressure. *Nav. Med. Bull.* 35: 373–380.

SMITH, E. B. 1969. The role of exotic gases in the study of narcosis. In: *The Physiology and Medicine of Diving and Compressed Air Work*, edited by P. B. Bennett and D. H. Elliott. London: Baillière, Tindall.

STERN, S. A., AND H. L. FRISCH 1973. Dependence of inert gas narcosis on lipid "free volume." *J. Appl. Physiol.* 34: 366–373.

F. Women and Diving

1. History

When women began to dive is not known, but the diving ama of Japan and Korea are the best-known example of diving women. The ama were referred to as early as 268 B.C., although the term *ama* originally applied to both men and women who dived (Nukada 1965). These early divers apparently used different techniques, depending on their sex; female divers collected shellfish and seaweed, while male divers used their hands or spears to catch fish. There is speculation that women began to dominate diving when the number of male divers decreased because of conscription into the armies of the sixth and seventh centuries (Nakamura 1962). The use of female ama may thus have arisen from necessity rather than from an increased tolerance to cold, as has often been suggested.

In the Western world, women have only recently begun diving. After the development of scuba, women gradually entered the sport diving field (Parry 1978), and by 1951 they were diving in significant numbers. The number of women presently certified to dive is estimated at 40,000 (Smith 1979), although many of these are not active. However, few women are engaged in commercial diving, although commercial diving schools do accept women students.

In scientific diving, however, the opportunities for women divers are much better. The first all-woman team of divers to carry out a saturation dive (in the Tektite II habitat at St. Croix, Virgin Islands) apparently performed as well as male divers (Beckman and Smith 1972). Differences in individual accomplishments between male and female divers engaged in other saturation research projects were shown to be related to factors other than the sex of the diver (R. Wicklund, personal communication). Women archeologist-divers working under the auspices of the Institute of Nautical Archaeology have conducted about 2500 decompression dives successfully (G. F. Bass, personal communication).

2. Physical Performance and Adaptability

In general, women do not have the muscular strength of men. This trait means that some commercial diving construction activities that require considerable physical strength, such as lifting, hauling, freeing bolts, or hanging on in a current cannot be performed by many women divers. On the other hand, many diving jobs call primarily for dexterity, judgment, and a working knowledge of mechanical devices, and these tasks can be performed as well by women as by men, since diving itself is well within the physical capability of women.

Several studies of the relative physiological adaptability of women and men to physical conditioning have been performed. Astrand and Rodahl (1970) have shown that oxygen consumption is based on lean body mass and is the same in men and women if the level of physical conditioning is the same for both sexes. Harris (1973) reports that maximum oxygen uptake in girls peaks between the ages of 9 and 14 and then declines gradually until the sixth decade of life. In males, this peaking takes place at about age 15. Allsen and co-workers (1977) have shown that menstruation does not affect oxygen uptake. The size and physical condition of the individual diver apparently plays a more important role in oxygen uptake than difference in the sex of the diver.

3. Decompression Sickness

The decompression tables in general use were developed to be used on young, healthy men. The procedures used to develop these tables were usually as follows: A preliminary table was created by extrapolating from another table or derived mathematically by using Haldane's basic concepts of tissue blood perfusion and gas solubility. These tables then were tested on healthy young men and were modified empirically until a high percentage of male divers could use them without developing clinical symptoms of decompression sickness. The process was repeated for each change in the table's depth or bottom time. The amount of safety factor built into a decompression table depends upon its intended use. For example, a table for commercial divers may be designed to minimize the amount of decompression time for economic reasons, particularly if a recompression chamber will be available at the dive site. On the other hand, a table for recreational divers requires a sufficient margin of safety to ensure that the likelihood of decompression sickness will be very small even if the table is used by the general public. The decompression tables recommended for nonprofessional scuba diving in the U.S. are based on the shallow water U.S. Navy Air Decompression tables revised by Workman (R. Workman, unpublished observations), or on tables very similar to them.

These tables have been widely used by female divers in sport and scientific diving. It has often been suggested in sport diving circles that the incidence of decompression sickness among female divers is slightly higher than that in males (Bangasser 1979; Bassett 1973). In fact, Meijne (1970) noted that European women divers were believed to be more susceptible to decompression sickness than males, but Meinje presented no supporting evidence. As yet, no rigorous studies have been carried out to determine if female divers are more susceptible to decompression sickness than male divers of similar age, fat burden, and physical conditioning. There has recently been some speculation about physiological differences that might make female divers more susceptible to decompression sickness than male divers. These are discussed below.

a. Extra Fat Burden

Behnke (1968) has pointed out that women have an average total body fat content of about 25%, while men have an average total body fat of 14%. Since it is well known that susceptibility to decompression sickness increases as the fat burden increases, it seems logical that women would generally be more susceptible to bends than men. However, female susceptibility to the bends cannot be satisfactorily quantified on the basis of records of decompression sickness incidents among recreational divers using the standard tables, because these tables have a large built-in safety factor. Thus, with the present tables women divers could actually be more susceptible and therefore closer to presenting clinical symptoms than male divers, and this would not be apparent, because it is impossible to tell how close a diver is to developing symptoms until these symptoms become clinical.

b. Oral Contraceptives

Some researchers have suggested that the use of oral contraceptives may increase a diver's susceptibility to decompression sickness because it may promote blood sludging, reduce venous tone, and cause hormonal changes in general. For this reason, the female aquanauts participating in the Tektite II saturation mission discontinued oral contraceptives 3 months before the mission began (Beckman and Smith 1972). Only one preliminary study (W. F. Fife, unpublished observations) has tested the effects of Brevicon (norethindrone/estradiol) on the decompression susceptibility of pigs; there was no evidence that this drug altered the susceptibility of these animals. If women are generally more susceptible to decompression sickness than men, taking contraceptives might increase their probability of incurring decompression sickness. However, unless oral contraceptives do create a clinical problem, there is no evidence to show that they alter female susceptibility to decompression sickness significantly, and their use for normal women divers is not contraindicated at this time.

c. Intrauterine Devices

There is no information to suggest that an intrauterine device increases susceptibility to decompression sickness. However, if the device permits the retrograde movement of fluid, the probability of infection may increase, because as much as 12 ml of water may cycle in and out the vagina during 10 min of active swimming (W. F. Fife, unpublished observations).

d. Premenstrual Fluid Retention and Menstruation

There is no experimental evidence to suggest that the retention of fluid in itself increases susceptibility to decompression sickness. Although female runners taking premenstrual diuretics have suffered an increased incidence of leg cramps, this phenomenon has not been reported in women divers. Bangasser (1979) reported that 3.8% of the women who made decompression dives while menstruating or taking oral contraceptives incurred decompression sickness. She also reported that 1.3% of women making no-decompression dives developed decompression sickness. These values are surprising, since virtually no decompression sickness would be expected for the diving population at large if standard procedures were observed. However, Bangasser's figures should be viewed with caution because of the difficulty of obtaining reliable data from untrained observers.

Two studies suggest that women divers may be more susceptible to decompression sickness than their male counterparts. The first of these was carried out by Bangasser (1979), who conducted a survey of 680 women divers. She found that female diving instructors reported a 3.3-fold increase in suspected or diagnosed decompression sickness compared to male instructors. Since these data were obtained from questionnaires, it was not possible to ensure that the responses of both sexes were equally objective, or that the same clinical standards were applied to all divers. On the other hand, a 3.3-fold difference cannot be ignored even with these reservations.

The second study involved healthy young U.S. Air Force flight nurses undergoing decompression in altitude chambers (Bassett 1973). Of the 3190 women tested, 7 developed decompression sickness after returning to surface pressure. Although the numbers in this study were small, this value represents a 10-fold increase in decompression sickness compared to the incidence in male subjects exposed to the same pressure changes. However, Air Force cadets are reported to have a higher incidence of altitude decompression sickness than older flight crew members on active duty, which raises the possibility that any increase in decompression sickness incidence seen in flight nurses may be due to factors other than the sex of the individual. For example, factors such as the stress of training were not eliminated in this study.

Experience in the Tektite II (Beckman and Smith 1972) and the Hydrolab (R.I. Wicklund, personal communication) underwater habitats did not demonstrate greater susceptiblity to decompression sickness among female divers, although the numbers involved were small. One of the 5 female divers in Tektite II developed decompression sickness, while 5 out of 50 male divers developed mild symptoms; none of the 285 male or 58 female divers in the Hydrolab program developed decompression sickness (Beckman and Smith 1972), although both habitats were located at nearly the same depth.

Bass (G. F. Bass, personal communication) now has conducted more than 15,000 decompression dives in connection with underwater archaeological excavations. Many of the divers on these expeditions carried out two decompression dives each day. Among the approximately 20% of the divers who were women, Bass reported no instances of decompression sickness, but there were two cases among the male divers. However, since Bass almost invariably works in remote locations, he uses more conservative tables to calculate decompression than the average sport diver, and he calculates depths and times precisely.

e. Summary

In summary, it is not clear whether women are more susceptible to decompression sickness than men. Most women divers continue to use the same decompression tables as men and consider them safe. However, when approaching the no-decompression limits, working hard, or diving in cold water, divers of both sexes are encouraged to calculate their decompression by using schedules for the next greater depth or the next longer bottom time. R. Workman (personal communication) suggested that divers on a no-decompression schedule make an arbitrary 2- to 5-min stop at 10 fsw. Employing either of these procedures would increase the safety of all divers. As a reasonable precaution, I believe that women diving while menstruating or taking oral contraceptives should use the next greater depth or next longer bottom time to calculate their decompression obligation.

I know of no instances in which decompression sickness treatment produced poor results simply because the patient was female, other than the report of Bassett (1973), which suggested that altitude decompression sickness was more frequent, more serious, and more refractory in women than man. Again, however, the numbers were very small. The concern of clinicians also arises because there are very few definitive studies of the effects of hyperbaric therapy on women, and there is therefore little basis on which to predict the effects of increased pressure on the female endocrine system, intrauterine devices, drug responses, the fetus, and other factors which may differentiate the female from the male patient.

4. Pregnancy and Diving

Understanding of the effects of diving on the pregnant woman and her fetus is rapidly advancing. Despite exhaustive discussion of the subject in an Undersea Medical Society Workshop report (Fife 1980), however, studies on pregnancy and diving have so far been preliminary and have raised more questions than they have answered (Brown 1979; Fife et al. 1978; McIver 1968; Stock et al. 1980).

In 1968, McIver exposed 28 pregnant dogs anesthetized with nembutal to a pressure equivalent to 165 fsw. Thirteen were exposed for 60, and 15 for 120, minutes of bottom time. All adult dogs presented marked and lethal disseminating intravascular bubbles. However, bubbles were found in only 2 of the 94 fetuses of the first group and in 2 of the 99 fetuses of the second group. In the 4 fetuses with bubbles, bubbles occurred only in the coronary arteries. Large bubbles were present in the amnionic fluid of all animals, but there was no evidence that these were detrimental to the fetuses. On the other hand, when 23 newborn pups from other litters were exposed to a simulated depth of 165 fsw for 60 min, 8 showed marked intravascular bubbles. The fetuses were apparently more resistant to decompression sickness than either the mothers or infants of approximately the same size as the exposed fetuses. These observations are strengthened by the work of Chen (1974), who noted that the fetuses of anesthetized pregnant rats did not show intravascular bubbles, even when the mother died of decompression sickness.

On the basis of these two studies and the belief that fetuses accumulated inert gas more slowly than mothers, it was initially felt that the fetus should be more resistant to decompression sickness than the mother, and that any dive that was safe for the mother would also be safe for the fetus.

In 1978, however, Fife and his co-workers noted that although dogs and rats have a countercurrent circulatory exchange between the mother and fetus, the exchange in humans is a concurrent system and is therefore probably less efficient. These workers instrumented seven pregnant sheep by placing Doppler flow probes around one of the umbilical arteries (Fife et al. 1978). In their early studies (W. P. Fife, unpublished observations) another probe also was placed around one of the maternal jugular veins. Table III-6 summarizes the results of 17 simulated dives made with these seven sheep.

As this table shows, even though no clinical symptoms of decompression sickness were noted in the mothers, the fetuses presented with circulating bubbles after simulated dives (100 fsw for 25 min) that are considered safe for humans. The fact that no circulating bubbles were detected in the maternal jugular veins should not be taken as proof that there were no bubbles anywhere in the maternal circulation; later studies (Brown 1979) showed that the jugular vein was a poor choice. Other subsequent studies (W. P. Fife, unpublished observations) showed that circulating bubbles were detected in the inferior vena cava by Doppler techniques after a dive to a simulated depth of 60 fsw for a bottom time of only 2.5 min, and in another 2.5-min dive to 100 fsw for a similar bottom time. In both instances these bubbles appeared when the animals struggled or when muscles in the rear legs were squeezed.

These results of studies on fetal susceptibility to decompression sickness should be viewed with caution because of results obtained subsequent to this initial study (Fife 1980; Stock et al. 1980). In at least two instances Doppler probes were placed on an umbilical artery of one fetal twin while the other twin was not surgically manipulated.

Table III-6
Dive Profiles

Dive No.	Depth, fsw	Time, min	Results Mother	Results Fetus
1	160	20	Neg.	Pos.**
2	145	20	Neg.	Pos.
3	145	20	Neg.	Pos.
4*	100	30	Neg.	Pos.
5	100	25	Neg.	Pos.
6	100	25	Neg.	Pos.
7	100	25	Neg.	Pos.
8	100	25	Neg.	Pos.
9	100	25	Neg.	Pos.
10	100	20	Neg.	Thresh.†
11	100	15	Neg.	Thresh.
12	100	10	Neg.	Neg.
13	80	40	Neg.	Thresh.
14	60	90	Neg.	Thresh.
15	60	70	Neg.	Neg.
16	60	60	Neg.	Neg.
17	40	200	Neg.	Neg.

* On this dive, the U.S. Navy Standard Air Decompression Table was followed.
** pos. (positive), Presence of massive bubbles in circulation that probably would have been fatal.
† Thresh. (threshold), Appearance of occasional acoustical events interpreted as probable circulating bubbles (however, treatment was not instituted).
[From Fife et al. (1978).]

In both of these instances the twin with the Doppler probe on one of its umbilical arteries developed intravascular bubbles, while no bubbles were detected in the untouched twin. This observation raised the possibility that the increased fetal susceptibility noted in the Fife et al. (1978) studies may have been due to surgical trauma or the presence of the Doppler probe on the umbilical artery. Whether the fetal bubbles were artifactual or not is unclear at this time. In one unpublished study, Fife and his co-workers have found that a third-trimester fetus that had had the probe implanted and then immediately removed from its umbilical artery did not develop decompression sickness, while the third-trimester fetus of a sheep that had undergone no surgery was stillborn 3 days after being subjected to a dive of the same depth and bottom time, and it had massive intravascular bubbles.

It is believed that bubbles are generally created when a diver surfaces even after a no-decompression dive to less than 60 fsw. Initially these bubbles may remain in or near the peripheral capillaries, particularly in muscle tissue. They can easily be forced into circulation by muscle action, including shivering. Normally, however, in the adult these venous bubbles are filtered out by the lungs and thus are prevented from becoming arterial gas emboli (Butler and Hills 1979). Contrary to earlier views, the mother may actually develop circulating bubbles before her fetus does (Brown 1979). However, on some dives the fetus may develop circulating bubbles before the mother presents clinical symptoms of decompression sickness. Because the fetus has a patent foramen ovale, its lungs are not able to serve as a bubble trap, and umbilical artery bubbles quickly become arterial gas emboli with potentially serious consequences. Thus umbilical artery bubbles should be regarded as a grave threat to the fetus, in contrast to the usually benign consequences of a modest number of venous bubbles in the adult.

There is little information on the effects of diving on pregnant women and their fetuses. In some instances, the ama of Japan and Korea continue their activities into the ninth month of pregnancy (Rahn and Yokoyama 1965), and there is no evidence that their fetuses suffer adverse consequences; however, these infants do tend to be smaller at birth. The children of ama are as healthy and as intelligent as the children of nondiving women of the same ethnic background and region. However, since the ama are engaged in breath-hold diving and remain on bottom for only 2-3 min before returning to the surface, they absorb less nitrogen than divers who remain on the bottom with scuba. Although it is possible for a breath-hold diver to develop decompression sickness by making a large number of dives in rapid succession with only short surface intervals (Rahn and Yokohama 1965), decompression sickness is unknown among the ama.

Bolton (1980) surveyed female scuba divers who dived while pregnant. Her initial study identified 136 such women. Among this group, six children were born with birth defects, a figure not significantly different from the 5% expected in the general female population. On the other hand, among the 24 pregnant women who dived to depths greater than 100 fsw there were three infants with birth defects. Although the numbers were small and the precise depths and times of each dive were not known, Bolton's study suggests that scuba diving to depths below 100 fsw may have caused birth defects in at least some infants.

It appears that the age of the fetus may affect its susceptibility to decompression sickness. Boycott, Damant, and Haldane (1908) noted that if pregnant sheep were subjected to dives to 168 fsw for periods of from 15 to 20 min, fetuses 4 in. or less in length did not present with bubbles, while those over 4 in. often did. Recent studies (Fife et al. 1978) also suggest that fetuses in the first trimester may be more resistant to decompression sickness than those in the third trimester. However, in early embryonic development destruction of even a single cell may result in serious or lethal abnormalities when growth and differentiation have taken place. For this reason, the consequences of decompression sickness in the embryo or early fetus may be worse than in the fetus near term.

Whether a pregnant woman is more susceptible to decompression sickness than a nonpregnant woman is an often-asked question. No studies designed to answer this question have been carried out. Willson (1978) has pointed out that female physiology is constantly changing, especially during pregnancy. There are major circulatory, hormonal, metabolic, and body compositional changes in pregnant women that could affect susceptibility, but since no studies have been conducted, the relationship of these changes to susceptibility is not known. For example, the increased blood flow associated with pregnancy might increase the rate of inert gas uptake and elimination from the tissues. However, since inert gas probably enters the tissues faster during compression than it later leaves during decompression, the increase in circulation may not provide protection against decompression sickness. Scientists reviewing this question (Fife 1980) felt that the standard decompression tables currently in use by sport divers probably are not optimal for pregnant females and may pose a risk to her health, particularly if the dive approaches the no-decompression limits.

There is no evidence that the exercise performed during diving is harmful to the pregnant diver. Pregnant women have swum (Rahn and Yokoyama 1965) and engaged in other active sports until late in pregnancy.

It is also unlikely that a pregnant scuba diver will develop hypoxia in the course of a shallow, uncomplicated dive with properly functioning equipment. However, unexpected problems such as loss of air, equipment malfunction, near-drowning, aspiration of seawater, or carbon monoxide poisoning might create a severe degree of hypoxia that could be passed on to the fetus. Recently the panel of diving physicians and physiologists convened by the Undersea Medical Society to study the question of diving and pregnancy recommended that until further studies are carried out, a woman who is or who thinks she might be pregnant should be discouraged from diving (Fife 1980).

5. Questions Frequently Asked

Physicians may be asked several questions by women divers. Many cannot yet be answered on the basis of rigorously controlled studies but may be answered on the basis of anecdotal information and common sense. Examples of these questions follow.

Will diving affect the sex of my baby? For years folklore supported the belief that divers produced more female than male offspring. This myth may have been based on an apparently apocryphal story about a team of Royal Navy divers rumored to have fathered 10 female and 1 male offspring. In any event, English diving clubs are rumored to advise their divers to father or conceive during nondiving months if they want a male child (Edmonds 1977). Two studies now suggest that there is no substance to this belief. One survey of divers of the Royal Australian Navy found that these men had fathered 112 male and 118 female offspring. A second survey was made (Bachrach and Holiman 1973) of U.S. divers who were members of the U.S. Navy Divers' Association. The 433 survey respondents reported that they had 165 girls and 173 boys in the period before they started diving, and that after diving 341 girls and 265 boys had been born. The pre- and post-diving male:female offspring ratios were not significantly different.

Are sharks attracted to menstruating females? Edmonds (1977) surveyed an Australian shark attack file covering 1000 incidents that had occurred along a recreational beachline and reported that although the swimming population was evenly divided between men and women, men were attacked 9 times more often than women. In addition, Edmonds reported that there was no record of a female scuba diver being attacked while swimming underwater. In summary, many women have dived while menstruating without experiencing problems with sharks.

WILLIAM P. FIFE

References

ALLSEN, P. E., P. PARSONA. AND G. R. BRYCE 1977. Effects of menstrual cycle on maximum oxygen uptake. *Phys. Sports Med.* July, p. 53–55.
ASTRAND, P. O., AND K. RODAHL 1970. *Textbook of Work Physiology*. New York: McGraw-Hill.

BACHRACH, A. J., AND M. HOLIMAN 1973. Diver offspring: miss or myth? *Sea Diver* December, p. 27.
BANGASSER, S. 1979. Incidence of decompression sickness in women scuba divers. In: *Proceedings of the Annual Scientific Meeting of the Undersea Medical Society*. Bethesda, MD: Undersea Medical Society.
BASSETT, B. E. 1973. Decompression sickness in female students exposed to altitude during physiological training. Paper presented at the 44th Annual Scientific Meeting of the Aerospace Medical Association, Las Vegas, NV.
BECKMAN, E. L., AND E. M. SMITH 1972. TEKTITE II, medical supervision of the scientist in the sea. *Tex. Rep. Biol. Med.*, Vol. 30.
BEHNKE, A. R. 1968. Physique and exercise, In: *Exercise Physiology*, edited by H. B. Falls. New York: Academic Press.
BOLTON, M. 1980. Scuba diving and fetal well-being: a survey of 208 women. *Undersea Biomed. Res.* 7: 183–189.
BOYCOTT, A. E., J. B. S. HALDANE. AND G. C. C. DAMANT 1908. The prevention of compressed air illness. *J. Hyg. (Camb.)* 8: 419–420.
BROWN, S. 1979. Comparison of fetal and maternal susceptibility to decompression sickness (Thesis). College Station: Texas A&M Univ.
BUTLER, B. D., AND B. A. HILLS 1979. The lung as a filter for microbubbles. *J. Appl. Physiol.: Respir. Environ. Exercise Physiol.* 47: 537–543.
CHEN, V. 1974. The prophylactic therapeutic treatment of decompression sickness by heparin and aspirin (Thesis). College Station: Texas A&M Univ.
EDMONDS, C. 1977. Female divers: facts and fallacies. *Scot. Diver*, May/June, p. 2–5.
FIFE, W. P. (chairman) 1980. Effects of Diving on Pregnancy. Bethesda, MD: Undersea Medical Society. (19th Workshop Nov. 1978.)
FIFE, W. P., C. SIMMANG. AND J. V. KITZMAN 1978. Susceptibility of fetal sheep to acute decompression sickness. *Undersea Biomed. Res.* 5: 287–292.
HARRIS, D. V. 1973. Women in sports; some misconceptions. *J. Sports Med.* March/April, p. 15–17.
MCIVER, R. G. 1968. Bends resistance in the fetus. Paper presented at the 1968 Annual Scientific Meeting of the Aerospace Medical Association, Bal Harbor, FL.
MEIJNE, N. G. 1970. *Hyperbaric Oxygen and Its Clinical Value*. American Lectures in Living Chemistry. Springfield, IL: Charles C Thomas.
NAKAMURA, Y. 1962. *The Women Sea Divers of Japan*. Tokyo: Chunichi Shinbun.
NUKADA, M. 1965. Historical development of the Ama's diving activities. In: *Physiology of Breath-hold Diving and the Ama of Japan*, edited by H. Rahn and T. Yokoyama. Washington, DC: Natl. Acad. Sci./Natl. Res. Council, p. 25–40.
PARRY, Z. 1978. The female ethic in diving history—poetry or prejudice. In: *Proceedings of the PADI Women in Diving Seminar*, edited by D. Graver. Santa Ana, CA: Professional Association of Diving Instructors.
RAHN, H., AND T. YOKOYAMA (editors) 1965. *The Physiology of Breath-hold Diving and the Ama of Japan*. Washington, DC: Natl. Acad. Sci./Natl. Res. Council.
RENNIE, D. W., B. G. COVINO, B. J. HOWELL, S. H. HONG, B. S. KANG. AND S. K. HONG 1962. Physical insulation of Korean diving women. *J. Appl. Physiol.* 17: 961–966.
SMITH, K. C. 1979. *The Woman Diver*. Sea Grant College Program. Rep. SG-79-803. College Station: Texas A&M Univ.
STOCK, M. K., E. H. LANPHIER, D. F. ANDERSON, L. C. ANDERSON, T. M. PHERNETTSON. AND J. H. G. RANKIN 1980. Responses of fetal sheep to simulated no-decompression dives. *J. Appl. Physiol.: Respir. Environ Exercise Physiol.* 48: 776–780.
WILLSON, J. R. 1978. Diving-in-pregnancy research possibilities. In: *Effects of Diving on Pregnancy*. Bethesda, MD: Undersea Medical Society, p. A6–A13. (19th Workshop Nov. 1978.)

G. Monitoring of Vital Signs; Doppler Monitoring

Humanistic, ethical, and cost considerations all encourage efforts to find ways to monitor divers at work. Ideally, monitoring a diver should (1) provide early warning to prevent the unexplained and sudden deaths that have occurred occasionally in the past; (2) prevent decompression sickness by sensing the physiological changes that precede clinical bends; and (3) maximize efficiency by pacing divers' exercise levels with respect to their decompression obligations. However, such monitors do not exist, although strides have been made in the past two decades toward meeting these goals. Monitoring of diving casualties during treatment is another diving-related application of this technology; this use of monitoring could indicate the need for further therapy or suggest abbreviation of a given treatment table, thereby reducing the risks associated with hyperbaric oxygenation.

Certain design requirements of monitors are obvious; they should be inexpensive, reliable, salt-water compatible, pressure and temperature independent, and capable of withstanding the rough physical environment typical of diving. In addition, they should not interfere with the diver's work or comfort. Other necessary characteristics of monitors are not so obvious. A monitor must accurately portray a physiological parameter in a manner that permits someone, either the diver or surface personnel, to make a decision based on the physiological information displayed. A monitor must sense a physiological change early enough to permit action to be taken to prevent an accident or a casualty. It may sometimes be preferable, therefore, to have a monitor read by the diver himself, rather than by topside personnel. In addition, results of monitoring should be simple enough to be interpreted by a nonphysician. Furthermore, a monitor should provide specific enough information to prevent action that would be contrary to the diver's safety from being taken. For example, the U.S. Navy Diving Manual (1973) formerly required that a stage diver be brought to the surface if diver-to-surface communication, the most basic of all monitors, was lost. However, after two men were killed by explosive decompression sickness because they were brought up from 300 fsw (9 ATA) when their radio failed, this requirement was changed to allow for interpretation of the significance of a monitor by topside personnel before action is taken. Finally, a monitor should provide a signal that can be recorded for later analysis should complications arise, performing a function similar to that of the "black box" on commercial jets today.

The U.S. Navy has pioneered the development of monitors for divers as part of its overall objective to assess man's performance capabilities at 2500 fsw (78 ATA) by 1985. (Naval Medical Research Institute 1977). Beginning in 1969 the Navy, in conjunction with NASA scientists, formulated the following list of preferred monitors:

1. Voice communication
2. Heart rate
3. Inspired P_{O_2}
4. Inspired P_{CO_2}
5. Hot water inlet temperature for heated suits
6. Depth and time

All of these sensors are available at this time. However, with the exception of depth/time and voice communication, these monitors are seldom used outside of research centers, for many reasons: expense, lack of durability, excessive maintenance requirements, and difficulty in translating the monitored response into a signal that can be interpreted by nonphysicians.

1. Voice Communication

No monitor has been as widely accepted and used as voice communications between the surface and the diver. The development of the helium unscrambler, which is used to make the speech of divers breathing helium-oxygen intelligible, has made on-line voice communication available to virtually all surface-supplied divers. Through proper use of this monitor, divers can receive topside guidance and information and inform surface personnel of incipient danger or other important occurrences. A considerable amount of subtle information may also be conveyed by a diver's voice, such as fatigue, confusion, or anxiety; these covert signals may lead surface personnel to terminate the dive. Even when all that is heard is the diver's breathing, this information is invaluable to the topside personnel.

The real advantages of two-way communication have been demonstrated in numerous operational diving situations. On one occasion a diver suffering from alternobaric vertigo of descent was close to panic until he was "talked down" by the master diver. On another, a trapped diver was reassured by the message that help was on the way. The fact that most diving fatalities occur in divers using scuba gear may be due not only to the lack of training of many scuba users but also to this mode's lack of voice communications. Clearly, on-line voice communication, supplemented by line-pull signals, is the first and most essential of all dive monitors. In the future, telemetry technology may allow even scuba divers to talk to surface personnel routinely.

2. Cardiovascular Monitors

Clinicians and diving medical officers have long searched for equipment that will adequately monitor cardiac function. Since cardiac output consists of the stroke volume times the heart rate, changes in one may be compensated for by changes in the other; an example is the well-known bradycardia associated with neck-out immersion, in which the decrease in pulse rate is more than compensated for by an increase in stroke volume, in accordance with Starling's law of the heart. The ideal parameter to measure would be cardiac output, but such invasive monitoring has never been performed even in diving casualties, using current thermodilution techniques, and could not be justified in healthy divers. This means that heart rate is the only measure of cardiovascular stability available in diving situations.

To date, heart rate is the most commonly measured physiological parameter, although all of its implications are not fully understood. More than 200 endogenous reflexes affect heart rate, and many of these reflexes are directly stimulated by diving. These reflexes are the bases for most technical procedures in monitoring. For example, exercise (measured as V_{O_2}) may cause an increase in pulse up to 215 beats per minute (bpm) at V_{O_2} levels of 4 liters/min (Astrand and Rodahl 1977). Superimposed upon this increase is the bradycardia known to occur with hyperoxia (Hesser et al. 1968), increased pressure, and gas density (Flynn et al. 1972), and apnea caused by cold water immersion (Pailer and Hansen 1972). Finally, the basic endocrine and autonomic control of heart rate, which involves the catecholamines, circulating thyroid hormone, core temperature, and so forth, provides for a highly individualized heart rate for various levels of exercise.

Very fast (>170 bpm) or very slow (<50 bpm) heart rates are a clear danger signal when compared to rates typical of the diver's operation situation. Heart rate monitoring can be accomplished by surface or subcutaneous electrodes with electrocardiogram (ECG) readout, digital or ear lobe pulse sensors, or precordial Doppler monitoring, which affords acoustic information as well.

Superficial electrodes applied with electrode gel, sealed with collodion, taped in place, and held securely by the diver's wet suit are well tolerated and can supply surface personnel with an on-line readout of the pulse. Three electrodes should be used for greater reliability and to decrease 60-Hz noise. Numerous studies have been conducted at the U.S. Naval Medical Research Institute and U.S. Navy Experimental Diving Unit using this method.

Pulse-rate monitoring is not currently done in operational diving, because the data cannot be accurately interpreted. Establishing absolute end points is not presently possible without restricting the diver's activity unduly, and it has never been shown that tachycardia or bradycardia per se predicts an unsafe situation. This method will probably be most useful to monitor the trend of an individual's heart rate, which could then be compared to his previous norm.

The future for cardiac monitoring is exciting, since research based on the clinician's need to assess cardiac output noninvasively is beginning to produce results. Research based on the principle that transthoracic impedance changes with variations in intrathoracic air and fluid volumes has used the electrical impedance cardiogram's first derivative (dZ/dt) to measure isovolumic contraction time and systolic time intervals, coupled with the standard ECG. These cardiac functions are thought to be even better sensors than cardiac output, because they suggest changes in myocardial efficiency. Recently, the technical obstacle of motion artifact has been overcome by use of the computerized ensemble averaging technique, which allows monitoring during exercise (Gollen et al. 1978).

The software to monitor cardiovascular function in the diver beyond the general assessment of pulse rate is not yet available. Until noninvasive means are available, invasive procedures such as central lines to measure central venous pressure (CVP) and cardiac output should only be used in diving casualties. Very often the situation typical of operational diving—bare chamber, minimal equipment, remote location—precludes even CVP monitors, despite the patient's fluid needs in cases involving either pulmonary decompression sickness or a paretic lesion. Pulmonary artery catheters have not been used in diving casualties. The Foley catheter, the "poor man's" measure of cardiac output, therefore, becomes an extremely important monitor in such situations.

3. Pulmonary Monitoring

Lung function may be divided into two distinct entities: ventilation and oxygenation. Ventilation, or the removal of carbon dioxide from the body, is perhaps the most critical of all functions, since hypercapnia predisposes divers to decompression sickness, central nervous system oxygen toxicity, and nitrogen narcosis. More importantly, hypercapnia is subjectively well tolerated by the diver under hyperoxic conditions but is exacerbated by the respiratory depression induced by hyperoxia, added dead space, increased gas densities, and immersion-induced changes in physiological dead space.

The importance of monitoring the "bellows" function of the lung has been demonstrated at the Naval Experimental Diving Unit, where divers with normal blood gases became dizzy from exercise-induced dyspnea while working underwater at 1600 fsw (50 ATA) (Spaur et al. 1977). In addition, dyspnea, which limited divers' work in another Navy-funded study, has been found to worsen after the cessation of exercise (Thalmann 1979). In addition, this dyspnea could not be predicted or related to any of the following monitored parameters: minute ventilation (MV), mixed-expired P_{O_2}, mixed-expired P_{CO_2}, end-tidal P_{O_2}, end-tidal P_{CO_2}, heart rate, respiratory rate, vital capacity, expiratory reserve volume, tidal volume, respiratory flow rate, esophageal pressure, mouth pressure, or midthoracic hydrostatic pressure. Despite these measurements, these researchers were unable to predict dyspnea in divers before its onset or to prevent its transient increase by having the divers exercise. Of the variables measured, only minute ventilation correlates somewhat with dyspnea; the usefulness of this measurement might be increased by knowing a diver's predive MV for a given level of work.

The U.S. Navy's recent development of a technique for measuring lung volumes by paired magnetometers may provide an accurate, on-line method of following minute ventilation and other ventilatory parameters (Robertson et al. 1978). The Navy is currently conducting research to apply these monitors to active, submerged divers; if this work is successful, a noninvasive, easily tolerated monitor without artifactual error will be available for ventilatory monitoring. However, ventilation monitoring is presently limited to listening to diver breathing patterns over voice communication systems.

Oxygenation monitoring has received much less attention because of the generally hyperoxic environment of most dives and the known thresholds for central nervous system oxygen toxicity. The Navy continues its development of P_{O_2} sampling in the inspiratory hose, with servofeedback to the oxygen delivery system in deep experimental closed-circuit rigs. However, such on-line sampling is not applied in shallow-water diving, despite the known hypoxia-producing effects of immersion: decreased functional residual capacity (Arborelius et al. 1972), increased air trapping (Dahlbäck and Lundgren 1972), and ventilation-perfusion mismatching (Litman et al. 1969).

4. Temperature Monitoring

Divers have been lost both to hyperthermia from equipment malfunction and to hypothermia, the insidious killer which, as well as being a direct cause of death, may distort the diver's judgment until he makes a fatal mistake. Much is known about the causes of hypothermia in the diving environment. The monitoring of core temperature remains a technical obstacle, but a solution to this problem may be close at hand.

Core temperature can be accurately followed by radio-pills or by placing thermal probes in the external auditory canal. Radio-pills will be practical when the cost of the pill decreases to the point where the pills can be disposed of after one use. The use of ear probes will depend on diver acceptance and the development of a nonocclusive way to hold the probe stationary in the external canal. Rectal probes are not well tolerated by divers, and the delay between body core and rectal temperature is notorious.

The development of a mathematical model to predict thermal stress and of more advanced methods of temperature monitoring awaits the future. Much of the research in this field has been done by the Yellow Spring Institute, in Yellow Springs, Ohio, and has been supported by the Office of Naval Research. This laboratory is currently investigating a device to heat an area of skin until negative heat flux is attained. The temperature gradient established by this method should be proportional to the underlying core temperature.

Accidents caused by hypothermia are often preceded by obvious signs of distress, such as shivering or confusion; in the future, these accidents will be prevented by core temperature monitoring.

5. Bubble Detection

Since Robert Boyle first described a bubble in the eye of a snake during decompression, scientists have assumed that the symptoms of decompression sickness are either directly or indirectly related to bubble formation and growth. Although this concept has never been proved scientifically, the overwhelming amount of data supporting this belief makes the search for *in vivo* bubbles attractive to the diving medical officer.

Although Behnke (1942) first coined the term "silent bubbles" to describe what he thought were asymptomatic bubbles during decompression, it was Franklin who popularized the use of the Doppler effect of reflected ultrasound from the moving bloodstream to detect these bubbles (Franklin et al. 1961). In 1968, Spencer and Campbell demonstrated that a Doppler flowmeter could detect gas emboli in the vena cava of sheep before the onset of decompression sickness (Spencer and Campbell 1968). Numerous animal and human experiments have been done subsequently to show that bubbles exist not only before the onset of decompression sickness but that divers routinely bubble when diving on standard U.S. Navy air tables, although these divers do not develop clinical bends. Spencer and Campbell (1972) detected asymptomatic venous gas emboli in the pulmonary vein using the Doppler technique in human volunteers exposed to 30 fsw on air for 12 hr and decompressed to the surface in 20 sec. Pain-only symptoms, relieved by recompression on USN Treatment Table 5, developed in five of these individuals (Spencer and Campbell 1972).

The detection of precordial bubbles by the Doppler technique was refined by the development of a bubble-scoring system (Spencer and Johanson 1974). This scoring system, originally an audiometric means to quantify bubble events, has been adapted to computer analysis by several other researchers. The scoring system is shown in Table III-7. This grading system continues to be refined; Johanson and Postles (1976) have identified an earlier, pre-Grade I signal, and Powell and Spencer (1977) have identified a more severe Grade "IV-plus" signal associated with severe decompression sickness in sheep.

Quantifying the precordial signal has enabled researchers to correlate high bubble scores with dives involving heavy work (Pilmanis et al. 1976), diver fatigue before the dive (Masurel et al. 1976), and injection of a vasodilator before experimental exposure of dogs (Pilmanis 1975). Neuman and his co-workers (1976) reported no statistically significant correlation between bubble scores and increased serum viscosity. These workers did note a correlation between sequential Grade IV scores and decompression sickness, although the high bubble scores were of no predictive value.

Table III-7
Doppler Bubble-Scoring System

Score	Bubble Signal
Zero	No bubbles heard
Grade I	Occasional bubbles
Grade II	Bubbles heard in less than half of the cardiac cycles
Grade III	Bubbles heard during more than half or all cardiac cycles
Grade IV	Bubble signal obscures normal heart sounds and is continuous

a. Ultrasound Research and Methods

Several areas of research involving ultrasound techniques have shown promise in recent years. Gross perfusion defects have been detected by radioisotopic lung scans used for screening purposes. Buckles and Knox (1969) used the interaction of a converging monochromatic light beam and a traveling acoustic wave, which produces Bragg diffraction that is detected by telescopic imaging, to identify bubbles. Changes in the speed of sound that occur when bubbles pass through a beam traversing a column of liquid may in the future be detected by ultrasonic velocimeters, and presently available flowmeters can be used to measure decreased vascular flow caused by intravascular bubbles. Research is being conducted to develop a technique to measure the change in electrical conductivity that occurs in the tissues after gas phase separation, and to develop computer-assisted ECG monitoring and phonocardiographic techniques to detect bubbles.

Four methods of ultrasound detection are presently in use. These include the attenuation of sound waves by bubbles, distortion of the sound beam traversing a bubble-containing tissue, beta scans or echography, and using the Doppler effect of moving bubbles on sound waves. Of these four methods, the last has been most successful in fetal heart monitoring and surgical situations. Although much smaller objects can be detected with the Doppler than with the beta scan, even the Doppler technique cannot detect stationary bubbles. Pulsed beam techniques and moving the sensor offer the greatest promise for detecting stationary bubbles. The most common technique involves two half-inch piezoelectrode crystals separated from each other by 1.3 cm and angled to provide maximum reception of a beam focused several centimeters below the skin. The exciter crystal emits a sound beam with a frequency of approximately 5 MHz, which is reflected to the receiving electrode; any frequency shift is detected by rather simple electronic equipment. The precordial probe is thus placed over the pulmonary outflow tract, and frequency shifts caused by bubbles are audible as "chirps" and "beeps."

This method still has many limitations. Anatomy limits the number of sampling sites accessible without using invasive techniques. Precordial monitoring detects only intravascular bubbles and offers no information about their point of origin. The presence of cardiac background noise makes location of the sensor critical and interpretation of the signal extremely difficult. It should be noted that a continuous exposure to energy in excess of 40 mW/cm^2 can cause cavitation in tissue; whether or not the Doppler itself can cause bubble formation in supersaturated tissue has never been studied. However, the effects of sonic-caused resonance on diffusion across the bubble/tissue interface makes bubbles grow faster.

There is a great deal of controversy about the significance of precordial bubbles in divers with peripheral symptoms. Classically, bubble scores have been equated with the formation of gas emboli in the tissue. However, bubble scores may correlate better with a tissue release curve, as Kindwall's inert gas elimination curves have demonstrated (Kindwall 1975; Kindwall et al. 1975), than with gas emboli.

b. Clinical Significance

Final evaluation of the clinical usefulness of the Doppler ultrasonic bubble detector must await an understanding of the complex relationships between the clinical signs and symptoms of decompression sickness and the physiological effects of bubbles in blood and tissue. Saturation divers using deep diffusion-limited tables for decompression have developed bends without evidence of precordial bubbles, and it is now generally agreed that divers bubble without bends. The occurrence and degree of precordial bubbling may depend on the physics of bubble growth and hematological transport. Further, symptoms may arise from secondary bubble effects, such as bradykinin and prostaglandin release by the lungs, changes in local tissue perfusion autoregulation, or electrochemical effects around the blood/bubble interface.

Little work of real clinical significance has been conducted to date. Tests of decompression tables have led some researchers to conclude that a 20% occurrence of venous gas emboli is safe and acceptable in a decompression profile. However, what Doppler-detected parameters should be used to design tables has not been established. For example, should a table be designed to permit a maximum allowable percentage of bubbles, a maximum depth or time of onset of bubbles, a maximum duration of bubbling, or should it take bubble location into account?

The most thorough operational tests of the Doppler detector were conducted by Pilmanis (1975) in a 5-year study sponsored by the Office of Naval Research. Dogs and scuba divers were studied at the Catalina Marine Science Center in Avalon, California. Pilmanis reported that dogs that had been given a vasodilator before a resting dive to 100 fsw for 20 min had significantly higher bubble scores than nonvasodilated animals. Bubble scores in both dogs and scuba divers rose precipitously when their tissues were near their calculated M-values (*see* Chapter IV for a discussion of M-values) on surfacing. Exercise during compression increased bubble scores over those of resting controls, although little change in scores was noted in subjects who exercised during decompression.

Neuman and his group (1976) showed that bubble scores in human divers could be decreased during chamber dives to 210 fsw for 50 min and to 170 fsw for 30 min by adding a 2- or 3-min stop 10 fsw below the deepest scheduled stop. The bubble scores of these divers were also lower than those of divers decompressed on the next deeper schedule (220 or 180 fsw, respectively). The Doppler technique may indicate when the initial decompression stop should be made during ascent from a dive, by signaling when bubbles begin.

Johanson and Postles (1976) used the Doppler detector to monitor men in working dives over Cobb Seamount off the Washington State coast. Asymptomatic venous gas emboli were heard after 17 of 29 dives (59%); there was a 10% incidence of pain-only decompression sickness in this series as a whole. The number of bends incidents was reduced to zero when the Doppler technique was used to determine when prophylactic surface oxygen breathing was indicated (D. C. Johanson, personal communication).

The U.S. Naval School of Salvage and Diving (Bayne 1978) after completing a two-year prospective blind analysis of bubble scores and clinical outcomes of chamber dives to 290 fsw for 10 min, reported that the Doppler technique had no predictive value when used without clinical information. In this study, precordial signals were taped and read at a remote location by a recognized expert, who was asked to score the signal at each decompression stop and at half-hour intervals on the surface, as well as to predict which divers were susceptible to decompression sickness. Divers were managed clinically by a physician with no knowledge of the results of the recordings. Only 4 of the 87 dives monitored yielded signals of quality too poor to be interpreted; on the 83 remaining dives, 36 divers were judged, based on bubble scores, to be "at risk." In this group, five cases of decompression sickness occurred; two involving pain-only bends, two skin bends, and one involving the spinal cord. In the 47 "safe" dives, as determined by bubble scores, there were three cases of bends: two pain-only cases, one of which occurred during decompression, and one case involving the spinal cord. The eight bends cases could not be distinguished, on the basis of either bubble scores or depth or time of onset, from the large number of asymptomatic bubblers. Clearly, in deep and short air dives the bubble signal alone, without clinical input, is too sensitive and nonspecific to be of operational use.

C. GRESHAM BAYNE

References

ARBORELIUS, M., JR., U. I. BALLDIN, B. LILJA. AND C. E. G. LUNDGREN 1972. Regional lung function in man during immersion with the head above water. *Aerosp. Med.* 43(7):701–707.

ASTRAND, P.-O., AND K. RODAHL 1977. *Textbook of Physiology* (2nd ed.). New York: McGraw-Hill.

BAYNE, C. G. 1978. Acute decompression sickness: 50 cases. *J. Am. Coll. Emerg. Phys.* 7: 351–354.

BEHNKE, A. R. 1942. Effects of high pressures; prevention and treatment of compressed air illness. *Med. Clin. N. Am.* July: 1213–1236.

BUCKLES, R. G., AND C. KNOX 1969. In vivo bubble detection by acoustical-optical imaging techniques. *Nature* 222: 771–772.

DAHLBÄCK, G. O., AND C. E. G. LUNDGREN 1972. Pulmonary air trapping induced by water immersion. *Aerosp. Med.* 43: 768–774.

FLYNN, E. T., T. E. BERGHAGE. AND E. F. COIL 1972. Influence of increased ambient pressure and gas density on cardiac rate in man. Rep. 4-72, Panama City, FL: U.S. Navy Experimental Diving Unit.

FRANKLIN, D. L., W. SCHLEGEL. AND R. F. RUSHMER 1961. Blood flow measured by Doppler frequency shift of back-scattered ultrasound. *Science* 134: 265–284.

GOLLEN, F. P., N. KIZAKEVICH. AND J. MCDERMOTT 1978. Continuous electrode monitoring of systolic time intervals during exercise. *Br. Heart J.* 40: 1390–1396.

HESSER, C. M., L. FAGRAEUS. AND D. LINNARSSON 1968. *Cardiorespiratory Responses to Exercise in Hyperbaric Environment*. Stockholm: Karolinska Institute.

JOHANSON, D. C., AND W. F. POSTLE 1976. Progression of VGE formation in open water diving. In: *Proceedings of the Third Annual Meeting of the North Pacific Chapter of the Undersea Medical Society*. Grand Forks: Univ. of North Dakota.

KINDWALL, E. P. 1975. Measurement of helium elimination from man during decompression breathing air or oxygen. *Undersea Biomed. Res.* 2: 277–284.
KINDWALL, E. P., A. BAZ, E. N. LIGHTFOOT, E. H. LANPHIER. AND A. SEIREG 1975. Nitrogen elimination in man during decompression. *Undersea Biomed. Res.* 2: 285–297.
LITMANN, M., P. CERETELLI, A. CHINET, J. P. FURBER, L. E. FARHI. AND D. W. RENNIE 1969. Redistribution of pulmonary blood flow during submersion. *Physiologist* 12: 285.
MASUREL, G., R. GUILLERM. AND P. CAVENEL 1976. Detection ultra-sonore par effect Doppler de bulles circulantes chez l'homme lars de 98 plongees a l'air. *Med. Aeronaut. Spat. Med. Subaquat. Hyp.* 15: 199–201.
NAVAL MEDICAL RESEARCH INSTITUTE 1977. Program for hyperbaric research and development. LAPROM Document No. 2. Bethesda, MD: Naval Medical Research Institute.
NEUMAN, T., R. GOAD. AND P. G. LINAWEAVER 1976. Changes in hematoligical and hemorrheological parameters following dives to 210 fsw and 132 fsw and their correlation with bubble score (Abstract). *Undersea Biomed. Res.* 3:A37–A38.
PAILER, P., AND H. G. HANSEN 1972. Cardiac response to apnea and water immersion during exercise in man. *J. Appl. Physiol.* 32: 193–198.
PILMANIS, A. A. 1975. Intravenous gas emboli in man after compressed air diving. Tech. Rep., O.N.R. Contract N00014-67-A-0269-0026. Washington, DC: Office of Naval Research.
PILMANIS, A. A., S. K. CHRISTOPERSON. AND H. J. DWYER 1976. The effect of "at depth" exercise on the formation of venous gas emboli in man during and after compressed air ocean diving. In: *Proceedings of the Third Annual Meeting of the North Pacific Chapter of the Undersea Medical Society*. Grand Forks: Univ. of North Dakota.
POWELL, M. R., AND M. P. SPENCER 1977. Physiological significance of Doppler-detected bubbles in decompression sickness (Abstract). *Undersea Biomed. Res.* 4:A25.
ROBERTSON, C. H., JR., M. E. BRADLEY, L. M. FRASER. AND L. D. HOMER 1978. Computerized measurement of ventilation with four chest wall magnetometers. Rep. No. NMRI 78-48. Bethesda, MD: Naval Medical Research Institute.
SPAUR, W. H., L. W. RAYMOND, M. M. KNOTT, J. C. CROTHERS, W. R. BRAITHWAITE, E. D. THALMANN. AND D. F. UDDIN 1977. Dyspnea in divers at 49.5 ATA: mechanical, not chemical in origin. *Undersea Biomed. Res.* 4: 183–198.
SPENCER, M. P., AND S. D. CAMPBELL 1968. Decompression of bubbles in venous and arterial blood during hyperbaric decompression. *Bull. Mason Clin.* 22: 1.
SPENCER, M. P., AND S. D. CAMPBELL 1972. Decompression venous gas emboli (Abstract). Program of the Fifth Symposium on Underwater Physiology, Freeport, Bahamas.
SPENCER, M. P., AND D. C. JOHANSON 1974. Investigation of new principles for human decompression schedules using the Doppler blood bubble detector. Tech. Rep., O.N.R. Contract N00014-73-C-0094. Washington, DC: Office of Naval Research.
THALMANN, E. D. 1979. Monitoring the diver's ventilatory situation. In: *Monitoring Vital Signs in the Diver*, edited by C. E. G. Lundgren. Bethesda, MD: Undersea Medical Society.
U.S. NAVY 1973. *U.S. Navy Diving Manual*. Washington, DC: U.S. Navy Dept.

H. Thermal Considerations

1. Heat Exchange in Air at One Atmosphere

In a normal person the temperature of the core of the body, i.e., the central nervous system and the thoracic, abdominal, and pelvic viscera, varies little in the face of large alterations in environmental temperature. On the other hand, skin temperature is extraordinarily variable. Under most conditions body temperature (average and deep) represents a balance between heat produced by the body and heat lost from the body.

In general, when a steady state exists, the exchange of heat between body and environment can be expressed by the following equation:

$$M - E \pm C \pm R = 0 \tag{1}$$

where M = rate at which heat is produced by metabolism; E = rate of heat lost by the evaporation of water; C = rate of loss (or gain) of heat by convection; and R = rate of loss (or gain) of heat by radiation. In the many instances of temporary non-steady state, the right side of Equation 1 (defined as "heat storage") is not zero. For instance, when, in vigorous exercise, metabolism for a time exceeds the loss of heat by evaporation, convection, and radiation, heat storage becomes positive. On the other hand, it will have a negative value when, on exposure to cold, heat loss is great and the compensatory increase in metabolism is somewhat delayed.

Evaporative heat loss depends on the fact that it requires a definite amount of heat to change a given amount of any liquid into vapor without changing the temperature. In the human body, each gram of water vaporized from the surface at room temperature entails the loss of about 580 cal. In general, evaporative heat loss (E) per unit body surface area is expressed as follows:

$$E = h_e \frac{(\overline{P}_{sk} - P_a)}{\gamma} \tag{2}$$

where h_e = evaporative heat transfer coefficient in cal/(m² · hr · °C), or W/(m² · °C); $\overline{P}_{sk}$ = mean water vapor pressure at the skin (saturated at skin temperature), in mmHg; P_a = water vapor pressure of the ambient gas, in mmHg; γ = the so-called psychrometer constant, introduced to give h_e the physical dimension of W/(m² · °C). At 20°C and 1 ATA air, γ has a value of 0.50 mmHg/°C.

The rate of evaporative heat loss is largely dependent on the rate of sweating (or the activity of the sweat glands). However, even in the absence of active sweating, evaporative heat loss continues because of insensible perspiration. Perspiration is the passage of water vapor through the skin by processes (including diffusion) that do not involve sweating. As discussed later, the efficiency of perspiration and sweating decreases with increasing ambient pressure (or gas density) because the evaporative mass transfer coefficient is related approximately inversely to barometric pressure (or gas density).

Convective heat transfer (gain or loss) is limited to fluids (liquids and gases); it is simply a mechanical process of mixing in which a cooler fluid comes into contact with a warmer fluid, becomes heated by conduction, and carries heat elsewhere. Thus, the forcing of a current of cool air over a heated body cools that body by convection. When a man sits in a draft, the air near his skin, air which has been warmed by conduction, is replaced by cold air that is warmed in turn; heat may thus be continually abstracted from the surface of his body. In general, convective heat loss (C) per unit body surface area is expressed as follows:

$$C = h_c (\overline{T}_{sk} - T_a) \tag{3}$$

where h_c = convective heat transfer coefficient (or convective heat conductance) in cal/(m² · hr · °C), or W/(m² · °C); $\overline{T}_{sk}$ = mean skin temperature in °C; T_a = ambient temperature in °C. The value of h_c is influenced by ambient pressure, velocity of air movement, and the density and specific heat of the fluid surrounding the body surface. In fact, the higher convective heat transfer capacity of water or a hyperbaric gas mixture is the main thermal problem associated with diving.

Radiant heat is transmitted by electromagnetic waves. Heat waves and light waves are identical except as regards wavelength, and they all travel at the same velocity (about 186,300 miles/sec). As a result of the heat liberated by metabolic processes, a person usually radiates energy through the air to other solid objects and not to the surrounding air. For instance, a man sitting in a heated room in the winter loses a good deal of heat toward a cold window pane and less heat toward the walls and ceiling. In general, the radiative heat loss (R) is proportional to the surface area of the body, to its emissive power, and to the difference in temperature between the radiating body and the body to which it is radiating.

Heat loss in man is effected mainly through the skin and partly through the respiratory tract and lungs. Heat is lost through the skin for the most part by radiation, convection, and evaporation of water. Through the respiratory tract and lungs, it is lost mainly by evaporation and partly by convection as the inspired air is warmed; increased ventilation augments the loss through the respiratory tract chiefly by increasing evaporation. On the other hand, increased density and the specific heat of a hyperbaric gas mixture augment the loss through the respiratory tract by increasing convection.

The relative amounts of heat lost from the body through the three avenues vary with conditions. When a person is seated in a room with air, walls, floor, and ceiling at a moderate temperature and with the surrounding air relatively dry and in slight motion, radiation and convection each account for about 40% and evaporation for about 20% of the total heat loss. Under such circumstances metabolic activities constitute the only source of heat, for the subject is not gaining any heat from the environment. As the air temperature decreases, the thermal gradient between the skin surface and the surrounding air increases. As a result, the percentage of heat lost to the environment through convection increases. On the other hand, when the air temperature increases to a level above the skin temperature, the heat gained through radiation and convection is added to the heat of metabolism, and the core temperature can be kept from rising only by the evaporation of sweat.

The zone of ambient temperature between 25°C and 30°C may be considered the zone of vasomotor regulation of body temperature in an unclothed man. In this zone, heat loss (radiation and convection) may be altered by changing the gradient ($\overline{T}_{sk} - T_a$) through skin and limb blood flow changes, and thermal equilibrium may be maintained without either sweating or increasing metabolism.

The overall human skin blood flow ranges from 150 to 200 milliliters (ml) per min in a cool environment and up to 2000 ml/min for conditions of heat stress. In some extremities the range of variation may be as high as 100-fold; this range is necessary to adjust the flow of heat from core to periphery. An expression of the delivery of heat from core to surface is the so-called tissue conductance (or whole-body conductance), calculated by a relation analogous to Ohm's law:

$$\text{cal/(hr} \cdot {}°\text{C)} = \frac{\dot{H}}{T_r - \overline{T}_{sk}} \qquad (4)$$

where cal/(hr · °C) = conductance; $\dot{H}$ = total heat loss from core to surface in cal/hr; T_r = core (rectal) temperature in °C; $\overline{T}_{sk}$ = mean skin temperature in °C.

Sometimes the tissue insulation (the reciprocal of conductance) is used to express the delivery of heat from core to surface. The lowest conductance of 5–10 kilocalories (kcal)/hr per °C is usually observed at the lowest end of the zone of vasomotor regulation; i.e., about 25°C in the ordinary air environment, which primarily represents the conductance of the subcutaneous fat. With heat exposure and maximum blood flows, the conductance may reach 150 kcal/hr per °C. There is thus about a 20-fold variation in conductance through the tissues. The lowest end of the zone of vasomotor regulation is called "the critical air temperature." Below this temperature, the core temperature cannot be maintained without increasing metabolic heat production, i.e., shivering. Unfortunately, however, convection increases because of the body movements during shivering, leading to an increase in total heat loss (and hence conductance).

The comfort zone is defined as the range of temperature in which heat loss and heat production are approximately the same and skin vessels are somewhat dilated. Below this zone peripheral vessels constrict, and above it they dilate progressively and vaporization suddenly increases because of sweating. In air at 1 ATA, the comfort zone is between 29°C and 31°C in an unclothed resting man and between 20°C and 30°C in a lightly dressed and mildly active man.

2. Thermal Balance in Water at One Atmosphere Absolute

That the human body cools faster in water than in air of the same temperature is well recognized. The main reasons for this are that the specific heat of water is 1000 times, and thermoconductivity 25 times, greater than those of air. This direct loss of body heat to the water is the dominant thermal problem of the diver and, in fact, dive duration is primarily determined by this body heat loss.

a. Heat Transfer Coefficient of Water and Critical Water Temperature

The primary avenue of heat transfer from the body surface to the surrounding water is convection and conduction; because of the long-wave infrared radiation of the body surface, and because water absorbs so effectively, radiation transfer is negligible. The combined heat transfer coefficient for convection and conduction varies from 44 W/(m² · °C) or 38 kcal/(m² · hr · °C) in still water to an average of 64 W/(m² · °C), or 55 kcal/(m² · hr · °C) in stirred water. Shivering in still water raises the heat transfer coefficient from 44 to 50 W/(m² · °C) (Boutelier et al. 1971). According to the analysis by Rapp (1971), the conductive heat transfer coefficient is about 11 W/(m² · °C) regardless of the degree of stirring, while the convective heat transfer coefficient increases from 94 W/(m² · °C) in still water to 400 W/(m² · °C) at a swimming speed of 0.5 m/sec. These values may be compared with the 1 to 2 W/(m² · °C) observed at 1 ATA air (26.5°C) by the U.S. Navy group (Raymond et al. 1975). Despite such a marked difference in the convective heat transfer coefficient between air and water, heat loss to water has been estimated to be only about two to five times that in air at the same temperature, indicating that heat loss in water is largely limited by the body (core-to-skin) tissue insulation and not by the skin-to-water heat transfer coefficient. Although the thermal comfort zone for a resting unclothed man immersed in water varies inversely with the subcutaneous fat thickness of the subject, it is reported to be 33°C–35°C (Craig and Dvorak 1966; Smith and Hanna 1975). Moreover, the critical water temperature, i.e., the lowest end of the zone of vasomotor regulation at which maximal peripheral vasoconstriction develops, is also as high as 29°C–33°C, depending upon subcutaneous fat thickness (Figure III-27). Since the water temperature most often involved in diving is much lower than this range, it is obvious that divers are exposed to considerable cold water stress.

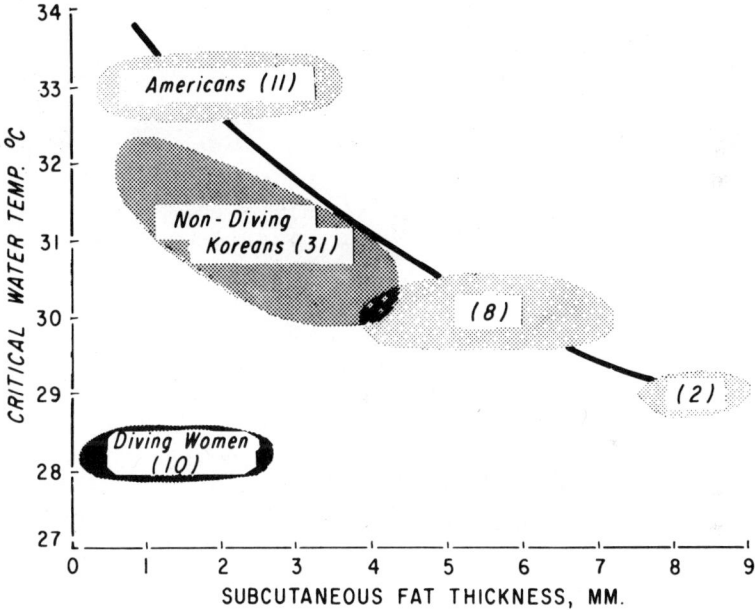

Figure III-27. Critical water temperature (defined as the coldest water subjects tolerate for 3 hr without shivering) as a function of mean subcutaneous fat thickness in U.S. men and women, nondiving Korean men and women, and Korean diving women. Areas encompass range of values for indicated number of subjects. Note the low critical water temperature for diving women relative to their subcutaneous fat thickness. [Adapted from Rennie (1965).]

b. Quantity of Heat Loss

The Korean women divers (ama) engaged in daily breath-hold diving through the year have been studied extensively. The temperature of the water in which these divers work varies from about 25°C in midsummer to 10°C in midwinter; however, the ama wear only a cotton bathing suit throughout the year, although their subcutaneous fat thickness is very small (0–2 mm). These divers stay in water until the rectal temperature decreases to about 35°C; this takes about 40 min and 20 min, respectively, in summer and winter (Figure III-28). By the time the rectal temperature drops to 35°C, they feel extremely cold, develop violent shivering, and come back to the shore to rewarm. Their oxygen consumption in the water increases about 2.5 times during the summer and 3.5 times during the winter. Based on these data, the cumulative extra heat loss per diving

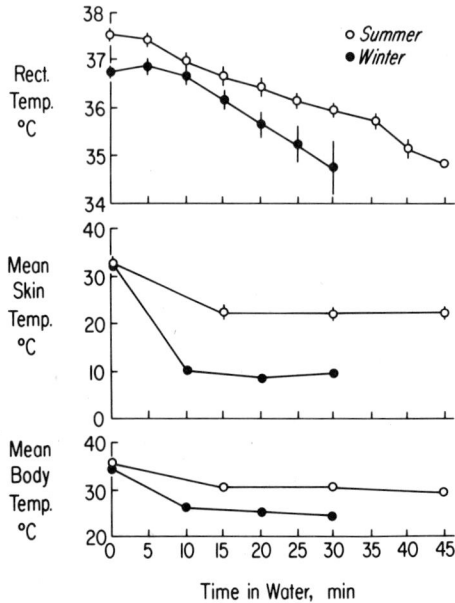

Figure III-28. Changes in rectal, mean skin, and mean body temperature during a diving work shift. [Adapted from Kang et al. (1965).]

work shift is estimated to be 388 kcal in summer and 557 kcal in winter. Since these divers work for two or three shifts a day in summer and only one or two in the winter, the total extra heat loss is estimated to be on the order of 1000 kcal/day (Kang et al. 1965). Because they are exposed to such severe cold water stress daily for many years, they have developed certain physiological adaptations to cold.

More recently, the magnitude of heat loss during immersion has been determined using direct calorimetry. According to Craig and Dvorak (1976), during 1 hr of immersion in water of 24°C the greatest heat loss occurred in the first 10 min and amounted to 84 kcal. The total net loss from body heat stores during the hour amounted to 183 kcal, 60% of which was lost in the first 20 min. Overall, the total heat loss during 1 hr of immersion in 24°C water amounted to 275 kcal. Webb (1978) conducted studies on three divers clad in lightweight dry suits who swam underwater in a tank at water temperatures of 5°C, 10°C, and 15°C until they reached a voluntary tolerance limit for cold. On the average, the subjects tolerated a loss of 210 kcal of body heat, with a drop of 0.3°C to 1.1°C in rectal temperature. In another series of similar studies, Webb reported a heat loss of 292 kcal in one subject during immersion in water of 5°C (Webb 1976). These results, obtained with direct calorimetry, indicate that a diver can voluntarily tolerate a loss of about 300 kcal of body heat.

The amount of heat loss measured by direct calorimetry is considerably less than that reported in the ama (Kang et al. 1965), which was calculated from increases in oxygen consumption and decreases in mean body temperature ($\Delta \overline{T}_b$). Using a conventional approach to calculate heat exchange in air, $\Delta \overline{T}_b$ during water immersion was computed as follows:

$$\Delta \overline{T}_b = 0.65 \, \Delta T_r + 0.35 \, \Delta \overline{T}_{sk} \tag{5}$$

However, applying this formula to human subjects immersed in water has not been validated. Direct calorimetry provides a more accurate determination of $\Delta \overline{T}_b$ using the following formula:

$$\Delta \overline{T}_b = \frac{\Delta \dot{H}}{0.83 \cdot BW} \tag{6}$$

where $\Delta \dot{H}$ = net heat loss for a specified period of time in kcal, determined by direct calorimetry; 0.83 = specific heat of the body in kcal/(°C · kg); and BW = body weight in kg.

Figure III-29 shows a comparison of $\Delta \overline{T}_b$ values obtained from calorimetry data (using Eq. 6) with those computed from ΔT_r and $\Delta \overline{T}_{sk}$ (using Eq. 5) during cooling in water (Webb 1978). The dashed line in the figure indicates the line of identity and the solid line the actual data. A linear relationship exists between the two values after cooling has produced a net heat loss of more than 100 kcal. However, it is important to note that the two $\Delta \overline{T}_b$ values are identical only at one point (approximately −4°C). Therefore, depending upon the degree of cooling, the net heat loss calculated from ΔT_r and $\Delta \overline{T}_{sk}$ could either overestimate or underestimate mean body temperature. This is important since most investigators do not have calorimeters and have to estimate heat loss from ΔT_r and $\Delta \overline{T}_{sk}$. Values obtained by estimation are acceptable only as first approximations. The reasons for the discrepancy between the values of $\Delta \overline{T}_b$ obtained by the two methods are not known. At least part of the discrepancy is caused by the lag in ΔT_r during cooling. During the early stages of cooling, T_r transiently rises, remains unchanged, or decreases only slightly. In general, the faster the cooling the greater the separation between T_r and $\Delta \dot{H}$.

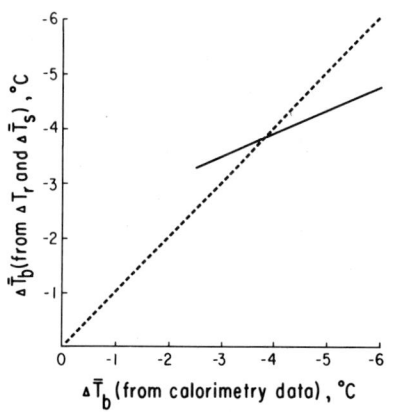

Figure III-29. Comparison of values of change in mean body temperature (ΔT_b) obtained from calorimetry data with those computed from changes in rectal and mean skin temperatures during immersion in water. [Adapted from Webb (1978).]

c. Protection by Wet Suits

When cold water stress is moderate (water temperature above 24°C), it is possible to maintain reasonable thermal equilibrium by increasing heat production through exercise. As stated earlier, thermoneutral water temperature is 33°C–35°C in a resting subject.

This decreases to 32°C when the subject is engaged in continuous underwater work that doubles oxygen consumption, and declines further to 26°C when continuous work triples oxygen consumption (Craig 1971).

However, as the water temperature decreases further (below 24°C), heat loss becomes so great that it becomes virtually impossible to maintain thermal balance without wearing a protective wet suit. Using direct calorimetry, Craig and Dvorak (1976) evaluated the protective effect of wearing a full wet suit during immersion in 24°C water. Figure III-30 shows the results of a typical experiment. Without a wet suit, this subject produced 90 kcal of heat during 1 hr of immersion while losing a total of 315 kcal; toward the end of the hour in water, the subject developed visible shivering. With the full wet suit both the rate of heat production and heat loss decreased by about 30%; by the end of 1.5 hr, both the cumulative heat production and total heat loss equaled that observed at the end of 1 hr without the suit. The most obvious difference with and without the protection of the suit was noted in the skin temperature (Figure III-31). Without protection, the mean skin temperature ($\overline{T}_{sk}$) of the immersed parts decreased rapidly, and at the end of the hour was only 1°C greater than the water temperature. With the jacket only, the $\overline{T}_{sk}$ remained considerably above the temperature of the water. Such a result might be expected, since four of the six sites at which the temperatures were measured were covered by the jacket. However, even the exposed upper and lower legs were 5°C warmer than without the suit. With the full wet suit on, the $\overline{T}_{sk}$ remained even higher. Figure III-31

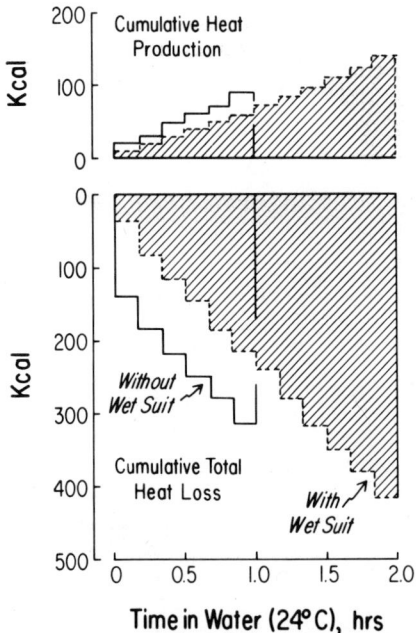

Figure III-30. Cumulative heat production and calorimetrically determined heat loss during immersion in water of 24°C with and without protective wet suits. [Adapted from Craig and Dvorak (1976).]

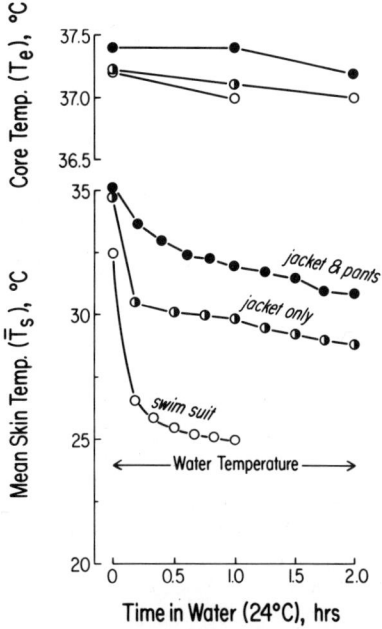

Figure III-31. Changes in core (esophageal) and mean skin temperature during immersion in water of 24°C with and without protective wet suits. [Adapted from Craig and Dvorak (1976).]

(*upper panel*) also shows the changes in core temperature (the esophageal temperature, T_e) during immersion with and without the protective suit. In all three cases, the T_e decreased by the same amount, 0.2°C. However, with the full suit on the decrease did not occur until the second hour. With jacket alone the rate of fall in T_e was about half that observed without this added protection. In both experiments with the suit, the subject was comfortable and felt cool only at the end of the 2 hr.

Using these data, Craig and Dvorak (1976) then computed the insulative value of the wet suit. Figure III-32 illustrates the approach they used, and Table III-8 gives various insulation values they computed. The total insulation (I_{total}) can be calculated from $(T_e - T_{H_2O})/\dot{H}$, or the reciprocal of conductance (C) (also see Eq. 4), and was about 0.11–0.13 (°C · m²)/W, regardless of whether the subject was protected by a wet suit during immersion. In the unprotected subject, this degree of insulation is provided by the peripheral tissues, i.e., the subcutaneous fat, nonperfused skin, and connective tissue, in the face of maximal peripheral vasoconstriction, i.e., $I_{total} = I_{tissue}$. On the other hand, in the subject with the full wet suit, there are two thermal conductivities or insulation indices in series, as depicted in Figure III-32. One part of the pathway for the heat loss to the water is from the core to the skin (I_{tissue}), and the other is from the skin through the suit to the water ($I_{wet\ suit}$). The former can be computed by using the gradient $(T_e - \overline{T}_{sk})$, and the latter using the gradient $(\overline{T}_{sk} - T_{H_2O})$. As shown in Table III-8,

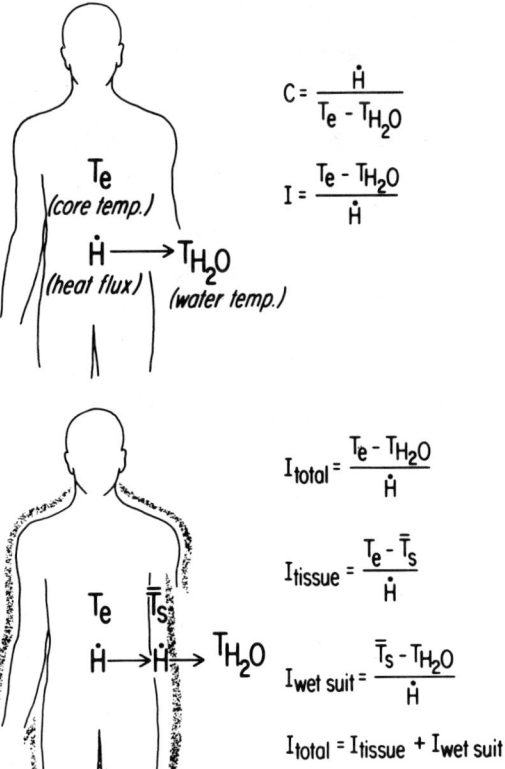

Figure III-32. Illustration of various components used to compute insulation values for tissue and wet suit.

Table III-8
Insulative Value of the Wet Suit during Immersion in 24°C Water[a]

	Insulation values		
	°C/(kcal·m²·hr)	(°C·m²)/W	clo[b]
$(T_e - T_{H_2O})/H$ at 1 hr (I_{total})			
Without wet suit	0.15	0.13	0.87
With wet suit	0.13	0.11	0.71
$(T_e - T_{sk})/H$ with wet suit (I_{tissue})	0.05	0.04	0.26
$(T_{sk} - T_{H_2O})/H$ with wet suit ($I_{wet\ suit}$)	0.08	0.07	0.45

[a] *See* Figure III-32 for definitions of various temperature and insulation terms. From Craig and Dvorak (1976).
[b] 1 clo = (0.155°C · m²)/W = 0.18°C/(kcal · m² · hr).

with the wet suit the I_{tissue} decreased to 0.04 (°C · m²)/W, while the suit provided additional insulation amounting to 0.07 (°C · m²)/W. In other words, wearing the suit keeps the skin warm and allows the subject to maintain blood flow to the periphery at a much greater rate than without the suit. In effect, the suit's major value seems to be maintaining the subject's comfort. Because the skin temperature is higher when wearing the wet suit, the subject did not shiver even though the core temperature decreased in 2 hr by the same degree as when the subject was without protection (Figure III-31).

d. Regional Heat Loss

As noted earlier, the critical water temperature (Figure III-27) is considerably higher than the critical air temperature. Since the maximal tissue insulation value is obtained at this critical water temperature, it is assumed that there is appreciable constriction of limb and skin blood vessels at this relatively high temperature. Rennie (1966) measured blood flow in the forearm and one finger and the rectal temperature of resting subjects during whole-body immersion in water of 35°C, 33°C, 32°C, and 30°C. In 35°C water, blood flow did not appreciably decline below control values, but in all cooler water both blood flows decreased dramatically. A similar result was obtained when the forearm alone was immersed in water. These results indicate that cutaneous cold receptor activity initiates vasoconstriction in water as warm as 33°C. These findings support the assumption that the maximal tissue insulation observed at the critical water temperature is indeed accompanied by marked constriction of the peripheral blood vessels.

To correlate blood flow and heat loss during immersion, Rennie (1966) determined heat flux from the forearm and finger during immersion. As expected, he found that finger skin heat flux and finger blood flow decreased by the same proportion during immersion in cooler water. Surprisingly, however, no such correlation between these two variables was observed for the forearm. Although resting forearm blood flow fell from an average of 15 to less than 1 ml/min per 100 ml tissue over a range of water temperature of 35.5°C–30°C, steady-state heat flux from the forearm did not decrease. These results imply that in cooler water, metabolic heat produced in the limb is conducted directly to the skin surface to be lost to the water environment at a rate equal to that of metabolic heat production. The limb circulation evidently contributes little to limb heat loss in water of critical temperature, although it may play an appreciable role in delivering heat to the skin in warmer water.

The quantity of heat lost from different body regions during the final 30 min of 3-hr immersions in water of critical temperature is summarized in Table III-9. It is interesting to note that skin heat loss is almost equally divided between trunk and limbs and to point out the importance of protecting the limbs during immersion in water. Although respiratory heat loss is not included in this table, it is estimated to be roughly 8%–10% of the total heat loss. Heat loss from the head is also not considered in Table III-9. It should be noted that the vessels of the head are uniquely unable to vasoconstrict in response to cold because of the absence of sphincteric control in scalp vessels (Bayne and Flynn 1982). Therefore, when diving in cold water the head should be well protected; it is interesting that the Korean and Japanese women divers do wrap their heads and necks.

Table III-9
Regional Heat Loss during Immersion in Water of Critical Temperature (30°C–31°C)[a]

Region	Fraction of surface area	Heat loss, kcal/hr/area	%
Thorax	0.18	10.5	29
Abdomen	0.18	9.0	25
Upper arms	0.08	1.8	5
Lower arms	0.08	3.7	10
Thighs	0.18	8.5	23
Lower legs	0.16	2.9	8
Total	0.86[b]	36.4	100

[a] From Rennie (1966).
[b] Excludes fingers, toes, and head.

e. Effects of Exercise

Exercise increases heat production and thus should reduce the rate at which body temperature falls during immersion in water. In fact, as noted above, thermoneutral temperature decreased to 26°C when the subject was engaged in continuous work that tripled oxygen consumption (Craig 1971). However, such beneficial effects of exercise seem to disappear in cold water. For instance, Pugh and Edholm (1955) observed that, in water at 16°C, the fatter of two men did indeed maintain his rectal temperature while swimming but the thinner man suffered a larger fall in temperature when he swam than when he kept still. In other words, exercise apparently had an adverse effect on temperature maintenance in the thin man.

A series of systematic immersion experiments carried out subsequently by Keatinge (1969) provided important conclusions about the paradoxical effect of exercise. The results of this study are shown in Figure III-33. Exercise increased these subjects' decreases in rectal temperature in both the 5°C and 15°C water, had no significant effect in 25°C water, and actually increased rectal temperature in 35°C water. It should be noted that

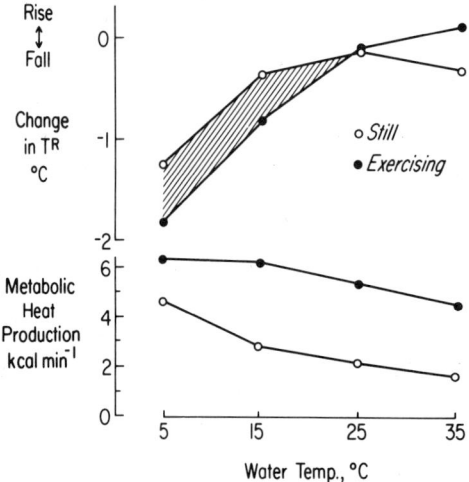

Figure III-33. Effect of exercise on body temperature and heat production in water at different temperatures. [Adapted from Keatinge (1969).]

the different effect of exercise on body temperature in water of different temperatures is not caused by exercise increasing heat production less in the cold than in the warm immersions; in fact, exercise increased heat production by as much in the 15°C immersions, and by only a little less in the 5°C immersion, than it did in the warmer immersion. This means that the adverse effect of exercise on body temperature in the cold water must be because exercise increases heat loss much more at the low than at the high water temperatures. Although additional data are needed to interpret these results, Keatinge (1969) states that "to a first approximation exercise can be assumed to have increased muscle blood flow, and therefore to have increased whole body conductance, by a comparable amount at all water temperatures." If we accept this assumption, it is possible to visualize a much greater increase in heat loss in cold water than in warm water because the temperature gradient ($T_r - T_{H_2O}$) increases as the water temperature decreases.

In another series of experiments, Keatinge observed that when the men were told to work as hard as possible in cold water (5°C and 15°C) they suffered smaller mean falls in rectal temperature than when they worked at the standard rate. This means that divers working in cold water can expect to maintain body temperature better if they work hard than if they work moderately. Another important observation made by Keatinge is the absence of an adverse effect of exercise on body temperature during brief immersions. For instance, the magnitude of the fall in rectal temperature in the first 10 min of cold immersion was always small and was not significantly increased by exercise. On the other hand, the adverse effect of exercise was increased in experiments that were prolonged beyond 20 min.

The core temperature is determined by the rate of heat loss relative to that of heat production. Since the rate of heat loss in cold water is inversely proportional to the subcutaneous fat thickness, it is of interest to find out if the adverse effect of exercise in cold immersions also occurs in fat men. The results of such an experiment are shown in Figure III-34. As expected, fat men were able to maintain their rectal temperatures quite well even in water of 5°C, but the adverse effect of exercise was still observed. In other words, exercise always increased the rate at which body temperature fell, regardless

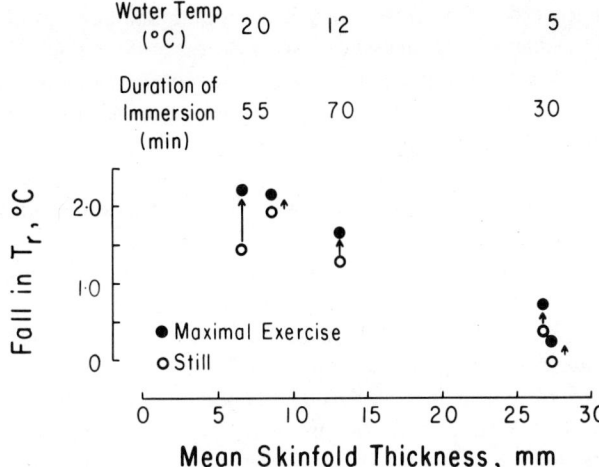

Figure III-34. Effect of maximal exercise on changes in rectal temperature of immersed subjects as a function of skinfold thickness. [Adapted from Keatinge (1969).]

of subcutaneous fat thickness. It should be stated, however, that the fat men had to be immersed in much colder water than the thin men before they were unable to stabilize their temperature when keeping still.

f. Symptoms of Severe and Prolonged Cold Exposure

Sudden cold water immersion of unclothed or lightly clad subjects leads to severe hypertension, cardiac arrhythmias (e.g., ventricular ectopic beats during the first few minutes), or even cardiac arrest (Keatinge 1969). Although the exact mechanism underlying the cardiac effect is not clear, it may be due to reflex-induced ventricular fibrillation. Another immediate effect of falling into very cold water is the gasping response in which, although the subject has a sense of difficulty in breathing, as much as 50–60 liters/min of air may be moved in and out of the lungs. This gasp effect lasts 1–2 min and is followed by a sustained hyperventilation lasting about 20 min, which results in a very considerable reduction in arterial P_{CO_2} and a marked respiratory alkalosis. In fact, some subjects show tetanic spasms during periods of immersion (Cooper 1976). It is likely that under these conditions there would be a significant reduction in cerebral blood flow (which is linked closely to the arterial P_{CO_2} level), and this could result in a clouding of judgment or loss of consciousness. The rapid onset of hyperventilation produced by cooling the skin clearly indicates that it is a reflex from cutaneous receptors. In this regard, it is important to note that habituation greatly reduces the hyperventilation produced by immersion in water (Keatinge 1969).

The reflex effects of cold on the circulation are bound to be much more dangerous to people with cardiovascular disease, e.g., coronary artery disease, hypertension. It is likely that cold causes angina by increasing the work and the oxygen requirement of hearts whose coronary arteries are too narrowed by disease to supply the extra blood to meet these requirements. In hypertensive patients, the sudden additional increase of pressure caused by cold immersion clearly carries the risk of rupturing a cerebral artery already weakened and dilated by the prolonged elevation of pressure.

During prolonged exposure to cold water stress, body heat storage decreases continuously. Various physiological mechanisms are activated during the early state to maintain the core temperature by both increasing heat production (i.e., shivering) and decreasing heat loss (i.e., peripheral vasoconstriction). However, these mechanisms cannot prevent the core temperature from continuously decreasing during prolonged exposure in cold water, as discussed above. The work of Hayward and co-workers (1975) has shown that the rate of rectal temperature decrease in subjects wearing light clothing and kapok life jackets is given by the equation $A = 0.0785 - 0.0034\ T_{H_2O}$, where A is the rectal temperature cooling rate in °C/min. As the degree of this hypothermia deepens, various cardiovascular, neuromuscular, and respiratory disturbances develop, eventually leading to loss of consciousness (at about 29°C–30°C of rectal temperature) and death (at about 25°C of rectal temperature). A tentative ordering of the symptoms of severe and prolonged cold exposure related to scales of body-heat loss and rectal temperature, as given by Webb (1976), is shown in Figure III-35. Admittedly, the list of symptoms and how they are related to the two scales is speculative at this stage, and perhaps future research will give substance and precision to such a chart. However, no one should be encouraged to let volunteer subjects be cooled below a final rectal temperature of 35°C or permit a heat loss of more than about 300 kcal.

g. Treatment of Immersion Hypothermia

Patients with mild cases of immersion hypothermia will recover if wet clothes are removed and they are wrapped in blankets or sleeping bags in a sheltered place and allowed to rewarm from their own metabolic heat production. Hot drinks and isometric exercise may be recommended. However, people with sufficiently severe immersion hypothermia (rectal temperatures below 34°C–35°C) to cause mental confusion or unconsciousness require immediate and active rewarming. Several means of active rewarming are available in the field: hot baths (40°C–44°C), portable hypothermic blankets, and supplying hot (40°C–44°C) humidified oxygen by mask. Of these, the hot bath is the most efficient, practical, and simple way to rewarm divers in the field.

Once the patient is removed from the cold exposure and external heat is applied, peripheral vasodilation develops, causing the cold, acidotic peripheral blood to enter the heart and visceral circulation while the warm central blood circulates through the cold skin. As a result, further heat loss occurs and the core temperature falls during the first 10–20 min of rewarming, a phenomenon known as *afterdrop*. Sometimes ventricular fibrillation occurs because of the continued reduction of core temperature, because of a temperature gradient across the myocardium, or because of hypovolemic shock secondary to blood loss to the periphery. Unfortunately, the use of hot baths is associated with the greatest afterdrop and the greatest danger of ventricular fibrillation. It is therefore recommended that the patient's trunk be placed in the bath with the limbs out of the water, to minimize afterdrop. Arterial blood pressure, core temperature (ear, esophageal, or rectal), and the electrocardiogram (if available) should be monitored continuously. In addition, the blood pH and glucose should be determined if the patient has poor respiration or is comatose. Severe acidosis or hypoglycemia, if present, should be treated.

As soon as the patient's heart beat and respiration are regular and increasing in frequency and his general condition is improving, or his deep body temperature is found

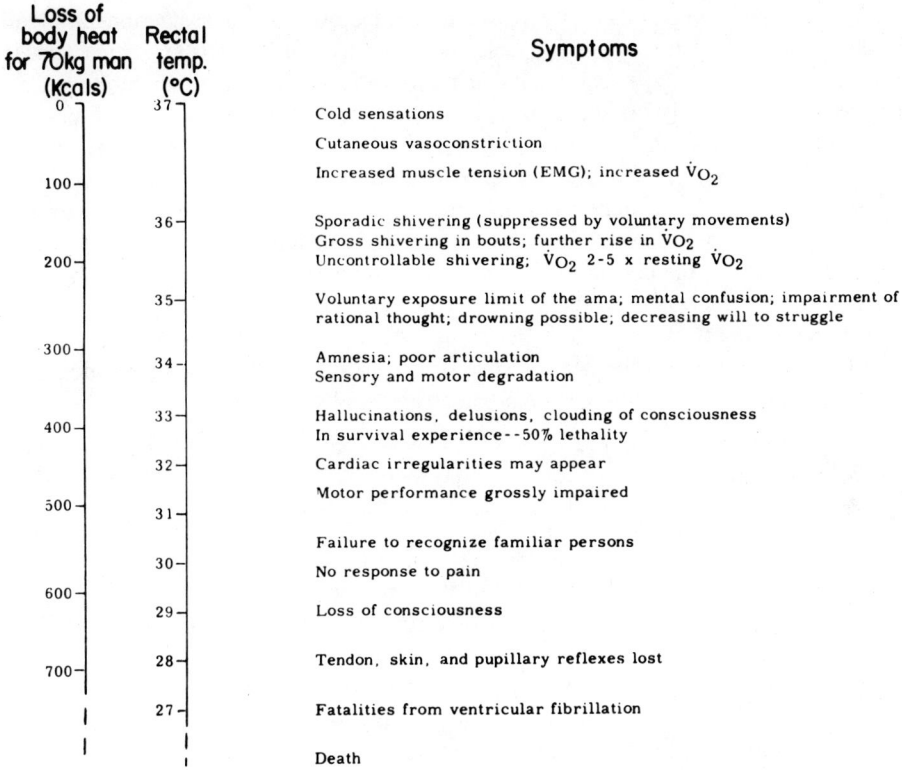

Figure III-35. A tentative ordering of symptoms of severe and prolonged cold exposure related to scales of body-heat loss and rectal temperature. The heat loss scale is linear, and the rectal temperature scale is nonlinear at the upper end, since rectal temperature does not reflect the large heat losses from the body shell. [From Webb (1976).]

to be above 32°C and rising steadily, the hot bath must be discontinued and the patient allowed to rewarm spontaneously under blankets.

h. Effects of Alcohol and Marijuana

It has been known for many years that alcohol tends even in moderate dosage to cause peripheral vasodilation in people in cold air. Theoretically, this should increase the rate of heat loss from the skin surface to the cold environment. Surprisingly, however, moderate amounts of alcohol have little effect on heat loss in cold water (Keatinge 1969). After drinking 75 ml of alcohol (diluted to 200 ml with water), 10 Navy men maintained higher blood flows during a 30-min immersion in 15°C water than in a control immersion without alcohol. The rate of heat loss was, however, very small even after alcohol, and the mean fall in rectal temperature after alcohol was not significantly greater than in the control immersion. Alcohol did have a dramatic effect on the subjective response to cold; the subjects reported that the water felt warmer after alcohol. On the basis of these findings, Keatinge states that alcohol could be dangerous to divers by making them unaware when body cooling has reached a dangerous level.

Marijuana and some of its derivatives have been known to increase peripheral blood flow and to induce hypothermia in animals. Should the hypothermia also be characteristic of man, divers who use marijuana might experience excessive hypothermia during a dive. Hanna and colleagues (1976) studied metabolic and thermal responses to a 60-min immersion in 28°C water in 10 subjects who smoked marijuana (0.739 g) or placebo immediately before immersion. They observed that the increase in heat production during immersion was significantly greater in the marijuana group than in the placebo group, or 117 vs. 91 kcal/(m^2 · hr). Despite this difference in metabolic response, rectal temperature at the end of the 60-min immersion was not different between the two groups, indicating that the extra heat produced after marijuana smoking was dissipated from the body surface. At least under these experimental conditions, marijuana did not seem to have any serious effects on the heat balance of divers in the water; however, additional studies involving colder and longer immersions are needed.

i. Cold Acclimatization

As stated above, the Korean women divers (ama) are daily engaged in diving in cold water, especially in winter when the water temperature is as low as 10°C. Extensive studies carried out on these divers revealed that they have developed various types of adaptation to cold (Hong 1973). The first type (metabolic adaptation) is manifested by a consistent reversible increase of about 20%–30% in the basal metabolic rate (BMR) in winter. The second type (insulative-hypothermic adaptation) is manifested by a significant elevation of shivering threshold (or significant lowering of the critical water temperature), which is observed throughout the year. For instance, the water temperature at which 50% of subjects shivered was 30°C for nondivers, as compared to 28°C in the divers (Figure III-36). Such a marked difference in the shivering threshold cannot be explained by the difference in the subcutaneous fat thickness (Figure III-27). Finally, the maximal tissue insulation in the ama at a comparable subcutaneous fat thickness is significantly greater than in nondivers through the year. Although these results are of considerable biological

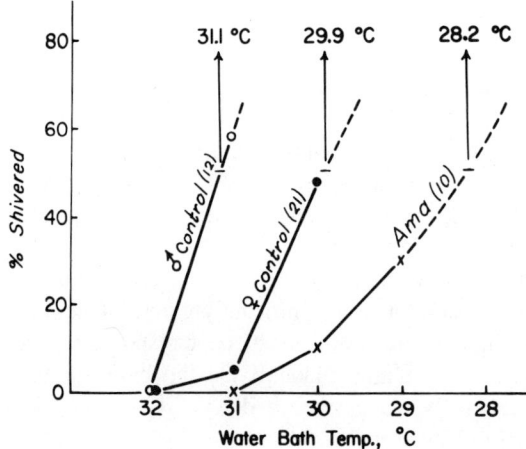

Figure III-36. Incidence of shivering at various water temperatures. Numerical figures in parentheses indicate number of subjects. [From Hong (1963).]

interest, it should be pointed out that these adaptive mechanisms do not play any significant role in the maintenance of core temperature when these divers work in water of 10°C, as the ama do in winter.

3. Thermal Balance in Dry Hyperbaric Environments

With the U.S. Navy's development of saturation diving techniques more than 20 years ago, divers can live in a hyperbaric environment for many days or even weeks. The most important physical characteristic of a hyperbaric environment in terms of thermal balance is the high gas density itself. However, another thermal factor occurs in the hyperbaric environment that is dependent on the physical characteristics of the diluent gas species. During a saturation dive to depths greater than 4–5 ATA, it is customary to pressurize the diving chamber primarily with breathing gases other than air to avoid oxygen toxicity and nitrogen narcosis. High gas density also causes increased ventilatory effort, with a consequent limitation on a diver's ability to perform work. It is therefore advantageous to use breathing gas with low density. As shown in Table III-10, both helium and hydrogen have a lower density than other gases. On the other hand, both the specific heat and thermoconductivity of helium and hydrogen are considerably greater than those of other gases, a circumstance that introduces thermal problems. In practice, helium is generally used as the diluent gas in saturation dives, although the use of hydrogen is being tested in several laboratories. More recently, the incidence of the high-pressure nervous syndrome (HPNS), which is often observed during the compression phase of deep dives (>600 fsw) is known to decrease markedly when nitrogen is added to the system (Bennett 1976). However, the fractional concentration of nitrogen in the chamber is much lower than that of helium; the thermal problems associated exclusively with helium-oxygen environments are discussed in this section.

Table III-10
Physical Properties of Various Gases at 28°C and 1 ATA[a]

Gas	Specific heat (c_p), cal/(g · °C)	Thermoconductivity (K), cal/(hr · cm · °C)	Density (ρ), g/liter	Heat capacity $(\rho \cdot c_p)$, cal/(liter · °C)
Air	0.256	0.225	1.15	0.294
Helium	1.242	1.292	0.20	0.248
Nitrogen	0.2486	0.2235	1.38	0.343
Neon	0.2460	0.420	0.99	0.243
Hydrogen	3.419	1.575	0.10	0.342

[a] Adapted from Morlock (1975).

a. Heat Transfer Properties

In the 1 ATA air environment, a lightly clad man moving around an environmental chamber is comfortable at temperatures between 20°C and 30°C. However, when the gas environment is changed from air to 80% He and 20% O_2 at 1 ATA, the comfort temperature range changes to between 23°C and 30°C. The main reason for this shift in comfort temperature range is the increased convective heat loss in the helium-oxygen environment. As indicated by Equation 2, convective heat loss is determined by the convective heat transfer coefficient (h_c) and the difference between mean skin and environmental temperatures ($\overline{T}_{sk} - T_a$). The absolute value of h_c is determined by many factors, some of which (such as the characteristic dimension of the body and the velocity of the fluid) are very difficult to estimate. Therefore, Webb (1970) has derived the following relative constants for various ambient media:

$$\text{Convective constant} = \frac{\rho \cdot c_p \cdot K}{\eta} \quad (7)$$

where ρ = density in g/liter; c_p = specific heat in cal/(g · °C); K = thermoconductivity in cal/(min · cm · °C); and η = viscosity in centipoise.

$$\text{Convective character} = \frac{\text{convective constant for ambient fluid}}{\text{convective constant for air (at 1 ATA)}} \quad (8)$$

Webb calculated these convective properties for seven fluids, and the results are shown in Table III-11. Note that the convective character of 80% He and 20% O_2 at 1 ATA is 2.6; this is because helium has a greater specific heat and thermoconductivity than nitrogen (Table III-10). In fact, the viscosity of helium is about 10% greater, and the density considerably lower, than those of nitrogen, which would tend to decrease the convective properties. Parenthetically, it may also be noted that the convective character of water is the highest of all fluids, amounting to 167.

Table III-11
Convective Characters of Several Fluids at 28°C[a]

Ambient fluids, %				Pressure, ATA	Convective constants	Convective characters
He	N_2	O_2	Others			
	80	20		1.0	0.61	1.0
80		20		1.0	1.57	2.6
78	18	4		7.2	17.2	28.2
90	8	2		14.6	36.6	60.0
98.3		1.7		20.7	52.0	85.2
			Water	1.0	102	167

[a] See Eqs. 7 and 8 for the definition of convective constants and characters. Adapted from Webb (1970).

In helium-oxygen saturation dives, the fractional concentration of helium increases with pressure, while that of oxygen decreases, to maintain a constant Po_2 at 0.3–0.4 ATA. Thus, the chamber gas at 31 ATA (1000 fsw) contains 96% helium and 1.3% oxygen. Such an increase in the concentration of helium, associated with greater increases in ρ, c_p, and K than in η in the hyperbaric environment (Morlock 1975), would accentuate the convective properties of the gas (Table III-11). This is the reason why convection from the body surface becomes the dominant heat loss pathway in hyperbaric and helium-rich environments.

Another unique aspect of heat transfer in the hyperbaric environment is the change in the evaporative heat loss. According to Rapp (1970), the evaporative heat transfer coefficient (h_e) is related to the mass transfer coefficient (h_D):

$$h_e = \frac{h_D \lambda}{R_w T} \qquad (9)$$

where h_D = mass transfer coefficient in m/hr; λ = latent heat of vaporization of water in kcal/kg; R_w = gas constant for water vapor; 3.47 mmHg · m³/kg · °K; and T = absolute temperature in °K. From this relationship it is evident that any change in h_D will cause a change in h_e and hence in the evaporative heat loss. As alluded to earlier, h_D is determined by the physical properties of the fluid surrounding the body, in accordance with the following relationship for laminar flow (Morlock 1975):

$$h_D = \frac{h_c \cdot (D_w)^{2/3}}{(\rho \cdot c_p)^{1/3} K^{2/3}} \qquad (10)$$

where D_w = water vapor diffusion coefficient in m²/hr. By substituting

$$h_e = \frac{h_c \cdot (D_w)^{2/3}}{(\rho \cdot c_p)^{1/3} \cdot K^{2/3}} \times \frac{\lambda}{R_w T} \qquad (11)$$

In this relationship it is important to note that both h_e and h_c are intimately related. According to the Chapman–Enskog theory (Reid and Sherwood 1966), D_w is inversely proportional to ambient pressure and also varies with the molecular species of the gases in the diffusion path. Recently, Paganelli and Kurata (1977) experimentally determined D_w under various conditions; representative results are shown in Table III-12. In general,

Table III-12

Water Vapor Diffusion Coefficients (D_W) at 25°C under Various Experimental Conditions[a]

Gas phase	Pressure, ATA	D_w, cm²/sec	Relative D_w
100% N_2	1	0.253	1.00
100% N_2	4	0.067	0.26
100% N_2	10	0.030	0.12
100% N_2	20	0.016	0.06
100% N_2	51	0.0075	0.03
100% He	1	0.836	1.00
100% He	4	0.209	0.25
100% He	10	0.085	0.10
100% He	20	0.044	0.05
100% He	51	0.019	0.02
74% He–26% O_2	1	0.52	1.00
74% He–26% O_2	4	0.14	0.27
74% He–26% O_2	20	0.031	0.06
98.4% He–1.6% O_2	1	0.80	1.00
98.4% He–1.6% O_2	20	0.042	0.05

[a]From Paganelli and Kurata (1977).

D_w decreased as an inverse function of pressure regardless of the gas composition. However, it is important to note that D_w increased markedly in helium or helium-oxygen environments, compared to nitrogen environments. Recently, Morlock (1975) computed theoretical values of h_c under various hyperbaric helium-oxygen environments and showed that they decrease rapidly between 1 ATA (air) and 10 ATA (330 fsw) (He-O_2); at pressures above 10 ATA, h_e decreased more modestly.

These analyses of the heat transfer properties of hyperbaric helium-oxygen environments indicate that convective heat loss would increase while evaporative heat loss would decrease progressively as ambient pressure increases. However, the degree of the increase in convective heat loss is far greater than that of the decrease in evaporative heat loss. As a result, the comfort temperature increases as the ambient pressure increases (Figure III-37). For instance, the chamber temperature should be raised to approximately 32°C at 61 ATA (2000 fsw) to keep the divers comfortable. Moreover, the comfort temperature range becomes very small, as in the case of immersion in water.

b. Heat Exchange

In most of the helium-oxygen saturation dives carried out in the early days, the chamber temperature was kept at a level lower than the comfort temperature shown in Figure III-37, and thus a marked increase in heat loss (mostly convective) occurred. More recently, attempts have been made to study the quantitative pattern of heat exchange through various avenues, e.g., convective, radiative, and evaporative, in thermally comfortable hyperbaric environments. One of the most comprehensive studies was carried out by the U.S. Navy in a 1973 dive to 49.5 ATA (1600 fsw) with 7 days of bottom time. The results obtained from this dive are shown in Figure III-38.

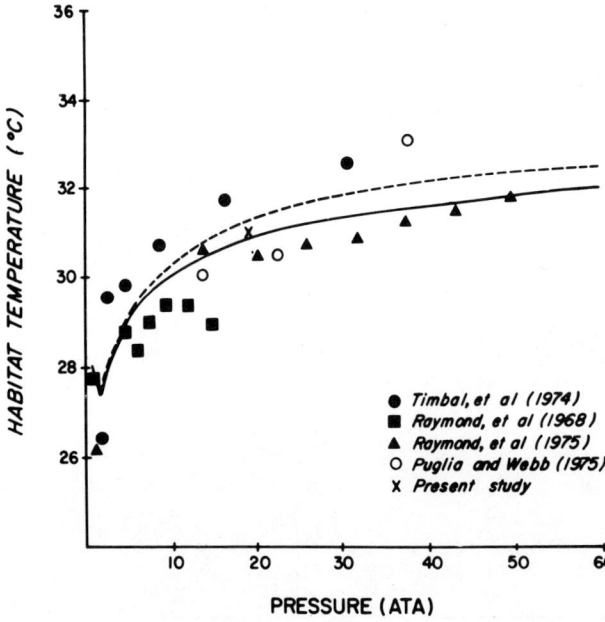

Figure III-37. Comfort temperatures for a prolonged stay in hyperbaric helium. Two prediction curves from Morlock (1975) are shown along with empirically determined temperatures from a number of saturation dives. *Solid line* predicts comfort temperature (equivalent to 28°C in air at 1 ATA) as a function of pressure if the Reynolds number of the gas is between 4 and 40; *dashed line* makes same prediction if the Reynolds number is between 4000 and 40,000. [From Webb et al. 1977).]

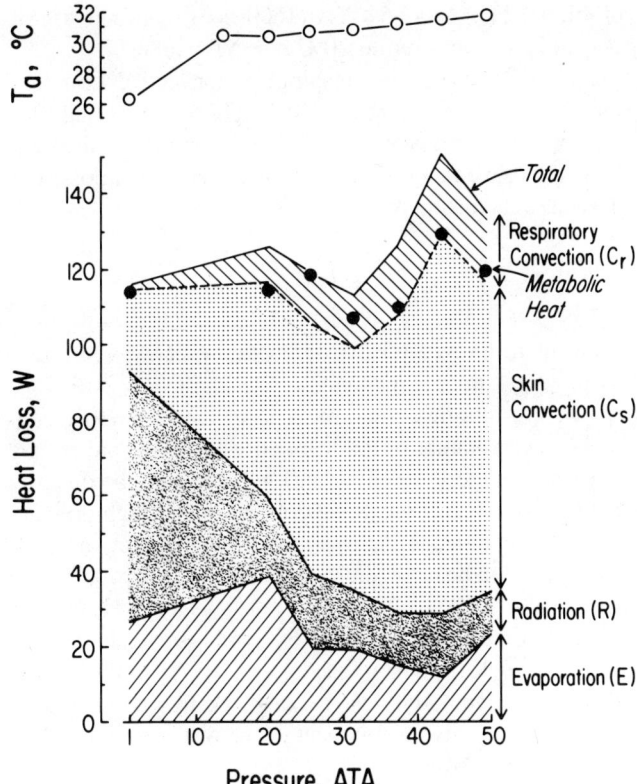

Figure III-38. Comfort temperature and heat loss through various avenues as a function of pressure. [Adapted from Raymond et al. (1975).]

Since the chamber temperature was raised as pressure increased to keep the divers comfortable, a reasonable thermal homeostasis was observed at all pressures. Thus total heat loss, which was approximately equal to metabolic heat production, remained almost unchanged at pressures between 1 and 49.5 ATA (33 and 1600 fsw). Rectal temperature was also maintained at around 37°C at all pressures. It was also noted that, despite the higher chamber temperature at higher pressures, there was no sweating and the mean skin temperature remained unchanged at all pressures. This indicates that the thermal gradient between the skin surface and the surrounding gas ($\overline{T}_{sk} - T_a$) became progressively smaller as pressure increased. Ordinarily, such a reduction in the thermal gradient should decrease heat loss because this gradient serves as the driving force for the loss. However, Figure III-38 shows that the heat loss by evaporation and radiation decreased, while that by convection increased markedly as chamber pressure increased. Since the relative humidity of the chamber gas at high pressures was slightly higher than at 1 ATA air (~70% vs. 60%), evaporative heat loss is expected to decrease at high pressures. As discussed above, the theoretical value of h_e decreased at high pressures, and thus the observed reduction in evaporative heat loss at high pressures could also be attributed in part to the low h_e. The reduction in radiative heat loss can be attributed to the decreased thermal gradient. The marked increase in the convective heat loss at high pressures is fully expected on the basis of the dependence of the convective properties of helium-oxygen mixtures on pressure (Table III-11). At 49.5 ATA (1600 fsw), convective heat loss accounted for 74% of total heat loss, compared to 20% at 1 ATA in air.

It is important to note in Figure III-38 that the respiratory convective heat loss increased from 1 W (0.8 kcal/hr) at 1 ATA air to nearly 20 W (17.2 kcal/hr) at 49.5 ATA (1600 fsw). In fact, respiratory convective heat loss accounted for 15% of the total heat loss at 49.5 ATA (1600 fsw). Experimentally, respiratory convective heat loss (C_r) can be determined from the following relationship:

$$C_r = \dot{V}_E \cdot \rho \cdot c_p \cdot (T_E - T_I) \qquad (12)$$

where $\dot{V}_E$ = minute ventilation in liter/min ATPS; T_E = temperature of expired gas in °C; and T_I = temperature of inspired gas in °C.

According to this equation, two factors determine the size of the respiratory convective heat loss at a given ρ and c_p: temperature of the inspired gas and the pulmonary ventilation. Any increase in $\dot{V}_E$ (due to exercise or shivering) will increase the quantity of C_r. It can be predicted that an exercising diver breathing cold gas under high pressure could incur a severe negative heat balance. According to a study conducted by the U.S. Navy (Hoke et al. 1976), a diver engaged in heavy exercise with an oxygen consumption of 3 liter/min (STPD) breathing cold gas (7°C) at 31 ATA (1000 fsw) lost 681 W (586 kcal/hr) through the respiratory system, which represents 65% of his metabolic heat production. Note that about 95% of this respiratory heat loss at 31 ATA (1000 fsw) represents convective loss, and the rest evaporative loss necessitated by humidification of the inspired gas. At 1 ATA air, the convective component of the respiratory heat loss represents about 10% (Moore et al. 1976).

As discussed earlier, h_c is expected to increase in hyperbaric helium-oxygen environments, as indicated by a marked increase in convective properties (Table III-11). Since Raymond and colleagues (1975) were able to determine the convective heat loss from the skin (C_{sk}) by subtracting respiratory convective heat loss (C_r) from total convective heat loss, they computed the values of h_c under different pressures by using Eq. 3. According to their analysis, h_c can be best expressed by the following power function:

$$h_c(W/m^2 \cdot °C) = 1.81 \, P^{0.63} \qquad (13)$$

where P = chamber pressure in ATA. Basically the same relationship ($h_c = 1.66 \, P^{0.71}$) was reported by a French group (Varène et al. 1976); overall, as the pressure increased from 1 ATA (air) to 49.5 ATA (He-O_2), h_c increased from about 2 to 20 W/m²·°C.

This information on h_c and respiratory convective heat loss has some practical importance in predicting the decrease in core temperature in unprotected divers at various temperatures. Under emergency conditions it is not always possible to provide the comfortable temperatures needed for thermal homeostasis; diving supervisors and medical officers are therefore often faced with the practical question of how rapidly body heat will be lost at a given chamber temperature and pressure if no special protective equipment is provided. Since convective heat loss (both skin and respiratory) represents the major avenue of heat loss, it is most important to estimate both C_{sk} and C_r. This can be done by making reasonable assumptions about $\overline{T}_{sk}$ and $\dot{V}_E$. With additional assumptions about metabolism and heat loss through radiation and evaporation, one should be able to estimate the net heat loss (ΔH), and then to calculate ΔT_r using Eqs. 5 and 6. Admittedly, this procedure is subject to a wide margin of error, but it still allows us to predict the degree of hypothermia likely in a given field condition. The results of such calculations, made by Raymond and his co-workers (1975), are depicted in Figure III-39. Note that unprotected divers would be rendered helpless by hypothermia in a few hours at chamber temperatures below about 25°C at 49.5 ATA (1600 fsw).

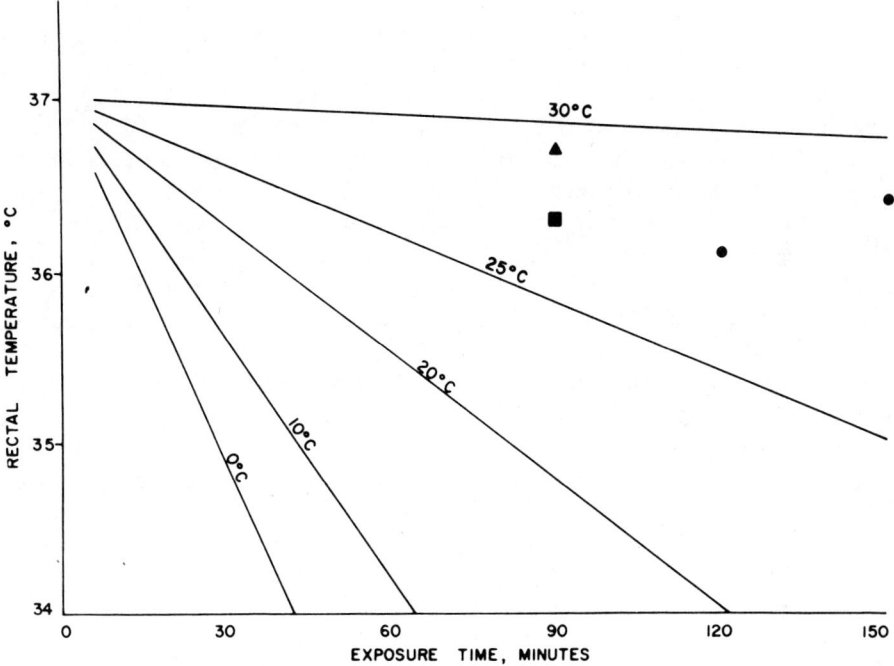

Figure III-39. Predicted fall in core temperature of unprotected resting males at various ambient temperatures in a still helium-oxygen atmosphere at 49.5 ATA (1600 fsw). A few measurements were made at that pressure in subjects A (■), B (●), and C (▲), and 31.0–31.7°C; their rates of cooling exceeded that predicted for 30°C. [From Raymond et al. (1975).]

4. Thermal Balance in Wet Hyperbaric Environments

Since the ultimate goal of a dive is to work in the open ocean where the diver is immersed in water under high pressure, it is important to consider thermal problems associated with the wet hyperbaric environment. As discussed in *Thermal Balance in Water* . . . , skin heat loss increases greatly during immersion even in water of modest temperature. For instance, 25°C subtropical Hawaiian water is considered stressful in terms of thermal balance (Figure III-30). In practice, therefore, all divers wear some sort of protective suits to minimize skin heat loss during exposure to water. For instance, the SeaLab III divers wore closed-cell foamed neoprene suits. However, pressure affects the insulative value of foamed neoprene adversely. In principle, a material's insulating efficiency is dependent on its thickness and thermal conductivity. A study conducted at the Naval Medical Research Institute (Rawlins and Tauber 1971) indicated that when a $^3/_{16}$-in wet suit was placed in a hyperbaric chamber and slowly pressurized with helium over 24 hr to 19.2 ATA (600 fsw), the suit's thickness decreased by about 50% until 4 ATA was attained, after which there was essentially no further change at greater depth. This compression effect is primarily caused by high hydrostatic pressure. In addition, there are secondary changes in the thickness of the wet suit caused by the movement of gas molecules between the neoprene and environment. During compression, helium diffuses into the neoprene, and oxygen and nitrogen diffuse out. After arrival at 19.2 ATA (600 fsw), the diffusion of helium continues, causing gradual reexpansion of the wet suit to about 65% of its initial thickness. Should a diver wearing such a wet suit filled with helium at high pressure enter the water (which contains no dissolved helium), the neoprene would rapidly outgas and lose thickness. Thus at 600 fsw (19.2 ATA), the insulation of a $^3/_{16}$-inch wet suit is approximately ¼ of its surface value after equilibration with helium, and decreases further as the dive continues.

The obvious solution to this problem is to use a suit made of incompressible material. In this regard, the constant-volume dry suit offers definite advantages. Dry suits eliminate the flushing of cold water around the body, and if the suit is inflated, its insulative capacity at the surface is not too different from that at depth (provided that an inflating gas with low heat capacity is used). According to a study conducted at the Japan Marine Science and Technology Center (Matsuda et al. 1978), the insulation provided by a dry suit over a thermal underwear-type suit made of 100% Polymid® material was adequate for a diver immersed in 15°C water to the neck at 1 ATA in air; however, its insulation value decreased markedly (by 70%) at 11 ATA in a helium–oxygen environment. Such losses in the insulation value of dry suits during cold water immersion in hyperbaric helium–oxygen environments could have been prevented had these workers used another inflating gas with a lower heat capacity. However, when the water temperature is very low, it is necessary to use electrically heated underwear.

Another potentially critical problem associated with wet saturation dives is respiratory heat loss. As discussed earlier, respiratory heat loss in a diver working in cold water at depth could lead to a severe negative heat balance. This problem can be eliminated only by heating the breathing gas. The U.S. Navy has published minimum acceptable temperatures of breathing gas for helium–oxygen dives of various depths (Table III-13).

Table III-13
Minimum Safe Temperature of Inspired Gas as a Function of Depth[a]

Depth		Gas temperature	
fsw	ATA	°C	°F
600	19.2	−1.0	30.2
700	22.2	4.0	39.2
800	25.2	7.8	46.1
900	28.3	10.8	51.5
1000	31.5	13.3	55.9

[a]Adapted from Braithwaite (1972).

References

BAYNE, D. G., AND E. T. FLYNN 1982. Immersion hypothermia and thermal protective garments for divers. In: *Diving Medical Officer's Student Guide* (2nd ed.), edited by E. T. Flynn, C. G. Bayne, and P. W. Catron. Washington, DC: U.S. Navy School of Diving and Salvage, U.S. Navy Technical Training Command.

BENNETT, P. B. 1976. The physiology of nitrogen narcosis and the high pressure nervous syndrome. In: *Diving Medicine*, edited by R. H. Strauss. New York: Grune and Stratton.

BOUTELIER, C., J. COLIN, AND J. TIMBAL 1971. Détermination du coefficient d'échange thermique dans l'eau en écoulement turbulent. *J. Physiol. (Paris)* 63: 207–209.

BRAITHWAITE, W. R. 1972. The calculation of minimum safe inspired gas temperature limits for deep diving. Rept. NEDU 12-72. Panama City, FL: U.S. Navy Experimental Diving Unit.

COOPER, K. E. 1976. Hypothermia. In: *Diving Medicine*, edited by R. H. Strauss. New York: Grune and Stratton.

CRAIG, A. B., JR. 1971. Heat exchange between man and the water environment. In: *Underwater Physiology IV. Proceedings of the Fourth Symposium on Underwater Physiology*, edited by C. J. Lambertsen. New York: Academic Press.

CRAIG, A. B., JR., AND M. DVORAK 1966. Thermal regulation during water immersion. *J. Appl. Physiol.* 21: 1577–1585.

CRAIG, A. B., JR., AND M. DVORAK 1976. Heat exchanges between man and the water environment. In: *Underwater Physiology V. Proceedings of the Fifth Symposium on Underwater Physiology*, edited by C. J. Lambertsen. Bethesda, MD: Fed. Am. Soc. Exp. Biol.

HANNA, J. M., R. H. STRAUSS, B. ITAGAKI, W. J. KWON, R. STANYON, J. BINDER, AND S. K. HONG 1976. Marijuana smoking and cold tolerance in man. *Aviat. Space Environ. Med.* 47: 634–639.

HAYWARD, J. S., J. D. ECKERSON, AND M. L. COLLINS 1975. Thermal balance and survival time prediction of man in cold water. *Can. J. Physiol. Pharmacol.* 53: 21–32.

HOKE, B., D. L. JACKSON, J. M. ALEXANDER, AND E. T. FLYNN 1976. Respiratory heat loss and pulmonary function during cold-gas breathing at high pressure. In: *Underwater Physiology V. Proceedings of the Fifth Symposium on Underwater Physiology*, edited by C. J. Lambertsen. Bethesda, MD: Fed. Am. Soc. Exp. Biol.

HONG, S. K. 1963. Comparison of diving and nondiving women of Korea. *Fed. Proc.* 22: 831–833.

HONG, S. K. 1973. Pattern of cold adaptation in women divers of Korea (ama). *Fed. Proc.* 32: 1614–1622.

KANG, D. H., P. K. KIM, B. S. KANG, S. H. SONG, AND S. K. HONG 1965. Energy metabolism and body temperature of the ama. *J. Appl. Physiol.* 20: 46–50.

KEATINGE, W. R. 1969. *Survival in Cold Water*. Oxford: Blackwell Scientific Publications.

MATSUDA, M., H. NAKAYAMA, H. ARITA, J. F. MORLOCK, J. CLAYBAUGH, R. M. SMITH, AND S. K. HONG 1978. Physiological responses to head-out immersion in water at 11 ATA. *Undersea Biomed. Res.* 5: 37–52.

MOORE, T. O., J. F. MORLOCK, D. A. LALLY, AND S. K. HONG 1976. Thermal cost of saturation diving: respiratory and whole body heat loss at 16.1 ATA. In: *Underwater Physiology V. Proceedings of the Fifth Symposium on Underwater Physiology*, edited by C. J. Lambertsen. Bethesda, MD: Fed. Am. Soc. Exp. Biol.

MORLOCK, J. F. 1975. Prediction of the various modes of heat loss from man in a dry and wet hyperbaric environment (Ph.D. Dissertation). Honolulu: Univ. of Hawaii.

PAGANELLI, C. V., AND F. K. KURATA 1977. Diffusion of water vapor in binary and ternary gas mixtures at increased pressures. *Respirat. Physiol.* 30: 15–26.

PUGH, L. G. C., AND O. G. EDHOLM 1955. The physiology of channel swimmers. *Lancet* 2: 761–768.

RAPP, G. M. 1970. Convective mass transfer and the coefficient of evaporative heat loss from human skin. In: *Physiological and Behavioral Temperature Regulation*, edited by J. D. Hardy, A. P. Gagge, and J. A. J. Stolwijk. Springfield, IL: Charles C Thomas.

RAPP, G. M. 1971. Convection coefficients of man in a forensic area of thermal physiology: heat transfer in underwater exercise. *J. Physiol. (Paris)* 63: 392–396.

RAWLINS, J. S. P., AND J. F. TAUBER 1971. Thermal balance at depth. In: *Underwater Physiology IV. Proceedings of the Fourth Symposium on Underwater Physiology*, edited by C. J. Lambertsen. New York: Academic Press.

RAYMOND, L. W., E. THALMANN, G. LINDGREN, H. C. LANGWORTHY, W. H. SPAUR, J. CROTHERS, W. BRAITHWAITE. AND T. BERGHAGE 1975. Thermal homeostasis of resting man in helium-oxygen at 1–50 ATA. *Undersea Biomed. Res.* 2: 51–68.

REID, R. C., AND T. K. SHERWOOD 1966. *Properties of Gases and Liquids* (2nd ed.). New York: McGraw-Hill.

RENNIE, D. W. 1965. Thermal insulation of Korean diving women and non-divers in water. In: *Physiology of Breath-Hold Diving and the Ama of Japan*, edited by H. Rahn and T. Yokoyama. Washington, DC: Natl. Acad. Sci./Natl. Res. Council

RENNIE, D. W. 1966. Body heat loss during immersion in water. In: *Human Adaptability and Its Methodology*, edited by H. Yashimura and J. S. Weiner. Tokyo: Japanese Society for the Promotion of Science.

SMITH, R. M., AND J. HANNA 1975. Skinfolds and resting heat loss in cold air and water. *J. Appl. Physiol.* 39: 93–102.

VARÈNE, P., J. TIMBAL, H. VIEILLEFOND, H. GUENARD, AND J. L'HUILLIER 1976. Energy balance of man in simulated dives from 1.5 to 31 ATA. In: *Underwater Physiology V. Proceedings of the Fifth Symposium on Underwater Physiology*, edited by C. J. Lambertsen. Bethesda, MD: Fed. Am. Soc. Exp. Biol.

WEBB, P. 1970. Body heat loss in undersea gaseous environments. *Aerosp. Med.* 41: 1282–1288.

WEBB, P. 1976. Thermal stress in undersea activity. In: *Underwater Physiology V. Proceedings of the Fifth Symposium on Underwater Physiology*, edited by C. J. Lambertsen. Bethesda, MD: Fed. Am. Soc. Exp. Biol.

WEBB, P. 1978. Calorimetric analysis of cold exposure in diving. In: *Underwater Physiology VI. Proceedings of the Sixth Symposium on Underwater Physiology*, edited by C. W. Shilling and M. W. Beckett. Bethesda, MD.: Fed. Am. Soc. Exp. Biol.

WEBB, P., S. J. TROUTMAN, JR., V. FRATTALI, R. H. DRESSENDORFER, J. DWYER, T. O. MOORE, J. F. MORLOCK, R. M. SMITH, Y. OHTA. AND S. K. HONG 1977. Hana Kai II: a 17-day dry saturation dive at 18.6 ATA. II. Energy balance. *Undersea Biomed. Res.* 4: 221–246.

I. Metabolism and Dietary Effects

A living animal carries on a continual exchange of materials and energy between its body and the environment. This exchange follows the conservation principle: none of the material or energy is lost in the exchange. The amount retained by the body is the difference between the intake and the output. The overall energy balance may be expressed by the following relationship:

$$E_{in} - E_{out} = \Delta E_S \tag{1}$$

where E_{in} = energy input, E_{out} = energy output, and ΔE_S = change in energy stores in the body.

The energy value of food consumed constitutes the sole source of energy input. Of all the chemical bonds in organic and inorganic compounds only one is significant as a source of energy: the bond between hydrogen and carbon that occurs in the compounds known as carbohydrates, lipids, and proteins. In the release of energy in biological reactions, carbon and hydrogen are oxidized to CO_2 and H_2O. The gas exchange, metabolizable energy, and water of oxidation of various organic compounds are shown in Table III-14; the values are markedly different for various compounds. Knowing the amounts of O_2 required (or CO_2 produced) and energy released by each compound permits one to calculate the caloric values for O_2 (or CO_2). These caloric values are often used to calculate energy consumption (see discussion below).

Table III-14

Numeric Factors for Carbohydrate, Fat, and Protein Metabolism in the Human Body[a]

	Carbohydrate, g	Fat, g	Protein, g
A. Gas Exchange			
$\quad O_2$ required (ml)	829	2,019	966
$\quad CO_2$ produced (ml)	829	1,427	782
$\quad$ Respiratory Quotient (RQ)	1.0	0.71	0.81
B. Metabolizable Energy	4.2	9.5	4.4
C. Caloric Values (kcal/liter)			
$\quad O_2$	5.05	4.69	4.60
$\quad CO_2$	5.05	6.63	5.68
D. Water of Oxidation (g)	0.60	1.07	0.41

[a] Adapted from Gemmill and Brobeck (1968).

The accurate determination of energy input requires corrections for fecal and urinary energy loss. Some of the food ingested is not absorbed by the gastrointestinal system, and thus there is a measurable loss of energy in the feces. Moreover, some of the oxygen and carbon of the constitutent amino acids continues to be combined with nitrogen and is excreted as nitrogenous compounds in the urine and feces. The energy content of food is quantified by burning a measured amount of material in a bomb calorimeter (direct calorimetry). In a recent saturation diving experiment, Webb and co-workers (1977) determined the fecal and urinary loss of calories by this technique, and they found that nearly 10% of food energy is lost in the feces and urine [337 kilocalories (kcal) out of 3552 kcal]. In practice, however, energy intake is indirectly estimated by using a food table, which agrees reasonably well ($\pm 10\%$) with directly measured values (Webb et al. 1977).

Energy output can be determined accurately by using a calorimeter to measure the heat liberated by the body. Again, output may be determined indirectly by measuring the amount of O_2 used or the amount of CO_2 given off and then converting these values into calories. However, as shown in Table III-14, caloric value varies with the type of organic compound being oxidized, and hence one has to know the composition of the food. One assumption underlying most calculations is that a nonprotein respiratory quotient (RQ) of 1.00 indicates an exclusive oxidation of carbohydrates, whereas one of 0.71 signifies an oxidation of fat alone; any RQ between these two values is caused by the burning of a mixture of fat and carbohydrate in definite proportions. The nonprotein RQ is calculated by deducting from the O_2 and CO_2 values of the total respiratory exchange the O_2 and CO_2 involved in the metabolism of protein. The urinary excretion of nitrogen reflects the quantity of proteins metabolized, and it has been determined that for every gram (g) of urinary nitrogen derived from protein, 5.94 liters of O_2 are consumed and

4.76 liters of CO_2 are produced. The caloric value of O_2 at various nonprotein RQs may be computed from the following relationship (Lusk 1928):

$$\text{Caloric value of } O_2 \text{ for non protein diet in kcal/liter} = 4.686 + \frac{(\text{nonprotein RQ} - 0.707) \cdot 0.361}{0.293} \quad (2)$$

Using these values and the fact that 1 g of urinary nitrogen is equivalent to 26.51 kcal, the total energy output (E_{out}) is obtained as follows:

$$E_{out} \text{ (kcal/hr)} = (26.51 \times U_N) + [(\dot{V}O_{2total} - \dot{V}O_{2protein}) \cdot CVO_2] \quad (3)$$

where U_N = urinary excretion of nitrogen in g/hr, $\dot{V}O_{2total}$ = total O_2 consumption in liter/hr STPD, $\dot{V}O_{2protein}$ = O_2 consumed to oxidize protein in liter/hr STPD (equal to ($U_N \cdot 5.94$)), and CVO_2 = caloric value of O_2 for nonprotein diet in kcal/liter (Eq. 2). In practice, however, we can estimate E_{out} by a much simpler relationship, using a caloric value of 4.8 kcal/liter:

$$E_{out} \text{ (kcal/hr)} = 4.8 \, \dot{V}O_{2total} \quad (4)$$

This simplified approach is based on the fact that the nonprotein RQ in a resting man maintained on a mixed diet is around 0.85. Although the value calculated by Equation 4 gives a reasonable approximation of E_{out}, Equation 3 should be used for accurate energy balance studies.

When E_{in} is equal to E_{out}, the body energy store (E_S) will stay constant, and body weight is expected to remain unchanged, provided that body fluid balance is also maintained. However, in situations in which the energy balance is disrupted, body energy store and body weight will change. In the case of a prolonged energy imbalance (especially a negative energy balance), one could expect a change of tissue protein store in addition to changes in carbohydrate and fat stores. However, it is generally assumed in energy balance studies lasting days or weeks that changes in body weight (when corrected for changes in total body water) involve fat stores rather than carbohydrate stores, especially if there is no evidence of a significant change in nitrogen balance.

Body fat content can be calculated from the value of the body volume. Whereas the fat of the body has a specific volume of about 1.10 ml/g, the remainder of the body has a specific volume of about 0.91 ml/g. This nonfat portion of the body is called the lean body mass. In principle, the body volume can be determined by immersing a subject in water and measuring the displacement volume. In practice, however, there is a problem of buoyancy caused by a force equal to the weight of the water displaced. [Readers are advised to consult the paper on this topic by Consolazio and colleagues (1963).] At any rate, once the measure of body volume is known, one can calculate the weight of body fat by the following relationship:

$$\text{Body volume (ml)} = 1.10 \, x + 0.91 \, (BW - x) \quad (5)$$

where x = weight of fat in grams, and BW = body weight in grams.

To enable investigators to estimate the fat content of the body more quickly and more easily than this method will permit, another technique is widely used: measurement of skinfold thickness. A fold of skin is elevated by gentle pinching, and its thickness is measured using calipers specially designed to close upon the skin with a standard force controlled by a spring. Measurements are made at certain standard locations over the body surface; this method assumes that fat is stored within the skin in proportion to its storage elsewhere in the body. In fact, many careful studies have shown that this method gives consistent results that correlate well with those obtained by means of Equation 5 (Brozek 1965). However, these judgments are based on average data and do not mean that in any given subject skinfold thickness will reveal subtle changes in body fat content.

1. *Energy Metabolism in Divers*

The major problem associated with energy balance in diving is the possible increase in E_{out} caused by the high convective heat transfer coefficient of the fluid surrounding the divers (see Section H of this chapter). Although such an increase in E_{out} can be counterbalanced by correspondingly increasing E_{in}, careful studies indicate that many saturation divers do not maintain the proper energy balance.

a. Energy Metabolism in the Ama

It is estimated that the ama, the women divers of Korea and Japan, subject themselves to a daily extra heat loss of approximately 1000 kcal by diving without protective suits in water considerably cooler than the thermoneutral level (Kang et al. 1965). Despite this high E_{out}, their body weight is maintained remarkably well, indicating that they must have a high E_{in}. Actual dietary surveys indicate that the average ama consumes approximately 3000 kcal a day, compared to a caloric intake among nondiving women of comparable age of 2000 kcal. This indicates that the ama counteract the high E_{out} by increasing E_{in} on a daily basis. However, these divers also develop a metabolic adaptation, indicated by a reversible increase in the basal metabolic rate (BMR) during the cold season (Figure III-40). In general, the level of BMR in the ama is comparable to that of nondivers during the summer but is approximately 30% greater than that of nondivers during the winter, when the seawater temperature is lowest (about 10°C or 50°F).

Metabolic adaptation to the cold has been observed in many animals, and a similar increase in BMR has been observed in Eskimos in the winter. However, the latter phenomenon is not related to cold stress but to a greater protein intake (Rodahl 1954). The measurement of urinary nitrogen excretion in the ama indicated that it does not vary with the season, which eliminates a higher protein intake as the underlying cause of the seasonal variation of BMR in these divers (Kang et al. 1963). There was also no evidence of anemia in the ama; anemia is also known to increase BMR. More recent studies on the ama (Hong 1973) showed that the elevated BMR in winter is not associated with an increased amount of thyroid iodine-131 (^{131}I) uptake; however, the rate of release of ^{131}I from the thyroid gland was significantly greater in the ama than in the nondivers, especially in winter. These and other findings suggest that the most likely reason for metabolic

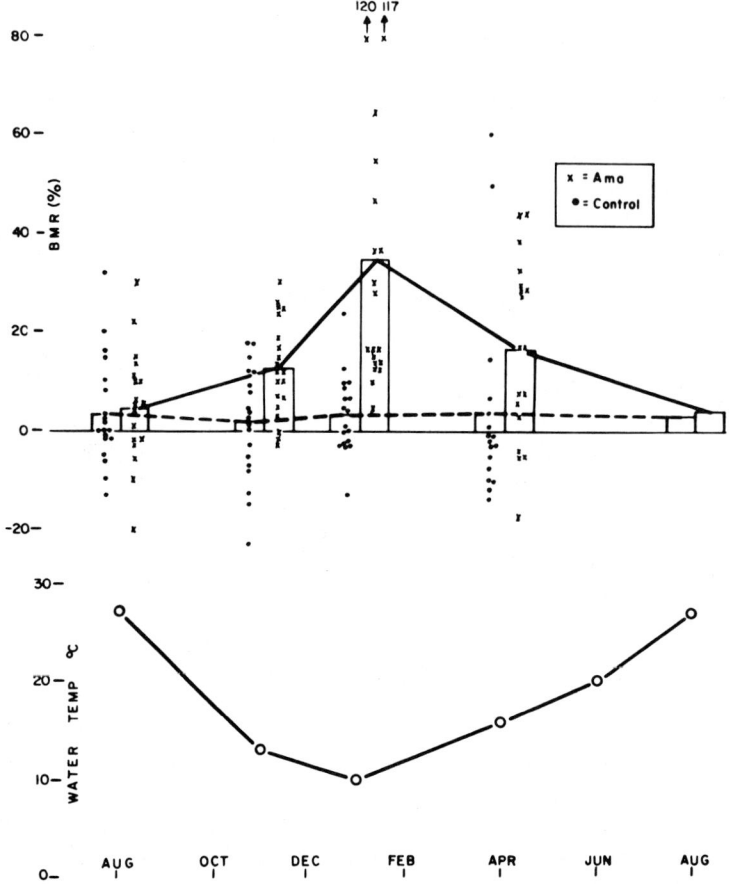

Figure III-40. Seasonal variations in basal metabolic rate. *Bar graph* represents average BMR for each group. *Lower part* of graph shows surface water temperature during the year. [Adapted from Kang et al. (1963).]

adaptation is increased utilization of thyroid hormone by the peripheral tissues (rather than increased thyroid function).

During exposures to severe cold stress, there is an increased release of norepinephrine (but not epinephrine) from the peripheral nerve endings (Weihl et al. 1978). Such an increase in norepinephrine release (as indicated by the increase in the urinary excretion of norepinephrine) was also found in the ama during the winter (Kang et al. 1970). In this regard, it should be pointed out that norepinephrine plays a central role in the development of nonshivering thermogenesis, a result of cold adaptation, in many species of animals. Many animal studies showed that the administration of exogenous norepinephrine to cold-adapted animals caused a marked increase in heat production (Hemingway and Price 1964). However, such calorigenic action of norepinephrine was rather small in the ama in the winter (Kang et al. 1970), suggesting that the development of nonshivering thermogenesis is not the main feature of cold adaptation in these divers.

Regardless of the mechanism(s) underlying the development of metabolic adaptation to cold, the higher BMR would require a higher E_{in} even when the ama are not exposed to cold, and this response is therefore not economical. In this respect, other types of cold adaptation manifested by the elevation of shivering threshold (see Figure III-36) and higher tissue insulation (Hong 1973) are more significant. The latter phenomena would tend to suppress the increase in E_{out} during exposure to cold, conserving energy to some extent. In fact, these types of adaptation are more common in man and are attributed to habituation.

b. Energy Metabolism in Saturation Divers

In the majority of saturation dives (both dry and wet) carried out in the early days of saturation diving, it was observed that most divers lost body weight under pressure despite high caloric intakes. Although this weight loss was greater when the divers were exposed to cold stress, it was evident even without it. The amount of body weight loss observed in different dives is shown in Table III-15. Overall, the average weight loss was roughly proportional to the mathematical product of pressure and the number of days of exposure without cold stress. Thus, the greatest weight loss was observed during the University of Pennsylvania's 1200-fsw (37 ATA) dive in 1971; a weight loss of 4 kg (8.8 lb) was observed on the last day at pressure (441 atm-days). In this dive, the average daily caloric intake was 3510 kcal, which should have prevented weight loss in young divers cooped up in the small hyperbaric chamber.

There are many plausible explanations for the persistent weight loss observed during saturation diving. The most likely seem to be: (1) caloric deficit caused by increased E_{out}; (2) loss of body water; (3) atrophy and tissue loss from confinement; (4) caloric deficit from poor absorption of food; and (5) some unidentified error in the caloric balance data, e.g., an overestimation of the caloric value of food taken in. A careful accounting of all the elements of energy balance and of fluid balance is therefore required to determine the cause of the weight loss. The most comprehensive studies to obtain this information were carried out in 1975 at the University of Hawaii (in collaboration with the Naval Medical Research Institute) during the 17-day dry saturation dive to 18.6 ATA (580 fsw) that is known as Hana Kai II (Hong et al. 1977b). In this dive, the magnitude of E_{in} was determined by directly measuring the caloric values of food, urine, and feces using a bomb calorimeter, and that of E_{out} by near-continuous 24-hr measurements of O_2 consumption and CO_2 production using a special method developed for saturation dives by Webb and Troutman (1970). At the same time, the thermal balance, nitrogen balance, body fluid balance, total body water volume, and total-body fat content were measured (Webb et al. 1977).

It was noted in the Hana Kai II dive that body weight decreased rapidly during the first five days at 18.5 ATA (580 fsw), after which it decreased more slowly (Figure III-41). Overall, body weight decreased by about 1.3 kg (3.1 lb) toward the end of the 18.6 ATA period. At the same time, a significant increase in urine flow was observed at 18.6 ATA without an increase in water intake, which led to a state of mild dehydration (Hong et al. 1977a). In fact, the rapid loss of body weight during the early period at pressure was probably caused by this dehydration, and even at the end of the 18.6 ATA period

Table III-15
Weight Loss in Saturation Diving as a Function of Depth and Duration of Dive

	Breathing gas and pressure (gas, ATA)	Duration at depth, days	Pressure exposure, atm-days	Mean weight loss, kg	Mean food intake, kcal/day	Reference
Helgoland (North Sea)	Air, 3.3[a]	10	23	4.0	6000	Webb et al. (1977)
Tektite II (Caribbean)	Air, 2.3	14–21	27	2.0	>3500	Webb et al. (1977)
U. Hawaii	HeO_2, 16.1	2	30	0.6	>4000	Webb et al. (1977)
JAMSTEC**	HeO_2, 7	7	42	0.0	2900	Webb et al. (1977)
Tekite I (Caribbean)	Air, 2.15	60	69	1.6	Ad lib.	Webb et al. (1977)
Genesis E	HeO_2, 7	12	72	0.6	4200	Webb et al. (1977)
SeaLab II (Bermuda)	HeN_2O_2, 7.2	15	93	2.0	>4000	Webb et al. (1977)
Aegir (offshore Hawaii)	HeO_2, 16.6[a]	6	94	2.9	Ad lib.	Webb et al. (1977)
USN, Experimental Diving Unit	HeO_2, 19.2	8	146	1.2	Ad lib.	Webb et al. (1977)
Sagittaire II	HeO_2, 49	4	192	1.5	2500	Webb et al. (1977)
U. Hawaii (Hana Kai II)	HeO_2, 18.6	17	282	0.8	3400	Webb et al. (1977)
USN, Experimental Diving Unit	HeO_2, 49.5	7	340	3.5	2900	Webb et al. (1977)
U. Penn.	HeO_2, 13,24, 28,37	17	441	4.0	3510	Webb et al. (1977)
Sagittaire III	HeO_2, 31	15	450	2.4	2580	Webb et al. (1977)
Sagittaire I	HeO_2, 31	17	510	2.4	2850	Webb et al. (1977)
U. Penn.	HeO_2, 37.3, 43.4	11	375	3.6	3193	Lambertsen et al. (1978)
AMTE	HeO_2, 31	7	210	−0.9 (gain)	3442	Hempelman (1978)
JAMSTEC[b]	HeO_2, 31	14	420	0.7	2900	Nakayama et al. (1980)

[a] Cold exposure during the dive.

[b] Japan Marine Science and Technology Center. Pressure exposure calculated as gauge pressure times days at bottom depth.

a slight dehydration was still present. When corrections were made for this reduction in total body water volume, a net weight loss of 0.8 kg was observed (Table III-15). The magnitude of E_{in} was kept high (>3000 kcal/day) throughout the dive. Although the size of E_{out} increased by about 10% at 18.6 ATA in the absence of cold stress (as indicated by the unchanged rectal and mean skin temperatures as well as by subjective sensation), it was always lower than the simultaneously determined E_{in}. Moreover, there was no evidence of negative nitrogen balance during the dive, indicating that no tissue was lost because of confinement. It thus appears that there was a small net loss of body fat (0.8 kg) during the 17-day exposure to the thermoneutral 18.6 ATA environment that cannot be accounted for by any of the mechanisms listed above.

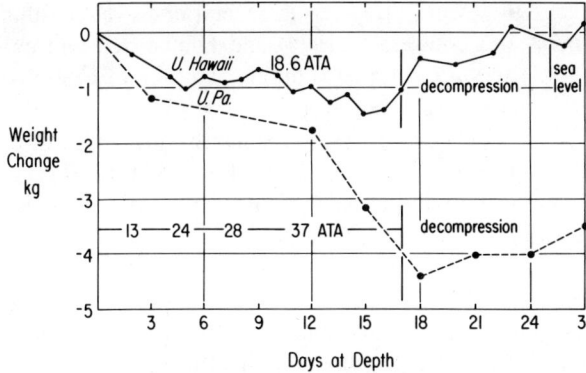

Figure III-41. Average weight changes for five subjects in the Hana Kai II dive (1975) and for four subjects in the University of Pennsylvania dive (1971). Weights corrected for buoyancy changes caused by increased gas density, but not for changes in total body water. [From Webb et al. (1977).]

According to the data in Table III-15, there was a net gain of body weight in the dive to 961 fsw (31 ATA) conducted by the Admiralty Marine Technology Establishment (AMTE) Physiological Laboratory (Hempelman 1978). Although the net gain of 0.9 kg (2 lb) was attributed to the corresponding increase in body fat, a more accurate measurement of body fat was needed. In this study, body fat content was calculated from skinfold thickness, a technique whose results show considerable variability and may not be sufficiently accurate for careful quantitative balance studies. Moreover, additional data on total body water volume are needed to support the AMTE conclusion.

In practically every saturation diving experiment carried out so far, a significant increase in urine flow has been noted (Hong 1975). According to a comprehensive study conducted during Hana Kai II (Hong et al. 1977a), this diuresis is not due to a greater water intake, and a weight loss caused by a negative water balance could not be induced. However, the mass transfer coefficient decreased in the hyperbaric environment, leading to a reduction in water vapor loss from the skin that would tend to prevent dehydration (see Section H of this chapter). In fact, studies show that dehydration, as shown by increases in plasma protein concentration, hematocrit ratio, and red blood cell counts, occurred only during the first 4 to 5 days of the hyperbaric period, after which it disappeared. Although total body water volume, as measured at the midpoint of the dive (Day 12), showed only a smaller net loss (0.5 kg or 1.1 lb) compared to the weight loss (1.3 kg), more systematic comparisons are needed to rule out body fluid loss as a factor in the loss of weight.

In a saturation dive to 961 fsw (31 ATA), Hempelman (1978) observed a marked increase in serum urea level without any evidence of renal failure and wondered if this indicated muscle wasting. In a more recent dive to 1333 fsw (43 ATA), Carlyle and associates (1978) found a dramatic increase in urea excretion in two divers maintained on a constant dietary intake, again suggesting a metabolic disturbance caused by pressure and helium. Although the fasting blood glucose level was reported to decrease at pressure (Carlyle et al. 1978), other investigators have reported no change (Hampelman 1978; Raymond et al. 1974). In this respect, Raymond and co-workers (1974) pointed out that although the fasting serum glucose level in hyperbaric helium-oxygen is often lower than predive values in air, most of this lowering in serum glucose levels was caused by artifacts incurred during decompression of the blood samples. Since serum insulin levels are closely associated with serum glucose levels, they were measured in several dives, but results are contradictory. Whereas Raymond and colleagues (1974) and Lambertsen and coworkers (1978) found no change in the serum insulin level during exposure to 1530 fsw (49.5 ATA), others reported a reduction during exposure to 961 fsw (31 ATA) (Hempelman 1978) and 1333 fsw (43 ATA) (Carlyle et al. 1978). Similarly, the serum level of free fatty acids shows no consistent pattern during deep dives. The serum triglyceride level has been shown to increase significantly during the early hyperbaric period (Lambertsen et al. 1978; Nakayama et al. 1980); however, the significance of this finding is not evident.

The serum level and urinary excretion of other hormones that have variable metabolic effects have also been determined in a limited number of saturation dives. These hormones include cortisol, epinephrine, norepinephrine, growth hormone, and thyroid hormones, but the results of this research are conflicting, and it is therefore impossible to make any definite conclusions at this time.

2. Electrolyte Metabolism in Divers

The development of a pronounced diuresis accompanied by natriuresis and kaliuresis during head-out immersion in water is well known (Epstein 1978). Moreover, similar renal responses were observed even during whole-body immersion with pressure breathing equipment (Graveline and Jackson 1962). Although it is beyond the scope of this chapter to deal with the still-disputed mechanisms underlying these responses to immersion, it should be noted that they are observed even during immersion in thermoneutral water and are potentiated in cold water (Matsuda et al. 1978; Reeves et al. 1965). Moreover, diuretic responses are dependent on the state of hydration. When subjects are immersed after overnight water deprivation, the increase in urine flow is slow and small, and its magnitude is proportional to the rate of excretion of osmotic substances. On the other hand, when hydrated subjects are immersed the increase in urine flow is rapid and greater, and its magnitude is proportional to the rate of excretion of free water. In other words, immersion appears to induce a water diuresis in hydrated subjects and an osmotic diuresis in dehydrated subjects.

The pattern of natriuresis and kaliuresis induced by immersion is dependent on the preimmersion sodium (Na) balance (Epstein 1978). For instance, in subjects in balance on low-Na (e.g., 10 mEq/day), the development of natriuresis is slow and it takes 2–3 hr before a significant increase in Na excretion is observed. On the other hand, in subjects in balance on high-Na (e.g., 150 mEq/day), a significant natriuresis develops in 1 hr and peaks in 3 hr; in some subjects, the increase in Na excretion was as great as 18 mEq/hr. On the other hand, the kaliuresis was much more marked in subjects in balance on low Na, in whom the rate of potassium (K) excretion has been shown to increase from the preimmersion level of 2–3 mEq/hr to between 7 and 8 mEq/hr within 2 hr of immersion. From these results a significant depletion of both Na and K can be predicted if the duration of water immersion is prolonged.

Electrolyte metabolism during dry saturation dives has not been investigated extensively in the past, and only a limited amount of information is available at present. As discussed above, hyperbaric diuresis has occurred in virtually all saturation dives carried out thus far. Unlike immersion diuresis, this diuresis is not usually accompanied by a corresponding increase in the excretion of osmotic substances, indicating that the increase in urine flow is caused primarily by the increase in free water excretion. In Hana Kai II, a careful balance study was conducted for Na and K (Hong et al. 1977a), and the results indicated that, despite the sustained diuresis at 580 fsw (18.6 ATA), neither the Na excretion nor the Na balance showed any change; on the other hand, the urinary excretion of K increased significantly at 580 fsw (18.6 ATA), and, in fact, a negative K balance (about 30 mEq/day) was noted throughout the hyperbaric period. A similar increase in K excretion has often been seen in other saturation dives (Hong 1975). The physiological significance of this observation is not yet clear.

The urinary excretion of other electrolytes such as calcium, magnesium, inorganic phosphate, and chlorine has been determined in some dives, but the results are conflicting and are difficult to interpret in the absence of data on the intake of these substances.

Since head-out immersion induces a marked diuresis and natriuresis, it can be used clinically to facilitate the elimination of water and Na from the body. In fact, Epstein and colleagues (1977) studied the immersion-induced alteration in renal water-handling in patients with alcoholic liver disease and found that immersion resulted in a dramatic but transient "normalization" of renal water excretion. Even in cirrhotic patients with more advanced "decompensation," these workers demonstrated that, despite an even greater impairment in renal water-handling in air, immersion caused a significant increase in urine flow compared to levels documented in normal control subjects. These observations strongly support exploring immersion as a clinical tool to treat certain patients suffering from abnormal body fluid and electrolyte balance.

3. Dietary Effects

Saturation divers should eat a well-balanced diet consisting of carbohydrates, fats, proteins, minerals, and vitamins. In most dives (dry or wet) carried out in the past, dietary regulation has rarely been enforced; the diver has been allowed to request whatever he wishes to eat, and poor records of intake have been kept. For relatively short nonsaturation dives, dietary regulation is not a major problem. The diver has easy access to a variety of foods and can be monitored without difficulty for evidence of any nutritional deficiency. In general, at least 2 hr should elapse between the last meal and a diving operation. Since lipemia may lead to thrombi and blockage of the circulation (Philp et al. 1967), it is particularly important to avoid a heavy ingestion of fat. If a prolonged, heavy exercise effort is anticipated in the dive, it is desirable to provide a supplementary diet heavy in carbohydrates.

For divers in a hyperbaric chamber for a long saturation dive, there are a host of problems involving food management. In many dives, hot meals are prepared by the support crew outside the chamber and are sent in through a small medical lock. However, high pressure has certain effects on the texture of food. For instance, bread becomes elastic, thick soup coagulates, fried foods diminish by one-third in volume, rice becomes lumpy, apples and pears bruise, and bananas spoil at once (but oranges undergo little change) (Segui and Conti 1972). In Hana Kai II, changes in divers' taste sensations were studied at 580 fsw (18.6 ATA) (O'Reilly et al. 1977). It was found that sweet sensitivity increased over time while sour sensitivity declined over the course of the dive; divers under pressure also became more sensitive to bitter stimuli but less sensitive to salt. A similar study conducted earlier by Elcombe and Tester (1973) in a 120 fsw (4 ATA) nitrogen-oxygen environment revealed no significant change in taste (or olfactory) sensitivity throughout the 14-day period of exposure to increased nitrogen pressures. It was also noted that when the divers were given considerable freedom of choice in the selection of meals, provided for the most part by a local restaurant, they preferred a lighter diet (e.g., fruits and salads) to heavy rich foods as the dive progressed (Hamilton et al. 1966). Despite these changes in food textures, taste sensitivity, and food preference under high pressure, divers appear to maintain good appetites and manage to eat an adequate amount of food, as indicated by the very high caloric intakes observed in some deep dives (Table III-15). Moreover, the composition of the diet (e.g., carbohydrates, fat, and protein) remained largely unchanged during exposure to high pressure (Matsuda et al. 1975; Hempelman 1978). Similarly, dietary intake of minerals such as iron, sodium, potassium, and calcium remained unchanged during exposure to 960 fsw (31 ATA) (Hempelman 1978).

During a U.S. Navy dive to a simulated depth of 850 fsw (27 ATA) with two excursions to 1000 fsw (32 ATA), Frattali and Robertson (1973) evaluated the nutritional status of two divers and noted that there was a marked decrease in thiamine excretion. This indicates a greater thiamine demand during exposure to high pressure. In another series of U.S. Navy dives at simulated depths of 1000 and 1600 fsw (32 and 51 ATA), Frattali and colleagues (1974) also observed a marked depression of serum vitamin C, which was attributed to a chamber gas P_{O_2} (0.3–0.35 ATA) greater than that at 1 ATA air (0.2 ATA). Petrovykh and co-workers (1977) conducted 15- to 18-day dives at 5 ATA nitrogen-oxygen using two divers with and without supplemental vitamin complex, and found that changes in nitrogen metabolism accompanied by an increase in blood sugar level occurred at high pressure only when vitamin complex was not given to the diver. These results clearly indicate that the vitamin requirement appears to change at high pressure, and that more critical studies are needed.

Alcoholic beverages are usually eliminated from the diet at high pressure, since it has been thought that they might aggravate the symptoms of the high pressure nervous syndrome (HPNS). In a 960-fsw (31 ATA) dive reported by Hempelman (1978), alcohol beverages were allowed in moderation (the maximal ingestion in any 24-hr period was limited to 16 g of ethanol as wine or ale); on examining the records, both objective and subjective, of HPNS symptoms on days when ethanol had been consumed, it was not possible to detect any effect of this quantity of ethanol on the development of the syndrome.

SUK KI HONG

References

BROZEK, J. 1965. *Human Body Composition: Approaches and Application.* New York: Pergamon Press.
CARLYLE, R. F., M. P. GARRARD. AND M. J. STOCK 1978. Observations on some metabolic and hormone levels in the blood of men during simulated saturation dives to 420 metres of sea water, 43 bar, in helium-oxygen mixtures. *J. Physiol. (Lond.)* 285: 44P–45P.

CONSOLAZIO, C. F., R. E. JOHNSON, AND L. J. PECORA 1963. *Physiological Measurements of Metabolic Functions in Man*. New York: McGraw-Hill.

ELCOMBE, D. D., AND J. H. TEETER 1973. Nitrogen narcosis during a 14-day continuous exposure to 5.2% O_2 in N_2 at pressure equivalent to 100 FSW (4 ata). *Aerosp. Med.* 44: 864–869.

EPSTEIN, M. 1978. Renal effects of head-out water immersion in man: implications for an understanding of volume homeostasis. *Physiol. Rev.* 58: 529–581.

EPSTEIN, M., R. LEVINSON, J. SANCHO, E. HABER, AND R. RE 1977. Characterization of the renin-aldosterone system in decompensated cirrhosis. *Circ. Res.* 41: 818–829.

FRATTALI, V., AND R. ROBERTSON 1973. Nutritional evaluation of humans during an oxygen-helium dive to a simulated depth of 1,000 ft. *Aerosp. Med.* 44: 14–21.

FRATTALI, V., L. W. RAYMOND, M. QUESADA, AND R. ROBERTSON 1974. Effects of hyperbaric helium-oxygen on caloric, fluid, mineral and nutrient requirements of saturation divers (abstract). *Undersea Biomed. Res.* 1: A29.

GEMMILL, C. L., AND J. R. BROBECK 1968. Energy exchange. In: *Medical Physiology* (12th ed.), edited by V. B. Mountcastle. St. Louis: C. V. Mosby.

GRAVELINE, D. E., AND M. M. JACKSON 1962. Diuresis associated with prolonged water immersion. *J. Appl. Physiol.* 17: 519–524.

HAMILTON, R. W., JR., J. B. MACINNIS, A. D. NOBLE, AND H. R. SCHREINER 1966. Saturation diving to 650 feet. Tech. Memorandum B-411. Tonawanda, NY: Ocean Systems, Inc.

HEMINGWAY, A., AND W. M. PRICE 1964. The calorigenic action of catecholamines in warm acclimated and cold acclimated nonshivering cats. *Int. J. Neuropharmacol.* 3: 495–503.

HEMPELMAN, H. V. 1978. Observations on men at pressures of up to 300 msw (31 bar). Rept. R78401. Gosport, Hants, U.K.: Admiralty Marine Technology Establishment.

HONG, S. K. 1973. Pattern of cold adaptation in women divers of Korea (ama). *Fed. Proc.* 32: 1614–1622.

HONG, S. K. 1975. Body fluid balance during saturation diving. In: *International Symposium on Man in the Sea*, edited by S. K. Hong. Bethesda, MD.: Undersea Medical Society.

HONG, S. K., J. R. CLAYBAUGH, V. FRATTALI, R. JOHNSON, F. KURATA, M. MATSUDA, A. A., MCDONOUGH, C. V. PAGANELLI, R. M. SMITH, AND P. WEBB 1977a. Hana Hai II: a 17-day dry saturation dive at 18.6 ATA. III. Body fluid balance. *Undersea Biomed. Res.* 4: 247–266.

HONG, S. K., R. M. SMITH, P. WEBB, AND M. MATSUDA 1977b. Hana Kai II: a 17-day dry saturation dive at 18.6 ATA. I. Objectives, design, and scope. *Undersea Biomed. Res.* 4: 211–220.

KANG, B. S., D. S. HAN, K. S. PAIK, Y. S. PARK, J. K. KIM, C. S. KIM, D. W. RENNIE, AND S. K. HONG 1970. Calorigenic action of norepinephrine in the Korean woman divers. *J. Appl. Physiol.* 29: 6–9.

KANG, D. H., P. K. KIM, B. S. KANG, S. H. SONG, AND S. K. HONG 1965. Energy metabolism and body temperature of the ama. *J. Appl. Physiol.* 20: 46–50.

KANG, B. S., S. H. SONG, C. S. SUH, AND S. K. HONG 1963. Changes in body temperature and basal metabolic rate of the ama. *J. Appl. Physiol.* 18: 483–488.

LAMBERTSEN, C. J., R. GELFAND, AND J. M. CLARK 1978. *Predictive Studies IV: Work Capability and Physiological Effects in He-O_2 Excursions to Pressures of 400-800-1,200 and 1,600 Feet of Sea Water*. Rept. 78-1. Philadelphia: Univ. of Pennsylvania, Institute for Environmental Medicine.

LUSK, G. 1928. *The Elements of the Science of Nutrition* (4th ed.). Philadelphia: W. B. Saunders.

MATSUDA, M., H. NAKAYAMA, H. ARITA, J. F. MORLOCK, J. CLAYBAUGH, R. M. SMITH, AND S. K. HONG 1978. Physiological responses to head-out immersion in water at 11 ATA. *Undersea Biomed. Res.* 5: 37–52.

MATSUDA, M., H. NAKAYAMA, A. ITOH, N. KIRIGAYA, F. K. KURATA, R. H. STRAUSS, AND S. K. HONG 1975. Physiology of man during a 10-day dry heliox saturation dive (SEATOPIA) to 7 ATA. I. Cardiovascular and thermoregulatory functions. *Undersea Biomed. Res.* 2: 101–118.

NAKAYAMA, H., S. K. HONG, J. CLAYBAUGH, N. MATSUI, Y. S. PARK, Y. OHTA, K. SHIRAKI, AND M. MATSUDA 1980. Energy and body fluid balance during a 14-day dry saturation dive at 31 ATA (Seadragon IV). In: *Underwater Physiology VII. Proceedings of the Seventh Symposium on Underwater Physiology*, edited by A. J. Bachrach and M. M. Matzen. Bethesda, MD: Undersea Medical Society.

O'REILLY, J. P., B. RESPICIO, F. K. KURATA, AND E. M. HAYASHI 1977. Hana Kai II: a 17-day dry saturation dive at 18.6 ATA. VII. Auditory, visual, and gustatory sensations. *Undersea Biomed. Res.* 4: 307–314.

PETROVYKH, V. A., O. A. SHOVKOPLYAS, D. A. MIKHELSON, AND E. N. ARANOVA 1977. Parameters of nitrogen, carbohydrate and lipid metabolism in man during prolonged exposure to hyperbaric conditions. *Kosm. Biol. Aviakosm. Med.* 11: 48–50.

PHILP, R. B., C. W. GOWDEY. AND M. PRASAD 1967. Changes in blood lipid concentration and cell counts following decompression sickness in rats and the influence of dietary lipid. *Can. J. Physiol. Pharmacol.* 45: 1047–1057.

RAYMOND, L., J. SODE, W. SPAUR, D. UDDIN, R. JOHNSONBAUGH, R. BRAUER, M. KNOTT. AND J. CROTHERS 1974. Glucose homeostasis of man in helium oxygen at 1-50 atmospheres absolute. *Undersea Biomed. Res.* 1: 325–334.

REEVES, E., J. W. WEAVER, J. J. BENJAMIN. AND C. H. MANN 1965. Comparison of physiological changes during long-term immersion to neck levels in water of 95°, 85° and 75°F. Rept. 9. Bethesda, MD: U.S. Naval Medical Research Institute.

RODAHL, K. 1954. *Eskimo Metabolism.* Oslo: Skrifto.

SEGUI, G., AND V. CONTI 1972. Compartement alimentaire de trois oceanauter au cours d'une experience de vie à saturation. *Bull. Medsubhyp.* 7: 15–18.

WEBB, P., AND S. J. TROUTMAN, JR. 1970. An instrument for the continuous measurement of oxygen consumption. *J. Appl. Physiol.* 29: 867–871.

WEBB, P., S. J. TROUTMAN, JR., V. FRATTALI, R. H. DRESSENDORFER, J. DWYER, T. O. MOORE, J. F. MORLOCK, R. M. SMITH, Y. OHTA. AND S. K. HONG 1977. Hana Kai II: a 17-day dry saturation dive at 18.6 ATA. II. Energy balance. *Undersea Biomed. Res.* 4: 221–246.

WEIHL, A. C., H. C. LANGWORTHY, R. P. LAYTON, P. F. HOAR. AND L. W. RAYMOND 1978. Metabolic responses of resting divers immersed in 25.5°C and 33°C water. *Undersea Biomed. Res.* 5:(Suppl.) 31–32.

J. Hyperbaric Arthralgia

Hyperbaric arthralgia includes a collection of joint symptoms that occur during compression to higher than normobaric pressures when nitrogen-oxygen or helium-oxygen mixtures are breathed (Bradley and Vorosmarti 1974). The prominent joint symptoms are joint pain and popping (cracking). The two frequently coexist, though either can occur independently during diving with helium-oxygen breathing mixtures. Joint pain is not prominent during air diving, although popping frequently occurs. This suggests that the mechanisms operative in helium-oxygen diving are also present in air diving. The perceived absence of joint pain during air diving is probably a result of the analgesia caused by nitrogen narcosis, which may mask mild degrees of pain.

Joints do not hurt if they are not moved. Rapid movements are more likely than slow movements to cause both joint pain and joint popping. This probably explains why hyperbaric arthralgia is usually not observed in divers while they are in the water but is primarily a syndrome of chamber or habitat diving. In the water, the diver is in a viscous medium with a protective suit that keeps him or her from making rapid movements.

In helium-oxygen diving there is an increase in the frequency of both joint popping and joint pain as depth increases. The frequency and severity of joint pain is, however, less during those dives in which slow compression rates are used. Joint discomfort and popping disappear or are ameliorated by returning to shallower depths or by waiting at bottom depth for a long enough period of time, which may be days.

The shoulder joint is the joint most frequently affected by hyperbaric arthralgia. In decreasing order of frequency, the knees, wrists, hips, and back are involved; fingers, ankles, and elbows are least often affected. Pain in the back, hips, and shoulders is often more severe and causes a greater limitation of motion than involvement of the other sites.

The remainder of this section attempts to answer three questions: What etiologic agent is responsible for hyperbaric arthralgia? By what means does it cause pain and popping of joints? What implications does this disorder have for the health of the diver? The discussion of these questions is necessarily speculative, since there has been little experimental work in this area.

One hypothesis of the origin of hyperbaric arthralgia has implicated increased hydrostatic pressure as the etiologic agent. This view can be criticized on the grounds that the fluids and structures of the body are compressed very little by the pressures encountered in modern deep diving. For example, the lubricating film between the articular surfaces of a joint in a diver compressed to 20 atm would retain 99.9% of its original thickness. On the other hand, structures such as bone and cartilage must have different compressibilities. Since cartilage is firmly affixed to bone, even small differences in the compressibilities of these structures might cause shear forces when hydrostatic pressure increases. This may explain how subchondral pain receptors are stimulated, which might be perceived in turn as the joint pain of hyperbaric arthralgia. It is less clear how these events would account for the joint popping that also occurs.

The other hypothesis considers osmotically induced shifts of fluid from the synovial cavities responsible for the syndrome of hyperbaric arthralgia. Kylstra et al. (1968) demonstrated that dissolved inert gases exert osmotic pressure and can cause shifts in fluid. When a diver is exposed to increased pressure, the partial pressure of gas in his or her blood temporarily exceeds the partial pressure of inert gas in poorly perfused tissues. Dissolved gas-concentration gradients may cause fluid to move from a squashy, water-filled tissue with no blood supply (such as articular cartilage) to the well-perfused adjacent ends of bones. Loss of water from the articular cartilage will interfere with the various modes of lubricating the joints and cause shear forces to become abnormally high. Additionally, there may be decreases in the elasticity and resiliency of the articular surfaces. In the presence of a cartilage layer that has been thinned by dehydration and of increased frictional resistance in the joints, pain receptors in the subchondral and synovial vascular plexus may be stimulated, causing the joint discomfort of hyperbaric arthralgia.

Osmotically induced shifts of water from articular cartilage may also be responsible for the popping of joints at depth. Joint popping normally occurs when joint surfaces are separated. It is caused by the formation and collapse of a cavitation bubble (cavitation is the formation of vapor and gas bubbles in a liquid caused by a reduction of total pressure). Whether a joint is susceptible to cavitation is apparently determined largely by the geometric configuration of the articulating surfaces. Joints that do not pop have concentric fits, while joints that pop have eccentrically configured articulations. There is an area in joints with eccentric configurations that is covered with a very thin film. When loads are applied to such joints, very low pressures are generated at the center of contact; when these low pressures occur in a fluid containing a high concentration of gas, cavitation occurs.

There are several means by which osmotic shifts of water from articular cartilage may cause joints to pop under hyperbaric conditions. The first is that loss of fluid from articular cartilage may deform the cartilage, thereby transforming a joint with a concentric fit to one with an eccentric fit. Second, loss of water from the fluid would decrease synovial fluid volume and bring articular surfaces closer, predisposing the fluid to cavitation. Third, interfering with various modes of joint lubrication may itself predispose the joint to cavitation phenomena.

What then are the implications of cavitation within joints? Cavitation is the formation of vapor and gas bubbles in a liquid followed by expansion of the cavitation bubble, which then collapses rapidly when it moves into areas of higher pressure. The fluid flowing in from all directions meets at a point and generates high impact forces, which are audible as noise. (Energy developed on a larger scale by the same forces is capable of eroding ships' propellers and damaging many types of hydraulic machinery.) In the joints of a diver, this energy is released by the collapse of the bubble when pressures increase. The large and sudden impact forces generated by the collapse of the bubble may stimulate synovial and subchondral pain receptors.

When inert gas is taken up by articular cartilage, water moves back into the cartilage; impaired joint lubrication and bubble formation generally then disappear. Indeed, joint pain, popping, and unpleasant arthresthesias eventually do disappear if the diver stays on the bottom.

Whether articular structures are damaged if joint lubrication is impaired and whether cavitation occurs when high energy is released is not known. There is, however, some reason to think that articular structures may be damaged, thereby predisposing the joint to degenerative joint disease. Until more information on the effects of hyperbaric arthralgia is available, the use of relatively slow compression rates for deep diving is advocated.

The author gratefully acknowledges the advice and superb editorial assistance of Ms. M. Matzen and Ms. R. Balenger.

MARK E. BRADLEY

References

BRADLEY, M. E., AND J. VOROSMARTI, JR. 1974. Hyperbaric arthralgia during helium-oxygen dives from 100 to 850 fsw. *Undersea Biomed. Res.* 1: 151–167.

KYLSTRA, J. A., I. S. LONGMUIR, AND M. GRACE 1968. Dysbarism: Osmosis caused by dissolved gas? *Science* 161: 289.

K. Vestibular and Auditory Function

Man, a terrestrial being, has evolved organs of hearing and balance that are well adapted to perform these functions in an air environment that is maintained within a relatively limited range of barometric pressures. Altering the density and pressure of man's environment causes significant physiological changes in these organs. Although man can usually adapt to gradual but small changes in barometric pressure, the relatively sudden and marked changes encountered in diving present significant problems.

The air-containing structures in the human organs of hearing, the external and middle ears, efficiently overcome the impedance mismatch of sound transmission between air and water. In wet and dry diving, which involves significant changes in the pressure and density of the surrounding medium, adequate pressure equilibration and ventilation between these cavities and the surrounding environment must be maintained; these air-containing structures thus become a liability. The effects of pressure and density changes upon the pressure-equilibrated external ear canal and middle ear transformer cause changes in the function of these structures and subsequently raise the auditory thresholds for sound transmitted in the aqueous and gaseous environments. With inadequate pressure equilibration in these structures, auditory thresholds are further elevated and the external ear canal, ear drum, contents of the middle ear, and inner ear may be injured. As discussed below, injuries of the external ear canal, ear drum, and middle ear frequently can be reversed with proper treatment; however, inner ear injuries involving nerve deafness and vestibular dysfunction frequently are not reversible.

1. Auditory Function

The organ of hearing (Figure III-42) is composed of three basic parts: the air-containing external ear, including the pinna and external auditory canal; the air-containing

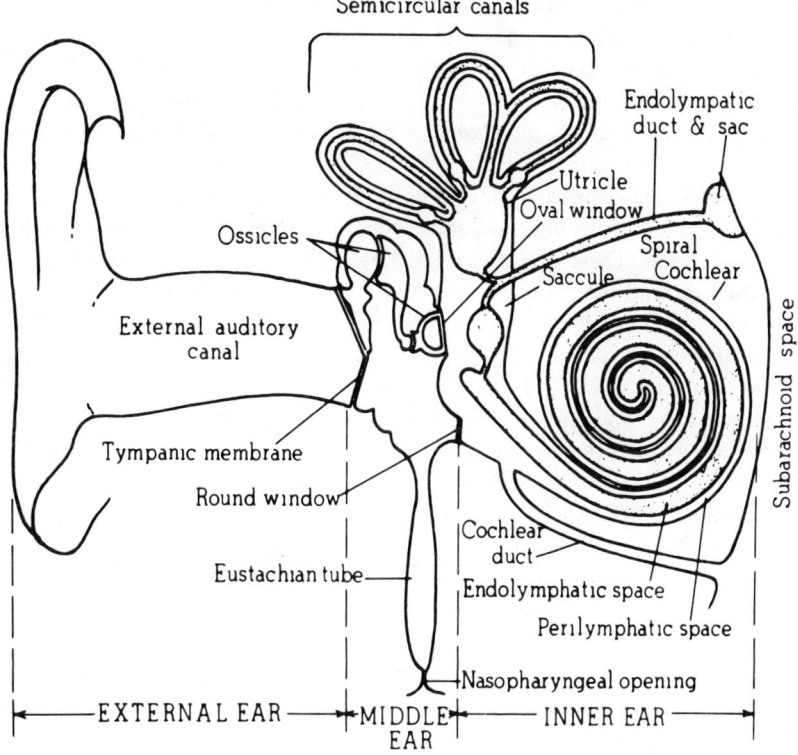

Figure III-42. Simplified diagrammatic drawing of the external, middle, and inner ear; the air-containing external auditory canal, middle ear, and eustachian tube are noted. The fluid-filled inner ear is subdivided into the perilymphatic and endolymphatic spaces, which connect to the subarachnoid space by the cochlear duct and endolymphatic duct, respectively. [From Farmer and Thomas (1976).]

middle ear, including the ear drum and ossicular chain; and the fluid-filled inner ear containing the auditory cochlear and vestibular organs. The middle ear is an irregularly shaped space connecting with variable air cell systems in other portions of the temporal bone (mastoid, petrous, and zygomatic areas). With an intact tympanic membrane, the only pathway for pressure equilibration between these air spaces and the ambient atmosphere is the eustachian tube. The ostium of the eustachian tube in the nasopharynx is normally closed except when opened by positive middle ear pressure or by the action of the palatine and pharyngeal muscles, as happens particularly during swallowing. Frequently, a positive nasopharyngeal pressure, such as that involved in a Valsalva maneuver, can force open the nasopharyngeal eustachian tubal ostium. However, adequate eustachian tubal patency is frequently not assured in diving (see Chapter IX, Section D). Any obstruction can lead to significant barotrauma in the middle ear or inner ear. Also, a Valsalva maneuver can cause an inner ear injury, particularly when performed at depth in the presence of an existing negative middle ear pressure. These injuries can be dangerous at the moment of occurrence because of the resulting vestibular dysfunction, and may also cause significant discomfort and permanent disability.

The physiology of the nontraumatized peripheral auditory system during diving in the absence of known barotrauma or decompression sickness has been studied by several investigators. Using tuning forks, Lester and Gomez (1898) noted decreased air and bone conduction in human subjects exposed to compressed air at 3.0 and 3.5 ATA. However, the persistence of these changes for one to two days after decompression suggests that otologic trauma had occurred. In 1966, Fluur and Adolfson (1966) published the results of well-performed audiometric threshold determinations made using calibrated transducers in divers exposed atraumatically to hyperbaric air in a chamber compressed to pressures of up to 11 ATA. Depth-related elevations of 30 to 40 dB in air conduction thresholds were found in the middle frequencies at the maximum depth. Bone conduction thresholds remained unchanged. These effects were believed to be caused by the increased density of compressed air and the resulting increased impedance of the middle ear transformer and decreased sound conduction to the inner ear. Farmer and colleagues (1971) studied the hearing of six asymptomatic divers pressurized in a chamber to 19.2 ATA (600 fsw) with helium-oxygen, and found that cochlear hearing thresholds and the ability to discriminate frequencies were not altered. However, gas conduction thresholds revealed low frequency hearing losses that disappeared gradually during decompression. These changes were considered secondary to a combination of an increase in ear resonance frequency due to an increase in the speed of sound in helium and an increased impedance of the middle ear transformer due to the increased gas density. Additional studies by Thomas and co-workers (1974) confirmed the presence of reversible, depth-related, and primarily low-frequency conductive hearing losses in a group of 33 asymptomatic divers during eight helium-oxygen chamber dives to simulated sea depths of up to 976 fsw (30 ATA or 305 msw). Again, no alterations in cochlear function were noted, and conductive hearing losses occurred primarily in the first 30.5 meters (98 fsw) of compression and did not increase significantly at deeper depths.

Measuring hearing thresholds in a dry compressed gas environment requires correction for the effect of this environment on the performance of earphones and microphones, essential equipment for psychoacoustic threshold determinations. These transducers must be carefully calibrated under similar gas and pressure conditions.

Several groups of investigators (Brandt and Hollien 1969; Hamilton 1957; Montague and Strickland 1961; Wainwright 1958) have measured auditory thresholds in the water at depths ranging from 3 to 32 meters (10 to 102 fsw). These workers found significant elevations in hearing thresholds that were not related to depth, but no alterations in cochlear function were observed. These results suggest that underwater hearing may occur primarily by bone conduction. Other mechanisms may also account for these elevated hearing thresholds obtained under wet conditions.

Thus, the auditory effects of diving, in the absence of barotrauma or decompression sickness, involve depth- and inert-gas–related conductive hearing losses without demonstrated changes in cochlear function up to simulated seawater depths of 1000 fsw (305 msw). Whether or not changes in cochlear function will be found at deeper depths remains to be determined. The conductive hearing losses thus far observed do not appear to significantly impair diving communication; the major communication problems are related to helium voice distortion during helium-oxygen compressions. Changes in the function of the peripheral auditory system do not appear to play a significant role in this problem.

2. Vestibular Function

In terrestrial environments, humans perceive spatial orientation, position, and motion by integration in the central nervous system of sensory inputs from three basic systems: the visual, proprioceptive, and vestibular systems. Visual and proprioceptive inputs are frequently distorted underwater because of murky water and buoyancy; thus, proper spatial orientation and motion perception become more dependent upon information received from the peripheral vestibular system located in the inner ears. In addition to hearing loss, dysfunction of this system may cause vertigo with nausea and, possibly, vomiting, thus presenting a potentially life-threatening danger to the affected diver.

Much of the previous diving literature on disturbances of equilibrium is not well documented or has discussed these problems only incidentally. Dizziness has not been defined specifically, and true vertigo has often not been differentiated from other vague balance disturbances such as light-headedness, unsteadiness, faintness, or swaying. Dizzy individuals have often not been evaluated adequately to differentiate primary disturbances of the vestibular system and end-organ or central vestibular injuries from other causes of disequilibrium. Also, divers who continue to have vertigo after apparent recovery are frequently not properly evaluated to determine their suitability for future diving. These deficiencies are understandable, because dizzy patients often present complex and perplexing diagnostic problems even for specialists. An understanding of vestibular physiology and a systematic approach to the evaluation of divers affected by disequilibrium should be developed.

Each semicircular canal, saccule, and utricle is paired with the same structure in the opposite inner ear. Head movements result in changes in resting neuronal discharge rates. In the case of the semicircular canals, angular acceleration causes a decrease or increase in the discharge rate of neuroepithelium in one canal, with an equal but opposite change in the paired canal of the opposite ear. The saccule and utricle in each inner ear respond similarly to linear acceleration. These changes are interpreted in the cerebral cortex as motion in a specific direction at a specific velocity. The eye muscle motor nuclei also receive this information and move the eyes in a compensatory manner to maintain the field of last gaze. Trunk and limb muscles are adjusted through the action on the anterior horn cells in the spinal cord by signals over the vestibulospinal tracts.

The cerebellum further modulates the system with adjustments in firing rates in the central vestibular system that allow for changes in muscle tone to compensate for any changes in position. The vestibular end organs in the inner ears thus are constantly discharging a resting pattern of signals to the brain; acceleration causes a change in this pattern of signals, which is distributed to the brain and then interpreted. If a sudden pathological decrease occurs in the neuronal firing rate of one of the vestibular end organs, the discharge rate to the paired central vestibular nuclei changes, and the brain perceives this information as hyperfunction of the noninjured side.

The cerebral cortex interprets this state as a condition of constant motion, which may be perceived as pitching, yawing, rolling, or rotating. A rotational component, vertigo, is usually present because of the predominance of the innervation from the six semicircular canals over the four otolithic organs. The eyes are rotated in the direction of last gaze to retain orientation. However, since the rotary sensation continues and the eyes cannot rotate indefinitely because of anatomical limitations, at the limit of gaze in any direction, inhibitor neurons in the reticular system around the eye muscle motor nuclei inhibit the incoming flow from the vestibular nuclei. Simultaneously, activation from the reticular activating neurons directs certain eye muscle motor nuclei to return the eyes quickly to the point of gaze from which the slow component originated. The slow and fast phases of vestibular nystagmus are generated in this manner.

Ataxia and staggering, nausea and vomiting, pallor, sweating, and other cardiovascular changes frequently occur because of connections in the central nervous system between the vestibular system and the spinal cord anterior horn cells, the dorsal motor nucleus of the tenth cranial nerve, and the hypothalamus. The cerebellum initially acts to compensate for these disorders by inhibiting the firing rates of the vestibular nuclei on the uninjured side, thus narrowing the difference in firing rates coming from each side and decreasing the magnitude of the symptoms (McCabe 1973).

With most vestibular end-organ injuries, the injured structures do not recover. However, compensation will occur over a period of time despite the continued hypofunction or lack of function of one vestibular end organ. This compensation is due to continued cerebellar suppression of the vestibular nuclei on the uninjured side and the gradual appearance of new resting electrical activity in the centrally located vestibular nuclei on the side of the injury. This new resting activity balances the unaffected and relatively hyperactive side, causing the symptoms to disappear in most positions and for most activities. The speed with which compensatory mechanisms develop depends on the severity of the original injury and the ability of the central nervous system to respond.

From these principles, several general concepts can be derived:

1. The first distinction that should be made in the evaluation of a dizzy diver is whether the diver has experienced dizziness related to dysfunction in other body systems or true vestibular vertigo related to dysfunction in the vestibular system.

2. With vestibular system dysfunction, classic labyrinthine nystagmus with well-defined fast and slow components is present. If a dizzy patient does not have nystagmus at the time of his dizziness, as detected either by visual observation or electronystagmography, the dizziness is usually not caused by vestibular system dysfunction.

3. Permanent inner ear vestibular injury does not produce continuous and nonepisodic dizziness for longer than 2 to 4 weeks. If dizziness is continuous for a longer period of time, the cause is usually not vestibular system end-organ dysfunction, because, as noted above, compensation usually occurs after such injuries. A possible exception to this rule would be a diver who has a persistent perilymph leak from a ruptured labyrinthine window (see Chapter IX, Section-D). Also, central vestibular system injury can cause continuous dizziness that is not vertiginous and that lasts for longer times.

4. Once it has been determined that dizziness is vertiginous in nature and perhaps caused by primary vestibular system dysfunction, the next distinction to be made is whether the damage is located in the end organ or the central vestibular pathways. Simultaneous nausea, vomiting, visual disturbance, presyncopy, and difficulty in standing or walking do not necessarily mean central nervous system injury. Auditory symptoms or signs or indications of damage to the tympanic membrane or the middle ear are more frequently associated with end-organ injury. The presence of other neurological signs or vertical nystagmus usually indicates central nervous system pathology.

5. The disappearance of vertigo over a period of days or weeks after an acute injury to the vestibular end organ is usually caused by the development of normal compensatory mechanisms in the central nervous system and does not necessarily mean that the vestibular end organ has recovered its previously healthy state. Therefore, all divers who have experienced vestibular system injury should be evaluated by specialists after their symptoms have apparently disappeared. Only in this way can rational judgments be made regarding an individual's suitability for future diving.

During most diving conditions, both vestibular end organs are stimulated appropriately and equally, and vertigo does not occur. However, in certain diving situations unequal stimulation occurs, and transient vertigo and nystagmus have been noted. Such occurrences, and occasionally nausea and vomiting, may be life threatening to divers.

The episodes of transient vertigo and dizziness noted in the literature during the breathing of nonphysiological gas mixtures were probably related to the effects of the breathing gas on the central nervous system rather than to primary vestibular system dysfunction (Edmonds et al. 1973). The unequal entry of cold water into the external ear canals after obstruction of one of the canals by cerumen, otitis externa, ear plugs, or bony exostoses may produce a caloric response. This is particularly true when the diver is oriented in a position in which the lateral semicircular canal is in a vertical plane (Edmonds et al. 1973). The unequal entry of cold water into the middle ear through tympanic membrane perforations may also cause transient vertigo from a caloric effect (Edmonds et al. 1973).

Transient vestibular dysfunction related to asymmetric middle ear pressure equilibration during ascent and descent has been described by Lundgren (1965), who coined the term *alternobaric vertigo*, and others (Edmonds et al. 1973; Terry and Dennison 1966; Vorosmarti and Bradley 1970). Tjernström (1973) has demonstrated actual nystagmus on electronystagmograph recordings that occurred in association with asymmetric middle ear pressure equilibration during ascent in shallow chamber dives.

Dizziness and vertigo have been described as one of the manifestations of the high-pressure nervous syndrome (HPNS) (Bennett and Towse 1971; Brauer 1968; Buehlmann et al. 1970). Further studies (Adolfson et al. 1972; Braithwaite et al. 1974; Farmer et al. 1974; Gauthier 1976) have shown that the dizziness of the HPNS is not accompanied by sustained vestibular nystagmus but is associated with decrements in postural equilibrium and bilaterally equal increases in the vestibuloocular reflex. Thus, the dizziness associated with HPNS does not appear to be related to unilateral dysfunction of the vestibular end organs or primary vestibular neurons, or both, but to central vestibular system dysfunction that does not have dominant unilateral effects.

JOSEPH C. FARMER, JR.

References

ADOLFSON, J. A., L. GOLDBERG. AND T. E. BERGHAGE 1972. Effects of increased ambient air pressures on standing steadiness in man. *Aerosp. Med.* 43: 520–524.
BENNETT, P. B., AND E. J. TOWSE 1971. The high pressure nervous syndrome during a simulated oxygen-helium dive to 1500 feet. *Electroencephalogr. Clin. Neurophysiol.* 31: 383–393.
BRAITHWAITE, W. R., T. E. BERGHAGE, AND J. C. CROTHERS 1974. Postural equilibrium and vestibular response at 49.5 ATA. *Undersea Biomed. Res.* 1: 309–323.
BRANDT, J. F., AND H. HOLLIEN 1969. Underwater hearing thresholds in man as a function of water depth. *J. Acoust. Soc. Am.* 46: 893–897.
BRAUER, R. W. 1968. Seeking man's depth level. *Ocean Industry* 3: 28–33.
BUEHLMANN, A., H. MATTHYS, H. OVERRATH, P. B. BENNETT, D. H. ELLIOTT. AND S. P. GRAY 1970. Saturation exposures of 31 ATA in an oxygen-helium atmosphere with excursions to 36 ATA. *Aerosp. Med.* 41: 394–402.
EDMONDS, C., P. FREEMAN, R. THOMAS, J. TONKIN. AND F. A. BLACKWOOD 1973. *Otological Aspects of Diving.* Sydney, Australia: Australian Medical Publishing Co.
FARMER, J. C., AND W. G. THOMAS 1976. Ear and sinus problems in diving. In: *Diving Medicine*, edited by R. M. Strauss. New York: Grune and Stratton, p. 109–133.
FARMER, J. C., W. G. THOMAS. AND M. J. PRESLAR 1971. Human auditory responses during hyperbaric helium-oxygen exposures. *Surg. Forum* 22: 456–458.
FARMER, J. C., W. G. THOMAS, R. W. SMITH. AND P. B. BENNETT 1974. Vestibular function during HPNS (abstract). *Undersea Biomed. Res.* 1: A-11.
FLUUR, E., AND J. ADOLFSON 1966. Hearing in hyperbaric air. *Aerosp. Med.* 57: 783–785.
GAUTHIER, G. M. 1976. Alterations of the human vestibulo-ocular reflex in a simulated dive at 62 ATA. *Undersea Biomed. Res.* 3: 103–112.
HAMILTON, P. M. 1957. Underwater hearing thresholds. *J. Acoust. Soc. Am.* 29: 792–794.
LESTER, J. C., AND V. GOMEZ 1898. Observations made in the caisson of the New East River Bridge as to the effects of compressed air upon the human ear. *Arch. Otolaryngol.* 27: 1–19.
LUNDGREN, C. E. G. 1965. Alternobaric vertigo—a diver's hazard. *Br. Med. J.* 2: 511–513.
McCABE, B. F. 1973. Vestibular physiology: its clinical application in understanding the dizzy patient. In: *Basic Sciences and Related Disciplines. Otolaryngology*, edited by M. M. Paparella and D. A. Schumrick. Philadelphia: Saunders, Vol. 1, p. 318–328.
MONTAGUE, W. E., AND J. F. STRICKLAND 1961. Sensitivity of the water-immersed ear to high and low level tones. *J. Acoust. Soc. Am.* 33: 1376–1381.
TERRY, L., AND W. L. DENNISON 1966. Vertigo amongst Divers. Special Rep. 66-2. Groton, CT: U.S. Navy Submarine Medical Center.
THOMAS, W. G., J. K. SUMMITT. AND J. C. FARMER 1974. Human auditory thresholds during deep saturation helium-oxygen dives. *J. Acoust. Soc. Am.* 55: 110–113.
TJERNSTRÖM, Ö. 1973. On alternobaric vertigo: experimental studies. *Försvarsmedicine* 9: 410–415.
VOROSMARTI, J., AND J. J. BRADLEY 1970. Alternobaric vertigo in military divers. *Mil. Med.* 135: 182–185.
WAINWRIGHT, W. N. 1958. Comparison of hearing thresholds in air and in water. *J. Acoust. Soc. Am.* 30: 1025–1029.

L. Vision

Vision underwater is profoundly altered from what it is in air for a variety of reasons. The majority of these reasons are physical, stemming from the fact that the eye is immersed in water and that light rays travel through the water rather than air. In addition, some physiological changes, either normal or pathological, may occur within the visual system underwater, which may further alter seeing.

1. Physical Factors in Underwater Seeing

a. Vision without a Face Mask

A submariner making an unhooded escape to the surface, a downed pilot, or a diver who has lost his mask suffers gross deterioration of vision caused by immersion of the eyes in water. Since the refractive index of the eye is very close to that of water, the loss of an air-corneal interface results in loss of most of the refraction of light rays needed for proper focus on the retina. The size of the change in vision is very large; individuals become in effect 40 to 50 diopters hyperopic.

Measures of acuity (Luria and Kinney 1969), made either underwater without a mask or in air by inducing hyperopia of up to 50 diopters, have shown that the vision of individuals is reduced to 20/100 or 20/200 under the best of conditions. Thus an air interface is essential for effective vision underwater.

b. Effects of Refraction

The diver's face mask usually provides this essential air interface, although other techniques are possible. Whatever the method, the additional interface between the air and the water causes various distortions of the visual image. The distortions are, of course, a physical consequence of the light energy passing from one medium (water) into another (air) in which its speed is greater. The refracted light rays form a virtual image of the object at three-quarters of the distance from the interface; the image (for a typical face mask) appears to be larger than the real object by a factor of about 1.27 and is transformed in shape, since greater refraction occurs at greater angles of incidence.

These changes in the effective retinal image may have several perceptual consequences: underestimations of distances underwater, overestimations of size, distortions of shape and position, and interference with hand-eye coordination. Empirical tests have been made of the extent to which divers suffered from these various perceptual distortions (Kinney et al. 1970). This research confirmed that distortions occur in the underwater perception of the distance, size, shape, and position of objects and in hand-eye coordination, and that some, but not all, of these changes can be predicted from the refractive changes in the visual image. In addition, this study showed that some perceptual distortions become smaller as the observer gains experience underwater.

Distance perception under water is affected by optical distortion, but water turbidity produces the opposite effect. This is illustrated in Figure III-43, which represents idealized

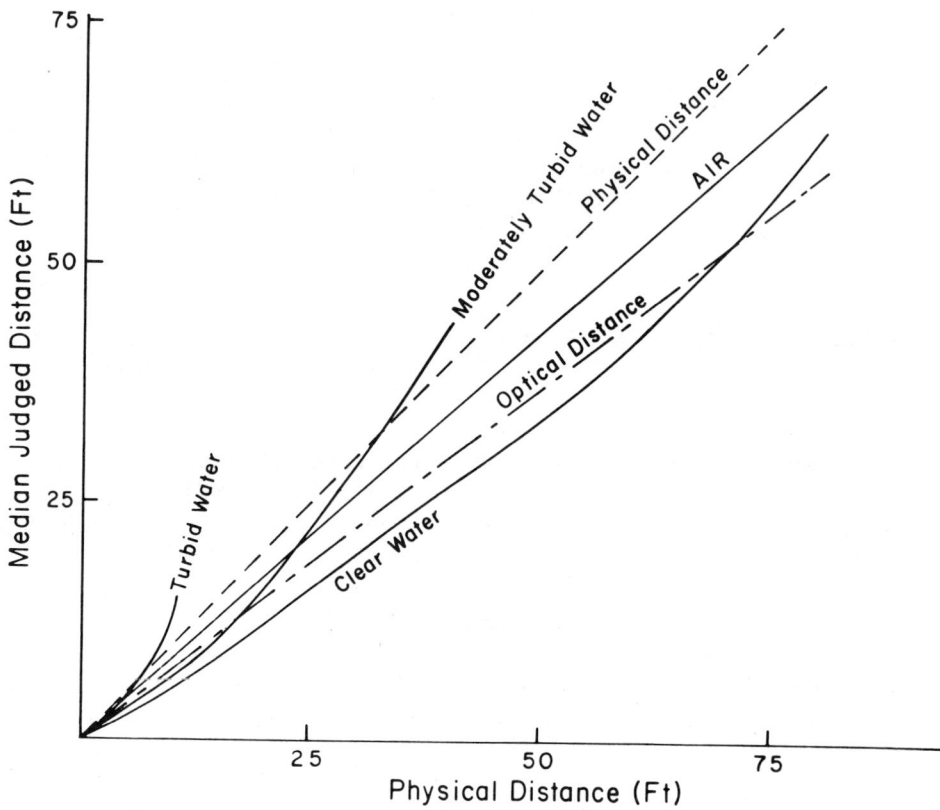

Figure III-43. Idealized functions for the perception of absolute distance in air, and in turbid, moderately turbid, and clear water. [From Ferris (1972b).]

data from many different experiments (Ferris 1972b). Divers are often told that objects will appear too close underwater; however, this is only true in clear water and at distances of a few feet (Ferris 1972a). In turbid water, on the other hand, the distance of an object is overestimated and the crossover from under- to overestimation varies with the turbidity of the water. Training can improve the ability of divers to estimate distance (Ferris 1973).

Objects underwater are also distorted in shape, which interferes with visual motor skills and hand-eye coordination, since objects are not located where they appear to be. Comparison of individuals with no underwater experience with those having various amounts of experience has shown that hand-eye coordination does improve with experience, although it is rarely as good as it is in air (Luria and Kinney 1970). The perception of size, however, does not improve with experience (Kinney and Luria 1970). The specific means of providing an air interface affects the type of distortion caused. Assessments of various commercially available face masks (Luria et al. 1974) and of hard hat diving systems (Kinney et al. 1972) have shown that each configuration has advantages and disadvantages. For example, it is possible to compensate optically for the increased retinal image caused by a normal face mask; compensating masks are effective in improving size and distance perception, but they reduce the size of the field of view. Thus, although it is possible to select the best mask for a given task, there is no single mask that is best for all tasks.

(i) Correction of Ametropia Underwater. The need for an air interface and the consequent effects of refraction apply to everyone underwater. However, many individuals (those with myopia, hyperopia, and astigmatism) require additional correction to see adequately. Since glasses cannot be worn with a face mask because of leakage around the temples, a variety of methods of providing the correction are available: for example, masks with apertures for lenses; lens holders within the mask; and large-sized lenses bonded to the faceplate.

Alternatively, one's regular contact lenses can be worn with a face mask; this technique provides the real advantages of good peripheral vision and no loss of vision when the diver gets out of the water and removes his or her mask. While many individuals wear contact lenses without problems, caution is advised. Simon and Bradley (1978) have observed small bubbles in the precorneal tear film of two divers after a 150-fsw chamber dive on air. Symptoms, which included soreness, halos, and decreased visual acuity, were not observed when divers wore soft contact lenses or put a tiny hole in the center of hard contact lenses.

c. Effects of Absorption and Scatter

The scattering and absorption of light energy or photons as they are transmitted through water have the greatest effect on underwater vision. Scattering occurs when the photons hit particles suspended in the water and change direction. Thus the more turbid the water, the greater the scattering and the consequent loss of contrast between an object and its background. There is a rough rule of thumb in vision that contrast must exceed 2% or an object will be invisible. This contrast limitation is rarely, except in severe smoke or fog, a factor in visual performance in air, where the size of an object is the major factor in its visibility. In water, however, contrasts commonly fall below 2% because of scatter; lack of contrast rather than size then becomes the limiting factor in visibility.

Visibility ranges can be calculated for specific conditions if sufficient data are available; in fact, Duntley (1958) has published a series of nomographs on which to base such predictions. Many variables are important, such as the size of the object, its inherent contrast, the general illumination or adaptation level, the line of sight, and, above all, the attenuation coefficients of the water. The latter reflect the amount of scatter in and absorption by a given body of water and may be sufficient to cause the range of visibility to change from less than 1 ft (30 cm) to more than 200 ft (60 m).

(i) Effect of Absorption. The amount of light transmitted through the water depends not only upon how much is scattered but also upon how much is absorbed by the water. The absorption characteristics of the specific body of water in which the diver is immersed therefore have a profound effect on what the diver can see. Clearest ocean water, like distilled water, does not absorb all wavelengths of light equally. Very short and very long wavelengths are absorbed to a greater extent than waves of other lengths, which causes peak transmittance for waves of about 480 nanometers (nm) in the blue-green portion of the spectrum. Since the amount of light energy absorbed varies exponentially with the distance the light travels through the water, all wavelengths except those around 480 nm are quickly lost at deeper depths. For the diver depending on natural light in

these waters, colors in the red-orange portion of the spectrum, such as those of blood or skin, are lost.

The transmittance of the water found in most bodies of water often differs greatly from that of distilled water because of silt, decomposed plant and animal material, pollution, and living organisms. Plankton are a common cause of change in transmittance. Plankton absorb short wavelengths of energy much more than long wavelengths, which causes the peak of the transmittance curve to shift to the yellow-green portion of the spectrum; the amount of shift depends on the density of the plankton.

Figure III-44 shows the spectral transmission curves for 1 m of water from several different bodies of water in which color vision was investigated (Kinney et al. 1967). Both the absolute percentage of light and the relative effectiveness of different wavelengths

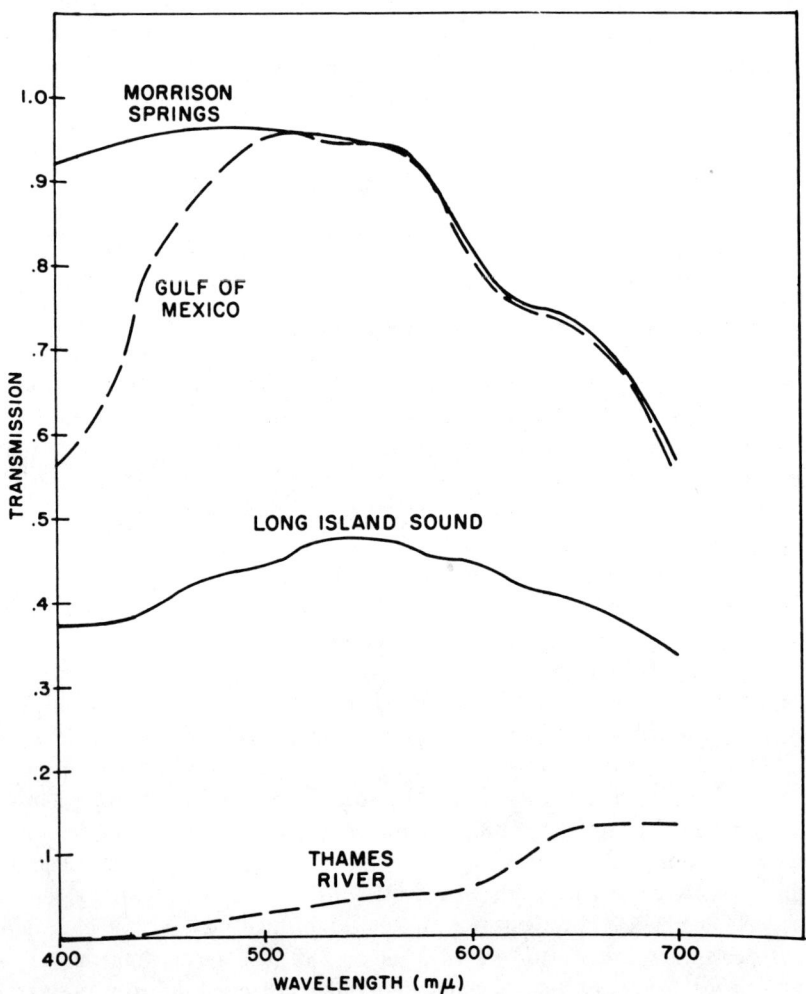

Figure III-44. Spectral transmittance of one meter of water from various bodies of water. [From Kinney et al. (1967).]

vary greatly from one body of water to another. As a consequence, the most visible colors can change dramatically underwater, depending on the type of water in which they are immersed. For example, the range of visibility in Morrison Springs was 85 ft, and the blues and greens were more visible than other colors. In the Thames River, on the other hand, the overall visibility range was only a few feet but oranges and reds were the easiest to see (Kinney et al. 1967).

It is possible to predict which colors will be perceived and which will be confused on the basis of information about the spectral transmittance curves of a particular body of water and the energy distribution of the light source, be it sunlight, tungsten, or mercury vapor (Kinney et al. 1969). In general, blues and greens are most effective in clearest water, greens and yellows in coastal water, and yellows and oranges in harbor waters.

2. Physiological Factors in Underwater Vision

Physiological changes in visual function during diving may be normal or adaptive, abnormal but reversible, or pathological and irreversible. All may be caused by the unusual pressures or breathing mixtures associated with diving; since the visual symptoms in many real-dive situations may be the same, determining whether pressure, the gas mixture, or a combination of factors caused the symptom may be difficult. Nonetheless, simulated dives performed in pressure chambers using controlled breathing mixtures have given some well-defined results.

a. Effect of Hyperbaric Oxygen

Breathing air at depth results in higher than normal partial pressures of oxygen which, if extreme, may have toxic effects. Nichols and Lambertsen (1969) have collated and summarized many studies that investigated the effects of breathing 100% oxygen. Constriction of the retinal blood vessels, one of the first changes to occur, is evident in people breathing 100% oxygen at atmospheric pressures. This constriction may be adaptive, however, since the supply of oxygen to the retina through the constricted vessels remains adequate for the tissues because the oxygen pressure is greater.

The visual symptoms of oxygen toxicity include diminution of acuity and constriction of the visual fields. The onset of these symptoms depends upon both the partial pressure of the oxygen and the length of time it is breathed. Although the use of oxygen partial pressures above 0.6 ATA is generally considered unwise for extended periods (National Oceanic and Atmospheric Administration 1975), 100% oxygen at 1 ATA apparently can be tolerated for 24 hr without adverse visual effects (Gallagher et al. 1963). Increased pressure may bring severe symptoms; Behnke and co-workers (1936) reported that the visual fields were constricted down to the central 10 degrees after breathing oxygen at a pressure of 3 ATA for 3.5 hr.

Air saturation diving, which by definition produces high partial pressures of oxygen for extended times, is of particular concern, but investigations of the upper limits of air saturation have thus far indicated that air exposures for 30 days at 50 or 60 fsw (2.5 or 2.8 ATA) are safe. Acuity, visual fields, night vision, and color vision showed no adverse effects at these pressures; however, blood vessel calibers were restricted, as expected (Kinney et al. 1974). Investigations at even higher partial pressures of oxygen have generally involved animals and have shown a variety of pathological changes, including retrolental fibroplasias (Patz 1965), hemorrhages, retinal detachments (Beehler et al. 1964), and visual cell death (Noell 1958).

Although most of these severe visual consequences of oxygen toxicity are not reversible, some are, if caught in time. A recent study (Kinney et al. 1977) that used fluorescein angiography to monitor oxygen toxicity showed early multifocal leakage and accumulation of dye in the retinas of monkeys exposed to 100% oxygen at 1 ATA for several days. The pathology appeared to be reversible, since angiograms 7 to 14 days after exposure showed the retinas returning to normal.

b. Effects of Nitrogen

The narcotic effects of high partial pressures of nitrogen on human beings are well known, but no specifically visual symptoms can be isolated from the general alterations of brain functioning that occur under these conditions. Measures of evoked cortical potentials under conditions conducive to nitrogen narcosis have shown alterations in normal auditory, visual, and somatic patterns (Bennett et al. 1969; Kinney and McKay 1971; Langley and Hamilton 1975). For example, measures of the visual evoked cortical potentials of 16 men at a simulated depth of 200 fsw breathing air showed specific changes in the normal response to a slow rate of stimulation, and losses of amplitude when stimulation was presented at a rapid rate; however, the etiology of these changes is unknown (Kinney et al. 1977).

c. Effect of Pressure

It is well known that the visual problems encountered during diving are caused either by high partial pressures of oxygen or of nitrogen and not by pressure itself, at least at normal operating depths. If helium is substituted for nitrogen and if the oxygen partial pressure is kept at or near its surface-air equivalent, vision generally remains normal. Thus Kelly and co-workers (1968) found no adverse effects on the visual function of divers at 825 fsw when the oxygen partial pressure was maintained at 0.3 ATA. Similarly, the divers at 1200 fsw in the first phase of studies at the University of Pennsylvania showed no adverse visual effects (Montabana and Lambertsen 1978).

However, it seems likely that some extreme limiting pressure will be found, as operating depths increase, at which visual function is affected. Indications of a minor amount of deterioration in acuity and accommodation were found after rapid compression to 1200 or 1600 fsw in the second phase of the University of Pennsylvania investigations (Montabana and Lambertsen 1978). In addition, increases in the latency of the visual evoked cortical potential have been noted at 1600 fsw and beyond (Kinney et al. 1978; Rostain and Dimov 1976).

JO ANN S. KINNEY

References

BEEHLER, C. C., N. L. NEWTON, J. F. CULVER, AND T. TREDICI 1964. Retinal detachment in adult dogs resulting from toxicity. *Arch. Ophthal.* 71: 665–670.

BEHNKE, A. R., I. S. FORBES, AND E. P. MOTLEY 1936. Circulatory and visual effects of oxygen at 3 atmospheres pressure. *Am. J. Physiol.* 114: 436–442.

BENNETT, P. B., K. N. ACKLES, AND V. J. CRIPPS 1969. Effects of hyperbaric nitrogen and oxygen on auditory evoked responses in man. *Aerosp. Med.* 40: 521–525.

DUNTLEY, S. Q. 1958. Nomographs for calculating visibility by swimmers. I. Natural light. Rep. 3-1. Project NS714-100, Task 3. Washington, DC: U.S. Navy Bureau of Ships.

FERRIS, S. H. 1972a. Improvement of absolute distance estimation underwater. *Percept. Mot. Skills* 35: 299–305.

FERRIS, S. H. 1972b. Magnitude estimation of absolute distance underwater. *Percept. Mot. Skills* 35: 963–971.

FERRIS, S. H. 1973. Improving absolute distance estimation in clear and in turbid water. *Percept. Mot. Skills* 36: 771–776.

GALLAGHER, T. J., R. E. MAMMEN, F. T. NOBREGA, AND T. TURAIDS 1963. Effects of various oxygen partial pressures on scotopic and photopic vision. Rep. United States Naval Aerospace Crew Equipment Laboratory.

KELLEY, J. S., P. G. BURCH, M. E. BRADLEY, AND D. E. CAMPBELL 1968. Visual function in divers at 15 to 26 atmospheres pressure. *Mil. Med.* 133: 827–829.

KINNEY, J. A. S., AND S. M. LURIA 1970. Conflicting visual and tactual-kinesthetic stimulation. *Percept. Psychophys.* 8: 189–192.

KINNEY, J. A. S., AND C. L. McKAY 1971. The visual evoked responses as a measure of nitrogen narcosis in Navy divers. Rep. 664. Groton, CT: U.S. Naval Submarine Medical Research Laboratory.

KINNEY, J. A. S., R. HAMMOND, R. GELFAND, AND J. CLARK 1978. Visual evoked cortical potentials in men during compression and saturation in $He-O_2$ equivalent to 400, 800, 1200 and 1600 feet of seawater. *Electroencephalogr. Clin. Neurophysiol.* 44: 151–171.

KINNEY, J. A. S., S. M. LURIA, S. H. FERRIS, AND H. M. PAULSON 1972. Optical and visual tests on the Navy prototype hard hat diving system. Rep. 731. Groton, CT: U.S. Naval Submarine Medical Research Laboratory.

KINNEY, J. A. S., S. M. LURIA, M. S. STRAUSS, C. L. McKAY, AND H. M. PAULSON 1974. Shallow Habitat Air Dive Series (SHAD I and II): The effects of visual performance and physiology. Rep. 793. Groton, CT: U.S. Naval Submarine Medical Research Laboratory.

KINNEY, J. A. S., S. M. LURIA, AND D. O. WEITZMAN 1967. Visibility of colors underwater. *J. Opt. Soc. Am.* 57: 802–809.

KINNEY, J. A. S., S. M. LURIA, AND D. O. WEITZMAN 1969. Visibility of colors underwater using artificial illumination. *J. Opt. Soc. Am.* 59: 624–628.

KINNEY, J. A. S., S. M. LURIA, D. O. WEITZMAN, AND H. MARKOWITZ 1970. Effects of diving experience on visual perception under water. Rep. 612. Groton, CT: Naval Submarine Medical Research Laboratory.

KINNEY, J. A. S., C. L. McKAY, AND R. A. GORDON 1977. The use of fluorescein angiography to study oxygen toxicity. *Ann. Ophthal.* 9: 989–995.

KINNEY, J. A. S., C. L. McKAY, AND S. M. LURIA 1977. Visual evoked responses and EEG's of 16 divers breathing air at 7 ATA. *Undersea Biomed. Res.* 4: 55–66.

LANGLEY, T. D., AND R. W. HAMILTON, JR. 1975. Somatic-evoked brain responses as indicators of adaptation to nitrogen narcosis. *Aviat. Space Environ. Med.* 46: 147–151.

LURIA, S. M., AND J. A. S. KINNEY 1969. Visual acuity under water without a face mask. Rep. 581. Groton, CT: U.S. Naval Submarine Medical Research Laboratory.

LURIA, S. M., AND J. A. S. KINNEY 1970. Underwater vision. *Science* 167: 1454–1461.

LURIA, S. M., S. H. FERRIS, C. L. McKAY, J. A. S. KINNEY, AND H. M. PAULSON 1974. Vision through various scuba facemasks. *Human Factors* 16: 395–405.

MONTABANA, D. J., AND C. J. LAMBERTSEN 1978. Visual function. In: *Predictive Studies IV: Work Capability and Physiological Effects in $He-O_2$ Excursions to Pressures of 400-800-1200 and 1600 Feet of Sea Water,* edited by C. J. Lambertsen, R. Gelfand, and J. M. Clark. Philadelphia: Institute for Environmental Medicine, Univ. of Pennsylvania.

NATIONAL OCEANIC AND ATMOSPHERIC ADMINISTRATION 1975. *The NOAA Diving Manual*. Washington, DC: U.S. Dept. of Commerce.

NICHOLS, C. W., AND C. J. LAMBERTSEN 1969. Effects of high oxygen pressures on the eye. *N. Engl. J. Med.* 281: 25–30.

NOELL, W. K. Effects of high and low oxygen tension on the visual system. Paper presented at the First International Symposium on Submarine and Space Medicine, New London, CT, 1958. In: *Environmental Effects on Consciousness: Proceedings*, edited by K. E. Schaefer. New York: Macmillan, 1962.

PATZ, A. 1965. Effect of oxygen on immature retinal vessels. *Invest. Ophthal.* 4: 988–999.

ROSTAIN, J. C., AND S. DIMOV, 1976. Potentiels évoqués visuels et cycle d'excitabilité au cours d'une plongée simulée à-610 m en atmosphère helium-oxygène (Physalie VI). *Electroencephalogr.Clin. Neurophysiol.* 41: 287–300.

SIMON, D. R., AND M. E. BRADLEY 1978. Corneal edema in divers wearing hard contact lenses. *Am. J. Ophthalmol.* 85: 462–464.

M. Breath-Hold Diving

Data recently published by the Center for Disease Control (1980) concerning underwater diving deaths in Florida for the period 1960–78 show that 15% of the total of 440 deaths, or 67 deaths, could not be linked definitely to air-supplied diving; presumably the bulk of these occurred during breath-hold (BH) diving. Craig (1976) summarized 58 cases of loss of consciousness during breath-hold underwater swimming and diving, 23 of which resulted in fatalities.

Although breath-hold diving is potentially dangerous, it is probably the most common type of diving because it is frequently practiced as part of snorkeling and free swimming. Furthermore, the moment any type of breathing gear ceases to function, its wearer instantly becomes a breath-hold diver.

1. Physiology

a. Mammalian Dive Reflex

Irving (1965) documents several profound changes that take place in true diving animals as a consequence of apnea and submersion. These include muscular relaxation (which of course can be overridden); astonishing levels of bradycardia, e.g., heart rates 13% of predive levels in harbor seals (Murdaugh et al. 1966); peripheral vasoconstriction; diminished blood supply to muscles with sparing of heart, brain, and lungs; reduced cardiac output (12% of predive levels); and depressed metabolism. All of these adaptations conserve the body's energy stores. Similar adjustments take place in man, but their extent is certainly less impressive than that in lower animals. In people, apnea and face immersion in cold water can slow the heart rate to 68% of control values (Speck and Bruce 1978). Interestingly, exercise potentiates the bradycardia that occurs during BH diving (Strømme and Blix 1976). This bradycardia is probably vagally mediated, because the response can be blocked by atropine (Heistad et al. 1968). Breath holding combined with cold water face immersion has been shown to be a potent means of treating paroxysmal atrial tachycardia (Wildenthal et al. 1975). However, cold water apneic immersion has induced various arrhythmias, including P-wave changes, heart block, nodal rhythm, wandering pacemaker, and premature ventricular contractions (Paulev 1968; Sasamoto 1965; Speck and Bruce 1978). Such factors as asphyxia, hypothermia, various respiratory maneuvers, vasocontriction, vagal stimulation, and acidosis have been suggested as contributing to the genesis of these arrhythmias (Sasamoto 1965). Mean arterial pressure increases by 14% during breath-holding diving in thermoneutral water and by 21% in 5°C water (Speck and Bruce 1978). There is no evidence that the diving response in man enhances his ability to perform BH diving.

b. Limits of Breath Holding

Mithoefer (1965b) defines the breath-hold breaking point as "the voluntary termination of breath holding in response to the development of a net ventilatory stimulus too strong to be further resisted by voluntary effort." In addition to psychological factors, at least four interdependent physiological elements orchestrate the onset of the breaking point: lung volume, P_{CO_2}, pH, and P_{O_2}. During breath holding, the lung volume may be reduced for diverse reasons, the main ones being that the respiratory exchange ratio ($R = \dot{V}_{CO_2}/\dot{V}_{O_2}$) may be less than 1.0 and that the pulmonary gas becomes compressed as diving depth increases. This is likely to enhance respiratory drive via the so-called deflation reflex. Thus, if a subject in a breath-holding experiment who has reached breaking point is allowed to reexpand his lungs with a gas mixture that does not change the alveolar P_{CO_2} and P_{O_2}, he will be able to prolong his breath hold (Fowler 1954). Furthermore, if a subject is allowed to rebreathe from an anesthesia bag initially filled with air delivered from the lung by a deep expiration, he will be able to sustain this activity much longer than a simple breath hold. He will also experience higher P_{CO_2} and lower P_{O_2} values on completion of rebreathing when compared with breath hold (Hill and Flack 1908). These observations indicate that both lung volume and movement of the respiratory muscles may increase the tolerance for hypercapnia and hypoxia. Figure III-45 shows that when breath holding is performed at larger lung volumes, one's ability to withstand high $P_{A_{CO_2}}$ levels increases.

Among the chemical factors controlling respiration, CO_2 appears to be the strongest (see Figure III-46). Although normal lung ventilation is regulated to keep $P_{A_{CO_2}}$ at about

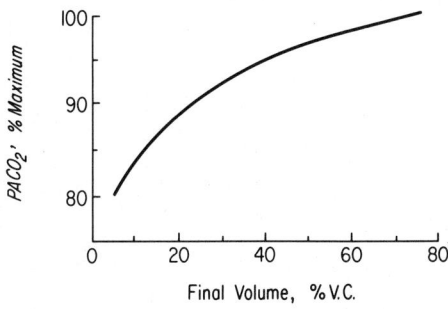

Figure III-45. Effect of lung volume (expressed as percent VC) at breaking point of breath holding with O_2 on tolerance for CO_2, expressing $P_{A_{CO_2}}$ at breaking point as percent of $P_{A_{CO_2}}$ when initial volume was at VC. [From Mithoefer (1965).]

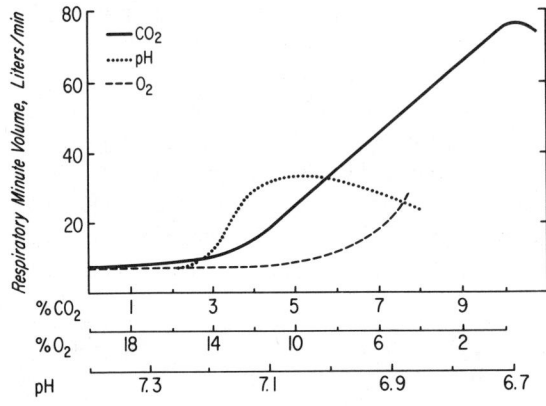

Figure III-46. Respiratory response to inhaled concentrations of CO_2 and O_2, and to blood pH. [From Comroe (1974) with permission.]

40 mmHg, breath holding may force it to exceed 50 mmHg. What levels are reached depends on the diver's determination, training (habituation), lung volume, $P_{A_{O_2}}$, physical activity, and, perhaps, other factors. As noted, Figure III-45 demonstrates that one is able to tolerate higher $P_{A_{CO_2}}$ if the breath is held at larger lung volumes. That an increased $P_{A_{O_2}}$ allows a higher $P_{A_{CO_2}}$ before the breaking point is reached is illustrated in Figure III-47, where the curves also show the effect of lung volume. It should be noted that as breath hold is performed at depth, $P_{A_{O_2}}$ levels may indeed be reached that far exceed the 120- to 130-mmHg range obtainable during air breathing at 1 ATA. The effect of high O_2 tensions on breath-hold time is shown in Figure III-48.

Directly to the point, Hesser (1965) has demonstrated that the maximum breath-hold time after breathing air increases as the ambient pressure increases. He also showed that nitrogen at high pressure (up to 3.8 ATA) has no significant influence on breath-holding ability under resting conditions.

Hyperventilation plays an important role in prolonging BH times. It is apparent that hyperventilation will decrease body stores of CO_2 as a function of time and alveolar ventilation. Therefore, one would expect that with lowered blood and tissue content initially, it will take longer for $P_{A_{CO_2}}$ to reach breaking point levels during the breath

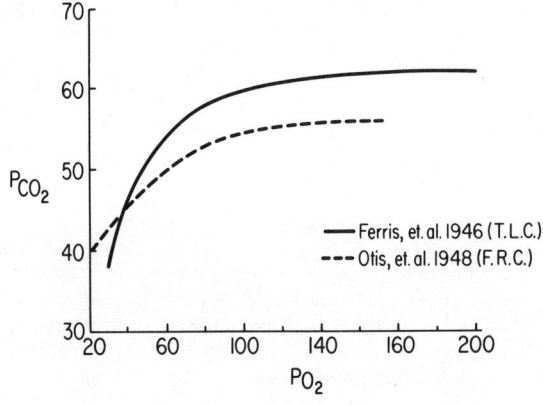

Figure III-47. Relationship between alveolar or arterial P_{CO_2} and P_{O_2} at breaking point of breath holding at two different lung volumes, VC, vital capacity, and FRC, functional residual capacity. [Adapted from Mithoefer (1965).]

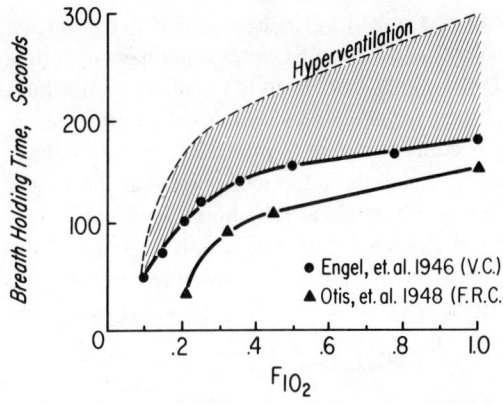

Figure III-48. Effect of inspired O_2 concentration (F_{IO_2}) on breath-holding time at two levels of inspired volume (VC and FRC). *Broken line* indicates predicted elevation of VC curve that would be produced by 2 min of hyperventilation. [Adapted from Mithoefer (1965).]

hold. Comroe (1974) found that hyperventilation for an hour may drop blood P_{CO_2} to 22 mmHg while elevating pH to 7.56. Since hemoglobin is almost fully saturated during normal breathing, no additional oxygen is sequestered by hyperventilation with air. Nevertheless, it would appear that for a given lung volume it will take longer to reach a breaking point P_{CO_2} and P_{O_2} combination if the breath hold has been preceded by hyperventilation. Stated in another way, the P_{AO_2}, which is time dependent, will be allowed to go much lower before a P_{ACO_2} level is reached that will provoke a sufficiently strong simulus to terminate the breath hold. There is an important implication here, namely that the P_{AO_2} may go below blackout levels (25–30 mmHg) before the breaking point is reached. If this happened during a BH dive, it could be fatal. In this situation the development of hypoxia is facilitated by falling alveolar P_{O_2} levels during ascent as a consequence of Boyle's law (discussed in more detail below). Craig (1961) was the first to describe the contribution of hyperventilation to hypoxia, unconsciousness, and drowning during underwater swimming. He has compiled a report of 58 cases of loss of consciousness during underwater swimming that lends strong support to this hypothesis (Craig 1976).

Oxygen availability is an important aspect of BH capacity, and the oxygen stores of the body therefore deserve attention. Rahn (1964) calculated the values in Table III-16 for a 70-kg (154-lb) man. In work on animals, Herber (1948) has shown that nearly all the oxygen stores will be utilized before death. Rahn (1964) shows that a 70-kg man at functional residual capacity (FRC), with a resting O_2 consumption of 300 ml/min,

Table III-16
Oxygen Stores for a 70-kg Man[a]

Form	Site	Oxygen store, ml. STPD
Hemoglobin	Venous blood	600
	Arterial blood	280
Myoglobin	Muscles	240
Physical solution	Tissues	56
Gas	Lung	370
	Total	1546

[a]From Rahn (1964), with permission from Pergamon Press.

would take 5 min (1546 ml ÷ 300 ml/min = 5 min) to exhaust his total body oxygen (having lapsed into coma a few minutes beforehand!). Furthermore, Rahn has taken data from the work of Otis and colleagues (1948) and has calculated the relative contribution to total body metabolism of the lung and blood oxygen stores during voluntary apnea in human subjects breathing different oxygen concentrations. Table III-17 presents these data; in reference to this table, Rahn (1964) makes the important point that the lung's contribution to metabolism during apnea is directly related to the initial lung volume. It is a straightforward proposition that the more oxygen a diver has within his lungs at the time of descent, the greater will be the lung's contribution to supporting overall body metabolism, and the longer the diver will be able to stay down (notwithstanding the increased work of overcoming an initially greater buoyancy).

Table III-17
Effects of Lung Volume and Exercise on the Relative Contribution of the Lung and Blood Stores to the Oxygen Consumed during Apnea

Condition	Lung vol, ml, BTPS	% of total O_2 consumed	
		From lung	From blood
Rest	3000	47	53
Rest	5300	80	20
Work[a]	5300	63	37

[a] Approximately twice resting O_2 consumption. From Rahn (1964), with permission from Pergamon Press.

What happens to $P_{A_{O_2}}$ and $P_{A_{CO_2}}$ during breath holding at 1 ATA is shown in Figure III-49. Not surprisingly, the fall in $P_{A_{O_2}}$ and rise in $P_{A_{CO_2}}$ are more marked when metabolism is bolstered by exercise. The disproportionately larger fall in O_2 tension compared to the rise in CO_2 tension reflects the fact that the capacity for O_2 storage is substantially less than that for CO_2. Other prominent features of the breath hold, illustrated in Figure III-50, are the time-related changes in gas exchange. Thus, the O_2 removal

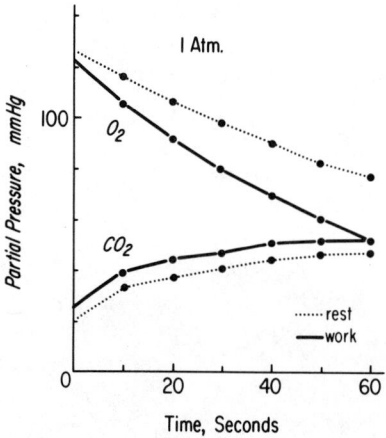

Figure III-49. Alveolar P_{O_2} and P_{CO_2} during breath holding with air. [From Lanphier and Rahn (1963).]

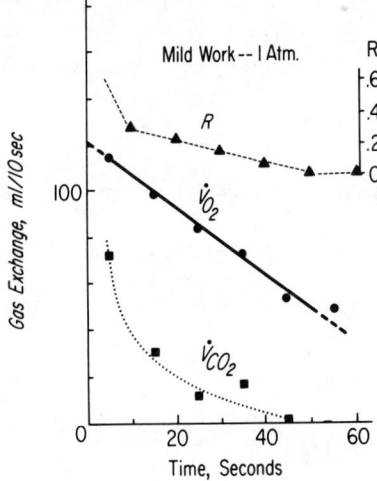

Figure III-50. Time course of $\dot{V}_{O_2}$, $\dot{V}_{CO_2}$, and interpolated values of respiratory exchange ratio (R) during breath holding in mild exercise. [From Lanphier and Rahn (1963b).]

from the lungs falls off linearly while CO_2 delivery diminishes in a curvilinear fashion. The net result of these two changes is a marked decline in the value of R.

The linear decrease in $\dot{V}_{O_2}$ seen in Figure III-50 only makes sense in light of the temporal constraints imposed on the physiological system by voluntary apnea in air. One must be aware that in an unstable system such as the body under enforced apnea, the $\dot{V}_{O_2}$ (or oxygen uptake by the blood) will not necessarily equal the oxygen consumption of the tissues, which is likely to remain stable (Hesser 1965). Under these conditions events transpire and are consummated in the course of one to two circulation cycles. Initially, as $P_{A_{O_2}}$ drops, less and less O_2 will be loaded into the venous blood, the oxygen content of which is at preapneic levels. After a circulation cycle, mixed venous blood that has a gradually declining O_2 content will arrive at the lungs. This would tend to enhance O_2 uptake again, while the fall in $P_{A_{O_2}}$ would counteract it, giving rise to a complex situation, depending on metabolism and the size of O_2 stores.

The reduction in CO_2 delivery to the lung reflects a fall in the blood-lung CO_2 diffusion gradient (Figure III-50). This is brought about by the CO_2 concentrating effect of lung shrinkage (due to $\dot{V}_{O_2}$), the Haldane effect, and, of course, the ongoing accumulation of CO_2 in the alveolar space. If the situation shown in Figure III-50 is extended, $\dot{V}_{O_2}$-caused shrinkage could make $P_{A_{CO_2}}$ exceed $P\bar{v}_{CO_2}$, at which instant CO_2 would be absorbed back into the blood (making the value of R negative). These effects will be further enhanced if the subject dives so that the lungs are compressed, causing $P_{A_{CO_2}}$ to increase according to Boyle's law.

Figures III-51 and III-52 depict a simulated diving situation in which the subject performs mild exercise combining breath holding with increased ambient pressures of 2 ATA; results from breath holding at 1 ATA are included for comparison (Lanphier and Rahn 1963a). During the descent phase of the dive (Figure III-51), the alveolar P_{O_2} and P_{CO_2} increase rapidly because of compression of the lungs. Once at 2 ATA, the P_{O_2} drops at a rate about double that for breath-holding at 1 ATA. This is explained partly by the fact that the higher $P_{A_{O_2}}$ at 2 ATA allows more complete saturation of the blood and partly by the fact that removal of an identical number of oxygen molecules at depth

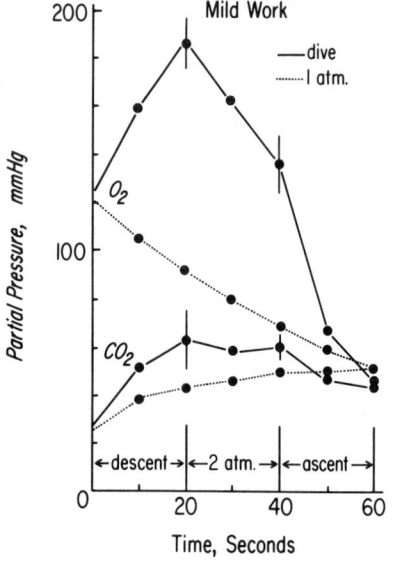

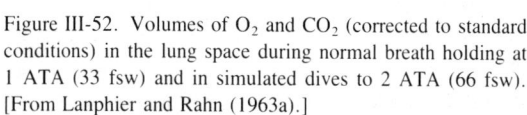

Figure III-51. Alveolar P_{O_2} and P_{CO_2} in breath holding with air at normal pressure and during simulated dives to 2 ATA (66 fsw). [From Lanphier and Rahn (1963a).]

Figure III-52. Volumes of O_2 and CO_2 (corrected to standard conditions) in the lung space during normal breath holding at 1 ATA (33 fsw) and in simulated dives to 2 ATA (66 fsw). [From Lanphier and Rahn (1963a).]

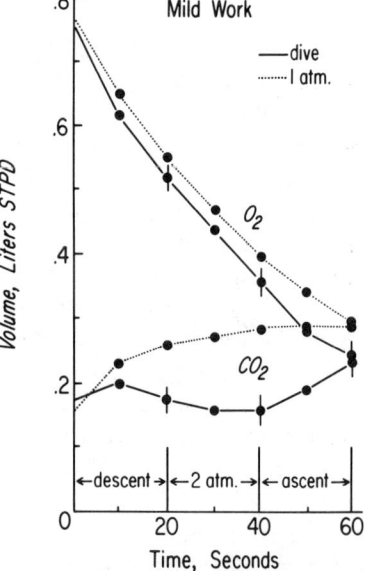

causes a larger drop in oxygen partial pressure than at the surface. The larger amount of O_2 remaining in the lungs at 1 ATA reflects the lower O_2 uptake at reduced pressures (Figure III-52).

During ascent the fall in total pulmonary gas pressure accounts for the fall in $P_{A_{O_2}}$, bringing it to below the 1-ATA level. Especially after somewhat longer bottom times, which are more easily achieved at greater depths, the fall in $P_{A_{O_2}}$ concomitant with ascent (also known as the "hypoxia of ascent") poses a grave threat to the diver (Craig 1968; Lanphier and Rahn 1963a).

The increase in $P_{A_{CO_2}}$ described earlier accounts for the fall in the CO_2 content of the lung at 2 ATA (Figure III-52) as CO_2 is reabsorbed into the blood. As for O_2, the fall in total pulmonary gas pressure during ascent accounts for the reduction in $P_{A_{CO_2}}$

(Figure III-51), which reestablishes the blood-air CO_2 pressure differential, thus allowing the CO_2 content of the lung to increase (Figure III-52). It should be noted that the data points on which Figures III-51 and III-52 were based were influenced by metabolism and, although to a small degree only, by nitrogen uptake and water vapor condensation at depth.

At this point it would be well to consider just how long an individual can hold his breath; this varies greatly and depends on a number of factors that have been discussed. For maximal performance one should hold one's breath at as large a lung volume as possible (this increases the lung O_2 store, allows greater CO_2 dilution, and retards the deflation reflex); after hyperventilation (to increase the CO_2 storage space, but note the danger of hypoxia); with the highest possible $P_{A_{O_2}}$ (this increases O_2 stores and reduces sensitivity to CO_2 and the deflation reflex).

In addition, breath-hold divers sometimes practice "tricks" that are alleged to enhance their BH time but which have not been systematically studied. These include blowing out moderate volumes of air when the breaking point is near, swallowing, and making Mueller and Valsalva maneuvers alternately.

Unquestionably, the subject's determination is a major factor in breath-hold capacity, and distracting factors probably also play a role. There have been reports of adolescent competitive swimmers, predominately breast strokers, who have lost consciousness during swim meets (Vaughan et al. 1975). Presumably, these young swimmers neglected to breathe because of excitement and intense concentration, and succumbed to hypoxia.

Mithoefer (1965b) has compiled some representative values for man's maximum breath-hold times at vital capacity at 1 ATA:

Conditions	Breath-hold times, sec
Moderate exercise, air	30
Rest, air, 3 min of hyperventilation	120
Rest, 100% O_2, 5 min of eupneic breathing	180
Rest, 100% O_2, 6 min of eupneic breathing	330
Rest, 100% O_2, 10 min of hyperventilation	700
Rest, 7 min of hyperventilation with air followed by several deep breaths of 100% O_2	1205 (unofficial record)

A comment on the remarkable breath-hold time of 1205 seconds (20 min 5 sec) is warranted. Provided that preparatory hyperventilation has reduced body CO_2 stores sufficiently, it is apparently possible to use up a full vital capacity of O_2 before breathing has to be resumed. Thus, in theory, a person with a large vital capacity, say 6.5 liters, which has been rinsed with O_2 while at rest with a $\dot{V}_{O_2}$ of 0.3 liters/min, should be able to hold his breath for 21.7 min (6.5 liters ÷ 0.3 liters/min). As a matter of fact the BH times recorded by Klocke and Rahn (1959) after quiet breathing and inspiration of a vital capacity of O_2 are quite impressive, reaching 7 to 8.5 minutes, with $P_{A_{CO_2}}$ levels ranging from 82 to 90 mmHg. Clearly, in these experiments the high O_2 tensions suppressed the CO_2 stimulus to breathe. Even in the experiments in the same study that employed hyperventilation and O_2 breathing, the final $P_{A_{CO_2}}$ values were of the same magnitude but the BH times reached maximums of 10 to 14 min, with lung volume reductions from 2.4 to 4.1 liters.

The high CO_2 tensions reached in these experiments might, under actual diving conditions, pose a threat to the diver. Moreover, attempting deep BH diving after hyperventilation with O_2 might create a risk of O_2 intoxication (especially in combination with hypercapnia, which causes cerebral vasodilation).

Water temperature has recently been identified as a factor that may have a marked effect on breath-hold capacity. Thus, while immersion in 35°C water may allow BH times somewhat longer than those seen in nonimmersed control experiments (C. E. G. Lundgren and J. Sterba, unpublished observations), gradually lowering the water temperature decreased BH time. At a water temperature of 15°C, BH time was typically 30% of the nonimmersed steady-state values (Sterba and Lundgren 1979). This was probably due to at least two different mechanisms, namely an intense stimulation of skin temperature receptors that is known to enhance breathing in the nonapneic situation, and an increase in metabolism.

c. Depth Limits of Breath-Hold Diving

Assuming that the world depth record for BH diving is not to be awarded posthumously, there appear to be two different considerations that bear on breath-hold diving tactics. The first is not to proceed beyond the depth at which barotrauma would supervene. The other is not to exceed the time limits set by the diver's tolerance for hypoxia and hypercapnia. With regard to thoracic barotrauma, the depth, i.e., pressure limit, is set by the relation between the initial lung volume and the minimal lung volume below which mechanical damage to the thoracic structures occurs. It would appear that this relation is defined by the quotient of Total Lung Capacity (TLC) and Residual Volume (RV). Consideration must be given to extrathoracic dead space, including that of a face mask (if worn), which requires pressure equilibration.

The spirometer values given for R. Croft, the U.S. Navy diver who in 1968 set a world record (later surpassed) of 73 m (240 fsw), were: TLC, 9.1 liters; RV, 1.3 liters (Schaefer et al. 1968). Assuming an extrathoracic dead space of 0.1 liter (no face mask used), and applying these values, Boyle's law yields the following equation for maximum attainable pressure:

$$(9.1 + 0.1) \times 1.0 = (1.3 + 0.1) P$$

and P = 6.6 ATA, i.e., a maximum depth of 56 m (183 fsw).

This theoretical limit is remarkably less than the depths actually achieved. The present world record is 100 m (328 fsw) set in 1977 by J. Mayol (Dr. P. Data, personal communication). Even if a few divers may have a somewhat more advantageous relationship between TLC and RV than Diver Croft, additional physiological mechanisms must be invoked to explain the great depths actually reached. This is especially the case, since limiting the calculations to the compression effects described by Boyle's law is an over-simplification that disregards the volume effect of gas exchange between blood and alveolar space.

The volume of gas in the lungs decreases during a BH dive not only in response to chest compression and gas uptake, but also because blood moves into the thorax. This happens partly because orthostatic effects on the circulation are balanced out by the external water column and partly because intrathoracic pressure falls below ambient pressure as the chest is compressed below FRC. The volume of redistributed blood may be substantial. There are no direct measurements, but thoracic impedance recordings on R. Croft in dives to 90 and 130 fsw indicated that a blood volume of between 850 and 1047 ml was redistributed from the periphery into the thorax (Schaefer et al. 1968). Head-out immersion studies employing a dye-dilution technique have shown intrathoracic blood pooling on the order of 700 ml subsequent to water entry (Arborelius et al. 1972).

The importance of the blood shifts becomes evident if the earlier computation based on chest compression alone [yielding a depth limit of 56 m (183 fsw)] is expanded to include a blood volume shift of 0.7 liter.

$$(9.1 + 0.1) \times 1.0 = (1.3 + 0.1 - 0.7) \times P$$

In this case, P = 13.1 ATA, i.e., a maximum depth of 121 m (398 fsw), which is 65% deeper than the depth actually reached by Croft.

Astonishingly, increasing the amount of redistributed blood to 1.0 liter yields a theoretical maximum depth of 220 m (722 fsw)! However, these theoretical computations have neglected gas absorption. Clearly, lung volume changes are dictated by O_2 uptake and the earlier described retardation of CO_2 off-gassing, which may progress to CO_2 uptake by the blood. This latter phenomenon is enhanced both by $\dot{V}O_2$ and by lung compression with increasing depth. Additional but less significant elements are water vapor loss and N_2 uptake. As a consequence there are both time- and depth-dependent components of lung volume shrinkage, and speed of ascent and descent will be rewarded by less volume loss. This insight is reflected in the techniques used by recent breath-hold world record holders for descent and ascent; high travel rates have been achieved by employing weights and inflatable flotation devices.

The question arises: what induces the diver to turn back and begin his ascent? If the warning signal is physiological not psychological, it could either be a sensation of chest discomfort caused by compression and/or blood pooling, or a respiratory urge caused by the deflation reflex and/or hypercapnia. At maximum depth, hypoxia is very unlikely because of the augmentation of $P_{A_{O_2}}$ by compression.

Theoretically, thoracic squeeze is the outcome of too-deep BH diving, although this condition apparently has never been unequivocally demonstrated. The squeeze mechanism would be activated if intrathoracic blood accumulation caused vascular engorgement severe enough to cause vascular damage. Overdistension of the heart is also a conceivable result. A case of heart dilation in connection with breathing through a long snorkel that produced a marked transthoracic pressure difference has been reported (Stigler 1911; see Chapter III-B).

Any respiratory urge felt at maximum depth is likely to be reduced during ascent. The expanding alveolar gas volume can accommodate more CO_2 (Figure III-52), allowing a reduction in $P_{A_{CO_2}}$ (Figure III-51), and will attenuate the deflation reflex. As pointed out by Lanphier and Rahn (1963a), the sense of relief this might give could encourage the diver to slow his ascent, thus increasing the danger of hypoxia.

Hypoxia may indeed be the major risk in deep BH dives. For example, assuming reasonable values for $\dot{V}O_2$ and oxygen stores of the body, it can be calculated that R. Croft arrived at his record depth of 73 m with a $P_{A_{O_2}}$ of about 700 mmHg. This high

O_2 pressure corresponds to an alveolar oxygen percentage of 11% at 8.3 ATA. Even assuming instantaneous return to the surface, this would have left him with a $P_{A_{O_2}}$ of only $0.11 \times (760 - 47\ P_{H_2O}\ vapor) = 78$ mmHg.

In reality Croft returned to the surface pulling himself up along the ascent line, consuming oxygen for an additional 68 sec. It is not surprising that some record attempts have ended with an unconscious diver floating to the surface (McWhirter 1980; Dr. P. Data, personal communication).

d. Acclimatization to Breath-Hold Diving in Man

Heath and Irwin (1968) have observed that BH times in air at 1 ATA become progressively lengthened over a short series of breath holds. They reported a prolongation of approximately 25% to 30% in BH time during six sequential BH attempts. The initial $P_{A_{O_2}}$ levels rose during serial BH attempts, and the initial $P_{A_{CO_2}}$ levels fell, suggesting that progressive hyperventilation may have contributed to breaking point prolongation. However, end-$P_{A_{CO_2}}$ increased toward the end of a BH series, while end-$P_{A_{O_2}}$ progressively fell. This implies that the breaking point stimulus was increasing steadily. Therefore, the authors concluded that the subjects had become acutely habituated to the stress of breath holding, aided to some extent by progressive hyperventilation. These effects are short-lived, however. Even after about 10 min of normal breathing this habituation is lost, although it can be reestablished by a new series of breath holds (C. E. G. Lundgren and J. Sterba, personal observations). Presumably the same mechanism is at work during BH diving.

Schaefer (1965) conducted a longitudinal study of physiological adaptation to BH diving in instructors at a U.S. Navy submarine escape training tower. When these instructors first reported for duty the majority could not make dives deeper than 60 to 70 fsw, but after several months of training most could reach a depth of 90 fsw. Vital capacities increased to volumes 20% greater than those predicted by a standard formula based on height, weight, and age. Additionally, TLC and Inspiratory Reserve Volume (IRV) increased, while RV decreased. The increase in TLC coupled with a decrease in RV allowed the divers to reach greater depths safely. Song and co-workers (1963) have also reported increased VC and IRV in Korean ama relative to nondiving controls.

Schaefer reported that BH divers have an increased tolerance (depressed ventilatory response) to elevated levels of CO_2 that is lost after a 5-month period of no diving. He reported increased plasma and red blood cell CO_2 content and decreased plasma pH during the period of heavy BH diving. Again, Schaefer's results were consistent with the findings of Song and co-workers (1963), who recorded a lower response to increased CO_2 in the Korean ama when compared with a nondiving native group.

Schaefer also compiled evidence suggesting that habituated BH divers have increased tolerance for hypoxia over nondiving controls. He tested the ventilatory response of resting subjects to a breathing mixture of 10.5% oxygen for 33 min. Although $P_{A_{O_2}}$ and $P_{A_{CO_2}}$ levels were identical for divers and controls, the divers demonstrated a smaller increase in minute ventilation. Schaefer determined that the divers used significantly less O_2 while exposed to hypoxia than the control subjects. He suggested that this could be explained either by the divers having shifted to anaerobic metabolism, or by a decrease in body metabolism requirements (a phenomenon known to occur in diving animals). He observed that this effect persisted in one subject even after a 33-min recovery period in air.

Schaefer has assembled evidence that suggests that the increased CO_2 tolerance seen in breath-hold divers is associated with a decreased adrenergic and stress response to CO_2 elevation. Subjects having high CO_2 tolerance showed smaller elevations of blood sugar and pulse rate when breathing hypercarbic mixtures than did individuals without such tolerance. Escape training tower instructors reported that they became capable of greater relaxation during BH diving as their experience grew. This observation is consistent with the hypothesis that subjects acclimatized to elevated CO_2 levels have a depressed autonomic response.

2. Medical Considerations

a. Drowning and Near-Drowning

As previously mentioned, most victims of drowning and near-drowning associated with breath-hold diving have a history of hyperventilation and acknowledged attempts at striving for maximum performance underwater. By hyperventilating, the diver reduces his body CO_2 stores without augmenting his O_2 stores, thereby retarding his most sensitive breaking point stimulus without compensating for it. Lung shrinkage plays a relatively minor role as the breaking point stimulus for divers breathing air (due to slow N_2 absorption), and therefore divers may become hypoxic without any premonitory signs. The problem is compounded by ascent to the surface, at which time $P_{A_{O_2}}$ falls precipitously: the hypoxia of ascent. Swimmers should be urged not to hyperventilate before diving. Oxygen breathing before diving should be discouraged because it could predispose to high $P_{A_{CO_2}}$ levels while lung volume is relatively large, a combination that could suppress the breaking point and allow buildup of $P_{A_{CO_2}}$ to dangerous levels, causing mental impairment, incoordination, and convulsions. If deep dives are attempted after oxygen breathing, there is the additional risk of O_2 intoxication, which may also lead to convulsions and loss of consciousness.

b. Cardiological Considerations

Sinus bradycardia, P-wave changes, AV block, AV nodal rhythm, sinus arrest followed by either nodal escape or ventricular escape, wandering pacemaker, premature ventricular and supraventricular beats, tented T-waves and negative T-waves have all been reported during breath-hold diving (Olsen et al. 1962; Paulev 1965; Sasamoto 1965; Speck and Bruce 1978). These arrhythmias have variously been attributed to asphyxia, hypothermia, vasoconstriction, hyperkalemia, acidosis, vagal stimulation, and combinations of these. Such arrhythmias do not appear to be pathological, in the sense that they are well tolerated by healthy young people, the segment of the population most likely to engage in BH diving. Nevertheless, if an individual with occult or known cardiac disease were to engage in BH diving, he could theoretically predispose himself to a fatal arrhythmia. In addition, the combination of exertion, hypoxia, and cold might precipitate myocardial infarction. Therefore, it is recommended that prospective or habitual BH divers be aware of the consequences and undergo regular cardiac evaluation.

c. Barotrauma

As is the case with any form of diving, pressure equilibration of the extrapulmonary air spaces (sinuses, middle ear, mastoid air cells, and nasal passages) must be accomplished during descent and ascent to preclude barotrauma (under- and overpressurization). The critical difference between BH diving and compressed air diving is that, in the former, the amount of gas available for equilibration is limited. The added dead space of a standard diving face mask increased this problem. Goggles of the noncompensated type should never be worn for BH diving because ocular squeeze could occur even on relatively shallow (3 m, or 10 fsw) dives (Rahn 1965). The ama have used goggles that have either small compensating bladders that expel air into the goggles as the diver descends or an oral inflation tube that accomplishes the same end. The Tuomotu pearl divers have approached the problem differently by constructing goggles of very small volume to minimize dead space. So equipped, dives of 40 m (120 fsw) are possible (Rahn 1965).

Theoretically, pulmonary barotrauma (thoracic squeeze) could occur during a breath-hold dive. Clinically the situation has only rarely been reported, and in view of the record depths achieved without injury the dearth of such histories is not surprising. Nevertheless, Strauss and Wright (1969) have reported a breath-hold diving accident that they consider suggestive of thoracic squeeze. A 28-year-old and experienced U.S. Navy diver had been performing BH dives to depths of 80 fsw and was seen "floating" face up at a depth of 40 fsw. He was unconscious and apneic, and frothy bright red blood was seen coming from his mouth. He developed intermittent clonic seizures within 10 min of the accident, in addition to frank hemoptysis. He gradually regained consciousness with supportive therapy, but subsequently lapsed into shock and died of cardiac arrest 3 hr after the accident. Postmortem examination revealed evidence of diffuse bilateral pulmonary vascular injury with intravascular congestion, interstitial edema, diffuse disruption of small vessels, and intra-alveolar hemorrhage. These findings were not felt to be consistent with drowning. However, barring an undetected physical abnormality in this diver, thoracic squeeze seems rather unlikely in view of the relatively shallow depth of diving, unless the diver began the dive on a small lung volume. Furthermore, Edmonds et al. (1976) note that the picture of heavy, edematous lungs that may be hemorrhagic and display pink or white froth in airways is consistent with drowning. Whether or not this case represents a true thoracic squeeze, this phenomenon probably constitutes only a remote hazard to the breath-hold diver.

Pulmonary overinflation with air embolism, pneumothorax, or mediastinal emphysema is usually a consequence of the intrapulmonary overpressure seen in compressed gas diving during ascent. Since the breath-hold diver's lungs are at a maximum volume on the surface before the dive, they can only lose volume subsequently, and therefore intrapulmonary pressure will of necessity be lower at the completion of a dive. Therefore, the problem of overinflation should not arise in BH diving under normal conditions. Nevertheless, it could happen in a BH diver who breathes compressed gas at depth. Such a diver would then have to vent the lungs during ascent, as would any scuba diver, and failure to do so could result in pulmonary overinflation.

d. Decompression Sickness

Cross (1965) has reported a malady related to the breath-hold diving practices of pearl divers in the South Pacific. Symptoms consist of a feeling of anguish, nausea, and vertigo, and the illness may or may not involve varying degrees of paralysis and other neurological involvement with residual deficits, unconsciousness, or death. The disease is called *taravana*, meaning "to fall crazily." The Paumotan divers hyperventilate from 3 to 10 min, make rapid weight-assisted descents, and remain submerged for an average of 1.5 min at depths as great as 40 m (140 fsw) or more. Ascent is hand-over-hand up a line. One diver who apparently succumbed to taravana appeared to have made 18 to 20 dives to 40 m in less than 2 hr. Although some of the manifestations of this disease can be explained by hypoxia, hypercarbia, and drowning, the neurological sequelae certainly suggest decompression sickness or air embolism (a lesion that is quite uncommon in BH diving). Taravana is unknown in a group of pearl divers from Mangareva whose *modus operandi* differs from that of the Paumotan divers only in that they space their dives over a period of 12 to 15 min instead of 4 to 10 min. Otherwise they dive to the same average depths for similar diving times. It may be that the long surface intervals prescribed by Mangarevan diving practice leave enough time for denitrogenation. Paulev (1965) has reported four cases of decompression sickness after repeated BH dives to 15 to 20 m (49 to 66 fsw) in a Norwegian submarine escape training tank. The signs, symptoms, and responses to therapeutic recompression were consistent with this author's interpretation. All four cases involved breathing compressed air at 20 m before the BH dives.

Lanphier (1965) has used a theoretical approach that allowed him to compare a series of BH dives with a single compressed air dive, using the U.S. Navy decompression tables. He concluded that some of the reported cases of taravana were probably incidents of decompression sickness, as were all the cases reported by Paulev. Among the inconsistencies in the occurrence of taravana Lanphier pointed out are: (1) Some cases occur at water depths where decompression sickness would be unlikely. (2) Incidence is not clearly related to length of bottom time or depth. (3) Typical bends pain is not a related symptom.

Lanphier points out that hypercarbia could be synergistic in the development of decompression sickness in BH divers, and he suggested the possibility of "silent bubbles" in these men. More recently, Spencer and Okino (1972) have studied an ama diver by means of a precordial ultrasonic bubble detector. The diver was examined after a 51-min period of 30 successive open ocean dives to 15 m, with dives averaging 53 sec. Asymptomatic venous gas emboli were detected for 1 hr after the last dive.

In summary, decompression sickness is a possible medical complication of breath-hold diving, but it should only be anticipated in circumstances of unusually frequent repetitive diving to relatively deep depths.

e. Vertigo and Disorientation

Perilymph fistula (round or oval window rupture), alternobaric vertigo, and caloric vertigo are ills that the BH diver shares with compressed gas divers. Since disorientation with a severely limited air supply could be particularly disastrous, individuals who are unusually susceptible to caloric stimulation of the ear canal or who, for whatever reason, have difficulty clearing their ears should be cautioned about the potentially deleterious consequences of breath-hold diving, particularly in cold water.

This section was written with partial support from the Office of Naval Research and the Naval Medical Research and Development Command through Office of Naval Research Contract N00014-78-C-0205.

DONALD D. HICKEY
CLAES E. G. LUNDGREN

References

ARBORELIUS, M., JR., U. I. BALLDIN, B. LILJA, AND C. E. G. LUNDGREN 1972. Hemodynamic changes in man during immersion with the head above water. *Aerosp. Med.* 43: 592–598.

CENTER FOR DISEASE CONTROL 1980. Underwater diving deaths—Florida. *Morbid. Mortal. Weekly Rep.* 29: 6.

COMROE, J. H., JR. 1974. *Physiology of Respiration* (2nd ed.). Chicago: Year Book Medical Publishers.

CRAIG, A. B., JR. 1961. Underwater swimming and loss of consciousness. *JAMA* 176: 255–258.

CRAIG, A. B., JR. 1968. Depth limits of breath hold diving. *Respirat. Physiol.* 5: 14–22.

CRAIG, A. B., JR. 1976. Summary of 58 cases of loss of consciousness during underwater swimming and diving. *Med. Sci. Sports* 8(3): 171–175.

CROSS, E. R. 1965. Taravana diving syndrome in the Tuamotu diver. In: *Physiology of Breath-hold Diving and the Ama of Japan*, edited by H. Rahn and T. Yokoyama. Washington, DC: Natl. Acad. Sci./Natl. Res. Council, p. 207–219.

EDMONDS, C., C. LOWRY, AND J. PENNEFATHER 1976. *Diving and Subaquatic Medicine.* Mosman, Australia: Diving Medical Centre.

ENGLE, G. L., E. B. FERRIS, J. P. WEBB, AND C. D. STEVENS 1946. Voluntary breath-holding. II. The relation of the maximum time of breath-holding to the oxygen tension of the inspired air. *J. Clin. Invest.* 25: 729–733.

FERRIS, E. B., G. L. ENGLE, C. D. STEPHENS, AND J. P. WEBB 1946. Voluntary breath-holding. III. The relation of the maximum time of breath-holding to the oxygen and carbon dioxide tensions of arterial blood, with a note on its clinical and physiological significance. *J. Clin. Invest.* 25: 734–743.

FOWLER, W. S. 1954. Breaking point of breath-holding. *J. Appl. Physiol.* 6: 539–545.

HEATH, J. R., AND C. J. IRWIN 1968. An increase in breath-hold time appearing after breath-holding. *Respirat. Physiol.* 4: 73–77.

HEISTAD, D. D., F. M. ABBOUD, AND J. W. ECKSTEIN 1968. Vasoconstrictor response to simulated diving in man. *J. Appl. Physiol.* 25: 542–549.

HERBER, F. J. 1948. Metabolic changes of blood and tissue gases during asphyxia. *Am. J. Physiol.* 152: 687–695.

HESSER, C. M. 1965. Breath holding under high pressure. In: *Physiology of Breath-hold Diving and the Ama of Japan*, edited by H. Rahn and T. Yokoyama. Washington, DC: Natl. Acad. Sci./Natl. Res. Council, p. 165–181.

HILL, L., AND M. FLACK 1908. The effect of excess CO_2 and of want of oxygen upon the respiration and the circulation. *J. Physiol. (Lond.)* 37: 77–111.

IRVING, L. 1965. Gas transport mechanism. In: *Handbook of Physiology, Respiration*, edited by W. Fenn and H. Rahn. Washington, DC: American Physiological Society, Sect. 3, Vol. I, p. 177–212.

KLOCKE, R., AND H. RAHN 1959. Breath holding after breathing of oxygen. *J. Appl. Physiol.* 14: 689–693.

LANPHIER, E. H. 1965. Application of decompression tables to repeated breath-hold dives. In: *Physiology of Breath-hold Diving and the Ama of Japan*, edited by H. Rahn and T. Yokoyama. Washington, DC: Natl. Acad. Sci./Natl. Res. Council, p. 227–236.

LANPHIER, E. H., AND H. RAHN 1963a. Alveolar gas exchange during breath-hold diving. *J. Appl. Physiol.* 18: 471–477.

LANPHIER, E. H., AND H. RAHN 1963b. Alveolar gas exchange during breath holding with air. *J. Appl. Physiol.* 18: 478–482.

MCWHIRTER, N. 1980. *Guiness Book of World Records*. New York: Sterling Publishing Co.
MITHOEFER, J. C. 1965a. Breath holding. In: *Handbook of Physiology, Respiration*, edited by W. Fenn and H. Rahn. Washington, DC: American Physiology Society, Sect. 3, Vol. II, p. 1011–1025.
MITHOEFER, J. C. 1965b. The breaking point of breath-holding. In: *Physiology of Breath-hold Diving and the Ama of Japan*, edited by H. Rahn and T. Yokoyama. Washington, DC: Natl. Acad. Sci./Natl. Res. Council, p. 195–205.
MURDAUGH, V. H, JR., E. D. ROBIN, J. E. MILLER, W. F. DREWRY, AND E. WEISS 1966. Adaptations to diving in the harbor seal: cardiac output during diving. *Am. J. Physiol.* 210: 176–180.
OLSEN, C. R., D. D. FANESTIL, AND P. F. SCHOLANDER 1962. Some effects of breath holding and apneic underwater diving on cardiac rhythm in man. *J. Appl. Physiol.* 17: 461–469.
OTIS, A. B., H. RAHN, AND W. O. FENN 1948. Alveolar gas changes during breath holding. *Am. J. Physiol.* 152: 674–686.
PAULEV, P. 1965. Decompression sickness following repeated breath-hold dives. In: *Physiology of Breath-hold Diving and the Ama of Japan*, edited by H. Rahn and T. Yokoyama. Washington, DC: Natl. Acad. Sci./Natl. Res. Council, p. 221–226.
PAULEV, P. 1968. Cardiac rhythm during breath holding and water immersion in man. *Acta. Physiol. Scand.* 73: 139–150.
RAHN, H. 1964. Oxygen stores of man. In: *Oxygen in the Animal Organism*, edited by F. Dickens and E. Neil. New York: Pergamon Press.
RAHN, H. 1965. The physiological stresses of the Ama. In: *Physiology of Breath-hold Diving and the Ama of Japan*, edited by H. Rahn and T. Yokoyama. Washington, DC: Natl. Acad. Sci./Natl. Res. Council, p. 113–138.
SASAMOTO, H. 1965. The electrocardiogram pattern of the diving ama. In: *Physiology of Breath-hold Diving and the Ama of Japan*, edited by H. Rahn and T. Yokoyama. Washington, DC: Natl. Acad. Sci./Natl. Res. Council, p. 271–280.
SCHAEFER, K. E. 1965. Adaptation to breath-hold diving. In: *Physiology of Breath-hold Diving and the Ama of Japan*, edited by H. Rahn and T. Yokoyama. Washington, DC: Natl. Acad. Sci./Natl. Res. Council, p. 237–252.
SCHAEFER, K. E., R. D. ALLISON, J. H. DOUGHERTY, C. R. CAREY, R. WALKER, F. YOST, AND D. PARKER 1968. Pulmonary and circulatory adjustments determining the limits in breathhold diving. *Science* 162: 1020–1023.
SONG, S. H., D. H. KANG, B. S. KANG, AND S. K. HONG 1963. Lung volumes and ventilatory responses to high CO_2 and low O_2 in the ama. *J. Appl. Physiol.* 18: 466–470.
SPECK, D. F., AND D. S. BRUCE 1978. Effect of varying thermal and apneic conditions on the human diving reflex. *Undersea Biomed. Res.* 5: 9–14.
SPENCER, M. P., AND H. OKINO 1972. Venous gas emboli following repeated breathhold dives (abstract). *Fed. Proc.* 31: 355.
STERBA, J. A., AND C. E. G. LUNDGREN 1979. Influence of water temperature on breath-holding time in submerged man (abstract). *Undersea Biomed. Res.* Suppl. 6: 29.
STIGLER, R. 1911. Die Kraft unserer Inspirations Muskulatur. *Pfluegers Arch.* 139: 234–254.
STRAUSS, M. B., AND P. WRIGHT 1969. A diving casualty suggesting a case of thoracic squeeze. Rep. 584. Groton, CT: Naval Submarine Medical Center.
STRØMME, S. B., AND A. S. BLIX 1976. Indirect evidence for arterial chemoreceptor reflex facilitation by face immersion in man. *Aviat. Space Environ. Med.* 47: 597–599.
VAUGHAN, V. C., R. J. MCKAY, AND W. E. NELSON 1975. In: *Nelson Textbook of Pediatrics* (10th ed.). Philadelphia: W. B. Saunders.
WILDENTHAL, K., J. M. ATKINS, S. J. LESHIN, AND C. L. SKELTON 1975. The diving reflex used to treat paroxysmal atrial tachycardia. *Lancet* 1: 12.

IV

Decompression Theory

A. *Introduction*

Following the commencement of the industrial revolution it became possible for human beings to manipulate the physics and chemistry of their environment on a grand scale. This led to the appearance of a large number of man-made disorders, for many of which the causative agent is easily established; the mechanism whereby the body reacts to these agents is, however, not sufficiently understood. Decompression sickness is such a disorder. It is provoked by our ability to change the pressure and chemical composition of the gases we breathe. One procedure for complete prevention of decompression sickness is therefore to not venture outside the limits of air composition and partial pressures normally encountered on the surface of the earth. A second way to eliminate the harmful effects of decompression sickness is to understand the responsible mechanisms and from this understanding to construct safe procedures. It is, of course, this second possibility that is examined in this chapter.

The first successful pump for exhausting the air from a container was invented in the 17th century by Von Guericke. Using his own version of this recently invented pump, Robert Boyle became in 1670 the first investigator in the field of decompression sickness when he decompressed a viper in his "exhausted receiver" and described the now-famous "bubble moving to and fro in the waterish humour of one of its eyes." From this and similar early experiments the idea arose that a rapid reduction of atmospheric pressure could lead to the release of bubbles into sensitive tissues of the body and that this could seriously impair their normal functions.

For work underwater, gases at pressures greater than atmospheric pressure are required, and it was some years before a pump could be used to raise the ambient pressure rather than lower it, as in the Boyle experiments described above. Many attempts had been made to descend into the sea by using a variety of diving apparatus, but until comparatively recent times all these devices were totally impractical for any reasonably prolonged underwater work and offered very little advantage beyond simple breath-hold diving. The diving bell was really the first successful underwater device, and it is generally agreed that Edmund Halley (of comet fame) designed, built, and used the first practical "bell" system

(Halley 1717). An artist's impression of this bell is given in Figure IV-1, and a brief description of this device serves to illustrate some of the difficulties facing the theoretician when he attempts to collect reliable data as a basis for his ideas. Halley's bell was constructed of wood and lined on the exterior surface with lead sheeting in order to give sufficient weight and stability to the bell when underwater. It had a cubic capacity of nearly 60 ft^3 (1.7 m^3) and was approximately 3 ft (0.9 m) in diameter at the top. It was realized that with two men in the bell when it was immersed in water the air contained within the bell would become foul. Drawing on more recent knowledge one can easily calculate that

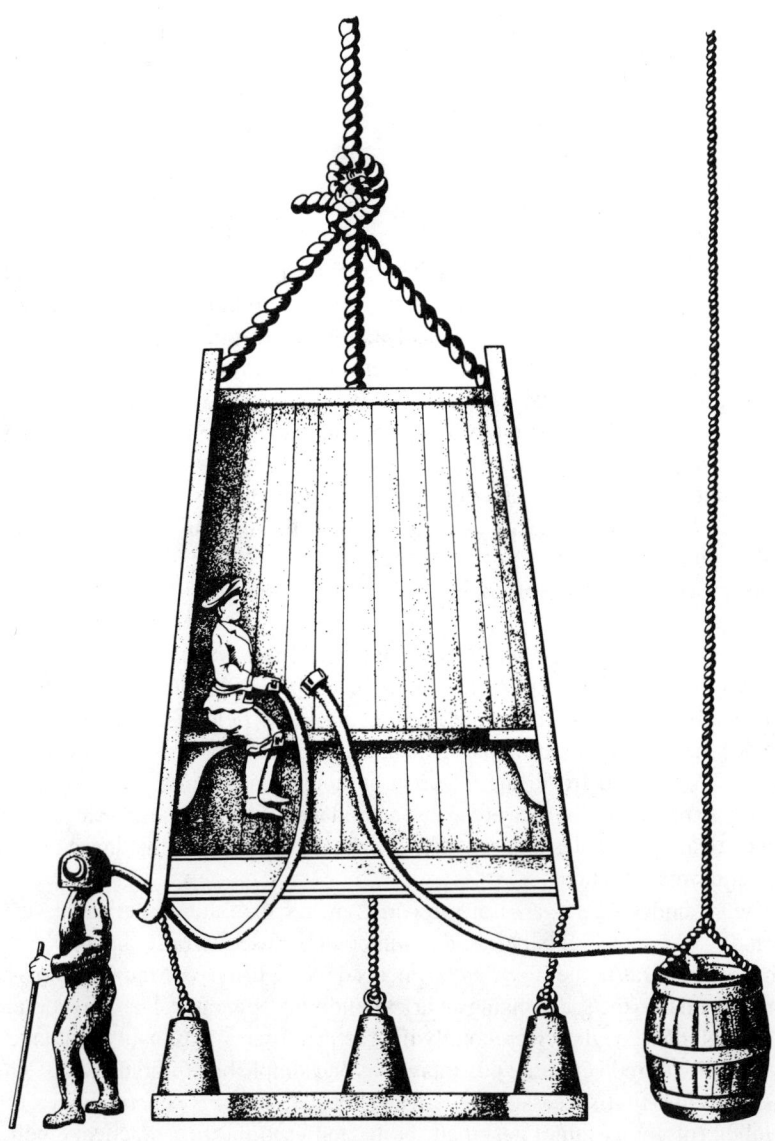

Figure IV-1. Artist's conception of Edmund Halley's diving bell (ca. 1717). [Adapted from Davis (1981).]

with two active men inside a bell the carbon dioxide concentration would reach about 3% in 1 hr, and this would be the useful duration for such a bell without some form of air replenishment. Fresh air, in this case, was supplied to the bell from lead-lined barrels having bung holes at the top and the bottom and a leather tube through which air could be forced from the barrels into the bell. After being emptied of air these barrels were hauled to the surface, where their air content was renewed, and thus the whole process was a continuous one. Depths as great as 60 ft (18 m) for dive durations as long as 1 1/2 hr were attained by using this particular technique.

Several important physiological points relevant to the theoretician should be noted. First, the nature of the breathing gas must be clearly defined; variability in the concentration of such physiologically active gases as carbon dioxide and oxygen could influence the validity of any decompression observations made. Second, the diver who leaves the bell at the end of his breathing tube is being subjected to a different environment from that of his companion seated within the bell. The diver may well be surrounded by quite cold water with the well-known ensuing physiological reactions to this. In addition he is attempting to draw fresh air for breathing purposes down a tube that is clearly giving added respiratory airflow "drag." He is rebreathing expired air. His head, neck, shoulders, and particularly his respiratory passages are at risk of squeeze effects if his helmet is attached to his suit. If his helmet is open ended and not equipped with a nonreturn valve he is in danger of drowning upon any lowering of his helmet below the water level of the bell. (In contrast, any raising of his helmet above the bell's water level will produce a free flow of air into the helmet, with relief from the foul air and possible squeeze effects.) And with immersion the hydrostatic relationships between blood pressure in the extremities and the pressure in the heart are altered and thus there are changes in the cardiovascular system. Third, some underwater workers are likely to be performing very little work (e.g., the seated attendant, who may or may not be pumping air into the diver's own hose by means of bellows), but others (e.g., the diver) are required to perform quite hard physical work. Fourth, human beings are very different in important factors such as stature, body composition, and level of physical fitness. Finally, and of extreme importance in studying the effects of exposure to raised pressures of air and other gases, it is necessary to know how long the subjects were exposed and to what pressure. With such a formidable list of variables to be brought under control in order to obtain consistent findings, it is hardly surprising that numerous and conflicting conclusions were reached from the data available in the early years of this discipline.

Placing human beings under raised pressures of air can conveniently be considered divisible into four separate phases, each of which has its own particular set of problems. The first phase is taking the person to pressure, and this compression phase sometimes causes the establishment of pressure differentials in body cavities such as the sinuses and the middle ear, producing in these instances sinus and ear pain and vertigo. The second phase comprises the sojourn at full pressure. Here, the compressed air worker (diver, caisson, tunnel) encounters the effects of raised pressures of oxygen, carbon dioxide, toxic gas contaminants such as carbon monoxide, and the inert gas nitrogen, any or all of which can give rise to numerous difficulties (e.g., oxygen toxicity, nitrogen narcosis, carbon dioxide intoxication, carbon monoxide toxicity), altered thermal balance, increased respiratory work, and communications problems. The third, or decompression, phase is the return to atmospheric pressure, which is followed by the fourth phase, or post-decompression period. It is these two latter phases that principally concern us. A note of caution must be introduced because, as becomes apparent later, the events occurring in phase 2 can profoundly influence the body's responses in the decompression and post-decompression periods. For the moment, however, let us consider only the evidence accumulated by the turn of the century concerning decompression and its consequences. It had become apparent that decompression could be followed by harmful effects varying in severity from death to mild itching of the skin. The prevention of these ill effects was soon seen to lie in pursuing a slow release of pressure. It would seem that everyone adopted some form of linear decompression procedure, i.e., the pressure was released at a certain number of bar (psi, kg/cm^2) per minute for the caisson and tunnel workers or a given number of meters (ft, fathoms) of ascent per minute for the diver. The practical problem in those days was to decide the most effective rate of pressure release.

B. Defining the Problem

An understanding of the basic processes producing the harmful effects of decompression was lacking until the time of Paul Bert (1878), who made numerous fundamental observations in a series of experiments between 1870 and 1890. He showed that the more serious forms of decompression sickness were provoked by the presence of large volumes of free gas, as opposed to dissolved gas, within body tissue. Furthermore, after careful analysis of the composition of these bubbles he concluded that nitrogen gas was the main constituent. Thus an outline picture of the etiology of decompression sickness could now be attempted: It is apparently caused by the release of gas emboli from nitrogen gas dissolved at pressure, and these nitrogen gas emboli then impair the functioning of the various tissues in which they lodge or are formed.

Meantime, a clearer clinical picture was also emerging. If the decompression was grossly inadequate, then the blood literally "frothed" and a condition descriptively termed *the chokes* was encountered, and this proved rapidly fatal unless promptly treated by recompression. If the decompression was not so provocative, then a condition known as *the staggers* was often seen; this too was a very serious manifestation of decompression sickness that could lead to permanent damage in the central nervous system, or even death. However, the most prevalent form of decompression sickness came to be termed *the bends*, so called by the workmen who constructed the bridge across the Mississippi River at St. Louis (1869–1874), the name referring to the affected gait that was fashionable among the young ladies of the time and apparently bore a resemblance to the behavior of those workmen who contracted the less serious, but painful, forms of decompression sickness (Jaminet 1871). The term nowadays refers to pain in or around a joint that can make itself felt either during the decompression or sometimes several hours post-decompression.

Although much early compressed air work was performed in Western Europe, most particularly France and England, it was the massive undertakings in the United States that provided a sound statistical basis for examining the frequency of occurrence of the various forms of decompression sickness. Table IV-1 gives the data on one such contract; these data, resulting from several years' work and involving more than one million decompressions, were reported in 1912 by Keays (see Keays 1912). As may be seen, by far the greatest number of decompression sickness incidents were attributed to the bends, and it would

Table IV-1
Frequency of Symptoms of Decompression Sickness[a]

Symptom	Number of incidents	Percent
Bends (joint pain)	3278	88.78
Bends with local manifestations	9	0.26
Pain with prostration	47	1.26
Central nervous system symptoms		
Hemiplegia	4	0.11
Spinal cord symptoms	80	2.16
Vertigo (staggers)	197	5.33
Dyspnea (chokes)	60	1.62
Partial or complete unconsciousness	17	0.46

[a]From data by Keays (1912).

seem a reasonable assumption that if the decompression procedures could be arranged to avoid attacks of bends, then decompression sickness in its various forms would become a rarity. By the turn of the century, therefore, the decompression problem had narrowed into one of understanding the physics and physiology of the initiation of the bends.

The most important period in the development of decompression theory commenced at the turn of the century when the navies of the world realized that underwater operations were about to become a necessary feature of modern warfare. Accordingly, research work was either performed by the navies themselves or was sponsored by them in external institutions, e.g., universities. The first (and some would say the most productive) of these navy-backed research efforts occurred in 1906 when the Royal Navy engaged the services of the renowned physiologist J. S. Haldane for a series of investigations specifically aimed at reaching regulations for the safe conduct of underwater work by divers. All serious students of decompression theory must read the original account by Haldane and his co-workers (Boycott et al. 1908), as it is the starting point for most modern treatments of decompression theory.

When Haldane commenced his pioneering studies the clinical features of decompression sickness were well documented, but in order to pursue a series of experiments that would certainly have a risk of the occurrence of serious decompression sickness from time to time, it was necessary to search for a suitable animal model. Consequently a great variety of animals were exposed to raised pressure of air in an attempt to assess their sensitivity to attacks of decompression sickness and their general suitability as experimental material. Two principal features of the animal model were vital. In the first place, whichever animal was chosen must exhibit a marginal form of decompression sickness that could be clearly identified as a pain in a joint and therefore could provide a realistic comparison with the principal human situation. After examining a wide spectrum of different animal species, Haldane and his co-workers decided that the goat most nearly satisfied their theoretical and practical requirements. The second essential characteristic of any suitable experimental animal was that the circulatory dynamics should be as near as possible to those of a human being. Once again, on the basis of body weight and composition (i.e., fat-to-water ratio) the goat was selected as the best experimental compromise. Clearly a large primate would have been more suitable, but anyone who has worked with these creatures realizes the tremendous problems they can bring; it is a tribute to Haldane's selection process that even nowadays the goat is still considered useful as an animal model for certain types of decompression sickness research. Relatively modern data on the relationship between body size and sensitivity to decompression sickness are shown in Figure IV-2, and as may be seen, the data give good support to considering the goat to be a suitable animal model.

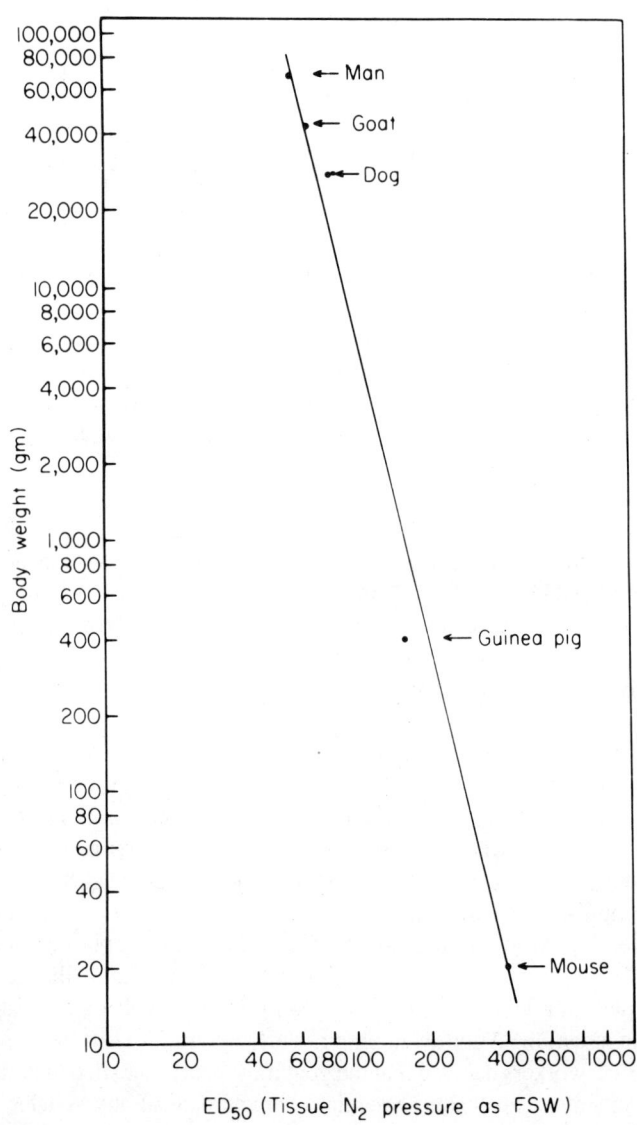

Figure IV-2. Relation of body weight (size) to sensitivity to decompression sickness. [From Flynn and Lambertsen (1971).]

C. The Haldane Concepts

Having chosen a suitable animal it was now necessary to discover the ground rules relating to the appearance and nonappearance of decompression sickness. If a beaker of water is exposed to a constant raised pressure of air, say P_1, and is stirred until no more gas will dissolve in the water at that pressure, then if the gas pressure above the liquid is now suddenly reduced to a new lower pressure, say P_2, the tendency to form bubbles could be described by the magnitude of the pressure drop, i.e., $P_1 - P_2$. It was thought sensible to check whether this supposition was true in the biological situation. If an animal was exposed for a prolonged period at some raised pressure, P_1, until all the tissues of its body had equilibrated with this pressure, then when the pressure was rapidly dropped to some new value, P_2, would the animal exhibit attacks of decompression sickness if $P_1 - P_2$ remained constant? Or perhaps some other relationship between P_1 and P_2 could be established. With this idea in mind Haldane and his co-workers exposed their goats for what they considered prolonged periods of time (1.5–2 hr) at raised pressures, then rapidly decompressed them to some lower pressure and awaited the outcome of this rapid pressure drop. They discovered that if they exposed their animals for such periods of time at a gauge pressure equivalent to pressure of about 45 fsw (2.36 ATA) and then rapidly decompressed these animals back to atmospheric pressure, some of them just began to exhibit mild joint pains (i.e., presumably bends) on surfacing or shortly afterward. It was decided therefore that a pressure difference of just over 1 atm pressure could be safely tolerated by all normal animals. The exposure pressure was next altered to 6 ATA (pressure of 165 fsw) and a rapid pressure drop of just over 1 atm (from 6 to 5) was indeed quite safe for all the animals, but so was a rapid pressure drop of 3 atm (from 6 to 3), and this result was clearly not consistent with the idea that a constant pressure drop defines the generation of bubbles and hence the appearance of decompression sickness. From these and similar experiments Haldane reached his first working hypothesis, which could be stated as follows: After prolonged exposure on air to pressures of 8 ATA it is quite safe to decompress rapidly to 4 ATA; similarly, after long exposure at 6 atm it is quite safe to ascend rapidly to 3 atm, and from exposure to 2 atm it is safe to decompress to 1 atm pressure. Put in simple mathematical terms, if P_1 is the exposure pressure and P_2 is the pressure to which decompression is taken rapidly, them P_1/P_2 is a constant and equal to 2. Clearly, as all tissues in the body are equilibrated following prolonged exposure to pressure, then the ratio value of 2.0 is applicable to all decompression situations for all tissues of the body. This ratio concept became a cornerstone of the Haldane calculation method.

The difficulties associated with deciding the rate at which various tissues acquired and eliminated dissolved inert gas had been avoided in these early experiments. All tissues had been brought to the same state, namely equilibrated to the pressure of gas being breathed. However, not all dives have prolonged bottom times, and in any case having decompressed safely from P_1 to P_2 on the ratio principle, how did one now proceed from the new pressure, P_2, back to atmospheric pressure? These problems demanded a knowledge of the rates at which various tissues of the body acquired dissolved inert gas when the pressures were raised and how they eliminated their excess inert gas content when the pressures were lowered.

Consider a man breathing pure air at normal atmospheric pressure who is suddenly at some time, $t = 0$, exposed to a raised air pressure of P_1 atm. This new pressure of air will be instantly transmitted to the lung surface in the alveoli, and gas will dissolve in the pulmonary tissues through which the pulmonary circulation passes. From relatively modern knowledge it is known that approximately 0.01 sec is required for the dissolved molecules in the alveolar lining to reach the underlying capillary bed. In view of the fact that it takes about 1.0 sec for blood to pass the length of a pulmonary capillary, it is quite certain that blood leaving the capillary bed is fully equilibrated with the gas pressure in the alveoli. For simplicity, therefore, let us assume that the arterial blood supplying the tissues is fully equilibrated with the pressure of gas being breathed and that whenever the gas being breathed changes, then the arterial blood instantly follows this change. Fortunately these simplifying assumptions would not lead to an error of more than a few percent, and providing the physiology of the body does not alter markedly during the course of a dive exposure, the errors will remain reasonably constant and therefore can be discounted.

Thus there is blood in equilibrium with the pressure of the gas breathed in the lungs that is being supplied via the arterial system to all the separate tissues of the body. The next stage of the problem is to decide how this dissolved gas in the arterial input is distributed within a particular tissue space. Histological examination of most tissues reveals a very large number of capillaries per unit volume; the figure varies from several hundreds in well-vascularized tissues to perhaps only one patent capillary per cubic millimeter in a tissue such as fat. The general point to be made, however, is that the intercapillary distance in nearly all tissues of the body is measured in fractions of a millimeter; accepting the normal diffusion coefficients for small gas molecules such as nitrogen and helium, it would be impossible to sustain large concentration gradients within a tissue space. Again, for simplicity, and without much error, let us assume that the concentration of dissolved gas throughout a tissue space is uniform. Given the acceptance of these various simplifying assumptions, the physics of the situation can be represented as in Figure IV-3.

Suppose the volume of arterial blood flowing in to the tissues is v ml/sec: then the volume of venous blood flowing out must also be v ml/sec; otherwise the tissue would progressively swell or shrink. Let the solubility of the inert gas in blood be s_1 ml (at

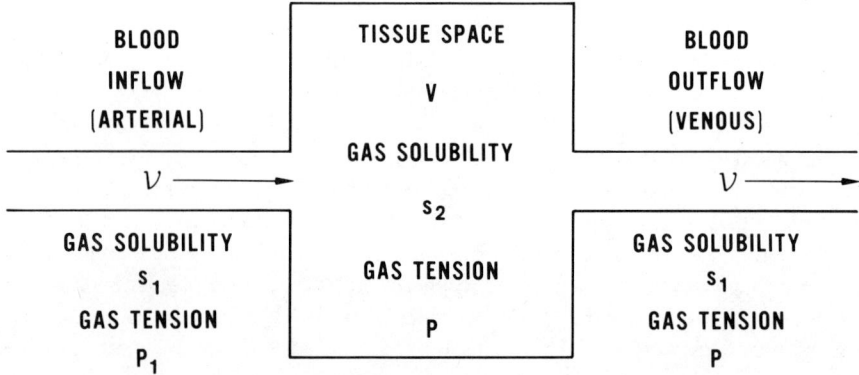

Figure IV-3. Concentration of dissolved gas in arterial, capillary, and venous blood. [(Adapted from Flynn and Lambertsen 1971).]

atmospheric pressure) per ml of blood (at 37°C). If the pressure of gas being breathed is kept at a steady value of P_1 atm, then the total quantity of dissolved gas entering the tissue per sec is $P_1 \cdot s_1 \cdot \nu$ ml. If the tissue is considered as possessing a dissolved gas tension of P atm where P is uniform throughout the tissue (as noted above) and is therefore also the tension in the outgoing venous blood, then the total quantity of dissolved gas leaving the tissue per second is $P \cdot s_1 \cdot \nu$ ml.

The quantity accumulating in the tissue per second is the difference between that entering and that leaving, i.e., $(P_1 - P)s_1 \cdot \nu$. Now this amount of dissolved gas is distributed per second in a tissue space of volume V and solubility s_2.

Suppose that a very small time Δt passes; then a small increase in tension ΔP will occur in the tissue, which will represent a volume of dissolved gas $\Delta P \cdot s_2 V$ ml. In this small time the blood has delivered $(P_1 - P)s_1 \nu \cdot \Delta t$ ml of dissolved gas. These two amounts must be equal, i.e.,

$$\Delta P \, s_2 V = (P_1 - P) \, s_1 \nu \cdot \Delta t$$

or

$$\Delta P / \Delta t = (P_1 - P)s_1 \, \nu / s_2 V$$

and s_1, ν, s_2, and V are all constants for any particular tissue; therefore $s_1 \nu / s_2 V$ is constant and will be called K:

$$\Delta P / \Delta t = K (P_1 - P)$$

as Δt becomes smaller,

$$dP/dt = K (P_1 - P) \tag{1}$$

Students of elementary calculus will know that the variables are separated

$$dP/(P_1 - P) = K \, dt$$

and then integrated

$$- \log (P_1 - P) = Kt + c_1$$

or, expressing this differently,

$$P_1 - P = c \, e^{-Kt} \tag{2}$$

But when $t = 0$, $P = 0$

$$\therefore P_1 = c \, e^0 = c$$

as $e^0 = 1$. Rearrange Equation 2 using this value of c,

$$P = P_1(1 - e^{-Kt}) \tag{3}$$

This is the fundamental equation of the original Haldane analysis, and it has become the basic mathematical expression for nearly all subsequent treatments of dissolved gas exchange in tissues. Continuous reference will be made to various aspects of this analysis and the often subtle hidden assumptions.

It is now opportune to examine how Haldane made use of this expression governing tissue inert gas exchange. Equation 3 refers to the situation where a tissue is acquiring excess dissolved gas through sudden imposition of a constant input pressure P_1 at time $t = 0$ and, as may be easily verified, when $t = \infty$, $P = P_1$, and the tissue has equilibrated with the arterial gas tension. The rate at which the tissue approaches this equilibrium state is entirely dependent on the K-value chosen, and $K = s_1 \nu / s_2 V$ requires a substantial knowledge of the tissue physics and physiology certainly not available in Haldane's day. Consequently he needed to make an "informed guess," and it is worth remarking that this practice of informed guessing has continued to the present day, since no one yet knows which tissue, or tissues, cause the bends, as becomes apparent later.

In common with many situations where exponential time constants are involved (e.g., radioactive decay) it is common practice to use the half time as a measure of the rate process. All exponential time courses have the same shape, and the simple property they have in common is that if t_1 is the time taken to reach half the value at $t\infty$, then 2 t_1 will be three-quarters of the way to this value, 3 t_1 will be seven-eighths, and so on. Each additional half time takes the value halfway between the previous value and the infinite value. A table of the percentage saturations of a Haldane-like tissue in terms of the number of half times is shown in Table IV-2. For the construction of his decompression table calculations Haldane chose tissue half times of 5, 10, 20, 40, and 75 min. One cannot help but notice the anomalous way he doubled up the half-time values from 5 to 40 and then called a halt at 75 instead of 80.

Let us now examine in some detail a typical decompression calculation according to the Haldane method.

In these early computations air was treated as a single gas. This is obviously incorrect for, as Haldane well knew, the bubbles responsible for decompression sickness are formed from excess dissolved nitrogen, but the proportion of nitrogen in air is always constant, so taking it as a single entity is therefore permissible and avoids multiplying every air pressure by a constant factor of 0.79, i.e., the proportion of nitrogen gas in air.

D. Using the Haldane Concepts

The best way to reveal how these decompression procedures were obtained is to give, in its original wording, an account by G. C. C. Damant (n.d.) of the calculation of two decompression profiles for use by compressed air workers. The method for divers is exactly the same in the main features, i.e., a pressure ratio principle to determine the permissible excess dissolved gas at any time during the decompression, and the use of pressure stages for off-loading this excess gas. In the case of the original diving tables the pressure units were feet of seawater and the pressure stages, or *stops* as they are frequently called, were placed at 10-fsw (3.05-msw) increments. When reading this account, bear in mind that 0.7 msw or 2.25 fsw is equivalent to 1 psi of pressure and therefore the two calculations that follow refer to 6 hr of exposure at 57 fsw or 17.5 msw and 1.5 hr at 68 fsw or 21 msw. One further important fact to be noted is that although the Haldane decompression ratio of 2:1 is much discussed by everyone studying this subject it was not used by Haldane for his calculations! These hidden oddities that occur in decompression table calculations have continued to the present day and are pointed out at the appropriate points in the subsequent considerations.

Haldane showed that it was safe and desirable, with working pressures up to about 80 lb/in^2 to begin decompression by rapidly reducing the air pressure to the equivalent of half (or a little less than half) the *absolute* working pressure. From this point onwards the air pressure should be gradually reduced at a rate slow enough to ensure that no part of the body is, at any time, supersaturated to such an extent as to cause risk of bubble formation. The processes of saturation and desaturation proceed at the same rate, following a logarithmic curve, but we cannot calculate for the body as a whole because some parts or groups of tissues saturate and desaturate more rapidly than others. In calculating we must take into account parts which become half saturated in 75, 40, 20, 10 and 5 minutes respectively. Table A [IV-2] tells us by what percentage each of these parts will become saturated or desaturated in a given number of minutes. The two last mentioned groups of tissues, called 10T and 5T, are only of importance when the time of exposure to pressure is short, as in diving work at very high pressures.

Table B [IV-3] gives, for various working pressures, the pressure to which the air lock may be reduced in the first rapid stage of decompression.

Table IV-2

TABLE A. Giving the Percentage Saturation at 1-min Intervals of Tissues (75T etc) That Become Half-Saturated in 75, 40, 20, 10, and 5 min[a]

		Time, in min			Saturation			Time, in min			Saturation
5T	10T	20T	40T	75T	percentage	5T	10T	20T	40T	75T	percentage
	0.14			1	1		4.74		19	36	28
	0.29		1	2	2		4.94			37	29
	0.44	1	2	3	3		5.14	10	20	38	30
	0.59			5	4		5.35		21	40	31
	0.74		3	6	5		5.56	11	22	42	32
	0.89			7	6		5.78		23	43	33
0.5	1.04	2	4	8	7	3	5.99	12	24	45	34
	1.20			9	8		6.21		25	46	35
	1.36		5	10	9		6.43	13	26	48	36
	1.52	3	6	11	10		6.66		27	50	37
	1.68			13	11		6.90	14	28	52	38
	1.84		7	14	12		7.13			53	39
1.0	2.01	4	8	15	13		7.37		29	55	40
	2.18		9	16	14		7.61	15	30	57	41
	2.34			18	15		7.85		31	59	42
	2.51	5	10	19	16	4	8.11	16	32	61	43
	2.68		11	20	17		8.36		33	63	44
	2.86			21	18		8.62	17	34	65	45
	3.04	6	12	23	19		8.89	18	36	67	46
	3.22		13	24	20		9.16		37	69	47
	3.40			26	21		9.43	19	38	71	48
	3.58	7	14	27	22		9.71		39	73	49
	3.77		15	29	23	5	10.0	20	40	75	50
2	3.96	8	16	30	24		10.3		41	77	51
	4.15			31	25		10.6	21	42	79	52
	4.34	9	17	32	26		10.9	22	44	82	53
	4.54	9	18	34	27		11.2		45	84	54

Table A—*Cont.*

\	Time, in min				Saturation percentage	\	Time, in min				Saturation percentage
5T	10T	20T	40T	75T		5T	10T	20T	40T	75T	
	11.5	23	46	86	55	11	21.8	44	87	163	78
	11.8		47	88	56		22.5	45	90	168	79
6	12.2	24	49	91	57		23.2	46	93	173	80
	12.5	25	50	94	58	12	23.9	48	96	179	81
	12.8	26	51	96	59		24.7	49	99	185	82
	13.2		53	99	60		25.5	51	102	191	83
	13.6	27	54	102	61	13	26.4	53	105	198	84
7	14.0	28	56	105	62		27.4	54	109	205	85
	14.3		57	107	63	14	28.4	56	113	213	86
	14.7	29	59	110	64		29.4	59	117	221	87
	15.1	30	60	113	65	15	30.6	61	122	230	88
	15.6	31	62	117	66	16	31.9	63	127	239	89
8	16.0	32	64	120	67		33.2	66	132	249	90
	16.4	33	66	123	68	17	34.7	69	138	260	91
	16.9	34	68	127	69	18	36.4	73	145	273	92
	17.4	35	70	130	70	19	38.3	77	153	287	93
9	17.9	36	72	134	71	20	40.6	81	162	304	94
	18.4	37	74	138	72	22	43.2	86	173	324	95
	18.9	38	76	142	73	23	46.4	93	185	348	96
	19.4	39	78	146	74	25	50.6	101	202	380	97
10	20.0	40	80	150	75	28	56.4	113	225	424	98
	20.6	41	82	154	76	33	66.4	133	265	498	99
	21.2	42	85	159	77						

[a] From Damant (n.d.).

ABBREVIATIONS

The following are used. All pressures are gauge pressures (i.e., above atmospheric) unless otherwise stated.

- WP *Working Pressure* to which a man has been exposed during his shift.
- SP *Saturation Pressure* of a man's body or a specified part of it. The solution pressure of dissolved nitrogen will be about 80% of the SP.
- LP *Lock Pressure* in a decompression lock or chamber at a specified stage of compression.
- DP *Difference of Pressure* between SP and LP at a given moment during decompression. It represents the stress under which desaturation is proceeding.
- "p" Highest working pressure from which a man can be rapidly (say in two minutes) decompressed to atmospheric pressure [147 psi] without danger of resultant compressed air illness, however long the shift may have been. [The term ''p'' was used, differently defined, by Boulton (1942).] Decompressions are calculated so that by the time LP reaches zero, SP will have fallen to 18 lb. Haldane considered 18 lb [a 2.2:1 ratio] a reasonable value for ''p''; this value has proved to be correct in the case of divers and is used in the following examples. Some people think it safe to shorten the decompressions of tunnel workers by using a higher value (e.g., 22 lb) [a 2.5:1 ratio] for ''p'', whilst others believe that a lower value is necessary to ensure complete safety [a strict 2.0:1 ratio, or 14.7 lb].
- 75T That group of tissues in a man's body which becomes half-saturated or reaches a SP of 50% of the WP in 75 minutes.
- 40T, Those faster saturating tissues which become half-saturated in the number of minutes
- 20T, indicated by the numeral . . .
- 10T,
- 5T

Decompression Theory

To illustrate the method, let us begin with the case of men who have been working for 6 hours or more at a WP of 25 lb. For practical purposes the bodies can be considered as fully saturated; that is to say, the SPs of 75T, 40T, 20T, etc., have all reached 25 lb. Our object is to reduce the LP at such a rate that by the time it has reached zero the SP in all parts of the body will have fallen to 18 lb ("p") or less. Since the process of desaturation follows the same course as that of saturation, 75T represents that part of the body which will be the last to reach the goal of SP 18 lb, and we may disregard 40T, etc., knowing that by the time 75T has reached 18 lb they will have fallen to some still lower SP.

Table B [IV-3] shows that we can begin the men's decompression by allowing the LP to fall rapidly from 25 lb to 5 lb when the situation will be: 75T has SP 25 lb, with LP 5 lb, makes DP 20 lb. Therefore, 75T must desaturate from SP 25 lb to SP 18 lb, or by 7 lb, which is 35% of the DP and (by Table A [IV-2]) would require 46 minutes' time if the LP remained steady at 5 lb.

But, in practice, instead of maintaining the LP at 5 lb, we allow it to fall at a uniform rate calculated to ensure that it will reach zero at the same time as the SP reaches 18 lb. In the present case, while the LP is falling by 5 lb, the SP must fall by 7 lb. To find the time required for this amount of desaturation, using only simple arithmetic, we may suppose that the LP falls in a series of 1-lb stages, remaining steady at each just long enough for the SP to fall by 1.4 lb. Thus:

1st Stage
    SP 25 lb   LP 5 lb   DP 20 lb   SP to fall 1.4 lb or 7% of DP takes 8 minutes
2nd Stage
    SP 23.6 lb   LP 4 lb   DP 19.6 lb   SP to fall 1.4 lb or 7% of DP takes 8 minutes
3rd Stage
    SP 22.2 lb   LP 3 lb   DP 19.2 lb   SP to fall 1.4 lb or 7% of DP takes 8 minutes
4th Stage
    SP 20.8 lb   LP 2 lb   DP 18.8 lb   SP to fall 1.4 lb or 7% of DP takes 8 minutes
5th Stage
    SP 19.4   LP 1 lb   DP 18.4 lb   SP to fall 1.4 lb or 8% of DP takes 9 minutes

Total time required   41 minutes

Taking the case of men who have become fully saturated under a WP of 40 lb. Table B [IV-3] shows that the LP may be rapidly reduced to 12 lb. Then, while it is slowly falling from 12 lb to zero, the SP must fall from 40 to 18 lb, or by an amount of 22 lb, which we can conveniently divide up into eleven decrements of 1.8 lb, and a twelfth of 2.2 lb, and the working, briefly expressed, becomes:

SP 40 lb	LP 12 lb	DP 28 lb	SP to fall 1.8 lb or 6.5% takes 7.5 minutes
SP 38.2 lb	LP 11 lb	DP 27.2 lb	SP to fall 1.8 lb or 6.5% takes 7.5 minutes
SP 36.4 lb	LP 10 lb	DP 26.4 lb	SP to fall 1.8 lb or 7 % takes 8 minutes
SP 34.6 lb	LP 9 lb	DP 25.6 lb	SP to fall 1.8 lb or 7 % takes 8 minutes
SP 32.8 lb	LP 8 lb	DP 24.8 lb	SP to fall 1.8 lb or 7 % takes 8 minutes
SP 31 lb	LP 7 lb	DP 24 lb	SP to fall 1.8 lb or 7.5% takes 8.5 minutes
SP 29.2 lb	LP 6 lb	DP 23.2 lb	SP to fall 1.8 lb or 7.5% takes 8.5 minutes
SP 27.4 lb	LP 5 lb	DP 22.4 lb	SP to fall 1.8 lb or 8 % takes 9 minutes
SP 25.6 lb	LP 4 lb	DP 21.6 lb	SP to fall 1.8 lb or 8.5% takes 9.5 minutes
SP 23.8 lb	LP 3 lb	DP 20.8 lb	SP to fall 1.8 lb or 8.5% takes 9.5 minutes
SP 22 lb	LP 2 lb	DP 20 lb	SP to fall 1.8 lb or 9 % takes 10 minutes
SP 20.2 lb	LP 1 lb	DP 19.2 lb	SP to fall 2.2 lb or 11.5% takes 13 minutes

Total time required   107 minutes

[It is of interest to note in this example that the decompression ratio (DR) from SP 40 to LP 12 is 2.05:1, or (40 + 14.7) ÷ 12 + 14.7), whereas that of SP 20.2 to LP 1, the last stop, is 2.22:1, or (20.2 + 14.7) ÷ 1 + 14.7).]

SHORT EXPOSURES

So far, we have only considered long exposures after which the desaturation of the slowest tissues, 75T, dominates the situation and the faster tissues may be disregarded. After short exposures they must be taken into account. Thus, after a shift of 1½ hours at WP 30 lb, Table A [IV-2] shows that the saturations of different parts of the body would be:

75T	57% of 30 lb or 17 lb
40T	79% of 30 lb or 24 lb
20T	96% of 30 lb or 29 lb

Since 75T has not reached the danger limit "p" of 18 lb, it need not be considered at all, but 40T and 20T will both need gradual decompression. Inspection or a rough calculation shows that, though 20T is the more highly saturated of the two at the start, its faster rate of desaturation will reduce it to the lower SP of the two during the course of decompression; therefore in this case we must base our calculation on 40T. Dropping to a LP of 7 lb, as shown by Table B [IV-3], we see that 40T has to fall from 24 to 18 lb, while LP is falling from 7 lb to zero.

Dividing the decompression up into seven 1-lb stages as before, we get:

40T SP 24 lb	LP 7 lb	DP 17 lb	with SP to fall by 0.5 lb, or 3% takes	2 minutes
40T SP 23.5 lb	LP 6 lb	DP 17.5 lb	with SP to fall by 0.5 lb, or 3% takes	2 minutes
40T SP 23 lb	LP 5 lb	DP 18 lb	with SP to fall by 1 lb, or 6% takes	3 minutes
40T SP 22 lb	LP 4 lb	DP 18 lb	with SP to fall by 1 lb, or 6% takes	3 minutes
40T SP 21 lb	LP 3 lb	DP 18 lb	with SP to fall by 1 lb, or 6% takes	3 minutes
40T SP 20 lb	LP 2 lb	DP 18 lb	with SP to fall by 1 lb, or 6% takes	3 minutes
40T SP 19 lb	LP 1 lb	DP 18 lb	with SP to fall by 1 lb, or 6% takes	3 minutes

Total time required   19 minutes

[In this example the 40T or from SP 24 to LP 7 is only 1.78:1, whereas that from SP 19 to LP 1, the last stop, is 2.14:1.]

Table IV-3

TABLE B. Initial Rapid Drops of Pressure in Decompression by the Late Professor J. S. Haldane's System in the Ratio of 2:1 (or Rather More) of Absolute Pressure.[a]

Working pressure, lb	May be reduced in 2 min to lb	Working pressure, lb	May be reduced in 2 min to lb
19	2	40	12
20	2	41	13
21	3	42	13
22	3	43	14
23	4	44	14
24	4	45	15
25	5	46	15
26	5	47	16
27	6	48	16
28	6	49	17
29	7	50	17
30	7	51	18
31	8	52	18
32	8	53	19
33	9	54	19
34	9	55	20
35	10	56	20
36	10	57	21
37	11	58	21
38	11	59	22
39	12	60	22

[a]From Davis (n.d.).

Haldane issued three separate air diving tables. The first table was for all those dives requiring a decompression time of less than 30 min. The second table was for all air dives requiring a decompression time of more than 30 min, and the third table was for deep air diving to depths of 330 ft (100 m). All his decompression procedures were characterized by a rapid ascent from depth to the first one or two stages, followed by a slow staged ascent to the surface. This decompression profile represented a radical departure from previous practice, which almost invariably consisted of raising the diver at a fixed rate of a certain number of feet per minute back to the surface, and it took the more conservative element in the diving world some years to recognize the value of Haldane's approach.

Haldane used some interesting auxiliary arguments to justify the rather dangerous-looking rush from depth to a first stage (or stop) and then the ever increasingly conservative ascent back to the surface via the shallower stages. He pointed out that as it is generally believed a bubble is responsible for decompression sickness, then if we consider a small bubble forming at, say, 100 ft or 30 m (4 ATA), it is easy to see that it will double its size if the diver ascends through the water a distance of 66 ft or 20 m, to a depth of 33 ft or 10 m, i.e., 2 ATA pressure. The pressure on the bubble has been halved and therefore the volume has been doubled (Boyle's law). Similarly, if we imagine a small bubble at 33 ft (2 ATA), then rapid ascent to the surface (1 ATA) will also double the bubble's size. In the first case, however, it had been necessary to ascend 66 ft or 20 m to achieve a double of size, whereas in the second case only an ascent of 33 ft or 10 m had been necessary. Clearly the nearer the surface, the more the rate of expansion of any bubbles. From this it follows that we must be much more careful when decompressing near the surface. A linear decompression, as Haldane emphasized, does not take into account such possible bubble expansions and is therefore potentially hazardous. The acid test of any procedure, however, is, "Does it work?" The answer became quite clear that for the range of depths and bottom times commonly used in those days the Haldane tables were remarkably successful and virtually eliminated all of the various manifestations of decompression sickness, including the bends.

The Royal Navy adopted the Haldane tables in 1908 and the first tables developed for the U.S. Navy, devised by French and Stilson in 1915 (see French 1916; Stilson 1915), were based on the Haldanian concepts of a decompression ratio and also used oxygen decompression to achieve depths between 200 fsw and 300 fsw. These tables were known as the Bureau of Construction and Repair tables (C & R tables). The C & R tables were used successfully in the 1915 salvage of the sunken submarine *F4* at a depth of 306 fsw.

E. *Post-Haldane Difficulties*

If the Haldane tables were so successful why are we not using them today for air diving? Paradoxically the demise of the Haldane approach was due in large measure to its success. In providing procedures that almost eliminated decompression sickness as a diving hazard it became part of the advancing front in underwater technology that was liberating the diver from many of the constraints of his environment. With the development of more-effective gas pumping and storage systems and of better-designed and more reliable diving suits, it became possible to descend deeper and stay longer on the bottom than had been contemplated at the turn of the century. The urge to exploit the divers' capabilities came from both military and commercial interests. From the military standpoint the advancing importance of underwater warfare clearly demanded an investment in diving technology. The commercial interests very largely stemmed from the considerable prizes available from successfully salvaging valuable cargoes in sunken vessels. The more the Haldane tables were used, the more their inadequacies began to emerge.

Haldane's "Table I" is reproduced in Figure IV-4. If a dive of duration and depth such as 25 min at 100 ft is planned, then it is seen that decompression stages are required at 30, 20, and 10 ft, involving a total decompression time of 19 min. Reference to the current U.S. Navy Standard Air Diving Tables reveals that 25 min at 100 ft can be safely followed by direct ascent to the surface at a generally applied rate of 25 ft/min. The knowledge that most of Haldane's "Table I" was indubitably safe, but unfortunately grossly oversafe, gradually accumulated with practical experience over the years.

If, on the other hand, one wishes to do a relatively long dive at 100 ft with a 2-hr bottom time, it is necessary to use Haldane's "Table II" (a page of which is reproduced in Figure IV-5), and it is seen that the total decompression time is 92 min for this particular dive. Again using the 1956 U.S. Navy Standard Air Diving tables for comparison with modern practice, it is seen that such a dive requires just over 132 min of decompression, although most diving supervisors faced with a dive of this nature will proceed one increment further on the diving table and give a decompression time of just over 202 min. The point to be noted is that the Haldane "Table II" (Figure IV-5) is clearly giving grossly inadequate decompression for the longer and deeper dives. In the years between the promulgation of these tables in 1908 and the early 1930s it had become apparent from practical usage that his "Table I" was mostly oversafe and his "Table II" was in many areas very undersafe. This led to a lack of confidence in the effectiveness of the Haldane tables and in turn promoted the next phase of diving research to define the nature of the problem more accurately.

Before embarking on the next stage of the development of concepts related to the etiology of decompression sickness, which were almost entirely confined to the diving situation, it is as well to be reminded that far greater numbers of men enter compressed air for work purposes in caissons and tunnels than for diving. In most countries the authorities promulgating regulations relating to work in compressed air by tunnelers and caisson workers are not the same as those responsible for diving regulations. Nevertheless, the medical and physiological problems encountered by men in these different areas of work are obviously very closely related. It is worth noting that between the two World Wars Haldane's principles for decompressing tunnel workers were adopted by several groups and, as with the diving situation, as long as the pressure was comparatively low (below 25 psi gauge) and the time at pressure not very great (not in excess of 4 hr), then Haldane's decompression profiles worked satisfactorily. When longer shifts and greater pressures became commercially desirable, the Haldane tables could not meet the challenge, and the incidence of bends (and indeed more serious forms of decompression sickness) became too great for acceptance by the contractors in the compressed air industry. It is seen later in this chapter that the problems encountered by compressed air workers began to influence the diving scene in more recent times.

TABLE I.

Depth.		Pressure Pounds per Square Inch.	Time under Water, i.e., from Surface to Beginning of Ascent.**	Stoppages in Minutes at different Depths.						Total Time for Ascent in Minutes.	Number of Cylinders needed †***	Revolutions of Pump per Minute.‡
Feet.	Fathoms.			60 ft.	50 ft.	40 ft.	30 ft.	20 ft.	10 ft.			
96–108	16–18	42½–48	20 to 25 mins....	—	—	—	1	5	10	19	4	20
			25 to 30 mins....	—	—	—	3	7	10	23		
			30 to 35 mins....	—	—	—	4	8	13	28		
			35 to 40 mins....	—	—	—	5	10	15	33		
108–120	18–20	48–53½	Up to 5 mins....	—	—	—	—	—	4	7	4	20
			5 to 10 mins. ...	—	—	—	—	2	6	11		
			10 to 15 mins....	—	—	—	2	3	7	15		
			15 to 20 mins....	—	—	—	3	5	8	19		
			20 to 25 mins....	—	—	—	5	5	10	23		
			25 to 30 mins....	—	—	—	5	8	12	28		
			30 to 35 mins....	—	—	—	5	10	15	33		
120–132	20–22	53½–59	Up to 5 mins....	—	—	—	—	—	5	8	4	25
			5 to 10 mins. ...	—	—	—	—	3	7	13		
			10 to 15 mins....	—	—	—	2	5	7	17		
			15 to 20 mins....	—	—	—	3	7	10	23		
			20 to 25 mins....	—	—	—	4	8	13	28		
			25 to 30 mins....	—	—	—	5	10	15	33		
132–144	22–24	59–64½	Up to 6 mins....	—	—	—	—	2	5	10	4	25
			6 to 12 mins. ...	—	—	—	3	5	5	16		
			12 to 16 mins....	—	—	—	4	7	5	21		
			16 to 20 mins....	—	—	1	4	8	10	26		
			20 to 25 mins....	—	—	2	5	10	12	32		
144–156	24–26	64½–70	Up to 5 mins....	—	—	—	—	2	5	10	4	25
			5 to 10 mins. ...	—	—	—	3	5	5	16		
			10 to 15 mins....	—	—	1	4	7	8	23		
			15 to 20 mins....	—	2	3	5	8	10	31		
156–168	26–28	70–75	Up to 5 mins....	—	—	—	—	2	5	10	4	30°
			5 to 10 mins. ...	—	—	2	3	5	5	18		
			10 to 13 mins....	—	1	2	4	6	8	24		
			13 to 16 mins....	—	2	3	5	7	10	30		
168–180	28–30	75–80½	Up to 5 mins....	—	—	—	—	3	5	11	4	30°
			5 to 9 mins. ...	—	—	2	3	5	5	18		
			9 to 12 mins. ...	—	—	3	4	6	8	24		
			12 to 14 mins....	—	2	3	5	7	10	30		
180–192	30–32	80½–86	Up to 5 mins....	—	—	—	1	3	5	12	6	25
			5 to 10 mins. ...	—	1	2	3	6	8	23		
			10 to 13 mins....	—	2	3	5	7	10	30		
192–204	32–34	86–91½	Up to 7 mins....	—	2	2	3	5	5	20	6	25
			7 to 12 mins. ...	2	2	3	5	7	10	32		

* If found difficult to maintain 30 revolutions, a second cylinder may be used.
† These figures are calculated on the supposition that the pump does not leak more than 20 per cent. at pressures up to 60 lbs. Instructions as to testing of Pumps are given on pages 65 and 66.
‡ i.e., using a Siebe-Gorman Two Cylinder Double-acting Pump.
** For instructions as to time for descent, see pages 89 and 90.
*** For actual quantities of air required at different depths, see page 87.

Figure IV-4. Replica of a page taken from Table I of a British diving manual BR 155/43, after data by Haldane. [From Davis (1935).]

TABLE II., showing Stoppages during Ascent after exceeding the Ordinary Limits of Time on the Bottom.

Depth.		Pressure in lbs. per sq. inch.	Time from leaving Surface to beginning of Ascent.	Stoppages at different Depths in Minutes.								Total Time for Ascent in Minutes.
Feet	Faths.			80 ft.	70 ft.	60 ft.	50 ft.	40 ft.	30 ft.	20 ft.	10 ft.	
66	11	29½	Over 3 hrs.	—	—	—	—	—	—	10	30	42
72	12	32	2 to 3 hrs.	—	—	—	—	—	—	10	30	42
			Over 3 hrs.	—	—	—	—	—	—	20	30	52
78	13	34½	1½ to 2½ hrs.	—	—	—	—	—	—	20	30	52
			Over 2½ hrs.	—	—	—	—	—	—	30	30	62
84	14	37	1¼ to 1½ hrs.	—	—	—	—	—	—	10	25	37
			1½ to 1¾ hrs.	—	—	—	—	—	—	10	30	42
			1¾ to 2 hrs.	—	—	—	—	—	—	15	30	47
			2 to 2¼ hrs.	—	—	—	—	—	—	20	30	52
			2¼ to 2½ hrs.	—	—	—	—	—	2	23	30	57
			2½ to 2¾ hrs.	—	—	—	—	—	3	27	30	62
			2¾ to 3 hrs.	—	—	—	—	—	5	30	30	67
			Over 3 hrs.	—	—	—	—	—	10	30	35	77
90	15	40	1 hr. to 1 hr. 12 mins.	—	—	—	—	—	5	10	20	37
			1 hr. 12 mins. to 1 hr. 20 mins.	—	—	—	—	—	5	15	20	42
			1 hr. 20 mins. to 1 hr. 30 mins.	—	—	—	—	—	5	15	25	47
			1 hr. 30 mins. to 1 hr. 44 mins.	—	—	—	—	—	5	20	25	52
			1 hr. 44 mins. to 2 hrs.	—	—	—	—	—	5	25	25	57
			2 hrs. to 2 hrs. 14 mins.	—	—	—	—	—	5	25	30	62
			2 hrs. 14 mins. to 2½ hrs.	—	—	—	—	—	5	30	30	67
			2½ hrs. to 2 hrs. 44 mins.	—	—	—	—	—	10	30	30	72
			2 hrs. 44 mins. to 3 hrs. 14 mins.	—	—	—	—	—	20	30	30	82
			Over 3 hrs. 14 mins.	—	—	—	—	—	20	35	35	92
96	16	42½	55 mins. to 1 hr. 12 mins.	—	—	—	—	—	5	10	25	42
			1 hr. 12 mins. to 1½ hrs.	—	—	—	—	—	5	15	30	52
			1½ hrs. to 1 hr. 54 mins.	—	—	—	—	—	5	25	30	62
			1 hr. 54 mins. to 2 hrs. 18 mins.	—	—	—	—	—	10	30	30	72
			2 hrs. 18 mins. to 2½ hrs.	—	—	—	—	—	10	30	35	77
			2½ hrs. to 2 hrs. 54 mins.	—	—	—	—	—	20	30	35	87
			Over 2 hrs. 54 mins.	—	—	—	—	—	30	35	35	102
108	18	48	40 to 50 mins.	—	—	—	—	—	8	10	20	41
			50 mins. to 1 hr.	—	—	—	—	—	10	15	20	48
			1 hr. to 1 hr. 18 mins.	—	—	—	—	—	10	20	25	58
			1 hr. 18 mins. to 1 hr. 44 mins.	—	—	—	—	—	15	20	35	73
			1 hr. 44 mins. to 2 hrs.	—	—	—	—	5	15	25	35	83
			2 hrs. to 2 hrs. 18 mins.	—	—	—	—	5	20	30	35	92
			2 hrs. 18 mins. to 2 hrs. 34 mins.	—	—	—	—	10	25	30	35	102
			2 hrs. 34 mins. to 2 hrs. 50 mins.	—	—	—	—	15	25	30	40	112
			Over 2 hrs. 50 mins.	—	—	—	—	15	30	35	40	122
120	20	53½	35 to 50 mins.	—	—	—	—	—	10	15	20	47
			50 mins. to 1 hr.	—	—	—	—	5	10	15	25	57
			1 hr. to 1 hr. 22 mins.	—	—	—	—	5	15	25	25	72
			1 hr. 22 mins. to 1 hr. 44 mins.	—	—	—	—	5	20	30	30	87
			1 hr. 44 mins. to 2 hrs.	—	—	—	—	10	20	30	35	97
			2 hrs. to 2 hrs. 22 mins.	—	—	—	—	15	25	35	35	112
			2 hrs. 22 mins. to 2 hrs. 44 mins.	—	—	—	—	20	30	35	40	127
			Over 2 hrs. 44 mins.	—	—	—	—	30	35	35	40	142

Figure IV-5. Replica of a page taken from Table II of a British diving manual BR 155/43, after data by Haldane. [From Davis (1935).]

From 1932 onward for the next 25 years diving research effort was almost entirely confined to the U.S. Navy. The names of A. R. Behnke, C. W. Shilling, J. A. Hawkins, O. D. Yarbrough, O. E. VanDerAue, T. L. Willmon, M. Des Grange, J. V. Dwyer and, more recently, R. D. Workman, are principally associated with a quite remarkable series of experiments, generally involving human volunteers, that helped to define some of the boundary conditions of the decompression problem in a quantitative manner for the first time.

To pursue a calculation using the Haldane method it is necessary to know the time constants (K-value of Eq. 1) for all tissues involved in the decompression problem. This in turn involves a knowledge of the rates of blood perfusion of these tissues and the solubilities of nitrogen in them. As remarked earlier such knowledge was certainly not available in Haldane's day, and indeed it is still very difficult to obtain reliable, accepted, data on many tissues even today. This means that Haldane's K-values are what one would term *informed guesses*. His value for the tissue with the longest half time was derived, in part, from a study of the behavior of his animals and, as he himself was well aware, it is always unsatisfactory to extrapolate from animal results and apply them to human beings.

Before proceeding with discussion of the human experimentation it would therefore be helpful to examine in greater detail the fundamental animal experiments from which the whole Haldanian set of ideas are derived. As will be recalled from the brief description of his experiments given earlier, he exposed animals to a constant raised pressure of air for periods of time as long as 2 hr and then decompressed them to some lower pressure in order to establish his rule of a ratio of 2:1. One of the first doubts that arises concerns the duration of exposure required to equilibrate all the tissues of a goat at a constant raised pressure. Haldane considered that 2 hr or thereabouts was quite sufficient, but investigators were soon led to enquire whether this was true. Many years later (Eaton and Hempleman 1962) this particular problem was investigated in the following manner. Goats were exposed to an excess pressure of air, say P_1, for a time, t min, and then rapidly decompressed to atmospheric pressure, where they were carefully watched to see whether an attack of bends followed this exposure. If no bends occurred, then on the next experiment some days later the same goat was given another exposure of duration t, but the pressure was increased to some new value, generally 5 ft (1.5 m) greater than the first. If bends did occur after the original exposure, the experiment was repeated at a pressure 5 ft (1.5 m) lower in an attempt to obtain a troublefree result. In this way it was possible to obtain a threshold bend pressure for that particular duration of exposure in a given animal. Repeating all these observations for numbers of different animals gives a response pattern for a population of goats. Such a curve of performance is reproduced in Figure IV-6. Several important points are immediately obvious from an examination of these results:

1. Deeper dives can only be safely performed if the duration of exposure is shortened.

2. After about 4 hr of exposure at pressure, and certainly after 6 hr, there seems to be no change in the levels of threshold bend pressure.

3. There is a wide variability in individual response at any particular combination of pressure and time.

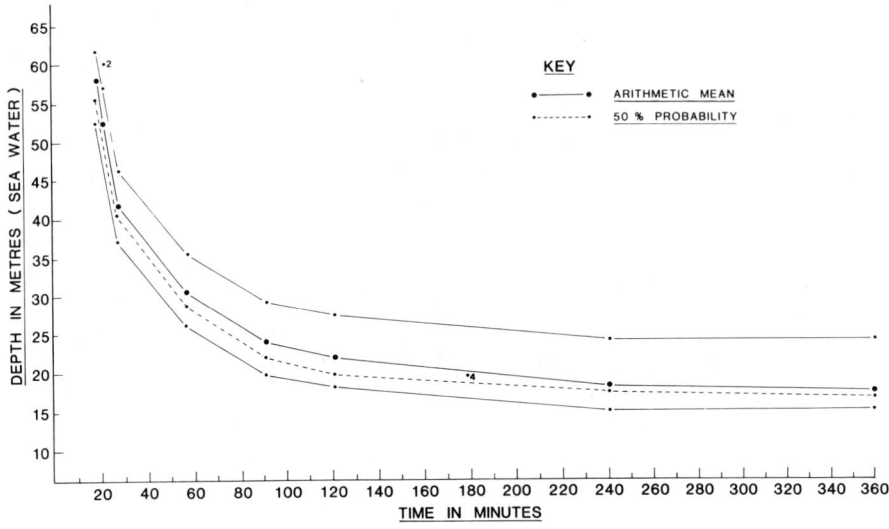

Figure IV-6. Population curve for goats, showing arithmetic mean and the 50% bend probablity. [From Eaton and Hempleman (1962).]

Such experimental results were not available to Haldane, and consequently his idea that 2 hr, or perhaps slightly more, would equilibrate all the tissues of a goat with gas at a constant raised pressure was unfortunately not correct, as can be seen by considering observation 2. There is clearly a difference between the threshold bend level at a 3-hr duration and the threshold level at 6 hr. This forces recognition of the fact that longer half times are involved in the decompression calculations than Haldane realized. In turn, this means that the decompression ratio concept was founded on the use of animals with some of their tissues not equilibrated with gas, which renders the whole theoretical framework somewhat dubious. Thus these later animal experiments revealed the underlying uncertainties in Haldane's concepts and offer one possible explanation of the reasons why his tables were impractical for both short-duration and long-duration air dives. The tissue half times had not been properly established, and the decompression ratio was probably not the value Haldane gave it.

F. U.S. Navy Initiative

By a different chain of reasoning these weaknesses in the Haldane approach became apparent to C. W. Shilling and his colleagues (Hawkins et al. 1935). In essence these U.S. Navy experimenters undertook in the mid-1930s a set of exposures using human volunteers; these were very similar to the much-later experiments with goats just described. Volunteers were exposed to raised pressures of air and then decompressed back to surface pressure without decompression stages. The results of these experiments are set out in Table IV-4. As with the goats, so with the men; it can be seen that short exposures allow a quite deep dive, whereas longer bottom times can only safely take place at shallower

Table IV-4
Summary of Results from Exposure of Human Volunteers to Air Dives of Varying Depths and Times[a]

No. of tests	Depth, ft	Individual exposures	Initial exposure time, min	Final time, min	Decompression sickness			No. of exposures	
					Time to 1st case, min	No. of cases	Before 1st case	After 1st case
75	100	600	8.5	34.5	—	0	600	0
18	100	75	14.5	39.5	37.5	3	56	19
50	100	127	32.5	51.5	40.5	5	46	81
59	100	429	3.0	48.0	43.0	5	408	21
28	150	70	18.5	24.5	18.5	5	4	66
34	150	117	10.5	22.5	19.5	8	80	37
18	150	71	9.5	21.5	20.5	2	56	15
18	150	54	18.0	27.0	26.5	2	42	12
74	150	214	10.0	28.0	28.0	5	206	8
38	167	141	6.5	22.5	17.5	6	95	46
9	185	72	6.5	15.5	14.5	3	56	16
23	200	173	7.5	16.0	13.5	2	133	40
		2143				46	178	361

[a] From data of Hawkins et al. (1935).

depths. This again suggests that perhaps there is a critical quantity of gas dissolved in the body tissues at pressure, and the longer one stays at a given pressure the more gas dissolves in body tissues and hence the more hazardous it becomes to lower the pressure. This, in outline, was Haldane's view, but whereas Haldane fixed every tissue half time with a 2:1 ratio, this was clearly not tenable when actual human diving performance was analyzed. Consequently after Hawkins, Shilling, and Hansen analyzed their findings in 1935, they concluded that each tissue half time was associated with a particular unique decompression ratio, and their theoretical analysis is given in Table IV-5.

A little later, in 1937, Yarbrough reissued his own analysis of the data and decided that the *fast* tissues, i.e., those with half times of 5 or 10 min, could tolerate such large decompression ratios that in effect they could be ignored, so he pressed ahead with his theoretical framework given in Table IV-5. Decompression tables based upon 20-, 40-, and 75-min half times, and using the lower value of the ratios for all dives to depths of 185 ft (55 m) or greater, were calculated by Yarbrough and issued for use by the U.S. Navy in 1937. The ratios Yarbrough used for the 20-, 40-, and 75-min half times were somewhat lower than those of Hawkins et al. because Yarbrough based them on dives involving exercise at depth; he concluded that this gave a greater loading of dissolved nitrogen to the tissues and dictated a more cautious decompression. This could now be said to represent the most significant step in the progress of decompression research since the original work of Haldane. These U.S. Navy tables gained worldwide acceptance alongside the original old Haldane tables, which were still in use despite their obvious deficiencies.

Table IV-5

Theoretical Analysis of Tissue Half Times[a] Determined From Exposures of Human Volunteers

Tissue half-time	Hawkins et al.[b]	Yarbrough[c]
5	4.35	—
10	3.56	—
20	2.21	1.94–2.21
40	1.58	1.38–1.58
75	1.42–1.58	1.38–1.58

[a] Time required for a tissue to absorb or eliminate one-half the equilibrium amount of inert gas.
[b] Data from Hawkins et al. (1935).
[c] Data from Yarbrough (1937).
These decompression ratios do not treat air as a single gas, as Haldane did, but use the nitrogen pressure in the tissue. On this basis Haldane's old ratio of 2.0 becomes 1.58.

Let us now ask the same question of these tables that we did for the Haldane tables: Why are we not using them today? Once again, as with Haldane's tables, their downfall was a measure of their success. These new tables gave a great extension to the amount of no-stop diving, with all the consequent benefits, including more useful work on the bottom and less air usage. Nevertheless, when they were required for long bottom times at deeper depths, these tables suffered the same fate as Haldane's "Table II" (Figure IV-5) because they just did not offer sufficient protection from decompression sickness. This defectiveness was first properly examined by VanDerAue and associates (1945) in a prolonged and extensive series of experiments designed to give the U.S. Navy the capability of performing safe surface decompression diving.

It will be helpful to understand the problem facing VanDerAue at that time. If a diver is sent down and works for a sufficient length of time so that he can no longer ascend to the surface without needing decompression stages in the water, then if an emergency occurs, like a storm blowing up or enemy action in the vicinity, he is in an extremely dangerous situation. It was decided that in such a situation the diver should be rapidly decompressed through the water and hauled up onto the deck of the support ship for surface decompression. Clearly, if he stayed on deck at atmospheric pressure in these circumstances, he was due to suffer a catastrophic attack of decompression sickness. The second part of this procedure was therefore to transfer the diver as rapidly as possible to a pressure chamber and recompress him as quickly as possible to avoid the impending attack of decompression sickness. This procedure presents three immediate problems: (1) How much time can be spent between leaving the bottom to starting recompression on deck? (2) To what pressure must the diver be recompressed in the deck chamber? Back to full pressure of his dive? Back to the pressure of what should have been first stop if he had not been hauled up? Or to some intermediate value between these two extremes? (3) What decompression is necessary after settling questions (1) and (2)?

In considering the last question first, two opposing views present themselves. It could be said that because the diver had been grossly underdecompressed for part of this procedure, he was near to being a bends patient and therefore required a decompression that ought to be very prolonged and close to a therapeutic recompression procedure. On the other hand it could be argued that the rapid pull to the surface had created a huge, although temporary, outflow of dissolved gas and that if the recompression had been quick enough to prevent significant bubble formation the diver would be in a much improved situation with far less nitrogen to remove during the subsequent decompression, which could therefore be shortened without loss of safety—an interesting dilemma that VanDerAue solved in his own way. The nature of his theoretical solution does not now concern us, but the practical procedure he used to justify his approach became the starting point for the next onslaught in the decompression battlefield. He decided to compare the effectiveness of his proposed surface decompression procedures with the existing standard air diving procedures (Yarbrough 1937) for the same bottom times and depths. The results of the comparison revealed that the Yarbrough tables were distinctly inadequate for dives such as 85 min at 100 ft (30 m), which gave 50% of his volunteers decompression sickness. Clearly this was an extremely bad result and, as pointed out by VanDerAue, it meant that the basis for the calculation of the Yarbrough tables needed urgent reappraisal. This important experimental work was completed in the period from the close of World War II to 1951.

Again, why did a set of procedures that are so patently inadequate manage to survive satisfactorily for so long? The answer is not far away when any official statistics on air diving accidents are examined. The vast majority of air dives are within the experimentally well-founded no-decompression limits, and almost all the remainder of the diving involves only a few mintues of decompression. Such dives do not represent a test for the adequacy of the total theoretical framework, as they only involve short-tissue half times. The great contribution of the group of Hawkins et al. (1935) was to delineate the limits of short bottom-time diving; hence, not surprisingly, the Yarbrough tables were troublefree with this type of diving. Unfortunately no similar experimental data had been assembled for long bottom-time dives, and therefore the calculations were necessarily informed guess-work. The guesses had clearly not been sufficiently near to the truth, as VanDerAue discovered. However, these long bottom-time and deep air dives were quite rare, although when tried they invariably gave an unacceptable incidence of bends, these results were submerged in any overall survey of the effectiveness of the Yarbrough tables because of the vast numbers of troublefree no-stop diving results. A mere glance at the statistics thus gives a false sense of security. Incidentally, this same weakness still applies to a great deal of data currently issued on the incidence of decompression sickness.

The next step was therefore fairly obvious. Some adjustment of the calculating procedures had to be made in order to keep the gains made by Yarbrough for the short bottom-time dives but render the decompression safer for long bottom times. A mathematician, Jolly V. Dwyer (1955), was brought into the small team of Des Granges, Dwyer, and Workman (Des Granges 1956); he analyzed the available diving data, and the Yarbrough calculations were completely revised. First, they concluded that deeper stops than previously used by Yarbrough were needed as the depth and duration increased; in other words, the supersaturation ratio must be depth and time dependent. (Yarbrough had introduced the idea that the ratio was only time dependent.) Second, they decided that Hawkins et al. (1935) had been correct in considering tissues with half-times as short as 5 min, and the spectrum of tissue half times was extended to 5, 10, 20, 40, 75, and

120. Significantly a tissue half time (120 min) considerably greater than the longest considered by Haldane and Yarbrough was now reintroduced after VanDerAue's earlier consideration of its theoretical existence. (O. E. VanDerAue, unpublished data on calculations made in 1946–1948 and used in dives at the Experimental Diving Unit, Washington, D.C., in 1951).

In outline the procedure they evolved for calculating the new tables was relatively simple, but the computations involved were exceedingly tedious, and because this really was not a task on which human beings should waste their lives, it was appropriately left to the computer. The tables can be calculated as follows: The nitrogen tension in a tissue is obtained by the method given earlier in the quoted Damant (n.d.) examples. Armed with this nitrogen tension and knowing the duration of the dive, it is possible to obtain the depth of the decompression stop from a relationship that Dwyer (1955) proposed between the tension of nitrogen in a particular tissue and the permitted supersaturation ratio. In essence, then, various tissue half times exist, each with a characteristic supersaturation ratio relationship that varies with the amount of dissolved gas in it. A notable difference between Yarbrough and Dwyer is that Yarbrough gave a single fixed ratio to each tissue but Dwyer gave a ratio relationship, dependent on depth, to each tissue. (This was also the conclusion of VanDerAue.) The calculation is therefore totally dependent on knowledge of the tissue half times and a set of ratio relationships and has now become a matter of following the tensions in each tissue as the decompression proceeds and discovering which is the controlling tissue at each of the stop values. This is easily stated, but if the calculations are done by traditional methods such as illustrated previously by the Damant examples, a vast amount of grinding arithmetic is involved.

Tables based on these concepts were adopted by the U.S. Navy in 1956 and are still in use today. In fact these tables have become the most widely used procedures to date.

Once again the question must be asked whether the air decompression problem has been solved by these 1956 procedures. Regrettably the answer must be no. They represent another step forward from the Yarbrough tables, but if long dives (e.g., 1 hr bottom time) are required at depths in excess of about 120 ft (36 m), then too great a number of bends occur. Beckmann (1976) has described a large air diving contract at depths of this order using the U.S. Navy air diving tables, and it is quite clear from his experience that a reexamination of the theoretical basis to these tables must be undertaken if air diving by the U.S. Navy is to be usefully extended in the future. To illustrate the point made previously, it should be noted, however, that when reporting on the 1956 tables the Naval Safety Center gave an overall incidence of bends of only 0.65% in 1976. Before leaving consideration of the present U.S. Navy tables it should be noted that there are separate calculations for exceptional exposures and that these calculations use additional half times of 160 and 240 min, with allowable supersaturation ratios lower than the standard 120-min tissue ratios. On testing the schedule calculated for a bottom-time dive of 360 min to a depth of 140 ft (43 m) there were two serious cases of bends among the U.S. Navy volunteer divers. Despite this somewhat discouraging result the tables were issued, but only for emergency use.

All the previous systems of calculation have used the concept of a maximum permitted supersaturation ratio. Now it is possible to regard this permitted supersaturation as a permitted excess pressure (pressure difference) rather than a pressure ratio. In view of the variation of allowable ratio values with both tissue half time and tissue gas tension it is not clear that a ratio concept is any better at expressing the controlling supersaturation value for a particular situation than a pressure difference. Clearly a fixed-pressure difference, as suggested by Rashbass (1955), will not suffice any more than will a Haldanian fixed ratio, but it may be easier to vary the pressure difference concept to suit the data than to vary the ratio. R. D. Workman (1965) investigated this possibility and evolved a calculating framework that has dominated many table calculations since he first advanced this system, and therefore this way of calculating schedules is given in some detail. Anyone wishing to understand the theoretical basis of the available tables, commercial or military, will find that the Workman ideas are extensively used.

If an exposure to raised pressure takes place, then it is easy to calculate any tissue inert gas tension, which we call Pti. Now, according to the Workman system there is for each tissue a unique value of Pti that will allow the diver to ascend safely to a particular stop value. Suppose we wish to ascend to a stop at a gauge depth D; extensive analysis of available data reveals that if these critical values of Pti referred to above are called M-values, then $M = M_0 + a \cdot D$, where M_0 is the maximum permitted excess tissue inert gas tension allowed when D (depth) = 0 (i.e., when the diver surfaces) and a is a constant that like M_0 depends on the tissue being considered.

The M-values for various tissue half times for any particular stop can easily be calculated from Table IV-6.

When calculating a decompression schedule for a particular dive Workman would make an allowance for the ascent time to the first stop. This refinement is omitted in this explanation of his method. The steps in the calculation follow:

1. Calculate the depth of the first stop, working to the nearest 10-ft (3-m) increment that is safe for the diver (see examples in Table IV-6).
2. Use the absolute depth of this stop to calculate its pressure (D + 33) in feet or (D + 10) in meters, and calculate the inert gas partial pressure present at the

Table IV-6
Equations for Calculating M-Values[a] of Various Tissues[b]

Half-time,[c] min	Equation
5	$M = 104 + (1.8 \cdot D)$[d]
10	$M = 88 + (1.6 \cdot D)$
20	$M = 72 + (1.5 \cdot D)$
40	$M = 56 + (1.4 \cdot D)$
80	$M = 54 + (1.3 \cdot D)$
120	$M = 52 + (1.2 \cdot D)$

[a] M-value, critical value of inert gas tension in tissue.
[b] Examples of use of equations: What is the M-value for the 80-min tissue at a 20-ft stop? Answer: $M = 54 + (1.3 \cdot 20) = 80$ ft. Or, if the 80-min tissue contains 80 ft of inert gas tension after completion of a dive, what is the stop to which this tissue can ascend safely? Answer: $(80 - 54)/1.3 = 20$ ft. [From Workman (1965).]
[c] Half time, time required for a tissue to absorb or eliminate one-half the equilibrium amount of inert gas.
[d] D, gauge depth in ft.

stop, i.e., (D + 33) · F, where F is the fraction of inert gas in the breathing gas; e.g., F = 0.79 for air.

3. Write down each tissue separately and note the value Pti (each tissue's inert gas tension) and each M value for the next lower stop. Find the inert gas "extraction" pressure gradient, i.e., Pti − (D + 33) F, which is, of course, merely the difference between the inert gas pressure value in the tissue and that on the stop to which the tissue has been decompressed.

4. Calculate how much gas each tissue loses and determine when this allows the diver to ascend to the next shallower stop. To accomplish this aim it is first necessary to assess what fraction (f) of the inert gas extraction pressure gradient needs to be lost by each tissue, i.e.,

$$f = \frac{Pti - M}{Pti - (D + 33) F}$$

When f is determined, see what time this means for each tissue. For example, if f = 0.5 (for simplicity in explanation) this means that the pressure gradient needs to be halved, which by definition each tissue will accomplish in its half time, i.e., 5 or 10 or 20 or 40 or 80 or 120 min. The greatest time required to accomplish this fractional reduction is therefore the safe stop duration. In the example just given this would be 120 min. Once the stop duration is known, use this to calculate the tissue gas tensions in each tissue. The controlling tissue will, of course, have a tension equal to its M-value, but all the other tissues will have values much less than their allowable M-values for ascent to the next stop.

5. Ascend 10 ft (3 m) to a stop value of D−10 and repeat the above calculations. Continue this procedure until the surfacing M-value for the controlling tissue is reached at the final 10-ft (3-m) stop.

The original M-values for using nitrogen gas or helium gas as the inert constitutent of the diver's breathing gas are given in Tables IV-7 and IV-8.

Air diving or helium diving tables can now be calculated with relative ease provided sets of M-values are available. If those calculating dive decompressions discover some inadequacy in the application of this system, then all they have to do is alter the table of M-values to take account of their problem. As a calculating system this is infinitely versatile and can, with appropriate manipulations, accommodate any results established by diving trials. Consequently this has become the most-used basis for those discovering the complexities of the decompression problem and requiring quick answers to particular diving situations, particularly those who serve commercial diving groups as advisers on decompression procedures.

G. Diffusion vs. Perfusion

While the U.S. Navy were engaged in revising the Yarbrough tables and preparing to introduce the 1956 tables an interesting development was being pioneered elsewhere. A simple single-tissue approach was suggested (Hempleman 1952) that could provide a

Table IV-7
Maximum Permissible Tissue Tensions in Use of Nitrogen Gas before Ascent to Next Stop[a]

Tissue half time,[b] min	Depth of decompression stop, fsw									
	10	20	30	40	50	60	70	80	90	100
5	104	122	140	158	176	194	212	230	248	266
10	88	104	120	136	152	168	184	200	216	232
20	72	87	102	117	132	147	162	177	192	207
40	56	70	84	98	112	126	140	154	168	182
80	54	67	80	93	106	119	132	145	158	171
120	52	64	76	88	100	112	124	136	148	160
160	51	63	74	86	97	109	120	132	143	155
200	51	62	73	84	95	106	117	128	139	150
240	50	61	72	83	94	105	116	127	138	149

[a] Data from Workman (1965).
[b] Time required for a tissue to absorb or eliminate one-half the equilibrium amount of inert gas.

Table IV-8
Maximum Permissible Tissue Tensions in Use of Helium Gas before Ascent to Next Stop[a]

Tissue half time,[b] min	Depth of decompression stop, fsw									
	10	20	30	40	50	60	70	80	90	100
5	86	101	116	131	146	161	176	191	206	221
10	74	88	102	116	130	144	158	172	186	200
20	66	79	92	105	118	131	144	157	170	183
40	60	72	84	96	108	120	132	144	156	168
80	56	68	80	92	104	116	128	140	152	164
120	54	66	78	90	102	114	126	138	150	162
160	54	65	76	87	98	109	120	131	142	153
200	53	63	73	83	93	103	113	123	133	143
240	53	63	73	83	93	103	113	123	133	143

[a] Data from Workman (1965).
[b] Time required for a tissue to absorb or eliminate one-half the equilibrium amount of inert gas.

satisfactory solution to the decompression problem. This idea, and some of the subsequent developments from it, are outlined to illustrate several further points of importance.

It seemed curious that whenever a marginal case of decompression sickness occurred, it resulted in a pain in or around a joint. Furthermore, these characteristic pains (bends) could follow a deep dive with short bottom time or a shallow dive of long duration. This was also true for animals, as was revealed in the goat experiments described earlier. This evidence strongly suggests that only one tissue type is principally involved and that there is a critical quantity of gas that this tissue can tolerate without pain.

If only one tissue is involved, however, and if the Haldane concept of tissue gas exchange described earlier is accepted, then the tissue saturates and desaturates with inert gas in a manner varying exponentially with time. If only one exponential, and therefore only one half time, is available for consideration it is quite impossible to fit the known data to such a model.

On examining a cross section of a joint it is striking to observe that perfusion of some parts is very sparse indeed, and cartilage, for example, is attached to the bone surface and would seem to rely almost entirely for its nutriment on diffusion of molecules from the synovial membrane and the surrounding fluid. Once the idea that diffusion is playing a dominating role in some tissues (rather than perfusion as postulated by Haldane), then the whole concept of tissue inert gas exchange alters radically. Suppose we simplify the physical factors involved and see where this leads. Let us consider cartilage as a slab of avascular tissue with one face of this slab well perfused by a network of blood vessels (synovial membrane). In essence this is a thin layer of blood in contact with a thick layer of cartilage, and the elementary physical laws of diffusion can be applied.

Suppose at time $t = 0$ the diver is suddenly exposed to a raised pressure of inert gas, which causes a step change in the concentration (tension) of inert gas being supplied to all organs of the body, and in particular to the blood flowing through the synovial membrane across the face of the slab of cartilage, then we know from Fick's Law of diffusion that, at some distance x from the blood layer inside the cartilage, the differential equation

$$\frac{\partial c}{\partial t} = K \cdot \frac{\partial^2 c}{\partial x^2}$$

(where K is the diffusion coefficient) describes the movement of dissolved inert gas (c) in the slab of tissue. It would not be appropriate to discuss the various solutions to this diffusion equation for different possible boundary conditions, as this can be found in any standard text book on differential equations. For the purposes of this model it was supposed that at time $t = 0$ the gas tension in the cartilage had some uniform value, and at this moment the tension in the blood was suddenly changed and maintained at some new raised level. The fractional saturation of the slab (α) after time t can be written as

$$\alpha = 1 - \frac{8}{\pi^2} (e^{Kt} + \frac{1}{9} e^{-9Kt} + \frac{1}{25} e^{-25Kt} + \ldots) \qquad (4)$$

As can be seen, after infinite time $\alpha = 1$, and after a very short time α is very nearly zero. Thus this more complex diffusion function has the same basic properties as the simple single-perfusion exponential function, but not the same time course. The K-value is constant for a given thickness of the slab and for a diffusion coefficient that has the same value throughout the thickness of the slab. This is a rather idealized situation but nevertheless worthy of consideration for modeling purposes.

When dissolved gas molecules diffuse uniformly from one face into a slab of tissue they behave as if they were in a semi-infinite space until they begin to reach the opposite face, at which time the diffusion gradients become influenced by the fact that the gas molecules cannot diffuse any further. Up to this time, and indeed for an appreciable time afterward, the quantity of gas diffusing into the tissue is proportional to the square root of the time. If this model is near enough correct for most practical purposes, and if there is a fixed and critical excess quantity of gas that can be tolerated on decompression, then for a dive to a depth P for a time t there will be some critical fixed quantity Q of dissolved gas such that

$$Q = P \sqrt{t} \quad (5)$$

So if a diver goes to P_1 for t_1, or to P_2 for t_2, then to remain marginally safe the following will be true:

$$P_1 \sqrt{t_1} = P_2 \sqrt{t_2} = Q \quad (6)$$

In fact, this relationship has been proved to give a remarkably good fit of the U.S. Navy no-stop dive data for all dives with bottom times of less than 100 min. Table IV-9 compares the prediction of the formula with the data given in the manual. This is very encouraging, especially when one looks back on the rather complex calculations that generated the data in the *U.S. Navy Diving Manual*. Consequently it was decided to use this model as the basis for calculating diving tables. It is much less versatile, however, than the Workman M-value treatment just described, but it has a certain appealing simplicity. Once the *K*-value is fixed in Eq. 1, then the fractional saturation is also fixed and is solely a function of time, whereas on the M-value scheme there are seven tissues available to fit the data!

Table IV-9

Bottom Time at Various Depths According to U.S. Navy Tables Compared with Hempleman Calculations[a]

Depth, ft	Bottom time, min	
	U.S. Navy table[b]	Q = 500 prediction[c]
50	100	100
60	60	69
70	50	51
80	40	39
90	30	31
100	25	25
110	20	21
120	15	17
190	5	7

[a] Table derived from equation in Hempleman (1952).
[b] Based on M-value scheme of Workman (1965).
[c] Expansion of equation developed by Hempleman (1952).

One other important feature of the Hempleman system of calculating is also worth attention. Anyone who has taken part in experimental diving observes that some dives can cause a persistent, low-level pain in a joint, which is called a *niggle* or *inkle*, for example. Such niggles can sometimes remain with the diver for 2 or 3 days. An extreme example was provided by an Ocean Systems diver reported by Hamilton et al. (1966) as sensitive to flight in an unpressurized aircraft 10 days after completion of his saturation helium dive. On conventional Haldane ideas it would be necessary to assign a half time to the tissue involved, which would be quite absurd. The dilemma is resolved by inferring that in such cases there is a bubble-tissue complex and that the half time in such a situation is not representative of the half time of the tissue when a bubble is not occluding the circulation. Now once this concept of a bubble-tissue complex is accepted, doubts arise whether such complexes are not also, but to a lesser degree, influencing the whole decompression process. In effect this would imply that the uptake and elimination of inert gases were not reversible processes. Therefore when acquiring dissolved gas during the compression and bottom time one K-value was used, but when decompression started it was supposed that there was a change in the physics of the situation and the elimination became much reduced, and the K-value was altered to account for this. Another argument was also used to support the idea of elimination being slower than uptake, and this was as follows: In any population there will obviously be those who acquire gas at pressure more rapidly than others, either because of their cardiovascular mechanisms and general physiology, or because they are exercising, or because of some similar external factor. Likewise, during decompression there will be those who eliminate dissolved gas rather more slowly than others. Because decompression tables are being designed for a large population of different people, it is essential to take some account of this obvious truth. The safest path is therefore to assume that the tables are dealing with the most rapid acquirers of gas and the slowest eliminators. Of necessity, therefore, an asymmetry must be introduced into the calculations.

The idea of a single-diffusion–limited tissue, as well as the view that the rate of uptake of dissolved gas at pressure and its release on decompression are not the same, was a radical departure from the current thinking. It might reasonably be expected that such a different theoretical basis would yield a vastly different set of decompression procedures, but as we have seen already, this model generates a set of no-stop dives almost identical with that of the U.S. Navy tables. The only noticeable differences arise when deeper, longer dives, e.g., 1 hr at 100 ft (30 m) are being undertaken. For such dives the diffusion-limited model gives a more conservative decompression, and indeed the 1968 air diving tables issued for general use by the Underwater Engineering Group of the United Kingdom have become very popular with contractors doing such arduous dives, as they undoubtedly lead to less decompression sickness than the U.S. Navy tables, especially if the version with oxygen stops is used.

The important point for the impartial observer to notice is that two philosophies are possible in approaching the decompression problem. The first philosophy can be summed up in the question, "What does the model matter as long as it works?" The second philosophy is, "If you don't understand what you're doing, it's potentially dangerous, and the model must therefore reflect the major features of the physiology during decompression." The first leads to a calculating system, e.g., M-values; the second leads to an attempt to identify a tissue or tissues responsible, e.g., the cartilage diffusion concept.

In order to satisfy the requirement that the tissue or tissues responsible for decompression sickness take several hours to equilibrate with gas at raised pressure it was necessary, with the diffusion-limited model, to assume it to be a relatively thick avascular piece of tissue, e.g., cartilage, tendon, bone. However, B. A. Hills (1966) challenged the accepted values of the diffusion coefficient for dissolved inert gas in tissues and used values a thousand times smaller than the generally accepted Krogh (1918) values. This drastically alters the K-values in the solution to the differential equation given above (Eq. 4). Such very low diffusion coefficients imply very slow inert gas exchange between the blood in the capillaries and the intercapillary tissue, and consequently the time scale of the decompression process can now be accommodated by relatively well-vascularized tissue as well as poorly vascularized tissue. Hills accordingly assumed for his model a central capillary with a surrounding cylinder of tissue. At time $t = 0$, when a dive commences, the blood in the capillary experiences a sustained step change in gas concentration, which then diffuses outward into the surrounding cylinder of tissue. The mathematical solution to this situation is rather more complex than for the tissue slab, but the square-root relationship will still hold, as noted previously, for short t-values.

It would seem that more recent measurements of the diffusion coefficient for dissolved inert gases in tissues do not support the very low values Hills used in his analysis, and consequently one is thrown back onto the original idea of a 2- or 3-mm-thick slice of avascular tissue in order to satisfy the time scales involved. In the course of his analysis, however, Hills also drew attention to several important points and some of these have become part of the current thinking.

When the gas tensions of the various dissolved gases in blood and tissue at atmospheric pressure are examined, an interesting feature emerges, as seen in Table IV-10. The partial pressure of nitrogen in the alveoli must be in equilibrium with the dissolved nitrogen gas tensions throughout the body, but oxygen is being used metabolically and its tension therefore drops noticeably. Some extra carbon dioxide is of course generated from the metabolic usage of this oxygen but does not replace the used oxygen tension. Consequently when the gas tensions are added together it is found that this total does not equal the hydrostatic pressure (760 mmHg, in this case) on the body. Any small bubble introduced into a tissue would rapidly equilibrate with the gas tensions in the surrounding tissue, and the total internal bubble pressure, being less than the outside pressure on the body, would cause such a bubble to start to shrink and continue shrinking until it disappeared completely under the influence of this excess hydrostatic pressure.

For simplicity the effects of surface tension have been ignored, but they would exert an extra pressure also tending to shrink the bubble.

The deficit in gas tensions in the various physiological situations, first noticed by Loeschcke (1956), was termed *the inherent unsaturation* by Hills. Quite independently, A. R. Behnke (1967) also drew attention to the fact that oxygen usage created a dis-

Table IV-10
Gas Pressures and Tensions in Blood and Tissue at Atmospheric Pressure

	Oxygen		Nitrogen		Carbon dioxide		Water vapor	
	Pressure, mmHg	Tension, mmHg	Pressure, mmHg	Tension, mmHg	Pressure, mmHg	Tension, mmHg	Pressure mmHg	Tension, mmHg
Air (dry)	152		608		—			
Alveolar gas	103		569		41		47	
Arterial blood		88		569		41		47
Venous blood		37		569		47		47
Tissue cells		10		569		49		47

equilibrium in gas tensions; he called the deficit *the oxygen window*. This idea of an oxygen window or inherent unsaturation has become a cornerstone in some of the attempts to quantify the decompression process. As has been pointed out, it should lead to bubble shrinkage and is therefore potentially very useful in opposing the bubble growth that leads to decompression sickness. At raised pressures of air, for example, the inherent unsaturation can be extremely large. Consider a dive to 66 ft (20 m) using air. The total pressure is near enough to 3 atm and the oxygen pressure is very nearly 0.6 atm, or 460 mmHg. Because nearly all oxygen is carried in blood as oxyhemoglobin, and very little is dissolved in the plasma, a simple calculation will show that although there has been a massive increase from the surface value of 0.2 to a level of 0.6 atm in the oxygen pressure of the breathing gas, very little extra oxygen is carried to the tissues.

The situation from the viewpoint of tissue oxygen tension is hardly affected, and consequently the inherent unsaturation or oxygen window value almost equals the oxygen pressure in the diver's breathing gas, i.e., 0.6 atm. If this concept is applicable to the decompression problem then a factor of primary importance is available for consideration.

Before leaving this diffusion-dominated treatment of the tissue inert gas exchange it is worth seeing how a fusion between perfusion-limited ideas and diffusion-limited ideas is now occurring. As was pointed out in 1963 (Hempleman 1963) and independently but earlier by Perl (1962), it can be misleading to think of a tissue as some isolated unit with a particular half time dependent upon its vascularity, as was supposed in the analysis given at the beginning of this chapter. If the whole body is sectioned one sometimes sees very well vascularized organs placed next to quite poorly vascularized ones. It is a matter of obvious elementary truth that if the well-vascularized tissue rapidly acquires dissolved inert gas and the poorly vascularized tissue only slowly acquires dissolved gas, then the fast tissue will begin to act as a source of dissolved gas for the slow tissue at the interface where the two tissues meet. The only way in which molecules can transfer from the fast to the slow tissue is by diffusion. Two points are apparent from this consideration. First, there are very few purely perfusion-limited or purely diffusion-limited processes in the body; and second, every slow tissue will have a fast component and every fast tissue will have a slow component. From a computational viewpoint this means that very few, if any, tissues of the body can be regarded as saturating exponentially with time and having a simple, single-characteristic exponential half time. It was lack of understanding on this point that led to the rejection of the single-tissue concept. If a single tissue has only half time, then indeed the diving data cannot be explained by using such a model; but if a single tissue is liberated from this constraint by intertissue diffusion, then a single-tissue perfusion-limited model is available for consideration.

H. *Data from Tunnel Workers*

So far the discussion on theoretical concepts underlying decompression procedures has been largely restricted to those used by divers. As mentioned earlier, however, there have been far more men breathing compressed air for caisson and tunnel work than for diving purposes. It is necessary to pay attention to their problems because they are closely interrelated to those of the diver. Furthermore, because of the large number of individual exposures to compressed air, the data tend to be more capable of statistical evaluation. A typical compressed air contract would have in excess of 250,000 entries into compressed air.

In 1954 W. M. D. Paton and D. N. Walder reported their findings from a compressed air contract concerned with the construction of a tunnel under the River Tyne, in England. The decompression tables used were those originally devised by Haldane, and the diving community would not be surprised to learn that large numbers of bends were encountered when shifts of a duration greater than 4 hr were undertaken at pressures exceeding 22 psi gauge (50 ft or 15 m). Accordingly, steps were taken to reduce the incidence of decompression sickness—for example, by lowering the threshold of 22 psi gauge (50 ft or 15 m) stated by Haldane as requiring only 2 min of decompression, i.e., virtually a no-step exposure, to 18 psi gauge (40 ft or 12 m). This is typical of the history of compressed air working in tunnels. A decompression procedure is adopted, it is tried and found inadequate in certain respects, and on-the-spot alterations are made to attempt to remove the difficulties. This contract would have therefore been one of a series of entirely unremarkable undertakings had it not been for the observation that the incidence of bends varied quite markedly with time even when the working conditions (e.g., pressure, temperature) were quite stable. A number of possibilities for this variation were examined. For example, it was thought that perhaps some decompressions terminated with the atmospheric pressure at a relatively low value, and thus the bubbles were expanding beyond their size at normal atmospheric pressure. This was quite a reasonable supposition, but barometric pressure showed no correlation with the fluctuations in the numbers of bends. After investigation of several such hypotheses it was found that the only one that could be strongly supported by analysis was the relationship between the influx of new laborers and the incidence of bends. It became apparent that "new starters" in compressed air were at a greater risk than those who had been regularly working in compressed air. Paton and Walder decided this increased resistance to decompression sickness was due to "acclimatization." Since then, other and perhaps more appropriate words (e.g., *adaptation*) have been used to describe this phenomenon, but the fact is well established that regular exposure of the work force can lead to a noticeable decrease in incidence of decompression sickness. Nevertheless, despite the unassailable evidence from this form of working, it would be highly speculative to assume that all forms of exposure to compressed gases will endow the same increased resistance.

In 1956 these same investigators were joined by a small additional team, and attention was turned to examining the evidence from the Dartford (River Thames) Tunnel (Golding et al. 1960).

Once again the acclimatization factor was confirmed as an influence on the incidence of the bends, and it was discovered that whenever there were long absences from regular work the men had lost their acclimatization. Opportunity arose to analyze more closely the time scale for this process of deacclimatization, and it was found that a 7- to 11-day half time would adequately describe it. That is, if a group of workers was absent from regular work for about a week, then the incidence of bends on return to work was about halfway between that of the new starters and the fully acclimatized workers. This was a very interesting finding, and although it added complications to understanding the etiology of decompression sickness, it was an important practical point for consideration when assessing the success of decompression schedules.

At first the ability to acclimatize men to working in raised pressures of air was seen as a highly desirable solution to the practical problem of keeping the bends incidence as low as possible. Nevertheless, doubts began to arise about the wisdom of such procedures. It is by no means certain that avoiding an attack of acute decompression sickness also avoids all tissue damage. Perhaps these acclimatized men should really be termed *desensitized*—men who are suffering gentle attacks of decompression sickness without feeling the pains they would have experienced if they were not acclimatized. Such thoughts receive considerable support from evidence, both indirect and direct (from ultrasonic bubble monitoring), that even when decompression does not lead to an attack of bends there are often silent bubbles circulating in the blood or lodged in tissues. Consequently, many investigators turned their attention to examining the chronic effects of decompression to uncover any adverse effects that had not presented during, or shortly after, the completion of decompression. There were two principal sources of concern. The first was the relationship between osteonecrosis and work in compressed air, and the second was the suggestion that the central nervous system was being irreversibly affected as a result of hyperbaric work.

Cases of painful and sometimes disabling osteonecrosis had been occasionally reported in caisson and tunnel workers from the turn of the century, but it was only the advent of large-scale radiographic surveys (Medical Research Council 1966) that established the fact that this disorder is widespread in these workers. This establishment of a link between hyperbaric exposure and subsequent osteonecrosis was one of the turning points in the history of hyperbaric medicine, and particularly of decompression procedures. Osteonecrosis became far more worrisome both to employers and employees than attacks of acute decompression sickness. The latter were relatively easily treated, and although a nuisance because they temporarily diverted the employers' resources onto nonproductive activities, they did not lead to the large claims for compensation that followed when an employee developed osteonecrosis. The discovery of large numbers of men with osteonecrosis in the tunnel and caisson industries naturally led to investigations of a similar nature in the diving industry. A rather different, and less worrisome, picture emerged here. It was apparent that vast numbers of ordinary divers never suffered either acute attacks of decompression sickness or osteonecrosis. The main source of osteonecrosis among divers was from either professional divers who indulged in repetitive air diving over many years (e.g., Japanese pearl fishers) or deep heliox divers using inadequately established procedures. Several surveys of such professional groups are given in Table IV-11.

At first glance these results in Table IV-11 are alarming, but two factors have since emerged that now render the problem less severe than might be thought from examining these gross data. First, there are various manifestations of osteonecrosis; only juxta-articular involvement is the real hazard to the worker, and even juxta-articular lesions will not always lead to breakdown of the articular surface and thus to the necessity for surgical intervention. The second feature that began to be noticed was that the incidence of the serious forms of this disorder is certainly not as great nowadays in either divers or tunnel workers. For example, there were no recorded cases of osteonecrosis from the Seattle, San Francisco, and Milwaukee tunnel projects, in the 1970–1980 decade (personal communications). The osteonecrosis problem drew attention to the way that decompression schedules had been constructed—with the objective of only the avoidance of bends.

Table IV-11
Incidence of Osteonecrosis Reported in Several Surveys

Survey	No. of divers	No. of divers with lesions	Incidence, %
Herget (1948)	90	29	32
Alnor (1963)	131	72	55
Ohta (1974)	301	152	50
Beckman (1976)	30	8	27
Totals	509	245	48

To avoid bend attacks is obviously highly desirable, and, as mentioned previously, if one can avoid the bends then almost all forms of acute decompression sickness are reduced to negligible proportions; but it has become clear from the identification of osteonecrosis as a serious threat to hyperbaric work that a closer look must be given to the possibility of delayed effects.

A further example of delayed effects from apparently "innocent" dives was afforded by the hematological investigation of J. Martin (Martin and Nichols 1971). Prior to his experiments it had been established by the Canadian workers Philp, Schacham, and Gowdey (1971) that there can be hematological changes during the course of exposure to diving pressures and sometimes shortly afterwards.

Martin, however, took these observations a step further. He used a standard dive that had always been troublefree from the viewpoint of the bends and that nevertheless was a substantial exposure to pressure, namely 1 hr at 100 ft (30 m). He used the Royal Navy Physiological Laboratory 1968 Air Diving Tables for his decompression procedure. No volunteers gave any indication of acute decompression sickness in the course of his experimentation, and therefore this schedule was considered adequately safe by normal standards. Nevertheless, the platelet count did exhibit changes, not during or shortly after the dive but about 1 or 2 days later, and several days were needed for a complete return to the predive levels. The time course is illustrated in Figure IV-7. These observations have since been confirmed by other workers, and it must now be realized that asymptomatic changes are taking place in the body despite apparently adequate decompression. More recently G. Nichols (1979) has been showing gross changes in the erythrocyte sedimentation rate (ESR) during the course of prolonged decompressions from both heliox and nitrox saturation diving. Some of these changes take as long as 3 weeks after completion of decompression before they return to predive values. It is now a question of deciding whether such platelet and ESR changes have any real significance from the viewpoint of assessing the adequacy of decompression procedures.

In addition to the changes taking place in the bones and blood, changes have been noted by I. Rozsahegyi (1959) attributable to central nervous system damage. It should be mentioned, however, that the old Hungarian decompression procedures that led to these findings are very inadequate when judged by any of the theoretical considerations outlined earlier in this chapter. Nevertheless, it is clear from the work of A. Palmer (1978) that animals (goats) given bend-producing schedules do exhibit spinal cord damage that can be seen histologically in animals killed several days, or even weeks, postdive. Thus there is further support for the view that hidden damage is taking place in a variety

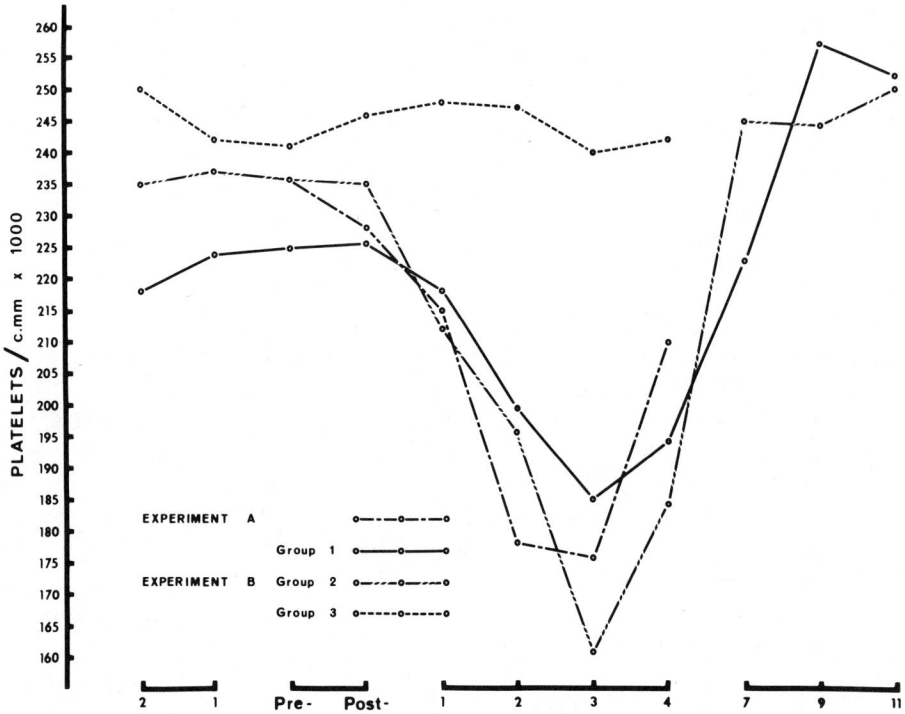

Figure IV-7. Platelet levels of several groups of divers (see text). The top curve is for a control group. [From Martin and Nichols (1971).]

of body tissues and that the adaptability of the body may be masking these problems except in those tissues where a pain results.

I. Bubble Generation and Growth

To some extent these features of the decompression problem could have been anticipated, because it had been concluded as early as 1951 by Bateman and by A. R. Behnke (1951) that asymptomatic bubbles must be produced from many diving procedures, and they termed such bubbles *silent*. For many years the evidence for silent bubbles remained circumstantial, but the advent of ultrasonic monitoring techniques showed that by using Doppler ultrasonic probes, asymptomatic bubbles could be detected in the bloodstream. The Seattle-based team headed by M. P. Spencer (Spencer and Campbell 1968) were foremost in establishing this technique as a major new contribution to the study of decompression procedures. Indeed the efficacies of various diving tables have been compared by obtaining the numbers of bubbles generated per unit time, or the total number of bubbles as a measure. The classification of types of bubbles *heard* has become more refined, and only certain types are considered to be significant by some investigators. It does seem, however, that although these ultrasonic techniques for bubble analysis are useful with relatively short exposures to raised pressure, they are not very helpful in assessing the likely outcome of saturation schedules. The summary statement by D. J. Kenyon (1974) at the May 1974 Undersea Medical Society effectively states the conclusion of many with experience in this field: "Doppler ultrasound monitoring of the divers was conducted. At no time were bubbles detected during either the saturation excursions or during ascent to the surface. This was found also in the case of decompression sickness." Before leaving the use of ultrasound it is worth noting that techniques other than Doppler, which requires moving bubbles for detection, are available. In particular there is ultrasonic imaging, pioneered by R. S. Mackay (Rubissow and Mackay 1973), which can detect stationary bubbles and as later adapted is available for both moving and stationary bubbles. However, these techniques require extremely careful experimental measurements, and such factors as very small movements by the subject can disturb the interpretation of the findings. The conclusion would seem to be that ultrasound is a promising but not yet proven tool for investigating decompression procedures.

One principal point of interest noted in the above account is that Doppler ultrasound seems to give good prognoses for nonsaturation divers but not for saturation exposures, whereas the ESR is in the reverse position, i.e., it gives a good indication of impending trouble for saturation diving but is useless for short bottom-time dives. The significance of these facts is not yet apparent.

In 1971 G. D. Blenkarn and co-workers (1971) at Duke University observed a curious skin rash developing as a result of what they termed "sequential breathing of various inert gases at 7 ATA." The explanation they offered for this urticaria was that each inert gas had its own characteristic diffusion and tissue solubility properties and that switching breathing mixtures at a constant raised pressure gave enhanced possibilities for generating large gas concentration gradients inside the body. Large concentration gradients imply large osmotic pressure effects with consequent movements of tissue fluid, and this was probably causing the effects on the skin.

The matter might well have rested on this explanation had it not been for some rather more dramatic experiments by C. J. Lambertsen and his co-workers (Graves et al. 1973), who in 1972 also subjected their volunteers to gas switching, but this time the pressure was much greater and equivalent to 1200 fsw (366 msw), and the gas being breathed within the chamber was heliox with switching to oxygen-neon or nitrox accomplished via a built-in breathing system. Thus men were breathing one inert gas mixture while surrounded by another—in this case, helium. After a quite long period of delay, sometimes 45 min, the men developed distressing symptoms and signs of vestibular disturbance. This was thought to be due to bubble formation caused by the presence of two inert gases diffusing in opposite directions and leading to a tissue supersaturation. The outline of their hypothesis is illustrated in Figure IV-8.

As may be seen it is possible to reach a steady state with gas diffusing through a lipid layer with different solubility and diffusion properties from the adjacent aqueous layer and to envisage a total gas tension at the interface that could exceed the hydrostatic pressure by as much as 30% according to these calculations. Following this initial explanation several other ingenious attempts have been made to account for isobaric bubble formation, and it has been well established that isobaric gas switching can lead to extensive and continuous bubble formation. For example, ultrasonic Doppler probes were used to detect circulating bubbles in volunteers exposed for several hours to raised (132 ft or 40

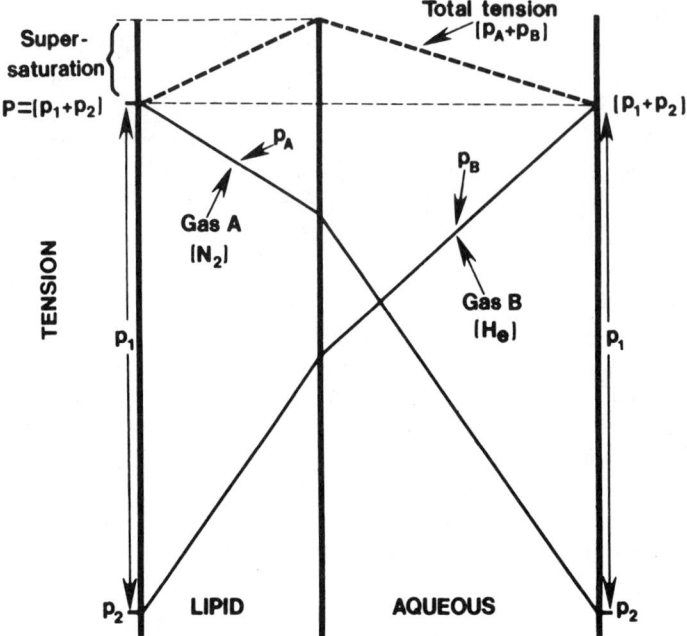

Figure IV-8. Initial explanation offered for isobaric decompression sickness signs caused by gas switching at pressure. For this idealized model the skin is bilayer with subcutaneous fat as the inner layer. The total ambient pressure is P, and the partial pressure of each inert gas is P_1. Gas A surrounds the body, Gas B is being breathed. When a steady state is reached Gas A diffuses linearly from the skin surface through each layer, and Gas B diffuses in the opposite direction. Both gases have different diffusion rates in the two layers, and their respective dissolved gas concentrations P_A and P_B are different in each layer. This could create supersaturation near to the lipid-aqueous boundary, as shown in the diagrammatic representation. [From Graves et al. (1973).]

m) pressures of air and then transferred with no change of pressure into a second chamber with an entirely new environment of heliox. After about 30 min in this second chamber circulating bubbles were readily detectable in the blood of all volunteers tested, and indeed one man developed bends from this procedure. Although various explanations of this phenomenon (which has come to be called *counterdiffusion supersaturation*) are available, the important practical point to note from the physician's viewpoint is that if the body is surrounded by helium gas at pressure, then it is very inadvisable to ask the diver, or patient, to breathe another inert gas mixture from a mouthpiece or helmet.

One matter that became unquestionably clearer from the isobaric counterdiffusion experimentation was that the release of free gas is the cause of decompression sickness and that not very large pressure differentials are needed to lead to large-scale bubble formation, provided a sufficient supply of dissolved inert gas is made available in the tissues. Obviously, if bubble formation could be prevented or rendered more difficult in some way, then decompression sickness would vanish or become a very rare disorder. A search for understanding the origins of bubble formation has therefore been one of the main lines of investigation in decompression research. Unfortunately, the matter has not been resolved, but a good deal of evidence has accumulated and some of this is relevant to increasing the physician's awareness of the nature of the problems facing him.

If a beaker of pure water at constant temperature is exposed to a raised pressure of a gas such as nitrogen or helium, and if sufficient time is allowed to elapse so that equilibrium is reached, then rapid decompression to a much lower pressure will have no visible effect—i.e., no bubbles will be formed. For a bubble to form in these circumstances, sufficient molecules have to come together in one small volume, and the chances of this happening can be shown to be unworthy of consideration. However, if a foreign surface is introduced into the beaker upon decompression, or if the liquid is stirred, then violent gas release takes place. All of this type of experimentation leads to the conclusion that a nucleus is necessary for promoting the formation of free gas from dissolved gas. In 1945 E. Newton-Harvey (Harvey 1945) demonstrated the same phenomenon in blood, namely that it is impossible to provoke bubble formation in supersaturated blood, but it can be made to effervesce profusely when stirred. He then went on to note that although he had demonstrated the virtual impossibility of producing bubbles in blood, it was, nevertheless, a matter of common observation that animals decompressed after exposure to only modest pressures of air often had bubbles visibly circulating in their vascular systems. This must mean, he decided, that the walls of the blood vessels have some property that promotes bubble formation, and he introduced the idea of crevices of gas within the vessel walls that remain permanently stable unless subjected to enormous pressures; these "gas nuclei" act as sources for the formation of bubbles when dissolved gas diffuses into them. Furthermore, from experimentation with excised lengths of blood vessels he decided that arterial vessels are most likely to be responsible.

At first thought it might seem dubious to implicate the arterial system as the source of bubbles in blood. When an animal is decompressed the arterial blood coming through the left side of the heart is in equilibrium, ignoring shunts with the alveolar gases, and therefore there is little or no supersaturation in such blood to promote bubble formation; as we saw earlier, this assumption is the basis of all the current decompression calculating systems. It must be remembered, however, that some arterial blood on its passage to those tissues which it supplied may pass through, or alongside, a tissue that contains a large concentration of dissolved inert gas. This dissolved gas will diffuse into the blood vessel, and the arterial blood in that particular vessel may reach a far from negligible level of supersaturation. Thus, it is not impossible to conceive that arterial blood could be a source of bubbles, in conformity with Newton-Harvey's suggestion.

The evidence is quite convincing that if bubbles are generated in water supersaturated with dissolved gas, then when the bubble redissolves (by reapplication of pressure or because the water becomes undersaturated) a small deposit of impurity is left behind (Liebemann 1957). Should there be a further decompression, then a new bubble will form, using this small deposit as its nucleus. D. M. J. P. Manley (1960) deduced that the deposit had a volume between 10^{-4} and 10^{-5} mm^3 and when the bubble was very small this deposit provided a "skin" around the free gas. The skin slows the diffusion rate from small (<0.1-mm-diameter) bubbles, and this slowing down can be readily demonstrated. Since this early work by Manley and the theoretical analysis of bubble growth and decay by P. S. Epstein and M. S. Plesset (1950) numerous refinements have been made in the observations, but basically there have been no major changes in the general conclusions. More recently, the experiments of D. E. Yount (1978), using specially prepared sections of gelatin, have supported the organic skin concept of Manley.

Perhaps some of the most significant experiments concerning bubble formation were those by Evans and Walder (1969), who took shrimps (*Crangon crangon*) at atmospheric pressure and decompressed them to 60-mmHg pressure, at which pressure all the shrimps could be seen through their translucent shells to have bubbles. They were then sealed in a polythene bag full of seawater and compressed hydrostatically to about 100 bars. On decompression from this pressure back to atmospheric pressure very few of the shrimps could be made to exhibit bubbles on a further decompression to 60 mmHg. It was concluded that the few minutes at high pressure had crushed most of the bubble nuclei and therefore prevented bubble formation. However, a very important further observation was made when it was found that if the shrimps were compressed and then decompressed hydrostatically but left about 4 hr to recover, they bubbled profusely when taken to the subatmospheric 60-mmHg pressure level. This shows that gas nuclei can be crushed out of existence but that either they re-form or new nuclei are born. This means that the whole process is (or can become) dynamic and that the body has a number of gas nuclei always present that it can replace or reconstitute every few hours. If these observations are confirmed, then interesting possibilities for the etiology of decompression sickness are opened.

Also considered by Evans and Walder was the possibility that fissile material such as uranium in the diet was providing the particle energy necessary to create a small bubble. This is an interesting suggestion, and doubtless some bubbles could be generated in this way, but it is not tenable as representing the principal etiologic mechanism.

Finally, there are those who believe that mechanical factors lead to bubble formation in supersaturated tissues. Two principal concepts dominate current thinking: First, it is possible that joint movement (Whitaker et al. 1945), which can involve very large shearing forces, or tribonucleation, i.e., movement of surfaces over one another (Ikels 1970), could bring gas out of solution. Second, it may be possible that vortical motion in the heart or at arterial bifurcations could cavitate the blood and cause regular injections of bubbles into the tissues (Laurens 1964). Both these suggestions are very reasonable. It will be necessary to complete a number of quite subtle experiments to establish which of the various explanations for bubble formation really satisfies the evidence.

Once a bubble is formed there is the further difficult problem of knowing how it grows or shrinks; for a given pressure gradient a helium bubble will probably grow more rapidly than a nitrogen bubble in aqueous tissue, but in fatty tissue the situation may be reversed. The problem with even attempting semiquantitative statements is that the diffusion coefficients and solubilities of the inert gases in the various tissues of the body are not known with sufficient accuracy. It is therefore possible to hold several views about bubble growth without any possibility of knowing which is nearest the truth. One of the main problems is that no one yet knows where the offending bubble is located. Given such major uncertainties it would not be sensible to enter into the detailed analysis, but a few simple physical points can be made. If the pressure on a bubble of diameter greater than 10 μm is doubled, then Boyle's law will hold true and the volume will be halved, but if the bubble is spherical, then the diameter will decrease by only about one-fifth. Should the gas be released as a long, cylindrical (sausagelike) embolus in a blood vessel, then of course the length will almost halve. On the other hand, if the gas is a combination of both these possibilities there could be considered change within the tissue (see Figure IV-9). One other point that must be mentioned is that if bubbles decrease to a diameter less than that of a capillary (about 10 μm), the surface tension inside such small bubbles starts to increase markedly unless surfactant substances are present, and this causes rapid dissolution of the bubble. Furthermore, if the bubble is trapped in a

Decompression Theory

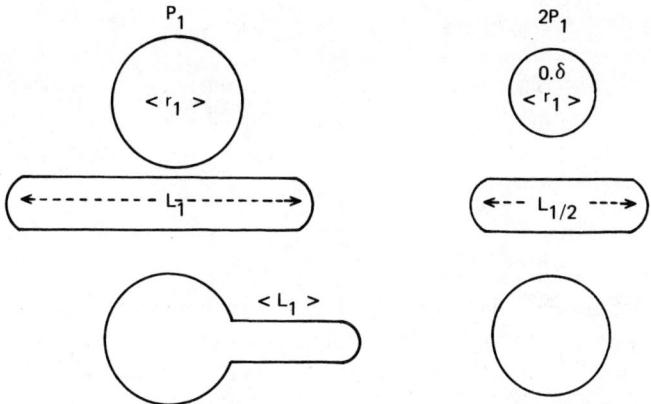

Figure IV-9. Three simplified tissue gas release possibilities showing that halving the volume can have quite different effects depending on the shape. Surface tension effects are being regarded as negligible.

blood vessel, then reducing its diameter to less than 10 µm will cause it to move through the capillary bed. The complexities of the problem can be seen, even from these simple considerations.

As seen earlier, the simple ratio principle of Haldane did not survive the test of usage and was replaced by mathematical manipulations designed to account for the undoubted fact that the permitted ratio was pressure dependent. Although 2:1 was satisfactory for low pressure values (around 1 atm) it was far from safe to use this same ratio value at several atmospheres of pressure. No controlled experimentation to discover the exact relationship between the ratio change and pressure was attempted until comparatively recently. In 1957 goats were exposed to raised pressures of air (P_1) for 6 hr, then decompressed rapidly to a new lower value (P_2), and held at P_2 to see whether a bend occurred (Hempleman 1957). In essence this repeated Haldane's old experiments but used a much longer time of exposure in order to ensure that all tissues of the goat were equilibrated (saturated) to the raised pressure before decompression took place. From these experiments the conclusion was that Haldane was (near enough for practical purposes) correct and that P_1/P_2 was constant over a wide range of pressure values. Hills (1966), however, examined the data critically and showed that a relationship of the form

$$P_1 = a\, P_2 \div b$$

much more accurately described the results. Since his original analysis there have been other experiments using human volunteers and there is little doubt that a similar relationship describes these results also. For dives on heliox to pressures as great as 10 bars (300 ft or 90 m) the equation

$$P_1 = 1.397\, P_2 + 5.7$$

satisfactorily describes the pressure P_2 (in meters) to which one can rapidly and safely decompress after exposure to pressure P_1 (in meters) for at least 24 hr with an oxygen partial pressure of 0.22 bar (i.e., normoxic). For deep helium diving the expression changes to

$$P_1 = 1.113 P_2 + 24.1$$

This different equation is necessary because the form of decompression sickness presenting at deep depths as a result of sudden drops in pressure changes from limb bends to mainly vestibular involvement.

For air the relationship is

$$P_1 = 1.361 P_2 + 3.4$$

In all these equations the values of P_1 and P_2 are expressed in absolute terms, i.e., when $P_1 = 10$ the pressure is 10 bars, or near enough 10 atm pressure. The various predictions for P_1 and P_2 using this formula, and previous estimations by others, are shown in Figure IV-10.

J. Diving Tables Today

There are, as can be seen, several successful ways of constructing decompression tables despite the unavailability of basic underlying physiological facts. No one yet knows the history of the origin of the bubble or bubbles that give rise to acute decompression sickness (Type I), nor is the site of action of these gaseous foreign bodies established. Added to these fundamental areas of ignorance are lesser but still important ones, such as whether an attack of the bends can lead to, or be an indicator of, impending bone necrosis or CNS damage. From the point of view of truly understanding the nature of the decompression problem the present level of knowledge is grossly inadequate.

Of the various tables available for use, the following account should be taken as guidance. Most of the air diving tables from the major navies of the world (U.S. Navy, French Navy, Royal Navy) are very satisfactory for the vast majority of air diving work (or sport). Indeed, if the bottom times, depths, and decompression times are compared, the similarity in international decompression requirements is obvious. However, if the decompression requirement exceeds about 1 hr, then all of these tables will begin to approach, or even greatly exceed, 1% incidence of bends. At this point it has been found by E. L. Beckmann (1976) that resort to extra decompression is mandatory, and he recommends following the 1968 air diving tables, which were issued in the United Kingdom by the Underwater Engineering Group of the Construction Industry's Research and Information Association, and using their Table II for oxygen breathing. Even these tables fail for really prolonged exposures to air pressures, and it is then necessary to consult the *NOAA Diving Manual* (Miller 1979).

Heliox diving is now largely a commercial offshore activity, and the various major diving firms have evolved their own decompression procedures generally designed around particular forms of diving practice. Their basic theories are most frequently some form of Workman's M-value concepts described earlier in this chapter. Experience has dictated which M-values give least trouble in a given set of circumstances. The U.S. Navy have had a set of bounce (i.e., short bottom time) helium diving tables for many years, but experience shows that use of these helium partial pressure tables is not successful at

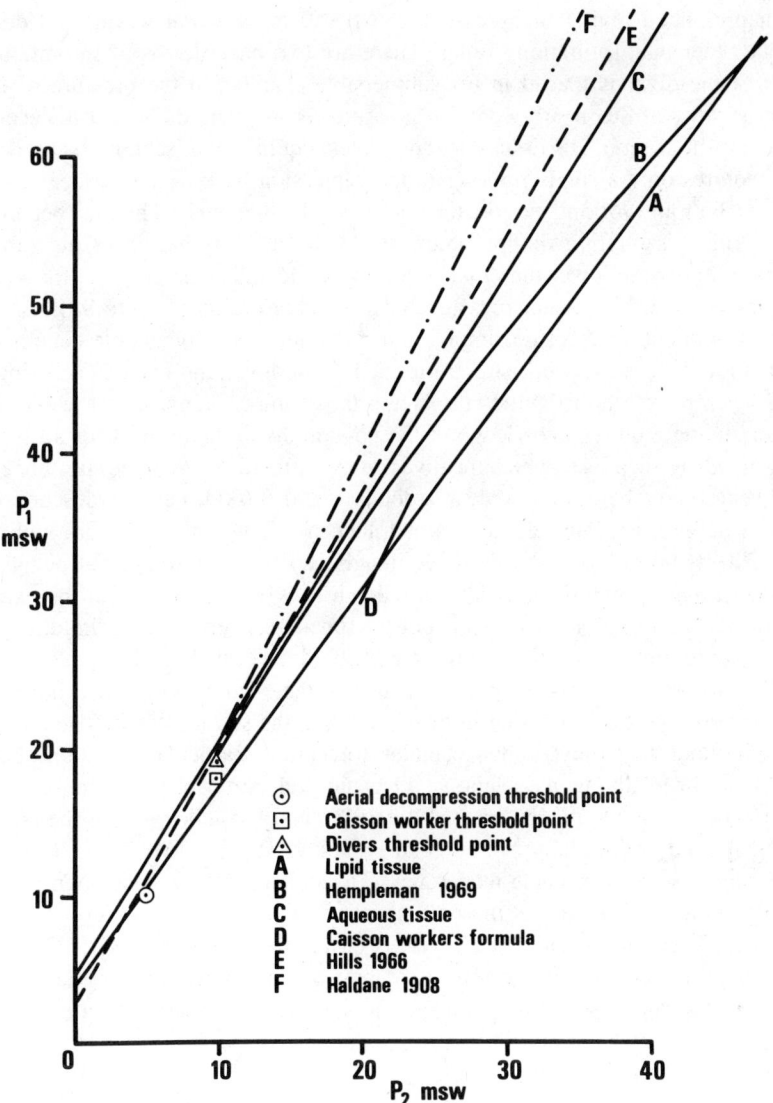

Figure IV-10. Absolute pressures are displayed. P_2 is the minimum pressure to which it is safe to ascend following a prolonged exposure to pressure P_1. Various estimates are tenable because insufficient direct evidence is available.

depths greater than about 300 ft (90 m) for bottom times in excess of 20 min. The commercial bounce tables appear better able to cope with this form of diving but they are normally labeled "commercial-in-confidence," and it is difficult to obtain any objective appraisal of their success. It does seem, however, that no groups perform regular bounce diving to depths in excess of 500 ft (150 m) and that bottom times exceeding 1 hr are not yet considered sufficiently troublefree at depths of 250 ft (80 m) or greater.

For prolonged diving in excess of 165 ft (50 m) it is not worth considering any technique other than saturation diving. There are two basic forms of saturation diving. In the first the diver is placed in his submersible chamber at the pressure of the work site and he stays at this nearly constant pressure for as many days as it is necessary for him to complete the job. His tissues are completely equilibrated (saturated) at this pressure and he requires only a single prolonged decompression back to the surface. Clearly the longer the bottom working period the more worthwhile this technique becomes. The second form of saturation diving occurs when the diver is placed in his submersible chamber at a pressure lower than that of the work site and as he goes out to work on the job he descends to this greater pressure for a working period of up to 8 hr, after which he returns, without need for decompression, back into the submersible chamber. These descents to and from the work site are termed *excursions,* and excursion diving is very popular when there are difficulties in placing the chamber alongside the work site. This excursion diving requires knowledge of the no-stop dive relationships for all the various *holding* or *storage* depths to which the diver returns after his work at the site. For example, if the diver is being held, or stored, at a depth of 200 ft (60 m) and he descends to work for 3 hr, what is the greatest depth at which he can safely work and return without stops back to 200 ft (60 m)? Suppose now we imagine such a 3-hr work shift being required four times a day. How does this alter the depth to which the diver can be expected to work safely? The variations in possible bottom times, rest periods at the holding pressure, and the holding pressure itself are infinite and could never be issued as tables for general uses. This becomes even more apparent if during the excursion the diver breathes a gas of different composition from that in the chamber at the storage depth. The complexities are so enormous that only guidance tables for certain particular situations have been issued. For nitrox diving the National Oceanic and Atmospheric Administration has evolved various suitable procedures (Miller 1979) and for heliox diving the U.S. Navy, Royal Navy, and various large commercial groupings (e.g., COMEX and Taylor Diving Oceaneering) also have suitable techniques. The student of this scene soon realizes that a suitable computer program is the only satisfactory solution to the very diverse set of possibilities: The real difficulty, however, is basing the computer program on a reliable mathematical model; this has been one of the principal topics of consideration in this chapter, and as can be seen there is as yet no sufficiently versatile theory available.

K. *General Observations*

It is not good enough just to reach a satisfactory calculating system that has no physiological basis. This may be illustrated by considering the cross section of the shoulder joint (Figure IV-11), which was used earlier to show that the synovial membrane or slab of cartilage was a reasonable model for consideration. It requires very little extra speculation, however, to suppose that inert gas would dissolve in other areas of the joint and in particular inside the bony capsule at the head of the joint, which is largely composed of fatty tissue and is relatively avascular. Such a tissue would take a very long time to saturate and desaturate with gas. It is inside a bony capsule, and a large pressure could be generated inside the bone that would indubitably cause pain. Indeed, bubbles inside

Decompression Theory 267

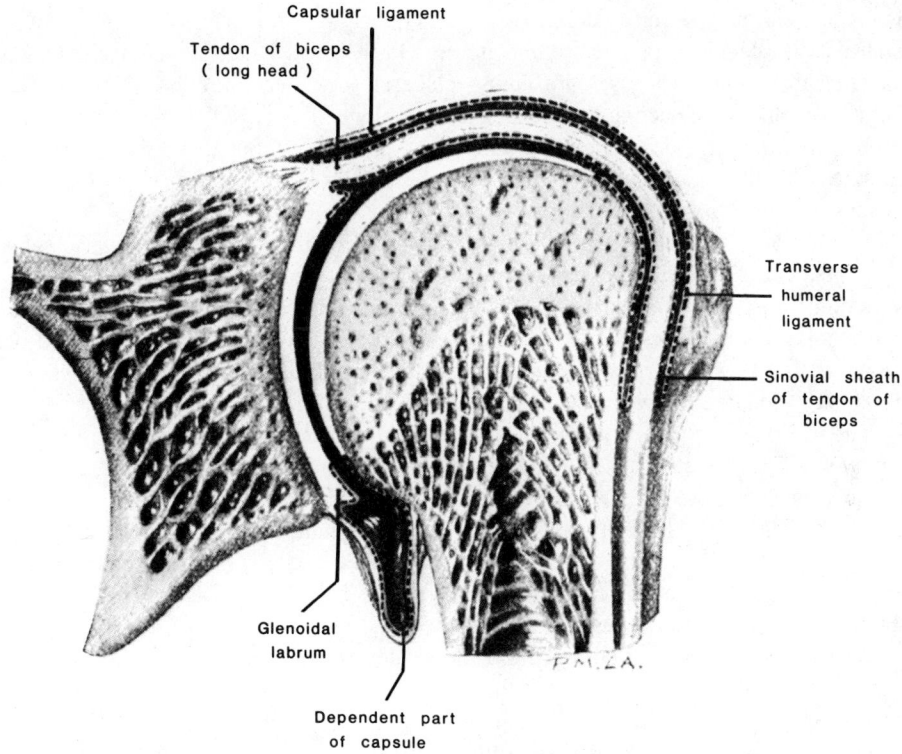

Figure IV-11. Section of shoulder joint to illustrate idea of viewing cartilage as a slab of tissue with a layer of blood along face of slab. See also reference in text to "whole joint" concept.

a bony capsule with long half times involved would explain why ultrasound does not detect the occurrence of decompression sickness from saturation diving. It is impossible to "see" inside a bone by using ultrasound, and the etiologic agent would therefore be undetectable by this technique. On the other hand, the presence of bubbles inside the bone, with the consequent generation of pressure and ischemia, would interfere with bone marrow function and lead to the hematological changes that have been observed. It could also be supposed that repeated insults of this type must lead to permanent bone damage, i.e., osteonecrosis. The whole picture can be seen to accord with most, if not all, the relevant available data, and it would be a trivial mathematical problem to generate several calculating systems from this basic model, one of which would doubtless be as good as any available at present!

Given this situation the physician must maintain a stance that does not adhere to any particular set of beliefs and yet offers a rational approach to decompression or any subsequent therapies involved. The best concepts to adopt are therefore the most conservative. It is safest to assume that every decompression, without exception, is accompanied by a bubble. This bubble may, or may not, manifest itself overtly, but silent bubbles are always present. If men work for several days on diving or tunnel procedures, and if it can be noticed that they are not having as many attacks of bends due to acclimatization or adaptation to work in compressed air, then it is safest to assume that this process can only occur by desensitizing and damaging some physiological response, which is not a desirable practice to encourage. On the other hand, if repetitive dives or exposures to compressed gases are taking place at such frequency that men begin to exhibit more and more decompression sickness problems, it is clear that the silent bubbles present after the first decompression are being gradually inflated by the subsequent exposures, and this again is malpractice. Both these latter situations (i.e., acclimatization and sensitization) do occur, regularly.

In addition to assuming that bubbles are always present in the body, it is also safest to assume that they can survive many days post-decompression and, unless there are clear contraindications, any abnormality occurring post-decompression is due to bubbles that could resolve if recompressed. In common with all such assumptions there will be occasions when following them will lead to failure, but until the etiology is better understood it is safest to assume the worst possible situation.

The technique of gas switching must be carefully examined and, for example, close scrutiny should be given to time-saving decompression procedures that rely on the breathing of nitrogen-rich mixtures when the body is surrounded by helium.

Finally, although all theorists agree that oxygen breathing speeds the elimination of inert gas from the tissues, it is also known that oxygen causes vasoconstrictive effects, and it is well established that oxygen breathing per se is not particularly effective if bubbles are hidden away in very slow tissues.

As has been mentioned before, the general idea behind breathing as large a partial pressure of oxygen as possible is that the inert gas contribution is thereby reduced and therefore the subsequent decompression problem is also reduced. It could be a false assumption, however, that oxygen is totally innocuous from the decompression standpoint. Reference to any standard textbook on physiology will reveal that the cardiovascular system responds markedly to large changes in arterial oxygen content. Many tissues suffer severe vasoconstrictive effects under high partial pressures of oxygen. For example, the exposed pial membrane of a cat can be seen to blanch when the animal is given raised oxygen pressures to breathe. The quantitative aspects of how the various tissue circulations respond to large changes in oxygen concentration is far from understood. Nevertheless, it can be said unequivocally that breathing pure oxygen or high partial pressures of oxygen does normally speed up the decompression. The only exception occurs when the schedule has given, or is close to giving, a bend. Oxygen on its own does not help here on most occasions. Only recompression, to remove or reduce the size of the offending bubbles, will be effective, and when accompanied by breathing of oxygen-rich mixtures is of course even more effective, but the possibility of oxygen toxicity must always be borne in mind. Limits for safe breathing of raised partial pressures of oxygen are given elsewhere in this book (see Chapter II).

Reference has been made earlier to the technique of surface decompression in attempts to shorten the "in water" decompression time required by the conventional diver. Although this is rarely used except by military divers, it is worth mentioning as a possible technique for emergencies, and clearly a physician will be involved at some point. A similar procedure is used by tunnel workers and is generally termed *decanting*. In this latter method the compressed air worker at the end of his shift period is rapidly decompressed to atmospheric pressure and then walks from the work chamber to a separate pressure chamber in which he is rapidly recompressed back to his former shift pressure.

He is normally then required to wait a few minutes at this maximum pressure, after which he is decompressed at the normal slow decompression rate demanded by his time at the full shift pressure. This procedure is used when for some technical reason it is not desirable to have the decompression lock directly attached to the main working chamber. Both surface decompression and decanting involve the highly undesirable practice of rapidly decompressing the man from his working pressure to atmospheric pressure, at which pressure he would suffer a serious attack of decompression sickness unless rapidly recompressed within a few minutes. Needless to say, for regular use these techniques require experienced teams to ensure success. Some groups attempt to render surface decompression less hazardous by completing one or two short deep stops in the water before surfacing directly, but although this is indubitably a move in the right direction, it still remains a technique for experienced teams of divers, and in any case is not to be encouraged except under compelling circumstances. As was pointed out when considering VanDerAue's testing of this technique, the areas of doubt about how the body is responding to the various violent pressure changes involved are too numerous for one to feel confident that lack of overt decompression sickness is necessarily accompanied by lack of hidden damage.

The day is not far distant when the theoretician will be able to offer divers or tunnel workers a set of versatile concepts that will render all forms of decompression sickness very rare events. It will be many years, however, before it is known whether these theoretical concepts are optimized for the great bulk of mankind and thus give the least time-consuming and the safest possible pressure-time courses for returning to atmospheric pressure. As may readily be appreciated, it is a monumental task to achieve optimized safe procedures for males or females, fat or thin, fit or unfit, working hard or resting, in cold or warm water, breathing various partial pressures of inert gases and oxygen, with short or long bottom times, during single or complex repetitive dive routines. Perhaps the practical answer will arrive with some device that can detect the very first indications of impending trouble. This would make it possible to monitor the pressure-time course on an individual basis and would make less essential the understanding of detailed physiological mechanisms.

H. V. HEMPLEMAN

References

ALNOR, P. C. 1963. Chronic changes in the bone structure of divers. *Bruns. Beitr. Klin. Chir.* 207: 475–485.
BATEMAN, J. B. 1951. Review of data on value of pre-oxygenation in prevention of decompression sickness. In: *Decompression Sickness*, edited by J. F. Fulton. Philadelphia: W. B. Saunders, Chap. 9, Pt. 1.
BECKMANN, E. L. 1976. Recommendations for improved air decompression schedules for commercial diving. Sea Grant Tech. Rep. UNIHI-SEA Grant-TR-76-02.
BEHNKE, A. R. 1951. Decompression sickness following exposure to high pressures. In: *Decompression Sickness*, edited by J. F. Fulton. Philadelphia: W. B. Saunders, p. 53–89.
BEHNKE, A. R. 1967. The isobaric (oxygen window) principle of decompression. In: *Trans. Third Annual Conference of the Marine Technology Society*. Washington, DC: Marine Technol. Soc.
BERT, P. 1878. *Barometric Pressure*, transl. by M. A. and F. A. Hitchcock. Columbus, OH: College Book Co., 1943, p. 5. (Republ. Bethesda, MD: Undersea Medical Society, 1978.)

BLENKARN, G. D., C. AQUADRO, B. A. HILLS. AND H. A. SALTZMAN 1971. Urticaria following sequential breathing of various inert gases at 7 ATA: a possible manifestation of gas-induced osmosis. *Aerosp. Med.* 42: 141–146.

BOULTON, G. O. 1942. The use of air locks. *J. Inst. Eng. Aust.* 14(1).

BOYCOTT, A. E., G. C. C. DAMANT, AND J. S. HALDANE 1980. Prevention of compressed air illness. *J. Hyg.* 8: 342–443.

CHRYSSANTHOU, C. P. 1973. Studies on the mechanism and prevention of decompression sickness. Progress Report of the Physiology Program. Arlington, VA: Office of Naval Research, p. 7–8.

DAMANT, G. C. C. (n.d.). *Calculating Decompressions on the Late Professor J. S. Haldane's System.* London: Siebe, Gorman and Co., Ltd.

DAVIS, R. H. 1935. In: *Siebe, Gorman & Co. Decompression Tables.* London: St. Catharine Press.

DAVIS, R. H. 1981. *Deep Diving and Submarine Operations* (8th Ed.). Gwent, Wales, U.K.: Siebe, Gorman and Co., Ltd.

DES GRANGES, M. 1956. *Standard Air Decompression Table.* Res. Rep. 5-57. Washington, DC: U.S. Navy Experimental Diving Unit.

DWYER, J. V. 1955. *Calculation of Air Decompression Tables.* Res. Rep. 4-56. Washington, DC: U.S. Navy Experimental Diving Unit.

EATON, W. J., AND H. V. HEMPLEMAN 1962. The incidence of bends in goats, after direct surfacing from raised pressures of air. Rep. 209. London: Medical Research Council, R.N. Personnel Research Committee, Underwater Physiology Sub-Committee.

EPSTEIN, P. S., AND M. S. PLESSET 1950. On the stability of gas bubbles in liquid-gas solutions. *J. Chem. Phys.* 18: 1505–1509.

EVANS, A., AND D. N. WALDER 1969. Significance of gas macronuclei in the aetiology of decompression sickness. *Nature (London)* 222: 251–252.

FLYNN, E. T., AND C. J. LAMBERTSEN 1971. Calibration of inert gas exchange in the mouse. In: *Underwater Physiology IV. Proceedings of the Fourth Symposium on Underwater Physiology*, edited by C. J. Lambertsen. New York: Academic Press, p. 179–191.

FRENCH, G. R. W. 1916. Diving operations in connection with the salvage of the USS "F-4." *U.S. Nav. Med. Bull.* 10: 74–91.

GOLDING, F. C., P. D. GRIFFITHS, W. D. M. PATON, D. N. WALDER. AND H. V. HEMPLEMAN 1960. Decompression sickness during construction of the Dartford Tunnel. *Br. J. Ind. Med.* 17: 167–180.

GRAVES, D. J., J. IDICULA, C. J. LAMBERTSEN. AND J. A. QUINN 1973. Bubble formation resulting from counter-diffusion supersaturation: A possible explanation for isobaric inert gas 'urticaria' and vertigo. *Phys. Med. Biol.* 18: 256–264.

HALLEY, E. 1717. The art of living under water. *Phil. Trans. R. Soc. London.*

HAMILTON, R. W., J. B. MACINNIS, A. D. NOBLE. AND H. R. SCHREINER 1966. Saturation diving at 650 feet. Technical Memorandum B-411. Tonawanda, NY: Ocean Systems.

HARVEY, E. N. 1945. Decompression sickness and bubble formation in blood and tissues. *Bull. N.Y. Acad. Med.* 21: 505–536.

HARVEY, E. N. 1951. Physical factors in bubble formulation. In: *Decompression Sickness*, edited by J. F. Fulton. Philadelphia: W. B. Saunders, p. 90–114.

HAWKINS, J. A., C. W. SHILLING. AND R. A. HANSEN 1935. A suggested change in calculating decompression tables for diving. *U.S. Nav. Med. Bull.* 33: 327–338.

HEMPLEMAN, H. V. 1952. Investigation into the decompression tables. A new theoretical basis for the calculation of decompression tables. Rep. III, Pt. A. London: Medical Research Council, R.N. Personnel Research Committee, Underwater Physiology Sub-Committee.

HEMPLEMAN, H. V. 1957. Investigation into the decompression tables. Further basic facts on decompression sickness. Rep. 168. London: Medical Research Council, R.N. Personnel Research Committee. Underwater Physiology Sub-Committee.

HEMPLEMAN, H. V. 1963. Tissue inert gas exchange and decompression sickness. In: *Proceedings of the Second Symposium on Underwater Physiology*, edited by C. J. Lambertsen and L. J. Greenbaum. Washington, DC: Natl. Acad. Sci./Natl. Res. Council.

HERGET, R. 1948. Recent observations of barotraumatic chronic joint complaints in divers. *Arch. Klin. Chir.* 261: 330–360.

HILLS, B. A. 1966. A thermodynamic and kinetic approach to decompression sickness. Adelaide: Libraries Board of South Australia. Thesis.

IKELS, K. G. 1970. Production of gas bubbles in fluids by tribonucleation. *J. Appl. Physiol.* 28: 524–527.

JAMINET, A. 1871. *Physical effects of compressed air and of the causes of pathological symptoms produced on man, by increased atmospheric pressure employed for the sinking of piers in the construction of the Illinois and St. Louis bridge over the Mississippi River at St. Louis, Missouri.* St. Louis: Ennis.

KEAYS, F. L. 1909. Compressed air illness, with a report of 3,692 cases. *Publ. Cornell Univ. Med. Coll.* 2: 1–55.

KEAYS, F. L. 1912. Compressed-air Illness. *Am. Labor. Legisl. Rev.* 2: 192–205.

KENYON, D. J., M. FREITAG, AND M. R. POWELL 1974. Efficient decompression procedure for 1000 foot diving. *Undersea Biomed. Res.* 1: A7.

KROGH, A. 1918. The rate of diffusion of gases through animal tissues, with some remarks on the coefficient of invasion. *J. Physiol.* 52: 391.

LAURENS, P. 1964. Considerations sur l'origine des bruits du coeur. *Acta Cardiol. (Brux.)* 19: 327–344.

LIEBERMANN, L. 1957. Air bubbles in water. *J. Appl. Phys.* 28: 205–211.

LOESCHCKE, V. H. 1956. Über die Diffusion von Gas in mit Gas untersättigte Lösungen mit Durchrechnung biologischer Beispiele. *Z. Naturforsch.* 11B: 613–620.

MANLEY, D. M. J. P. 1960. Change of size of air bubbles in water containing a small dissolved air content. *Br. J. Appl. Phys.* 11: 38–42.

MARTIN, K. J., AND G. NICHOLS 1971. Changes in platelets in man after simulated diving. Rep. 5/71. Orpington, Kent, England: R. N. Physiological Laboratory.

MEDICAL RESEARCH COUNCIL DECOMPRESSION SICKNESS PANEL 1966. Bone lesions in compressed air workers with special reference to men who worked on the Clyde Tunnels 1958 to 1963. *J. Bone Joint Surg. (Lond.)* 48B: 207–235.

MILLER, J. W. (editor) 1979. *NOAA Diving Manual.* Washington DC: National Oceanic and Atmospheric Administration, U.S. Dept. of Commerce.

NICHOLS, G. 1979. Changes in erythrocyte sedimentation associated with saturation diving. *Annual Scientific Meeting, European Union of Biological Sciences Fifth Scientific Meeting, Bergen, Norway.*

OHTA, Y., AND O. SHIGETO 1974. *Symposium on Dysbaric Osteonecrosis,* edited by E. L. Beckmann and D. H. Elliott. Washington, DC: National Institute of Occupational Safety and Health.

PALMER, A. C., W. F. BLAKEMORE, J. E. PAYNE, AND A. SILLENCE 1978. Decompression sickness in the goat: nature of brain and spinal cord lesions at 48 hours. *Undersea Biomed. Res.* 5: 276–286.

PATON, W. D. M., AND D. N. WALDER 1954. Compressed air illness—An investigation during the construction of the Tyne Tunnel, 1948/1950. Spec. Rep., Ser. No. 281. London: Medical Research Council.

PERL, W. 1962. Heat and matter distribution in body tissues and the determination of tissue blood flow by local clearance methods. *J. Theor. Biol.* 2: 201–235.

PERL, W., H. RACKOW, E. SALANITRE, G. L. WOLF, AND R. M. EPSTEIN 1965. Inter-tissue diffusion effect for inert fat-soluble gases. *J. Appl. Physiol.* 20: 621–627.

PHILP, R. B., P. SCHACHAM, AND C. W. GOWDEY 1971. Involvement of platelets and microthrombi in experimental decompression sickness; similarities with disseminated intra-vascular coagulation. *Aerosp. Med.* 42: 494–502.

RAHN, H., AND W. O. FENN 1955. *A Graphical Analysis of the Respiratory Gas Exchange.* Washington, DC: Am. Physiol. Soc.

RASHBASS, C. R. 1955. Investigation into the decompression Tables. Rep. VI New Tables. Rep. 151. London: Medical Research Council, R. N. Personnel Research Committee, Underwater Physiology Sub-Committee.

ROZSAHEGYI, I. 1959. The late consequences of the neurological forms of decompression sickness. *Br. J. Ind. Med.* 16: 311–317.

RUBISSOW, G. J., AND R. S. MACKAY 1974. Decompression study and control using ultrasonics. *Aerosp. Med.* 45: 473–478.

SPENCER, M. P., AND S. D. CAMPBELL 1968. The development of bubbles in the venous and arterial blood during hyperbaric decompression. *Bull. Mason Clin.* 22: 26–32.

STILSON, G. D. 1915. *Report on deep diving tests-USN.* Washington, DC: U.S. Department of the Navy, Bur. of Construction and Repair.

U.S. NAVY 1978. *U.S. Navy Diving Manual (Change 2), Air Diving.* Washington, DC: U.S. Navy Dept., Vol. 1. (NAVSEA 0994-LP-001-9010.)

UNDERWATER ENGINEERING GROUP 1968. *Air Diving Tables*. London: Her Majesty's Stationery Office.
VANDERAUE, O. E., E. S. BRINTON, AND R. J. KELLER 1945. Surface decompression and testing of decompression tables with safety limits for certain depths and exposures. Res. Rep. Washington, DC: U.S. Navy Experimental Diving Unit.
WHITAKER, D. M., L. R. BLINKS, W. E. BERG, V. C. TWITTY, AND M. HARRIS 1945. Muscular activity and bubble formation in animals decompressed to simulated altitudes. *J. Gen. Physiol.* 28: 213–223.
WORKMAN, R. D. 1965. Calculation of decompression schedules for nitrogen-oxygen and helium-oxygen dives. Res. Rep. 6-65. Washington, DC: U.S. Navy Experimental Diving Unit.
YARBROUGH, O. D. 1937. Calculation of decompression tables. Res. Rep. Washington, DC: U.S. Navy Experimental Diving Unit.
YOUNT, D. E. 1978. Responses to the twelve assumptions presently used for calculating decompression schedules. In: *Decompression Theory*. Bethesda, MD: Undersea Medical Society. (Decompression Workshop.)

V

Immediate Medical Evaluation of the Diving Casualty

A. *Introduction*

Of particular importance in diving accidents is the immediate and appropriate care of the victim. Proper initial management frequently makes the difference between complete recovery and permanent crippling or death. The most dramatic and life-threatening condition is air embolism, but even so simple a thing as a few hours' delay in recompression of a diver who has missed proper decompression may precipitate aseptic necrosis of the bone (dysbaric osteonecrosis) years later.

The following are emergency conditions a diving physician is likely to encounter. All are covered in detail elsewhere in this book and are mentioned here to emphasize the need for careful diagnosis of often complex conditions.

- Air embolism, which usually results from holding the breath during ascent and which may occur from as shallow a depth as 4 ft. Immediate recompression is required.
- Decompression sickness (bends), which may be pain only (Type I) or even paralysis (Type II). Usually is slower to develop than air embolism but also must be treated by recompression.
- Barotrauma to the middle ear, sinuses, and, less commonly, rupture of the round or oval window of the ear, face squeeze, or, very rarely, whole-body squeeze.
- Atelectasis or other evidence of pulmonary barotrauma may be seen but is not life threatening unless it occurs during decompression, where expansion of the air in the chest of the collapsed side may press on the mediastinum, in which case it has been known to cause death.
- Hypoxia may occur due to faulty life-support equipment but is not seen except at the site of the dive.
- Contamination of the breathing gas also causes dramatic problems, but it is only at the site of the dive. You may be called, though, and you should know the possibilities.

- Injury from trauma or the bites, stings, and lacerations from marine organisms.
- Natural illness such as heart attack, stroke, or epileptic seizure must be remembered as possibilities.

B. *Emergency Care*

1. *General Statement*

Although you, as a diving physician, may not be in a hands-on position, the odds are that you will be called for advice and thus should be familiar with the diagnostic problems and the treatment facilities available.

2. *Divers Alert Network (DAN)*

The Divers Alert Network was developed by the Undersea Medical Society with support from the National Institute of Occupational Safety and Health and the National Oceanic and Atmospheric Administration; the network is now operated by Duke University. All that is necessary is to call (919) 684-8111 and say DAN, and a direct connection is made with a knowledgeable physician who not only may give advice on treatment but will indicate the nearest pressure chamber facility and the best method of emergency transportation.

3. *Diving Medics*

The diver medics are also known as Emergency Medical Technicians/Diver (EMT/D), Diver Emergency Medical Technicians, Diver First-Responders, or Diver Medics.

It is well for the physician to recognize that these men are well trained and capable. In fact, with the advent of this group the injured diver faces better prospects of recovery than ever. The diver medic communicates with the designated physician as quickly as possible, and he is capable of doing the following immediately or upon medical advice: "Making rapid assessment of the degree of injury; stabilization by CPR; control of hemorrhage; splinting of fractures; hydration with intravenous fluids; catheterizing the patient to closed drainage in bladder injury; working in the chamber with the patient and giving standard nursing care; assisting in the chamber control of temperature, oxygen supply, and carbon dioxide removal; keeping accurate medical records even during crises" (Keith Van Meter, personal communication).

It is interesting to note that in the commercial diving field the divers themselves are receiving first aid instruction. Other groups are doing the same thing through furnishing pamphlets, such as that of Rutkowski (1982) of the National Oceanic and Atmospheric Administration and the Florida Underwater Council.

4. Immediate Action

Aside from natural illness such as heart attack, stroke, or epileptic seizure, the diver who becomes incapacitated or develops symptoms of pain or paralysis after surfacing from a dive is most likely suffering from cerebral air embolism or decompression sickness. Very possibly it will not be immediately known what the patient's difficulty is, but regardless of what he may be suffering from, the most immediate thing is to have him lie down. If the victim has symptoms related to his lungs (coughing, hemoptysis) or central nervous system (convulsions, unconsciousness, numbness, unequal pupils, blindness, or paralysis), he should be placed in Trendelenburg's position at an angle of at least 20° to 30°. The patient should be rotated to either side if he is unconscious or obtunded, as this will tend to prevent aspiration in case of vomiting. Once this maneuver has been performed, it should be definitely determined that the patient has a free airway. Mouth-to-mouth resuscitation should be started immediately if he is not breathing on his own, and if the carotid pulse is absent, cardiopulmonary resuscitation (CPR) should be instituted by a second person. Throughout the period of diagnosis and transportation to the ultimate center, the patient should be kept head down in this position as much as possible. Personnel should be instructed not to cease any resuscitative attempts until the patient is pronounced dead by a licensed physician.

Placing the patient in Trendelenburg's position is the recommended initial treatment for cerebral air embolism. Meanwhile the procedure does no great harm if this is not the underlying cause of the problem. In the event that air embolism is subsequently ruled out, the patient can then be returned to normal position.

C. Diagnosis

1. Background

It is important for an accurate diagnosis to be made quickly to determine if emergency recompression in a hyperbaric chamber is necessary. In some cases the diagnosis may influence the choice of facility to be used. The physicians manning the chamber can then be given much more information prior to the arrival of the patient. Immediate diagnosis will also make possible more rational treatment before the patient reaches a chamber.

The following facts are all important in making the diagnosis;
- A diving accident victim can be any person who has been breathing air or other gas mixture under water, regardless of depth.
- Gas or air embolism can occur in as little as 2 to 4 ft (70 mmHg) if one ascends holding his breath.
- Decompression sickness can occur in any individual who violates the decompression tables either willingly or unintentionally when surfacing from depths greater than 30 ft.
- "Bubble trouble" can happen to anyone, anywhere, at anytime, far out at sea, in lakes, rivers, and even in the home swimming pool.

- For any patient who exhibits any of the signs or symptoms of a diving accident the one crucial question is, "Did the subject breath air under water?" If yes, treat as a diving accident victim and move to a hyperbaric facility at once.
- If patient is paralyzed get him out of the emergency room at once and on the way to the nearest hyperbaric facility, breathing oxygen on the way.
- If patient is unconscious initiate CPR if necessary and send at once to the nearest hyperbaric facility.

2. Air Embolism

a. General Statement

Air embolism is treated in detail elsewhere in this book, so the cause of the condition need not be discussed. However, the symptomatology and therapy are considered in some detail, since they are so directly related to the emergency handling of most diving accidents.

b. Signs and Symptoms

The symptom picture may include sudden unconsciousness, convulsions, paralysis, bleeding from the mouth, or death within minutes. The onset is immediate within a minute or two of surfacing. Symptoms occurring as late as 5 min after a normal surface interval usually are not air embolism. Other signs to look for are mottling of the tongue (Liebermeister's sign), unequal pupils, subcutaneous emphysema above the clavicles and in the neck, swelling of the neck, a change in voice quality, chest pain, or nausea. Pneumothorax may be a possible but rare concomitant. All of these signs and symptoms are included in the "burst lung syndrome." Occasionally patients will have subcutaneous emphysema and complain of fullness around the neck along with chest pain and nausea; mediastinal air and/or pneumopericardium will be visible on radiographs. The aftereffects of cerebral air embolism can be subtle, however, and may only manifest themselves as a personality change that may not be noticed by the examining physician. It is therefore important to ask the patient's diving companions, friends, or relatives, whether he "seems his normal self."

Rutkowski has given the symptomatology of arterial gas embolism for the layman as follows: "Unconsciousness, paralysis, weakness, confusion, headache, or other neurological deficit. Can be associated with pneumothorax or air under the skin of the neck [emphysema]. Can result from as shallow as 4 feet of water depth."

c. Emergency Treatment

(i). Place in the Trendelenburg Position. Use of the Trendelenburg position has been shown by research and clinical experience to be effective (Kruse 1963), and my own clinical experience bears this out. Three patients regained consciousness within 20 to 30 min after being placed in this position (unpublished observations). One had some residual confusion on arrival at the chamber, but the other two appeared normal. All

patients were treated with recompression, however, and were found to have normal neurological and mental examinations following treatment. One patient developed transient 4+ proteinuria after chamber treatment; this cleared in a few days.

(ii). Administer Oxygen. Oxygen should be administered through a tightly fitting mask. The object is to denitrogenate the patient by excluding nitrogen from his lungs, not to provide the patient with more oxygen per se. The mask seal is tight enough if the patient could theoretically breathe from the mask while lying on his back under water.

(iii). Transfer to Hyperbaric Facility. The diagnosis of cerebral embolism carries with it the obligation to transport the victim as quickly as possible to a recompression facility with the capability of recompressing the patient to 6 ATA or an equivalent 165 fsw (50 msw). Arrangements should be made immediately to transport the patient to such a facility no matter how far away it is, for remarkable results have been achieved after hours of delay (as many as 21 hr) in recompression in cases of embolism.

3. *Decompression Sickness*

a. General Statement

As in the case of air embolism, decompression sickness (DCS) is discussed in detail in several places in this book, so the etiology is not considered here. However, both symptomatology and therapy are presented in some detail.

b. Symptoms

Ninety percent of all cases of decompression sickness include pain (Rivera 1964). The pain may appear anywhere in the body, but commonly it is located in one of the limbs and often is in an arm or leg that has been exercised a great deal during the dive. It also tends to appear at the site of a recent injury or sprain. The pain is usually steady, is not made worse by movement, and often does not throb. There is nothing the patient can do to ease or change the pain. Localized edema may also be a feature of pain-only decompression sickness, but it usually responds promptly to oxygen therapy.

Approximately 25% of all cases of bends in divers involve neurologic symptoms (Rivera 1964). These symptoms may be numbness or paralysis of an arm or leg, vertigo (staggers), or visual distortions or blindness. If the spinal cord is involved, the most common site is the upper lumbar and lower thoracic region, which typically produces a paralysis from T10 down. If the diver complains of a pins-and-needles feeling in his lower extremities or buttocks, consider it cord decompression sickness until proved otherwise. The paralysis or numbness may be limited to one extremity, however, and often cord lesions are patchy, giving the neurologist the impression he may be dealing with hysteria. Girdling abdominal pain should be considered to be associated with cord involvement until proved otherwise.

About 2% of DCS patients develop respiratory symptoms or *chokes* (Rivera 1964). If, after surfacing from a dive, a diver develops wheezing and a troublesome cough with rapid respirations, it may be inferred that his lungs are involved.

Rutkowski's statement for the layman is as follows: "Decompression Sickness ('Bends'). Joint pain, back or abdominal pain, paralysis, numbness, tingling, inability to control bowels or urine, headache, dizziness, partial blindness, confusion, shortness of breath, chest pain, cough, shock."

c. Treatment

(i). General Statement. Immediate recompression in the nearest pressure chamber and then controlled decompression is the treatment of DCS, and it should be the choice even if the nearest chamber is more than an hour away. All patient with symptoms of DCS except mild skin itch or marbling or mottling (termed *skin bends*) should receive recompression treatment with as little delay as possible. Skin bends, particularly skin mottling, may possibly be a precursor to very serious symptoms later on, and the patient should be kept under observation.

The following measures should be taken if transfer to a recompression chamber is not feasible and also should be observed during the period until transportation is available.

(ii). Denitrogenation. Nitrogen bubbles can theoretically be reduced in size by increasing the gradient for the nitrogen leaving the bubbles. This is accomplished by letting the patient breathe oxygen to eliminate the nitrogen. With the partial pressure of nitrogen reduced in the blood stream, the nitrogen bubbles will dissolve more rapidly. It must be remembered that oxygen is given, not to oxygenate the patient, but to denitrogenate him, so for that reason the mask must be extremely tight in fit. The rule to follow for effective denitrogenation is that the mask must seal well enough to theoretically allow the patient to breathe, were he lying on his back underwater. Anything less than this will be inadequate.

An additional advantage of oxygen administration is that reduced blood sludging is observed as soon as the Po_2 is increased (Swindle 1937). Sludging of the blood is a concomitant of decompression sickness, and this stagnation in the epidural venous plexis may be responsible for some of the symptoms and signs of spinal cord decompression sickness.

(iii). Hydration. Hallenbeck, et al. (1975) have observed that, at least for the first 30 min or so in experimental animals, stagnation and stasis of the blood in the epidural venous plexis can be greatly reduced by adequate hydration. Wolkiewicz and Plante-Longchamp, quoted by Fructus (1979), have presented evidence that patients who were hydrated early after the onset of symptoms had a decrease in their symptoms compared to unhydrated patients prior to actual recompression. If the patient is conscious and capable of doing so, have him drink a liter of fluid each hour for the first 2 hr. Forcing oral fluids (isotonic or slightly hypertonic, if possible) in the conscious patient, or preferably using an intravenous infusion of Ringer's lactate/5% dextrose in saline, or normal saline to ensure good urine flow, is of crucial importance in the immediate treatment of decompression sickness. The use of plain 5% dextrose in water is discouraged, as the glucose will be metabolized away, leaving water, which may worsen neural tissue edema. The patient may be dehydrated or low on fluids due to inadequate water intake in a tropical environment or perhaps post-alcoholic dehydration. An adequate urine output is 1 to 2 ml/kg per hr (Kindwall 1979). It is important to place a urinary catheter if the patient is unable to urinate or appears to have a neurogenic bladder.

In bends shock, fluid volume replacement is absolutely mandatory. Low molar dextran (dextran-40) and its heavier analogue (dextran-70) are useful as plasma expanders. Dextran-40 is lost quickly through the kidneys but exerts a stronger osmotic pressure because of its smaller molecular size. Because of its rapid excretion, dextran-70 should probably be given after the unit of dextran-40 if blood volume needs to be continuously bolstered. Plasma will also be of use in decompression sickness shock.

Of more recent interest is the plasma colloid osmotic pressure. This determination can be made in some institutions, and if it falls below 19 to 20 mmHg, albumin should be administered until colloid osmotic pressure is restored. Pulmonary and generalized edema becomes evident at pressures of 15 to 16 mmHg, and there is no survival if colloid osmotic pressure drops below 11 mmHg. In decompression sickness shock, the fluid is not lost from the body; it is simply extravasated into the tissues, from where it theoretically may be retrieved and returned to the vascular compartment. Maintaining plasma colloid pressure to prevent extravasation is superior to simple volume replacement, especially in patients where pulmonary edema is a concomitant. In shock, colloid osmotic pressure does not bear a simple relationship to the amount of circulating albumin.

(iv). Drugs. (a) Steroids. If it is anticipated that there will be a long interval until the chamber can be reached, and if the patient is suffering from severe decompression sickness, steroids are indicated. These drugs are given because they tend to stabilize vascular endothelium and have an antiedema effect that has been noted by neurosurgeons. Early experimental work has suggested that steroids exascerbate oxygen toxicity, but clinically this has not been observed even in the presence of high dosages of steroids. Pretreatment with steroids has not increased the risk of convulsions on U.S. Navy oxygen treatment tables 5 and 6 (Kindwall 1979). The recommended dosage would appear to be 1 g of rapidly acting steroids such as hydrocortisone hemisuccinate given intravenously in a bolus, with 4 mg of dexamethasone 21-phosphate given concomitantly intramuscularly. The latter drug is continued in 8-mg dosage every 6 hr for 2 to 3 days. It should be remembered that any drug given intramuscularly will be poorly absorbed if the patient is being treated with oxygen under pressure.

(b) Glycerol. The value of glycerin in the treatment of cerebral edema was demonstrated by Tourtelotte (1972), Matthew (1972), and Reinglass (1974). It is given orally, 0.8 ml/kg body wt in a 50% solution of water, which may be flavored with lemonade to make it more palatable. Glycerol would appear to have many advantages for the diver when compared with other edema-reducing agents, as summarized by Saper and Yosselson (1975). It is superior to mannitol and urea in that it does not derange electrolyte balance, and it exerts maximal effect in 1 hr with a duration of effect of 6 hr; this is faster than all other agents. It does not cause rebound edema and, of particular advantage to the diver who may be remote from the services of a paramedic or physician, it can be given orally by a layman. It may, however, cause nausea and vomiting because of its unpalatability; in such case it can be given via nasogastric tube. J. C. Davis (personal communication) described a case of spinal cord decompression sickness where glycerol produced immediate and dramatic improvement.

(c) Aspirin. Aspirin has theoretical value because it appears to inhibit platelet aggregation. Two tablets taken orally will exert maximal effect in this regard in 30 min. However, once platelet aggregation is complete and vessel blockage has been established it has no theoretical value. For this reason, to have an effect aspirin would have to be given immediately after the earliest symptoms appear. Although there are no experimental data to demonstrate its prophylactic value when taken before decompression, there is essentially no risk in giving a couple of aspirin tablets early in illness to a conscious patient with no shock—the only type of patient to whom aspirin should be given.

(d) Narcotic analgesic. The use of opiates is usually contraindicated unless there is some overriding necessity such as concomitant traumatic injury. Potent analgesics mask symptoms and hinder evaluation of response to eventual treatment in the recompression chamber. Use of them may also produce a rise in the arterial P_{CO_2} which in turn brings on early central nervous system oxygen toxicity during oxygen therapy in the chamber. It should be noted parenthetically that hyperbaric oxygen therapy produces an intense vasoconstriction that may slow the absorption of intramuscular narcotics. If a repeat dose is then given in the chamber, when the patient is subsequently decompressed he will be receiving an effective overdose of narcotics upon relief of vasoconstriction.

(e) Sedatives. If the patient is extremely agitated or restless and requires sedation during transport, or if agitation is so great that sedation is required to carry out treatment, diazepam is the preferred drug. The intravenous route is best and the dosage is the same as indicated for convulsion suppression.

(f) Other Measures. At the present time there are no theoretical or clinical data to suggest the use of additional adjuctive agents in the immediate emergency treatment of decompression sickness. While the above measures are being taken, another individual should be assigned to locating and contracting the nearest chamber, determining its operational status and staffing, and arranging for transportation.

4. Determining the Cause of the Accident

If a diving death has occurred, there is always reason to investigate its cause. The same holds true of course for any serious accident. The Emergency Room physician can be very helpful in this regard if he obtains the names and addresses of the patient's diving companions and any witnesses to the accident. It is also important that the diving gear involved be preserved for subsequent examination and testing, and any gas remaining in the patient's air tank should be saved for analysis. Chapter XV, "Diving Accident Investigation," details these procedures.

ERIC P. KINDWALL

References

FRUCTUS, X. 1979. Treatment of serious decompression sickness. In: *Treatment of Serious Decompression Sickness and Arterial Gas Embolism*, edited by J. C. Davis. Bethesda, MD: Undersea Medical Society, p. 37–43. (Workshop, Duke Univ., Jan. 1979.)

HALLENBECK, U. M., A. A. BOVE, AND D. H. ELLIOTT 1975. Decompression sickness studies. In: *Underwater Physiology V. Proceedings of the Fifth Symposium on Underwater Physiology*, edited by C. J. Lambertsen. Bethesda, MD: Fed. Am. Soc. Exp. Biol.

KINDWALL, E. P. 1979. Adjunctive treatment methods. In: *Treatment of Serious Decompression Sickness and Arterial Gas Embolism*, edited by J. C. Davis. Bethesda, MD: Undersea Medical Society, p. 45–49. (Workshop Rep. No. 34.)

KRUSE, C. A. 1963. Air embolism and other skin diving problems. *Northwest Med.* 62: 525–529.

MATHEW, N. T., V. M. RIVERA, J. S. MEYER, ET AL. 1972. Double-blind evaluation of glycerol therapy in acute cerebral infarction. *Lancet* 2: 1327–1329.

REINGLASS, J. L. 1974. Dose response curve of intravenous glycerol in the treatment of cerebral edema due to trauma: a case report. *Neuro. Minneap.* 24: 743.

RIVERA, J. C. 1964. Decompression sickness among divers: an analysis of 935 cases. *Mil. Med.* 129: 314.

RUTKOWSKI, D. 1982. *Diving Accident Manual*. Miami, FL: Florida Underwater Council and National Oceanic and Atmospheric Administration.

SAPER, J. R., AND S. YOSSELSON 1975. Raised intra-cranial pressure. *Postgrad Med.* 57: 89–94.

SWINDLE, P. F. 1937. Occlusion of blood vessels by agglutinated red cells mainly seen in tadpoles and very young kangaroos. *Am. J. Physiol.* 120: 59.

TOURTELOTTE, W. W., J. L. REINGLASS, AND T. A. NEWKIRK 1972. Cerebral dehydration action of glycerol. I. Historical aspects with emphasis on the toxicity and intravenous administration. *Clin. Pharmacol. Ther.* 13: 159–171.

VI

Diagnosis and Treatment of Decompression Sickness

A. General Survey

1. History

Decompression sickness has in the past been defined as an overt illness that may appear in a human being while diving or following a reduction in environmental pressure sufficient to cause bubble formation and/or growth from the gases dissolved in the tissues. Other terms have been legitimized by use to have an equivalent meaning, despite the opinions of experts that it would be more desirable either to not use such terms at all or else to use them only in relation to a particular type of decompression sickness: such terms include *caisson disease, compressed air illness,* and *the bends*. The diving medical community has been fairly successful in discouraging the use of the term *dysbarism*, which really could refer to any one of the many disorders that might result from a change in pressure, and the term *aeroembolism*, which was confusing because it was often unclear whether the reference was to air embolism or to aviators' decompression sickness. At any rate the classic definition of decompression sickness (DCS), while still applicable in the majority of cases, is no longer strictly correct. For example there is now serious doubt that DCS is overt in all cases. Although Behnke (1951) had hypothesized the "silent bubble" as early as 1951, it has only been since ultrasound detectors have achieved prominence over the past decade that a number of investigators have actually demonstrated that bubbles do exist in the venous circulation during any significant decompression, whether overt symptoms of DCS are present or not. This implies that DCS develops when there is some critical bubble effect (due to the amount of bubbles and their secondary interactions) rather than a critical supersaturation as classically defined. Furthermore, it has recently been recognized that an isobaric form of counterdiffusion can lead to bubble formation without a reduction in environmental pressure.

Robert Boyle demonstrated in 1670 that a reduction in pressure could lead to bubble formation in living tissue, and it is perhaps surprising that the significance of his findings was not appreciated for more than two centuries, since references to the problems, diseases, and deaths of early human divers date back to well before the Christian era. It was not until the development of the first practical deep-sea diving outfit by Augustus Siebe in 1819 and the large-capacity compressors that allowed the use of caissons in securing bridge foundations on river bottoms (first used by Triger in 1841) that large numbers of men had the means to work at raised environmental pressures for significant periods of time. While a boon for construction, salvage, and other projects, it was not long before the human costs began to be appreciated. Of the Greek sponge divers who began to use the fully closed helmeted diving suit designed by Siebe in 1837, it is said that 50% died during the first year; prior to this they had for the most part used the simple expediency of breath-hold diving and, over a period of 100 generations or so, appeared to have acquired a remarkable degree of freedom from the physiological hazards of their profession. In the early 1840s, symptoms of DCS were first described by Triger, a French mining engineer, in coal miners working in shafts that were pressurized to prevent flooding (Triger 1841). Early attempts to explain the development of DCS symptoms included theories such as reflex spinal cord damage secondary to exhaustion and cold, frictional electricity caused by compressed air, toxemia secondary to increased tissue catabolism, stasis and congestion of internal organs caused by blood forced internally by the pressure, or alternatively by hypovolemia in internal organs secondary to a rapid return of blood peripherally during decompression.

In 1847 (although this work was not published until 1854), Pol and Watelle realized there was a relationship between the onset of symptoms, the depth and duration of exposure, and the rapidity of decompression. They also observed in 1847 that symptomatic relief could sometimes be obtained by returning the victim to an increased pressure environment, and they therefore suggested that gas bubbles might be involved in the development of DCS. Nonetheless, it was to be the early 1900s before the "new" treatment modes for DCS victims gained widespread acceptance as a result of these and similar observations by a number of physiologists and physicians involved in major engineering projects. In the meantime, the literature was replete with anecdotal accounts of DCS cases throughout the world and measures routinely taken for the affliction—measures that today make us shudder. For example, Dr. Graham Blick from 1900 to 1908 was an Australian district medical officer with medical responsibility for a large pearling center employing more than 400 divers who daily harvested oysters at depths from 40 to 120 ft. In reviewing more than 200 cases of "diver's palsy" Blick writes, "The most troublesome cases were those complicated by cystitis and deep sloughing. The former complication is very frequently set up by imperfectly cleaned catheters used by the diver's friends, often for several days, while making for port. The paralysis of micturition is so well known among the men themselves that no diver would consider his outfit complete without a soft catheter." (Blick 1909). Those must have been the days when men were men! Perhaps even more revealing of the attitude toward DCS before the early 1900s are the words in 1871 of A. Jaminet, a physician who had medical responsibility during the construction of an arched bridge across the Mississippi river at St. Louis, Missouri. The caissons for this huge undertaking were sunk in as deep as 115 ft of water, by far the greatest depth at which this type of work had ever been performed. Between February 10 and February 19, 1870, Dr. Jaminet made three visits to the working chamber at depths ranging from 69 ft to 81 ft (21–25m). With each decompression he was increasingly affected by "severe epigastric pain" and a "feeling of great fatigue and depression of the system." He was unable to make a scheduled visit on

February 22 because he was so "feeble," and he elected to wait until the caisson touched bedrock. Rock was hit at 95 ft (29 m) on February 28, and Dr. Jaminet entered the caisson once more. His communication reveals that

> . . . having terminated our experiments, which lasted two hours . . . we were ready to return . . . I remained three quarters of an hour longer . . . the door of the air-chambers was closed, the equalizing valve was freely opened, the compressed air escaping very rapidly . . . I was taken with a violent pain in the head. We were only three minutes and a half in the air-lock, to return into the shaft or normal atmosphere . . . . After resting four times in ascending the stairs, I arrived at the surface of the pier, almost exhausted. I sat down a few minutes, but did not feel any better. I was taken again with the same epigastric pain as in my former visit. I was dizzy, so that no sooner was I on board the boat which crossed us to shore than I had to sit down on the stairs of the cabin to prevent myself from falling: my pulse grew weaker, and after reaching the shore, I had to use great exertions to reach my buggy, only half a square distant. I succeeded in getting in.
>
> During that time the epigastric pain increased. I had nothing to take to relieve me, an accident in the caisson having deprived me of my flask containing the cordial which I intended to use in case of necessity, if suffering as before from the same pain.
>
> In the course of a few minutes I drove home, which I reached at half-past two o'clock P.M., three-quarters of an hour after leaving the air-chambers or caisson. The last effort brought me to my office, where in a few minutes I became paralyzed.
>
> This concluded my fourth systematic regular observation.
> Home 28 February 2:30 o'clock P.M.
>
> Being in my office paralyzed and unable to speak for a few minutes, but conscious of what was passing around, I made signs to my wife and persons with her at the time not to move me at all, but to lower my head and raise my feet as high as possible. In the course of a few minutes, I was able to articulate a few words, but with great effort, and to say what should be done to me. I was to be left perfectly quiet on my back or my right side, my head on a level with my body, my legs stretched, and my feet elevated two feet above my head.
>
> Then I took a teaspoonful of old Jamaica rum every five minutes three times in succession, and kept a small piece of ice in my mouth to quench my thirst. A few minutes after I commenced taking two large tablespoonsful of beef tea every five minutes. I was suffering from profuse cold perspiration, every effort to speak caused great suffering and fainting, my pulse was 106 per minute, both legs and my left arm were paralyzed, still I was suffering in both with excruciating pains which I can only compare to pains felt after a fracture of the left leg, which I experienced some years ago. During the pains in my limbs, which increased at intervals, my pulse was 115 per minute.
>
> I knew well that in my situation, as I said to my wife, that after doing all I directed to be done, if I was no better by half-past five o'clock that same evening that nothing more could be done. (Jaminet 1871)

The narrative continues and relates that about a week later Jaminet began to recover. This case is interesting not only because it demonstrates accepted treatment of the day for DCS (liberal amounts of alcohol, taken internally, is even today the self-remedy for several abalone divers I know in Southern California and, I suspect, for other groups of divers elsewhere), but it is also one of the few first-person accounts of a physician describing the symptomatology and course of severe neurological DCS in himself.

After the mid-19th century progress toward an understanding of DCS gained momentum. In 1857 Seyler demonstrated that bubbles blocked the pulmonary circulation. In 1861 Bucquoy (cited in Bert, 1878, p. 460) published probably the first full accounts of the hazards of compressed air work and pointed out the need for slow decompression. In 1872 Friedburg commented on similarities between severe DCS and surgical air embolism. In 1878 Paul Bert, a French physiologist of an incredibly wide range of interests, carried out experiments demonstrating to his satisfaction that DCS was due to the liberation of nitrogen in the form of bubbles in the blood and tissues of experimental animals. Bert (1878) recommended recompression (and subsequent decompression) with oxygen as treatment for DCS but did not specify decompression rates. Up until 1900 there were no widely promulgated tabulated decompression tables that could minimize the occurrence of DCS. The Greek sponge divers and undoubtedly other groups had by this time developed their own tables by trial and error, but such tables may not have worked for anyone but themselves, since even today the Greek sponge divers are reputed to stay at depth longer and require less decompression than any other hard hat divers. In 1900, Heller, Mager, and von Schrötter recommended linear decompression at a rate of 20 min for each 33 ft of ascent, a procedure that proved adequate for short dives to as much as 160 fsw (49 msw), but not for long dives. Then in 1908 the British Admiralty commissioned J. S. Haldane to compose decompression schedules to be used by Royal Navy divers, and virtually all schedules devised since that time have been based on empirical modifications of Haldane's concepts (Boycott et al. 1908). These modifications and how they fit into modern decompression theory are the subject of much of Chapter IV, "Decompression Theory." Suffice it to say that with the adoption of Haldane's tables and hypotheses by most groups involved in diving work, the hazards of decompression were substantially reduced, though not completely eliminated.

Strangely, these tables were not adopted for tunnel and caisson work. The first medical recompression lock was apparently installed at a construction site in 1889 and certainly the symptoms of DCS were well known by that time, the term *bends* having been coined from the "Grecian bend," an affected way of walking favored by fashionable ladies of the era, which reminded the caisson workers of the stoop affected by men afflicted with the painful symptoms of DCS. In 1909 Keays showed there was no doubt that recompression was the treatment of choice in handling DCS casualties, and in 1912 Hill published a paper compiling the many accounts of earlier victims of DCS from civil engineering contract reports, thereby emphasizing the high risks of permanent disability and death to workers in pressurized environments. Nevertheless, a number of years were to pass before acceptable decompression schedules and therapeutic regimes for DCS were routinely instituted by the majority of caisson and tunneling companies.

Even though the basic pathophysiological mechanisms underlying DCS remain obscure, decompression tables from the models that have been manipulated over the years have been able to prevent overt DCS in the majority of divers. However, there remain far too many seemingly paradoxical situations and unanswered questions to let us believe that our mathematical models give us an accurate picture of the true processes underlying decompression and DCS. Likewise, much of the treatment of DCS is by and large empirical, in part due to the difficulties involved in establishing suitable animal research models and the ethical impossibility of doing controlled human studies to assess different therapeutic regimes, at least as regards pressure and oxygen, the two fundamental aspects of DCS treatment.

As would be expected, the early development of effective therapeutic regimes for treating DCS roughly paralleled the growing awareness that separation of gas from solution was the primary insult in all forms of DCS as well as the concurrent development of decompression tables that called for gradual reduction in pressure depending on the duration and depth of exposure. In the last two decades of the 19th century, medical locks (pressure chambers to allow the victim of DCS to undergo recompression treatment attended by a physician) were installed and in use during the construction of the Brooklyn Bridge, the Hudson River Tunnel, and other civil engineering contracts. At least one schedule called for recompression to the original pressure at which the victim had been working, followed by slow decompression to the surface after the pain was relieved (some 30 years later this treatment philosophy was officially endorsed by the New York Public Service Commission). Generally, however, there was no standardization of treatment schedules or procedures, just as there was no standardization of decompression schedules.

Standard recompression treatment procedures published in the *U.S. Navy Diving Manual* in 1924 were not fully successful, since more than 50% of those treated experienced a recurrence of symptoms. Unfortunately, results appeared to be no better by 1945, whether using the new oxygen treatment tables that had been promulgated by the U.S. Navy Bureau of Medicine and Surgery in 1944 or the air treatment tables in the 1942 edition of the *U.S. Navy Diving Manual*. Accordingly a series of tests were undertaken by VanDerAue and associates (1945) at the Naval Medical Research Institute and the Navy Experimental Diving Unit, and as a result of this work the U.S. Navy Air Recompression Tables 1 through 4 were promulgated in 1945. These tables were widely accepted and became the standard for the U.S. Navy, several foreign navies, and many commercial companies worldwide for the next 20 years. Initially these tables were much more successful than previous tables, but by 1964 a review by Rivera confirmed that the failure rate for initial recompression had been increasing drastically in recent years. Even worse, the failure rate in treating severe cases of DCS had risen nearly back to the 50% level. The primary reason for this was felt to be the fact that many more amateur divers were being treated at Navy facilities, and many of these grossly disobeyed standard decompression procedures and experienced long delays before arriving at a treatment chamber. This led in 1964 to reinvestigation of oxygen breathing treatment tables by two U.S. Navy medical officers (Goodman and Workman 1965). Use of these tables over the next 2 years resulted in overall failure rates as well as failure rates for serious cases of less than 4%. These tables subsequently have been shown by Erde and Edmonds (1975) to have as high as a 13%–15% chance of failure with initial recompression in cases where there has been more than a 3-hr delay between the onset of symptoms and the initiation of therapy, a situation that occurs frequently when the victim is a nonmilitary or nonprofessional diver (a description of most divers). In a more recent series reported by J. C. Davis (1979) the figure was an overall 10% failure rate for cases with long delays between onset and treatment. For most cases of DCS these oxygen treatment tables are the most effective therapeutic tables available and thus they have become the treatment of choice throughout the world.

2. Symptoms and Signs

It used to be said that if a physician was well versed in all the manifestations of syphilis, he probably had a pretty fair grasp of general internal medicine. A similar analogy might be made between decompression sickness and diving medicine. The clinical manifestations of this fascinating disorder are myriad. They can frequently be bizarre and misleading, mimicking other diseases related or unrelated to diving. Each case seems to be unique in pattern, combination, and severity of signs and symptoms. One of the most highly respected pioneers of diving medicine, Dr. Albert R. Behnke, after reviewing a series of 55 cases in 1951 (see Behnke 1951), concluded that "on no single point do all cases agree." The objective of this section is to discuss a number of the many possible consequences that can occur if decompression procedures are ignored or prove inadequate for a given pressure exposure, to help the physician better recognize and differentiate any cases of DCS he or she might encounter in practice or be asked to advise on.

As mentioned previously, most workers in the field now feel that the primary event leading to DCS is the formation of bubbles from gases dissolved in the tissues, either by random bubble nucleation or by the activation of preexisting nuclei. Whichever the case, once bubbles are present they can lead to the many different manifestations of DCS or they may remain asymptomatic, depending on such factors as bubble distribution, individual variability of response to the bubbles, and the relative importance of direct mechanical effects of the bubbles versus secondary bubble-induced effects. Symptoms can appear during or immediately after decompression or after a delay of several hours. Most cases will present within 6 hr of the dive—in one series more than 50% of all divers with DCS developed symptoms within 1 hr of the dive and 90% within 6 hr. When delay in symptom onset occurs it is most likely due to the gradual progression of edema and secondary blood-bubble interactions. (See Griffiths 1969; Kidd and Elliott 1969; Rivera 1964; Slark 1962.)

To more easily standardize the identification, prognosis, and therapy of DCS, a clinical classification is frequently used that divides the symptoms into a Type I or Type II category, the former describing musculoskeletal, pain-only, bends and the latter being reserved for symptoms other than pain as well as for any patients who exhibit abnormal physical signs. While the term Type I may be reasonably clear when applied to acute DCS affecting the musculoskeletal system, the term Type II is not completely satisfactory because it covers such a conglomeration of symptoms ranging all the way from small patches of hypesthesia to complete cardiovascular collapse. It would be clearer to actually designate the organ or organ system or systems affected: for example, "This patient is suffering from DCS affecting the inner ear and the musculoskeletal system."

a. Cutaneous and Lymphatic Symptoms

Cutaneous and lymphatic manifestations can range from being very localized and innocuous at one end of the spectrum to quite generalized and ominous at the other. Simple itching is a common complication occurring for the most part after short, deep, dry-chamber dives and is usually considered to be an essentially local reaction and not a serious manifestation of DCS. This pruritus, which generally affects the hands, wrists, nose, and ears, can be quite intense and may or may not be associated with a slight transient folliculitis. (The symptoms are attributed to small gas bubbles in the superficial dermal layers.) A red punctate rash is sometimes seen predominantly over the chest, shoulders, back, and upper abdomen and may be associated with some sort of tissue histamine release. This rash can last from a few minutes to several hours. A more serious, papular, erythematous rash can occur over the same distribution when there is enough endogenous gas present to interfere with venous drainage. This rash becomes angry looking and lumpy as the collections of papules merge to form placques with flat, firm borders. Coughing, or in any other way increasing the intrathoracic pressure, will accentuate this rash (Mellinghoff's sign). Alternately, marbling of the skin can occur, generally beginning as a small, pale area with cyanotic mottling and then spreading peripherally with extension of the cyanotic areas. The edematous mottled areas are warmer than the surrounding skin, and even when the marbling disappears with recompression the affected areas often become tender to palpation within a few hours. The reader should consult the discussion of this topic in Edmonds et al. (1976).

Subcutaneous emphysema sometimes occurs in localized areas or along tendon sheaths and has the typical crepitus sensation on palpation (not to be confused with the supraclavicular subcutaneous emphysema extending from the mediastinum as a result of pulmonary barotrauma).

Bubbles will obstruct lymphatics in about 5% of patients and cause pain and swelling of discrete groups of lymph nodes or lymphedema of the tissues drained by the involved nodes, or both. This manifestation is usually seen over the trunk and more rarely over the head and neck. Recompression normally gives prompt relief, though the swollen nodes often continue to recede for days after treatment.

b. Musculoskeletal Symptoms

Limb bends is a term commonly applied to the musculoskeletal form of DCS that occurs in approximately 85%–90% of all cases; although it is the most common type of DCS, it is also among the types we know the least about. It is a localized pain that can vary widely in its intensity, and apart from the pain in one or more limbs, the victim often neither looks nor feels particularly ill. Though sometimes localized within the joint, the pain is usually periarticular and limited to those parts of the body primarily concerned with locomotion, i.e., certain joints such as the sternoclavicular joints, the temporomandibular joints, and the joints of the vertebral column are normally not affected. Ferris and Engel (1951) and Haymaker (1957) have demonstrated that ischemic injury (as through use of a tourniquet) to a limb during decompression predisposes the involved limb to DCS. Logically, old injuries, if resulting in compromised tissue perfusion, would predispose to DCS in the same way. Apart from this, the shoulder is the most commonly affected joint in divers, followed by the elbows, wrists, hands, hips, knees, and ankles. Involvement is seldom symmetrical when two or more joints are affected, and often adjoining joints on the same extremity are affected. Limb bends are more common in the hips and knees of saturation divers, aviators, and caisson workers, and perhaps this is related to impaired circulation caused by cramped positions in chambers, cockpits, or tunnels (see B. A. Hills 1977, p. 33). It could also be related to the nature of the work and the selective exercise undertaken in the different pressure-related occupations.

Sometimes musculoskeletal DCS only consists of a mild, barely detectable discomfort (called a *niggle* by divers) but more frequently the syndrome starts with discomfort around a joint that rapidly proceeds to a deep, dull ache. A good description of limb bends was offered by Behnke in 1951 when he described it as "a dull, throbbing type of pain, progressive and shifting in character, and frequently felt around the joints, or deeply in muscles and bones." At first, movement may provide some relief, but once the pain is well established, movement will aggravate it, so the involved extremity is usually held flexed in a position of maximum comfort. If untreated, the pain frequently becomes excruciating over the next few hours and then gradually abates to a dull ache throughout the next week. This residual aching may persist for weeks and occasionally is accompanied by erythema and edema over the area (which has led to confusion with some forms of arthritis). It is very important to remember that somewhere between 20% and 30% of these cases are associated with more serious manifestations of DCS, a percentage that would probably be even higher if a careful examination to rule out CNS involvement was performed in every case.

Various mechanisms for the musculoskeletal pain of limb bends have been proposed, including vascular occlusion by circulating bubbles and products of blood-bubble interactions, and mechanical deformation of nerve fibers in tendons and ligaments by development and growth of bubbles in these relatively poorly perfused tissues where they have little room for expansion.

c. Central Neurological Symptoms

Central neurological DCS can manifest itself in a number of ways. The results of complete or partial occlusion of a cerebral vessel depend on the area affected and the collateral arterial supply just as in cerebrovascular accidents from other causes. Neurological manifestations can include paralysis (usually hemiparalysis), various visual disturbances, aphasia (receptive or expressive), severe headache, impaired cerebration in general, loss of consciousness, seizures, and death. When the cerebellum is involved, speech difficulties, tremor, and ataxia (called *the staggers* by divers) may be seen. Spinal cord lesions not infrequently begin with only local spinal or girdle pains of the lower extremities, but the condition can rapidly proceed to paraplegia (often with urinary retention and fecal incontinence), unconsciousness, and ultimately death.

Traditionally damage to the central nervous system (CNS) caused by decompression was attributed to occlusion of the systemic arterial circulation by gas emboli. While this seems to offer an adequate explanation for cerebral symptoms and their relatively infrequent occurrence, a more likely mechanism in spinal cord involvement (which is seen in nearly 80% of cases of neurological DCS) has been shown to be interference with venous drainage from the cord by bubbles, both directly and indirectly. The symptoms, pathophysiology, and treatment of spinal cord DCS are fully detailed in Section C of this chapter. Complex hematological and hemorrheological interrelationships are also described in that section.

d. Peripheral Neurological Symptoms

Decompression sickness involving the peripheral nervous system is sometimes seen as a patchy kind of sensory deficit predominantly involving the lower extremities; it is attributed to bubble formation in the myelin of peripheral nerves. It can be difficult to differentiate from an incomplete spinal lesion, but the distinction is important, since the spinal cord injury is potentially much more disabling if not recognized and treated appropriately (if in doubt, treat for the more serious injury).

e. Audiovestibular Symptoms

Audiovestibular DCS signs and symptoms such as tinnitus, nystagmus, complete or partial deafness, vertigo, nausea, vomiting, and ataxia have recently been recognized as occurring independently of other manifestations of DCS. Where otitic barotrauma can reasonably be ruled out, these patients are now felt to be afflicted with a form of DCS related to bubble formation in the perilymph or endolymph or in the small end-type nutrient blood vessels supplying the cochlear and labyrinthine apparatus. This form of DCS has been under intensive investigation recently and has taken on new importance with recognition that the overall incidence is probably significantly higher than previously thought. Research in this area also includes investigation of similar symptoms occurring during or after a switch of breathing gases at fixed depths. The symptoms, pathophysiology, and treatment of audiovestibular DCS are the subjects of Section B of this chapter.

f. Respiratory and Cardiovascular Symptoms

Respiratory and cardiovascular manifestations are of course indicative of serious DCS. The lungs are a very efficient bubble filter and it seems reasonable to assume that pulmonary response to bubbles will depend on the total number of bubbles and their rate of arrival. That is, a few gas bubbles may be efficiently trapped until the gas inside them can diffuse out, and so they produce no symptoms, but when the defense mechanisms of the lung are overcome by large numbers of bubbles arriving in relatively short periods of time, the direct mechanical effects and a number of secondary bubble-induced effects can lead to airway constriction, decreased pulmonary blood flow, increased pulmonary vascular resistance, alterations in the ventilation-perfusion ratio, chest pain, coughing (called *the chokes*, a triad of respiratory signs and symptoms described fully in Section C of this chapter), tachypnea, hypoxia, and shock with marked increases in the swings of intrathoracic pressure. A secondary detrimental effect of the raised pulmonary arterial pressure occasioned by the multiple pulmonary gas emboli may be to predispose an individual to paradoxical embolism through a patent foramen ovale, an atrial septal defect, or some type of intrapulmonary arteriovenous shunt. Bubbles could then enter the cerebral circulation, leading to symptoms already described, or the coronary arteries, leading to symptoms indistinguishable from those of a myocardial infarction—chest pain, arrhythmias, or sudden death.

g. Shock and Other Manifestations

Shock or sudden collapse that occurs as a manifestation of DCS is frequently accompanied by the chokes and indicates a fulminant form of DCS. A number of mechanisms may contribute to the development of shock in DCS, including loss of vascular tone as a result of spinal cord involvement, myocardial depression from hypoxemia and acidosis, pulmonary embolization and hypovolemia secondary to a diffuse increase in capillary permeability resulting in a loss of plasma water and hemoconcentration.

Miscellaneous manifestations of DCS such as pain in the back, abdomen, or chest, in contrast to limb pain, may represent spinal cord involvement and should be considered as such, especially because acute lower abdominal pain has been a principle feature in a few patient fatalities. Diver fatigue more extreme than that occurring routinely after a dive has long been recognized as a part of the DCS syndrome.

h. Aseptic Bone Necrosis

Aseptic bone necrosis is commonly seen in compressed air workers and certain groups of divers and is now felt by many scientists to be a delayed type of DCS that is due to primary or secondary occlusive effects of bubbles. These effects may include physical obstruction of small vessels, dissolved gases bringing about a change in osmotic properties and hence circulation, damage to vessel walls with biochemical and clotting abnormalities, extravascular bubble growth in unexpandable bone leading to vascular occlusion, and disruption of fat cells by intracellular bubbles with subsequent showers of fat emboli. Dysbaric osteonecrosis is a current research priority, since avoidance of long-term disability due to bone damage is as important as avoidance of the classic forms of DCS. Since there is some measure of doubt in attributing this disease completely to inadequate decompression, it is usually considered separately from DCS and is the subject of Section B of Chapter IX of this book.

3. *Diagnosis*

One of the most important things that can be said about decompression sickness is that it is a condition that must be considered in the differential diagnosis of anyone becoming ill after a dive. This may seem obvious, but despite poor record keeping and frequent instances of failure to follow repetitive dive techniques and standard ascent rates, victims (as well as the victim's friends) will frequently proclaim that the dive was neither deep enough nor long enough to produce DCS. Such claims should always be viewed with skepticism. As mentioned in the discussion of symptoms, a real problem in the differential diagnosis of DCS is that it can easily be confused with a number of other illnesses. It must also be remembered that DCS can be induced or aggravated by flying too soon after diving, due to the reduced atmospheric pressure and associated expansion or formation of bubbles.

Most cases of DCS will not present diagnostic difficulty to a physician; however, there are occasions when various diagnostic techniques not now generally available at a work site or treatment site would be most advantageous. This lack of facilities is less of a problem where the distinction between DCS and arterial gas embolism does not radically alter the initial therapeutic compression selected. It is unfortunate that the latest in advanced life-support techniques are generally unavailable to the physician called to attend a diving accident, although the problem is beginning to be addressed in the offshore diving industry.

The diagnostic value of history taking and clinical examination, as in most areas of medicine, cannot be overstressed. The ability to reach an accurate diagnosis may not always affect the initial compression but certainly becomes important when adjuvant and supportive therapy are considered. The cardiovascular, pulmonary, and biochemical pathophysiology in acutely ill patients suffering from DCS are for the most part still ill defined, thus a careful baseline physical examination with particular attention to any subsequent changes in the victim's neurological status is the basic monitor of DCS. It is worth emphasizing that when eliciting a history from the patient or when taking information about a patient, answers to the following questions (I keep them as a reminder beside the phone) are important in reaching a differential diagnosis and influencing advice given regarding therapy:

> *Name* of person you are talking to; *name* and age of victim; *primary physician's name; telephone number* you can ring back (if cut off, need more information, etc.); *geographical location* of caller and victim (to help with directions to nearest chamber). *Time interval* between surfacing and symptom onset; *time of onset* of presenting signs and symptoms (as well as their *location*,

severity, and *course*); *pressure exposure history* (both the day of the accident and the previous few days); *type* of diving; *depth and bottom time; amount of decompression* received and on what gases; *result* of physician's initial exam; any *lab results* obtained; *test of pressure results* if one was done. Was victim diving in *fresh or salt water*, at *altitude or at sea level;* and was he on any *medications?* Finally, advice on *adjunctive* measures to be taken on the way to the chamber (position, fluids, steroids, oxygen, aspirin, etc.).

The most common error in treating DCS is failure to diagnose the seriousness of the condition. While unnecessary to discuss performance of the physical examination for the intended readership of this book, it is not presumptive to say that diagnosis can be much more difficult in a hot, noisy, cramped chamber, and attention to small things can be of great help, e.g., using a short, taped, double-tube stethoscope to make auscultation easier in a dense atmosphere, ear defenders during compression to prevent temporary decreases in auditory acuity, "crash bag" for acute diagnosis and therapy kept fully stocked and available.

For diagnosis of audiovestibular DCS, otoscopic examination, audiometry, and caloric and Romberg testing do not take up a great deal of time and should be done if possible. Of greater importance is the need for prompt action in recompressing a diver who, while undergoing decompression, suddenly develops vertigo, nausea, deafness, or ringing in the ears.

It would seem prudent in cases of serious DCS to routinely take blood for hematocrit. Often reports of hypotension and tachycardia have accompanied case reports of serious DCS in the literature. Hypovolemia is further evidenced by high hematocrits (as high as 72% in one severely ill patient who ultimately survived) and decreased urinary output. Routine measurements of hematocrit and urinary output, however, while perhaps of some diagnostic help, are really most valuable as easily obtainable objective parameters to guide management in replacement of fluids. It would be valuable if some *quick* hematological test could differentiate between mild and serious DCS. If the events at the blood-bubble interface are significant in determining the severity of DCS, one possible test of value would be an assay of fibrinogen degradation products (FDP). Inwood (1973) and other authors suggest that raised FDP levels are of significance in serious DCS, and a reliable 2-min slide test is commercially available. This form of investigation may be worth doing if results are to influence management of the case; however, none of the many other possibly significant hematological changes described in DCS lend themselves to easy assay within a time limit that could influence the course of therapy.

A combination of clinical judgment and awareness of the diagnostic recommendations that have been passed along by word of mouth from some of the experienced diving physicians is not without value. A few of these hints have been recorded by Flynn and Bayne (1977) in the course syllabus for medical officers at the U.S. Navy School of Diving and Salvage:

- Hot showers or hot compresses sometimes make bends pain worse, perhaps aiding a doubtful diagnosis.

- Inflating a blood pressure cuff above arterial pressure around an affected extremity joint, either on the surface or at depth, may totally relieve a limb bend, again helping confirm the diagnosis. Both of the foregoing maneuvers do not give very reproducible results in my experience. A far more effective diagnostic procedure is a test of pressure that involves taking the patient to 60 ft (2.8 ATA) and having him or her breathe pure oxygen for 20 min. If there is no change in the quality, intensity, or location of the pain, a diagnosis of limb bends is probably incorrect and the patient can be surfaced, nothing having been lost, i.e., no more inert gas has been added to the tissues.

- Hyperreflexia with clonus is not infrequently seen with what for all other purposes, is pain-only bends. These findings disappear when the pain disappears.

- In a patient with paraplegia secondary to a severe lower spinal cord bends, the presence of a bulbocavernosus reflex is a very good prognostic sign.

- Irritative cord lesions may show pain only initially but can progress to neurological dysfunction if treatment is delayed.

- Cerebral lesions, unless massive as in a blowup, are normally pure sensory or pure motor, thus helping to differentiate cerebral gas embolism from cord DCS. Cord DCS usually shows combined sensory motor defects, due to the anatomical relationship of motor nuclei and sensory tracts in the cord as well as to the diffuse nature of the damage.

- Cord lesions generally present with bilateral neurological symptoms, whereas cerebral lesions of gas embolism are more likely to be unilateral. So a paraplegic diver with sensorimotor deficits is more likely to be suffering from DCS than a hemiplegic diver with pure motor or pure sensory deficits.

- A roaring tinnitus associated with sudden hearing loss and vertigo is more likely to be associated with a perilymph fistula than with inner ear DCS.

- A delay of more than 10 min between surfacing and symptom onset is nearly always inconsistent with diagnosis of gas embolism from pulmonary barotrauma.

In 1976 the multiagency-sponsored National Plan for the Safety and Health of Divers (Shilling and Beckett 1976) listed the techniques applicable to diving illnesses that might require more sophisticated aids than are generally available. (Asterisks indicate those techniques that are technically easy but presently not readily available at most work and treatment sites.)

* Bacterial culture and sensitivity determination
  Blood hemoglobin determination
  Blood pressure determination
  Body temperature determination (oral, rectal)

* Electrocardiography

* Electroencephalography

* Electronystagmography
  Fluorescein staining of eye
  Hematocrit determination

* Microscopic studies (blood, urine)
  Ophthalmoscopy
  Otoscopy

* pH determination (blood, urine)
* Blood electrolytes determination
  Rhinoscopy

So, ignoring highly sophisticated technological aids to diagnosis, there are a number of routine methods capable of being adapted for use under pressure. Ultimately, perhaps, a standard range and form of electrical penetrations can be recommended for all chambers so that the physician will be assured of compatability with any monitoring or diagnostic equipment he may care to use. But at present, on most sites, adjunctive diagnostic devices are generally limited to a reflex hammer, a stethoscope, and a blood pressure cuff. Nevertheless, with a few simple and basic diagnostic maneuvers and with a good history (and a test of pressure if there is still doubt) diagnosis of the vast majority of DCS cases, as well as other diving disorders, can be readily sorted out.

4. Therapy

> There is something fascinating about science. One gets such wholesale returns of conjecture out of such a trifling investment of fact.
> ———Mark Twain.
> *Life on the Mississippi,* 1874

> Half of what we've taught you is wrong; unfortunately we don't know which half.
> ———Medical School Professor, 1969

Although the physician responsible for diving accident management may (not unjustly) feel that such witticisms as these are particularly applicable to the empirical nature of DCS therapy, he or she can at least take comfort in the knowledge that such treatment can be dramatically effective. While not all patients arriving alive at the chamber can be cured of the sometimes irreversible damage to the nervous and/or cardiovascular systems, it is still well known that DCS leading to venous stasis, cord edema, and cellular ischemia that results in loss of function and apparently fixed lesions (which would have an extremely poor prognosis if from any other cause) not infrequently are completely reversible with repeated hyperbaric oxygenation and "tincture of time." Thus, what follows in this section can be prefaced by the remark that an aggressive and optimistic attitude in the diagnosis and treatment of DCS is both justifiable and desirable.

In a more perfect world, our therapy for decompression sickness would be, in the words of Barnard, "a system of treatment, based on sound theory, upon firm experimental evidence, and extensive clinical trials; flexible enough to suit the many different types of cases which will continue to occur as a result of our efforts to understand the etiology of the disease and to achieve its prevention." Unfortunately, this is not the case and, as already pointed out, "methods are often based on unproven theories and scanty experimental evidence, without the benefits of controlled clinical trials." (Barnard 1978). Still, current methods have proved to be effective in many different situations worldwide. A favorable outcome is particularly likely if diagnosis is early and treatment is early and thorough, as shown by Bayne (1979) in a recent series of cases from the U.S. Naval School of Diving and Salvage. The information in this section, while believed to be a consensus of the best available, is only for guidance, since every situation cannot be predicted and experienced physicians in diving medicine still have some differences of opinion on details of treatment.

The primary treatment of DCS has been and remains recompression therapy. A variety of recompression schedules are available that are quite effective when DCS occurs at a shallow depth or at atmospheric pressure and treatment is begun early. U.S. Navy Treatment Tables 5 and 6 (Tables VI-1 and VI-2), which provide hyperbaric oxygen and minimal recompression (to 2.8 ATA or 60 fsw) for varying periods of time, have been in use since the mid-1960s and are examples of such regimens. They are useful in nearly all circumstances and can be used successfully to treat the primary occurrence of DCS as well as recurrences during and subsequent to initial treatment. The use of hyperbaric oxygen and minimal recompression has for practical purposes replaced the use of recompression regimes using extensive recompression with air for DCS occurring near surface pressure, for several reasons: First, with oxygen breathing the gradient for elimination of inert gas from tissues is maximized, so bubbles resolve more quickly than during air breathing. Second, CNS edema frequently occurs as a consequence of neurological DCS or arterial gas embolism, and hyperoxia reduces this edema. Third, minimal recompression oxygen breathing tables are more effective in treatment cases where treatment has been delayed, though whether this is due to the antiedema effect, or to the maximized oxygen gradient to hypoxic tissues, is unclear. Fourth, since no additional inert gas is absorbed by the tissues during oxygen breathing, a patient can be decompressed to the surface with greater safety from an oxygen table should the need arise. Finally, since these tables are much shorter than the air tables, the length of time that patients and tenders must be confined to the chamber is shortened, and patients who need further intensive care can be transferred to a hospital setting much sooner.

Table VI-1

U.S. Navy Recompression Treatment Table 5
(Oxygen Treatment)[a]

Depth		Time, min	Breathing medium	Total elapsed time	
ft	m			hr	min
60	18	20	Oxygen		20
60	18	5	Air		25
60	18	20	Oxygen		45
60–30	18–9	30	Oxygen	1	15
30	9	5	Air	1	20
30	9	20	Oxygen	1	40
30	9	5	Air	1	45
30–0	9–0	30	Oxygen	2	15

[a] Used for treatment of pain-only decompression sickness when oxygen can be used and symptoms are relieved within 10 min at 60 ft. Patient breathes oxygen from the surface. Descent rate is 25 ft/min. Ascent rate is 1 ft/min. Do not compensate for slower ascent rates. Compensate for faster rates by halting the ascent. Time at 60 ft begins on arrival at 60 ft. If oxygen breathing must be interrupted, allow 15 min after reaction has entirely subsided, and resume schedule at point of interruption. If oxygen breathing must be interrupted at 60 ft, switch to Table 6 upon arrival at 30-ft stop. The tender breathes air throughout. If treatment is a repetitive dive for the tender or if the table is lengthened, tender should breathe oxygen during the last 30 min of ascent to the surface. [From *U.S. Navy Diving Manual* 1978.]

Table VI-2
U.S. Navy Recompression Treatment Table 6
(Oxygen Treatment)[a]

Depth		Time,	Breathing	Total elapsed time[b]	
ft	m	min	medium	hr	min
60	18	20	Oxygen		20
60	18	5	Air		25
60	18	20	Oxygen		45
60	18	5	Air		50
60	18	20	Oxygen	1	10
60	18	5	Air	1	15
60–30	18–9	30	Oxygen	1	45
30	9	15	Air	2	0
30	9	60	Oxygen	3	0
30	9	15	Air	3	15
30	9	60	Oxygen	4	15
30–0	9–0	30	Oxygen	4	45

[a] Used for treatment of decompression sickness when oxygen can be used and symptoms are not relieved within 10 min at 60 ft. Patient breathes oxygen from the surface. Descent rate is 25 ft/min. Ascent rate is 1 ft/min. Do not compensate for slower ascent rates. Compensate for faster rates by halting the ascent. Time at 60 ft begins on arrival at 60 ft. If oxygen breathing must be interrupted, allow 15 min after the reaction has entirely subsided and resume schedule at point of interruption. Tender breathes air throughout. If treatment is a repetitive dive for the tender or the table is lengthened, the tender should breathe oxygen during the last 30 min of ascent to the surface. [From *U.S. Navy Diving Manual* (1978).]

[b] Does not include descent time.

Once a diagnosis of DCS has been made, treatment is always initiated (with the exceptions discussed later) by placing the patient on oxygen by mask, compressing to 60 fsw (18 msw), and completing the first oxygen treatment period. If the victim had pain-only musculoskeletal DCS and has by now obtained complete relief, treatment is completed on U.S. Navy Table 5 (Table VI-1). If relief of pain is not complete, or if any serious signs or symptoms had been present initially, Table 6 is used. Extra oxygen sessions can be given at 60 fsw and again at 30 fsw (9 msw) if relief is not yet complete (if such sessions are given, any inside attendants should also breathe oxygen during the final 30-min decompression to atmospheric pressure from 30 fsw, and another, air-breathing, observer should be locked in).

The flow chart in the U.S. Navy Diving Manual for DCS treatment (Figure VI-1) allows for further compression to 165 fsw (50 msw) in case of either worsening symptoms or need for deeper recompression. Deeper recompression should not be taken lightly but may be necessary in cases of blowup or in cases of serious DCS of recent onset where the patient is still deteriorating after the first 20 min of oxygen breathing at 60 fsw. In the Royal Navy, the patient is never compressed beyond 60 fsw when more than 5 hr have elapsed before treatment is initiated, and this seems a reasonable procedure. After this amount of time, the feeling is that the patient's condition is primarily due to the initiation of pathological processes that are no longer susceptible primarily to the beneficial physical effects of pressure (i.e., reduction in bubble size).

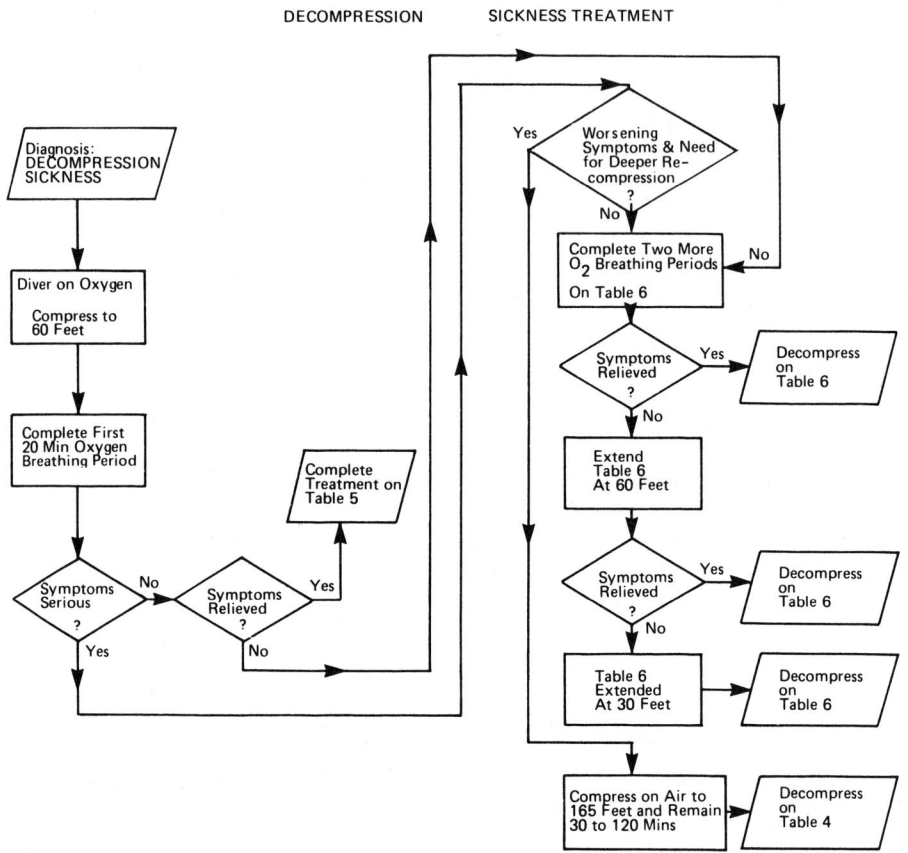

Figure VI-1. Flow chart for treatment of decompression sickness. [Adapted from *U.S. Navy Diving Manual* (1978).]

If it does become necessary to recompress to 165 fsw due to worsening symptoms, the flow chart (Figure VI-3) calls for completion of treatment on U.S. Navy Table 4 (Table VI-3) once the bottom time at 165 fsw exceeds 30 min (if complete relief was obtained in less than 30 min, the patient could be decompressed on U.S. Navy 6A; see Table VI-4). Again, with this regime an air-breathing observer must be locked in and the original attendant treated on U.S. Navy Table 6 as well.

The air breathing tables in the U.S. Navy Diving Manual (Table VI-3) are less effective than the short-duration oxygen Tables 5 and 6, are more apt to produce Type I DCS symptoms in the attendant (at least U.S. Navy Table 4 is), and should only be used when oxygen is not available for treatment. Use of the air tables is outlined in Table VI-3 and in the list of U.S. Navy recompression treatment tables (Table VI-5).

When DCS occurs at great depth, during an excursion from a saturation base, or explosively as in blowup (explosive decompression), heroic measures may be necessary to treat the victim; however, the basic philosophy behind treatment remains the same. The use of high partial pressures of oxygen (i.e., 1.5–2.8 ATA) forms the basis of

Table VI-3
U.S. Navy Air Recompression Tables

Stops	DCS, pain only		DCS, serious symptoms
Rate of descent 25 ft/min Rate of ascent 1 min between stops	Pain relieved at depths less than 66 fsw	Pain relieved at depths greater than 66 fsw If pain does not improve within 30 min at 165 ft, the case probably is not DCS; decompress on Table 2A	Serious symptoms include any of the following: 1. Unconsciousness 2. Convulsions 3. Weakness or inability to use arms or legs 4. Air embolism 5. Any visual disturbances 6. Dizziness 7. Loss of speech or hearing 8. Severe shortness of breath or chokes 9. Bends occuring while still under pressure Symptoms relieved in 30 min at 165 ft, use Table 3; if not relieved, use Table 4

Pressure, psi	ft	Table 1A[a]	Table 2A[a]	Table 3[a]	Table 4[a]
73.4	165		30 (air)	30 (air)	30 to 120 (air)
62.3	140		12 (air)	12 (air)	30 (air)
53.4	120		12 (air)	12 (air)	30 (air)
44.5	100	30 (air)	12 (air)	12 (air)	30 (air)
35.6	80	12 (air)	12 (air)	12 (air)	30 (air)
26.7	60	30 (air)	30 (air)	30 (O_2) or (air)	6 hr (air)
22.3	50	30 (air)	30 (air)	30 (O_2) or (air)	6 hr (air)
17.8	40	30 (air)	30 (air)	30 (O_2) or (air)	6 hr (air)
13.4	30	60 (air)	2 hr (air)	12 hr (air)	First 11 hr (air) Then 1 hr (O_2) or (air)
8.9	20	60 (air)	2 hr (air)	2 hr (air)	First 1 hr (air) Then 1 hr (O_2) or (air)
4.5	10	2 hr (air)	4 hr (air)	2 hr (air)	First 1 hr (air) Then 1 hr (O_2) or (air)
SURFACE		1 min (air)	1 min (air)	1 min (air)	1 min (O_2)

[a] Time at all stops in minutes unless otherwise indicated

treatment, together with rapid recompression ranging from 30 ft to the depth of relief. This may actually be equal to or greater than the depth of the dive, since a diver who is explosively decompressed from the bottom on a deep, long dive, say 300 fsw (92 msw) for 30 min, will have such massive bubbling that recompression to 165 fsw (50 msw) will be inadequate to restore circulation. The oxygen therapy usually consists of breathing an appropriate gas mixture by mask in cycles (20 min breathing the high P_{O_2} mix alternating with 5 min breathing the regular diving mixture) to minimize the occurrence of oxygen toxicity in the pulmonary and nervous systems. Up to six cycles are commonly used, and this may be repeated after a 6-hr "hold" at treatment depth. The patient would generally be maintained at treatment depth for 12–24 hr, or longer if necessary. Clearly after such a long treatment at a fixed depth, subsequent decompression must be according to a saturation profile, and appropriate help should be sought from an individual who is well informed on decompression from saturation. Obviously such treatment schemes can

Table VI-4

U.S. Navy Recompression Treatment Table 6A
(Oxygen Treatment)[a]

Depth		Time,	Breathing	Total elapsed time	
ft	m	min	medium	hr	min
165	50	30	Air		30
165—60	50–18	4	Air		34
60	18	20	Oxygen		54
60	18	5	Air		59
60	18	20	Oxygen	1	19
60	18	5	Air	1	24
60	18	20	Oxygen	1	44
60	18	5	Air	1	49
60–30	18—9	30	Oxygen	2	19
30	9	15	Air	2	34
30	9	60	Oxygen	3	34
30	9	15	Air	3	49
30	9	60	Oxygen	4	49
30–0	9–0	30	Oxygen	5	19

[a] Used for treatment of gas embolism when oxygen can be used and symptoms moderate to a major extent within 30 min at 165 ft. Descent rate is as fast as possible. Ascent rate is 1 ft/min. Do not compensate for slower ascent rates. Compensate for faster ascent rates by halting the ascent. Time at 165 ft includes time from the surface. If oxygen breathing must be interrupted, allow 15 min after the reaction time has entirely subsided and resume schedule at point of interruption. Tender breathes air throughout. If treatment is a repetitive dive for the tender or the table is lengthened, the tender should breathe oxygen during the last 30 min of ascent to the surface. [From *U.S. Navy Diving Manual* (1978).]

only be used when a chamber is available with a life-support system capable of monitoring and maintaining the oxygen, carbon dioxide, temperature, humidity, and trace contaminants within predetermined limits.

Driven primarily by the oil industry, development of procedures for nonsaturation diving at depths in excess of 400 ft has been much in evidence in recent years. These procedures are normally developed for a specific job (thus a specific depth and bottom time), often using specific equipment. During development, decompression tables for these dives are empirically modified until a certain number of symptomfree dives have been made on them; the tables may then be used operationally, but they usually require further modification after initial use. So while there exist acceptably safe tables for a certain number of depths, bottom times, and jobs deeper than 400 ft (122 m), no available theory allows one to safely extrapolate from one successful table to a new depth and bottom time. In 1975 an Undersea Medical Society workshop (Hamilton 1975) indicated that a high proportion of the total number of DCS cases occurring during this type of diving initially present with audiovestibular symptoms. As already indicated, the pathophysiology of this form of DCS may be quite different from that involved in other forms of DCS, and it is important to remember that in this situation recompression must be accomplished immediately and must be carried to the point at which relief begins to occur, or to the deepest depth of the dive, whichever is less.

Table VI-5
List of U.S. Navy Recompression Treatment Tables[a]

Table No.	Table title	Use
5	Oxygen treatment of pain-only decompression sickness	Treatment of pain-only decompression sickness when symptoms are relived within 10 min at 60 ft
6	Oxygen treatment of serious decompression sickness	Treatment of serious decompression sickness or pain-only decompression sickness when symptoms are not relieved within 10 min at 60 ft
6A	Air and oxygen treatment of gas embolism	Treatment of gas embolism; use also when unable to determine whether symptoms are caused by gas embolism or severe decompression sickness
1A	Air treatment of pain-only decompression sickness—100-ft treatment	Treatment of pain-only decompression sickness when oxygen unavailable and pain is relieved at a depth less than 66 ft
2A	Air treatment of pain-only decompression sickness—165-ft treatment	Treatment of pain-only decompression sickness when oxygen unavailable and pain is relieved at a depth greater than 66 ft
3	Air treatment of serious decompression sickness or gas embolism	Treatment of serious symptoms or gas embolism when oxygen unavailable and symptoms are relieved within 30 min at 165 ft
4	Air treatment of serious decompression sickness or gas embolism	Treatment of worsening symptoms during the first 20-min oxygen breathing period at 60 ft on Table 6, or when symptoms are not relieved within 30 min at 165 ft using air treatment Table 3

[a] This chart presents oxygen treatment tables before air treatment tables as the oxygen breathing method is preferred. Use of Decompression Table 5A-Minimal Decompression, Oxygen Breathing Method for Treatment of Decompression Sickness and Gas Embolism, has been discontinued. [From U.S. Navy Diving Manual (1978).]

Recurrence of DCS signs or symptoms either during treatment or after treatment can be managed as illustrated in the flow charts from the *U.S. Navy Diving Manual* (Figures VI-2 and VI-3). Recurrences can be difficult to differentiate from residual effects or incomplete relief. What appears to be a recurrence may actually be the onset of cerebral or spinal cord edema, and if this is suspected, pharmacological treatment of edema and hyperbaric oxygen therapy are called for. The patient should be observed for a further 6 hr beyond initial successful treatment or after treatment of a recurrence.

Attention should always be paid to prevention of pulmonary oxygen toxicity, particularly when repetitive treatments are given with the oxygen breathing tables. The higher the oxygen partial pressure, the greater the rate at which pulmonary oxygen toxicity occurs, and the shorter the latent period between initiation of oxygen breathing and onset of symptoms. Early signs of oxygen toxicity include tunnel vision, tinnitus, nausea, small-muscle fasciculation (especially of the hands and perioral areas), and dizziness, in addition to sore throat, coughing, and substernal pain. One method of measuring the damaging effects of total oxygen exposure uses the UPTD (Unit Pulmonary Toxic Dose) to calculate overall oxygen exposure (Wright 1972). One UPTD is defined as the effect

302   Chapter VI

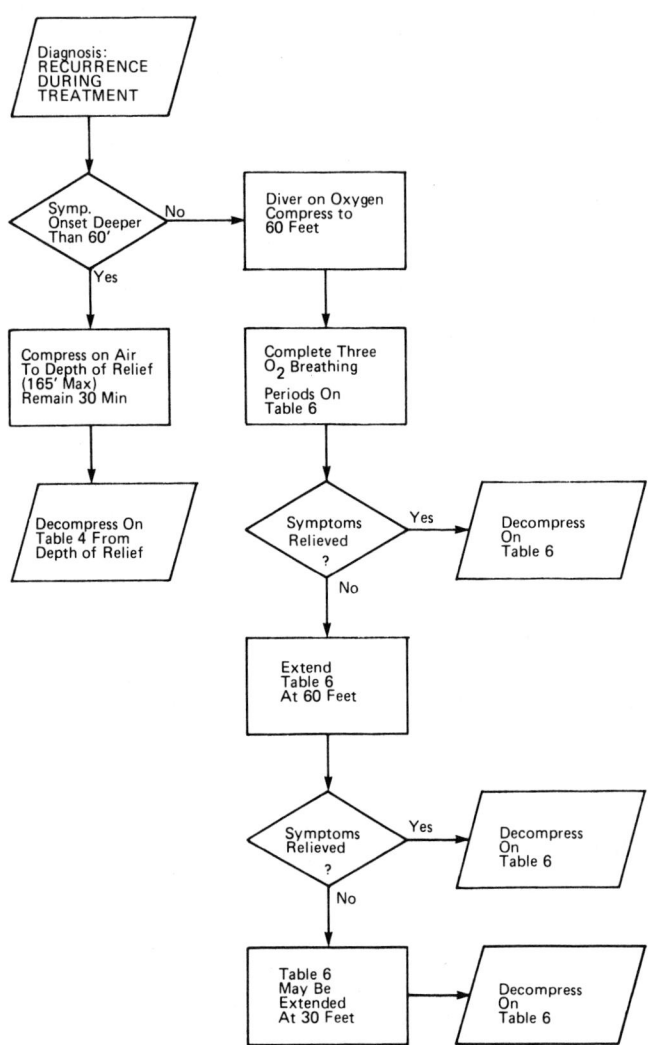

Figure VI-2. Flow chart for treatment of recurrence of decompression sickness during treatment. [Adapted from *U.S. Navy Diving Manual* (1978).]

of breathing a mixture with an oxygen partial pressure of 1 ATA for 1 min (for example, 100% oxygen at the surface for 1 min or a 50% oxygen mixture at 33 fsw (10 msw) for 1 min). The system is not fully reliable, however, and in the meantime clinical observations remain the diagnostic procedure of choice, remembering that in some cases pulmonary symptoms are acceptable if the overall benefit of oxygen outweighs the reversible lung trauma.

Not infrequently the question of using monoplace chambers for treating DCS is raised. These units have been used for on-site treatment of DCS, usually not without

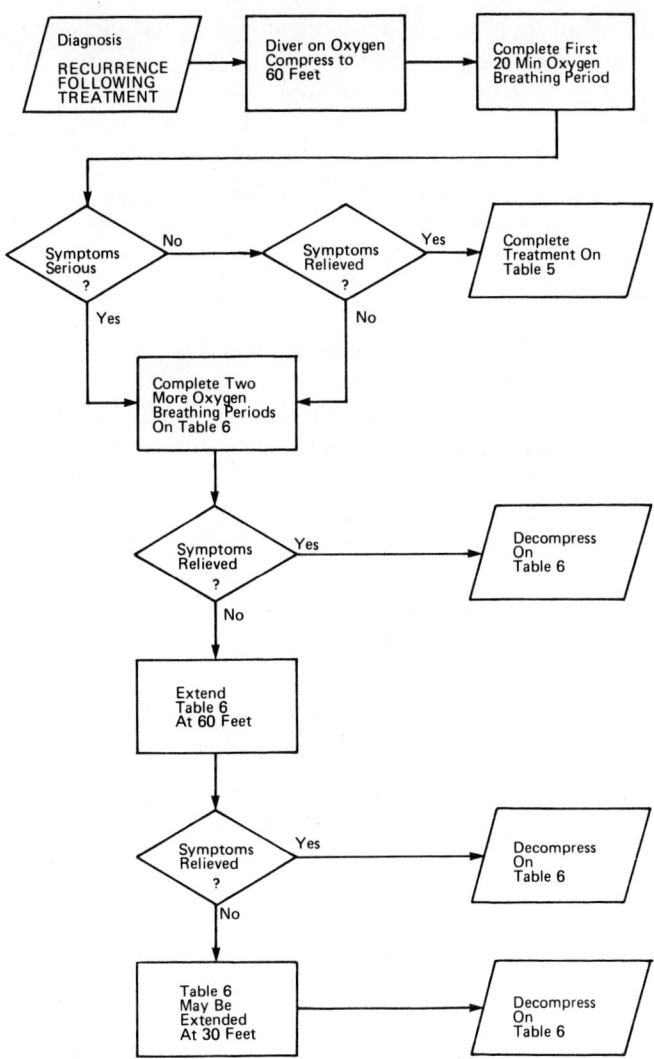

Figure VI-3. Flow chart for treatment of recurrence of decompression sickness following treatment. [Adapted from *U.S. Navy Diving Manual* (1978).]

significant problems. Originally, portable one-man chambers were intended for use in serious cases in remote areas, primarily as a way to transport patients under pressure to a larger chamber for definitive care, but difficulties have become apparent. Few larger chambers are able to accept or mate with one-man chambers. The one-man chambers are limited to short air tables (such as U.S. Navy Tables 1A and 2A), since they are not equipped for oxygen delivery or for prolonged treatment on air. Serious cases of DCS or arterial gas embolism are the worst risks for one-man chambers because there is no way to get to the patient (for airway clearing, anticonvulsive medication, cardiopulmonary resuscitation, etc.) once treatment has been initiated.

Several makes of one-man oxygen-filled chambers are in use in hospitals and clinics worldwide for the treatment of various nondiving disorders, and though of value for the disorders they were intended for, most authorities feel they are inadequate for treatment of DCS and arterial gas embolism, again primarily because the patient is inaccessible for supportive and sometimes lifesaving care. Also, with these chambers oxygen toxicity considerations limit the time a patient can be kept at pressure, even in cases where decompression to the surface would be contraindicated. In the rare instance when a life-threatening emergency occurs in a remote location where a one-man oxygen chamber is available, Kindwall has given the following guidelines: take the patient to a pressure of 59 fsw (18 msw) and hold there for 30 min. Then decompress over a 30-min period to 33 fsw (10 msw) and hold at that pressure for 60 min. Then decompress to the surface over another 30-min period. Repeat the complete procedure, after the patient has had a 30-min break breathing air on the surface, if complete relief has not been obtained. Avoid the use of these one-man oxygen chambers if at all possible, since large multiplace chambers have greater depth capabilities, allow breathing of gases other than pure oxygen, and are both safer and more effective in treating diving-related disorders.

In-water oxygen treatment of DCS, or use of oxygen supplied in water at a maximum depth of 30 fsw (9 msw), has been used successfully in remote regions of the Indian and Pacific Oceans (see Edmonds et al. 1981); the procedures, experienced personnel, and equipment that are mandatory before in-water decompression on air can be used are formidable: the victim must be conscious and able to care for themselves (otherwise even simple airway patency cannot be assured); the patient must have a full face mask or helmet (scuba with a mouthpiece is unacceptable); there must be a sufficient supply of gas for treatment of the victim, for attendants, and for backup; thermal protection must be assured, weather conditions good, and an experienced attendant with the victim at all times. If all these conditions cannot be met, the mildly ill patient should be put on oxygen by mask and transported to the nearest recompression facility, no matter how far away. The technique of in-water oxygen recompression is a treatment of last resort and is not suitable for worldwide or even widespread use. For example even in the subtropical waters of the Caribbean the dangers of hypothermia would be a very real problem. As for in-water recompression therapy with compressed air, virtually all experts strongly advise against it, not least because of the many tragic experiences that have resulted from such attempts.

While early recompression, oxygen, and time are the proven ingredients in successful management of DCS, adjunctive therapy (by and large pharmacological) is receiving increased attention and can be used in association with all recompression treatment regimens, though perhaps the most effective area of use, as covered in Chapter V, is during the immediate medical evaluation and transport of the diving casualty. The drugs that are most commonly used are blood volume expanders, anticoagulants, and anti-inflammatory agents.

To start with volume expanders, the dextrans (low-molecular-weight dextran-40 as well as its heavier analogue, dextran-70) have been recommended for use in DCS for many years. They expand intravascular volume osmotically and were thought to reduce blood viscosity and decrease platelet adhesiveness. Recent work indicates that the decrease in blood viscosity associated with their use can be attributed to hemodilution and that they do not really decrease platelet adhesiveness. So any plasma volume expander should be as effective as the dextrans for treatment of DCS without carrying the added risk of allergic reactions that are associated with its use. In any event, plasma volume expansion is clearly of therapeutic benefit. General advice is to treat pain-only DCS solely with recompression and high oxygen partial pressure, unless more than 3 to 5 hr have elapsed prior to treatment, in which case it is reasonable and prudent to give the patient 500–1000 ml of a balanced electrolyte solution. Advances in the knowledge of the importance of the microcirculation have made the administration of volume expanders routine in all cases of DCS complicated by serious symptoms or shock.

Recompression without adequate volume expansion may be insufficient in some cases to completely eliminate the symptoms of DCS. Similarly, with the administration of adequate intravenous therapy and the reconstitution of plasma volume, symptoms may subside.

Anticoagulants are the next drugs to mention in the pharmacological arsenal. Heparin has been postulated to be useful in the treatment of DCS. It interferes with and prevents blood clotting and also clears lipids from the blood. Heparin administered to animals prior to a decompression stress results in a lower incidence of DCS in these animals than in the untreated control animals. However, no controlled work has been done in human beings that shows that heparin is useful in the treatment of already established DCS, and it should never be used in audiovestibular DCS. Additionally, there are theoretical arguments that would indicate that the use of heparin in active central nervous system DCS might aggravate the lesion.

In addition to its analgesic and anti-inflammatory properties, aspirin, although not strictly an anticoagulant, does decrease platelet adhesiveness. Again, although assumed to be true from a theoretical viewpoint, there are no well-controlled studies indicating that aspirin is of benefit in acute DCS, and there are some indications that animals pretreated with aspirin prior to compression-decompression stress may have a higher incidence of aseptic bone necrosis. Aspirin has never been given to patients with DCS in a dose high enough to evaluate its anti-inflammatory effects in DCS.

The only other type of anti-inflammatory drugs that have been used extensively are the corticosteroid agents. Dexamethasone has been used frequently in the therapy of central nervous system DCS in the belief that it might reduce the spinal cord edema that may play a role in DCS. Once again there is no evidence currently available absolutely proving that these agents have a beneficial effect on the course of DCS, but they are often used on the advice of neurosurgeons and on the strength of the experience in that surgical subspecialty. Several regimens have been advocated. An example of one in widespread use is 100 mg of hydrocortisone i.v. and 12 mg of dexamethasone i.m. initially, followed by 6–8 mg of dexamethasone i.m. every 6 hr for an additional 48–72 hr. It can then be stopped abruptly, and although with this schedule steroid peptic ulcer is not felt to be a danger, I think it is still wise to cover a patient in a stress situation on steroids with a drug like cimetidine, which has been shown to be highly effective in affording protection from hyperacidity. Another reminder to tuck away, now that the use of corticosteroids has become so common, is that dexamethasone can exacerbate latent diabetes.

Several other agents, including mannitol, urea, and glycerol, have on occasion been used to treat DCS felt to be complicated by cerebral edema. Theoretically, glycerol would be preferable, since it reportedly does not cause rebound edema or derange electrolyte balance, and it exerts maximal effect in an hour (even intravenous corticosteroids have a minimum lag time of 4–6 hr before an effect can be demonstrated). Glycerol in a 50% solution of water flavored with lemonade for palatability can be given orally in a dosage of 0.8 ml/kg body wt. If medication cannot be given orally (or via a nasogastric tube), mannitol, 100 g in 500 ml fluid, can be run in intravenously over a period of an hour.

Intravenous Valium in 10-mg doses as necessary has been useful in controlling convulsions due to CNS damage. When a patient's nervous system is supressed pharmacologically, extreme care must be taken not to exceed depth-time limits relating to development of CNS oxygen toxicity.

A well-reported case by Norman et al. (1979) brings into focus all the modalities currently considered useful in the management of a complex diving accident—including recompression, oxygen, time, and intensive and adjunctive drug therapy.

Most of the practical aspects of managing patients in a hyperbaric chamber are covered elsewhere in the book. Here it will suffice to say that even with training (which is mandatory) the role of a diving physician should be largely advisory, and he or she will generally be much more effective outside a chamber than inside it. The decision to enter a chamber should not be taken lightly, and if necessary, the shorter and shallower the stay, the better. The length of stay can be facilitated by briefing both inside and outside personnel before being compressed, i.e., have the inside attendant prepare the patient for examination in advance, take all necessary equipment to avoid time-wasting lock-in maneuvers later on, etc. Note-cards and other "peripheral brains" can be very helpful in the confusing and distinctly non-hospitallike setting of the standard dive site or treatment site chamber (use pencils at depth; ballpoints and fountain pens tend to get DCS and make a mess). Consult another diving physician for advice and/or corroboration on all but the most simple cases. Even the most experienced offshore physicians do this for protection of their patients and of themselves. In making the decision to enter a chamber, a reasonable knowledge of your own narcotic limitations at various treatment depths is helpful, as is an awareness of your own repetitive dive limitations in planning subsequent entries for examinations or drug administration. Ensure that inside attendants are aware of the early signs of oxygen toxicity (tunnel vision, tinnitus, nausea, small-muscle fasciculation, especially of the hands and perioral regions, dizziness) and appropriate emergency measures (remove oxygen mask, wait 15 min, then resume treatment; if symptoms recur treatment can be continued at a lower oxygen partial pressure). In case of an oxygen convulsion, management is the same as for grand-mal–type convulsions from other causes, paying particular attention to protecting the patient from injury on the numerous hard projections in a chamber. If you are a consultant for a recompression facility in your area, check that a fully stocked, in-date crash bag is maintained at the site (for suggested equipment see Table VI-6).

From the point of view of the medical practitioner first called to give help, priority management of the patient will involve successful transfer to a recompression facility without delay. Some useful telephone numbers (subject to change) for medical advice on diving accidents or for advice concerning location of nearest recompression facility are as follows:

In the United States

- U.S. Navy Experimental Diving Unit, Panama City, Florida. Duty Medical Officer: (904) 234-4355 (24-hr diving accident watch).

Table VI-6
Equipment for the Treatment of Decompression Illnesses*

1. Surgical equipment and instruments 2 Small dressing bowls 2 Self-retaining catheters with sealed drainage bag attached 2 Intravenous giving sets with long drip chambers (e.g."xter) 4 20-ml syringes 4 2-ml syringes 4 10-ml syringes 10 No. 21 1½" hypodermic needles 10 No., 25 1" hypodermic needles 1 Laerdal resuscitator bag with a 100% oxygen fitting and with fitting to bib system 4 Medicut cannulae size 12 4 Medicut cannulae size 16 1 Disposable oro-pharyngeal airway (size 4) 1 No. 9 endotracheal tube 1 No. 9.5 endotracheal tube 1 Laryngoscope 1 Tourniquet 1 Mouth-to-mouth resuscitation tube 1 Pair of 7" mayo scissors 1 Foot operated sucker 2 Sucker catheters 1 Mouth gag 4 Pairs of 5" spencer wells 2 Pairs of 8" spencer wells 1 Sequestrene bottle 1 Plain blood bottle **2. Dressings** 2 Pairs sterile disposable gloves 12 Mediswabs 1 Roll 1" adhesive plaster 1 Tube urethral anaesthetic cream	2 Large shell dressings 100 g Cotton wool (sterile) 2 Sterile standard dressing packs **3. Drugs** 4 5 ml 1% xylocaine 50 ml hibitane solution 2 500 ml bottles macrodex in saline 2 1-liter bottles dextrose saline 3 Injections morphia 15 mg 1 Phial heparin, 5000 units/cc 25 Tablets diazepam 5 mg 50 Tablets prednisone 6 2-cc Injection frusemide 40 mg 6 2-cc Injection dexamethasone 5 mg/ml. 60 Soluble aspirin tablets 4 Injections diazepam 10 mg **4. Diagnostic instruments** 1 Pencil torch with batteries 1 Thermocouple thermometer 1 Stethoscope 1 Aneroid sphygmomanometer with a hole drilled in the outer case 1 Auriscope with spare batteries 1 Reflex hammer **5. Pneumothorax equipment** (to be packed in a separate container and labeled **"For Pneumothorax"**) Mediswabs 2-ml syringe and 21 G needle 2-ml of 2% xylocaine Disposable scalpel Argyle trochar catheter, No. 10, 23 cm Heimlich chest drain valve, No. 3460— Bard Parker Blenderm surgical tape

[a] Recommendations of Medical Equipment Sub-Committee of the European Undersea Bio-Medical Society, Dr. R. A. F. Cox, Chairman.

- Naval Medical Research Institute, Bethesda, Maryland. Duty Diving Medical Officer: (301) 295-0283 (24-hr diving accident watch).

- U.S. Air Force, San Antonio, Texas (24-hr consultative service in diving medicine and general hyperbaric medicine). Duty Hyperbaric Medical Officer: (512) LEO-FAST.

- Divers Alert Network (DAN), Duke University Medical Center, Durham, North Carolina. Switchboard operator at (919) 684-8111 will respond to word DAN by supplying information on closest regional diving accident center or satellite treatment facility (24-hr service).

- University of Southern California Medical Action Center (medical cover for recompression facility on Catalina Island west of Los Angeles): (213) 226-7087.

- U.S. Coast Guard (East Coast): (212) 264-8743 (for advice on chamber locations).

- U.S. Coast Guard (West Coast): (415) 556-5326.

In Canada

- Defence and Civil Institute for Environmental Medicine, Toronto, Ontario. Duty Diving Medical Officer: (416) 633-4240.

In the United Kingdom

- Royal Navy: HMS *Vernon*, Portsmouth: (0705)22351. (In working hours ask for The Superintendent of Diving, Ext. 872375, 872366, 872376. Out of working hours ask for the Duty Lieutenant Commander, Ext. 872413, 872414, 872415.)

- Offshore Medical Support, Aberdeen, Scotland: (0224) 871848. Telex 73677(Casvac).

- North Sea Medical Centre, Ltd., Great Yarmouth. (0493) 63264. Telex 975118 (Normed G).

In the Indo-Pacific

- Royal Australian Naval School of Underwater Medicine, HMAS *Penguin*, Balmoral, Sydney. Duty Medical Officer: (02)960-0444.

There is undoubtedly room for improvement in the investigation of DCS following therapy, even if the therapy has been overtly successful (since healing probably requires weeks and even then may not be complete). Apart from uncomplicated mild DCS, all cases deserve full investigation following therapy. Such investigation should be concentrated on providing relevant information on the etiology of the accident, in-hospital management of any alterations in pulmonary, cardiovascular, or other organ system status, and prognosis with regard to future diving. This kind of assessment and investigation after initial therapy has on occasion indicated the need for further active hyperbaric oxygen therapy. Two recent cases of vestibular DCS were ostensibly free of signs and symptoms following therapy. Immediate and full follow-up ear, nose, and throat investigation revealed a unilateral canal paresis in each case, and further hyperbaric oxygen therapy was successful in achieving normality.

When there are residual manifestations of DCS, major or minor, it has become standard practice to continue hyperbaric oxygenation once or twice daily for as long as definite improvement is seen with each session (most commonly Table 5 or 6 or their equivalents are used). There is no proof that this treatment effects the ultimate outcome but the consensus is that recovery is probably hastened. The benefits of physiotherapy should not be overlooked.

Coincidental illnesses such as myocardial infarctions, diabetes, appendicitis, and ruptured spleens have occurred along with DCS, and though they are easy to miss when thinking in terms of a diving illness, such conditions should be excluded as far as possible, since most recompression chambers are totally unsuitable for major surgery (see the chapter on emergency surgery and anesthesia at high pressure).

5. New Ideas

The prognosis when decompression sickness occurs in a sport diver is often less favorable than that for DCS occurring in the military or professional setting where treatment facilities and knowledgeable people are always immediately available. In contrast, the sport diver's case may be diagnosed correctly only after long delays and even then, transportation problems frequently cause further procrastination in treatment. Furthermore, although the U.S. Navy treats more than 100 nonmilitary divers every year, the procedures laid down in the *U.S. Navy Diving Manual* for treating DCS were developed for U.S. Navy divers, diving with U.S. Navy equipment, under U.S. Navy circumstances. While better care during transport to recompression facilities, combined with the use of the standard treatment tables already discussed, will result in satisfactory outcomes in the majority of cases (even most of the delayed cases and many cases improperly managed initially), there will be some difficult cases where the patient deteriorates either during or upon completion of standard treatment.

Present evidence is minimal, but alternative approaches are being investigated in several centers with the aim of developing superior treatment procedures for these difficult cases. These alternative approaches generally utilize recompression to between 100 and 165 fsw (30.5 and 50 msw), a stay at maximum pressure in excess of 2 hr, the use of enriched oxygen mixtures with one or more inert gases, and a saturation type of final decompression. Fluid resuscitation and pharmacological treatment of central nervous system edema are also important facets of these approaches. Evaluations of the therapeutic use of indomethacin and heparin and of prostaglandin inhibitors are examples of other current experimental therapeutic approaches.

The U.S. Navy is pursuing the option of being able to remain at 60 fsw (18 msw) indefinitely when the victim does not respond satisfactorily to standard therapy or deteriorates on attempted decompression. At 60 fsw the chamber can be maintained on air with intermittant 100% oxygen breathing periods until maximum benefit has been obtained; then saturation decompression on air to the surface can be undertaken. No special gas mixtures are required. To facilitate this procedure a new type of multiplace chamber has been designed, and modifications are planned for existing chambers. Such modifications include an oxygen analyzer to ensure continuous safe oxygen levels in the chamber, an oxygen overboard dump system to reduce ventilation requirements and fire hazard, a fan-driven CO_2 scrubber to reduce the ventilation required for control of metabolically produced carbon dioxide, and a heat exchanger or alternate cooling device for use in hot climates (serious consequences have been reported from tropical climes when no provisions were made to protect chamber occupants from overheating and dehydration). If these modifications and new generation of chambers are supported, a great deal more flexibility in the treatment of DCS will be possible.

Late in 1978 the Undersea Medical Society (1980) held a workshop on the effects of diving on pregnancy. As regards therapy of DCS, it is evident that oxygen partial pressures far greater than 1.0 ATA would be encountered if the need to be treated for

DCS arose in a pregnant patient. Since the teratogenic effects of high oxygen partial pressures are well documented, this possibility (of potential treatment and the risks involved) should be pointed out to pregnant women. It is only one of several reasons that one of the workshop's final recommendations was that women who are or may be pregnant are advised not to dive.

In conclusion, although DCS is a fascinating affliction from the viewpoint of the physiologist trying to understand it and the physician treating it, it is a potentially extremely serious condition that should (and could) be a rarity in diving. Because of the possible severity of DCS and the difficulties of treatment, the sport diver's first interest should be to prevent DCS by limiting exposure; this has always been the emphasis in military diving.

ROBERT F. GOAD

References

ALBANO, G. 1972. Hyperbaric oxygen therapy of decompression neuropathies and epiphyseal bone infarcts. Twenty-seven cases of gas embolism. *Ann. Med. Nav. (Rome)* 77: 497–534.

BARNARD, E. E. P. 1978. The use of oxygen and pressure as independent variables in the treatment of decompression sickness. In: *Congress Proceedings on Medical Aspects of Diving Accidents, Commission of the European Communities, Mines Safety and Health Commission, Luxembourg.*

BASSETT, B. E. 1979. The woman diver. *Sport Diver* Summer: 152–155.

BAYNE, C. G., W. S. HUNT, P. G. BRAY, AND D. C. JOHANSON 1979. Doppler diagnosis: a prospective clinical trial in human decompression sickness (Abstract). *Undersea Biomed. Res.* 6 (Suppl.):17.

BEHNKE, A. R., JR. 1951. Decompression sickness following exposure to high pressures. In: *Decompression Sickness*, edited by J. F. Fulton. Philadelphia: Saunders, p. 53–89.

BEHNKE, A. R., JR. 1974. Marine and other hyperbaric environments. In: *Environmental Physiology*, edited by N. B. Slouim. St. Louis: Mosby, p. 399–436.

BENNETT, P. B., AND D. H. ELLIOTT (editors) 1975. *The Physiology and Medicine of Diving and Compressed Air Work* (2nd ed.). London: Ballière, Tindall.

BERGHAGE, T. E., J. VOROSMARTI, JR., AND E. E. P. BARNARD 1978. Recompression treatment tables used throughout the world by government and industry. Rep. No. 78-16. Bethesda, MD: Naval Medical Research and Development Command.

BERT, P. 1878. *Barometric Pressure* (transl. by M. A. and F. A. Hitchcock). Columbus, OH: College Book Co., 1943. (Republ. Bethesda, MD: Undersea Medical Society, 1978.)

BLICK, G. 1909. [Correspondence.] *Br. Med. J.* December.

BORNMANN, R. C. 1967. Experience with minimal recompression, oxygen breathing treatment of decompression sickness and air embolism. Memorandum Rep. Washington, DC: U.S. Navy Experimental Diving Unit.

BOYCOTT, A. E., G. C. C. DAMANT, AND J. S. HALDANE 1908. Prevention of compressed air illness. *J. Hyg.* 8: 342–443.

BRUNNER, F. P., P. G. FRICK, AND A. A. BÜHLMANN 1964. Post-decompression shock due to extravasation of plasma. *Lancet* May: 1071.

BUCKLES, R. G., AND C. KNOX 1969. In vivo bubble detection by acoustic-optical imaging techniques. *Nature (Lond.)* 222: 771–772.

DAVIS, J. C. 1979. Treatment of decompression accidents among sport scuba divers with delay between onset and compression. In: *Treatment of Serious Decompression Sickness and Arterial Gas Embolism*, edited by J. C. Davis. Bethesda, MD: Undersea Medical Society. (Undersea Med. Soc. Workshop Rep. No. 34.)

DAVIS, J. C. (editor) 1979. *Treatment of Serious Decompression Sickness and Arterial Gas Embolism*. Bethesda, MD: Undersea Medical Society. (Undersea Med. Soc. Workshop Rep. No. 34.)

DAVIS, J. C., AND T. K. HUNT (editors) 1977. *Hyperbaric Oxygen Therapy.* Bethesda, MD: Undersea Medical Society.
DAVIS, R. W. 1962. *Deep Diving and Submarine Operations* (7th ed.). Chessington, Surrey, U.K.: Siebe-Gorman.
EDMONDS, C., C. LOWRY, AND J. PENNEFATHER 1981. *Diving and Subaquatic Medicine.* Mosman, Australia: Diving Medical Centre.
ELLIOTT, D. H. 1967. The bends—current concepts in the treatment of decompression sickness. *J. Bone Joint Surg. (Lond.)* 49B: 588–590.
ELLIOTT, D. H., J. M. HALLENBECK, AND A. A. BOVE 1974. Acute decompression sickness. *Lancet* (Occasional Survey) p. 1193.
ERDE, A., AND C. EDMONDS 1975. Decompression sickness. A clinical series. *J. Occup. Med.* 17(5): 324–328.
FERRIS, E. B., AND G. L. ENGEL 1951. The clinical nature of high altitude decompression sickness. In: *Decompression Sickness*, by J. F. Fulton. Philadelphia: Saunders.
FLYNN, E. T., AND C. G. BAYNE 1977. *Diving Medical Officer Student Guide* (manual for U.S. Naval School of Diving and Salvage, Course No. A-6A-0010).
GOAD, R. F., AND T. S. NEUMAN 1977. Decompression sickness: state of the art 1977. *Mar. Technol. Soc. J.* 11: 8–12.
GOODMAN, M. W., AND R. D. WORKMAN 1965. Minimal-recompression, oxygen-breathing approach to treatment of decompression sickness in divers and aviators. Rep. No. 5-65. Washington, DC: U.S. Navy Experimental Diving Unit.
GRIFFITHS, P. D. 1969. Clinical manifestations and treatment of decompression sickness in divers. In: *The Physiology and Medicine of Diving and Compressed Air Work*, edited by P. B. Bennett and D. H. Elliott. London: Ballière, Tindall, p. 451–463.
HAMILTON, R. W. (editor) 1975. *Development of Decompression Procedures for Depths in Excess of 400 Feet.* Bethesda, MD: Undersea Medical Society. (9th Workshop 2-28-76.)
HAYMAKER, W. 1957. Decompression sickness. In: *Handbuch des speziellen pathologischen Anatomie und Histologie*, edited by O. Lubarsch, F. Henke, and R. Rossie. Berlin: Springer-Verlag, Vol. XIII, Pt. I, p. 1600–1672.
HELLER, R., W. MAGER, AND H. VON SCHRÖTTER 1900. *Luftdruckerkrankungen mit besonderer Berucksichtigung der sogenannten Caissonkrankheit.* Vienna: Holder. [Engl. title: Air pressure illnesses with particular emphasis on the so-called caisson's disease.]
HILL, L. 1912. *Caisson Sickness and the Physiology of Work in Compressed Air.* London: Edward Arnold.
HILLS, B. A. 1977. *Decompression Sickness. The Biophysical Basis of Prevention and Treatment.* New York: John Wiley, Vol. 1.
INWOOD, M. J. 1973. Experimental evidence in support of the hypothesis that intravascular bubbles activate the hemostatic process. In: *Proceedings, Symposium on Blood-Bubble Interaction in Decompression Sickness*, edited by K. N. Ackles. Downsview, Ontario: Canadian Defense Research Board. (Canada DCIEM Conf. Proc. 73-CP-960.)
JAMES, P. B. 1977. The detection of pneumothorax by ultra-sound. In: *Proceedings of the Seventh International Hyperbaric Congress, Aberdeen, Scotland.*
JAMINET, A. 1871. *Physical effects of compressed air and of the pathological symptoms produced in man, by increased atmospheric pressure employed for the sinking of piers in the construction of the Illinois and St. Louis Bridge over the Mississippi River at St. Louis, Missouri.* St. Louis: R. and T. A. Ennis, p. 135.
KEAYS, F. L. 1909. Compressed air illness, with a report of 3,692 cases. *Publ. Cornell Univ. Med. Coll.* 2: 1–55.
KENT, M. B. (editor) 1978. *Effects of Diving on Pregnancy.* Bethesda, MD: Undersea Medical Society. (19th Workshop.)
KIDD, D. J., AND D. H. ELLIOTT 1969. Clinical manifestations and treatment of decompression sickness in divers. In: *The Physiology and Medicine of Diving and Compressed Air Work*, edited by P. B. Bennett and D. H. Elliott. London: Ballière, Tindall, p. 306–413.
KINDWALL, E. P. 1975. Medical aspects of commercial diving and compressed air work. In: *Occupational Medicine Principles and Practical Applications*, edited by C. Zenz. Chicago: Year Book Medical Publ.
MILES, S., AND D. MACKAY 1976. *Underwater Medicine.* Philadelphia: Lippincott.
MILLER, J. N., L. FAGRAEUS, P. B. BENNETT, D. H. ELLIOTT, T. G. SHIELDS, AND J. GRIMSTAD 1978. Nitrogen-oxygen saturation therapy in serious cases of compressed-air decompression sickness. *Lancet* 2: 169–171.

NEUMAN, T. S., D. A. HALL, AND P. G. LINAWEAVER 1976. Gas phase separation during decompression in man: ultra-sound monitoring. *Undersea Biomed. Res.* 3: 121–130.

NORMAN, J. M., C. M. CHILDS, C. JONES, J. A. R. SMITH, J. ROSS, G. RIDDLE, A. MACINTOSH, N. I. P. MCKIE, I. I. MACCAULEY, AND X. FRUCTUS 1979. Management of a complex diving accident. *Undersea Biomed Res.* 6: 209–216.

PEARSON, R. R., AND R. DE G. HANSON 1979. Diving accidents. *Practitioner* 222: 793–797.

PEARSON, R. R., AND D. R. LEITCH 1979. Treatment of air or oxygen/nitrogen mixture decompression illness in the Royal Navy. *J. R. Nav. Med. Serv.* 65: 53–62.

PENZIAS, W., AND M. W. GOODMAN 1973. *Man Beneath the Sea—A Review of Underwater Engineering*. New York: John Wiley.

POL, B., AND T. J. J. WATELLE 1854. Memoire sur les effects de la compression de l'air. *Ann. Hyg. Publ. Med. Legale Paris* 1: 241–279.

RIVERA, J. C. 1964. Decompression sickness among divers; an analysis of 935 cases. *Mil. Med.* 129: 316–334.

ROYAL NAVY 1972. *Royal Navy Diving Manual*. London: Her Majesty's Stationery Office. (BR 2806.)

SHILLING, C. W., AND M. W. BECKETT (editors). 1976. *National Plan for the Safety and Health of Divers in Their Quest for Subsea Energy*. Bethesda, MD: Undersea Medical Society.

SHILLING, C. W., M. F. WERTS, AND N. R. SCHANDELMEIER (editors). 1976. *The Underwater Handbook: A Guide to Physiology and Performance for the Engineer*. New York: Plenum Press.

SLARK, A. G. 1962. *Treatment of 137 cases of decompression sickness*. RNPRC Rep. 63-1030. London: Medical Research Council.

SPAUR, W. H. 1979. U.S. Navy treatment methods. In: *Treatment of Serious Decompression Sickness and Arterial Gas Embolism*, edited by J. C. Davis. Bethesda, MD: Undersea Medical Society. (Undersea Med. Soc. Workshop Rep. No. 34.)

STRAUSS, R. H. (editor) 1976. *Diving Medicine*. New York: Grune and Stratton.

STRAUSS, R. H. AND D. E. YOUNT 1977. Decompression sickness. *Am. Scientist* 65: 598–604.

TRIGER, M. 1841. Memoire sur un appareil à air comprimé, pour le percement des puits de mines et autres travaux, sous eaux et dans les sables submergés. *C.R. Acad. Sci. (Paris)* 13: 884.

U.S. NAVY 1975. *U.S. Navy Diving Manual. (Change 2). Air Diving*. Washington, DC: U.S. Department of the Navy, Vol. 1. (NAVSEA 0994-LP-001-9010.)

U.S. NAVY 1978. *U.S. Navy Diving Manual (Change 2). Air Diving*. Washington, DC: U.S. Department of the Navy, Vol. 1. (NAVSEA 0994-LP-001-9010.)

VANDERAUE, O. E., W. A. WHITE, R. HAYTER, E. S. BRINTON, J. R. KELLAR, AND A. R. BEHNKE 1945. *Physiologic factors underlying the prevention and treatment of decompression sickness*. Rep. No. 1. Washington, DC: U.S. Navy Experimental Diving Unit.

WRIGHT, W. B. 1972. *Use of the University of Pennsylvania, Institute for Environmental Medicine procedure for calculation of cumulative pulmonary oxygen toxicity*. Rep. No. 2-72. Washington, DC: U.S. Navy Experimental Diving Unit.

B. Inner Ear Decompression Sickness

1. Introduction

Several 19th and early 20th century investigators noted otologic injuries in divers. A. H. Smith, in his 1873 description of so-called caisson disease, noted severe deafness and vestibular problems among other injuries in compressed air workers. Heller et al. (1895) and Alt et al. (1897) described both middle and inner ear injuries during compression and decompression. These investigators were among the first to suggest that inner ear injuries occurring during decompression were related to nitrogen bubble formation in the labyrinthine vasculature. Vail (1929) also noted that middle and inner ear injuries could occur in compressed air workers during compression and decompression. He performed animal studies with histological observations and concluded that otologic injuries occurring during decompression were related to nitrogen bubbles causing emboli or necrosis in the inner ear.

In the 1930s and 1940s safety procedures for air diving improved, and the frequency of inner ear injuries in diving apparently decreased. Indeed, most of the diving literature concerning decompression sickness (DCS) noted symptoms suggestive of inner ear injury only in association with what was thought to be central nervous system decompression sickness, where the inner ear symptoms were relegated to secondary importance and frequently considered related to lesions located in the central nervous system (CNS). Hearing loss and tinnitus, with or without vertigo, occurring during or shortly after decompression were often not treated, for isolated inner ear decompression sickness was not thought likely to occur, or, at most, to be rare. Such conclusions made at that time are understandable now: isolated inner ear injuries are usually not life threatening unless a diver experiences severe vertigo with nausea and vomiting while underwater; the vestibular symptoms resulting from destruction of one inner ear will usually subside after a few weeks even though no recovery of inner ear function has occurred, as noted in Chapter 3-K; and the frequency of isolated inner ear decompression sickness appears to be much greater with deeper helium-oxygen diving than with the air diving, the major diving medium during those decades.

During the 1960s and 1970s, exposures to deeper depths using mixed helium atmospheres became frequent. Isolated symptoms were described of inner ear dysfunction occurring during or shortly after decompressions from dives in which decompression sickness is possible, and the syndrome of inner ear decompression sickness was recognized. Buhlmann and Waldvogel (1967), describing 82 decompression accidents from a series of dives ranging in bottom depths from 11 ATA to 23 ATA, noted that the only neurological symptoms of the entire series consisted of vertigo, nausea, vomiting, and tinnitus in 11 divers, with hearing loss being present in 2 of these divers. These cases apparently were only noted during decompressions from dives with deeper bottom depths, 147–221 m. In a later publication, Buhlmann and Gehring (1976) described 12 cases of inner ear symptoms after 24 decompressions from depths ranging from 42.05 to 305 m.

a. Recent Human Studies

Farmer and colleagues (1976) have described 23 cases of isolated inner ear symptoms occurring during or shortly after decompression from 4 air and 19 helium-oxygen exposures. Ten of these cases had been previously noted by Rubenstein and Summitt (1971). None of these cases were associated with symptoms suggestive of middle ear barotrauma during compression, otologic symptoms while at the maximum depth, uncontrolled or rapid ascents, nor with other symptoms or signs suggestive of central nervous system decompression sickness. Ten of these divers were noted to have vertigo only, 7 were noted to have hearing loss and tinnitus only, and 6 exhibited hearing loss, tinnitus, and vertigo.

In this series, a significant correlation between prompt recompression treatment and recovery was noted. The 11 divers who were recompressed within 42 min after the onset of otologic symptoms experienced relief during recompression, and subsequent studies revealed no residual inner ear dysfunction. Three divers were recompressed within 60 to 68 min after symptom onset; one of these experienced relief of symptoms. The remaining

2 divers had only partial or no relief and demonstrated significant residual inner ear dysfunction after treatment. In the remaining cases, recompression treatment was either delayed longer than 68 min after symptom onset or was not given, and the divers experienced residual inner ear dysfunction.

Thirteen of the nineteen helium dives in this series involved a switch to an air atmosphere at depths ranging from 60 to 150 ft (18 to 53 m) during the latter stages of decompression. In one of these patients the symptoms began before the air switch but became more severe after the diver had entered the air atmosphere. The authors postulated that the sudden decrease in helium partial pressure possibly contributed to formation of helium gas bubbles in inner ear tissues during decompression. Another speculated pathophysiological mechanism involved the formation of bubbles at inner ear tissue boundaries resulting from the counterdiffusion of two different gases between inner ear fluid compartments, similar to the counterdiffusion mechanism suggested by Lambertsen and Idicula (1975) to explain the inner ear injuries noted at stable deep depths after inert gas changes.

b. Recent Animal Studies

Recent animal studies have increased our understanding of the pathophysiology of inner ear decompression sickness. McCormick et al. (1975) showed that guinea pigs subjected to rapid decompression developed bubble formations and hemorrhages in the labyrinthine fluid spaces and decreases in cochlear potentials, along with other manifestations of decompression sickness. McCormick and his colleagues also observed that the deficiencies in inner ear electrical function in decompressed guinea pigs could be lessened by treatment of the animals with heparin prior to the dives. This suggested that a key mechanism of inner ear decompression sickness may be hypercoagulation in the inner ear microvasculature, as described by Philp (1974) in his investigations of coagulation changes in decompression sickness, or lipid emboli, or both. Recent extensive investigations by Landolt et al. (1980) using squirrel monkeys have revealed that the inner ear in the squirrel monkeys, apparently similar to the inner ear in man, is unusually susceptible to decompression sickness. Clinical observations, electronystagmographic recordings, and postdive histological studies revealed that the symptoms of inner ear dysfunction occurred during the latter stages of decompression and were related to inner ear abnormalities. Central nervous system decompression sickness did occur in some animals and most frequently involved the spinal cord. Histological studies demonstrated varying degrees of hemorrhagic lesions and granular precipitate in the labyrinth. Inner ears of monkeys killed 38 to 383 days following decompression showed the appearance of connective tissue and new bone growth in the damaged regions of the semicircular canals. No apparent differences in the inner ear injuries were noted with different ambient gases, with switching of gases during the latter stages of decompression, nor with the type of diving profile.

2. Management of Inner Ear Decompression Sickness

As a result of the human investigations, the following principles of management of inner ear decompression sickness were proposed by Farmer et al. in 1976 and, thus far, appear to be effective:

1. Vertigo, nausea, vomiting, and tinnitus with or without hearing loss that begins during or shortly after the decompression phase of dives in which decompression sickness is possible should be considered as likely to represent inner ear decompression sickness. Prompt recompression is essential. Divers who experience such symptoms during or shortly after a switch to an air environment during decompression from deep helium oxygen exposures should be switched back to the presymptom helium oxygen atmosphere and recompressed promptly.

2. The optimum treatment depth or depth of recompression has not been established. Theoretically, the optimum recompression depth is the lesser of the depth of relief or the bottom depth. Nevertheless, labyrinthine trauma from inner ear bubble formation may result in hemorrhage or structural deformities, and prompt relief will not be seen, even though an adequate depth of recompression to drive the bubbles back into solution is achieved. Returning to the bottom depth in some situations may be hazardous or impractical. Therefore it was arbitrarily suggested that the optimum treatment depth in these situations should be at least 3 atm deeper than the depth of symptom onset. This seems to be adequate; future studies are needed, however, to more precisely define the optimum recompression profile. When symptom onset occurs after surfacing, prompt recompression using recompression tables suitable for treatment of central nervous system decompression sickness should be used.

3. Drugs that supposedly increase intracranial and inner ear blood flow are generally not effective in this regard and may result in shunting of blood flow to the periphery. Also, if labyrinthine hemorrhage has occurred, as indicated by animal studies, anticoagulants may result in additional intracochlear bleeding. Thus, these agents are considered potentially harmful and not recommended once DCS has started.

4. Diazepam, 5 to 15 mg i.m., has been noted to result in significant relief of vertigo, nausea, and vomiting during otologic decompression sickness. This drug can suppress the nystagmus accompanying such injuries and thus mask a sign of optimum treatment. In many cases, however, the symptoms are so severe that relief is essential. Monitoring of respiratory rate and blood pressure is desirable after parenteral administration of this drug.

5. Fluid replacement and other measures such as the administration of oxygen-enriched treatment gases (advocated in the treatment of general decompression sickness) are indicated. Whether or not steroids and salicylates are beneficial in the management of inner ear decompression sickness is not known. Certainly, if significant hemorrhage has occurred, the use of salicylates would not be desirable because of an additional anticoagulation effect. In addition, salicylates are potentially ototoxic.

6. A complete otologic examination as soon as possible after adequate recompression therapy is essential. This includes a complete history, physical examination including neurological evaluation, audiometry, and electronystagmography. A disappearance of vestibular symptoms several weeks after the injury does not usually mean that recovery of inner ear function has occurred, for central nervous system compensation will take place and cause individuals who have completely lost inner ear vestibular function on one side to become essentially asymptomatic provided a normal inner ear is present on the uninjured side.

7. Divers who suffer permanent inner ear dysfunction as a result of inner ear decompression sickness should not be returned to diving. Further inner ear injury to the same ear is felt by some to be more likely and could result in extreme danger at depth

from the associated vertigo and possible nausea and vomiting. Also, injury to the opposite ear during further diving could result in significant disability for nondiving activities in occupational or life skills involving communication or balance.

JOSEPH C. FARMER, JR.

References

ALT, F., R. HELLER, W. MAGER. AND H. VON SCHROTTER 1897. Pathologie der Luftdruckerkrankungen der Gehörorgans. *Monatsschr. Ohrenheilkd. Laryngorhinol.* 31: 229–242. (Pathology of Air Pressure Diseases of the Auditory Organs, transl. by A. Woke. Naval Medical Research Institute, 1972.)

BÜHLMANN, A. A., AND H. GEHRING 1976. Inner ear disorders resulting from inadequate decompression—"vertigo bends." In: *Underwater Physiology V, Proceedings of the Fifth Symposium on Underwater Physiology*, edited by C. J. Lambertsen. Bethesda, MD.: Fed. Am. Soc. Exp. Biol. p. 341–347.

BÜHLMANN, A., AND W. WALDVOGEL 1967. The treatment of decompression sickness. *Helv. Med. Acta* 33: 487–491.

FARMER, J. C., W. G. THOMAS, D. G. YOUNGBLOOD. AND P. B. BENNETT 1976. Inner ear decompression sickness. *Laryngoscope.* 86: 1315–1327.

HELLER, R., W. MAGER AND, H. VON SCHROTTER 1895. Vorlaufige Mittheilung über Caissonarbeiter. *Wien, Klin. Wochenschr.* 8: 475–476. (Introductory Report on Caisson Workers, transl. by A. Woke. Medical Research Institute, 1972.)

LAMBERTSEN, C. J., AND J. IDICULA 1975. A new gas lesion syndrome in man, induced by "isobaric gas counterdiffusion." *J. Appl. Physiol.* 39: 434–443.

LANDOLT, J. P., K. E. MONEY, E. D. L. TOPLIFF, A. D. NICHOLAS, J. LAUFER. AND W. H. JOHNSON 1980. Pathophysiology of inner ear dysfunction in the squirrel monkey in rapid decompression. *J. Appl. Physiol.* 49: 1070–1082.

MCCORMICK, J. G., W. B. HOLLAND, R. W. BRAUER. AND I. L. HOLLEMAN, JR. 1975. Sudden hearing loss due to diving and its prevention with heparin. *Otolaryingol. Clin. N. Am.* 8: 2: 417–430.

PHILP, R. B. 1974. A review of blood changes associated with compression-decompression: relationship to decompression sickness. *Undersea Biomed. Res.* 1: 117–150.

RUBENSTEIN, C. J., AND J. K. SUMMITT 1971. Vestibular derangement in decompression. In: *Underwater Physiology IV. Proceedings of the Fourth Symposium on Underwater Physiology*, edited by C. J. Lambertsen. New York: Academic Press, p. 287–292.

SMITH, A. H. 1873. *The Effects of High Atmospheric Pressure, Including the Caisson Disease.* Brooklyn, NY: Eagle Print, p. 1–53.

VAIL, H. H. 1929. Traumatic conditions of the ear in workers in an atmosphere of compressed air. *Arch Otolaryngol.* 10: 113–126.

C. Neurological Forms of Decompression Sickness

1. Overview and Introduction

Approximately 10%–35% of those cases of decompression sickness that come to active treatment will show some signs of central nervous system involvement (Rivera 1966; Slark 1965). Rarely will such patients show central nervous system involvement exclusively. The majority of the patients will also exhibit musculoskeletal symptoms; in addition, other systems commonly may be involved (Slark 1965).

The patients exhibiting central nervous system involvement present the most difficult treatment problems, and a significant number will never achieve a complete cure in spite of all known treatments.

Prodromal indications of neurological decompression sickness may include pain in conjunction with cardiopulmonary and constitutional upset. This may take the form of a cardiopulmonary embarrassment known as *the chokes*, which may progress to clinical shock. The prelude may be only a severe fatigue disproportionate to the preceding exertion, but it may lead to peripheral vasoconstriction, nausea, sweating, hypotension, and malaise.

The chokes are a triad of signs and symptoms: (1) There is a burning substernal pain of increasing severity. At first, it may be apparent only on coughing, but it progresses to frank inspiratory and expiratory pain. (2) A cough, intermittent at first and readily provoked by smoking, develops into uncontrollable paroxysms. (3) There is progressive dyspnea and respiratory distress. The cause is presumed to be the combined effects of gaseous embolization of the pulmonary artery and the release, within blood and from lung, of smooth-muscle–active substances causing vasoconstriction and possibly bronchoconstriction (Chryssanthou et al. 1970). The vasoconstriction can raise capillary hydrostatic pressure leading to pulmonary edema.

Shock, with which the chokes is sometimes associated, may be due to a combination of mechanisms. Contributing factors may be a loss of vascular tone caused by cord involvement, myocardial depression from hypoxemia and acidosis, and pulmonary embolization. A major mechanism is hypovolemia. The hypovolemia probably results from a widespread increase in capillary permeability and cell sludging, which leads to loss of plasma water and a consequent increase in hematocrit (Cockett and Nakamura 1964a, 1964b).

As decompression sickness is caused by vascular obstruction arising from random *in situ* bubble formation within the vascular system, presentation of neurological decompression sickness is largely unpredictable. However, the spinal cord is the area most frequently afflicted, because of the peculiar physiology of the epidural vertebral venous system and comparatively tenuous blood supply of the spinal cord (Woollam and Miller 1958).

Aviators frequently suffer cerebral lesions presenting in protean ways, but commonly manifested by migrainelike headaches with visual disturbances and, occasionally, hemiparesis (Fryer and Roxburgh 1965).

Spinal lesions are more common than cerebral lesions in divers, presenting classically as regional sensory disturbances, paraplegia, and paralysis of bowel and bladder with urine retention and fecal incontinence. Less commonly, radicular trunk pain may also indicate cord involvement.

These various forms of decompression sickness tend to develop rapidly after the offending decompression and, because of the dominantly vascular nature of the disease, the first aid measures and subsequent treatment include circulatory support and measures to counteract sludging and stasis, in addition to recompression and hyperbaric oxygen administration for the removal of the root cause.

The following example observed by one of us (D. Leitch) illustrates the complexity and duration of a very severe case, with spinal and supraspinal involvement:

An "experienced" professional diver carried out an energetic wreck survey in about 180 ft (55 m) of water. After 25 min, he surfaced directly. While getting another diving set ready in order to complete his task, he developed shoulder pain, which disappeared when he dived again. After another 20 min, he again surfaced directly, but was so fatigued that he had to be lifted into the boat for transport to the nearby ship to undergo surface decompression. Within 5 to 10 min of surfacing, while on his way across the deck to the chamber, he became unsteady and had to be assisted into the chamber. The surface decompression table was commenced and during the initial decompression to 40 ft (12 m), he became aphasic, lost the coordination of both arms, and developed severe tremor in both legs. During several unorthodox treatment maneuvers, and before expert help was summoned, he twice lost consciousness and briefly lost the sight in one eye. After a subsequent stormy course that was managed by means of pressure, oxygen, drugs, and fluids, he was left with an almost complete paraplegia; various sensory deficits, mostly below T8, although one arm was patchily involved; asymmetric weakness of both forearms and hands; a paralyzed bladder; and fecal incontinence. Subsequent intensive rehabilitation enabled him to walk without aid after 8 months. Bladder control returned within 8 weeks, and he even regained the capacity for sexual intercourse, although there was some residual sensory deficit.

2. Clinical Presentation

a. Onset

It should be remembered that neurological decompression sickness is often preceded by musculoskeletal pain, chokes, general malaise, or any combination of these. A number of observers have reported the occurrence of respiratory problems as a precursor to neurological decompression sickness (Behnke and Shaw 1937; Hallenbeck et al. 1975b; Heller et al. 1900).

The latency for development of serious forms of DCS tends to be shorter than that of pain-only bends. In a detailed series of cases monitored by Kidd and Elliott (1975), all of the neurological cases had presented within about 90 min of surfacing; the pain-only cases had continued to occur for up to 15 hr.

Failure to diagnose neurological decompression sickness is a recurrent problem because a subtle neurological deficit may be less apparent than joint pain, which is distressing but less likely to leave a permanent sequela. There is often some functional power loss associated with severe pain, and the differentiation between the two problems is never easy, even with experience. Thus, there is a risk of overlooking what is in fact the main problem and, consequently, undertreating it. Slark (1965), in a retrospective survey of cases treated by the Royal Navy, suggests that his apportioning of serious cases into categories may, in fact, be an underestimate of their frequency for this very reason. In addition, many patients are seen and treated by medically unskilled personnel who are unable to make fine discriminations on the physical examination and may fail to perceive subtle signs of neurological disease.

b. Signs and Symptoms

A summary of perhaps the three best-known surveys of decompression sickness in divers is given in Table VI-7. Although it is not obvious from the surveys in the format presented in Table VI-7, neurological cases are dominated by cord lesions, but involve-

Table VI-7
Distribution of Signs and Symptoms in Serious Decompression Sickness

	Percentage of all cases surveyed
Rivera 1966 ($N = 935$)	
Numbness/paresthesia	21.2
Muscular weakness	20.6
Paralysis	6.1
Urinary disturbance	2.5
Muscular twitching	1.2
Incoordination	0.9
Dizziness/vertigo	8.5
Nausea/vomiting	7.9
Visual disturbance	6.8
Headache	3.9
Unconsciousness	2.7
Personality change	1.6
Agitation/restlessness	1.3
Convulsion	1.1
Equilibrium disturbances	0.7
Auditory	0.3
Cranial nerves	0.2
Aphasia	0.2
Dyspnea	2.0
Fatigue	1.2
Slark 1965 ($N = 137$)	
Disorder of sensation	8.0
Disorder of power	11.0
Vertigo	4.4
Nausea/vomiting	5.1
Visual disorder	2.2
Headache	3.6
Unconsciousness	2.9
Shock	5.8

	Percentage of serious cases only
Kidd and Elliott 1975 (total $N = 250+$)	
Sensory impairment	25
Motor impairment	13
Dizziness	19
Nausea/vomiting	5
Visual disorder	10
Confusion/disorientation	14
Dysarthria	3
Dyspnea/coughing	17

ment of the vestibular system, the cranial nerves, the brain stem, or the cerebrum is not rare.

Because virtually any area of brain can be affected, there are many possible manifestations of cerebral decompression sickness, among them: behavioral disorders (moodiness, change of affect, loss of judgment), psychoses, visual blurring, diplopia, scotomata, hemianopsia, fortification spectra, migrainous headaches (usually in those with a history of migraine), speech disorders, motor weakness, sensory disturbances, incoordination, unconsciousness, and frank convulsions (Rivera 1966).

The development of cord lesions is often insidious, with slowly developing paresthesias and slight limb weakness that may be overshadowed by localized pain or the chokes, until well advanced. A pins-and-needles sensation may be felt in the feet, which later feel woolly and cold. The subsequent evolution of the disease may be slow or fast and may lead to paraplegia with loss of bladder and sphincter control. Several different cord segments may be affected at once, giving patchy neurological deficits; unilateral involvement can occur. The lower extremities commonly are more affected than the arms. Lesions may not be strictly segmental, and cases of "glove-and-stocking" sensory deficit have been seen.

Back, chest, and abdominal girdle pain may herald a cord problem. Care must be taken either not to attribute the pains to simple musculoskeletal bends or to pass them off as colic resulting from visceral gas.

The diversity and multifocal nature of the lesions make careful neurological examination important in all cases. However, this should not be allowed to cause significant delays in treatment. Occasionally, some previous condition or injury may predispose the patient to the onset of DCS and even determine the site of the lesion. We have seen cases where a prolapsed intervertebral disk was a contributing factor. The following case described by Kidd and Elliott (1975) is a good example:

> As part of an investigation into the cause of an epileptiform convulsion while diving, a 25-year-old diver had a lumbar puncture. The results were normal, though during the procedure, his right leg had twitched for a second or two, indicating some nerve root irritation. Six days later, having been declared fully fit to resume diving, he dived on air to 50 ft (2.5 ATA) for 25 min. This is a very safe dive, yet for 2 hours afterwards, he noticed a strip of tingling down the length of the back of his right leg, though he did not report this. Some 20 days after the lumbar puncture, he dived on air to 180 ft (6.5 ATA) for 15 min, another safe dive but requiring some decompression stoppages. After 45 min since surfacing, he noticed the onset of analgesia in patches down the back of his right thigh and knee extending down to the outer aspect of his right foot. On examination, there was an area of impaired sensation corresponding to the distribution of S1 & 2 from the gluteal region to the foot. There were no other physical signs. He was treated by recompression with complete relief and suffered no recurrence. After treatment, the diver stated that during this incident he had felt quite fit "in himself" in contrast to the definite "off color" feeling which he has experienced during previous limb bends.

c. Diagnosis

The diagnosis of decompression sickness should be considered in anyone developing evidence of neurological dysfunction within a day or two of exposure to a decompression. Decompression sickness can only follow decompression. In view of the frequency with which prodromal symptoms and signs usher in neurological decompression sickness, care must be taken not to trivialize apparent pain-only bends. Evidence should be sought for nervous system involvement by doing a careful history and physical examination. In like manner, musculoskeletal pain should not be automatically ascribed to trauma or strain during the dive.

Several points serve to distinguish decompression sickness and arterial gas embolism if a good history can be obtained. Arterial gas embolism usually follows some unplanned surfacing maneuver and may or may not involve omitted decompression. The onset tends to be within 10 min of surfacing and the symptoms and signs are referable to brain dysfunction. Decompression sickness in all of its forms can follow apparently safe dives, although some cases that are attributed to decompression sickness may be the result of small arterial gas emboli arising from some disregarded or unobserved pulmonary lesions ranging from acute bronchitis to carcinoma of the bronchus.

In two retrospective studies of cases of decompression sickness, Rivera (1966) and Slark (1965) both found that some case reports were inadequately detailed. In addition, different prevalence rates for conditions such as shock and dyspnea suggested that different populations were sampled in the two series or that they reflected different biases in their reporting; either way, the possibility of missed symptomatology arises. The cases arising from closely monitored experimental dives will be different from those arising from sport diving, in which delay in treatment allows more advanced syndromes to develop.

The high proportion of cases affecting the brain in series reported by Rozsahegyi (1959) and by Peters et al. (1977), and some of the bizarre findings attributed to cord lesions by other authors, suggest that there may be a higher incidence of brain involvement in divers than is generally believed. Nevertheless, follow-up surveys may be vulnerable to a biased sampling procedure that would select a disproportionate number of severe cases. Cases with residual problems may be easier to identify retrospectively because of more meticulous record-keeping, and individuals with persistent deficits are probably more willing to participate in long-term follow-up studies than those without evident problems.

3. Mechanisms of Neurological Decompression Sickness

The basic cause of decompression sickness is bubble formation. The exact site in which the bubbles initially arise and develop remains unknown. On the basis of Guyton and Coleman's (1968) view that interstitial fluid pressure and intralymphatic pressure are slightly lower than ambient pressure at 1 atm, these regions would be reasonable sites for bubble nucleation. Certainly, ultrasonic monitoring indicates that the first circulating bubbles are usually detected in the venous rather than the arterial circulation (Spencer et al. 1975).

The bubbles cause mechanical disruption and vascular obstruction, but they also set in train a series of far-reaching pathological reaction through the surface activity at the blood-gas interface (boundary).

The surface activity results from the interface-generated electrokinetic forces distorting the circulating globular proteins of the plasma. Ordinarily, these proteins are oriented so that the hydrophobic part is on the inside of the molecule and the hydrophilic part is in aqueous blood. The blood-gas interface causes this configuration to be altered so that the hydrophobic part points across the boundary into the bubble (Lee and Hairston 1981). Enzyme activation or protein denaturation may occur. Hageman factor is activated, and active sites on enzymes may be exposed. These events can lead to some proteins becoming lyophobic with resultant clumping of red cells and the adherence, release, and aggregation of platelets (Hallenbeck et al. 1973).

Interfacially denatured lipoproteins release bound lipid, which can then coalesce into globules. Fat emboli develop from such coalescence of intravascular lipid as well as intravasation of depot fat (Bergentz 1961). The tendency for sludging of red cells, intravascular bubbles, and fat emboli contribute to reduced organ perfusion rates with a consequent decrease in shear-strain rate and an increase in viscosity that is most pronounced in postcapillary segments. This process effectively increases intracapillary pressure, which, in turn, induces vascular fluid loss into the tissues. The consequent hemoconcentration generates a vicious circle, which with time becomes increasingly difficult to break while fibrinogen concentration increases and cell agglutination occurs. Bubble-released substances cause increased capillary permeability, which causes further fluid loss. If the process is sufficiently widespread, venous return declines and so, in its turn, does cardiac output. The process rapidly produces a marked increase in hematocrit, which may easily exceed 50% (Cockett and Nakamura 1964a).

The participating mechanisms are tightly interlocked and vasoactive amines, kinins, and complement are among the many substances that are released and activated. The resultant hastening of coagulation in the area of stasis leads to fibrin deposition, which reinforces the vascular obstruction started by the platelet and red blood cell aggregates and bubbles. The resulting local ischemia causes synthesis of prostaglandins, which can contribute to further stasis and fluid loss.

Postmortem examination of the cord in dogs has shown the neurological lesions resulting from decompression sickness to be largely confined to the white matter (Hallenbeck et al. 1975a). The lesions were found scattered throughout the spinal cord; no lesions were found in the brain. The infarctions showed perivascular hemorrhages of variable degree, and with the gray matter sparing, this suggested venous rather than arterial obstruction (Henson and Parsons 1967).

Studies of the cords of goats that had been dived and treated for decompression sickness gave similar findings, with lesions mainly in the white matter at the watershed of the arterial supply, adjacent to the gray matter (Palmer et al. 1977). The main area affected was the cervical region. Interestingly, a large proportion of the goats with lesions had never been treated for nor had they shown signs of neurological involvement. Again, no lesions were found in the brain.

The possibility of extravascular bubbles in the cord remains. Such bubbles were observed by Boycott et al. (1908) in goat cords, but Catchpole and Gersh (1947) were unable to confirm this finding in their series.

Spinal cord damage induced by decompression sickness had long been thought to be the result of arterial embolization with bubbles (Catchpole and Gersh 1947). Several arguments militate against this as the primary process. In systemic arterial embolization, the brain is the main target organ, and cord embolization is rare. In one large survey of neurological vascular disease, no cases of cord embolization were found (Blackwood 1958). This finding is not surprising when one considers that the human brain constitutes about 98% of the central nervous system (Truex and Carpenter 1969), receives 75 to 85 times more blood flow than the cord (Kety 1960), and should receive proportionately more of any emboli distributing arterially. In divers, it is largely the cord that is affected by DCS, and arterial gas embolism resulting from pulmonary barotrauma affects the brain. Although both pathological processes are mediated by intravascular bubbles, the factors determining their selection of a target organ are clearly different.

Some understanding of the cord vasculature sheds light upon the mechanism of cord DCS. According to Batson (1940), the epidural vertebral venous system (EVVS) in man is a large, valveless plexiform lake. It is connected at each intervertebral foramen with ascending lumbar veins in the abdomen, with azygous and hemiazygous veins in the thorax, and with the vertebral veins in the neck. The EVVS also communicates with cranial dural sinuses via ventral occipital sinuses and with posterior bronchial and parietal pleural veins. The direction of flow in the EVVS changes frequently in response to respiration and fluctuations in intracavity pressure. Radicular veins drain the cord into the EVVS and, like the arterial supply, it is nonsegmental and rather tenous (Woolam and Miller 1958). Clemens (1970) states that the volume of the system is some 20 times greater than the arterial supply to the region it drains, so that only about 5% of the EVVS blood volume needs to be flowing at any one time.

The EVVS thus differs from other veins in that it is not just a unidirectional duct returning blood toward the heart, but it more closely resembles a stagnant pool with an ordinarily sluggish flow that frequently changes direction. By virtue of its peculiar physiology it is vulnerable to obstruction by bubbles, and the stasis can rapidly proceed into the sequence of coagulation previously described.

The situation has been clarified in a dog model of cord decompression sickness (Hallenbeck et al. 1975a, 1976). The dog EVVS is less complex than the human system, being basically a pair of venous trunks extending from skull to sacrum within the spinal column. It joins the cranial dural sinuses and anastomoses with the azygous and hemi-azygous veins (Miller et al. 1964).

The presence of the epidural fat, which stores inert gas, and the transmission of intrapleural negative pressures to the EVVS may render these vessels a site of predilection for early bubble formation. Furthermore, the communication between the EVVS and the cavity veins potentially allows the access of bubbles and the products of blood-bubble interaction from other regions to the EVVS.

In the serious forms of decompression sickness (DCS) considered here, the bubbles begin to accumulate in the EVVS. The bubbles may be of local or distant origin, or both, but because of the peculiarities of the EVVS already described they tend to coalesce and grow without being carried away (Hallenbeck 1976).

Some of these studies have shown that bubbles and the products of blood–gas interface activity form peripherally and return to the lungs via the heart. So-called silent bubbles (they do not cause clinically apparent DCS) have been detected en route to the lungs by the use of ultrasonics (Spencer et al. 1975). The absence of decompression sickness in these cases suggests that the lungs can cope with some dose rate of bubbles, and it is known that they can inactivate many of the products of the bubble surface activity (Fishman and Pietra 1974a, 1974b). Nevertheless, if the bubble assault becomes too great, the lung mechanisms will be overwhelmed; vascular obstruction will occur, causing a rise in pulmonary artery pressure and, in turn, of central venous pressure. The increased pressure in central veins reflects back into the EVVS, further facilitating congestion and stasis to a point of complete occlusion. If the stasis lasts longer than the silicone clotting time, fibrin formation will occur, reinforcing the obstruction (Botti and Ratnoff 1964). However, it is quite possible for the obstruction of the EVVS to develop without the facilitatory influence of the cardiovascular and pulmonary changes and for the whole process to continue to the point of infarction.

In dogs decompressed from a deep dive there often was a rise in right ventricular pressure associated with some respiratory distress, which indicated bubble embolization of the pulmonary artery. The pulmonary hypertension generally appeared within 20 min of the decompression. Usually, this hypertension was followed immediately by a rise in cerebrospinal fluid pressure, which was disproportionate to an accompanying central venous pressure rise. Signs of neurological deficit appeared immediately thereafter. In a number of cases the cord lesions developed without the preceding cardiopulmonary changes. The obstruction of the EVVS noted in these cases indicates that the EVVS may become blocked in the absence of pulmonary hypertension and central venous congestion (Henson and Parsons 1967). These findings may explain why not all clinical patients with DCS-induced cord damage complain of pulmonary disturbances.

Once the hemostatic process has been initiated, fibrin is laid down and the consolidation of the obstruction begins. The resulting ischemic damage initiates the mechanisms implicated in a process termed *post-ischemic impairment of microvascular perfusion* (Hallenbeck and Furlow 1978). Prompt treatment is essential to avoid permanent damage.

The pathophysiological process previously described would not explain the occasional episodes of supraspinal involvement observed in clinical cases of DCS. But, because the brain is a frequent target of arterial embolic episodes, it seems possible that a sufficiently great rise in pulmonary artery pressure could open up arteriovenous shunts, which would allow bubbles to embolize cerebral vessels and cause focal vascular stasis. Some of the episodes may also be migrainlike attacks precipitated by the decompression (Anderson et al. 1965).

The question of extravascular bubbles remains, and this mechanism offers a possible explanation for cases such as that described by Kidd and Elliott (1975) in their section Signs and Symptoms.

4. Prognosis

Case surveys clearly show that delay between onset and treatment decreases the likelihood of complete recovery and frequently complicates the treatment (Kidd and Elliott 1975; Rivera 1966; Slark 1965). Consideration of the mechanisms outlined previously would lead to the prediction that any delay in restoration of circulation would adversely affect prognosis.

Rivera (1966) observed that an onset of symptoms within 15 min of surfacing was associated with more residual defects than an onset of the disease after a longer interval. This difference is presumed to be because the earlier the onset, the more severe the case. During his follow-up of tunnel workers who had been treated for neurological decompression sickness, Rozsahegyi (1959) found that after 2.5 to 5.5 years, many of the workers had significant neurological disturbances, even the ones who had been sign free and symptom free on completion of the compression therapy. Additionally, Rozsahegyi (1959) found that those who were not completely free of problems within 6 weeks of treatment were likely to have problems for several years at least. Of those with an incomplete response to recompression therapy only 4% were completely clear after 2.5 years. He stated that progress over the first 6 months can be good, and thereafter small improvements may continue for several years although complete recovery is highly unlikely.

A contribution to the problem of late sequelae may be the failure to make a correct judgment about the seriousness of a case when it arrives for treatment. The most commonly noted sequelae are varying degrees of sensory and motor loss that may be associated with bladder control problems and impotency; occasionally, there may be various cerebral changes.

5. Concepts of Treatment

a. Philosophy

A useful conceptual approach to the treatment of spinal cord decompression sickness is to consider, in the order of their priority, the mechanisms underlying development of the disturbance: (1) Arrest the causative process, i.e., the formation and growth of bubbles; (2) prevent the onset of less treatable processes such as coagulation and progressive impairment of microcirculatory perfusion; (3) protect against tissue hypoxia and ischemia; (4) remove the offending bubbles; (5) return to atmospheric pressure.

If the causative process can be arrested quickly, the problem of coagulation, and progressive circulatory stasis probably will not arise. Current practice is to breathe oxygen and compress to 60 fsw (2.8 ATA) as soon as possible. In cases occurring at depth similar recompression with or without the breathing of oxygen-rich mixtures is employed. These maneuvers cause some reduction in bubble size by compression and improve tissue oxygenation, while also accelerating the disappearance of the gas phase by increasing the pressure gradient for diffusion. The third mainstay of the basic treatment, time, will allow the gas to be reabsorbed and decompression to the surface to be carried out.

The selection and use of appropriate therapeutic compression tables is described in part A of this chapter.

b. Initial Treatment

The watchwords in treatment of serious decompression sickness are *compression without delay*. Delay in the starting of treatment allows the secondary, but more refractory, pathological processes to develop. Any delay in the implementing of recompression increases the likelihood that additional measures will be required. For instance, intravenous fluid administration may be necessary. At the most basic level, liberal quantities of fluid may be given by mouth. The introduction of an intravenous line is advisable at any early stage in most cases. Ringer's Lactate or 5% dextrose-saline are appropriate fluids at this point (Kindwall 1979). Oxygen breathing is probably of benefit even without additional pressure. The antiplatelet properties of aspirin may also be beneficial if two tablets are given at the start. (See Chapter V.) Saumarez et al. (1973) report on a DCS patient who could not be brought to a compression chamber, but whom they treated successfully with oxygen and drug therapy exclusively.

c. Adjuvant Therapy

The volume of fluid required can be decided from the hematocrit before and during treatment. The extent of the problem is evident from the very high hematocrits that have been reported (Cockett and Nakamura 1960a).

Low-molecular-weight dextrans (40 and 70) have been widely used for some years in the dose of 2 liters every 24 hr for 2 to 3 days. Although dextrans purportedly have antiagglutination properties, they have not been proved superior to crystalloid solutions in practice, and current opinion would favor the crystalloids already mentioned (Davis 1979).

To what extent tissue edema is present remains unclear, but the use of steroids is advocated by many for an alleged protective effect in tissue hypoxia and for the ability to stabilize membranes. Dexamethasone in the dose of 12 mg at once with 8 mg every 6 hr for 24 hr and 4 mg every 6 hr for a further 2 or 3 days has been recommended.

Other drugs may be employed as appropriate to combat other medical conditions. Heparin in subanticoagulant doses (2000 IU) has occasionally been used for its antilipemic properties. Whether or not this is beneficial in treatment remains unknown.

In the future it may become possible to reverse the secondary effects of hemostasis by the use of drug combinations such as indomethecin, PGI_2, and heparin (Hallenbeck and Furlow 1979).

d. Clinical Management

With the risk of bladder paralysis present, a fluid balance chart should be kept and at the first sign of urine retention, an indwelling catheter should be introduced.

In severe cases, it is likely that regional circulation has been greatly compromised from the loss of plasma water and hypercoagulability. This point is made only to emphasize that this is a serious medical condition and that, regardless of its exotic origin, it should be treated as such by established principles of medical care. Pressure and oxygen may well remove the causative insult and alleviate some of the ischemia, but the subsequent processes may continue and can lead to apparent relapses and failure to respond.

Most physicians who treat divers have seen cases in which there were delays of from hours to days between onset and treatment; many of these patients have shown considerable improvement on receiving compression therapy. Therefore, no matter what the delay, pressure and oxygen should be tried.

Patients that do not fully recover with a single therapeutic recompression often improve with repeated oxygen treatments, either as U.S. Navy Table 5 or with 1 hr at 2 ATA. Whether or not the outcome has been influenced may never be ascertained, but many patients will show improvement that is temporally associated with the extra treatments repeated over a few days.

Vigorous physical rehabilitation is obligatory in all disabled cases and will commonly produce very satisfactory return of function.

DAVID R. LEITCH
JOHN M. HALLENBECK

References

ANDERSON, B., A. HEYMAN, R. E. WHALEN, AND H. A. SALTZMAN 1965. Migraine-like phenomena after decompression from hyperbaric environment. *Neurol. Minneap.* 15: 1035–1040.

BATSON, O. V. 1940. The function of the vertebral veins and their role in the spread of metastasis. *Ann. Surg.* 112: 138–149.

BEHNKE, A. R., AND L. A. SHAW 1937. The use of oxygen in the treatment of compressed air illness. *Nav. Med. Bull.* 35: 61–73.

BERGENTZ, S. E. 1961. Studies on the genesis of posttraumatic fat embolism. *Acta Chir. Scand. Suppl.* 282: 1–72.

BLACKWOOD, W. 1958. Discussion on vascular disease of the spinal cord. *Proc. R. Soc. Med.* 51: 543–547.

BOTTI, R. E., AND O. D. RATNOFF 1964. Studies on the pathogenesis of thrombosis: an experimental "hypercoagulable" state induced by the intravenous injection of ellagic acid. *J. Lab. Clin. Med.* 64: 385–398.

BOYCOTT, A. E., G. C. C. DAMANT, AND J. S. HALDANE 1908. The prevention of compressed air illness. *J. Hyg.* 8: 342–443.

CATCHPOLE, H. R., AND I. GERSH 1947. Pathogentic factors and pathological consequences of decompression sickness. *Physiol. Rev. 27: 360–397.*

CHRYSSANTHOU, C., F. TEICHNER, G. GOLDSTEIN, J. KALBERER, AND W. ANTOPOL 1970. Studies on dysbarism. III. A smooth muscle-acting factor (SMAF) in mouse lungs and its increase in decompression sickness. *Aerosp. Med.* 41: 43–48.

CLEMENS, H. J. 1970. *Intraosseous Spinal Venography.* Baltimore: Williams & Wilkins, p. 13.

COCKETT, A. T. K., AND R. M. NAKAMURA 1964a. A new concept in the treatment of decompression sickness (dysbarism). *Lancet.* 1: 1102.

COCKETT, A. T. K., AND R. M. NAKAMURA 1964b. Newer concepts in the pathophysiology of experimental dysbarism—decompression sickness. *Am. Surg.* 30: 447–451.

DAVIS, J. S. (editor) 1979. *Treatment of Serious Decompression Sickness and Arterial Gas Embolism.* Bethesda, MD: Undersea Medical Society. (Workshop Rep. No. 34.)

FISHMAN, A. P., AND G. G. PIETRA 1974a. Handling of bioactive materials by the lung I. *N. Engl. J. Med.* 291: 884–890.

FISHMAN, A. P., AND G. G. PIETRA 1974b. Handling of bioactive materials by the lung II. *N. Engl. J. Med.* 291: 953–959.

FRYER, D. I., AND H. L. ROXBURGH 1965. Decompression sickness. In: *Textbook of Aviation Physiology*, edited by J. A. Gillies. Oxford, UK: Pergamon Press, p. 122–151.

GUYTON, A. C., AND T. G. COLEMAN 1968. Regulation of interstitial fluid volume and pressure. *Ann. NY Acad. Sci.* 150: 537–547.

HALLENBECK, J. M. 1976. Cinephotomicrography of dog spinal vessels during cord damaging decompression sickness. *Neurology Minneap.* 26: 190–199.

HALLENBECK, J. M., A. A. BOVE, AND D. H. ELLIOTT 1975a. Mechanisms underlying spinal cord damage in decompression sickness. *Neurology Minneap.* 25: 308–316.

HALLENBECK, J. M., A. A. BOVE, R. B. MOQUIN, AND D. H. ELLIOTT 1973. Accelerated coagulation of whole blood and cell free plasma by bubbling in vivo. *Aerosp. Med.* 44: 712–714.

HALLENBECK, J. M., D. H. ELLIOTT, AND A. A. BOVE 1975b. Decompression sickness studies in the dog. In: *Underwater Physiology V. Proceedings of the Fifth Symposium on Underwater Physiology*, edited by C. J. Lambertsen. Bethesda, MD: Fed. Am. Soc. Exp. Biol., p. 273–286.

HALLENBECK, J. M., AND T. W. FURLOW 1978. Influence of several plasma fractions on post-ischemic microvascular reperfusion in the central nervous system. *Stroke* 9: 375–382.

HALLENBECK, J. M., AND T. W. FURLOW 1979. Prostaglandin I2 and indomethacin prevent impairment of postischemic brain reperfusion in the dog. *Stroke* 10: 629–637.

HELLER, R., W. MAGER, AND H. VON SCHRÖTTER 1900. *Luftdruckerkrankungen, mit besonderer Berucksichtigung der sogenannten Caissonkrankheit.* Vienna: A. Holder.

HENSON, R. A., AND I. M. PARSONS 1967. Ischemic lesions of the spinal cord: an illustrated review. *Q. J. Med.* 36: 205–222.

KETY, S. S. 1960. The cerebral circulation. In: *Handbook of Physiology, Neurophysiology*, edited by J. Field and H. W. Magoun. Washington, DC: Am. Physiol. Soc., Sect. 1, Vol. III, p. 1751–1760.

KIDD, D. J., AND D. H. ELLIOTT 1975. Decompression disorders in divers. In: *The Physiology and Medicine of Diving and Compressed Air Work*, edited by P. B. Bennett and D. H. Elliott. London: Baillière, Tindall, p. 472–495.

KINDWALL, E. P. 1974. Adjunctive treatment methods. In: *Serious Decompression Sickness and Arterial Gas Embolism*, edited by J. C. Davis. Bethesda, MD: Undersea Medical Society, p. 45–49. (Workshop Rep. No. 34.)

LEE, W. H., AND P. HAIRSTON 1971. Structural effects on blood proteins at the blood-gas interface. *Fed. Proc.* 30: 1615–1620.

MILLER, M. E., G. C. CHRISTENSEN, AND H. E. EVANS 1964. *Anatomy of the Dog*. Philadelphia: Saunders, p. 424.

PALMER, A. C., W. F. BLACKEMORE, AND A. G. GREENWOOD 1977. Pathological changes in the spinal cord of goats with experimental decompression sickness. *Undersea Biomed. Res.* 4(1):A33.

PETERS, B. H., H. S. LEVIN, AND P. J. KELLY 1977. Neurologic and psychologic manifestations of decompression illness in divers. *Neurol. Minneap.* 27: 125–127.

RIVERA, J. C. 1966. Decompression sickness among divers: an analysis of 935 cases. *Mil. Med.* 129: 314–334.

ROZSAHEGYI, I. 1959. Late consequences of neurological forms of decompression sickness. *Br. J. Ind. Med.* 16: 311–317.

SAUMAREZ, R. C., J. F. BOLT, AND R. J. GREGORY 1973. Neurological decompression sickness treated without decompression. *Br. Med. J.* 1: 151–152.

SLARK, A. G. 1965. Treatment of 137 cases of decompression sickness. *J. R. Nav. Med. Serv.* 50: 219–225.

SPENCER, M. P., D. C. JOHANSON, AND S. D. CAMPBELL 1975. Safe decompression with the Doppler ultrasonic blood bubble detector. In: *Underwater Physiology V. Proceedings of the Fifth Symposium on Underwater Physiology*, edited by C. J. Lambertsen. Bethesda, MD: Fed. Am. Soc. Exp. Biol., p. 311–326.

TRUEX, R. C., AND M. B. CARPENTER 1969. Origin and composition of the nervous system. In: *Human Neuroanatomy*, by O. S. Strong. Baltimore: Williams & Wilkins, p. 59–88.

WOOLLAM, D. H. M., AND J. W. MILLER 1958. Discussion on vascular disease of the spinal cord. *Proc. R. Soc. Med.* 51: 540–543.

D. *Delay after Decompression Sickness before Diving Again*

The wide diversity of opinion about the amount of time after a diver has had decompression sickness (DCS) that he should "stand down" before diving again suggests that there are no clear medical indications to direct the choice.

The guidelines given here are intended to serve as operating rules until more definitive and universally accepted criteria become available. They are based in part on a workshop conducted by the Undersea Medical Society in 1980. (The workshop, "Post Decompression Sickness Return to Diving," was held in Belle Chasse, LA, in May 1980 under a contract with the National Oceanic and Atmospheric Administration.) Each case is different, so judgment has to be used in implementing the stated rules. Guidelines are given in Table VI-8. The times recommended are considered to be adequate for the diver to rest and recover and also to allow the diver to be observed for further symptoms, and in particular to allow for a proper medical examination should it be indicated.

Current thinking holds that the nature of a pain-only bend (described in section B of this chapter) is different from those involving the nervous system. It is likely that an easily relieved pain-only limb bend will not predispose the diver to any subsequent injury,

Table VI-8
Recommended Delay following Decompression Sickness before Diving Again

Case	Situation	Time to Resume Diving After End of Treatment	Physician Involvement
A	Pain-only symptoms, cleared completely and without remission	1 day or 24 hr[a]	None[b]
B	1. Difficult pain-only cases, or those substantially relieved but with some residual pain, swelling, or tenderness 2. Recurrence of pain-only symptoms after initial treatment or during decompression 3. Pain occurring while still under pressure on U.S.N. air/mixed-gas tables 4. Chokes[c] or extreme fatigue, promptly treated and without additional symptoms	24 hr after complete relief[a]	Contacted for opinion during treatment, if difficult, or afterward in any case[b]
C	Neurological involvement (CNS, sensory, or vestibular), easily and completely resolved	1 week[a] following complete relief	Examines diver before he resumes diving
D	1. Difficult neurological cases, those which require extensive treament or do not resolve completely (minor deficit, not disabling) 2. DCS resulting in sensory deficit, definitive residual paralysis, etc., following normal dive with proper decompression 3. Embolism resulting in similar symptoms from routine dive with normal surfacing	6 weeks[a]	Takes part in treatment; examines diver after treatment and approves resumption of diving[d,e]
E	Embolism or DCS resulting from blowup, accident, or other irregular procedure	Dealt with according to symptoms, course of treatment, and residual effects as recommended in Cases A–D, above	
F	Skin involvement	No delay, but diver should be examined and watched	None[f]

[a] Times given are guidelines for supervisor and must be interpreted on the basis of prevailing conditions; they are not intended to be strict minimums. For example, a diver treated easily and successfully for pain-only bends in the afternoon may dive the following morning after a good night's sleep. These periods are intended for rest and recovery, and also allow for observation of the diver for further symptoms, and for medical examinations where appropriate.

[b] In difficult pain-only cases diver should be seen by physician if operationally practical; if diver is in a remote location he should be monitored by supervisor or medic until 24 hr after pain has subsided. Physician should be contacted if practical. In cases of residual inflammation anti-inflammatory drugs can be given (under supervision of physician), or other therapy appropriate to the symptoms.

[c] *The chokes* is a condition discussed in section C of this chapter and defined in the Glossary.

[d] Hyperbaric oxygen therapy may be beneficial in cases where relief is not complete during treatment.

[e] In some cases it will be necessary to "ground" the diver permanently. Clear guidelines for this decision have not been worked out, and few cases are alike. The diver and his employer are both involved with the physician in considering all pertinent factors.

[f] A diver with skin symptoms should be examined at the time of their occurrence and watched carefully after the dive. (Adapted from "Post Decompression Sickness Return to Diving," A Workshop held by the Undersea Medical Society in Belle Chasse, LA, in May 1980 under a contract with the National Oceanic and Atmospheric Administration.)

but that if it does the most likely result will be no more than a pain-only bend in the same place. On the other hand, most authorities feel that after a central nervous system (CNS) injury, the diver may be more susceptible to DCS than usual, and also that a subsequent dive may do further damage to the same site.

It is important to note that there is no fixed relation between the treatment used and the delay before returning to work; the waiting period is based only on the nature of the symptoms and their response to treatment.

Some physicians, to be conservative, have in their individual practices called for longer times for recuperation before advising the diver to go back to work. At the UMS workshop mentioned, all participants endorsed the times given in Table VI-8 and agreed that only the experience of widespread use of a single set of criteria like these would settle the issue.

The diver who has had any audiovestibular symptoms—e.g., loss of hearing or ringing in the ears, or vertigo with nystagmus—and even if the treatment was successful, must before diving again be examined by an ear specialist experienced in diving medicine. Loss of one vestibular organ will be compensated and probably not noticed, but loss of both will be disabling. Special tests can ascertain the extent of the injury.

Serious symptoms not completely relieved during treatment (Table VI-8, Case D) call for at least a temporary grounding of the diver by the physician. Up to 2 weeks of posttreatment hyperbaric oxygen therapy (daily on U.S.N. Table 5) has been found to be effective in some cases and is recommended, at the discretion of the treating physician.

Occasionally a diver receives an injury serious enough to prevent him from diving again for some time, possibly not ever again. This is a complex decision involving many variables. This decision is up to the responsible physician in consultation with the diver and possibly may involve the diver's personal physician as well. While there is no hard and fast rule, it is also generally agreed that a diver who has had two cases of embolism should be considered for grounding. All cases of embolism, regardless of cause, should be followed by a thorough medical exam.

Once an injury is stable, the diver may be able to resume diving after a brief convalescence, provided the injury has not limited the diver's performance, that is, it will not restrict his ability to do his job or jeopardize his own safety or that of others. Most divers recover from neurological DCS injuries after a few weeks or at most a few months. The nature of his anticipated exposure should be considered in making the judgment of whether the diver should be grounded. This decision process, as stated earlier, is indeed complex and should definitely involve the diver. If he is allowed to resume diving he should be warned about his potential susceptibility.

If a diver has received a definitive neurological injury from an otherwise routine dive, whether a result of DCS or embolism, then he may be unusually susceptible and the physician will normally advise him to stop diving. If he is allowed to resume diving, he should be warned about his potential susceptibility. He may also be grounded if it appears that a subsequent injury might be debilitating. For example, a diver who has lost one vestibular organ will recover essentially normal function, but if he loses the other he will be disabled; he should give up diving.

It should be noted that numbness in the fingertips, a feeling that they are "full of sawdust," is a common sequel to an extensive treatment involving oxygen breathing. This is not neurological decompression sickness and should not preclude the resumption of diving. Complete remission usually takes several weeks; diving may be resumed 14 days after the treatment if numb fingertips is the only involvement. Needless to say, a thorough medical workup would be given before making this diagnosis.

R. W. HAMILTON

VII

Diagnosis and Treatment of Gas Embolism

A. *Pulmonary Barotrauma and Arterial Gas Embolism*

As with most aspects of underwater medicine the terminology related to pulmonary barotrauma and associated arterial gas emboli is often confused. For the purpose of this chapter, pulmonary barotrauma is synonomous with *burst lung* and *pulmonary overinflation syndrome* and refers to decompression-induced trauma to lung tissue. This decompression-induced lung damage must be distinguished from compression-induced pulmonary barotrauma, which is often known as *lung squeeze*. Compression-related pulmonary barotrauma is relatively rare and occurs when lung volumes contract as a result of compression to less than residual volume. Such an occurrence is only found in breath-hold diving and other forms of diving where the breathing mixture is not adjusted to compensate for an increase in the depth of the diver. Theoretically, very rapid initial compression rates during the initial phases of compression from atmospheric pressure are capable of causing compression pulmonary barotrauma. In practice, such compression rates cannot be achieved by the diver descending in water.

Conversely, decompression pulmonary barotrauma is not only of importance in its own right but is also the precursor of arterial gas embolism which, with decompression sickness, is a principal form of dysbaric illness.

B. *Pulmonary Barotrauma*

1. *Introduction and Definitions*

Pulmonary overinflation, the cause of decompression pulmonary barotrauma, occurs in a wide variety of situations and may be associated with an equally wide variety of disease processes. Pulmonary overinflation may be the result of gas trapping during decompression or sudden uncompensated rises in intrathoracic presure. The effect of pulmonary overinflation may be limited to localized damage to the alveolar walls but may also result in alveolar rupture and give rise to pulmonary interstitial emphysema as alveolar gas escapes into pulmonary interstitial tissues. The truly encyclopedic work of Macklin and Macklin (1944) not only listed the wide variety of possible causes of pulmonary interstitial emphysema but introduced the concept of alveoli of different types in regard to their potential as a source of interstitial emphysema. Partitional alveoli were described that are entirely surrounded by other alveoli, and these were contrasted with marginal or nonpartitional alveoli, whose bases rest upon or against some other lung structure such as bronchioles, connective tissue septa, pleural tissue, or blood vessels. Partitional alveoli are not the principal cause of interstitial emphysema, because they have intercommunicating pores, the so-called pores of Kohn, and when rupture occurs may only release gas into adjacent alveoli. Equally, marginal alveoli resting upon bronchioles will encounter the same degree of distending force as exists within the bronchioles, and it is the marginal alveoli resting upon blood vessels that are the source of interstitial gas in pulmonary overdistension. The intra-alveolar gas escapes into the perivascular sheaths of pulmonary blood vessels, a process that is directly related to the inability of the vascular lumen to expand to counteract and balance the increasing surrounding alveolar pressure. A pressure gradient is created, and the gas takes the line of least resistance by tracking along perivascular sheaths toward the hilum of the lung. Lymphatic pathways within the lung are not involved in this process but, as described later, the gas may rupture into the pulmonary venous vasculature and enter the arterial circulation via the left heart. Ignoring this possibility, the gas, having tracked along the perivascular tissues to the hilum of the lung, gives rise to mediastinal emphysema, sometimes referred to as *pneumomediastinum*. From the mediastinum, the gas may extend to various sites that are diagramatically represented in Figure VII-1.

Several of the sequelae are of particular interest. It is important to realize that pneumothorax occurring as a result of pulmonary overinflation is almost always the result of secondary rupture of gas into the pleural cavity from the hilum of the lung and the mediastinum. Direct rupture of gas into the pleural cavity through the visceral pleura is rare, although possible if there are preexisting cysts or subpleural bullae. Further, pneumothorax as a result of pulmonary overinflation is frequently bilateral, thus emphasizing the central nature of the site of rupture of gas into the pleural cavity.

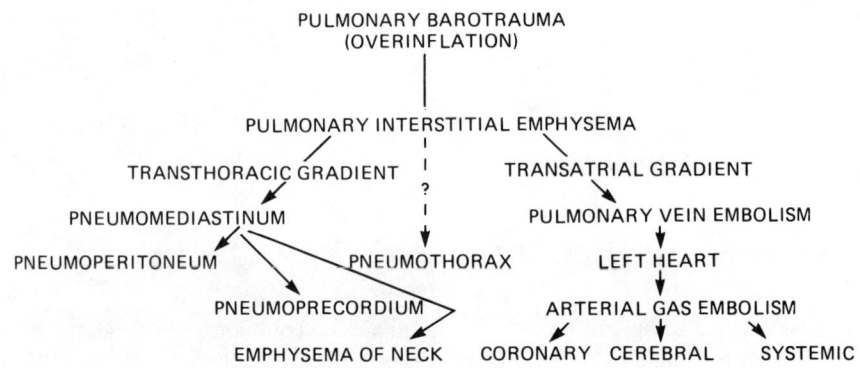

Figure VII-1. Routes taken by extra-alveolar gas following pulmonary barotrauma.

Extension of mediastinal emphysema into the subcutaneous tissues of the root of the neck and upper anterior chest wall is common and not infrequently given the clearly incorrect definition of *surgical* emphysema. A further question of terminology arises with extension of mediastinal gas into the pericardial and precordial tissues. *Pneumoprecordium,* known as Hamman's sign, is not uncommon and, by definition, refers only to gas lying between the anterior surface of the heart and the chest wall. Palpable subcutaneous gas may occasionally be felt precordially. *Pneumopericardium* is a feature often reported in the literature. It does not refer to gas within the pericardial sac; the gas is merely an extension of mediastinal gas into tissues between parietal pericardial and pleural membranes. As cardiac tamponade has been reported on at least one occasion as a result of mediastinal emphysema, the exact location of the gas has added clinical significance.

Additional symptomatology may result from the lung damage itself, and the significance of chest pain, cough, and hemoptysis is discussed later.

Macklin and Macklin (1944) also differentiate between benign and malignant mediastinal emphysema, and while this distinction appears to have fallen into disuse, the current tendency to regard mediastinal emphysema somewhat lightly neglects to acknowledge the occasions when benign emphysema may become malignant. These occasions may be summarized under three headings: (1) When a tamponade effect interferes with cardiac function or blood flow in major intrathoracic blood vessels; (2) when bilateral pneumothorax occurs with consequent respiratory embarrassment; (3) when the intrapulmonary element of the emphysema "splints" the lungs in the inspiratory phase and impairs ventilation.

The first few "submarine lung" training deaths in the U.S. Navy were diagnosed as compressed air illness. This was not logical, and the first to call attention to the problem was Behnke (1932), who hypothesized correctly that it was air embolism from ruptured lung tissue. Then Polak and Adams (1932) demonstrated in animal experiments that intrapulmonary pressure plus distension allows the air to escape into the circulation, usually by rupture of lung tissue. Shilling (1933) in his work on expiratory force demonstrated that pressure alone was not the cause of air embolism.

Schaefer et al. (1958) introduced the term *transpulmonic pressure* to describe the driving force behind the alveolar gas once it has escaped into perivascular tissues. Transpulmonic pressure is the difference between intratracheal and intrapleural pressures. Intrapleural pressure may be regarded as equal to the systemic venous pressure within the great veins. Schaefer and colleagues also demonstrated in experimental animals that thoracic and abdominal binding protected against artificially raised intratracheal pressure, and this effect can be attributed to the increased intrapleural pressure conferred by thoracic binding, which gives some extra resistance to the effect that overinflation has of forcing blood out of the large systemic veins within the thorax. Schaefer et al. also introduced the term *transatrial pressure* to describe the driving force behind gas that has ruptured into the pulmonary venous system. Transatrial pressure is defined as the difference between intratracheal and pulmonary venous pressure.

Malhotra and Wright (1959, 1960, 1961) quantified the pulmonary overpressure necessary to cause pulmonary barotrauma with alveolar rupture. Using animals and fresh unchilled cadavers, they showed that overpressures of as little as 80 mmHg would give alveolar rupture. Schaefer and colleagues' findings on abdominal and thoracic binding were confirmed by values of 133 mmHg (1 case) and 190 mmHg (2 cases) when the cadavers received such protection. Malhotra and Wright also demonstrated that when experimental animals were given muscle relaxants, the pressures necessary to produce alveolar rupture were reduced.

In work with dogs that were exposed to rapid decompression to altitude after tracheal clamps had been applied, Harvey (1954) showed that lung rupture occurred when lung volumes approached three times functional residual volume.

The most common cause of air embolism associated with diving is panic or emergency movement to the surface with a lung full of compressed air and the breath being held. It is interesting that a lung rupture from an overpressure of as little as 80 mmHg translates into an ascent of only 3.2 ft, so it is obvious that when the lungs are filled with compressed air, even at the bottom of a swimming pool, it is not safe to hold the breath and come to the surface.

In addition to the modest overpressures necessary, gas trapping may occur in localized areas of lung because of locally reduced compliancy as a result of some pathological lesion or scarring. Equally, obstructive airways disease of various types may cause quite local gas trapping. These features are discussed under the etiology of pulmonary barotrauma in diving accidents.

It is possible to make some observations from both animal experimental work and clinical experience regarding factors that may be involved in determining which route is taken by gas once alveolar rupture has occurred. These may be summarized as follows:

1. The volume of gas escaping from alveoli is not in itself a determining factor in the route it takes after entering the perivascular sheaths. Large volumes of gas may accumulate in the mediastinum without evidence of pulmonary vein embolization. Conversely, relatively large amounts of gas may become intravascular without evidence of mediastinal emphysema. In reviewing 199 cases involving unequivocal evidence of arterial gas embolism following pulmonary barotrauma with entry of gas into the pulmonary venous circulation, I found that only 21% of these cases had any evidence of mediastinal gas.

2. The rate of transfer of gas into pulmonary interstitial tissue is a factor of importance in that a sudden short rise in intra-alveolar pressure, whether part of localized gas trapping or a reflection of a more general rise in intratracheal pressure, seems much more likely to give invasion of the pulmonary venous circulation than does a slower, more-sustained overpressure. In the latter case, often a result of the diver's free-flowing demand valves giving rise to relatively modest overpressures, large amounts of mediastinal gas may accumulate without any evidence of pulmonary venous embolization.

3. The combination of pneumothorax, either unilateral or bilateral, and arterial gas embolization is rare. The series of cases previously referred to showed that only 5% of the cases had such a combination. Despite such a low incidence, the possibility of such a combination has obvious therapeutic implications.

2. Intravascular Gaseous Emboli

Before discussing the specific effects of arterial gas embolism it is well worth considering intravascular gas embolism in more general terms. Boyle (1670a, 1670b), in decompression experiments with animals in vacuums created by his 1659 invention of the vacuum pump, was perhaps the first scientist to demonstrate and describe intravascular gas emboli. He was the forerunner of generations of scientists who have produced intravascular gas emboli in experimental animals by various means. These experiments may be divided into systemic venous embolization with a variety of gases and systemic arterial embolization via the pulmonary vein or isolated arteries such as the femoral, mesenteric, and carotid arteries. The difference between systemic venous gas emboli and their arterial counterpart is not always clear from reports of research, and there is added confusion from the use of such terms as *aeroembolism,* which has been variously used to describe decompression sickness occurring from hypobaric conditions attendant upon simulated or real high altitude exposure, or true arterial gas emboli composed of air. For this reason, the term *aeroembolism* should be avoided.

In general, much greater tolerance is shown to systemic venous gas emboli, whatever their constituents, than to systemic arterial gas emboli. The somewhat macabre 19th century experiment of Cormack, Hare, and Magendie are all quoted by Moore and Braselton (1940). Cormack twice exhaled fully in quick succession into the jugular vein of a horse before it is described as becoming "uneasy." Hare rapidly injected 60 ml of air into the jugular vein of a 12-lb dog without harmful effect, and Magendie, "threw 40–50 pints of air" into the jugular vein of an old horse, which is said not to have "died immediately." Of possible comfort to the internist worried by bubbles of air in the tubes of intravenous drips is the calculation of Barthelmy (which is quoted by Moore and Braselton) that suggests than an average man could tolerate as much as two-thirds of a liter of air introduced quite rapidly into a systemic vein. This figure clearly ignores the disastrous possibility of gas becoming arterialized through a patent foramen ovale.

The effects of systemic venous gas emboli may be summed up as a dose-and-rate–dependent sequence of elevated pulmonary arterial pressure, rising right ventricular pressure, rising central venous pressure, and falling systemic arterial pressure. Extremes of venous gas embolization (with complete obstruction of the pulmonary arterial circulation by gas emboli and foaming within the right ventricle) lead to right heart failure said to be secondary to diminished coronary perfusion. The published works of Durant's group (1947, 1954), Holt et al. (1966), Thomas and Stephens (1974), Van Allen and Hrdina (1929), and Verstappen et al. (1977a–1977d), to name but a small number of authors, contain both quantitative and qualitative data of interest to the student of this particular aspect of intravascular gas emboli.

The proven existence of inert gas systemic venous emboli as a result of decompression is of much more than academic interest in a study of systemic arterial gas emboli. A great deal of literature exists describing the various ways in which venous inert gas emboli may initiate overt signs and symptoms of decompression sickness, but it is less well documented how easily such venous gas emboli may become arterialized by migration. Three possible routes of migration exist within the lungs and heart alone: (1) Transpulmonary migration through the pulmonary capillary bed; (2) migration through arteriovenous shunts in the pulmonary circulation; (3) migration from right to left auricles through a patent or potentially patent foramen ovale.

Further, Marchand et al. (1950) describe the existence of bronchopulmonary arteriovenous shunts, and Batson (1942) suggests the vertebral venous system as a potential bypass between portal, caval, and pulmonary venous systems. With the exception of the last-mentioned possibility, all the other potential sources of migration of systemic venous emboli would have even greater potential in the presence of pulmonary hypertension with raised right ventricular and pulmonary arterial pressures. Bert (1878) postulated that, in decompression breathing air, a small number of nitrogen bubbles will become arterialized. Since then many studies have shown this possibility to be real. Spencer et al. (1965) suggested that a pulmonary arteriolar pressure in excess of 29 mmHg was necessary for migration of gas bubbles in the human lung. The earlier animal work of the Curtillets (1939a) had suggested a somewhat higher figure of 60 mmHg for migration of bubbles in dogs. Both these figures refer to measurable emboli, and Rangell (1942), together with Butler and Hills (1979), are but two of several authors whose work with dogs suggests that gas emboli of less than 20–30 μm have little trouble passing through the lungs. The work of Prinzmetal et al. (1948) showed that solid emboli of up to 500 μm may pass through the lung circulation and such evidence may, at least in part, support the description of Von Hayek (1960) of subpleural "giant" capillaries and other potential arteriovenous shunts in the lung through which up to one-tenth of the pulmonary arterial blood flow may pass. Larger and potentially deformable gas emboli may be expected to migrate in similar fashion.

Clinical evidence for such migration has been provided from accidental venous embolization during neurosurgical procedures in cases described by Vourch (1971) and Chandler et al. (1974). Both these authors specifically excluded a patent foramen ovale as the source of arterialization, and this raises another possibility. Various authors such as Lubarsch (1924), Kaufmann (1924), and Friedburg (1956) report postmortem findings giving the incidence of patent foramen ovale as anything from 20%–32.5%. Again, the role of pulmonary hypertension in exposing such a defect is easily imagined, and Haymaker and Johnston (1955) quote two fatal cases of decompression sickness where arterialization of nitrogen emboli had certainly occurred via a patent foramen ovale. Certain authors such as Wagner (1945), Lever et al. (1966), and Buckles (1968) have suggested that systemic arterial gas emboli appear before venous gas emboli in decompression events affecting the peripheral vascular field. There is little doubt that this is not a true reflection of events, and Lever (1967) altered his views by reporting the preexistence of venous gas emboli. However, whereas there is a great deal of supporting evidence that in most cases of frank decompression sickness there is little or no evidence for arterialization of the inert gas emboli, a growing body of opinion suggests that so-called cerebral decompression sickness is caused by migration of systemic venous emboli, thus giving rise to what has been termed a "paradoxical" situation. On one occasion I surveyed 127 cases of decompression sickness for which detailed clinical evidence was available, and I found that only 8% of the cases had clear-cut evidence of cerebral involvement and only a single case showed evidence of both cerebral and spinal cord lesions. In all those cases the cerebral involvement was manifested by lesions suggestive of diffuse cortical involvement. All the cases resulted from dives that grossly exceeded accepted time-depth limits, and the onset was always within 15 min after the diver had surfaced. Although all were held to be undoubted cases of decompression sickness, the differential diagnosis of cerebral arterial gas embolism may seem equally appropriate despite the consistent lack of both evidence of problems during ascent and objective evidence of pulmonary barotrauma.

Before returning to consideration of arterial gas embolism as a result of pulmonary barotrauma, it is necessary to mention two other sources of arterialized gas emboli that have been suggested on somewhat theoretical grounds as being a possible outcome of decompression. Lever et al. (1966) postulated that turbulence within the left heart could cause bubbles within blood supersaturated with inert gas, a theory akin to that of several authors who suggest cavitation as a causative factor. Hempleman (1967) suggested that systemic arterial microemboli could be generated within the lung during decompression as inert gas is released from relatively poorly perfused areas of lung tissue. While it may be possible to entertain these various theories as possible causes of arterialized gas in hyperbaric exposures of sufficient magnitude to cause decompression sickness, they are largely unacceptable in those cases of pulmonary barotrauma and arterial gas embolism associated with the briefest of hyperbaric exposures.

Many other sources of nonhyperbaric-associated arterial gas emboli have been reported, of which the most common used to be various intrathoracic surgical procedures for which Durant and his group (1949) provided a powerfully argued case that disasters arising from such procedures were not due to "pleural shock," as described by Capps (1937), but were due to arterial gas embolism. More recently, with the decline of turberculosis, such causes of arterial gas embolism have also declined and have been replaced by open heart surgery, neurosurgery, kidney dialysis, and the use of extracorporeal oxygenators as the most common causes of problems arising from arterial gas emboli. Much work has been published on these aspects of arterial gas embolism, and it is sufficient to cite the work of Brierley (1963, 1967), Gallagher and Pearson (1973), Kessler and Patterson (1970), F. C. Spencer et al. (1965), and M. P. Spencer et al.(1969) in this respect. Indeed, Kessler and Patterson quantified the degree of arterial oxygen emboli from nonmembrane type of extracorporeal oxygenators as anything from 500–15,000/min of a size between 50–150 μm. Although they termed the measured emboli as *particles,* at least 50% altered size on compression and must have been gaseous.

a. Effect on Pulmonary Circulation

A great deal of experimental work exists to show that the principal impact of gas emboli reaching and passing through the left heart is upon the heart and brain as a result of embolization of the coronary and cerebral arterial circulations. This is not to deny that embolization of other parts of the systemic arterial circulation does not occur, but clinical experience indicates it is most rare.

Van Allen and Hrdina (1929), in an extensive series of experiments with dogs using direct injection of air into the pulmonary vein, produced clear evidence that the bodily position of the dog was of critical importance in deciding the distribution of the gas emboli after their passage through the left ventricle. He was able to achieve selective sparing of either coronary or cerebral circulations, and the conclusion was that the buoyance of the gas emboli was a vital factor in deciding their distribution. This finding, still valid and unchallenged, is of extreme importance to the diver whose erect, head-up position as he ascends through the water virtually ensures that the majority of gas emboli resulting from pulmonary barotrauma will enter the cerebral circulation. Van Allen and Hrdina also described cardiac responses that were dose dependent in terms of rate and total amount of air introduced into the pulmonary vein. He described rapid cardiac arrest within 2–3 min of injection of relatively large amounts of air in contrast to a delayed (but equally severe) reaction up to 30 min after injection of smaller amounts of air. By using bubble traps inserted into the common carotid arteries, Van Allen was able to isolate purely cardiac responses from cerebral responses of a reflex cardiovascular and primary neuromuscular nature. Rukstinat (1931) injected air directly into the coronary arteries of dogs and demonstrated that rate of injection was more important than total amount of gas in producing myocardial ischemic lesions directly equivalent to those produced by other experimental methods of coronary artery occlusion.

The Durant group (1949), again using direct injection of air into the left anterior descending coronary artery of dogs, detected ischemic electrocardiographic (ECG) changes resulting from as little as 0.05 ml of air and showed that these changes could be temporary with apparent full recovery and without lasting cardiac damage. Alternatively, they found that higher doses could give ventricular fibrillation and death. Geoghegan and Lam (1953) added to the understanding by describing arteriovenous progression of air bubbles in the carotid arteries of artificially embolized dogs. These bubbles moved forward with each systolic pressure wave, although, with sausage-shaped bubbles, there was a damping effect with the proximal end moving more than the distal end. Much other work has not only confirmed Van Allen and Hrdina's observations on the importance of buoyancy of bubbles but also demonstrated the qualitatively similar effects of emboli from various gas sources such as oxygen, nitrogen, helium, and carbon dioxide. Quantitatively (and not surprisingly, due to its high solubility), carbon dioxide is always found to be tolerated better than other gases. In summary, the great deal of research that has been done confirms that coronary artery gas embolization may be a fatal outcome of pulmonary barotrauma with sudden death from acute cardiac ischemia with arrest or fibrillation. Equally, sublethal amounts of gas in the coronary circulation may be tolerated with full recovery. These points are well illustrated by available case histories. Secondary or reflex cardiac arrhythmias may, however, result from cerebral arterial gas emboli. Greene (1978) discussed the difficulty of analyzing available histories of cases of arterial gas embolism that resulted in sudden death from cardiac arrest or arrhythmias and deciding whether the cause was primary coronary artery involvement or was secondary to brain stem involvement following cerebral arterial embolization. A well-documented case of death following diving-induced coronary artery gas embolism is that described by Harveyson et al. (1956).

b. Cerebral Arterial Gas Embolism

Before detailing the specific effects of gas emboli on the cerebral circulation, it is useful to consider some general features of the effects of gas emboli on arterial vessels. Chase (1934), using aortic injection of air to visualize the effect of gas microemboli on the arteriolar bed of the mesenteric artery, described a short-lived initial vasoconstriction followed by prolonged intense hyperemia with dilation of arterioles. Chase did not see gas microemboli progressing beyond the arteriolar bed, although he did describe perivascular hemorrhage in the capillary bed and venules. Duff and colleagues (1954) injected various gases into the brachial arteries of human volunteers and, measuring blood flow in the forearm, confirmed the condition of initial vasoconstriction followed by a sustained period of vasodilation. Baird and Miyagishima (1966), in dogs, again confirmed that gas emboli do not proceed as far as the capillary bed and either arrest in arterioles or pass through arteriovenous anastomotic channels. The work of these authors and of Bond et al. (1965), who studied femoral artery gas embolization in dogs, also clearly demonstrated that the vasoconstriction and vasodilation were mechanical effects of gas emboli that were not associated with altered tissue metabolism or lowered oxygen tension in tissues. The vascular changes occurred in chronically denervated limbs, were unaffected by antihistamine substances, resulted from brief contact between gas emboli and the endothelium of arterioles, and the subsequent vasodilation continued for at least several hours after the gas emboli had dispersed.

Interpreting these results in terms of the cerebral arterial circulation must be done with caution in view of the difficulty in visualizing the cerebral circulation in experimental animals in areas other than the superficial pial arterial system. Nevertheless, a great deal of evidence is available from animal work where carotid embolization has been used in association with direct visualization of the pial arteries. The great majority of this work confirms the initial transient vasoconstriction followed by a passive vasodilation in those parts of the arteriolar network actually embolized. The studies of Naquet et al. (1974), using baboons, are typical of the work showing the initial vasoconstriction visualized in pial arterioles. There is every reason to believe that these events are mirrored in the cortical gray matter supplied by the pial circulation through penetrating arterioles, which, in man, typically divide two or three times before the capillary bed is reached. Again, the arrest of gas emboli at the precapillary arteriolar level without invasion of the capillary bed is confirmed by various authors using cranial windows in a variety of experimental animals. While considerable emphasis has been placed by various researchers on the form in which gas emboli are introduced into the cerebral circulation (e.g., a single bolus of gas or a foam preparation), the process of bubble splitting described by the Curtillets (1937b) almost certainly ensures that the cerebral microcirculation is presented with a wide variety of bubble sizes, a factor further modified by the ability of bubbles to coalesce into long sausage shapes within blood vessels. The dynamics and the physical properties of intravascular gas emboli are indeed complex and may be summed up as follows:

1. Small bubbles, of a size below the diameter of the containing blood vessel, may lose velocity by collision with other bubbles or the vessel wall, and blockage may occur from a foam of small bubbles.

2. Bubbles slightly larger than the diameter of the containing blood vessel form sausage-shaped bubbles with convex ends. These bubbles may slowly progress with systolic pressure waves or may arrest with important consequences in terms of the loss of a fluid film along the contact between the bubble and blood vessel endothelium.

3. Either foamed collections of bubbles or chains of sausage-shaped bubbles may coalesce to allow quite long occluding bubbles.

Perhaps the best descriptions of these events are those of Eiseman et al. (1959) and Grulke (1975).

The impact of arterial gas emboli reaching the cerebral circulation via the carotid arteries is mainly in the gray matter of the cortex with relative sparing of the subcortical white matter. The evidence for this comes from both human clinical evidence and experimental animal work. Janke and Esfahani (1970) describe the cerebral damage resulting from gas emboli produced by extracorporeal oxygenators as being supratentorial rather than subtentorial. This feature has been described in various postmortem findings following death from cerebral arterial gas embolism. Fries et et al.(1957) and De la Torre et al. (1962) are typical of authors whose animal work confirms the sparing of the white matter. Further, the lesions tend to occur in the so-called boundary zones between the cortical areas supplied by the three principal branches of the circle of Willis. Although anatomical differences exist among the animals used by various authors, a circle of Willis with anterior, middle, and posterior branches is common to all except cats. These boundary zones in cortical gray matter have profuse arterial anastomotic pathways but also may be considered as areas where gas emboli lodging in blood vessels lose the "push" from systolic pressure waves because they are, in effect, in a zone of conflicting vascular pressures and flow. It is therefore possible that oscillation and then arrest is more likely to happen to gas bubbles in these areas despite the very profuse arterial anastomotic pathways in all areas and levels of the cortex. In contrast, arteriovenous anastomoses at cortical level are said by Hasegawa et al.(1967) to be rare.

It is probable that this distribution of emboli to the gray matter is a function of size. Swank and Hain (1952) showed that paraffin emboli with a diameter of between 4 and 60 μm, when injected into carotid arteries of dogs, tended to give concentrations of emboli of more than 15 μm in the gray matter. Kennedy et al. (1974), with baboons, and the Curtillets (1939b), with dogs, showed that air emboli tended to lodge mainly in the pial and cortical arteriolar vessels of the 20- to 40-μm-diameter range. It is interesting to contrast this relative sparing of cerebral white matter with spinal cord decompression sickness lesions, which are described by Hallenbeck et al. (1975) and Palmer et al.(1976) as being predominantly in the white matter.

The lesions produced by arteriolar obstruction due to gas emboli tend to be ischemic infarcts as opposed to hemorrhagic or "red" infarcts. Fazio and Sacchi (1954), using dogs, were only able to produce a predominance of red infarcts by using vasopressor substances 30 min after experimental embolization. All the evidence from experimental work and human clinical experience shows that whatever the degree of damage to cerebral tissue, the effect is multifocal.

The blood-brain barrier (BBB), one of several "blood-tissue" barriers that exist in the body and have permeability properties that tend to be exclusive for each organ, is also affected by gas emboli and the effect has been much studied. Using vital dyes and colloids and drugs, either on their own or in combination with isotopes for labeling purposes, authors such as Broman (1966), Johansson (1974), Lee (1974), and Rozdilsky and Olszewski (1957) all support the fact that gas emboli, when compared with other insults known to affect the BBB, have a truly unique effect. Further, this effect is evident after the briefest of contact between the gas bubble and the endothelium. Johansson noticed alterations in the BBB in the cerebral arteries and arterioles of rabbits in which the exposure to gaseous emboli had only been 2–3 sec. The effects on the BBB are ascribed by both Broman et al. (1966) and Johansson (1974) to separation of the blood vessel endothelium from the intravasal liquid phase. Although the alteration of permeability is a complex interaction of several factors, either in association with, or as a result of the primary insult of the gas emboli, the concept of a graded response is well established. In simple terms, minor damage to the BBB will lead to extravasation of fluid and electrolytes, whereas severe damage may result in permeability to large protein molecules. Ah See (1977) demonstrated a leakage of isotope-labeled dextran molecules (FITC Dextran) within 30 min of artificially embolizing rabbits. Ah See's work is of interest in that it would suggest that if the concept of vasogenic and cytotoxic cerebral edema, as described by Reulen (1976), is valid, the edema consequent upon cerebral arterial gas embolization is predominantly vasogenic in character. This distinction is of potential importance in the therapeutic approach to cerebral arterial gas embolization and is referred to later.

Of interest to the argument that cerebral decompression sickness may be a form of cerebral arterial gas embolism is the work of Chryssanthou et al. (1977), who were able to alter the BBB in rabbits by a single pressure exposure with a 23-min decompression after 12 min at the equivalent of 202 fsw. All the rabbits showing altered permeability of the BBB to trypan blue had visible intravascular gas emboli in the cerebral circulation.

Human clinical experience tends to confirm the fact that frontoparietal cortical lesions are the most common outcome of gas embolization, but there is no doubt that other areas of the brain may be involved. Of particular interest are the cardiorespiratory responses. Certainly, cardiovascular responses may be a result of brain stem embolization, and De la Torre and associates (1962), by selective clipping of various arteries leading from the circle of Willis, were able to produce transient rises in systolic blood pressure and significant tachycardia in dogs when the brain stem was embolized. Fries et al. (1957) had produced similar effects in dogs and was able to grade the cardiovascular responses into *acute* and *chronic,* depending on the severity of the insult. Evans et el.(1977), using cats, distinguished between the cardiovascular effects of coronary artery gas embolization (hypotension and rapid left ventricular failure) and cerebral artery gas embolization (hypertension and arrhythmias). Simms et al. (1971), described ECG changes in dogs that had had carotid embolization, but there are many reported intracranial events and lesions that can give ECG changes and arrhythmias. The reflex elevation of systemic blood pressure in association with a rise in intracranial pressure is well known.

Both Fries et al. (1957) and De la Torre et al. (1962) also described apnea followed by bradypnea or Cheyne-Stokes respiration following gas embolization of dogs. De la Torre felt that such responses were distinct from cardiovascular responses, although both were mediated in the brain stem, whereas Babcock and Netsky (1960), using solid emboli, claimed to show that the cardiovascular responses in dogs were secondary to the cerebral hypoxia that resulted from the apnea. Babcock also postulated that the respiratory changes he produced were a function of the total volume of cerebral tissue made ischemic and was unable to demonstrate any evidence of brain stem embolization in his animals. It is widely reported that an increase or decrease in respiratory rate may follow electrical stimulation of very circumscribed areas of brain such as the anterior sigmoid gyrus or the posterior cingulate area. Thus a deree of contradiction exists from which only one certain conclusion of importance may be applied to the human situation, namely, that early and adequate ventilation is necessary for cases for arterial gas embolism with apnea.

One final point of interest arising from De la Torre's work is that he felt that brain stem embolization only occurred when the anterior cerebral circulation became full of bubbles and an unphysiological blood flow occurred in the circle of Willis, thus allowing bubbles to reach the brain stem. Whether brain stem embolization in the human situation similarly reflects a severe embolic insult reaching the circle of Willis via the internal carotid arteries, or whether it is the result of direct embolization via the vertebrobasilar system, is not clear from available evidence, and both mechanisms must be considered possible.

A further feature of animal work that throws some light on the immediate impact of gas emboli comes from the work of several authors studying postembolic cerebral blood flow (CBF), using a variety of animals. The work of Meldrum et al. (1971) is typical and, using xenon-133 isotope clearance techniques to study baboons in the postembolic phase, he demonstrated a total arrest of regional blood flow in approximately one-quarter of the animals studied. Simms et al. (1970) had also reported a similar initial fall in regional CBF, using the same technique in dogs, and also showed that the effect was transient. Simms showed an impressive subsequent rise in regional CBF, which he described as *supernormal perfusion,* and this is convincing evidence of the vasodilation previously referred to. This vasodilation and supernormal perfusion is comparable in many respects to the so-called luxury perfusion syndrome that follows other types of acute cerebrovascular lesions. Indirect confirmation of these events came from the simultaneous electroencephalographic (EEG) monitoring of the animals used by Meldrum et al.(1971), which showed postembolic changes ranging from bilateral EEG silence for as long as 80 sec to symmetrical depression for as long as 8 hr. It is of note that bilateral changes occurred even with unilateral carotid embolization. In longer-term studies on baboons, Naquet et al. (1966) demonstrated postembolic focal irritative ECG changes coming on within 1 to 12 hr.

Various authors have looked at postembolic events in the cerebrospinal fluid (CSF). De la Torre (1962) and Simms et al. (1972) both described dramatic increases in cisternal pressure after carotid embolization of dogs. This event is, of course, significant in the possible causes of postembolic hypertension. Another feature of interest from animal work is the often-reported rise in oxygen tension of cerebral venous blood and cisternal CSF following cerebral arterial gas embolism in experimental animals. Simms et al. (1972) showed a significant rise in oxygen tension in both CSF and cerebral venous blood in dogs as early as 4 min after embolization. He attributed this to a variety of factors, including vasodilation with an increased CBF providing oxygen in excess of tissue needs, tissue damage reducing oxygen utilization, arteriovenous shunting of blood with bypass of the cerebral capillary bed, and limited oxygen diffusion due to increase in intercapillary distances when blocking occurs in the capillary bed. Whatever combination of these factors occurs, it is quite clear that increased CBF does not prevent the adverse effect of loss of functional capillary perfusion, a fact evidenced by the incidence of cerebral tissue damage in experimental animals exhibiting such CBF responses.

An expected corollary of cerebral ischemia is the occurrence of lactic acid accumulation due to anaerobic metabolism. This feature is reflected in the postembolic lactic acidosis observed by various authors in CSF. Also, as Simms and colleagues observe, such metabolic factors may have an important part to play in cerebral perfusion and at least modify the physical effects of gas emboli on brain vasculature. It is equally clear, however, that in this respect the effect of gas emboli is little different from the many other possible causes of cerebral ischemia.

Despite the occasionally contradictory nature of experimental animal work, of which it has been possible to give only a limited representative sample, a study of such work gives an insight and some understanding into the features of cerebral arterial gas embolism in the human situation.

3. Etiology of Pulmonary Barotrauma

In addition to considering pulmonary barotrauma and its sequelae arising from diving, it is necessary to include submarine escape training accidents, for they are much more extensively reported on in relevant literature and involve an identical type of decompression accident. Dealing first with the incidence of pulmonary barotrauma in diving, it is only possible to give a fairly general view of the extent of the problem. In the United

States, the total number of cases of pulmonary barotrauma among sport divers is largely unknown, although some measure of the problem can be gained from figures given by the National Underwater Accident Data Center, University of Rhode Island, at an Undersea Medical Society Workshop on Emergency Ascent Training held in 1977 (Samson and Miller 1979). These figures indicated that emergency ascent training alone accounted for 25 out of 80 diving deaths during the 1970–1976 period. By implication it would seem that the majority of these training fatalities involved arterial gas embolism, although no breakdown of the figures is available.

In the United Kingdom, where a much smaller population of divers exists in a geographically small area, the treatment of sport diving accidents is almost exclusively carried out by the Royal Navy. A review I made of 382 sport diving accidents resulting in decompression-related illnesses treated by the Royal Navy in the period 1970–1980 gave the following breakdown:

Decompression sickness of all types	297 (77.7%)
Pulmonary barotrauma	11 (2.9%)
Pulmonary barotrauma with arterial gas embolism	74 (19.4%)

These figures should be regarded with some caution because it is certain that a number of undiagnosed cases of asymptomatic and uncomplicated pulmonary barotrauma must have occurred together with a lesser number of unreported cases where symptoms and signs did occur but were of insufficient severity to merit attention or therapy.

Available figures for military diving during the period 1970–1980 suggest that the problem is very minor.

Of the 74 cases of arterial gas embolism dealt with by the Royal Navy in the period 1970–1980, 11 deaths resulted, of which 4 occurred before therapy of any kind could be given. The causes of these 74 cases and the 11 cases of uncomplicated pulmonary barotrauma may be further classified:

Apparently normal ascent	22 (25.9%)
Emergency ascent using artificial buoyancy	32 (37.6%)
Emergency ascent without artificial buoyancy	22 (25.9%)
Free flowing demand valves (pulmonary barotrauma only)	5 (5.9%)
Normal ascent complicated by lung pathology	4 (4.7%)

Only 7 of the 85 cases resulted from emergency training procedures. The most common cause of this type of accident was inadvertent or intended use of artificially buoyant life jackets (ABLJs) combined with inadequate exhalation during ascent. The growing use of ABLJs throughout the last decade is reflected in the rising number of accidents associated with their use, but it must be stressed that this comment is not a condemnation of these jackets, for it is not known what would have been the outcome of some of these accidents if artificially buoyant aids had not been used to counter the original emergency. Also, there are no reliable figures known to the author relating to the successful emergency use of these devices.

Much more accurate and detailed statistics exist for submarine escape training procedures carried at two United States Navy (USN) centers (Groton and Pearl Harbor) and a single Royal Navy (RN) center (H.M.S. *Dolphin*). Similar training is carried out by the Swedish, Norwegian, and Federal German navies. A variety of techniques of escape from submarines have been taught in the past, and various modifications have occurred over the years. Initially, underwater closed-circuit oxygen breathing sets such as the

Momsen lung (USN) and the Davis submarine escape breathing apparatus (RN) were used, but World War II experience showed that they were inherently dangerous for a variety of reasons and, more recently, escape procedures have concentrated on buoyant ascent with a hood attached to a stole, such as the Steinke hood (USN) or a hood attached to an allover buoyant suit that acts as a survival suit on the surface (RN). During ascent, the escapee breathes from air entrapped within the hood during the process of escape from the submarine. Detailed accounts of the U.S. Navy methods of submarine escape and associated accidents are given in the work of Polak and Adams (1932), Behnke (1932), Liebon et al. (1959), Moses (1964), Van Genderen and Waite (1967, 1968), and Waite et al. (1967). Royal Navy experience is obtainable from the work of Lambert (1958), Elliott et al. (1975), Donald (1979), and Pearson (1981).

The overall incidence of pulmonary barotrauma and arterial gas embolism is of the order of 1 in 2900 ascents in Royal Navy training. The only comparable available U.S. Navy figures relate to experience at Groton and suggest an incidence rate of approximately 1 in 5000 (Van Genderen 1967), if early training with the Momsen lung is excluded. The difference in the incidence rates for the two navies is, at least, partly due to the deeper buoyant nonhooded ascent training carried out by the Royal Navy prior to 1974.

Several interesting features arise from studying case histories of accidents arising in submarine escape training. As with diving, a relatively high number of accidents result from apparently normal ascents with unremarkable exhalation or breathing patterns during ascent. In the case of Royal Navy training, no less than 67% of the accidents appeared to have normal respiratory function during ascent. Moses (1964) reported that 35 out of 62 casualties at Groton (i.e., 56%) appeared to make normal ascents. Of interest in this respect is the finding of Ingvar et al.(1973) that in Swedish submarine escape training, frankly abnormal focal EEG changes occurred in 3.5% of trainees, some of them after apparently normal ascents. Adolfson and Lindemark (1973), when reporting work complementary to that of Ingvar et al., stated that 3.1% of the same group of trainees had typical chest x-ray changes of pulmonary interstitial and mediastinal emphysema. Of 14 trainees showing EEG changes, 5 were free from neurological signs and symptoms. While none of Adolfson and Lindemark's cases showing x-ray changes were free from both signs and symptoms, Reese (1968) demonstrated chest x-ray changes with varying amounts of extra-alveolar air in asymptomatic and sign-free submarine escape trainees.

It is important to stress again that, in the human situation, localized gas trapping may occur in the lungs rather than a generalized overpressure such as occurs in breath holding or failure to exhale correctly. Thus it is possible to state that any lung disease or abnormality that reduces lung compliance, in both a local as well as a general sense, should be carefully assessed in potential divers and submarine escape trainees. Also, any potential form of obstruction of airways should be similarly regarded. While it is impossible to quantify the risk from any particular condition, it is equally possible to cite a wide variety of causative lung disorders that have given rise to pulmonary barotrauma in normal ascents quite apart from the accelerated ascent rates of emergency buoyant ascent or submarine escape training where ascent rates of 9 ft/sec (2.7 m/sec) are essential to the techniques of escape from depths in the 650-ft (200-m) range. Therefore it is considered essential that divers are subject to medical screening that carefully assesses lung function in light of medical history, large-plate chest roentgenograms, and clinical examination. It is also the practice in the United Kingdom to screen both commercial and military divers by establishing the ratio of forced expiratory volume in 1 sec (FEV_1)

to forced vital capacity (FVC). An FEV_1/FVC ratio of less than 75% of predicted values will automatically disqualify new-entry candidates from diving until fuller pulmonary function testing can be carried out. For trained divers having their annual medical examinations, a ratio of 70% or more is allowed. It is possible to argue that such a relatively crude test of pulmonary function may be open to misinterpretation, but it is a simple initial screening procedure capable of being used without resort to expensive equipment. Experience seems to indicate that further testing of divers with a ratio lower than 70% does in fact reveal a significant amount of potentially dangerous obstructive airways disease.

It is not within the scope of this chapter to detail all the possible lesions that may give rise to gas trapping, but a selection of causes of fatal cases of arterial gas embolism in divers reveals such features as lung cysts, emphysematous bullae, unresolved pneumonic consolidation, bronchogenic carcinoma, scarring from healed tubercular lesions, and bronchial plugging—a variety of reasons. One of the first reported cases of fatal arterial gas embolism from bronchial obstruction was that described by Liebow et al. (1959) where a broncholith of tuberculous origin had obstructed a main bronchus. While there is no doubt that conscientious medical screening is necessary for both diving candidates and practicing divers and will be able to identify high-risk factors, it must also be admitted that despite the most careful medical screening and training, casualties will still occur involving both pulmonary barotrauma and arterial gas embolism. The experience of submarine escape training gives ample support to the need for continuing research into the possibility of identifying further risk factors and developing more accurate practical screening procedures. In this respect, the retrospective survey of six cases of pulmonary barotrauma in divers carried out by Colebatch et al. (1973) is of interest, for he found significantly higher postaccident levels of maximum transpulmonary pressures and lower "static" pulmonary compliances when they were compared with a control group of divers.

Before leaving etiological factors, it is necessary to remember underwater blast as a cause of pulmonary barotrauma in divers; two such cases (unpublished) come to mind, one of which resulted in arterial gas embolism, although it was not possible to decide whether the subsequent inevitable decompression or pulmonary blast damage was the cause of the arterial gas embolism.

4. Presentation and Diagnosis

Although pulmonary barotrauma may lead to arterial gas embolism, with some inevitable masking of symptoms either way, the presentations of both conditions are dealt with separately in this chapter.

Pulmonary barotrauma, identified by both subjective and objective evidence, but without evidence of arterial gas embolism, occurred in only 12.9% of the previously mentioned diving accidents and in 4.5% of the Royal Navy submarine escape training accidents that resulted from pulmonary overinflation. As has been stressed previously, these figures only relate to cases where signs and symptoms were of sufficient severity to attract attention.

The most common single symptom associated with pulmonary barotrauma is, without doubt, chest pain. In a majority of cases, the chest pain will be lateralized and localized, but more general or retrosternal pain may occur. Chest pain is an early symptom and, in the most cases, comes on within 5 min of surfacing. Although normally of a totally different character, the girdle pain of decompression sickness affecting the thoracic spinal cord should always be considered as an alternative diagnosis.

Hemoptysis, classically described in cases of pulmonary barotrauma as "frothy, bloody sputum," is by contrast, less commonly encountered. If it a feature of the symptomatology, it is usually an early feature occurring in the first 5 min. Dyspnea of troublesome proportions is quite rarely encountered. Obviously, it is principally a function of the degree of lung damage resulting from the barotrauma and the impression is that a degree of pulmonary barotrauma sufficient to cause troublesome dyspnea would almost certainly give rise to arterial gas embolism of sufficient severity to mask dyspnea or impose other CNS-induced respiratory alterations. A further feature of the dyspnea caused by pulmonary barotrauma is that it needs to be distinguished from the type of decompression sickness called *chokes*. While chokes will only normally result from dives where safe time-depth increments have been grossly exceeded, they typically occur shortly after surfacing, and the differential diagnosis between chokes and pulmonary barotrauma may be hard, even impossible, to establish. The symptoms of chokes are classically described as retrosternal burning pain with spasms of coughing that may lead to tachypnea, shock, severe hypoxia, laryngospasm, and what has been described as "tussive syncope." Although some controversy has existed in the past, there is little doubt that chokes result from massive invasion of the pulmonary microcirculation by microbubbles of inert gas and may be the precursor of arterialization of inert gas emboli, which in turn then give rise to cerebral manifestations of decompression sickness. Such a process may be positively assisted by the coughing that accompanies chokes. A startling worsening of this cough occurs if the victim attempts to smoke a cigarette. Some diagnostic help may be available from observation of the frequency with which chokes are accompanied by some other early and distinctive manifestation of decompression sickness. This feature was highlighted by Fryer and Roxburgh (1965).

An objective manifestation of pulmonary barotrauma is palpable subcutaneous emphysema, which is typically first noticed in the root of the neck as the gas extends upward from the mediastinum. Although the time of onset of cervical subcutaneous emphysema is to a certain extent dependent on the amount of gas that invades the mediastinum, the onset of such a symptom is usually relatively late, occurring typically some 2–4 hr after surfacing. However, cases are known to the author where this sign has been evident in as little as 15 min. Not infrequently, such a presentation may be the first and only sign of pulmonary barotrauma, and these cases tend to occur later rather than earlier. Voice changes, characteristically giving the voice a "tinny" quality and ascribed to what has been termed *submucous emphysema*, are a relatively common accompaniment of cervical subcutaneous emphysema and are another symptom that tends to have a late onset.

The cervical emphysema may be very extensive and spread upward in the tissue planes of the neck or over the clavicles to the anterior chest wall. Rarely, precordial emphysema may be palpable as gas extends from the mediastinum to give pneumoprecordium or Hamman's sign. Such precordial gas, however, is sometimes only diagnosed from the characteristic sound heard on auscultation. While pneumopericardium has been previously discussed and is probably merely an extension of mediastinal gas into the tissues between the pleura and the pericardium rather than frank gas in the pericardial sac, cardiac tamponade has been reported with its characteristic clinical signs.

Pneumoperitoneum is a further possible extension of mediastinal gas, but it is rarely if ever a cause of symptoms and is only occasionally diagnosed from roentgenograms.

Pneumothorax, in addition to its accompanying subjective complaint of chest pain, whether localized or widespread, may give rise to dyspnea of varying severity and, in severe cases, hypoxia, cyanosis, tachypnea, and shock. The diagnosis of pneumothorax is always possible from chest roentgenograms and, on occasion, may be a surprise finding for which no symptomatic evidence was available. In the Royal Navy series of submarine escape training accidents, the 109 nonfatal accidents showed 4 cases of uncomplicated mediastinal and cervical emphysema, 1 case of uncomplicated unilateral pneumothorax, 15 cases of arterial gas embolism with x-ray evidence of mediastinal emphysema, and 7 cases of arterial gas embolism with associated pneumothorax (3 bilateral, 4 unilateral). The association between arterial gas embolism and pneumothorax is fortunately rare in view of the therapeutic implications of pneumothorax, which is discussed later.

In view of the frequency of chest pain of various types as a presentation of pulmonary barotrauma and pneumothorax, it is not surprising that the diagnosis of coronary artery gas embolism is exceedingly difficult to make without resort to ECG tracings, which must in any case be viewed with some caution if cerebral arterial gas embolism has occurred. All the evidence suggests, however, that in divers and submarine escape trainees coronary artery gas embolism is rare. The series of submarine escape training accidents previously referred to gave only five cases where there was unequivocal evidence of ischemic ECG changes, and these were all transient. Similarly, diving-related cases of pulmonary barotrauma and arterial gas embolism show a very low incidence of associated coronary artery gas embolism. It must be remembered, however, that the fatal cases of pulmonary barotrauma where early death has occurred from cardiac arrest (or presumed fibrillation) rarely yield evidence at postmortem that positively allows coronary artery embolization to be incriminated. Many of these cases have had attempted recompression therapy that, as is seen later, considerably alters the significance that may be attached to intravascular gas found at postmortem. The case previously referred to that was described by Harveyson et al. (1956) is one of the very few fatal cases that has been written up of coronary artery gas embolism resulting from diving. This case resulted in the delayed death of an 18-year-old diver who collapsed following a training free ascent from 20 ft. The initial symptoms and signs were of a general and profound nature, and death ensued in 28 hr. No recompression therapy was attempted, and a postmortem revealed multiple myocardial infarcts secondary to occlusion of coronary arteries by gas emboli. No evidence of cerebral arterial embolization was found. More commonly, where ECG changes suggestive of myocardial ischemia have been described with other manifestations of pulmonary barotrauma, the findings seem to have been of a chance and transient nature.

C. Arterial Gas Embolism

1. Presentation

The presentation of cerebral arterial gas embolism has been described as protean, a description that acknowledges the complex events involved. Reference has already been made to research work in animals, which tended to allow a broad classification into cardiorespiratory and neuromuscular responses. Gillen (1968), in reviewing 83 cases of what he termed *cerebral gas embolism*, classified the presentation into five types:

Type 1. Abrupt loss of consciousness with varying degrees of asymmetrical limb signs, scattered cranial nerve defects, and dramatic cardiorespiratory collapse. Such cases were ascribed to a severe degree of embolization affecting both the carotid and vertebrobasilar arterial systems.

Type 2. Unilateral signs and symptoms, both motor and sensory, that were attributed to unilateral embolization of an internal carotid artery.

Type 3. Signs and symptoms attributable to single lesions in the brain stem.

Type 4. Functional disorders attributable to emboli affecting only fragments of extramedullary portions of cranial nerves.

Type 5. Minor disturbances of the central nervous system in association with evidence of mediastinal emphysema.

Such classifications serve to emphasize the vast range of possible presentations, and another description of presenting signs and symptoms prepared from Royal Navy submarine escape training accidents and Royal Navy-treated diving accidents produces a similarly diverse spectrum. Only the initial dominant presenting features are classified and are based on a classification broadly similar to that used by Greene (1978) when reporting on Royal Navy submarine escape training accidents between 1954 and 1976.

Inevitably, some of the Royal Navy cases in Table VII-1 showed multiple presenting signs and symptoms, although such multiplicity was not often seen. All the cases showing visual disturbances had other neurological signs and symptoms. Visual disturbances, whether a presenting symptom or developing after an interval, generally seemed associated with a severe degree of cerebral arterial embolization and signs of diffuse damage to the brain.

Table VII-1 shows that *coma*, defined for these purposes as "unresponsive unconsciousness," was easily the most common presentation. Almost as common a presentation was *stupor and confusion*, whose definitions are largely self-explanatory and have been used to describe a variety of presentations that involve some remaining degree of responsiveness. This category includes three cases of aphasia. *Collapse* is a term often used by eyewitnesses but, for the purpose of Table VII-1, has been restricted to accident victims who fell to the ground and, although unable to assist themselves, retained awareness. It is accepted that some of these cases involved sudden loss of postural tone and might have involved paretic signs, whereas others in this category could possibly be included in the category of stupor.

Of considerable importance is the predominance of unilateral and unimodal motor and sensory changes. This is in contrast to the frequent bilaterality and bimodality of the signs and symptoms resulting from spinal cord decompression sickness. This feature is of diagnostic importance and is referred to later. Also of interest is the paucity of cases involving headache as a presenting symptom.

Progression of the presenting signs and symptoms in the two series of cases was very different because all the submarine escape training accidents were recompressed with a minimum of delay, whereas the diving accidents, with one exception, involved a delay before recompression therapy was possible. While the results of therapy are discussed later, it is worth noting that 42 of the 79 cases of arterial gas embolism resulting from diving showed some degree of spontaneous improvement in the period before therapy was commenced. Indeed, of the 31 diving cases of coma listed in Table VII-1, 24

Table VII-1
Presenting Signs and Symptoms in 114 Royal Navy Submarine Escape Training Accidents and 74 Diving Accidents Involving Arterial Gas Embolism[a]

Signs and symptoms	Percentage of incidence	
	Submarine escape training	Diving
Coma with convulsions	7	18
Coma without convulsions	29	22
Stupor and confusion	14	24
Collapse	8	4
Vertigo	14	8
Visual disturbance	6	9
Headache	2	1
Unilateral motor changes	17	14
Unilateral sensory changes	10	8
Unilateral motor and sensory changes	6	1
Bilateral motor changes	1	8
Bilateral sensory changes	1	1

[a] List compiled from case histories and records of initial postaccident medical examinations. In the case of submarine escape training accidents the examinations were always carried out within 5 min of onset of symptoms.

recovered some degree of responsiveness before therapy; a typical pattern of events involved coma, which lightened after 10–15 min (or less) and unmasked focal motor or sensory disturbances as consciousness and awareness returned. Such a spontaneous improvement also occurred in 11 cases involving an initial presentation of focal neurological deficits of one kind or another. Twelve cases, including 4 that initially presented as coma, had a complete and spontaneous resolution of signs and symptoms within periods ranging from 15 min to 4 hr. These spontaneous improvements were not always sustained, however, and this therapeutic consideration is discussed later.

The relationship of the onset of signs and symptoms of arterial gas embolism to the causative decompression is a further feature of diagnostic importance. In the 188 cases of arterial gas embolism described in Table VII-1, the longest interval to onset of signs and symptoms after a completed decompression was 8 min. This was an atypically long interval, and all the other cases showed evidence of arterial gas embolism within 5 min. In those cases where coma was a presenting sign, the time interval was never more than 30 sec, although a small number of cases progressed to coma less than a minute after exhibiting some other presenting feature. With few exceptions, the cases reviewed reinforced the trend for serious cases to show very early and profound disturbances, whereas less severe and localized disturbances of motor or sensory function may present after a relatively longer interval of up to 5 min. Any evidence of arterial gas embolism occurring more than 5 min after a completed decompression is rare. This rapid onset of signs and symptoms is in contrast with decompression sickness, which, although capable of giving rise to very early signs and symptoms if acceptable time-depth limits are grossly exceeded, more often involves a delay in excess of 5 min before giving rise to neurological dysfunction. It is also important to note that while musculoskeletal pain is by far the commonest presenting feature of decompression sickness and is not one of the normal presentations of arterial gas embolism, divers may have coexisting decompression sickness and arterial gas embolism. This possibility should always be considered where apparent cases of arterial gas embolism exhibit musculoskeletal pain.

Of the cases reviewed, 17 had a fatal outcome (5 from submarine escape training). Eight of these cases involved immediate and irreversible cardiorespiratory collapse despite the fact that 4 were immediately recompressed. Greene (1978) highlights the difficulty of establishing whether these cases were due to direct coronary artery involvement or a reflex inhibition of cardiac function secondary to brain stem embolization. Unfortunately, postmortem evidence in these 8 cases did not conclusively establish which of these factors might have been responsible. It must be added that recompression of casualties who are in cardiorespiratory arrest may lead to unreliable postmortem findings because of further intravascular inert gas bubble formation during decompression. Both Hempleman (1972) and Smith-Sivertsen (1973) have given attention to this possibility.

The series of diving-related arterial gas embolism contains 3 divers who had two separate episodes of arterial gas embolism. None of these cases demonstrated any underlying lung pathology and none involved unusually stressful decompressions. As it is common practice in the United Kingdom to prohibit further diving after a proven decompression-induced arterial gas embolism, it is impossible to attach any significance to this finding.

The erect attitude of ascent through the water leads to a predominance of cerebral arterial involvement in contrast with iatrogenic cases of arterial gas embolism where the victim is usually recumbent at the time of embolization. Coronary artery embolization is most likely to occur in the recumbent position. Therefore, it is not surprising that only five of the submarine escape training victims showed ECG evidence of myocardial ischemic changes. These ECG changes were detected by in-chamber monitoring shortly after the initial embolization and, with one exception, were transient. The one exception had changes that outlasted compression therapy but reverted to normal within 48 hr. Very few of the diving accidents had such monitoring immediately after the onset of signs and symptoms. Two divers had ECG changes on admission to hospital after compression therapy, and again those proved transient. Therefore it seems that coronary artery embolization is relatively uncommon in decompression-induced arterial gas embolism.

Evidence of arterial gas embolization in other organs and body sites is very hard to find in the literature dealing with decompression accidents. In the cases reviewed here, a single case of unequivocal embolization of the spinal cord occurred in a diver. It resulted in clear evidence of a severe segmental lesion.

Electrocardiographic examination was only routinely carried out on submarine escape training accidents on admission to hospital after completion of recompression therapy; only 15 cases exhibited EEG abnormalities consistent with focal neurological damage. As with the ECG changes, these EEG abnormalities were fortunately transient. In all cases, the EEG changes were characterized by an unusual degree of slow-wave activity, which in some cases was localized and in others was extensive and bilateral.

2. Diagnosis

The diagnosis of arterial gas embolism resulting from decompression may be easy or it may be particularly difficult. Nevertheless it is important to try to establish such a diagnosis for therapeutic reasons in view of the existence of special therapeutic compression regimes for arterial gas embolism. It is especially necessary to try to distinguish arterial gas embolism from decompression sickness, although as mentioned previously they may coexist in the same patient if the time-depth profile of the pressure exposure has been adequate to give rise to decompression sickness. Blowups from deep or saturation diving may give extreme examples of such a combination.

The presentation of pulmonary barotrauma and its sequelae other than arterial gas embolism has already been dealt with, but it is important to remember that associated arterial gas embolism is always a possibility in such cases and may not be eliminated without a searching examination and careful observation of seemingly uncomplicated cases of pulmonary barotrauma. The association of evidence of pulmonary barotrauma with neurological signs and symptoms of a cerebral nature or origin is, for all practical purposes, diagnostic of arterial gas embolism.

The history of the dive or pressure exposure leading to signs and symptoms is of fundamental diagnostic importance in all decompression illnesses. A history of dives to less than 30 ft (9 m), or to time-depth limits short of those expected to give rise to decompression sickness, is of diagnostic significance, as is a history of precipitate or abnormally rapid ascent. The story of breath holding during artificial buoyancy is all too familiar as a cause of pulmonary overinflation accidents, particularly in sport divers.

The time to onset of symptoms following decompression is of obvious importance, for signs and symptoms of arterial gas embolism should always have become manifest within 10 min.

The neurological evidence for arterial gas embolism presents a much more difficult diagnostic problem. The unusual cerebral signs and symptoms of arterial gas embolism are equally common to so-called cerebral decompression sickness, although this similarity is not surprising in view of the probability that this form of decompression sickness is due to venous gas emboli becoming arterialized. However, the more common form of neurological damage in decompression sickness involves the spinal cord in a relatively diffuse fashion and tends to produce bilateral and bimodal motor and sensory disturbances. In contrast, cerebral arterial gas embolism gives focal brain damage and has a tendency to produce unilateral and unimodal neurological disturbances, but this feature is not always present and, at best, is only an aid to diagnosis.

Coma, with or without convulsions, following shortly after a decompression must be regarded as indicative of cerebral arterial gas embolism and treated appropriately. Alternative diagnoses obviously may exist in such cases, but the possible sequelae of failure to treat a case of cerebral arterial gas embolism are of paramount importance.

As has been described, other nonspecific or poorly localized cerebral symptomatology does occur and the previously listed categories of collapse and vertigo can all be confused with the vertigo of vestibular decompression sickness. In particular, certain features of brain stem embolization may be impossible to distinguish from vestibular decompression sickness without resort to complex investigation.

A useful guide to some of the differential diagnostic points between the two major decompression illnesses is given in the *U.S. Navy Diving Manual* and also by Gillen (1968). Certain other diagnostic features have been described that are of varying practical value. Durant et al. (1949) and Schlaepfer (1972) both list marbling of the skin as a specific sign due to embolism of dermal blood vessels, and they describe it as more common over the upper part of the body. Durant and associates also list visible gas emboli in retinal blood vessels, x-ray evidence of gas in cerebral blood vessels, and a somewhat impractical sign called *air bleeding*. This latter sign, attributed to Van Allan and Hrdina (1929), involves making a "small incision in the skin over the most superior portion of the body" and subsequently observing the gas bubbles in the escaping blood. Another, somewhat bizarre, observation was that of Liebermeister (1929), who noted sharply defined areas of pallor in the tongue and believed this sign, if present, was diagnostic of arterial gas embolism. He held that it was equally indicative of freedom from arterial gas if the tongue was normal. It is pertinent to observe that the time taken to establish most of these accessory diagnostic features is rarely present in view of the urgency to provide definitive therapy.

3. Therapy

There can be no doubt that the primary therapy for decompression-induced arterial gas embolism is recompression as soon as possible. This need for recompression is equally true for cases of arterial gas embolism arising from other accidents, particularly those arising from diagnostic and surgical procedures, and it is unfortunate that many such cases do not receive recompression therapy.

Because diving accidents frequently occur in remote situations, first-aid measures are important and potentially life saving. Certainly cardiopulmonary resuscitation may be effective in enabling survival of the initial impact of arterial gas embolism. Caution should be exercised with whatever method is used for ventilation in view of the possible hazard of further gas embolism from the site of the pulmonary barotrauma, and while this risk is probably theoretical, it should prevent overenthusiastic attempts at ventilation.

If available, 100% oxygen should be given by means of a well-fitting oral-nasal mask and continued until recompression therapy becomes possible.

The victim should, if possible, be placed in a head-down position to avoid the possibility of further embolization from gas still trapped in the left heart. Atkinson (1963), in a study to confirm the importance of body position on the route taken by arterialized gas, described two cases where placing the patient in a head-down position seemed in itself to effect a cure from signs of cerebral arterial gas embolism.

Adjuvant drug and fluid therapy is routinely employed in the therapy of arterial gas embolism and is described later. If circumstances permit, such therapy ought to be instituted as a first-aid measure.

When transport to a recompression facility is necessary, it is important to minimize the further potentially damaging decompression that could occur with flying. It is therefore recommended that helicopters fly as low as possible and always remain below 1000 ft (300 m) if the accident occurred at sea level. For accidents at altitude, every effort should be made to avoid further decompression. The use of pressurized aircraft is possible for transport over longer distances, but it should be remembered that the cabins in such aircraft are normally only pressurized to the equivalent of 8000 ft above sea level and must be suitably adjusted.

Much interest has been aroused in the use of transportable hyperbaric chambers for evacuation of diving accidents. The majority of such chambers are single-person, single-compartment chambers that may have the additional capability of being locked onto larger two-compartment chambers, thus allowing transfer of the patient under pressure. It is argued later that single-person (monoplace) chambers are not suitable for the optimum therapy of decompression illnesses and if used for emergency therapy or transport should only be used for minimal recompression therapeutic tables using 100% oxygen breathing at a maximum of 2.8 ATA.

It is preferable for single-person chambers to have a built-in breathing system (BIBS) to allow the oxygen to be breathed in an air-filled chamber that should be flushed through at regular intervals to prevent buildup of oxygen in the chamber atmosphere. The majority of the NATO navies are equipped with such chambers. Careful patient assessment should occur before use of such chambers, and it is very doubtful whether circumstances ever warrant their use with unconscious patients. The restriction of the therapy used in single-person chambers to minimal recompression oxygen tables ensures that, in the event that some emergency occurs to the patient, the chamber may be safely and quickly surfaced to allow patient care. Such a safety factor does not exist with the use of therapeutic tables calling for the breathing of higher pressure air or oxygen-nitrogen mixtures except during the early stages of therapy when there is no risk from decompression sickness.

It is conventional to describe the therapeutic approach to arterial gas embolism in terms of pressure, oxygen, and adjuvant drug therapy, although pressure and oxygen are not entirely independent variables.

a. Pressure

Recompression to an arbitrary depth is the keystone of therapy, although the amount of recompression remains the subject of continuing debate.

The aim of using pressure is to compress bubbles and allow them to clear the microcirculation. While the dynamics involved in compression of sausage-shaped bubbles is complex, there is no doubt that pressure can be dramatically effective in this respect. Animal experiments using cranial windows have been used to demonstrate the effect of recompression on intravascular gas emboli produced artificially by carotid injection of gas. The typical experiments described by Waite et al. (1967) and Grulke (1975) amply confirm the ability of pressure to compress gas bubbles in the pial arterial vessels. Many other factors are involved if the pressure is to be successful in this respect, not the least of which is the presence of an adequate systemic arterial blood pressure to give a "push" to the bubbles and ensure their onward progress. Other events such as bubble coalescence and the deposition of platelets, fibrin, and lipid material at the gas-blood boundary, as described by Warren et al. (1973), tend to stabilize gas bubbles with associated endothelial damage to the embolized blood vessels. These events take time, but those involving the gas-blood boundary are described by Adebahr (1972) as demonstrable within 5 min. Therefore, the rapidity with which recompression is carried out is of critical importance.

In terms of volume reduction of bubbles there is little extra to be gained by recompression to more than 6 ATA, and most therapeutic recompression regimes for arterial gas embolism are based on an initial arbitrary recompression to 6 ATA. Until the work of Waite et al. (1967) no special tables existed for the therapy of arterial gas embolism, and 6 ATA air-breathing tables normally used for the treatment of decompression sickness were used with varying amounts of time spent at 6 ATA. Waite and colleagues, using dogs, demonstrated that resolution of bubbles in the pial vessels was complete in all six of his experimental animals after recompression to 4 ATA; they concluded that there was insufficient evidence to warrant changing the standard procedure of recompression to 6 ATA, but the possible efficacy of more modest pressures was clearly demonstrated. It should be noted that the dogs in the Waite study were recompressed immediately on development of clinical signs of arterial gas embolism. From the experiments of Waite and colleagues came two therapeutic recompression tables that allowed for recompression to 6 ATA for 15 min or 30 min, depending on the time taken for relief of major signs and symptoms. The 15-min stay at 6 ATA was followed by the "short" minimal recompression oxygen treatment table of Goodman and Workman (1965), and the 30-min stay at 6 ATA was followed by a "long" minimal recompression oxygen treatment table. These minimal recompression oxygen treatment tables involve breathing of pure oxygen at 2.8 ATA and 1.9 ATA with short air-breathing breaks. Listed as U.S. Navy Tables 5 and 6, they became U.S. Navy Tables 5A and 6A if preceded by an air-breathing period at 6 ATA. Van Genderen and Waite (1968) described the value of this new therapeutic approach for arterial gas embolism, as did Bornmann (1967). U.S. Navy Table 5A has now been dropped from the *U.S. Navy Diving Manual*, and U.S. Navy Table 6A remains as the initial choice of therapeutic table. A metricized version of U.S. Navy Table 6A exists in the *Royal Navy Diving Manual* (Royal Navy Table 63) that also allows for intermittent breathing of 32.5%–67.5% oxygen-nitrogen mixtures in an air-filled chamber at 6 ATA. This routine is an attempt to combine the beneficial effect of pressure with a raised partial pressure of oxygen (P_{O_2}). In this case, the P_{O_2} would be 1.96 ATA.

Failure to respond to recompression to 6 ATA within 30 min may be followed by an extended stay at 6 ATA for up to 2 hr followed by a long staged decompression on U.S. Navy Table 4 or some equivalent decompression. The Royal Navy Table 73 uses a similar staged decompression to a pressure of 2.8 ATA followed by a change to a "slow-bleed" type of decompression to the surface. Both these tables allow for intermittent breathing of 100% oxygen at pressures of 2.8 ATA or less. A full description of all the available therapeutic recompression tables is given in a review by Berghage et al. (1978). It should be remembered that the ability to keep patients at 6 ATA and to use high partial pressures of oxygen is limited by the possibility of pulmonary oxygen toxicity, which is a time-and-dose–related disorder encountered with breathing mixtures with a P_{O_2} in excess of 0.5 ATA.

A small series of cases of decompression illness has been reported by Miller et al. (1978) where, for a variety of reasons that included the onset of acute pulmonary oxygen toxicity during recompression therapy, resort was made to oxygen-nitrogen saturation therapy with a chamber atmosphere containing less than 0.4 bar P_{O_2}. From this experience it has been proposed that oxygen-nitrogen saturation should be used as an elective procedure at 4 ATA should patients fail to respond to 2 hr of pressure at 6 ATA. Should relapse occur at some lower pressure, oxygen-nitrogen saturation may be used at some lesser pressure down to 2.5 ATA, where saturation on air is feasible. The current evidence for this procedure is unconvincing and research is needed to establish its place as an elective therapeutic procedure, notwithstanding its value when pulmonary oxygen toxicity has occurred.

In summary, the majority of opinion favors recompression to 6 ATA for 30 min followed by decompression to 2.8 ATA where breathing of pure oxygen may start. Oxygen-nitrogen mixtures may be used at 6 ATA to give a higher P_{O_2} that may be of therapeutic value. Failure to respond to recompression to 6 ATA may necessitate holding the patient at 6 ATA for 2 hr, after which decompression should commence on a recognized decompression schedule.

b. Oxygen

As has already been discussed, the pressure or partial pressure of oxygen in breathing mixtures is a product of overall pressure. Air at 6 ATA has a P_{O_2} of 1.26 ATA in contrast to the 2.8 ATA available when breathing pure oxygen at the equivalent depth of 60 fsw, which is recommended in the minimal recompression oxygen tables.

The role of an increase in P_{O_2} in the therapy of arterial gas embolism is threefold:

1. The gradient for diffusion of the inert gas in the intravascular gas emboli to be absorbed into solution in the surrounding plasma will be increased. This is due to the lowering of the partial pressure of inert gas in the blood that comes from breathing pure oxygen or hyperoxic mixtures. This effect will clearly be of less significance if therapy is delayed and events at the blood-gas boundary add a degree of permanency to bubbles. Similarly, coalescence will change the surface area of bubbles in contact with blood, making it smaller for any given volume of intravascular gas.

2. Irrespective of whatever embolic gas leads to complete or partial vascular occlusion, the initial cerebral insult in arterial gas embolism is due to hypoxia. Any raising of arterial P_{O_2} in blood going to the brain can only be beneficial in such circumstances. Although Bergofsky and Bertun (1966) and Jacobson and Lawson (1963) have suggested that such an effect would be negated by a diminished cerebral blood flow secondary to the vasoconstriction induced by a raised arterial P_{O_2}, three factors negate this argument. Sukoff et al. (1968) is typical of a number of authors who point out that the additional arterial oxygen is very largely dissolved in plasma and that breathing pure oxygen at 3 ATA allows a 100% increase in the potential arteriovenous extraction of oxygen by tissues. Further, the secondary passive vasodilation in blood vessels that have been embolized is not responsive to oxygen-induced vasoconstriction, and enhanced oxygen delivery to areas of hypoxic brain damage may be possible. Kety (1957) also adds to this argument by drawing attention to the contributory effect of locally raised carbon dioxide levels in areas of hypoxic damage and the antagonistic effect that will be exerted on any potential vasoconstriction. A final mechanism for enhanced oxygen delivery to areas of hypoxic damage is by diffusion. Peirce and Jacobson (1977) draw attention to this possibility, and it has been shown by Altman and Dittmer (1971) that maximum diffusion distances in cortical brain tissue is 20 μm with 56 μm possible in white matter. These distances are relatively large compared to the 6 μm possible in cardiac muscle.

3. The vasoconstriction secondary to increased arterial P_{O_2} may be, in itself, of very significant value. Secondary cerebral edema of some degree is certainly a possible sequel of cerebral arterial gas embolism. The cerebral edema has been shown by Ah See (1977) and other authors to have a large vasogenic component in contrast to the cytotoxic type of edema. Klatzo (1967) differentiated between vasogenic and cytotoxic edema in both etiological and pathological terms. The extracellular nature of vasogenic edema, which is secondary to vascular endothelial damage, implies that it would be responsive to a reduction in cerebral blood flow (CBF). Sukoff et al. (1968) gives a detailed account of the protective effect of hyperbaric oxygen in experimental animals and a very great deal of work has been done on quantifying the reduction in CBF that is possible. Some caution

is necessary in interpreting this work, and although many authors suggest that a 30% reduction in CBF may be possible with oxygen breathing up to 3 ATA, J. D. Miller et al. (1970) demonstrated that this effect reached a plateau at 2 ATA in his animal experiments. Using cats, he showed that with levels higher than 2 ATA there seemed to be increasing antagonism by accumulation of carbon dioxide in tissues subject to reduced blood flow. A further finding by Miller and colleagues was that when oxygen breathing ceased, the rebound effect, which gives an enhanced CBF, was particularly exaggerated when oxygen breathing at 3 ATA was used. It is for this reason that the Royal Navy allows for use of 32%–67% oxygen-nitrogen mixtures at 6 ATA during the initial stages of recompression therapy. The P_{O_2} of 1.95 ATA given by this mixture at 6 ATA seems more prudent than other available oxygen-nitrogen mixtures.

Apart from the therapeutic recompression tables mentioned previously, some authors have reported satisfactory results using minimal recompression oxygen tables without an initial compression to 6 ATA. Hart (1974), in reporting on a series of cases of arterial gas embolism, claimed that therapy with pure oxygen at 3 ATA was more successful than his experience with U.S. Navy Table 6A. This observation is of importance in that it would suggest that the monoplace chambers normally used for the more routine application of hyperbaric oxygen therapy are also suitable for the treatment of arterial gas embolism. Because such chambers often use an oxygen atmosphere, no air-breathing breaks are possible to ameliorate the problems of oxygen toxicity, and Hart suggested a routine involving 30 min at 3 ATA followed by 60 min at 2.5 ATA. Wattel et al. (1975) reported on successful use of oxygen at 2.1 ATA for therapy of arterial gas embolism in monoplace chambers. It is known that research is currently being conducted to establish the suitability of this type of therapy, but there is no doubt that initial compression to 6 ATA must be used if at all possible, and a body of opinion represented by Kindwall (1976) maintains that 6-ATA treatment is imperative enough to warrant taking patients to chambers capable of such therapy even if monoplace chambers are more accessible.

The therapeutic attractions of oxygen as opposed to pressure should be taken into account when patients have failed to respond to recompression to 6 ATA or when they relapse during decompression in the range of pressures in excess of 2.8 ATA. Provided there is no complication from pulmonary oxygen toxicity, the continuation of decompression to 2.8 ATA, where pure oxygen may be used, seems logically more attractive than embarking on a complicated extension to therapy involving saturation at a P_{O_2} of less than 0.5 ATA.

c. Adjuvant Therapy

The selection and use of adjuvant therapy is perhaps the most controversial aspect of the treatment of arterial gas embolism. One reason for this is the inability to judge the efficacy of adjuvant drug and intravenous fluid therapy in clinical situations where the two variables of pressure and oxygen already exist. It is clear that much more research is required to establish the true value of adjuvant therapy, and some advocated forms of such therapy can only have, at best, an empirical basis.

The most widely used form of adjuvant therapy is administration of steroids, particularly glucocorticoids such as dexamethasone. There is little disagreement that steroid administration can be of dramatic value in relieving raised intracranial pressure due to conditions such as metastatic cerebral tumors and, equally, it is generally accepted that they are of little or no value in the stroke situation. In work of relevance to the therapy of cerebral arterial gas embolism, glucocorticoids have been shown by Pappius and McCann (1969), Go (1971), and Yamaguchi et al. (1975), together with several other authors, to favorably influence vasogenic edema formation following various types of experimental brain injury in animals. Fishman (1975) suggested that dexamethasone was unlikely to influence cytotoxic edema such as results from severe degrees of cerebral hypoxia, and it is also relevant that cytotoxic edema is rarely responsible for significant rises in intracranial pressure. Conversely Fishman suggested that dexamethasone was likely to be beneficial in vasogenic edema secondary to blood-brain barrier (BBB) damage. Reulen (1976) added to the supporting evidence and suggested that dexamethasone has a multiple action on vascular endothelial permeability, electrolyte and water transport across cell membranes at the capillary-glial boundary, a reduction in cerebrospinal fluid production and, last, a stabilizing effect on lysosomal activity within cell membranes.

Dexamethasone has been used routinely by the Royal Navy since 1977 for all suspected or confirmed cases of cerebral arterial gas embolism. It is given intravenously in loading doses of 16 mg. To date, 36 diving and submarine escape training accidents have been treated this way, and there is growing evidence that the incidence of relapse, particularly late relapse, is much reduced. Therapy with dexamethasone may be continued for up to 72 hr with intramuscular doses of 6–8 mg every 6 hr.

Even early use of flucocorticoids may be unable to prevent severe degrees of relapse or deterioration due to cerebral edema. Various diuretics, including mannitol and frusemide, have been advocated for use in such cases. Royal Navy experience of two such cases suggests that 500 mg mannitol may be effective. Both Shenkin and Bouzarth (1970) and Fishman (1975) recommended mannitol as the diurectic of choice for cerebral edema even though the diuretic action is short lived and repeated administration is not possible. Kindwall (1979) has described some success with hypertonic solutions and recommends oral administration of 50% glycerol in water on the basis that rebound edema is less common and the diuretic action of a single dose may be prolonged for as long as 6 hr. The recent report by Goad et al. (1981) of the successful testing of a ventilator capable of reliable operation under pressure raises the possibility of controlled hyperventilation to produce a hypocapnic reduction in CBF as a means of controlling cerebral edema. Although in routine nonhyperbaric clinical use, such a method raises considerable logistic problems in hyperbaric surroundings, and its use in a condition originating from pulmonary barotrauma needs careful evaluation.

The role of anticoagulent therapy for this condition has not been researched or used in a controlled way, although Kindwall (1979) has suggested that iatrogenic arterial gas embolism appears to have a less dramatic impact on patients who are already heparinized for other clinical reasons. As a result of animal research, several other miscellaneous substances have been suggested as having potential value. Eiseman et al. (1959) drew attention to the prophylactic action of agents that reduce surface tension in dogs subject to experimental carotid embolization with air. Several substances were tried, of which Dow-Corning Anti-Foam A was the most successful. There is no recorded clinical experience with such drugs. The dramatic cardiovascular effects of experimental brain stem embolization in cats have been shown by Evans et al. (1980) to be prevented by prophylactic use of intravenous lidocaine. Much earlier work by Cadenat and Monsaingeon (1946) claimed dramatic success for intravenous procaine given to four patients with iatrogenic cerebral arterial gas embolism. Popovic et al. (1976) has claimed a significant protective action against mortality for levodopa (10 mg/kg) given into the descending aorta of rats 2 min after embolization with air into the same part of the aorta. Clinical applications for these various drugs await much further research, and these and other drugs of potential value would only seem of value in a prophylactic sense, thus imposing a severe limitation on their use.

4. Relapse after Initial Response to Therapy

A little-described feature of the therapy of cerebral arterial gas embolism is relapse following an initial response to recompression. Of 199 well-documented cases of cerebral arterial gas embolism treated by the Royal Navy, some degree of relapse was seen in 32% of cases. This figure seemed little affected by treatment delays, although more recent use of dexamethasone and tables based on U.S. Navy Table 6A seems to be of value in reducing the relapse incidence. Careful scrutiny of other reported cases from a wide variety of sources reveals relapse to be a common problem, although only Elliott et al. (1975), Gillen (1968), and Hallenbeck and Furlow (1977) make specific mention of it when discussing therapy. The degree of relapse may be profound and delayed by as much as 6–8 hr. Royal Navy experience includes two cases where death followed an apparently complete initial recovery on compression to 6 ATA. Conversely, relapse may be minor and not life threatening. The clinical features of severe relapse are very suggestive of increasing intracranial pressure, and postmortems on the two fatalities described showed very severe degrees of cerebral edema. It is also of interest that spontaneous recovery without specific therapy is not uncommon and relapse also occurs in approximately one-third of these cases.

Regrowth of persisting arterial gas emboli during decompression and reembolization from the initial causative lung lesions have both been advanced as etiological factors in relapse. Neither theory is wholly acceptable in view of the form and onset in time observed in relapses that, in any case, not infrequently occur without any change in pressure. Royal Navy experience also shows that relapse during decompression treated by simple recompression rarely exhibits any marked response. Indeed, decompression has continued in two recent cases showing relapse while resort was made to adjuvant therapy, and neither showed any continued worsening as a result of decompression. Much more satisfactory explanations for the etiology of relapse are vasogenic edema secondary to BBB permeability changes caused by arterial gas emboli or the "no-reflow" phenomenon initially described by Ames et al. (1968) and the subject of much recent work by Hallenbeck (1977, 1979) and Hallenbeck and Furlow (1977, 1979). Neither explanation is mutually exclusive. Although vasogenic edema is possible after the briefest of exposures of cerebral arteriolar vascular endothelium to arrested gas emboli, both Fischer (1972) and Little et al. (1975) suggest that transient ischemia of nervous tissue does not lead to a no-reflow phenomenon. This would suggest that this phenomenon is a less-likely explanation for relapse in cases where recompression therapy is immediate and full relief occurs rapidly. Clearly, such cases do not suffer from significant and sustained ischemia. However, Hallenbeck has shown that endothelial damage is an initiating factor in the complex chain of events leading to progressive failure of perfusion following an initial restoration of perfusion after the original ischemic insult. It is possible to postulate a vicious circle of events in which vasogenic edema itself may lead to sufficient ischemia to initiate the no-reflow phenomenon. While vasogenic edema may be favorably influenced by hyperbaric oxygen, steroids, and diuretics, Hallenbeck et al. (1979) have suggested that a combination of ibuprofen, PGI_2, and heparin may be of use in avoiding the no-reflow phenomenon. This important work may have a significant bearing on the use of adjuvant therapy.

5. Other Considerations

The therapy of cerebral arterial gas embolism is often complicated by other associated clinical problems, which in themselves may give rise to extreme therapeutic difficulties within the confines of a hyperbaric chamber. Ideally, patient monitoring should be provided, and various methods exist of obtaining ECG, EEG, and electronystagmography (ENG) recordings from patients under pressure. The Royal Navy has considerable experience of taking chest roentgenograms through the glass viewports of chambers, and the quality is certainly adequate to eliminate the possibility of pneumothorax. Recently, a safe method of electrical defibrillation has been developed for Royal Navy chambers.

In general, careful thought ought to be given to the provision of intensive and supportive care in hyperbaric facilities used for therapeutic purposes. Any case of suspected or confirmed arterial gas embolism should be admitted to a hospital after completion of initial recompression therapy. Investigations should include completion of initial recompression therapy. Investigations should include chest roentgenograms, ECG, EEG, and brain scan together with a full neurological assessment. Ventilation and perfusion studies of the lungs may be considered on an individual basis.

Any residual neurological problems should be actively treated with continued hyperbaric oxygen therapy on at least a daily basis. Formal therapeutic tables may be used, although recompression to 2 ATA on pure oxygen for 1 hr followed by decompression over 30 min has often been advocated. Pearson and Leitch (1979) have reported favorably on the use of continuing hyperbaric oxygen therapy until no sustained clinical or subjective improvement occurs.

Finally, although it is often supposed that long-term sequelae are very rare following cerebral arterial gas embolism, such is not the case, and the diffuse nature of the insult to the brain suggests that long-term follow-up of severe cases should always be attempted and special care given to assessment of the less tangible areas of mood, memory, personality, and intellectual capability. Only when a sufficient number of cases are followed up in this way can the present (perhaps overoptimistic) views on the therapy of cerebral gas embolism be supported.

R. R. PEARSON

References

ADEBAHR, G. 1972. Morphologic shock equivalents in air embolism, diving accidents and decompression sickness. *Beitr. Gerichtl. Med.* 28: 87–91.
ADOLFSON, J. A., AND C. LINDEMARK 1973. Pulmonary and neurological complications in free escape. In: *Proceedings of First Annual Scientific Meeting of the European Undersea Biomedical Society*, edited by C. M. Hesser and D. Linnarson. *Forsvarmedicin* 9: 244–246.

AH SEE, A. K. 1977. Permeability of the blood-brain barrier to FITC labelled Dextran in massive cerebral air embolism. In: *Workshop on Arterial Air Embolism and Acute Stroke*, edited by J. M. Hallenbeck and L. J. Greenbaum. Bethesda, MD: Undersea Medical Society, p. 43–48.

ALTMAN, P. L., AND D. S. DITTMER 1971. *Respiration and Circulation*. Bethesda, MD: Fed. Am. Soc. Exp. Biol., p. 453.

AMES, A., R. L. WRIGHT, M. KOWADA, J. M. THURSTON, AND G. MAJNO 1968. Cerebral ischemia II. The no-reflow phenomenon. *Am. J. Pathol.* 52: 437–453.

ATKINSON, J. R. 1963. Experimental air embolism. *Northwest Med.* 62: 699–703.

BABCOCK, R. H., AND M. J. NETSKY 1960. Respiratory and cardiovascular responses to experimental cerebral emboli. *Arch. Neurol. Chicago* 2: 556–564.

BAIRD, R. J., AND R. T. MIYAGISHIMA 1966. The nature of vasodilation which follows arterial gas embolization. *Can. J. Surg.* 9: 6–15.

BATSON, O. V. 1942. The role of vertebral veins in metastatic processes. *Ann. Intern. Med.* 16: 38.

BEHNKE, A. R. 1932. Analysis of accidents occurring in training with the submarine "lung." *U.S. Nav. Med. Bull.* 30: 177–185.

BERGHAGE, T. E., J. VOROSMARTI, JR., AND E. E. P. BARNARD 1978. Recompression treatment tables used throughout the world by government and industry. Rep. No. 78-16. Bethesda, MD: Naval Medical Research and Development Command, Naval Medical Research Institute.

BERGOFSKY, F. H., AND P. BERTUN 1966. Response of regional circulations to hyperoxia. *J. Appl. Physiol.* 21: 567–572.

BERT, P. 1878. *La Pression Barometrique. Recherches de Physiologie Experimentale*. Paris: Masson. (Transl. by M. A. and F. A. Hitchcock). Columbus, OH: College Book Co, 1943. (Republ. Bethesda, MD: Undersea Medical Society, 1978.)

BOND, R. F., T. DURANT. AND M. J. OPPENHEIMER 1965. Hemodynamic alterations produced by intra-arterial gas emboli. *Am. J. Physiol.* 208: 984–992.

BORNMANN, R. C. 1967. Experience with minimal recompression oxygen breathing: treatment of decompression sickness and air embolism. Memorandum Report Project SF0110605, Task 11513-2. Washington, DC: U.S. Navy Experimental Diving Unit.

BOYLE, R. 1670a. New pneumatical observations about respiration. *Phil. Trans. R. Soc.* 5: 2011–2031.

BOYLE, R. 1670b. Continuation of the observations concerning respiration. *Phil. Trans. R. Soc.* 5: 2035–2056.

BRIERLEY, J. B. 1963. Neuropathological findings in patients dying after open-heart surgery. *Thorax* 18: 291–304.

BRIERLEY, J. B. 1967. Brain damage complicating open-heart surgery: a neuropathological study of 46 patients. *Proc. R. Soc. Med.* 60: 34–35.

BROMAN, T., P. I. BRANEMARK, B. JOHANSSON, AND O. STEINWALL 1966. Intravital and post-mortem studies on air embolism damage of the blood-brain barrier tested with trypan blue. *Acta. Neurol. Scand.* 42: 146–152.

BUCKLES, R. G. 1968. The physics of bubble formation and growth. *Aerosp. Med.* 39: 1062–1069.

BUCKLES, R. G., AND C. KNOX 1969. In vivo bubble detection by acoustic-optical imaging techniques. *Nature* 222: 771–772.

BUTLER, R. D., AND B. A. HILLS 1979. The lung as a filter for microbubbles. *J. Appl. Physiol.* 47: 537–543.

CADENAT, M. M., AND A. MONSAINGEON 1946. Embolie gazeuse du cerveau. Heureuse action de novocainisation intraveineuse. *Mem. Acad. Chir.* 72: 355–359.

CAPPS, J. A. 1937. Air embolism versus pleural reflex as the cause of pleural shock. *JAMA* 109: 852–854.

CHANDLER, W. F., D. G. DIMCHEFF, AND J. A. TAREN 1974. Acute pulmonary oedema following venous air embolism during a neurosurgical procedure. *J. Neurosurg.* 40: 400–404.

CHASE, W. H. 1934. Anatomical and experimental observations on air embolism. *Surg. Gynecol. Obstet.* 59: 569–577.

CHRYSSANTHOU, C., M. SPRINGER, AND S. LIPSCHITZ 1977. Blood-brain and blood-lung barrier alteration by dysbaric exposure. *Undersea Biomed. Res.* 4: 117–129.

COLEBATCH, H. J. H., M. M. SMITH, AND C. K. Y. NG 1973. Increased elastic recoil as a determinant of pulmonary barotrauma in divers. *Respir. Physiol.* 26: 55–64.

CURTILLET, E., AND A. CURTILLET 1939a. L'Embolie gazeuse. La traversée des anastomoses arterio-veineuses. *C.R. Soc. Biol. Paris* 130: 647–650.

CURTILLET, E., AND A. CURTILLET 1939b. Étude experimentale de l'embolie gazeuse. *J. Physiol. Pathol. Gen.* 40: 573–584.

DE LA TORRE, E., J. MEREDITH, AND M. J. NETSKY 1962. Cerebral air embolism in the dog. *Arch. Neurol.* 6: 307–316.

DE LA TORRE, E., O. C. MITCHELL, AND M. G. NETSKY 1962. The seat of respiratory and cardiovascular responses to cerebral air emboli. *Neurol. Minneap.* 12: 140–147.

DONALD, K. W. 1979. Submarine escape breathing air. A review and analysis of animal experiments by the Royal Navy. *Bull. Europ. Physiol. Pathol. Resp.* 15: 739–754.

DUFF, F., A. D. M. GREENFIELD, AND R. W. WHELAN 1954. Observations on the mechanism of the vasodilation following arterial gas embolism. *Clin. Sci.* 13: 365–376.

DURANT, T. M., J. LONG, AND M. J. OPPENHEIMER 1947. Pulmonary (venous) air embolism. *Am. Heart J.* 33: 269–281.

DURANT, T. M., M. J. OPPENHEIMER, M. R. WEBSTER, AND J. LONG 1949. Arterial air embolism. *Am. Heart J.* 38: 481–500.

DURANT, T. M., M. J. OPPENHEIMER, P. R. LYNCH, G. ASCIANO, AND D. WEBBER 1954. Body position in relation to venous air embolism. A roentgenologic study. *Am. J. Med. Sci.* 227: 509–518.

EISEMAN, B., B. J. BAXTER, AND K. PRACHUABMOH 1959. Surface tension reducing substances in the management of coronary air embolism. *Ann. Surg.* 149: 374–380.

ELLIOTT, D. H., J. A. B. HARRISON, AND E. E. P. BARNARD 1978. Clinical and radiological features of 88 cases of decompression barotrauma. In: *Underwater Physiology VI. Proceedings of the Sixth Symposium on Underwater Physiology*, edited by C. W. Shilling and M. W. Beckett. Bethesda, MD: Fed. Am. Soc. Exp. Biol., p. 527–535.

EVANS, D. E., E. HARDENBERGH, AND J. M. HALLENBECK 1977. Cardiovascular effects of arterial air embolism. In: *Workshop on Arterial Air Embolism and Acute Stroke*, edited by J. M. Hallenbeck and L. J. Greenbaum. Bethesda, MD: Undersea Medical Society, p. 20–23.

EVANS, D. E., A. I. KOBRINE, E. T. FLYNN, AND M. E. BRADLEY 1980. Treatment of cardiovascular dysfunction resulting from cerebral air embolism. In: *Program and Abstracts, 7th Symposium on Underwater Physiology*. Bethesda, MD: Undersea Medical Society, p. 14.

FAZIO, C., AND U. SACCHI 1954. Experimentally produced red softening of the brain. *J. Neuropathol. Exp. Neurol.* 13: 476.

FISCHER, E. G. 1972. Studies on mechanisms of impairment of cerebral circulation following ischemia: effect of haemodilution and perfusion pressure. *Stroke* 3: 538–542.

FISHMAN R. A. 1975. Brain edema. *N. Engl. J. Med.* 293: 706–711.

FRIEDBURG, C. K. 1956. *Diseases of the Heart* (2nd ed.). Philadelphia: W. B. Saunders.

FRIES, C. C., B. LEVOWITZ, S. ADLER, A. W. COOK, ET AL. 1957. Experimental gas embolism. *Ann. Surg.* 145: 461–470.

FRYER, D. I., AND H. L. ROXBURGH 1965. Decompression sickness. In: *Textbook of Aviation Physiology*, edited by J. A. Gillies. Oxford: Pergamon Press. p. 121–151.

GALLAGHER, E. G., AND T. D. PEARSON 1973. Ultrasonic identification of source of gaseous microemboli during open-heart surgery. *Thorax* 28: 295–305.

GEOGHEGAN, T., AND C. R. LAM 1953. The mechanism of death from intracardiac air and its reversibility. *Ann. Surg.* 139: 351–359.

GILLEN, H. W. 1968. Symptomatology of cerebral gas embolism. *Neurology Minneap.* 18: 507–512.

GOAD, R. F., C. SCOTT, A. M. SAYWARD, AND R. HOWARD 1981. Function of the Oxford ventilator at high pressure. Rep. No. 9/81. Alverstoke, Hants, UK: Institute of Naval Medicine.

GO, K. G., F. VAN WOUDENBERG, H. BEEKHUIS, T. SCHUT, AND H. DOORENBOS 1971. Effect of hydrocortisone on cold induced edema in rat brain. *Neurochirurgia* 14: 232–240.

GOODMAN, M. W., AND R. D. WORKMAN 1965. Minimal recompression, oxygen breathing approach to the treatment of decompression sickness in divers and aviators. Rep. No. 5-65. Washington, DC: U.S. Navy Experimental Diving Unit.

GREENE, K. M. 1978. Causes of death in submarine escape training casualties: analysis of cases and review of the literature. AMTE(E) Rep. R78-502. Alverstoke, Hants, UK: AMTE Physiological Laboratory.

GRULKE, D. C. 1975. Experimental cerebral air embolism: a physical and physiological study using uniform microbubbles of known size. Thesis in Physiology. London: Univ. of London.

HALLENBECK, J. M. 1977. Prevention of post-ischemic impairment of microvascular perfusion. *Neurol. Minneap.* 27: 3–10.

HALLENBECK, J. M. 1979. Factors influencing the extent and degree of spinal cord damage in decompression sickness. In: *Decompression Sickness and Its Therapy,* edited by C. J. Lambertsen. Allentown, PA: Air Products and Chemicals, Inc., p. 7–17.

HALLENBECK, J. M., A. A. BOVE, AND D. H. ELLIOTT 1975. Mechanisms underlying spinal cord decompression sickness. *Neurology Minneap.* 25: 308–316.

HALLENBECK, J. M., AND T. W. FURLOW, JR. 1977. Impaired microvascular perfusion and secondary deterioration in dysbaric cerebral embolism. In: *Workshop on Arterial Air Embolism and Acute Stroke,* edited by J. M. Hallenbeck and L. J. Greenbaum. Bethesda, MD: Undersea Medical Society, p. 76–86.

HALLENBECK, J. M., AND T. W. FURLOW, JR. 1979. Prostaglandins influence on nutrient perfusion in brain during the post-ischemic period. In: *Prostaglandin,* edited by J. R. Vane and S. Bergstrom. New York: Raven Press. p. 299–310.

HALLENBECK, J. M., L. J. GREENBAUM, AND D. R. LEITCH 1979. The influence of Ibuprofen, PGI_2 and heparin on evoked response recovery after air embolism. *Undersea Biomed. Res. Suppl.* 6: 36–37. (Program and Abstracts, Undersea Medical Society Annual Scientific Meeting.)

HART, G. B. 1974. Treatment of decompression illness and air embolism. *Aerosp. Med.* 45: 1190–1193.

HARVEY, R. B., AND J. A. SCHILLING 1954. Relationship between lung pressures and volumes and traumatic air embolism. *Fed. Proc.* 13: 68.

HARVEYSON, K. B., B. E. E. HIRSCHFELD, AND J. I. TONGE 1956. Fatal air embolism resulting from the use of a compressed air diving unit., *Med. J. Aust.* 1: 658–660.

HASEGAWA, T., J. R. RAVENS, AND J. F. TOOLE 1967. Precapillary arteriovenous anastomoses. *Arch. Neurol. Chicago* 16: 217–224.

HAYMAKER, W., AND A. D. JOHNSTON 1955. Pathology of decompression sickness: a comparison of lesions in airmen with those in caisson workers and divers. *Mil. Med.* 117: 285–306.

HEMPLEMAN, H. V. 1972. The site of origin of gaseous emboli produced by decompression from raised pressures of air and other gases. In: *Proceedings of Third International Conference on Hyperbaric Medicine and Underwater Physiology,* edited by X. Fructus. Paris: Doin, p. 160–162.

HOLT, E. R., JR., M. D. WATTS, R. WEBB, W. A. COOK, AND M. O. UNAL 1966. Air embolism: Hemodynamics and therapy. *Ann. Thorac. Surg.* 2: 551–560.

INGVAR, D. H., J. ADOLFSON, AND C. O. LINDEMARK 1973. Cerebral air embolism during training of submarine personnel in free escape: an electroencephalographic study. *Aerosp. Med.* 44: 628–653.

JACOBSEN, I., AND D. D. LAWSON 1963. The effect of hyperbaric oxygen on experimental cerebral infarction in the dog. *J. Neurosurg.* 20: 849–859.

JANKE, W. H., AND A. A. ESFAHANI 1970. Air embolism following open heart surgery. *Mich. Med.* 69: 761–762.

JOHANSSON, B. 1974. Damage to the blood-brain barrier in experimental gas embolism. In: *Collque en l'embolie gazeuse du système carotidien,* edited by G. Arfel and R. Naquet. Paris: Doin, p. 165–170.

KAUFMANN, A. 1924. Quoted by H. Steindl. *Wein. Klin. Wochenschr.* 37: 206.

KENNEDY, J. H., N. H. C. WANG, G. V. MILLER, AND A. HARTMAN 1974. Factors influencing distribution of cerebral gas embolism. *Cryobiology* 11: 483–492.

KESSLER, J., AND R. H. PATTERSON, JR. 1970. The production of microemboli by various blood oxygenators. *Ann. Thorac. Surg.* 9: 221–228.

KETY, S. S. 1957. Determinants of tissue oxygen tension. *Fed. Proc.* 16: 666–670.

KINDWALL, E. P. 1976. *Hyperbaric Medicine Procedures.* Milwaukee, WI: St. Luke's Hospital.

KINDWALL, E. P. 1979. Role of adjunctive drug and fluid therapy. In: *Treatment of Serious Decompression Sickness and Arterial Gas Embolism,* edited by J. C. Davis. Bethesda, MD: Undersea Medical Society, p. 45–50. (Workshop.)

KLATZO, I. 1967. Neuropathological aspects of brain edema. *J. Neuropathol. Exp. Neurol.* 26: 1–14.

LAMBERT, R. J. W. 1958. Submarine escape. *Proc. R. Soc. Med.* 51: 824–827.

LEE, J. C. 1974. The blood-brain barrier and cerebral air embolism. In: *Colloque en l'embolie gazeuse du système carotidien,* edited by G. Arfel and R. Naquet. Paris: Doin, p. 158–164.

LEVER, M. J. 1967. Personal communication quoted by D. H. Elliott. In: *The Physiology and Medicine of Diving and Compressed Air Work,* edited by P. B. Bennett and D. H. Elliott. London: Ballière, Tindall, p. 423.

LEVER, M. J., K. W. MILLER, W. D. M. PATON, AND E. B. SMITH 1966. Experiments on the genesis of bubbles as a result of rapid decompression. *J. Physiol. London* 184: 964–969.

LIEBERMEISTER, G. 1929. Anamisches Zungenphanomen, ein Fruhsymptom der arteriellen Luftembolie. *Klin. Wochenschr.* 8: 21.

LIEBOW, A. A., J. E. STARK, J. VOGEL, AND K. E. SCHAEFER 1959. Intrapulmonary air trapping in submarine escape training casualties. Rep. No. 330. *U.S. Armed Forces Med. J.* 10: 265–289.

LITTLE, J. R., F. W. L. KERR, AND T. M. SUNDT 1975. Microcirculatory obstruction in cerebral ischemia. *Mayo Clin. Proc.* 50: 264–270.

LUBARSCH, O. 1922. Quoted by H. Steindl. *Wien. Klin. Wochenschr.* 37: 206.

MACKLIN, M. T., AND C. C. MACKLIN 1944. Malignant interstitial emphysema of the lungs and mediastinum as an important occult complication in many respiratory diseases and conditions; an interpretation of the clinical literature in the light of laboratory experiments. *Medicine* 23: 281–358.

MALHOTRA, M. S., AND H. C. WRIGHT 1959. Air embolism during decompression and its prevention. Admiralty Report RNPL 9/59. London: Ministry of Defence, R.N. Physiological Laboratory.

MALHOTRA, M. S., AND H. C. WRIGHT 1960. Arterial air embolism during decompression and its prevention. *Proc. R. Soc. Lond. Ser. B* 154: 418–427.

MALHOTRA, M. S., AND H. C. WRIGHT 1961. The effects of a raised intrapulmonary pressure on the lungs of fresh unchilled cadavers. *J. Pathol. Bacteriol.* 82: 198–202.

MARCHAND, P., J. C. GILROY, AND V. H. WILSON 1950. An anatomical study of the bronchial vascular system and its variation in disease. *Thorax* 5: 207–221.

MELDRUM, B. S., J. J. PAPY, AND R. A. VIGOROUX 1971. Intracarotid air embolism in the baboon: effects on cerebral blood flow and electroencephalogram. *Brain Res.* 25: 301–315.

MILLER, J. D., W. FITCH, I. MCA. LEDINGHAM, AND W. B. JENNETT 1970. The effect of hyperbaric oxygen on experimentally raised intracranial pressure. *J. Neurosurg.* 33: 287–296.

MILLER, J. N., L. FRAGRAEUS, P. B. BENNETT, D. H. ELLIOTT, T. G. SHIELDS, AND J. GRIMSTAD 1978. Nitrogen-oxygen saturation therapy in serious cases of compressed air decompression sickness. *Lancet* 2: 169–171.

MOORE, R. M., AND C. W. BRASELTON 1940. Injections of air and carbon dioxide into a pulmonary vein. *Ann. Surg.* 112: 212–218.

MOSES, H. L. 1964. Casualties in individual submarine escape. *U.S. Nav. Submar. Med. Cent. Rep.* 438.

NAQUET, R., G. ARFEL, M. CHOUX, D. DUBOIS, AND D. RICHE 1966. Étude experimentale de l'embolie gazeuse par voie carotidienne chez le chat. *Electroencephalogr. Clin. Neurophysiol.* 20: 181–196.

NAQUET, R., M. CHOUX, C. BAURAND, J. C. GUILLERMIN, AND R. P. VIGÖROUX 1974. Étude comparative de l'embolie cerebrale provoquee par divers gaz ou mélanges gazeux. In: *Colloque en l'embolie gazeuse du système carotidien*, edited by G. Arfel and R. Naquet. Paris: Doin, p. 78–84.

PALMER, A. C., W. F. BLAKEMORE, AND A. C. GREENWOOD 1976. Neuropathology of decompression sickness (dysbarism) in the goat. *Neuropathol. Appl. Neurobiol.* 2: 145–156.

PAPPIUS, H. M., AND P. W. MCCANN 1969. Effects of steroids on cerebral edema in cats. *Arch. Neurol. Chicago* 20: 207–216.

PEARSON, R. R. 1981. A review of submarine escape training accidents with reference to the use of slowed or interrupted training ascents. Rep. 15/81. Alverstoke, Hants, UK: Institute of Naval Medicine.

PEARSON, R. R., AND D. R. LEITCH 1979. Treatment of air or oxygen/nitrogen mixture decompression illnesses in the Royal Navy. *J. R. Nav. Med. Serv.* 65: 53–62.

PEIRCE, E. C., II, AND J. H. JACOBSON 1977. Cerebral edema. In: *Hyperbaric Oxygen Therapy*, edited by J. C. Davis and T. K. Hunt. Bethesda, MD: Undersea Medical Society, p. 287–301.

POLAK, I. B., AND B. H. ADAMS 1932. Traumatic air embolism in submarine escape training. *U.S. Nav. Med. Bull.* 30: 165–177.

POPOVIC, P., V. POPOVIC, AND R. SCHAFFER 1976. Injectable agent for the treatment of air emboli induced paraplegia in rats. *Aviat. Space Environ. Med.* 47: 1073–1075.

PRINZMETAL, M., E. M. ORNITZ, B. SIMKIN, AND H. C. BERGMAN 1948. Arteriovenous anastomoses in liver, spleen and lungs. *Am. J. Physiol.* 152: 48.

RANGELL, L. 1942. Cerebral air embolism: the question of arterialization of intravenous air across the barrier of the pulmonary capillaries. *J. Nerv. Ment. Dis.* 96: 542.

REESE, E. J. 1968. Extra-alveolar air resulting from submarine escape training: a post-training roentgenographic survey of 170 submariners. *U.S. Nav. Submar. Res. Lab. Rep.* 550.

REULEN, H. J. 1976. Vasogenic brain oedema: new aspects in its formation, resolution and therapy. *Br. J. Anaesth.* 48: 741–752.

REULEN, H. J., A. HADJIDIMOS, AND U. HASE 1973. Steroids in the treatment of brain oedema. In: *Advances in Neurosurgery I,* edited by K. Schurmann, M. Brock, H. J. Reulen, and D. Voth. New York: Springer-Verlag, p. 92.

ROYAL NAVY 1964. *Royal Navy Diving Manual.* BR155. London: Her Majesty's Stationery Office.

ROYAL NAVY 1972. *Royal Navy Diving Manual.* BR2806. London: Her Majesty's Stationery Office.

ROZDILSKY, B., AND J. OLSZWESKI 1957. Permeability of cerebral blood vessels studied by radioactive iodinated bovine albumin. *Neurol. Minneap.* 7: 270–279.

RUKSTINAT, G. J. 1931. Experimental air embolism of the coronary arteries. *JAMA* 96: 26–28.

SAMSON, R. I., AND J. W. MILLER (chairmen) 1979. *Emergency Ascent Training.* Bethesda, MD: Undersea Medical Society. (Workshop Dec. 1977.)

SCHAEFER, K. E., W. P. MCNULTY, C. R. CAREY, AND A. A. LIEBOW 1958. Mechanisms in development of interstitial emphysema and air embolism in decompression from depth. *J. Appl. Physiol.* 13: 15–29.

SCHLAEPFER, K. 1972. Air embolism following various diagnostic procedures in diseases of the pleura and the lung. *Bull. Johns Hopkins Hosp.* 133: 321–330.

SHENKIN, H. A., AND W. F. BOUZARTH 1970. Clinical methods of reducing intracranial pressure. *N. Engl. J. Med.* 282: 1465–1471.

SHILLING, C. W. 1933. Expiratory force as related to submarine escape training. *U.S. Nav. Med. Bull.* 31: 1–7.

SIMMS, N. M., G. S. KUSH, D. M. LONG, M. M. KOKEN, AND L. A. FRENCH 1970. Regional cerebral blood flow alterations following arterial air embolism. *Surg. Forum* 21: 427–429.

SIMMS, N. M., G. S. KUSH, D. M. LONG ET AL. 1971. Increase in regional cerebral blood flow following experimental arterial air embolism. *J. Neurosurg.* 34: 665–671.

SIMMS, N. M., D. M. LONG, J. H. MATTHEWS, AND S. N. CHOU 1972. Hyperoxia of cerebral venous and cisternal cerebrospinal fluid following arterial air embolism. *J. Neurosurg.* 37: 30–35.

SMITH-SIVERTSEN, J. 1973. The origin of intravascular gas bubbles produced by decompression of rats killed prior to hyperbaric exposure. RNPL Rep. No. 10/73. Alverstoke, Hants, UK: Royal Naval Physiological Laboratory.

SPENCER, F. C., N. P. ROSSI, S. C. YU ET AL. 1965. The significance of air embolism during cardiopulmonary by-pass. *J. Thorac. Cardiov. Surg.* 49: 615–634.

SPENCER, M. P., G. H. LAWRENCE, AND G. I. THOMAS 1969. The use of ultrasonics in the determination of arterial air embolism during open-heart surgery. *Ann. Thorac. Surg.* 8: 489–497.

SUKOFF, M. H., S. A. HOLLIN, O. E. ESPINOSA, AND J. H. JACOBSON II 1968. The protective effect of hyperbaric oxygenation in experimental cerebral edema. *J. Neurosurg.* 29: 236–241.

SWANK, R. L., AND R. L. HAIN 1952. The effect of different sized emboli on the vascular system and parenchyma of the brain. *J. Neuropathol. Exp. Neurol.* 11: 280–299.

THOMAS, A. N., AND B. G. STEPHENS 1974. Air embolism: a cause of morbidity and death after penetrating chest trauma. *J. Trauma* 14: 633–638.

U.S. NAVY 1978. *U.S. Navy Diving Manual (Change 2). Air Diving.* Washington, DC: U.S. Navy Department, Vol. 1. (NAVSEA 0094-LP-001-9010).

VAN ALLEN, C. M., AND L. S. HRDINA 1929. Air embolism from the pulmonary vein. *Arch. Surg. Chicago* 19: 567–599.

VAN GENDEREN, L. 1967. Study of air embolism and extra-alveolar accidents associated with submarine escape training casualties. *U.S. Nav. Submar. Med. Cent. Rep.* 500.

VAN GENDEREN, L., AND C. L. WAITE 1968. Evaluation and treatment of traumatic cerebral air embolism. *Aerosp. Med.* 39: 709–713.

VERSTAPPEN, F. T. J., J. A. BERNARDS, AND F. KREUZER 1977a. Effects of pulmonary gas embolism on circulation and respiration in the dog. *Pfluegers Arch.* 368: 89–96.

VERSTAPPEN, F. T. J., J. A. BERNARDS, AND F. KREUZER 1977b. Effects of pulmonary gas embolism on circulation and respiration in the dog. II. Effects on respiration. *Pfluegers Arch.* 368: 97–104.

VERSTAPPEN, F. T. J., J. A. BERNARDS, AND F. KREUZER 1977c. Effects of pulmonary gas embolism on circulation and respiration in the dog. III. Excretion of venous gas bubbles in the lung. *Pfluegers Arch.* 370: 67–70.

VERSTAPPEN, F. T. J., J. A. BERNARDS, AND F. KREUZER 1977d. Effects of pulmonary gas embolism on circulation and respiration in the dog. IV. Origin of arterial hypoxaemia during pulmonary gas embolism. *Pfluegers Arch.* 370: 71–75.

VON HAYEK, H. 1960. *The Human Lung.* New York: Hafner Publishing Co.

VOURCH, G. 1971. Paradoxical air embolism. *N. Engl. J. Med.* 293: 184–185.
WAGNER, C. E. 1945. Observations of gas bubbles in pial vessels of cats following rapid decompression from high pressure atmospheres. *J. Neurophysiol.* 8: 29–32.
WAITE, C. L., W. F. MAZZONE, M. E. GREENWOOD, AND R. T. LARSEN 1967. Cerebral air embolism. I. Basic studies. *U.S. Nav. Submar. Med. Cent. Rep.* 493.
WARREN, B. A., R. B. PHILP, AND M. J. INWOOD 1973. The ultrastructural morphology of air embolism: platelet adhesion to the interface and endothelial damage. *Br. J. Exp. Pathol.* 54: 163–172.
WATTEL, F., B. GOSSELIN, C. CHOPIN, E. LEPOUTRE, AND S. FLIPO 1975. Les embolies gazeuses et leur traitement par l'oxygene hyperbare. *Lille Med.* 20: 91–95.
YAMAGUCHI, M., S. SHIRAKATA, K. TAOMOTO, AND S. MATSUMOTO 1975. Steroid treatment of brain oedema. *Surg. Neurol.* 4: 5–8.

VIII

Near-Drowning

Drowning is a major cause of the accidental death of young people. Approximately 6000 persons drown in the United States each year; half of the victims are less than 20 years of age (U.S. Dept. Health and Human Services 1980). The vast majority are male (Kruis et al. 1979; Modell et al. 1976; Orlowski 1979), and at least 35% of the victims have been accomplished swimmers (Modell 1971).

Because reporting of "near-drowning" is not required, how many persons near-drown is not really known. It has been estimated that eight persons near-drown for each one drowned (Schuman et al. 1976); this injury is thus significant. The current enthusiasm for scuba diving and other water-related sports makes it imperative that physicians be well versed in the pathophysiology and management of near-drowning.

A. Definitions

To understand the statistics and literature of drowning and near-drowning, definitions are necessary. Webster's dictionary defines "drown" as "to suffocate by submersion, especially in water" (Websters 1979). Cot (1931) demonstrated that approximately 10%–15% of drowned persons die from hypoxia (suffocate) due to laryngospasm or breath holding without also aspirating. Modell has offered a classification of the injuries of drowning and near-drowning (Modell 1971, 1981); by use of this system drowned persons may be categorized into two subgroups: those who aspirate water and those who do not.

"Near-drowned" describes those persons who survive submersion, at least temporarily. This group is also divided into those who aspirate and those who do not. In one study, 12% of near-drowned victims did not evidently aspirate (Modell et al. 1976).

"Delayed death subsequent to near-drowning" describes those who are resuscitated but die later due to the injury or to secondary complications, such as unrecognized pulmonary insufficiency, secondary bacterial infection, or irreversible anoxic damage to the central nervous system. Because the primary cause of death and the time until delayed death vary, it is difficult to determine the number of delayed deaths that occur.

B. Modifying Factors

The circumstances of the injury influence the nature of the lesion. The chemical content and the amount of the water aspirated differ with each accident. An infinite variety of potentially pathogenic water contaminants, such as bacteria and algae, have an impact on a victim's clinical course that usually cannot be foreseen. Similarly, the duration and severity of hypoxia or of circulatory collapse determine the damage to the central nervous system; yet no one can predict what that impact will be, even when the exact details of the accident are known.

The effect of water temperature on the duration of submersion that a human being can survive has long been of interest (Conn 1979; Conn et al. 1978; Fleetham and Munt 1978; Nemiroff 1977a, 1977b; Nemiroff et al. 1977). Reports of complete recovery after prolonged submersion in very cold water have appeared in the literature, the longest recorded submersion being 40 min (Siebke et al. 1975). These reports are encouraging and should stimulate the clinician to continue aggressive resuscitation of and intensive care for victims of such accidents. The core body temperature must be determined in all near-drowned victims; while the rapid onset of hypothermia may protect the brain from anoxic damage, hypothermia also causes abnormal neurological and cardiovascular functions (Fleetham and Munt 1978). While some authors advocate maintaining mild to moderate degrees of hypothermia for brain resuscitation (Conn et al. 1978, 1980), severe hypothermia must be corrected simultaneously with therapy for near-drowning. Since blood gas tensions are measured at 37°C, correction of these values to the patient's body temperature is often necessary to assess the results of therapy (Fleetham and Munt 1978).

The *diving reflex*, which has been well documented in diving mammals, has also been described in other animals and in the human being (Anderson 1966; Campbell et al. 1969; Gooden 1972, Hunt 1974). During immersion of the head this reflex appears to protect vital organs against hypoxia. The reflex is initiated by stimulation of the mandibular division of the trigeminal nerve and is mediated by the vagus, resulting in bradycardia and intense vasoconstriction (Anderson 1966; Campbell et al. 1969). The culmination is that the circulating blood is shunted primarily to the brain and to the heart. The intensity of the reflex varies in different subjects, but it appears to be greatest when the subject has taken a deep breath of air immediately before facial immersion and when the water is cold (less than 20°C) (Campbell et al. 1969). Thus the duration of submersion that can be tolerated without central nervous system damage may be prolonged by the diving reflex.

C. History

The resuscitation of drowned victims has been attempted for many centuries. Examples of such measures have been documented by ancient murals and scrolls (Schechter 1969). Tracheotomy was first described around 100 B.C. and was probably used to resuscitate drowned victims. Europeans learned fumigation techniques from American Indians, who used tobacco smoke blown into the mouth and rectum to revive the victim (Schechter 1969).

In the late 18th century the Royal Humane Society was formed in Great Britain. The Society promoted current resuscitation techniques, provided equipment for rescue, and distributed educational pamphlets to the public (Redding 1977, Schechter 1969). In 1788 Kite offered a device for tracheal cannulation called "Kite's apparatus for the resuscitation of the partially drowned" (Sykes 1972).

The number of techniques for artificial ventilation promoted during the 19th century indicates the inadequate results of each. The Schafer prone chest-pressure technique was introduced in 1904 but was replaced by the prone, back-pressure, arm-lift technique offered by Neilsen in 1932 (see Comroe 1979). This technique was widely endorsed by many agencies teaching rescue and first-aid techniques (Redding 1977).

In 1958 Safar et al. (1958) introduced the mouth-to-mouth technique of ventilation and demonstrated the superiority of this method over previously recommended ones. Techniques to provide effective cardiopulmonary resuscitation by rescuers at the scene of the accident were finally completed with the rediscovery of closed-chest cardiac massage in 1960 (Kouwenhoven et al. 1960). Redding et al.(1961) demonstrated the effectiveness of these techniques for the resuscitation of near-drowned experimental animals soon thereafter.

In spite of the many centuries of interest in drowning, only in the past three decades have the details of the pathophysiology of the injury come to light. Early experimental studies evidenced hypoxia in animals that aspirated fresh water or seawater, but the studies suggested that changes in blood volume and serum electrolyte concentrations were critical in cardiac arrest due to drowning (Swann and Brucer 1949; Swann et al. 1947). This led many clinicians to focus on electrolytes in treating the near-drowned human. In 1963, however, Fuller (1963a, 1963b), reporting on a large series of drowned and near-drowned humans, determined that significant electrolyte abnormalities did not occur. Modell and co-workers, by studying drowned and near-drowned humans and experimental animals (Modell and Davis 1969; Modell et al. 1968a; Modell and Moya 1966; Modell et al. 1966, 1967) provided insight into the differences between drowned humans and previous animal models and refined the experimental animal model with which drowning and near-drowning could be examined in the laboratory. Since that time numerous studies have defined the temporal and quantitative changes in blood volume (Modell and Moya 1966; Modell et al. 1967), serum electrolyte concentrations (Modell and Davis 1969; Modell et al. 1968a; Modell and Moya 1966; Modell et al.1966, 1967), acid-base balance (Modell et al. 1966), and arterial oxygenation (Modell et al. 1968b; Modell et al. 1972; Ruiz et al. 1973) and have determined the physiological changes that occur in the lungs and the cardiovascular system after experimental near-drowning (Modell et al. 1968b; Modell et al. 1972, 1974; Ruiz et al. 1973; Bergquist et al. 1980) and the effects of various modes of ventilatory support (Bergquist et al. 1980; Modell et al. 1974; Ruiz et al. 1973). Reports of large series of near-drowned humans, which support the information gained from experimental animal studies, have become available in the past 10 years (Fandel and Bancalari 1976; Modell et al. 1976; Orlowski 1979; Pearn et al. 1979; Peterson 1977). Recent investigations have concentrated on the prevention and reversal of anoxic brain damage and the effects and treatment of ventilation-perfusion abnormalities secondary to near-drowning (Bergquist et al. 1980; Conn et al. 1980; Modell et al. 1980).

D. Physiological Changes

1. Oxygenation and Acid-Base Balance

The primary injury in both drowning and near-drowning is respiratory insufficiency with impaired arterial oxygenation and altered acid-base balance (Fuller 1963b; Modell 1971). Other organ damage that has been described after near-drowning is frequently due to hypoxia and acidosis. While the victim who near-drowns without aspirating has no structural pulmonary injury and may not have abnormal arterial oxygenation upon evaluation in the hospital, he may have suffered hypoxemia from a lack of ventilation long enough to damage the central nervous system. Cot (1931) demonstrated in 1931 that 10% of drowned humans on whom autopsies were performed did not evidence aspiration. Modell et al. (1976) reported that 12% of a large series of near-drowned patients did not show clinical, chemical, or roentgenographic evidence of aspiration. An experimental study to determine the effects of airway obstruction (such as would result from larynogospasm) on the arterial oxygenation and acid-base balance of dogs demonstrated that arterial carbon dioxide tension (Pa_{CO_2}) increased approximately 6 mmHg/min and arterial pH (pHa) decreased approximately 0.05 U/min, but that the arterial oxygen tension (Pa_{O_2}) decreased dramatically from a base-line average of 92 mmHg to 40 mmHg after 1 min of tracheal obstruction, to 10 mmHg after 3 min and to 4 mmHg after 5 min (Modell et al. 1972). In spite of the extreme hypoxemia after 5 min of tracheal obstruction, 80% of the animals were successfully resuscitated by a brief period of positive pressure ventilation and, in some cases, closed chest cardiac massage. The Pa_{O_2} and Pa_{CO_2} approached base-line values 10 min after the experiment began.

If a near-drowned victim has not aspirated and ventilation and circulation are promptly restored, complete recovery usually follows without further therapy. This does not happen, however, when the victim has aspirated a significant quantity of water or gastric contents. In an experimental study of dogs that aspirated 22 ml/kg of fresh water or saline, Pa_{O_2} decreased to an average of 40 mmHg within 1 min and remained essentially unchanged during the 1-hr study (Modell et al. 1966). In the same animals, pHa decreased to its lowest value within 5 min, then improved but did not return to normal after 1 hr; Pa_{CO_2} increased transiently, peaked after 5 min, but returned to normal within 1 hr. Several studies of human victims have documented that some patients may suffer severe arterial hypoxemia in spite of mechanical ventilatory support and high concentrations of inspired oxygen (Fandel and Bancalari 1976; Modell et al. 1976). Indeed, some patients die from pulmonary insufficiency during the course of aggressive respiratory support.

The severity of hypoxemia or acidemia found from the initial analysis of arterial blood gas tensions and pH does not allow a prediction of the outcome; some patients with severe hypoxemia and acidemia recover, while others with near-normal blood gas tensions and pHa when admitted to the hospital die (Fandel and Bancalari 1976; Kruus et al. 1979; Modell et al. 1976; Orlowski 1979). The reestablishment of spontaneous ventilation or the institution of mechanical ventilation reverses the respiratory acidosis, but metabolic acidosis usually persists for a longer time due to hypoxia and cardiovascular depression (Modell et al. 1966, 1976). When the metabolic acidosis is severe, the intravenous administration of sodium bicarbonate may be necessary. Otherwise, metabolic acidosis is usually reversed with the restoration of oxygenation and the stabilization of cardiovascular function.

The etiology of hypoxemia in near-drowning in fresh water differs from that after seawater near-drowning. When fresh water is aspirated it is absorbed from the lungs into the circulation (Modell and Moya 1966). Fresh water, however, alters the surface tension properties of pulmonary surfactant; after experimental aspiration of fresh water the minimal surface tension reached at maximal compression of the surfactant extracted from the lung is higher than normal (Giammona and Modell 1967). Because of the abnormal surface tension properties, alveoli become unstable and tend to collapse, producing areas of low- but-finite ratios of ventilation to perfusion and areas of complete atelectasis that result in relative and absolute intrapulmonary shunting of blood, respectively (Modell et al. 1968b).

After seawater near-drowning the hypertonic fluid aspirated into the lung causes intra- vascular fluid to move into the lung and results in fluid-filled alveoli that are perfused but not ventilated (Modell et al. 1967; Modell et al. 1968b). This, in turn, results in absolute intrapulmonary shunting of venous blood. As opposed to aspiration of fresh water, seawa- ter aspiration does not change the surface tension properties of pulmonary surfactant, but it does reduce the quantity of surfactant (Giammona and Modell 1967). After seawater aspiration in experimental animals, approximately 1.5 times the volume of water aspirated can be recovered from lungs drained 5 min after aspiration, whereas no significant quantity of fluid can be drained from the lungs of animals that aspirate fresh water (Modell et al. 1974).

The aspiration of either fresh water or seawater reduces pulmonary compliance (Hal- magyi and Colebatch 1961). Similarly, both types may result in pulmonary edema, but by different mechanisms (Modell et al. 1966). After seawater aspiration, body fluids drawn into the alveolar space by the hypertonic seawater cause pulmonary edema (Modell et al. 1974). With aspiration of fresh water, damage to the pulmonary surfactant may contribute to the development of pulmonary edema (Giammona and Modell 1967).

The danger of hyperventilation before swimming was emphasized by Craig (1961), who studied the effects of breath holding on alveolar oxygen and carbon dioxide tensions after hyperventilation and after excerise. He found that after hyperventilation, breath holding accompanied by exercise dramatically reduced alveolar oxygen tension whereas carbon dioxide tension was not increased to the point of stimulating inspiration. Because hypoxia is a poor respiratory stimulant in otherwise healthy persons, this appears to be a likely explanation for competent swimmers' drowning during underwater swimming. Once consciousness is lost, victims may or may not aspirate before being removed from the water.

2. Anatomical Pulmonary Changes

The pathologic changes in the human lung after drowning were well described by Fuller (1963a, 1963b). In a large series of drowned humans he found that 70% evidenced aspirated particulate matter, such as mud, sand, algae, and vomitus. In victims who succumbed 12 to 72 hr after the accident, examination of the lungs frequently revealed bronchopneumonia, lung abscesses, pulmonary edema, mechanical injury, and deposition of hyaline membranes in the alveoli. Butt et al. (1970) evaluated survivors' pulmonary function tests and arterial oxygen tensions and reported that there was no consistent permanent abnormality in these tests after clinical recovery.

Investigations of acute pathologic changes in the lungs of experimental rats after the aspiration of small quantities of fresh water revealed essentially no anatomical changes, whereas similar volumes of aspirated seawater caused alveolar hemorrhage and increased the lung weight (Halmagyi 1961). After large quantities of fresh water were aspirated, electron microscopy of rat lung revealed widened alveolar septa, collapsed capillaries, enlarged endothelial and septal cell nuclei, swollen mitochondria, and obliterated cell outlines. With similar volumes of aspirated seawater the changes were less marked. The septal and endothelial nuclei were small, and structural integrity was preserved (Reidbord and Spitz 1966).

Hyperexpanded lungs and acute emphysema have been described in both humans and experimental animals that die soon after the injury (Fuller 1963b; Miloslavich 1934). This is believed to be caused by alveoli ruptured by a widely fluctuating transpulmonary pressure due to ventilatory efforts against a closed glottis or a column of water obstructing the airway during submersion.

3. Blood Volume and Electrolyte Concentrations

Early studies by Swann and Brucer and colleagues (1947, 1949) demonstrated a large increase in blood volume with severely reduced concentrations of serum sodium and serum chloride when experimental dogs were drowned by total immersion in fresh water. Another group of dogs drowned by immersion in seawater had reduced blood volume and elevated serum sodium and serum chloride concentrations. These findings influenced the therapy of near-drowned humans for more than a decade even though similar changes in electrolyte concentrations in humans had not been reported (Fuller 1963b). Modell and Davis (1969) observed that 85% of autopsied drowned humans had either normal serum electrolyte concentrations or only mild derangements.

When water was aspirated by experimental dogs, it was determined that, after 3 min, the serum electrolyte changes reflected the volume of fluid aspirated, with reduced serum sodium and serum chloride concentrations after aspiration of fresh water and elevated concentrations after seawater aspiration (Modell et al. 1967). With aspiration of fresh water, the serum electrolyte concentrations returned to normal without therapy within 10 to 60 min after aspiration, but with seawater aspiration the electrolyte concentrations remained slightly elevated after 1 hr (Modell and Moya 1966). Ventricular fibrillation occurred frequently in animals that aspirated 44 ml/kg of fresh water, but it did not occur in animals aspirating 22 ml/kg or less. Serum potassium was elevated transiently after aspiration of fresh water but returned to normal after 10 min. The temporary nature of the electrolyte changes that occur after the aspiration of water by experimental animals explains the failure to find such changes in human victims at the time of admission to the hospital (Fandel and Bancalari 1976; Modell et al. 1968a, 1976).

Blood volume also changes after experimental near-drowning. After aspiration of fresh water, blood volume increases transiently but returns toward normal after 10 min (Modell and Moya 1966); it decreases after aspiration of seawater (Modell et al. 1967; Swann and Brucer 1949; Swann et al. 1947). The nature of these changes suggests that the movement of fluids between tissue compartments assists in the maintenance of homeostasis. After aspiration of either fresh water or seawater the effective circulating blood volume is frequently reduced some time after the injury and may be due to pulmonary edema, redistribution of fluid, decreased venous return secondary to positive pressure ventilation, or a combination of factors (Bergquist et al. 1980).

4. Cardiovascular System

Although early studies of dogs drowned in fresh water by total immersion suggested that death was due to ventricular fibrillation (Swann and Brucer 1949; Swann et al. 1947), this finding has rarely been reported in humans (Modell et al. 1976), probably because humans rarely aspirate enough water to cause the degree of hyponatremia necessary for ventricular fibrillation. Instead, the cardiovascular changes seen after near-drowning with fresh water or seawater are most likely due to hypoxemia and acidosis. Bradycardia is a common arrhythmia found early in near-drowned humans and experimental animals and may be due either to hypoxia or to the diving reflex (Gooden 1972; Modell and Moya 1966; Modell et al. 1967). Almost every arrhythmia known has been described in near-drowned humans and animals (Fandel and Bancalari 1976; Modell and Moya 1966; Peterson 1977; Swann et al. 1947).

Intense vasoconstriction may result from near-drowning and may be due to a number of causes, including the diving reflex, hypothermia, hypoxia, catecholamine release, or a combination of these factors. The vasoconstriction may be so intense that a pulse may be difficult to palpate at the scene of the accident even when spontaneous cardiac activity is present.

In addition to arrhythmias, a number of other electrocardiographic (ECG) changes have been reported after near-drowning (Modell and Moya 1966; Modell et al. 1967; Swann et al. 1947). These include elevation or depression of the ST wave, changes in T-wave amplitude, increased P-R interval, and widening of the QRS complex. These changes are usually due to myocardial hypoxia and possibly hypothermia as well. Correction of hypoxia, acidosis, and hypothermia should return the ECG to normal.

A recent animal study has demonstrated an immediate reduction in cardiac output along with bradycardia, hypotension, and increased systemic vascular resistance after aspiration of fresh water (Bergquist et al. 1980). These parameters returned toward normal within 30 min in the untreated animals. Cardiac output then decreases with the institution of controlled mechanical ventilation (CMV) with or without positive end-expiratory pressure (PEEP) or continuous positive airway pressure (CPAP) greater than 15 cmH$_2$O. This is probably due to an absolute or relative reduction in the effective circulating blood volume. In such cases cardiac output should return to normal if the intravascular volume is increased with supplemental fluid.

Arterial blood pressure may be normal, increased, or decreased after near-drowning and may vary with the time elapsed since the injury (Modell et al. 1966, 1967; Rivers et al. 1970; Swann and Brucer 1949). Central venous pressure (CVP) rises briefly after the aspiration of small volumes of fresh water or seawater but rapidly returns to normal (Modell and Moya 1966; Modell et al. 1967).

Pulmonary artery pressure and pulmonary artery occlusion pressure have been monitored in experimental animals after aspiration of fresh water, and both have been found to increase transiently (Bergquist et al. 1980). Systemic and pulmonary vascular resistances were calculated in the same study and were found to be elevated even after other parameters had returned to normal.

5. Hematology

Near-drowning has not been shown to significantly affect the hemoglobin concentrations and hematrocrits of humans or experimental animals unless very large volumes of either fresh water or seawater are aspirated (Fandel and Bancalari 1976; Modell and Moya 1966; Modell et al. 1966, 1967, 1968a, 1976). The degree of hemolysis necessary to significantly increase plasma hemoglobin concentration in human victims is rare; even when plasma hemoglobin is elevated it rarely causes renal damage (Fuller 1963a; Modell et al. 1968a).

The white blood cell (WBC) count is frequently elevated early after near-drowing (Fuller 1963a; Gauto et al. 1979; Gilfoil and Carvajal 1977; Modell 1963; Rivers et al. 1970). Later elevations of the white blood cell count must be considered a possible indication of infection.

There are few reports of platelet counts or clotting function after near-drowning. A single case of disseminated intravascular coagulation after near-drowning was reported in a patient who also had severe hypoxemia, acidosis, and hemolysis (Culpepper 1975).

6. Renal Function

Renal dysfunction is uncommon after near-drowning (Grausz et al. 1971; Kvittingen and Naess 1963). Fuller (1963b) reported in his study that 12 out of 50 who near-drowned had transient albuminuria, cylindruria, or both. One of these patients also had transiently elevated blood urea nitrogen. These changes were thought to be due to renal hypoxia, but none of these patients suffered significant renal dysfunction. One victim who died had acute tubular necrosis that was attributed to prolonged hypotension.

Plasma hemoglobin secondary to hemolysis might be expected to cause renal dysfunction after near-drowning. Fuller (1963b) reported two cases of hemoglobinemia and hemoglobinuria, one after the aspiration of fresh water and the other after seawater. Neither patient evidenced renal dynsfunction. Modell et al. (1968a) reported a patient with a plasma hemoglobin level of 500 mg/100 ml without evidence of renal damage. In such cases, it is prudent to keep urinary output brisk. If oxygenation, acid-base balance, and intravascular volume are adequate, renal failure after near-drowning is unlikely.

7. Central Nervous System

Survival after the pulmonary injury of near-drowning has improved since the advent of arterial blood gas analysis and of sophisticated methods of monitoring and ventilatory support (Conn et al. 1980; Fuller 1963a; Modell et al. 1976, 1980). However, anoxic central nervous system damage is significant and is a major concern in current investigations. Peterson (1977) reported that 21% of survivors in his study had evidence of some brain damage. Other investigators have reported a 0–12% incidence of brain damage in survivors and encourage an optimistic and aggressive approach to all near-drowned victims (Conn et al. 1980; Fandel and Bancalari 1976; Modell et al. 1980; Pearn et al. 1979).

There is no evidence suggesting the etiology of brain damage after near-drowning is other than anoxia (Fuller 1963a, 1963b; Miles 1968). Fuller (1963b) reported that brain lesions of different ages may be found at autopsy and may be secondary to cerebral edema.

A number of investigators sought clues for the prognosis of near-drowned patients that might help guide initial management. There appears to be no firm correlation between outcome and initial values of arterial oxygen tension, pH, electrolyte concentrations, EEG recordings, or temperature nor between outcome and duration of submersion, initial resuscitative measures, or need for mechanical ventilation (Conn et al. 1980; Fandel and Bancalari 1976; Kruus et al. 1979; Modell et al. 1976, 1980; Orlowski 1979; Pearn et al. 1979; Peterson 1977). Level of consciousness at the time of admission to the hospital provided some prediction of outcome in two retrospective series reported by Conn et al. (1980) and Modell et al. (1980). In Conn's series (1980) of 96 children, 53% were awake and 6% had "blunted" (described as confused, combative, lethargic, or semicomatose) levels of consciousness at the time of admission; all survived with normal brain function. Thirty-nine patients were described as comatose at the time of admission. Of these, 43.5% had normal survival, 23% survived with brain damage, and 33.5% died. Overall, 77% of the 96 patients survived with normal function, 9% survived with brain damage, and 13.5% died. When the comatose children were categorized as "decorticate," "decerebrate," or flaccid, Conn found that 66% of "decorticate," 56% of "decerebrate," and 14% of flaccid patients survived with normal function. Eighteen of the comatose patients received aggressive measures for cerebral resuscitation, including hyperventilation, dehydration, muscle paralysis, active cooling, corticosteroids and barbiturates, and had intracranial pressure monitored. Ten of eleven "decorticate" or "decerebrate" patients who were so treated survived with normal function; one survived with brain damage. Of seven flaccid patients so treated six died, and one survived with normal function.

The series of 121 patients reported by Modell et al. (1980) included adults as well as children. All of the 61 patients who were alert at the time of admission recovered with normal function, even though some had suffered cardiopulmonary arrest at the time of the accident. Thirty-one patients with "blunted" consciousness on admission either survived normally (90%) or died from pulmonary insufficiency (10%). Twenty-nine patients were comatose at the time of admission; 55% of these survived with apparently normal brain function, 10% survived with brain damage, and 34% died. Overall, 87% survived with apparently normal function, 2% survived with brain damage, and 11% died. In this study no specific protocol for cerebral resuscitation was used, although many of the comatose patients received corticosteroids and were hyperventilated for presumed brain edema. As a result of these studies Conn and Modell (1980) have recommended that a prospective study be undertaken to further evaluate the effects of aggressive brain resuscitation on comatose near-drowned victims.

8. Infection

Infection after near-drowning has not been widely reported, possibly because of the difficulty in making a precise diagnosis in many cases. Fuller (1963b) reported that 22 of 50 near-drowned survivors in his series had fever and leukocytosis that persisted longer than 2 days after the accident. He did not report how many of these victims had pulmonary infiltrates or received antibiotics. In all victims with delayed deaths after near-drowning Fuller reported varying degrees of bronchopneumonia or multiple lung abscesses. Peterson (1977) reported that 4 of 72 patients in his series had "aspiration pneumonia" but, again, the criteria for diagnosis and the treatment given were not further documented. Modell et al. (1976) did not report the incidence of infection in a series of 91 patients but did report that the use of prophylactic antibiotics did not improve the survival rate of those patients who received them and, thus, recommended that antibiotics be given only to treat active infections.

E. Treatment

1. Immediate First Aid

Because hypoxia is the major cause of death and injury from drowning and near-drowning, the primary goal of the rescuer is to restore oxygen delivery as rapidly as possible after the accident. Resuscitation is facilitated by airway control, artificial ventilation, and chest compression with the victim on a firm surface, so rescue from the water must be prompt. Occasionally this may not be possible, and artificial ventilation must be started while the victim is still in the water. This maneuver may be difficult, even for experienced swimmers but may restore oxygenation if an apneic victim still has some effective circulation. A method for providing both closed chest massage and artifical ventilation, using a scuba regulator, for victims still in the water has been described (March and Matthews 1980). This method, intended for use when divers near-drown where a boat or land is not readily accessible, should not be used when the victim can be rapidly removed from the water.

Without sophisticated rescue equipment, mouth-to-mouth and mouth-to-nose ventilation have been proven the most effective emergency modes available (Safar et al. 1958) and may be done in the water, if necessary, or immediately on reaching land. The maintenance of a patent airway, such as by maneuvers described by the American Heart Association (1980), is critical in providing emergency ventilation.

Although recommended in the past, attempts to drain water from the lungs and the stomach should not be undertaken (Ruben and Ruben 1962). Studies have documented that after 3 min no water can be drained from the lungs of animals that aspirate fresh water (Modell et al. 1968b); similar results have been reported in humans (Ruben and Ruben 1962). While as much as 1.5 times the volume of aspirated fluid may be drained from the lungs of experimental animals near-drowned in seawater (Modell et al. 1974), studies of humans suggest that few people aspirate the volumes used in animal studies (Modell and Davis 1969). Besides delaying cardiopulmonary resuscitation, draining the lungs or stomach may result in regurgitation and the aspiration of gastric contents.

As in other cases of cardiopulmonary resuscitation, once ventilation is instituted, the rescuer must determine whether spontaneous circulation is present. Because of the intense vasoconstriction that may occur after near-drowning, the heart may be beating though a peripheral pulse may not be palpable. The rescuer has no way to determine this, however, so cardiac arrest must be presumed. Closed chest massage is continued, along with artificial ventilation, until spontaneous circulation and ventilation are restored or until the rescuer can be relieved or can no longer continue (American Heart Association 1980).

If a victim near-drowns without aspiration and if he is resuscitated before cerebral hypoxia occurs, recovery is usually rapid. Such a victim may appear to be perfectly normal within minutes of rescue. If cerebral hypoxia has occurred, severe or fatal brain damage may result in spite of normal cardiopulmonary function after resuscitation. If aspiration has occurred, the pulmonary lesion may be severe and may cause profound hypoxemia even after the restoration of spontaneous ventilation and circulation (Modell et al. 1968a, 1976). The patient's appearance at the scene of the accident may not accurately reflect hypoxia, particularly when the victim is cold, vasoconstricted, and stressed. There is no way at the scene of the accident to determine whether the victim has aspirated or is hypoxemic, so all victims should be transported to a hospital for further evaluation.

2. Emergency Transportation

Frequently, emergency transportation services can provide personnel trained in advanced life support and the medical supplies needed for such therapy. Since hypoxia and acidosis are major concerns in all near-drowned victims, these abnormalities should be corrected promptly. Supplemental oxygen should be provided in the highest concentration possible as soon as possible. Low concentrations of supplemental oxygen should not be used in the fear of removing the "hypoxic ventilatory drive," which would be extremely unusual in a near-drowned victim, and such therapy is ineffective for severe hypoxemia.

If the victim is awake and breathing spontaneously, supplemental oxygen may be provided by a face mask. If the victim is unconscious or does not respond to cardiopulmonary resuscitation, supplemental oxygen should be provided by mechanical ventilation through an endotracheal tube. Since the unconscious or arrested patient cannot protect himself from the aspiration of gastric contents, endotracheal intubation will prevent this, and it also prevents distension of the stomach during mechanical ventilation. Many emergency medical technicians can perform endotracheal intubation in the field; when endotracheal intubation is not feasible, an esophageal obturator airway may be used to facilitate the ventilation of a deeply comatose or arrested patient, provided that the operator is familiar with its placement as well as the benefits and risks involved.

Other advanced resuscitative procedures should be performed before or during transport whenever possible. These include the placement of a large-bore intravenous catheter for fluid and drug therapy and the monitoring of the electrocardiogram for arrhythmias. Specific drug therapy, such as the intravenous administration of sodium bicarbonate, may be recommended if the emergency rescue team is in radio contact with the hospital physician. While positive end-expiratory pressure (PEEP) is frequently needed to decrease intrapulmonary shunting and improve arterial oxygenation after near-drowning (Bergquist et al. 1980; Modell et al. 1974, 1976; Ruiz et al. 1973), this form of therapy is usually not available before admission to hospital.

3. Emergency Room Care

Upon admission to the emergency room, evaluation of oxygenation takes priority, since initial therapy must correct hypoxemia. Arterial blood should be obtained and analyzed for pH, Pa_{CO_2} and Pa_{O_2}. The highest possible concentration of supplemental oxygen should be given until arterial blood gas analysis demonstrates that it is no longer needed.

Approximately 70% of near-drowned victims have significant metabolic acidosis at the time of admission and many require at least partial correction by the intravenous administration of sodium bicarbonate (Modell et al. 1976). As oxygenation improves and as cardiovascular stability is achieved further bicarbonate therapy usually becomes unnecessary.

Some patients may incur trauma along with near-drowning, such as from a motor vehicle accident. A victim who near-drowns while diving may suffer a cervical spine fracture that may result in quadriplegia. The scuba diver may near-drown secondary to a cerebral air embolus or, if a scuba diver has near-drowned at depth, decompression sickness may develop after rescue. Thus, rapid and thorough physical examination, including a detailed neurological evaluation, of all near-drowned patients soon after admission is important and may indicate specific roentgenograms, laboratory tests, and further therapy.

In addition to arterial blood gas and pH measurements, laboratory tests on admission should include a complete blood cell count, a determination of serum electroyte concentrations, and a urinalysis. Although the latter tests are usually normal at the time of admission, they may reveal other problems and will help to determine appropriate fluid therapy. A 12-lead electrocardiogram should be obtained to evaluate possible hypoxic myocardial damage or arrhythmias. A chest roentgenogram alone should not be used to evaluate the degree of pulmonary insufficiency or the results of therapy but it should always be obtained in the emergency room to provide baseline information, to document the placement of the endotracheal tube or central venous catheter, and to rule out barotrauma. While the chest roentgenogram may appear normal, it usually reveals pulmonary edema, infiltrates, or atelectasis (Fuller 1963a, 1963b; Modell et al. 1976).

4. Respiratory Care

The degree of arterial hypoxemia and intrapulmonary shunting after near-drowning varies widely in both humans and experimental animals. Intrapulmonary shunting in excess of 70% of the cardiac output has been described in both (Bergquist et al. 1980). Studies of dogs that aspirated 22 ml/kg of either seawater or fresh water have demonstrated the efficacy of PEEP to reduce intrapulmonary shunting and to improve arterial oxygenation (Bergquist et al. 1980; Modell et al.1974; Ruiz et al. 1973). After seawater aspiration, intrapulmonary shunt and Pa_{O_2} consistently improved with either spontaneous ventilation with PEEP or mechanical ventilation with PEEP (Modell et al. 1974). After aspiration of fresh water some dogs demonstrated marked improvement in intrapulmonary shunting with spontaneous ventilation and continuous positive airway pressure (CPAP), while others improved little without the addition of mechanical ventilation (Bergquist et al. 1980). Due to the altered surfactant activity after aspiration of fresh water, mechanical ventilation may be needed to reinflate collapsed alveoli before PEEP or CPAP can maintain alveolar inflation. Seawater aspiration reduces the amount of surfactant but does not change its compression characteristics, so spontaneous ventilation with PEEP or CPAP would be expected to maintain alveolar inflation without the addition of mechanical ventilation. These effects have been observed in both humans and experimental animals after seawater near-drowning (Modell et al. 1974, 1976).

Mechanical ventilation decreases cardiac output after dogs aspirate fresh water and PEEP further reduces cardiac output. While CPAP lower than 15 cmH$_2$O does not significantly reduce cardiac output, higher levels of CPAP may cause significant reduction. The decrease in cardiac output with spontaneous ventilation with CPAP was not as severe as that caused by mechanical ventilation with similar levels of PEEP (Bergquist et al. 1980). Since mechanical ventilation and PEEP increase intrathoracic pressure and decrease venous return to the heart, increasing the intravascular volume with supplemental fluid should overcome these effects so that the necessary amount of mechanical ventilation or positive airway pressure can be applied.

Clinically, the amount of PEEP or CPAP necessary to lower intrapulmonary shunt and to optimize arterial oxygen tension while maintaining cardiovascular stability must be individualized. The optimal level produces the lowest intrapulmonary shunt without adversely affecting cardiac output (Downs and Modell 1977; Downs et al. 1973). If the patient is alert, cooperative, and normocarbic, up to 15 cmH$_2$O of CPAP may be provided through a tight-fitting face mask, such as an anesthesia mask. A face mask is not recommended with higher than 15 cmH$_2$O, because an adequate seal that will prevent fluctuations in the level of CPAP is difficult to maintain and because higher levels may open the gastroesophageal sphincter and distend the stomach. If the patient is obtunded, comatose, or hypercarbic, or requires more than 15 cmH$_2$O, then CPAP is provided through an endotracheal tube.

Mechanical ventilation can be added as needed with intermittent mandatory ventilation (IMV) by adjusting the number of mechanical breaths necessary to maintain an acceptable pHa and Pa$_{CO_2}$ while allowing the patient to continue breathing spontaneously (Downs and Modell 1977). After dogs aspirate fresh water, controlled mechanical ventilation (CMV) with PEEP has lowered intrapulmonary shunt more consistently than spontaneous ventilation with CPAP (Bergquist et al. 1980). In humans, CMV may be needed only rarely to achieve similar results. Although it has not been proved in a controlled fashion, the addition of a few breaths per minute of IMV to a given level of CPAP may improve ratios of ventilation to perfusion by reexpanding alveoli that tend to collapse; this should be tried if spontaneous breathing and CPAP do not achieve the desired effect.

There is often concern that increasing PEEP or CPAP may significantly reduce cardiac output, particularly if mechanical ventilation is added. However, this reduced cardiac output is due to an absolute or relative hypovolemia, and cardiac output can be maintained with fluid therapy. A Swan-Ganz catheter optimizes therapy: the amount of fluid necessary to improve cardiac output is best determined by evaluating pulmonary artery wedge pressure and cardiac output, while the amount of CPAP necessary is best determined by calculating the intrapulmonary shunt fraction. In fact, as oxygenation is improved by PEEP, cardiac output may be secondarily improved (Downs et al. 1973).

As PEEP or CPAP is optimized and intrapulmonary shunting is reduced the inspired oxygen fraction ($F_{I_{O_2}}$) should be lowered; a high $F_{I_{O_2}}$ (i.e., > 0.5) for a prolonged period may result in pulmonary oxygen toxicity (Clark 1974). In addition, absorption atelectasis may result from a high $F_{I_{O_2}}$ and may convert an area with low ratios of ventilation to perfusion into one with absolute intrapulmonary shunting of blood (Douglas et al. 1976). At the opposite end of the spectrum, $F_{I_{O_2}} < 0.3$ may increase the calculated intrapulmonary shunt or may reduce Pa_{O_2} more than might be expected in light of previous changes in the $F_{I_{O_2}}$. This phenomenon may be explained by the "unmasking" of intrapulmonary shunt in areas of low ratios of ventilation to perfusion that respond to increases in alveolar oxygen tension and, thus, may not indicate a worsening of the patient's condition (Douglas et al. 1976).

Pulmonary edema frequently occurs after aspiration of both fresh water and seawater (Fuller 1963b; Modell et al. 1976). The therapy of choice is to titrate PEEP or CPAP. Once achieved, the optimal level should not be lowered rapidly or discontinued abruptly, since pulmonary edema may recur within seconds. Pulmonary edema should not be suctioned, because it may recur or hypoxemia and atelectasis may result. When the patient is being treated for pulmonary edema with PEEP or CPAP, suctioning should only be performed to remove plugs of mucus and maintain airway patency.

When the hypoxemic near-drowned victim requires PEEP or CPAP, it should be applied in the emergency room and continued in the intensive care unit. Therapy is guided by the analysis of arterial blood gas tensions or intrapulmonary shunt fraction after incremental increases of 3–5 cmH$_2$O CPAP. Occasionally, pulmonary edema may be so severe that CPAP is increased more than that before an arterial blood specimen is analyzed. This type of therapy requires constant and careful evaluation of the clinical results, including observation of changes in the respiratory rate, the severity of retractions, and the amount of pulmonary edema present in the airway. In such cases, systemic arterial and pulmonary artery catheterization should be performed as soon as feasible.

The procedure of removing CPAP or PEEP is similar to that of its application. When the intrapulmonary shunt is minimized (less than 15% of cardiac output) and stabilized, CPAP is reduced 2–3 cmH$_2$O at a time, and the arterial blood gas analysis or intrapulmonary shunt fraction is repeated after each reduction in CPAP. If arterial oxygenation or intrapulmonary shunting does not worsen after the reduction, the maneuver is repeated. If the intrapulmonary shunt fraction increases or the arterial oxygen tension decreases after a reduction in CPAP, then the previous level is still necessary. After a while, the reduction in CPAP can be repeated to determine whether further weaning is possible.

Bronchospasm may occur after near-drowning. If mild, bronchospasm may be treated with an aerosol of a bronchodilating agent. More severe cases may require an intravenous infusion of aminophylline. Therapy should be optimized by physical examination and determination of serum drug levels.

5. In-Hospital Monitoring and Therapy

All near-drowned victims should be taken to the hospital for an evaluation. If the patient is asymptomatic and has normal arterial blood gas tensions and chest roentgenogram at the time of admission, he is observed for 12–24 hr and, if a repeat physical examination and blood gas analysis are normal, discharged. A follow-up visit should be arranged for several days later.

If the patient has only mild hypoxemia that requires only small amounts of supplemental oxyen, hospitalization is usually brief; however, the patient should be monitored intensely, in case the condition worsens. The patient may be monitored in the intensive care unit for 24 hr and then, if stable, be transferred to the ward until supplemental oxygen is no longer necessary. Follow-up evaluation should be performed 1 or 2 days after discharge and continued as necessary.

The patient with significant hypoxemia or with an abnormal level of consciousness requires admission to an intensive care unit for aggressive monitoring and support. Blood pressure, pulse, respiratory rate, and temperature are monitored frequently or continuously. Careful recording of intake and output are necessary. In addition to continuous electrocardiographic (ECG) monitoring, an indwelling arterial catheter should be used; it facilitates the monitoring of arterial blood pressure and provides an access to sample arterial blood for pHa, Pa_{CO_2}, and Pa_{O_2}. A nasogastric tube and a urinary catheter are often necessary in the seriously ill patient. While a central venous catheter may be helpful in assessing intravascular volume in some patients, a pulmonary artery catheter is frequently necessary to measure intrapulmonary shunting, to assess the effects of CPAP, and to evaluate the cardiovascular system.

6. Brain Resuscitation

With appropriate respiratory care and cardiovascular support, normal survival should result in a greater number than 90% of the patients who either are alert or have a "blunted" level of consciousness when admitted (Conn et al. 1980; Modell et al. 1980). The prognosis for comatose patients is uncertain. Specific measures for brain resuscitation have not been fully evaluated and have some intrinsic risks. Moderate hyperventilation (Pa_{CO_2} approximately 30 mmHg) has been shown to reduce intracranial pressure secondary to brain edema, although the duration and degree of this effect may be inadequate if swelling is severe (Severinghaus and Lassen 1967). Most clinicians use pharmacologic doses of steroids to treat cerebral edema, although experimental evidence for beneficial results after global anoxia has not been demonstrated (Fishman 1975). Hypothermia and barbiturate coma have been advocated by some authors on the grounds that these measures reduce cerebral metabolism and, therefore, cerebral edema; but this has not been proved in a large series of patients (Conn et al. 1980). Maintenance of high Pa_{O_2} has also been promoted on the basis that oxygen diffusion into the brain may be improved, but again firm scientific evidence is lacking (Conn et al. 1980). In determining which, if any, of these maneuvers to use as therapy for the comatose near-drowned victim, the clinician must recognize that further investigation in this area is needed and that the dangers of certain types of therapy may be greater than the benefits (Conn and Modell 1980).

7. Corticosteroids and Antibiotics

Corticosteroids and prophylactic antibiotics for near-drowned patients were initially recommended in 1968 because they were thought to be beneficial for aspiration pneumonitis (Modell et al. 1968a). Since that time a number of studies have failed to demonstrate benefits from either class of drugs when used for this purpose after near-drowning. Experimentally, dogs that aspirated fresh water showed no improvement in oxygenation or survival rate when pharmacologic doses of corticosteroids were given (Calderwood et al. 1975). A large clinical series demonstrated similar results (Modell et al. 1976). Recently, Wynn et al. (1979) have demonstrated that corticosteroids may interfere with long-term pulmonary healing after the aspiration of foodstuff by animals. At present, administering corticosteroids for their anti-inflammatory effect is not recommended for near-drowned victims.

Prophylactic antibiotic therapy for near-drowned humans has also been shown to have no benefit (Modell et al. 1976). Whereas secondary pulmonary infection may develop in the near-drowned victim, prophylactic antibiotics may worsen the situation by allowing resistant organisms to develop. Appropriate management consists of careful observation for the development of infection by following Gram stains and cultures of the sputum, frequent temperature recordings, daily white blood cell counts, and chest roentgenograms as indicated. If the patient evidences pulmonary infection, such as by fever, leukocytosis, or infiltrates on chest roentgenograms, sputum and blood cultures should be obtained and antibiotic therapy should be prescribed without delay. Infection frequently manifests on the second or third hospital day, a time when pulmonary edema should have resolved. Then, in addtion to antibiotic therapy, vigorous pulmonary toilet should also be instituted.

Care must be exercised when using invasive monitors, such as pulmonary artery catheters and even urinary catheters, as septicemia may result from their prolonged use. When a catheter is no longer necessary it should be removed. Prolonged use may necessitate the replacement of the catheter, always by sterile technique.

8. Hyperbaric Oxygen Therapy

Hyperbaric oxygen therapy is indicated for the near-drowned scuba diver who also suffers cerebral air embolus or decompression sickness. If the patient is comatose at the time of admission it may be impossible to determine the exact cause, and a trial of recompression therapy is indicated. Even when the victim is alert and complaining only of joint pain, more serious manifestations of decompression sickness may occur later if it is left untreated. These patients require a level of care that can only be provided in a multiplace hyperbaric chamber that encompasses intensive respiratory and cardiovascular support services. In addition to pulmonary and neurological injuries that may be quite severe, these patients frequently suffer severe dehydration as well and may require massive volumes of fluid and invasive monitoring to guide therapy. In evaluating a near-drowned scuba diver every attempt must be made to ascertain whether hyperbaric oxygen therapy is indicated and, if so, to keep the patient stable during transportation to the appropriate facility.

9. Summary

Prompt resuscitation and aggressive respiratory and cardiovascular intensive care are crucial for the optimal survival of near-drowned persons. While pathophysiology is related to the type and quantity of fluid aspirated, the severity of the injury cannot be predicted from the history of the accident or the victim's apparent condition at the scene of the accident. The primary injury is pulmonary, resulting in arterial hypoxemia and secondary hypoxic damage to other organ systems, of which the central nervous system is the most critical in terms of surviving normally.

All near-drowned victims should be evaluated and observed in the hospital. Therapy must be individualized; invasive monitoring and intensive support facilitate successful treatment. While much is yet to be learned about techniques of cerebral resuscitation, the outcome of a comatose, near-drowned patient may depend on an optimistic and aggressive approach.

Case Histories

1. Case No. 1: DD, 1972

A 20-year-old man was diving in a freshwater spring with a friend. Their first dive was to 90 ft for 30 min. Later they made a second dive to 90 ft, again for 30 min, after which they began to surface slowly. At 45 ft, one of the divers hit the side of the spring and caused a mud slide. Another group of divers found the patient unconscious at the surface, without his air regulator. The patient received cardipulmonary resuscitation for approximately 5 min, after which he gradually awakened. He was awake, alert, and in no acute distress upon arrival of the rescue team. The friend was not rescued, and his body was recovered the following day.

Upon arrival at the hospital 4 hr later, the patient complained of substernal "tightness," coughed occasionally, and was moderately short of breath. Coughing produced clear sputum tinged with blood and mud. He denied any joint discomfort or central nervous system complaints. The initial vital signs were blood pressure 110/80 mmHg, pulse 80 beats/min, respiration 20 breaths/min, and temperature 38°C. Physical examination was completely normal except for decreased breath sounds in the entire left thorax. Laboratory test results at the time of admission included a white blood cell count of 7700, hematocrit of 45%, and normal serum electrolyte concentrations. An analysis of arterial blood drawn while the patient breathed room air revealed a pH of 7.50, a Pa_{CO_2} of 17 mmHg, and a Pa_{O_2} of 100 mmHg. The chest roentgenogram showed a left lung infiltrate. The electrocardiogram was normal.

An intravenous catheter was inserted for maintenance fluids and 2 g of methylprednisolone was given intravenously. The patient was admitted to the intensive care unit (ICU) for observation.

Four hours after admission the patient complained of bilateral hip pain and an "aching sensation" in the left knee. The substernal discomfort persisted and was not relieved by antacids. The patient was taken to a monoplace hyperbaric chamber and treated according to a U.S. Navy Treatment Table 5, with complete relief of his chest and joint pain. The patient then returned to the ICU, where repeat arterial blood gas analysis revealed a pH of 7.39, a Pa_{CO_2} of 35 mmHg and a Pa_{O_2} of 74 mmHg. After 24 hr of observation in the ICU the blood gas tensions were unchanged. He was asymptomatic, so he was transferred to the ward.

On the third day after the accident, the patient had a shaking chill associated with a temperature of 39.7°C. Although the white blood cell count was not elevated, chest roentgenogram showed a persistent left lower lobe infiltrate, and the patient received a 5-day course of penicillin (5 million U i.v. every 6 hr) and kanamycin (500 mg i.m. every 12 hr). Sputum cultures taken at that time grew normal flora, and blood cultures failed to demonstrate bacteremia. After the institution of antibiotic therapy, the patient remained afebrile and the infiltrate gradually improved. The patient was discharged after he was afebrile for 48 hr without antibiotic therapy. He was asymptomatic at that time and the pulmonary infiltrate had nearly resolved.

2. Case No. 2: VYW, 1979

A 25-year-old woman was learning to swim in a pool. She was left alone by her friends for 3 to 5 min; when they returned they found her unconscious and floating in the water. She was removed from the pool and given mouth-to-mouth ventilation. She rapidly returned to consciousness and seemed to be oriented.

In the emergency room, she was noted to be awake and alert. Vital signs were blood pressure 102/70 mmHg, pulse 136 beats/min, respiration 24 breaths/min, and temperature 36.8°C. Physical examination was normal except for decreased breath sounds in both lower lung fields. Arterial blood gas analysis while the patient breathed room air revealed a pH of 7.29, a Pa_{CO_2} of 34 mmHg, and Pa_{O_2} of 51 mmHg. The white blood cell count was 10,200 and hematocrit was 39%. Serum electrolyte concentrations were within normal limits. Chest roentgenogram revealed bilateral lower lobe infiltrates.

The patient was admitted to the ICU and, because she was alert, continuous positive airway pressure (CPAP) was given through a tight-fitting mask. With room air and 5 cmH_2O of CPAP, arterial blood gas analysis revealed a pH of 7.37, a Pa_{CO_2} of 35 mmHg, and a Pa_{O_2} of 70 mmHg. The CPAP was titrated in 3-cmH_2O increments to 11 cmH_2O and the Pa_{O_2} increased with each increment in CPAP. At 11 cmH_2O of CPAP, arterial blood gas analysis revealed a pH of 7.35, a Pa_{CO_2} of 39 mmHg and a Pa_{O_2} of 90 mmHg. Because the patient complained of nausea and vomited several times during her initial treatment, nasotracheal intubation was performed 6 hr after admission. The CPAP was continued at 11 cmH_2O for another 10 hr and then gradually decreased without deterioration in arterial oxygenation. After the arterial Pa_{O_2} was unchanged with 5 cmH_2O of CPAP, the patient was extubated. She was observed in the ICU for another 24 hr and she remained asymptomatic and afebrile. The chest roentgenogram appeared normal the morning after admission. She was discharged from the hospital after another 24 hr of observation on the ward.

3. Case No. 3: CV, 1980

A 3-year-old boy, left unattended by his mother for a few minutes, was found at the bottom of a neighbor's pool. He was removed from the pool and was found to be cyanotic and apneic. He was given three breaths of mouth-to-mouth ventilation, after which he began spontaneous breathing, and "a large amount of fluid" poured out of his mouth. Mouth-to-mouth ventilation was continued, in spite of spontaneous breathing, until the rescue squad arrived. They noted that he began crying shortly after their arrival.

During evaluation in the emergency room the patient was awake and speaking. Vital signs were blood pressure 130/80 mmHg, pulse 120 beats/min, respiration 32 breaths/min, and temperature 36.5°C. Physical examination was normal except for minimal intercostal retractions and diffuse rhonchi heard in both lung fields. Analysis of arterial blood drawn while the patient breathed room air revealed a pH of 7.19, a Pa_{CO_2} of 32 mmHg and a Pa_{O_2} of 75 mmHg. The white blood cell count was 16,400 and hematocrit was 37%. Serum electrolyte concentrations were within normal limits. The chest roentgenogram revealed diffuse interstitial infiltrates. An intravenous catheter was inserted, and the patient was given 10 meq of sodium bicarbonate, after which the pH returned toward normal.

The patient was admitted in the ICU for further evaluation and monitoring. An indwelling arterial catheter was placed to facilitate monitoring of arterial blood gases. Three hours after the accident arterial blood gas analysis showed a pH of 7.42, a Pa_{CO_2} of 32 mmHg, and a Pa_{O_2} of 85 mmHg while the patient breathed room air. Eight hours after the accident the pH was 7.39, Pa_{CO_2} was 38 mmHg, and Pa_{O_2} was 101 mmHg. The patient was observed in the ICU another 12 hr. Because his blood gas tensions remained unchanged, his chest roentgenogram had cleared, and he remained afebrile, he was transferred to the ward. Twenty-four hours later the patient was discharged from the hospital and had no further complications.

BARBARA B. TABELING

References

AMERICAN HEART ASSOCIATION 1980. Standards and guidelines for cardiopulmonary resuscitation (CPR) and emergency cardiac care (ECC). *JAMA* 244: 453–512.
ANDERSEN, H. T. 1966. Physiologic adaptations in diving vertebrates. *Physiol. Rev.* 46: 212–243.
BERGQUIST, R. E., M. M. VOGELHUT, J. H. MODELL, S. J. SLOAN, AND B. C. RUIZ 1980. Comparison of ventilatory patterns in the treatment of freshwater near-drowning in dogs. *Anesthesiology* 52: 142–148.
BUTT, M. P., A. JALOWAYSKI, J. H. MODELL, AND S. T. GIAMMONA 1970. Pulmonary function after resuscitation from near-drowning. *Anesthesiology* 32: 275–277.
CALDERWOOD, H. W., J. H. MODELL, AND B. C. RUIZ 1975. The ineffectiveness of steroid therapy for treatment of freshwater near-drowning. *Anesthesiology* 43: 642–650.
CAMPBELL, L. B., B. A. GOODEN, AND J. D. HOROWITZ 1969. Cardiovascular responses to partial and total immersion in man. *J. Physiol. (Lond.)* 202: 239–250.

CLARK, J.M. 1974. The toxicity of oxygen. *Am. Rev. Respir. Dis.* 110: 40–500.
COMROE, J. H., JR. 1979. ". . . In comes the good air." Part I. Rise and fall of the Schafer method. *Am. Rev. Respir. Dis.* 119: 803–809.
CONN, A. W. 1979. Near-drowning and hypothermia (Editorial). *Can. Med. Assoc. J.* 120: 397–400.
CONN, A. W., J. F. EDMONDS, AND G. A. BARKER 1978. Near-drowning in cold fresh water: current treatment regimen. *Can. Anaesth. Soc. J.* 25: 259–265.
CONN, A. W., AND J. W. MODELL 1980. Current neurological considerations in near-drowning (Editorial). *Can. Anaesth. Soc. J.* 27: 197–198.
CONN, A. W., J. E. MONTES, G. A. BARKER, AND J. F. EDMONDS 1980. Cerebral salvage in near-drowning following neurological classification by triage. *Can. Anaesth. Soc. J.* 27: 201–210.
COT, C. 1931. Les asphyxies accidentelles (submersion, electrocution, intoxication, oxycarbonique): Étude clinique, therapeutique, et preventive. Paris: N. Maloine Éditions Médicales.
CRAIG, A.B., JR. 1961. Causes of loss of consciousness during underwater swimming. *J. Appl. Physiol.* 16: 583-586.
CULPEPPER, R. M. 1975. Bleeding diathesis in fresh water drowning. *Ann. Intern. Med.* 83: 675.
DOUGLAS, M. E., J. B. DOWNS, F. J. DANNEMILLER, M. R. HODGES, AND E. S. MUNSON 1976. Change in pulmonary venous admixture with varying inspired oxygen. *Anesth. Analg. Clevel.* 55: 688–695.
DOWNS, J. B., E. F. KLEIN, JR., AND J. H. MODELL 1973. The effect of incremental PEEP on Pa_{O_2} in patients with respiratory failure. *Anesth. Analg. Cleve.* 62: 210–214.
DOWNS, J. B., AND J. H. MODELL 1977. Patterns of respiratory support aimed at pathophysiologic conditions. *ASA Refresher Courses in Anesthesiology* 5: 71–85.
FANDEL, I., AND E. BANCALARI 1976. Near-drowning in children: clinical aspects. *Pediatrics* 58: 573–579.
FISHMAN, R. A. 1975. Brain edema. *N. Engl. J. Med.* 293: 706–711.
FLEETHAM, J. W., AND P. W. MUNT 1978. Near-drowning in Canadian waters. *Can. Med. Assoc. J.* 118: 914–917.
FULLER, R. H. 1963a. The clinical pathology of human near-drowning. *Proc. R. Soc. Med.* 56: 33–38.
FULLER, R. H. 1963b. The 1962 Wellcome prize essay. Drowning and the postimmersion syndrome. A clinicopathologic study. *Milit. Med.* 128: 22–36.
GAUTO, A., J. A. MAJESKI, AND J. W. ALEXANDER 1979. Drowning and near-drowning: current concepts and neutrophil function studies. *South. Med. J.* 72: 690–692.
GIAMMONA, S. T., AND J. H. MODELL 1967. Drowning by total immersion. Effects on pulmonary surfactant of distilled water, isotonic saline, and sea water. *Am. J. Dis. Child.* 114: 612–616.
GILFOIL, M. P., AND H. F. CARVAJAL 1977. Near-drowning in children. *Tex. Med.* 73: 39–44.
GOODEN, B. A. 1972. Drowning and the diving reflex in man. *Med. J. Aust.* 2: 583–587.
GRAUSZ, H., W. J. C. AMEND, JR., AND L. E. EARLEY 1971. Acute renal failure complicating submersion in seawater. *JAMA* 217: 207–209.
HALMAGYI, D. F. J. 1961. Lung changes and incidence of respiratory arrest in rats after aspiration of sea and fresh water. *J. Appl. Physiol.* 16: 41–44.
HALMAGYI, D. F. J., AND H. J. COLEBATCH 1961. The drowned lung. A physiological approach to its mechanism and management. *Austr. Ann. Med.* 10: 68–77.
HUNT, P. K. 1974. Effect and treatment of the "diving reflex." *Can. Med. Assoc. J.* 111: 1330–1331.
KOUWENHOVEN, W. B., J. R. JUDE, AND G. G. KNICKERBOCKER 1960. Closed chest cardiac massage. *JAMA* 173: 1064–1067.
KRUUS, S., L. BERGSTROM, T. SUUTARINEN, AND R. HYVONEN 1979. The prognosis of near-drowned children. *Acta Paediatr. Scand.* 68: 315–322.
KVITTINGEN, T. D., AND A. NAESS 1963. Recovery from drowning in fresh water. *Br. Med. J.* 5341: 1315–1317.
MARCH, N. F., AND R. C. MATTHEWS 1980. Feasibility study of CPR in the water. *Undersea Biomed. Res.* 7: 141–148.
MILES, S. 1968. Drowning. *Br. Med. J.* 3: 597–600.
MILOSLAVICH, E. L. 1934. Pathological anatomy of death by drowning. *Am. J. Clin. Pathol.* 4: 42–49.
MODELL, J. H. 1963. Resuscitation after aspiration of chlorinated freshwater. *JAMA* 185: 651–655.
MODELL, J. H. 1971. *Pathophysiology and Treatment of Drowning and Near-Drowning.* Springfield, IL: Charles C Thomas, p. 8–9, 13.
MODELL, J. H. 1981. Drown versus near-drown: a discussion of definitions (Editorial). *Crit. Care Med.* 9: 351–352.

MODELL, J. H., H. W. CALDERWOOD, B. C. RUIZ, J. B. DOWNS. AND R. L. CHAPMAN, JR. 1974. Effects of ventilatory patterns on arterial oxygenation after near-drowning in sea water. *Anesthesiology* 40: 376–384.

MODELL, J. H., AND J. H. DAVIS 1969. Electrolyte changes in human drowning victims. *Anesthesiology* 30: 414–420.

MODELL, J. H., J. H. DAVIS, S. T. GIAMMONA, F. MOYA. AND J. B. MANN 1968a. Blood gas and electrolyte changes in human near-drowning victims. *JAMA* 203: 337–343.

MODELL, J. H., M. GAUB, F. MOYA, B. VESTAL. AND H. SWARZ 1966. Physiologic effects of near drowning with chlorinated fresh water, distilled water and isotonic saline. *Anesthesiology* 27: 33–41.

MODELL, J. H., S. A. GRAVES. AND A. KETOVER 1976. Clinical course of 91 consecutive near-drowning victims. *Chest* 70: 231–238.

MODELL, J. H., S. A. GRAVES. AND E. J. KUCK 1980. Near-drowning: correlation of level of consciousness and survival. *Can Anaesth. Soc. J.* 27: 211–215.

MODELL, J. H., E. J. KUCK, B. C. RUIZ, AND H. HEINITSH 1972. Effect of intravenous vs. aspirated distilled water on serum electrolytes and blood gas tensions. *J. Appl. Physiol.* 32: 579–584.

MODELL, J. H., AND F. MOYA 1966. Effects of volume of aspirated fluid during chlorinated fresh water drowning. *Anesthesiology* 27: 662–672.

MODELL, J. H., F. MOYA, E. J. NEWBY, B. C. RUIZ. AND A. V. SHOWERS 1967. The effects of fluid volume in seawater drowning. *Ann. Intern. Med.* 67: 68–80.

MODELL, J. H., F. MOYA, H. D. WILLIAMS. AND T. C. WEIBLEY 1968b. Changes in blood gases and A-aDO2 during near-drowning. *Anesthesiology* 29: 456–465.

NEMIROFF, M. J. 1977a. Accidental cold-water immersion and survival characteristics. In: Program and abstracts. Undersea Medical Society Annual Scientific Meeting, May 1977, Toronto, Canada. *Undersea Biomed. Res.* 4:A56.

NEMIROFF, M. J. 1977b. Resuscitation following cold-water near-drowning. In: *Proc. Ninth International Conference on Underwater Education*. Colton, CA: National Association of Underwater Instructors, p. 168.

NEMIROFF, M. J., G. R. SALTZ, AND J. C. WEG 1977. Survival after cold-water near-drowning: the protective effect of the diving reflex. *Am. Rev. Respir. Dis.* 115: 145.

ORLOWSKI, J. P. 1979. Prognostic factors in pediatric cases of drowning and near-drowning. *J. Am. Coll. Emerg. Phys.* 8: 176–179.

PEARN, J. H., R. D. BART, JR., AND R. YAMAOKA 1979. Neurologic sequelae after childhood near-drowning: a total population study from Hawaii. *Pediatrics* 64: 187–191.

PETERSON, B. 1977. Morbidity of childhood near-drowning. *Pediatrics* 59: 364–370.

REDDING, J. S. 1977. Historical vignettes concerning resuscitation from drowning. In: *Advances in Cardiopulmonary Resuscitation*, edited by P. Safar. New York: Springer-Verlag, p. 276–280.

REDDING, J. S., R. A. COZINE, G. C. VOIGHT. AND P. SAFAR 1961. Resuscitation from drowning. *JAMA* 178: 1136–1139.

REIDBORD, H. E., AND W. U. SPITZ 1966. Ultrastructural alterations in rat lungs. Changes after intratracheal perfusion with freshwater and seawater. *Arch. Pathol.* 81: 103–111.

RIVERS, J. F., G. ORR. AND H. R. LEE 1970. Drowning. Its clinical sequelae and management. *Br. Med. J.* 702(2):157–161.

RUBEN, A., AND H. RUBEN 1962. Artificial respiration. Flow of water from the lung and the stomach. *Lancet* 1: 780–781.

RUIZ, B. C., H. W. CALDERWOOD, J. H. MODELL. AND J. E. BROGDON 1973. Effect of ventilatory patterns on arterial oxygenation after near-drowning with fresh water: a comparative study in dogs. *Anesth. Analg. Clevel.* 52: 570–576.

SAFAR, P., L. A. ESCARRAGA. AND J. O. ELAM 1958. A comparison of the mouth-to-mouth and mouth-to-airway methods of artificial respiration with the chest-pressure arm-lift methods. *N. Engl. J. Med.* 258: 671–677.

SCHECHTER, D. C. 1969. Role of the humane society in the history of resuscitation. *Surg. Gynecol. Obstet.* 129: 811–815.

SCHUMAN, S. H., J. R. ROWE, H. M. GLAZER. AND J. S. REDDING 1976. The iceberg phenomenon of near drowning. *Crit. Care Med.* 4: 127–128.

SEVERINGHAUS, J. W., AND N. LASSEN 1967. Step hypocapnea to separate arterial from tissue P_{CO_2} in the regulation of cerebral blood flow. *Circ. Res.* 20: 272–278.

SIEBKE, H., H. BREIVEK, T. ROD. AND B. LIND 1975. Survival after 40 minutes' submersion without cerebral sequelae. *Lancet* 1: 1275–1277.

SWANN, H. G., AND M. BRUCER 1949. The cardiorespiratory and biochemical events during rapid anoxic death. VI. Freshwater and sea water drowning. *Tex. Rep. Biol. Med.* 7: 604–618.

SWANN, H. G., M. BRUCER, C. MOORE, AND B. L. VEZIEN 1947. Freshwater and sea water drowning: a study of the terminal cardiac and biochemical events. *Tex. Rep. Biol. Med.* 5: 423–437.

SYKES, W. S. 1972. *Essays on the First Hundred Years of Anaesthesia.* Huntington, NY: Robert E. Krieger Publ. Co., vol. II, p. 97–98.

U.S. DEPT. OF HEALTH AND HUMAN SERVICES 1980. *Vital Statistics of the United States 1976. Mortality.* Hyattsville, MD: National Center for Health Statistics, vol. II, pt. A, p. 1–245.

WEBSTER'S NEW COLLEGIATE DICTIONARY 1979. Springfield, MA: G. and C. Merriam Co., p. 347.

WYNNE, J. W., J. C. REYNOLDS, C. I. HOOD, D. AUERBACH, AND J. ONDRASICK 1979. Steroid therapy for pneumonitis induced in rabbits by aspiration of foodstuff. *Anesthesiology* 51: 11–19.

IX

Diagnosis and Treatment of Other Diving-Related Conditions

A. *The Unconscious Diver*

A diver who loses consciousness while under water creates a serious and potentially disastrous situation, especially in a deep dive. However, careful planning has made possible many successful rescues, even under the most difficult situation of diving from a bell. This section considers the probable causes of unconsciousness and suggests appropriate responses, including a plan of action for recovering the unconscious diver and performing resuscitation. Since each situation is different and a single plan cannot cover all possible circumstances, the guidelines given here should be reviewed and discussed by diving groups and used as a starting point for team planning, training, and action.

1. *Factors Leading to Loss of Consciousness*

An understanding of the physiological mechanisms involved in loss of consciousness may help to prevent its occurrence or to deal with it most effectively should it occur. In a study (Childs 1976) in Aberdeen, Scotland, of some 150 episodes of partial or complete loss of consciousness by a diver, it was found that in more than half the cases the diver had no advance warning, although in some of these cases the supervisor noted changes in behavior. Of those wherein some warning signs were noted, the main problem lay in some aspect of respiration; in other cases neurological symptoms were noted that could be classed as precursors to unconsciousness—namely, dizziness, faintness, or blurred vision.

a. Relevant Physiology

Consciousness is maintained by the higher centers of the brain. For these centers to function properly, the brain cells must continuously generate metabolic energy, and to do this they need a continuous supply of glucose and oxygen; both are delivered by the blood.

Very little energy can be stored in the brain tissue. Anything that disturbs the delivery of oxygenated nutrient-rich blood to the blood supply of the brain will affect consciousness.

The control system for the blood supply to the brain is remarkably effective, and it has a lot of reserve capability and redundancy; it takes a relatively big disturbance to render the system ineffective. The system depends on complex interactions to make it work properly; however, it can be quite vulnerable when several factors act in combination.

In addition to disruption of brain metabolism, which in turn is due to a reduction in blood flow to the brain, other incidences of loss of consciousness are caused by drugs, anesthetics, and toxic agents or by trauma such as a blow to the head.

b. Predisposing Conditions

While loss of consciousness may be brought on by a specific environmental or physiological situation, the condition of the diver at the moment can have a significant effect on his vulnerability. Several factors might make an otherwise healthy diver more susceptible:

(i) *Low Blood Sugar.* Hypoglycemia can result from fasting or very hard work.

(ii) *Fatigue.* Extreme fatigue may occur as a result of either hard work or loss of sleep.

(iii) *Hypothermia.* Consciousness is clouded as body temperature approaches 4°C below normal (33°C or 91°F) and is lost about 2°C below that (31°C or 87°F).

(iv) *Overheating.* A diver can get overheated when working in water or in a helium atmosphere at or near body temperature. This can lead to heat exhaustion and increase the diver's vulnerability to other factors.

(v) *Dehydration.* Dehydration is not a common problem in diving, but it would result from inadequate fluid intake and from living in a chamber that is too warm.

(vi) *Drugs.* Alcohol, barbiturates, marijuana, and certain medicines can leave a diver extremely vulnerable.

(vii) *Emotional States.* A diver who is preoccupied or afraid may be at risk. This is probably a much more important factor than is generally realized. (See Chapter XII, "Stress Physiology and Behavior Underwater''.)

(viii) *Inexperience.* Surveys have shown that the inexperienced diver has a greater chance of being involved in an episode of loss of consciousness.

c. Environmental Factors

A number of causative factors are primarily a function of the diver's working environment and his encounter with it. Treatment tailored to the cause will be more effective, so any environmental factor that could have caused the loss of consciousness should be considered when planning the rescue and treatment of each case. For example, a diver who has been in water of moderate temperature for only a short time and has not complained of being cold is not likely to have passed out because of hypothermia.

(i) *Hypoxia.* Because divers are usually exposed to high partial pressures of oxygen (P_{O_2}), the role of low oxygen is often underrated. It is most likely to occur with use of some type of closed-circuit breathing or life-support equipment or as the result of an improper gas mixture. Susceptibility to hypoxia is influenced by many other factors, especially hard work, cold, CO_2, and low blood glucose. Useful consciousness may be lost between 0.14 and 0.08 ATA P_{O_2}, depending on circumstances and individual susceptibility. Asphyxia is the result of not being able to breathe and results in a combination of both hypoxia and CO_2 retention. It might be caused by strangulation or a loss of gas supply.

An interesting example concerns the experienced sport diver who went to his basement to get his tanks for his first dive of the spring and found to his satisfaction that because there was plenty of pressure, the tanks would not have to be charged. On his dive he lost consciousness when he had barely gotten into the water, and he sank to the bottom. Fortunately his buddy pulled him out at once, and resuscitation was easy. Analysis of the air in his tank revealed less than 4% oxygen instead of the expected 20%—during the long winter the oxygen had formed iron oxide inside the tank (Temple et al. 1975).

(ii) Carbon Dioxide Retention. Retention of CO_2 can result from failure of a life-support system to remove CO_2 or from exercise that is excessive for the breathing system in use—especially where the gas is dense. An increasing level of CO_2 will lead to an increased breathing rate, headache, nausea, and possibly convulsions before unconsciousness. It takes a very high level of CO_2 to actually cause unconsciousness in the normally healthy individual. It should be noted, however, that some individuals are themselves carbon dioxide retainers and this may lead to problems. For example a young man was demonstrating the use of scuba gear at a northern Michigan summer resort; working at about 30 ft he felt very dizzy and nauseated. Fortunately he still had enough consciousness to immediately come to the surface. Upon examination he was found to retain carbon dioxide to a marked degree.

(iii) Oxygen Toxicity. A high partial pressure of oxygen can cause a convulsion that will be followed by a few minutes of unconsciousness. This can happen at oxygen levels as low as 1.8 ATA during heavy exercise, whereas P_{O_2} at 3.8 ATA can be tolerated at rest. Once again this depends on individual oxygen tolerance, which varies markedly from individual to individual. An attendant administering hyperbaric oxygen therapy to a patient went into convulsions himself from the increased oxygen that spilled from the mask of the patient. He was found to have a very low tolerance for oxygen.

(iv) Toxic Gases. Carbon monoxide reduces the capacity of the blood to carry oxygen and can resemble hypoxia in most of its effects. (Note, however, that the skin is pink instead of blue.) Before unconsciousness occurs, most other gases likely to be encountered in diving will cause nausea or irritation of the lungs. An exception is the asphyxiants (that is, those that displace oxygen). At high pressure, oxygen or even air may become toxic, but under these conditions it ought to be suspected because of the high density. Carbon monoxide poisoning is easily treated by hyperbaric oxygenation. But prevention is most important and is not too difficult, yet the literature is replete with reports of divers being furnished compressed breathing gas contaminated with carbon monoxide because the air intake of the compressor was downwind from the engine exhaust.

(v) Near-Drowning. It may take only a small amount of water to cause a drowning death. This could be due either to a reflex constriction of the glottis or to heart failure—the real reason is seldom known. Many of the fatalities associated with diving have the diagnosis "death from drowning," but what led up to the inhalation of water is seldom recorded, and that is what we really need to know. Chapter VIII of this book discusses near-drowning.

(vi) Strangulation (Choking). The trachea can be constricted by external pressure or can be mechanically blocked, or a reflex spasm of the larynx (laryngospasm) can result from irritation by any material, even a liquid. Vomiting, for whatever reason, can thus cause choking or, essentially, drowning.

(vii) Cold. Hypothermia is not likely to be the primary cause of unconsciousness in a well-supervised dive, but it will be a contributing factor in most episodes. It takes time for hypothermia to develop, and the diver will show other signs before he is cold enough to lose consciousness. It has been suggested that a very cold diver doing heavy work might need more oxygen than the blood can deliver. Sudden immersion in cold water can disable the unprotected individual and result in gasping and uncoordinated movements that can lead to drowning, but unconsciousness is not likely to be a direct effect of cold.

(viii) Overheating. The effects of hyperthermia may be heat exhaustion, which results from excesses in the body's attempts to maintain proper temperature, and heat stroke, a collapse of the temperature control mechanism. Both can lead to unconsciousness, but hyperthermia, like hypothermia, takes time to develop. Incidents have been reported of divers in hot water suits who passed out on reentering the bell; this reaction is considered to result from peripheral vasodilation due to the warmed skin plus the sudden loss of the hydrostatic support that had been provided by immersion.

(ix) Electric Shock. Electric current passing through the body can cause (1) cardiac arrhythmias including ventricular tachycardia, ventricular fibrillation, and cardiac standstill; (2) paralysis of respiratory muscles; and (3) seizures with loss of consciousness. Alternating current in the frequency range of 50–150 Hz is particularly dangerous.

(x) Physical Injury. A blow to the head can knock a person out, and other injury can cause shock that leads to unconsciousness.

(xi) Rapid Decompression. After abrupt surfacing or too rapid decompression two factors operate: (1) The diver who "blows up" or otherwise surfaces out of control is a prime candidate for embolism and explosive decompression sickness and should be handled accordingly. (2) If the oxygen pressure is near normal on bottom it could become inadequate when the pressure is reduced.

(xii) Shallow-Water Blackout. This condition is associated with breath-hold swimming and is the cause of many swimming pool deaths. A swimmer who has hyperventilated so as to hold his breath for a longer underwater swim may reduce his body content of CO_2 enough to reduce his inherent drive to breathe; when his blood oxygen is used up he will lose consciousness and drift to the bottom.

d. Physiological Factors

Since consciousness is physiological by definition, all of the environmental factors in the preceding section have a physiological element. Some loss of consciousness can also be due to factors more or less unrelated to the environment. A few of these are discussed here. It must be emphasized again that there is often a great deal of interaction between the various factors.

(i) Hyperventilation. If the amount of lung ventilation is so great that the CO_2 is eliminated faster than the body produces it, then the level of CO_2 in the blood will be lowered by this flushing action. When the blood CO_2 is lowered to less than half the normal level, a variety of disturbances in the body are created. One of these is a constriction of blood vessels in the brain, which leads to dizziness and other symptoms strikingly similar to those of hypoxia. Hyperventilization can lead also to incapacitation as a result of muscle spasm and (very rarely) unconsciousness. Anxiety causes many people to increase their breathing frequency, and some do this also when breathing by mask, but traditionally divers

do the reverse and slow down their breathing. Because of this training and the restrictions imposed by dense gas and the breathing equipment, enough hyperventilation to cause incapacitation seems quite unlikely in the diving situation. Furthermore, hyperventilation is essentially self-correcting, since the diver's breathing rate will slow down as soon as he loses consciousness. In a strict sense hyperventilation is any fast breathing, and it may very well be a normal and proper response to exercise, inspired CO_2, or other cause. A related situation is discussed in the next paragraph.

(ii) Inability to Control Breathing Rate. Another phenomenon, which divers sometimes call "hyperventilation," is an excessively fast breathing rate when using demand apparatus. Both exercise and a slight buildup of CO_2 stimulate breathing; that is, they call for an increase in lung ventilation. It is felt that if the diver increases his breathing rate (or frequency) but not depth of each breath, then the dead space ventilation becomes a greater proportion of the total breath. His lung ventilation becomes less effective and CO_2 increases still further, and this vicious circle continues until consciousness is lost because of excessive CO_2. Divers should consciously take deeper breaths when they feel an increased urge to breathe; with tended divers the supervisors should listen for rapid breathing and, when it appears to be coming on, warn divers to breathe more deeply and slow down their work level.

(iii) Fainting (Psychogenic Shock). Fainting can result from fear, bad news, the sight of blood, and other similar patterns. It may also result from a subconscious desire to escape from the prevailing situation.

(iv) Diving Reflex. Sudden contact of the body (particularly the face) with very cold water can cause a marked slowing of the heart rate that could precipitate unconsciousness.

(v) Prevailing Medical Problems. Epilepsy, stroke, heart failure, infection, and similar spontaneous and unpredicted reactions have been found to account for a large number of otherwise unexplained diving accidents. Thorough medical examination and a high level of personal fitness help to prevent this type of problem. Heart failure is suspected in many otherwise unexplained cases and seems to be provoked by such things as CO_2 or O_2 convulsions, hypoxia, cold, thermal shock, embolism, and strangulation.

(vi) Carbon Dioxide Retention. As mentioned in the preceding section, if an individual is a carbon dioxide retainer at a pathological level, problems in diving may result.

2. *Recovering an Unconscious Diver*

It is imperative to get an unconscious diver out of the water as quickly as possible. It is true that almost every case is different, but in an emergency it is critical for a set of procedures to be known and rehearsed, so that prompt and decisive action can be taken without having to take time to think.

a. Unconscious Diver in the Water

If a diver in the water is unresponsive, then he will have to be pulled to the surface or brought back into the bell or habitat. No time can be wasted. If a diver is unconscious, assume he will need to be resuscitated; to be fully effective, resuscitation must begin within 3 min of the time the diver stopped breathing. It should be a one-to-one operation, a rescuing diver being constantly with the unconscious diver and directing operations. The rate of ascent should be consistent with the emergency; it is preferable to deviate from decompression tables rather then delay needed resuscitation. When decompression is compromised or embolism is likely, then treatment should be performed after the diver is safely in the chamber and being resuscitated. If an unconscious diver has been hauled to the surface the rescuers should assume that he has embolism and treat accordingly.

b. Unconscious Bell or Habitat Diver

Additional problems are associated with dragging and then hoisting the unconscious diver into a bell or habitat. Also, resuscitation in water or in the bell presents additional difficulties, but they can be and have been successfully worked out.

3. Resuscitation

The priorities are the same in water or in the bell or habitat as they are on land: check for vital signs, assure a clear airway, restore breathing, assure heart function, and stop bleeding.

a. Check Vital Signs

If there is a carotid pulse and the diver is breathing, no emergency attempts at resuscitation are necessary. If neither pulse nor breathing is found, start emergency treatment at once as noted below.

b. Insert Airway

Clear the mouth and insert the oropharyngeal airway. If the head is hanging forward, try to support the chin.

c. Mouth-to-Mouth Resuscitation

Begin respiratory resuscitation as soon as possible, filling the lungs once every 5 sec.

d. Cardiac Resuscitation

Begin cardiac compression if needed. Try a few relatively sharp blows in an attempt to start the heart; follow each with a few breaths. Check for heartbeat before repeating, as another blow could stop the heart again. If the heart does not start after a few tries, attempt to support the circulation with cardiac massage (standard CPR) until either the diver revives or it is clear that the situation is hopeless. Cardiac compression can be performed on a diver hanging by his harness by holding his shoulders and applying chest compression with either the head or knee, but practice is required, and the technique will not be effective unless the diver is at least partially immersed.

e. Treat Significant Bleeding

Apply a compression dressing or a tourniquet as appropriate to control bleeding.

f. Transfer Injured Diver

If the diver has regained consciousness (and depending on his condition and other circumstances), put him in a deck decompression chamber or transfer him ashore to either a hyperbaric unit or a hospital.

g. Report the Incident

All cases of a diver's loss of consciousness for any reason whatsoever must be reported at once to higher authority, and a detailed record should be prepared to include all events surrounding the incident. (See Chapter XV, "Diving Accident Investigation.")

R. W. HAMILTON

References

CHILDS, C. M. 1976. *Investigation Into Loss of Consciousness in Diving.* Second Report. Aberdeen, U.K.: Department of Energy.
TEMPLE, J. D., JR., R. T. BOSSHARDT, AND J. H. DAVIS 1975. SCUBA tank corrosion as a cause of death. *J. Forensic Sci.* 20: 571–575.

B. *Osteonecrosis*

1. *Introduction*

The first report of a suited diver developing osteonecrosis appeared in 1941 (Grutzmacher). It had been recognized for some years that men working at pressure in caissons, tunnels, and bells might suffer from bone damage, but all the early papers were concerned with case reports about men with advanced lesions, and no effort was made to determine the prevalance of the condition in symptomless divers until some years later. Part of the reason for this delay was that although bone necrosis in its gross form is easily recognized on a radiograph, the more subtle changes of the early stages of the disease are not so generally appreciated.

There are, of course, many conditions with which osteonecrosis may be associated (Table IX-1), and indeed an idiopathic variety has been described. Most of these conditions can usually be eliminated as a likely cause by considering the patient's age and past history and by the use of suitable screening tests.

Table IX-1
Some Conditions Reported to Be
Associated with Osteonecrosis

Hyperbaric exposure	Trauma
Steroid therapy	Rheumatoid arthritis
Sickle cell anaemia	Gout
Diabetes	Ionizing radiation
Chronic alcoholism	Syphilis
Cirrhosis of the liver	Alcaptonuria
Hepatitis	Arteriosclerosis
Pancreatitis	Hyperlipidaemia
Gaucher's disease	

The osteonecrosis seen in compressed air workers and divers mainly involves the humerus, femur, and tibia, and it is rarely found elsewhere. The sites affected in these bones can be separated into those adjacent to an articular surface and known as juxta-articular lesions (JA), and those that are clear of the articular surface and known as head, neck, and shaft lesions (HNS).

Experience has shown that whereas in compressed air workers the shoulders and hips are affected roughly in equal proportion, in divers the JA lesions mainly affect the shoulder joints and only rarely the hip joints.

The start of naval diving interest in this condition was sparked off by the rather unexpected finding that the prevalence of osteonecrosis in a group of 241 apparently fit compressed air workers on a site in Great Britain was found to be as high as 19% (9.5% JA lesions and 9.5% HNS lesions), in spite of use of a lengthened statutory decompression table (McCallum et al. 1966). In 1970 Elliott and Harrison reported the results of radiologically surveying 350 British Royal Navy divers; they found an overall percentage of 4%, with 1.1% having JA lesions. This was followed by a report from the United States Navy in 1976 (Harvey and Sphar) about 611 divers; in this the overall prevalence was 2.4%, with 1.9% having JA lesions.

As far as commercial diving is concerned, in 1974 Ohta and Matsunga reported the prevalence of osteonecrosis in a group of 301 professional Japanese shellfish divers and found that about 50% had osteonecrosis, 14.6% having JA lesions. Fortunately the figures for the commercial divers operating in the North Sea are not nearly so alarming in spite of the heavy economic pressures and often severe diving conditions. Through the co-operation of the Approved Diving Doctors, the Medical Research Council Decompression Sickness Central Registry in Newcastle upon Tyne, England, has been able to keep a close watch on the development of osteonecrosis in these men. At present the overall prevalence in the 4744 divers known to have been passed medically fit to work in the North Sea is 4.1%, and 1.2% have JA lesions.

2. Diagnosis by Radiology

At the moment the diagnosis of osteonecrosis usually rests solely on radiographic findings, since clinical signs and symptoms only appear at a stage when severe and possibly irreparable damage has already been done to the skeleton. Even so, a considerable time, probably at least 3 months, must pass between the causal insult and the appearance of the first radiologically detectable changes.

It is now generally accepted that when screening divers for evidence of osteonecrosis only the shoulders, hips, and knee regions need be radiographed. The basic skeletal survey then should include anteroposterior projections of the heads and proximal shafts of both humeri and both femora, and anteroposterior and lateral projections of the distal two-thirds of both femora and proximal one-third of both tibiae, including the knee joints.

The radiographic diagnosis of early lesions of aseptic bone necrosis requires high quality radiographs that demonstrate the bone trabeculae clearly. The optimum screen-film combination (using rare-earth intensifying screens, if available) and good screen-film contact are required, together with a grid of adequate ratio and a focal spot of 0.6 to 1.2 mm. A tube with a high-speed rotating anode and 0.6-mm target, if available, is ideal.

Exposures should always be adequate. Probably the greatest fault lies in underpenetration of the bone tissue. Increased penetration by as much as 5–10 kV above normal is recommended.

In Great Britain the recommendation of the *Code of Practice for the Protection of Persons against Ionizing Radiation Arising from Medical and Dental Use* (1972) should be followed. Gonads must always be protected by a lead shield when radiographing the hips. Estimation of the radiation dose received by the patient indicates that this basic survey can safely be repeated at intervals of not less than 6 months. The practical details of an acceptable procedure are given in the Appendix to this section.

In 1966 the Medical Research Council Decompression Sickness Panel (McCallum et al. 1966) first described its system of recognizing and classifying the various radiological changes of both early and late osteonecrosis so that it became possible to record succinctly the relevant lesions and to make reasonable comparisons between various surveys. This classification is set out in Table IX-2 and the categories are defined in the text that follows. Illustrations of these lesions are to be found in Davidson (1976).

a. Juxta-articular Lesions

(i) A1. Dense areas with an intact articular cortex occur in the head of the humerus or femur close to or involving the articular cortex. In their earliest stage lesions may be difficult to detect in the femoral head because of the acetabular shadows, but tomography or a magnification film may demonstrate them more clearly.

(ii) A2. Spherical segmental opacity is seen typically in the humeral head and is shaped like the segment of a sphere.

(iii) A3. Linear opacity is found typically in the humeral head as a curved or serpiginous shadow of varied thickness and density, and there may be other small, dense areas distal to it.

(iv) A4. Structural failure. Structural failure may follow A1, A2, or A3 and is accompanied by pain and stiffness in the joint. There are three main appearances: (1) A4a. A fine transradiant subcortical line under the articular cortex of the humeral or femoral head. The cortex and underlying bone have not collapsed. (2) A4b. Collapse of the articular cortex, which may involve up to half of its extent, sometimes with a stepped depression in the head of the bone. A large triangular opacity is usually present in the

Table IX-2
Medical Research Council Classification of Osteonecrosis

Juxta-articular lesions	
Dense areas with an intact articular cortex	A1
Spherical segmental opacities	A2
Linear opacity	A3
Structural failure	
Transradient subcortical band	A4a
Collapse of the articular cortex	A4b
Sequestration of part of the cortex	A4c
Osteoarthritis	A5
Head, neck, and shaft lesions	
Dense areas	B1
Irregular calcified areas	B2
Transradiant areas	B3

adjacent bone. (3) A4c. Sequestration of part of the cortex may occur by fracture through the necrotic area in the subchondral zone.

(v) A5. Osteoarthritis. Osteophyte formation occurs at the lower part of the articular cortex of the humerus and in the hip at the margin of the femoral head. It is typical of bone necrosis with osteoarthritis that the width of the joint space remains normal in the earlier stages. At an advanced stage the picture is similar to that of osteoarthritis from a variety of other causes.

b. Head, Neck, and Shaft Lesions

(i) B1. Dense areas are commonly sited in the neck and proximal shaft of the femur and humerus, but they also occur elsewhere in the long bones.

(ii) B2. Irregular calcified areas are often large, bilateral, and prominent because of extensive irregular calcification, but in their early stages they present as vague shadows seen best in the distal femur in lateral views. They also occur in the proximal part of the humerus and tibia.

(iii) B3. Transradiant areas are found in the distal shaft of the femur and proximal shaft of the humerus occupying the whole width of the medulla, and they are several centimeters long, with scalloping of the endosteum.

Sometimes doubts are raised about regarding the presence of bone islands and cysts as forms of osteonecrosis. Bone islands are small areas of cortical bone, round or oval in shape, that lie in the medulla and are partly connected with the cortex. They are probably developmental in origin, rarely change in size or shape, and like the small cysts occasionally seen in the neck of the femur are probably not related to diving (Davidson et al. 1977).

3. *Other Methods of Diagnosis*

Since radiological investigation is not always possible or even desirable at a time appropriate to detect damage after every dive, it is usually impossible to identify the particular dive responsible for the damage to a bone.

Research has therefore been directed to see if it is possible to identify a marker in either urine or blood that can be immediately associated with damage to a bone, that is, within a few hours, or at least within a few days.

Of the factors so far studied, serum ferritin appears to be the most promising (Gregg et al. 1977).

Bone scanning using bone-seeking radioisotopes is also under trial as a sensitive method of discovering areas of disturbed bone physiology following diving, but at the moment it appears as though both it and serum ferritin level may be so sensitive that they perhaps indicate degrees of damage so minor that they will be corrected without leaving any permanent indication of their existence. For practical purposes, then, diagnosis of osteonecrosis rests on radiology at this time.

4. Clinical Management and Treatment

As a general principle it is usual to strive for as early a diagnosis as possible on the grounds that it will be in the best interests of the patient. There is no doubt that it would be very helpful if the diagnosis could be made early enough to identify the dives that resulted in osteonecrosis. With this information it would then be possible to study within a day or two all the factors applying to those dives and possibly to identify exactly the cause of bone damage. By studying the rather crude data at present available it can be seen that vulnerable individuals are those who dive to depths greater than 50 m and those who undertake dives of longer than 4-hr duration. It is for this reason that the bones of such individuals should be radiographed regularly; for practical purposes this means at approximately yearly intervals. Provided that proper techniques are used, particularly with respect to protecting the gonads, the dose of irradiation from such an investigation is very small and certainly acceptable in Great Britain.

Juxta-articular lesions must be regarded as serious, because if they are in the direct line of weight-bearing across a joint, they may collapse and give rise to an irregular articular surface, which in all probability will result in pain on movement, limited mobility, and a risk of the development of a secondary osteoarthritis. It is thought that about 8% of JA lesions may break down in this way and eventually require surgical treatment.

Unfortunately, at the moment there is no way of telling which JA lesions will break down and which will remain stable. Neither can a time scale be estimated for the deterioration of a JA lesion. Some have been known to remain unchanged for 10 to 15 years, while occasionally a lesion will progress from first recognition to sequestrum formation in 3 months. Because continuation of diving may increase the risk of a serious outcome, because other joints may become affected, and because the treatment of the serious form of the condition in such young men is not entirely satisfactory, divers in Great Britain with JA osteonecrosis are usually stopped from further diving.

Head, neck, and shaft lesions, on the other hand, are probably harmless in that they rarely if ever give rise to symptoms and certainly never seem to result in weakness of the bone. Occasionally a man with a shaft lesion will complain of pain, but so far it has not been possible to establish for certain that this is associated with the underlying lesion. Finally, and just for completeness, it must be admitted that it has been suggested that there is a very remote possibility that neoplastic changes could occur in such a lesion at some time in the distant future. Supporting evidence for this hypothesis is, however, scarce. At present only four cases have been described in the world literature, and these were all in elderly, former compressed air workers.

The question is often asked: Does the presence of an HNS lesion indicate that a diver is more likely to suffer from a JA lesion subsequently than a diver who does not have a JA lesion? The data at present available are such that this question cannot be answered in a statistically significant way, and the accumulation of more data must be awaited. In Great Britain divers with HNS lesions are not stopped from diving but are, of course, followed up by regular radiographic bone examinations.

5. Underlying Pathological Changes

Since the radiological appearances of osteonecrosis have formed the basis for diagnosis over the years, it is obviously important to have some idea of the pathological changes underlying them.

Fortunately, due to the work of Kahlstrom et al. (1939) and others up to and including McCallum et al. (1966), it is possible to build up a reasonably good correlation between the radiographic appearances and the underlying histological changes. Basically a juxta-articular area of osteonecrosis is recognized histologically by acellularity of the bone marrow and by the absence of osteocytes in the bone lacunae. When revascularization occurs the marrow may return virtually to normal, but recognizable unresorbed dead bone cores remain for a long time in the center of trabeculae newly covered by laminar bone. When these reach a critical thickness they can be detected on radiographic examination as an area of increased density. That some repaired trabeculae do not reach this critical thickness results in an often very much greater area of damaged bone than can be suspected from the x-ray picture. Another interesting finding is that the repair process often appears to stop short of completion, leaving a band of dense fibrous tissue between the repaired area and that remaining necrotic. The trabeculae adjacent to the fibrous tissue on the revascularized side are often very broad, and this accounts for the dense linear opacity sometimes seen on a radiograph. Third, even over unrevascularized dead bone the articular cartilage of a joint surface is usually viable and of normal thickness. This accounts for the persistence of the normal joint space seen on radiographs of even extensive lesions.

Head, neck, and shaft lesions consist of a central area of dead fatty marrow (shown by the absence of cell nuclei) surrounded by a well-developed fibrous capsule on the inner surface of which is a very cellular layer. The overlying inner half of the cortex shows evidence of bone death with spicules of new living bone deposited on the endosteal surface (Gregg et al. 1980).

6. Etiology

At the moment bone necrosis is thought to result from embolization of the blood supply by bubbles that occur during decompression. The condition can be mimicked in rabbits by the use of glass microspheres to simulate bubbles. It has to be admitted that there is not always a clear relationship between the site of bone necrosis lesions and the site of a previous attack of Type I decompression sickness, but since the existence of silent bubbles is now clearly established, perhaps this is not surprising. In addition it should be remembered that decompression schedules are not expected to be 100% effective, so that not all osteonecrosis should necessarily be assumed to be the consequence of a badly executed decompression schedule. If the schedule used was inappropriate for the dive, or if the schedule was not accurately followed, then clearly the risk of causing bone damage would have been increased.

In recent years a good deal of doubt has been voiced from time to time about whether the osteonecrosis seen in divers and compressed air workers really is due to the occurrence of bubbles. For instance, it has been pointed out that because one of the recognized causes of osteonecrosis is chronic alcoholism, perhaps this factor is more important among divers than their exposure to pressure.

Other factors claimed to be responsible for the initiation of osteonecrosis are fat embolism, blood changes in decompression such as intravascular agglutination, platelet aggregation, and gas-induced osmosis (McCallum 1975).

Unfortunately the evidence that any of these has a crucial role is lacking. Nevertheless, the bubble embolism hypothesis has many weaknesses. For example, to result in the death of an osteocyte a bubble embolus would have to persist for 6–21 hr, and this seems to be a long time. However, the probability that it will occur in man, who has a relatively long circulation time, is certainly greater than the probability that it will occur in small laboratory animals, which have a short circulation time, and may explain why the latter do not get osteonecrosis but man does.

At present it seems to me that for osteonecrosis to occur may require the concurrence of two or more factors; one of these is probably the presence of a bubble, but the other factor or factors are not yet evident.

D. N. WALDER

APPENDIX

A1. *Recommended Procedure for X-Ray by Medical Research Council Decompression Sickness Panel*

Aa. Shoulder: Anteroposterior Projection

The area to be examined is the head and neck of the humerus, including the proximal third of the shaft.

The radiograph should show the articular surface of the humeral head unobscured by overlying bony structures and should give good definition of the trabeculae of the head and shaft.

A 24-by-18-cm screen film is recommended with high definition or rare-earth intensifying screens and a moving grid.

The examination is best carried out on a horizontal table.

From the supine position the patient is rotated through about 45° toward the side under examination until the blade of the scapula is parallel to the table top. The raised shoulder is supported on sandbags.

The arm under examination should be straight, supinated, and abducted 10°. An extending pull should be applied to the arm so that the humeral head is clear of the bony processes of the scapula.

The x-ray beam should be at right angles to the film and centered over the head of the humerus. A beam should be collimated to show only the head and proximal third of the humerus.

The patient should hold his breath while the exposure is made.

Ab. Hip Joint and Proximal Third of Shaft of Femur: Anteroposterior View

The radiograph should show good definition of the articular surface of the femoral head and of the trabeculae of both head and shaft. The underlying acetabulum cannot be avoided.

A separate radiograph of each hip is required.

A 30-by-24-cm screen film is recommended with fast tungstate or rare-earth intensifying screens and a moving grid. Fast tungstate screens are recommended in this situation to reduce the radiation dose. To increase penetration, 2.5 to 5 kV more power than normal should be used.

The gonads must be protected, but care should be taken to ensure that the protection does not obscure the femoral head.

With the patient supine the plane across the anterior superior iliac spines should be horizontal. The foot of the side under examination should be at right angles to the table top and sandbagged into position.

The x-ray beam should be at right angles to the film, centered over the head of the femur, and collimated to show the head and proximal third of the femur.

Ac. Knee Joint: Anteroposterior Projection to Show Distal Two-Thirds of Femur and Proximal Third of Tibia

The radiograph should show clear trabecular detail in the lower two-thirds of the femur and the upper third of the tibia.

There is a variation of density between the middle and lower thirds of the femoral shaft so that it is necessary to increase the kilovoltage, reduce the milliamperage, and use a moving grid to produce a radiograph of even contrast. Care should be taken not to underpenetrate the shaft of the femur.

A 40-by-15-cm screen film is recommended with high definition or rare-earth intensifying screens and a moving grid.

The patient should sit on the x-ray table with both legs extended.

Each knee should be examined separately.

The x-ray beam should be at right angles to the table top. In order for the lower two-thirds of the femur to be included, the beam should be centered at the upper border of the patella—not through the joint space. The beam should be collimated to show only the area under examination.

Ad. Knee Joint: Lateral Projection to Show Distal Two-Thirds of Femur and Proximal Third of Tibia

A lateral radiograph of the lower femur and upper tibia may demonstrate slight variations in bone density and trabeculae detail which are not apparent in the anteroposterior projection.

The requirements of definition are the same as for the anteroposterior projection. The gradation of density along the femoral shaft is also evident in the lateral projection and the exposure should be adjusted to give a radiograph of even contrast.

Either a 40-by-30-cm or a 40-by-15-cm screen film is recommended with a high definition or rare-earth intensifying screens and a moving grid.

Using the wide film, positioning should be as for a normal lateral projection of the knee, with the knee flexed and the tibia parallel to the long axis of the film. Care should be taken to include the distal two-thirds of the femur.

If the narrow film is used, the leg should be straight and parallel to the long axis of the film in order to include the distal two-thirds of the femur.

The x-ray beam should be at right angles to the film and centered over the femur level with the upper border of the patella. The beam should be collimated to the area under examination.

References

Code of Practice for the Protection of Persons against Ionizing Radiations Arising from Medical and Dental Use 1972. London: Her Majesty's Stationery Office.

DAVIDSON, J. K. 1976. *Aseptic Necrosis of Bone*. New York: American Elsevier, Ltd.

DAVIDSON, J. K., J. A. B. HARRISON, P. JACOBS, T. E. HILDITCH, M. CATTO, AND W. T. HENDRY 1977. The significance of bone islands, cystic areas and sclerotic areas in dysbaric osteonecrosis. *Méd. Aeronaut. Spat. Méd. Sub. Hyp.* 16(64): 407–410.

ELLIOTT, D. H., AND J. A. B. HARRISON 1970. Bone necrosis—an occupational hazard of diving. *J. R. Nav. Med. Serv.* 56: 140–161.

EUROPEAN DIVING TECHNOLOGY COMMITTEE 1980. *Guidelines for the Evaluation of Medical Fitness to Dive*. London: CIRIA Underwater Engineering Group.

GREGG, P. J., E. J. EASTHAM, J. I. BELL. AND D. N. WALDER 1977. Serum ferritin and dysbaric osteonecrosis. *Undersea Biomed. Res.* 4: 75–79.

GREGG, P. J., D. N. WALDER. AND I. RANNIE 1980. Caisson disease of bone: a study of the Göttingen minipig as an animal model. *Br. J. Exp. Pathol.* 61: 39–54.

GRUTZMACHER, K. T. 1941. Veranderungen am Schultergelenk als Folge von Drucklufterkrankung. *Roentgenpraxis (Leipzig)* 13: 216–218.

HARVEY, C. A., AND R. L. SPHAR 1976. Dysbaric osteonecrosis in divers. A survey of 611 selected navy divers. *U.S. Nav. Submar. Med. Res. Lab. Rep.* 832: 55.

KAHLSTROM, S. C., C. C. BURTON. AND D. B. PHEMISTER 1939. Aseptic necrosis of bone. I. Infarction of bones in caisson disease resulting in encapsualted and calcified areas in diaphyses and in arthritis deformans. *Surg. Gynecol. Obstet.* 68: 129–146.

MCCALLIUM, R. I. 1975. Dysbaric osteonecrosis: aseptic necrosis of bone. In: *The Physiology and Medicine of Diving and Compressed Air Work* (2nd ed.), edited by P. B. Bennett and D. H. Elliott. London: Baillière, Tindall, p. 504–521.

MCCALLUM, R. I., D. N. WALDER, R. BARNES, M. E. CATTO, J. K. DAVIDSON, D. I. FRYER, F. C. GOLDING. AND W. D. M. PATON 1966. Bone lesions in compressed-air workers with special reference to men who worked on the Clyde Tunnels 1958 to 1963. *J. Bone Joint Surg. (Lond.)* 48B:207–235.

OHTA, Y., AND H. MATSUNAGA 1974. Bone lesions in divers. *J. Bone Joint Surg. (Lond.)* 56B:3–16.

C. Microbes and the Diver

1. Introduction

The relationship between man and his environment is always important but never more so than when one considers man and his indigenous microflora and also the microorganisms in the environment. This is particularly true when considering confining a man in a habitat for long periods of time, but it is also true when one considers the familiar diving practice of sharing and exchanging equipment—even buddy breathing—which may facilitate cross-infection.

2. Cross-Infections

Upper respiratory infections (colds, sore throat, sinusitis) are highly undesirable in a closed space such as a habitat, for these infections are easily transferred to others. In World War II during the first 10 days on a submarine patrol, upper respiratory infections of all personnel were exchanged, and then there was a period of freedom from infection until another person was brought aboard, as a downed aviator or a prisoner. Thus in planning for habitat activity it is important to consider the interaction of the individuals with each other as well as with the environment.

Sciarli et al. (1973) reported on the condition of four divers in a French diving program who lived at a depth of 300 m (984 ft) for 8 days. Although the atmosphere of the chamber was disinfected and the divers used local disinfectants, they still developed conjunctivitis and skin rash and had earaches. In fact, painful inflammation and secretion in the auditory canals, without involvement of the tympanum, seemed to be the most common problem. High relative humidity (86%) was believed to be the cause, for in subsequent dives when the relative humidity was kept between 40% and 50% these conditions did not occur.

Oser (1972) reports a similar experience in the German habitat *Helgoland*, where aquanats lived under conditions involving a pressure of 2.0 atm. The health of the aquanats was medically supervised, and "infections involving the ear made necessary almost daily medical inspections."

The bacteriological aspects of the TEKTITE I program were presented by Cobet et al. (1970); once again the primary problem was otitis externa. In fact otitis externa is the most common complaint of swimmers, divers, and aquanauts.

3. Diving with an Infection

Diving with a preexisting infection is more common and more important than infection due to diving. As pointed out by Edmonds et al. (1981) in their chapter on infections, upper respiratory infections are particularly bad for the diver, since swelling and blockage of the mucus-lined drainage passages leads to barotrauma of the middle ear and of the several sinuses. But respiratory infection involving the lungs is more likely to cause serious damage. For example, a mucus plug may obstruct smaller airways and act as a ball valve or flap valve allowing the air to enter the alveolae distal to the valve during descent but blocking the air from escaping during ascent. This may lead to pulmonary barotrauma with its various sequelae—pulmonary tissue damage, emphysema, pneumothorax, or air embolism.

4. Local Infections Associated with Diving

Otitis externa, the most common infection associated with diving, and otitis media due to diving are both covered in Section D of this chapter.

a. Sinusitis

The paranasal or accessory nasal sinuses (frontal, ethmoidal, and maxillary) may become a problem for the diver because of failure to equalize pressure within the sinus with the changing ambient pressure. It is well to remember that these sinuses are drained into the nasal cavity through small ostia lined with mucous membrane that responds to external trauma by swelling and thus closing the opening. An adequate amount of ventilation and pressure equalization in the paranasal sinuses is important in diving, both during compression and during decompression.

The cause of the problem is usually nasal congestion, which in turn may be due to infection (common cold), allergies, smoking, chronic irritation from prolonged and excessive use of nose drops, or anatomical deviation (deviated nasal septum, polyps, or mucosal folds).

The predominant symptom is pain. In one series studied (Edmonds et al. 1981) the sinuses involved were frontal (68% of the patients), ethmoidal area (16%), and maxillary area (6%).

The most common sign is bloody discharge from the nose, but radiography of the sinuses performed within 24 hr of an incident showed "the maxillary sinus was affected with either mucosal thickening or fluid level, in 74% of cases, the frontal in 24%, and the ethmoidal in 15%. A fluid level was present in the maxillary sinus in 12% of the cases" (Edmonds et al. 1981).

Therapy is not neccesary in most cases, as the patients spontaneously recover. Short-term use of nasal decongestants speeds the return to normal. Antibiotics are rarely indicated, and neither sinus lavage nor surgery is required or advisable.

Prevention consists of not diving with an upper respiratory infection or when the nasal passages are blocked. Occasionally repair of a deviated nasal septum or the removal of nasal polyps may be indicated.

b. Skin Infection

Athlete's foot (tinea pedis) is a dermatophytosis due to a *Trichophyton* or *Epidermophyton floccosum* and is common in swimmers and divers. It is spread by moist environment, such as bare feet on wet decks or on floors of communal showers. Athlete's foot is usually only a nuisance, but if it gets out of hand it may lead to secondary infection and lymphadenitis.

Divers who are continually exposed to salt water, especially in the tropics, with no freshwater showers available, are quite likely to develop a generalized dermatitis that can be quite bothersome because of the itching and burning sensation. To prevent this from happening it is important to not wear clothing soaked with salt water for long periods of time and to use a freshwater shower after a saltwater swim or dive, and also to rinse the swim or diving suit in fresh water after use in salt water and dry it thoroughly.

c. Infections from Wounds, Bites, Stings

The effects of harmful marine organisms and the treatment of wounds from them are discussed in some detail in Section F of this chapter. Each is unique in some respect, and the only treatment common to all is a general antiseptic procedure to prevent spreading of the infections.

5. *Systemic Infections*

a. Disease from Polluted Water

Hepatitis, typhoid, paratyphoid, cholera, and schistosomiasis have been reported following swimming or scuba diving in bacterially contaminated water. The possibility of bacterial pollution of water must be carefully checked and no diving allowed except in case of emergency, and then care must be taken to minimize possible contamination. In addition to careful bathing after the dive, the suit, helmet, and gloves must be cleaned and dried.

b. Leptospirosis

Leptospirosis has been reported from swimming in polluted fresh water. The organism may gain entry through a break in the skin or mucous membrane, or from swallowing polluted water.

c. Pharyngoconjunctival Fever

Pharyngoconjunctival fever is an acute illness caused by several types of adenovirus and has been reported in association with swimming in polluted water. It is characterized by fever, malaise, pharyngitis, cervical lymphadenopathy, cough, conjunctivitis, and sometimes diarrhea. Treatment is symptomatic.

d. Near-Drowning

Near-drowning may lead to secondary pulmonary infection due to aspiration of either polluted fresh or salt water. This is one of the reasons why all near-drowning patients should be hospitalized for observation for a few days. Chapter VIII deals with all aspects of this problem.

CARL EDMONDS
CHARLES W. SHILLING

References

COBET, A. B., D. N. WRIGHT, AND P. I. WARREN 1970. Tektite I program: bacteriological aspects. *Aerosp. Med.* 41: 611–616.
EDMONDS, C., C. LOWRY, AND J. PENNEFATHER 1981. *Diving and Subaquatic Medicine.* Mosmon, Australia: Diving Medical Centre.
OSER, H. 1972. Medizinische Erfahrungen beim Einsatz des Unterwasserlaboratorium 'Helgoland' in Herbst 1971. *DFVLR-Nachrichten,* p. 307–308.
SCIARLI, R., F. F. SICARDI, C. KEMAIRE, AND D. PROSPERI 1973. Mycobacteriologie et plongée à saturation. *Bull. Medsubhyp.* 9: 15–21.

D. Ear and Sinuses

As described in Chapter III, in the section on vestibular function, the air-containing middle ear spaces and paranasal sinus cavities become liabilities for humans during exposures to the compressed gas environments encountered in diving. Proper pressure equilibration between these cavities and the ambient atmosphere must occur during all phases of diving. Lack of proper pressure equilibration results in significant injury to the tissues adjacent to these air-containing cavities; this injury is commonly termed *barotrauma*.

1. Otologic Barotrauma

a. Middle Ear Barotrauma

Middle ear barotrauma is the most common medical problem encountered in diving. Numerous previous publications have described and discussed this entity in detail; particularly noteworthy are works by Shilling and Everly (1942), Taylor (1959), Edmonds et al. (1973), and Farmer and Thomas (1976).

Middle ear barotrauma results from inadequate pressure equilibration between the middle ear-temporal bone air-containing spaces and the external environment. It occurs most often during compression or descent when middle ear pressure becomes negative relative to increasing ambient pressure. With an intact eardrum, the only route for adequate equilibration of middle ear pressure is through the eustachian tube. The nasopharyngeal ostium of the eustachian tube is normally closed, and it opens with swallowing, primarily through the actions of the tensor and levator muscles of the palate. During the rapid pressure changes encountered in diving, the nasopharyngeal ostium of the eustachian tube

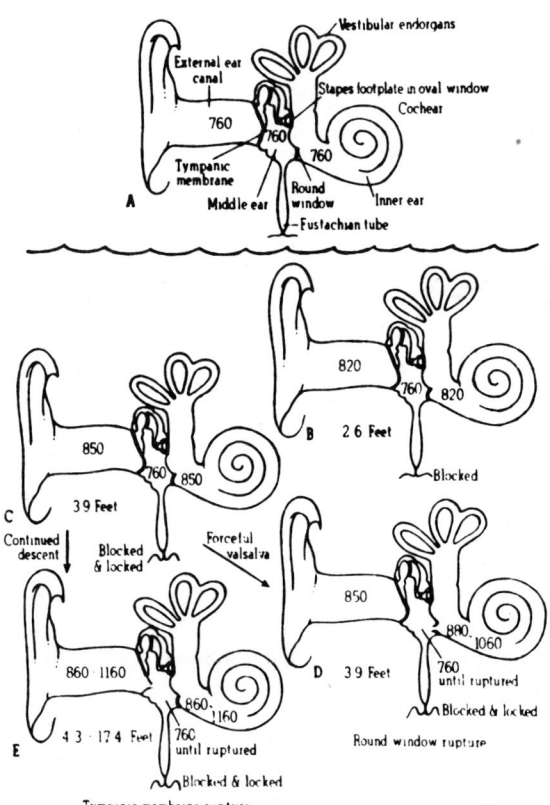

Figure IX-1. Otologic barotauma during descent. Theoretical sequence of events in right ear of diver who does not equilibrate middle ear pressure during descent. Pressures shown in mmHg. *A:* Surface condition with equal pressures (760 mmHg) throughout and patent eustachian tube with normally closed nasopharyngeal ostium. *B:* Depth of approximately 2.6 ft (0.79 m) after diver failed to open eustachian tube upon entering water. Pressure differential of 60 mmHg exists (820 − 760 = 60). Tympanic membrane and round window are bulging into middle ear. Diver notices pain and pressure in ear, with conductive hearing loss and possible vertigo. *C:* Depth of approximately 3.9 ft (1.19 m) with 90 mmHg pressure differential and blocked and locked Eustachian tube. *D:* Forceful Valsalva's manuever can lead to rupture of round window with resulting leak of perilymph into middle ear. Exact pressure differential at which rupture occurs in humans is unknown. Studies in cats have indicated that round window ruptures occur when pressure of 120–300 mmHg is applied to the cerebrospinal fluid space at 1 ATA. *E:* Continued descent can lead to tympanic membrane rupture at pressure differentials of 100–499 mmHg or depths of 4.3–17.4 ft (1.31–5.30 m). Actual rupture point is quite variable. (Reprinted with permission from Farmer, J. C., and W. G. Thomas. Ear and sinus problems in diving. In: *Diving Medicine,* edited by R. M. Strauss. New York: Grune and Stratton, 1976. p. 118.)

can fail to sufficiently open if the diver does not make active attempts by swallowing or if local inflammation and swelling, usually resulting from nasal inflammatory disease, prevents opening. With increasingly negative middle ear pressure, eustachian tubal opening becomes more difficult because of a nasopharyngeal valve effect (Figure IX-1, *B* and *C*).

With descent and the absence of middle ear pressure equilibration, a pressure differential of approximately 60 mmHg between the middle ear and inner ear as well as the ambient environment will occur at a depth of approximately 2.6 ft or 0.8 m (Figure IX-1, *B*). Ear fullness and pain are usually noted (Keller 1958). Possible vertiginous sensations, particularly if only one ear is involved, can also occur. Continued descent to a depth of 3.9 ft (1.2 m) results in a pressure differential of 90 mmHg. The eustachian tube becomes blocked and usually cannot be opened voluntarily (Keller 1958; see also Figure IX-1,*C*). The tympanic membrane has been noted to rupture at varying pressure differentials ranging from 100 to 500 mmHg, equivalent to depths of 4.3 to 17.4 ft (1.3

to 5.3 m) (Keller 1958; see Figure IX-1, *E*). A forceful Valsalva maneuver during these conditions can result in an increase in the already existing pressure differential between the inner ear and middle ear and can lead to rupture of the round or oval window with leakage of perilymph and injury of the inner ear (Figure IX-1, *D*). This has been termed *inner ear barotrauma* and is discussed in a later section.

With inadequate middle ear pressure equilibration during descent, a diver may notice mild tinnitus. A conductive hearing loss is always present, but it is frequently not noted during underwater conditions. Severe pain is usually felt with tympanic membrane rupture. Predive nasal dysfunction with obstruction and congestion or discharge, or both, increases the likelihood of inadequate eustachian tubal function and middle or possible inner ear barotrauma. The absence of predive nasal symptoms does not, however, rule out the possibility of such barotrauma. Also, the occurrence of middle ear barotrauma is dependent on the descent rate in addition to eustachian tubal function.

Pathological changes during middle ear barotrauma occur in the entire middle ear as well as the eardrum and include edema and hemorrhages in the middle ear mucosa plus inflammation and collection of serous fluid or blood, or both, in the middle ear. Eardrum perforations, if present, may be obvious or small and obscure. Blood in the external ear canal indicates that an eardrum perforation has occurred. Occasionally, minimal or no sign of middle ear barotrauma is seen with initial otoscopic examination, and obvious signs of negative middle ear pressure with eardrum retraction and inflammation and/or middle ear effusion will develop within the subsequent 24 hr.

The best treament of the middle ear barotrauma is caution and prevention. An adequate prediving otolaryngologic examination that emphasizes nasal and eustachian tubal function should be done. Particular attention should be paid to those individuals who have preexisting signs and symptoms of middle ear and nasal disease. Frequent bouts of ear infection or drainage, or both, a history of middle ear surgery, the presence of a healed or patent eardrum perforation, and the existence of a cholesteatoma—all suggest poor eustachian tubal function during nondiving conditions. Such individuals are more likely to be unable to tolerate the pressure changes encountered in diving.

Other important factors in the prevention of middle ear and possible inner ear barotrauma include avoiding diving in the presence of significant nasal inflammatory disease, not continuing descent without adequate ear clearing every 2 ft, slowing the descent rates, and avoiding performance of a Valsalva maneuver at depth. Once middle ear barotrauma has occurred, the first task of the examining physician is to rule out inner ear dynsfunction that suggests possible labyrinthine window rupture or inner ear barotrauma. Nerve deafness or loud tinnitus or severe vertigo suggests inner ear injury.

Divers should be aware of various safe maneuvers to aid middle ear pressure equilibration. The simplest maneuver is a modified yawn and swallowing. This maneuver is accomplished by thrusting the lower jaw anteriorly and slightly opening the jaw while maintaining the lips pursed around the regulator. This may be followed by a swallow if ear clearing has not occurred. Another nontraumatic way of ventilating the middle ear is called the Frenzel maneuver. This consists of voluntarily closing the glottis, mouth, and nose while contracting the muscles of the floor of the mouth and the superior pharyngeal constrictors. With the nose, mouth, and glottis closed, the elevated tongue can be used as a piston to compress air in the nasopharynx and thus into the eustachian tube. The mass of the tongue is strongly driven backward and acts to compress the nasopharyngeal air space both directly and indirectly through the soft palate.

Another method of middle ear pressure equilibrium consists of activation of the palatal muscles by raising the soft palate. With experience, this technique can be mastered without the need to swallow or move the jaw.

The Toynbee maneuver consists of swallowing with the mouth and nose closed; it is the inverse of the Valsalva maneuver and has some use in relieving middle ear overpressure rather than underpressure.

These maneuvers for eustachian tubal opening and middle ear pressure equilibrium during diving are safe in that they are not likely to induce significant changes in the fluid pressures of arterial, central venous, or cerebrospinal fluid, or of the inner ear, as would tend to occur with a Valsalva maneuver. Thus, dangerous overpressures in these spaces with subsequent pulmonary or inner ear barotrauma are less likely with these maneuvers than with the Valsalva maneuver. Also, these maneuvers, in contrast to the Valsalva maneuver, involve contraction of the tensor palatine muscle, which acts to open the nasopharyngeal orifice of the eustachian tube. Thus less pressure is required for tubal opening than with the Valsalva maneuver.

Once inner ear injury has been ruled out, treatment principles depend on the degree of injury and, in particular, on the presence or absence of eardrum perforation. A previous classification or grading of middle ear barotrauma has been presented by Teed (1944) and consists of these categories: Grade 0, normal appearance; Grade 1, retraction of the eardrum with redness over the pars flacida and along the long process of the malleus; Grade 2, retraction and redness of the entire eardrum; Grade 3, same as Grade 2 plus evidence of fluid in the middle ear; Grade 4, blood in the middle ear or perforation of the eardrum, or both.

This classification has limited value, for the otoscopic findings in middle ear barotrauma frequently include combinations of changes in different grades. Previous eardrum perforations or scarring can obscure the current middle ear findings. Most importantly, treatment is not completely dependent upon which of the five grades are present. Therefore, patients should be classified as follows: (1) those with symptoms but without otoscopic signs, (2) those with symptoms and otoscopic signs but without eardrum perforations, (3) those with symptoms and otoscopic signs including eardrum perforations (Farmer and Thomas 1976). Discussion of these categories follows.

1. For those patients with symptoms but without otoscopic signs, further diving should be avoided until any preexistng nasal symptoms have cleared, all ear symptoms have cleared, and the individual can easily autoinflate both middle ears at the surface. Long-acting topical nose drops can be used. These drops should be administered to the patient in the supine position and with the head hyperextended. Systemic decongestant or antihistamine preparations, or both, can be used; however, caution should be observed as regards the sedative effects of the antihistamines and undesirable adrenergic effects of the decongestant compounds.

2. Divers suffering middle ear barotrauma who have symptoms and otoscopic findings (usually a retracted and injected eardrum with a middle ear effusion) but not eardrum perforation should observe rest and avoid further diving until complete resolution of the otoscopic findings has occurred, and until both ears can be easily autoinflated at the surface. This usually requires 5 to 10 days and depends on the severity of the injury and the presence of coexisting nasal disease. Topical nasal preparations and systemic decongestants and antihistamines can be used as noted above. The use of systemic antibiotics

should be definitely considered if signs of bacterial infection such as purulent nasal discharge, cough with purulent sputum production, or fever are present. Appropriate cultures are desirable before the antibiotics are given; however, antibiotic administration should not be delayed until culture reports are available. Topical ear drop preparations containing antibiotics, steroids, or anesthetic agents are of little or no benefit with an intact eardrum. These substances do not readily cross the outer squamous epithelial layer of the tympanic membrane. Inert ear drops such as glycerin or mineral oil warmed to body temperature may provide partial pain relief. These substances should be used only when the physician is sure that an eardrum perforation does not exist. Sufficient pain relief usually requires systemic analgesic medications.

3. Patients with symptoms and ostoscopic findings including eardrum perforations should be treated in a manner similar to that described for cases with ostoscopic findings but without eardrum perforation. In addition, ear cleansing with 1.5% hydrogen peroxide irrigations warmed to body temperature can be used if significant amounts of blood and other debris are present in the ear canal. Such a solution is prepared by mixing commercially available 3% hydrogen peroxide with equal amounts of water that has been warmed so that the temperature of the resulting solution approaches body temperature. Irrigation of the ear with a solution that is significantly warmer or cooler than body temperature can result in a caloric effect on the inner ear with vertigo and possible nausea and vomiting. Such irrigations can be accomplished by using a small rubber-bulb ear syringe or a 20-to-50-ml hypodermic syringe connected to soft plastic tubing. Once blood, purulent material, and other debris have been cleared from the ear canal, the peroxide irrigations can be discontinued. Solutions containing alcohol or acids should not be used when an eardrum perforation exists because of a significant irritating effect on the middle ear mucosa. Most commercial antibiotic ear drop preparations contain drugs that are ototoxic to the inner ear. These should not be used in the presence of an eardrum perforation. Also, otic solutions containing topical anesthetics are usually inadequate for analgesia. As described above, if purulent discharge is noted from the nose, the tracheobronchial tree, or the ear, these drainages should be cultured and systemic antibiotics should then be administered. If the eardrum does not heal after 1 to 2 weeks of appropriate therapy, referral to an otolaryngologist should be done. In addition, further diving should be avoided until healing with or without surgical repair of the eardrum has taken place, and until adequate middle ear ventilation is present. Fortuantely, most eardrum perforations that result from middle ear barotrauma heal spontaneously and surgical repair is not required. Poor eustachian tubal function resulting from nasal disease can delay healing.

Inadequate middle ear pressure equilibration during ascent, resulting in a relative positive pressure in the middle ear, can occur, but this is infrequent because the eustachian tube usually opens without difficulty in response to a positive middle ear pressure. Transient vertigo secondary to asymmetrical middle ear pressure equilibration during ascent has been described (Terry and Dennison 1966; Vorosmarti and Bradley 1970) and particularly studied by Lundgren et al.(1974) and Tjerstrom (1973). This phenomenon, termed *alternobaric vertigo,* is related to increased middle ear pressure in one ear during ascent with resulting unequal vestibular end-organ stimulation. Many individuals who have encountered this problem during diving also note unilateral middle ear pressure equilibration problems during descent. The vertigo encountered during ascent has been noted to disappear by stopping the ascent, by descending again, or in association with a sudden hissing of air in one ear.

Vertigo during underwater exposures can be quite hazardous. The resulting spatial disorientation accompanying nausea and vomiting can be fatal. The best treatment of this problem is prevention. Divers who have difficulties with ear clearing or who experience vertigo when performing a Valsalva maneuver at the surface should not dive. Ear fullness, blockage, or vertigo during descent should signal divers to halt further compression and ascend until the symptoms disappear. If such symptoms are noted during ascent, the ascent should be stopped and the diver should descend until the symptoms disappear, provided gas supplies and other conditions permit. To always dive with a companion will reduce the hazard of these incidents.

b. External Ear Canal Barotrauma

External ear canal obstruction that occurs during ascent or descent can result in barotrauma to the canal and eardrum. Congestion, hemorrhage, and outward or inward bulging of the tympanic membrane occurs. With marked pressure changes, tympanic membrane rupture can occur. The best treatment of external ear canal barotrauma is prevention. Accumulated masses of cerumen in the ear canal, which can potentially obstruct the ear during diving, should be removed by irrigating the ear with water warmed to body temperature. The use of tight-fitting diving hoods, solid ear plugs, or phones that can completely seal the external ear canal during diving should be avoided. Once external ear canal barotrauma has occurred it should be treated similarly to the treatment described above for middle ear barotrauma. If significant swelling of the external ear canal has occurred, the treatment described in a subsequent section for otitis externa should be observed (Farmer and Thomas 1976).

c. Inner Ear Barotrauma

Inner ear injuries that occur in association with relatively shallow diving or show onset of otologic symptoms during the compression phase of deeper diving have been termed inner ear barotrauma. These injuries were first documented and named by Freeman and Edmonds in 1972 and have been related to labyrinthine window ruptures (Edmonds et al. 1974). Implosive and explosive mechanisms for such ruptures were postulated by Goodhill et al. (1973). The explosive mechanism, depicted in Figure IX-1, D, suggests that with inadequate middle ear clearing during descent, middle ear pressure becomes negative relative to intralabyrinthine pressure as well as ambient pressure. Either straining or a Valsalva maneuver results in a further increase in the pressure differential between the labyrinth and the middle ear as a result of transmission of increases in cerebrospinal fluid pressure to the inner ear. Rupture of the round or oval window membrane into the middle ear and a subsequent perilymph fistula can occur. The implosive mechanism suggests that with a sudden Valsalva maneuver that does result in middle ear ventilation, the rapid increase in middle ear pressure can result in rupture of the round or oval window into the intralabyrinthine space. Another possible implosivelike mechanism suggests that in the presence of a negative middle ear pressure, inward displacement of the eardrum, ossicular chain, and stapes footplate occurs. With a significant negative middle ear pressure, the footplate can sublux into the vestibule and an oval window fistula can occur. Simmons (1978) has suggested that the pressure changes encountered with inadequate equilibration of middle ear pressure during the descent phase of diving may result in intralabyrinthine membrane breaks without specific labyrinthine window rupture. Most of the described cases of labyrinthine window ruptures in association with diving have involved the round window. A few cases have been noted to involve the oval window (Caruso et al. 1977).

A diver who experiences persistent vertigo with or without sensorineural hearing loss or loud tinnitus following dives in which decompression sickness is unlikely should be considered as possibly having a case of inner ear barotrauma and labyrinthine window fistula. These patients should not be subjected to recompression therapy, because such therapy exposes the patient to the same pressure changes that contributed to the injury. Instead, these divers should be placed on bed rest with head elevation, and any maneuvers that may increase the pressure of cerebrospinal fluid and perilymphatic fluid should be avoided. Medications that supposedly increase intracranial and inner ear blood flow are generally not effective and may result in a decrease of intracranial blood flow due to shunting of the axial circulation to the periphery and skin. Anticoagulants are potentially harmful because of possible hemorrhage from traumatized otologic tissues. Ear drops containing ototoxic antibiotics should be avoided. A complete otologic evaluation by a knowledgeable physician, to include an otoscopic examination, proper audiometric testing, a complete neurological examination, and tests for vestibular function, should be accomplished as soon as feasible.

The need for immediate exploratory tympanotomy is controversial. Some authors have advocated immediate exploratory surgery in all suspected incidents (Pullen et al. 1979). Others have suggested reserving surgery for those who do not improve after 48 to 72 hours of bed rest with head elevation (Goodhill et al. 1973). Caruso et al. (1977) note that although the majority of labyrinthine window ruptures may heal spontaneously with conservative treatment, such treatment may be associated with progressive hearing loss. They suggest that when the diagnosis is fairly certain surgery be performed without delay to prevent further inner ear deterioration. The best management principles may include conservative treatment, with exploratory surgery being reserved for those who demonstrate no improvement after 4 to 5 days (Singleton et al. 1978) or worsening of inner ear function after 24 to 48 hr, or a combination of these conditions.

In some cases, the differential diagnosis of inner ear barotrauma and inner ear decompression sickness is difficult. Some of the related dives involve exposures close to the no-decompression limits. Divers occasionally do not know when during the dive the symptoms began, and signs of middle ear barotrauma suggesting the possibility of inner ear barotrauma or other systemic signs of decompression sickness may not be present. An accurate, prompt diagnosis is essential, because the proper treatment of each of these two entities is significantly different: recompression therapy should be avoided in cases with labyrinthine window rupture; prompt recompression therapy is essential for the proper management of inner ear decompression sickness. Usually, an accurate history and physical examination will allow one to easily differentiate these two entities, but other factors that should be considered in the differential diagnosis include the following:

1. The time of symptom onset. Divers who indicate that their otologic symptoms started during compression are likely to be suffering from inner ear barotrauma; whereas

divers whose symptoms start during or shortly after decompression are likely to be suffering from inner ear decompression sickness.

2. Knowledge of the dive type and profile. Symptoms of inner ear dysfunction associated with shallow dives in which decompression sickness is unlikely should not be suspected to result from decompression sickness, but inner ear barotrauma is certainly likely in these instances. Also, dives associated with rapid descents are more likely to result in inadequate middle ear pressure equilibration during compression (especially with inexperienced divers) and subsequent inner ear barotrauma. Inner ear barotrauma seems to be more common with air diving; whereas inner ear decompression sickness appears more common with deeper helium diving.

3. The presence or absence of associated symptoms should be noted. Divers experiencing ear pain, blockage, or fullness during compression are more likely to have inner ear barotrauma (Freeman 1978). Divers who have noted symptoms of decompression sickness involving other organ systems certainly should be suspected of having their inner ear symptoms secondary to inner ear decompression sickness.

4. The presence or absence of associated physical findings should be noted. Divers who exhibit physical findings compatible with middle ear barotrauma should certainly be suspected of having a possible labyrinthine window rupture as an explanation of their inner ear symptoms. Dives who show other signs of decompression sickness, such as neurological deficits, should be suspected of having their inner ear symptoms as a result of inner ear decompression sickness.

All cases of inner ear injury during diving should have a follow-up otoneurological evaluation after treatment. This should be done even though symptom relief has occurred. Individuals who exhibit permanent inner ear deficits should not be returned to diving, since future injury, especially to the uninvolved ear, can result in significant and permanent disability.

2. Otitis Externa

Otitis externa is a frequent and painful, sometimes debilitating, malady encountered in all types of diving. The external ear canal is lined with squamous epithelium and has a slightly acid pH. Cerumen is produced in the outer cartilaginous ear canal and contains water-soluble, bacteriostatic fatty acids in addition to the oil-soluble fatty acids. These factors along with the constant outward migration of the squamous epithelium provide a natural cleansing mechanism and protection from infection in this skin-lined cul-de-sac. Excessive exposure to water or humid atmospheres can produce maceration of the squamous epithelium and can dissolve or dilute the water-soluble fatty acids of cerumen, resulting in a shift of pH toward alkalinity and providing a good medium for bacterial growth. Collections of ceruminous debris, local trauma, the presence of seborrheic dermatitis, and poorly fitting or improperly cleaned ear plugs can contribute to otitis externa. The bacteria present in otitis externa in divers is frequently mixed with organisms among which *Pseudomonas* and *Proteus* predominate. *Staphylococcus aureus* and other Gram-positive organisms are also seen.

The symptoms of otitis externa include pain with itching or burning. A thin or serous discharge may be present. Examination shows an inflamed, swollen, and extremely tender external auditory canal. With progression of the process, erythema of the pinna and surrounding skin plus cervical lymphadenitis can be seen. Less frequently, complete obstruction of the ear canal can occur, with abscess formation and possible involvement of bone and cartilage. Fortunately, this complication is rare and practically never seen in the absence of other debilitating illness, such as poorly controlled diabetes, an unlikely situation in the usual diving population.

The best treatment of otitis externa is prevention. Ear canals should be cleaned of ceruminous debris, and local trauma should be avoided. Adequate control of any seborrheic conditions should be achieved before diving. If ventilated ear plugs are to be used, these devices should be properly fitted and cleaned. Yet in spite of these precautions, otitis externa frequently occurs in a number of types of diving. A useful, prophylactic topical ear solution for use during exposures to humid and aqueous environments is one containing a buffered weak acid, as 2% acetic acid in aluminum acetate. These solutions should be used several times daily. Alcohol has been used as a prophylactic measure with variable success. On the other hand, alcohol will dissolve the ceruminous fat-soluble fatty acids that are considered to be protective, and ear solutions that contain alcohol can be irritating to skin that is already inflamed; these solutions are therefore not recommended.

Once otitis externa is present, treatment principles include relief of pain, cleansing the external auditory canal, and specific therapy to provide topical antibiotics and a more normal pH to the canal. Narcotics are usually required for adequate pain relief. Cleansing is best accomplished by ear irrigation using lukewarm tap water, care being taken to dry the ear canal afterward. A stream of warm air from a hair dryer blown into the canal is useful for this purpose. If an eardrum perforation exists, irrigation with water should be avoided. Suction and gentle cotton wipes should be used instead.

Specific therapy should consist of an ear drop preparation that is on the neutral or acid pH side and contains topical antibiotics. Several such commercial preparations also contain steroids, which are not contraindicated and are felt by some authorities to significantly add to pain relief because of their anti-inflammatory actions. Adequate amounts of these agents should be used three to four times daily. If debris or other material has accumulated in the canal, repeat cleansing should be accomplished before each application of ear drops. If the ear canal swelling is of such a degree that the medications can not easily be instilled into the entire auditory canal, a cotton wick or commercially available methylcellulose sponge wick should be inserted and the medication instilled onto the wick several times daily. These wicks can usually be removed in about 3 to 5 days, once the canal swelling has subsided. All swimming and diving should cease until the otitis externa has cleared.

Systemic antibiotics can be used in the management of severe cases. One should keep in mind, however, that the causative bacterial organisms are frequently in the *Proteus* or *Pseudomonas* families and are resistant to many antibiotics. Therefore, for the management of severe cases, appropriate cultures are important in the choice of systemic antibiotics.

3. *Inner Ear Injuries at Stable Deep Depths*

In the previous sections, inner ear injuries have been described during descent, where such injuries represent inner ear barotrauma, and during ascent, where such injuries are inner ear decompression sickness. Inner ear injuries have also been described on one occasion at stable deep depths (Sundmaker 1973). These occurred at a dive at the University of Pennsylvania in the late summer of 1971. Three divers who had been breathing an oxyhelium atmosphere noted the sudden onset of vertigo, nausea, and nystagmus shortly after starting to breathe by mask a gas mixture containing a second inert gas (neon or nitrogen) at a depth of approximately 600 ft (183 m). Follow-up evaluations after the dive revealed permanent end-organ vestibular dysfunction in two of the three affected subjects. No changes in auditory function were noted. The likely mechanism of these injuries appears to be related to bubbling at tissue boundaries in the inner ear fluid compartments that had resulted from the counterdiffusion of the dissolved inert gases across these membranes (Graves et al. 1973). Increased pressure in the endolymphatic space from the osmotic flux of water has also been suggested as a possible cause of these injuries (Farmer 1977). The best treatment of such injuries is prevention—i.e., avoidance of inert gas changes at stable deep depths.

4. Inner Ear Injuries and High Background Noise during Diving

Excessive noise exposure is a definite cause of sensorineural deafness. The degree of inner ear injury from noise exposure is directly proportional to the intensity of the noise as well as the duration of exposure. A previous survey of Royal Navy divers (Coles and Knight 1961) concluded that sensorineural deafness seen in the usual diving population could be explained as resulting from previous nondiving noise exposures, and that the incidences of such deafness in divers were no greater than that incidence in the overall nondiving population when allowances were made for age. Other studies (Summitt and Reimers 1971) have shown that excessive and potentially damaging noise levels do exist in various diving conditions, especially in chambers and helmets. Whether the reversible, depth-related conductive hearing losses seen in diving that are related to decreased sound transmission by the eardrum and ossicles in compressed gas (Fluur and Adolfson 1966, Thomas et al. 1974) are sufficient to provide protection from excessive noise during diving is not yet known. Temporary shifts in the threshold of bone conduction indicating early inner ear injury have been noted in air helmet dives (Summitt and Reimers 1971). This would suggest that the conductive losses do not provide sufficient attenuation to protect divers from cochlear injury due to the excessive noise that may be encountered in multiple phases of diving. At this time appropriate criteria for risk of damage from noise exposure in diving are not known. Until such criteria are established, diving helmets and chambers should be designated to avoid excessive noise exposure.

5. Paranasal Sinus Barotrauma

Paranasal sinus barotrauma has been well described in fliers (Wright and Boyd 1945; Campbell 1945) and in divers (Idicula 1972, Fagan et al. 1976). The mechanisms and pathophysiology of the barotrauma are similar in diving and flying. Inadequate pressure equilibration between the air-containing paranasal sinus cavities can occur during ascent or during descent; it is usually related to chronic nasal dysfunction, with secondary inflammation and congestion of the nasal mucosa that result in blockage of the paranasal sinus ostia. Cysts or polyps within the nose or within the sinus cavity can also cause such obstruction. When this obstruction occurs in the absence of ambient pressure change, the air contained within the sinus cavities becomes partially absorbed and a relative vacuum develops. Swelling, engorgement, and inflammation of the sinus mucosa with a transudate in the sinus cavity may then appear. When this obstruction occurs during descent while diving or flying, the relative vacuum in the sinus cavity and the resultant mucosal damage are greater, and actual hemorrhage into the submucosal layers and sinus cavities can occur. Paranasal sinus barotrauma can also occur during ascent, when the pathological mechanism is frequently related to a one-way valve blockage of the sinus ostium by inflamed mucosa, cysts, or polyps located within the sinus cavity. Thus, pressure equilization can occur during descent but is impaired during ascent.

Chronic nasal and sinus disease can predispose a diver to paranasal sinus and middle ear barotrauma. The common underlying etiologies of such chronic disease can be attributed to a number of causes: (1) allergy, either intrinsic or extrinsic; (2) chronic irritation from smoking, excessive or prolonged use of nose drops or nasal sprays, or exposures to toxic or irritating chemical vapors; (3) mechanical obstruction from internal and external nasal deformities, polyps, or neoplasia; (4) vasomotor causes from chronic tension, stress, or anxiety.

In many patients with chronic nasal and sinus disease, more than one of the above factors is involved. Exposure to cold, dry air normally results in increased nasal blood flow and congestion and increased mucous secretion. Thus, worsening of these underlying conditions is frequently seen during the winter months. Secondary bacterial infection not uncommonly occurs and is indicated by the appearance of purulent discharge. Frequently, and especially in patients with allergies (asthma) or chronic irritation from smoking, there is associated chronic inflammation of the lower respiratory tract.

Normally, the total volume of nasal and sinus mucous secretion in a healthy adult is approximately 1 liter per day. Approximately one-half of this volume is evaporated by the inspired and expired air; the remaining half is carried as a protective mucous blanket by the microscopic motile cilia located on the surface of the nasal and sinus mucosa to the posterior aspect of the nose and nasopharynx, whence it is swallowed. Thus, some postnasal discharge is a normal phenomenon. In the presence of underlying chronic disease or secondary infection, or both, a significant change occurs in the character and volume of this discharge. Attempts should be made during prediving physical examinations, as well as during the examination of divers who have experienced paranasal sinus and otologic barotrauma, to identify and specifically manage any chronic nasal problems found. Individuals who cannot be adequately managed and who cannot adequately ventilate the middle ear or sinus cavities during atmospheric pressure changes should not engage in diving.

In a study of 50 consecutive cases of documented paranasal sinus barotrauma in divers, Fagan et al. (1976) noted that the symptoms developed during or immediately after descent in 68% of the divers and during or immediately after ascent in 32%. Pain was the predominant symptom being noted in all cases of descent and in 75% of the cases of ascent. It was most commonly noted in the frontal area. This is perhaps explained by the fact that the nasofrontal duct is longer and more tortuous, whereas the communications for the maxillary, ethmoid, and sphenoid sinuses with the nasal cavity are short ostia. Epistaxis was the second most common symptom, occurring in 58% of the cases. A history of previous sinus barotrauma was reported by 32% of the patients, and 50% had a history of recent upper respiratory tract infections. A history of chronic nasal and sinus problems was also reported by 50% of the patients. Associated signs of middle ear barotrauma were noted in 48% of the divers.

Additional symptoms that may be seen in addition to pain and epistaxis include pain in the upper teeth and occasional paresthesias and decreased sensation over the infraorbital nerve distribution (Newman et al. 1975). Purulent nasal discharge suggests secondary infection.

Treatment consists of the use of topical and systemic adrenergic agents. With purulent nasal discharge, cultures and appropriate antibiotics should be used. Further atmospheric pressure changes should be avoided until recovery. Fortunately, most cases recover within 5 to 10 days with medical therapy alone. Individuals who have symptoms persisting for longer periods or who have other signs of systemic illness should be referred for otolaryngological evaluation and radiographs of the sinuses.

Most of the patients in the series reported by Fagan et al. (1976) required no treatment. The few that did require treatment responded to nasal decongestants alone; only occasional patients required antibiotics. No patient required sinus lavage or surgery.

The use of systemic and topical adrenergic agents can improve nasal function and paranasal sinus and middle ear ventilation. Such agents should be used cautiously, however. A rebound phenomenon when the effect of the drug wears off, especially with topical nose drops, can lead to even greater nasal congestion and increased problems of pressure equalization in the ears and sinuses. All topical nasal decongestants cause varying degrees of paralysis of the microscopic cilia and dissolution of the protective mucous blanket. Thus, prolonged use of these agents can result in chronic nasal irriation and mucosal inflammation with problems of pressure equalization in the ears and sinuses during diving. The antihistamine components of the combination systemic medications can unpredictably have an effect of drowsiness. Also, the adrenergic components in these medications can cause systemic adrenergic effects that may be detrimental in some diving conditions.

JOSEPH C. FARMER, JR.

References

CAMPBELL, P. 1945. Aerosinusitis, a resume. *Ann. Otol. Rhinol. Laryngol.* 54: 69–83.
CARUSO, B. G., P. E. WINKELMANN, M. J. CORREIA, G. E. MILTENBERGER, AND J. T. LOVE 1977. Otologic and otoneurologic injuries in divers: clinical studies on nine commercial and two sport divers. *Laryngoscope* 87: 508–521.
COLES, R., AND J. KNIGHT 1961. Aural and audiometric survey of qualified divers and submarine escape training instructors. *Med. Res. Council Ser. Rep.* 61/1011. London: Royal Naval Physiological Laboratory.
EDMONDS, E., P. FREEMAN, R. THOMAS, J. TONKIN, AND F. A. BLACKWOOD 1973. *Otological Aspects of Diving.* Sidney: Australian Medical Publishing Co.
EDMONDS, C., P. FREEMAN, AND F. TONKIN 1974. Fistula of the round window in diving. *Trans. Am. Acad. Ophthalmol. Otolaryngol.* 78: 444–447.
FAGAN, P., B. MCKENZIE, AND E. EDMONDS 1976. Sinus barotrauma in divers. *Ann. Otol. Rhinol. Laryngol.* 85: 61–64.

FARMER, J. C. 1977. Diving injuries to the inner ear. *Ann. Otol. Rhinol. Laryngol.* 86 *Suppl.* 36.
FARMER, J. C., AND W. G. THOMAS 1976. Ear and sinus problems in diving. In: *Diving Medicine,* edited by R. H. Strauss. New York: Grune and Stratton, p. 109–133.
FLUUR, E., AND J. ADOLFSON 1966. Hearing in hyperbaric air. *Aerosp. Med.* 57: 783–785.
FREEMAN, P. 1978. Rupture of the round window membrane. *Otolarynol. Clin. N. Am.* 11: 81–93.
FREEMAN, P., AND C. EDMONDS 1972. Inner ear barotrauma. *Arch. Otolaryngol.* 95: 556–563.
GOODHILL, V., I. HARRIS, AND S. BROCKMAN 1973. Sudden deafness and labyrinthine window ruptures. *Ann. Otol. Rhinol. Laryngol.* 82: 2–12.
GRAVES, D., J. IDICULA, C. LAMBERTSEN, AND J. QUINN 1973 Bubble formation in physical and biological systems: a manifestation of counterdiffusion in composite media. *Science* 179: 582–584.
HARKER, L., J. NORANTE, AND J. RZU 1974. Experimental rupture of the round window membrane. *Trans. Am. Acad. Ophthalmol. Otolaryngol.* 78: 448–452.
IDICULA, J. 1972. Perplexing case of maxillary sinus barotrauma. *Aerosp. Med.* 43: 891–892.
KELLER, A. 1958. A study of the relationship of air pressure to myringorupture. *Laryngoscope* 68: 2015–2029.
LUNDGREN, C., O. TJERNSTROM, AND H. ORNHAGEN 1974. Alternobaric vertigo and hearing disturbances in connection with diving: an epidemiologic study. *Undersea Biomed. Res.* 1: 251–258.
NEUMAN, T., H. SETTLE, G. BEAVER, AND P. G. LINAWEAVER 1975. Maxillary sinus barotrauma with cranial nerve involvement: case report. *Aviat. Space Environ. Med.* 46: 314–315.
PULLEN, F. W., G. J. ROSENBERG, AND C. H. CABEZA 1979. Sudden hearing loss in divers and fliers. *Laryngoscope* 89: 1373–1377.
SHILLING, C. W., AND I. A. EVERLEY 1942. Auditory acuity in submarine personnel, Part III. *U.S. Nav. Med. Bull.* 40: 664–686.
SIMMONS, F. B. 1978. Fluid dynamics in sudden sensorineural hearing loss. *Otolaryngol. Clin. N. Am.* 11: 55–61.
SINGLETON, G. T., M. C. KARLAN, K. N. POST, AND D. G. BOCK 1978. Perilymph fistulas. Diagnostic criteria and therapy. *Ann. Otol. Rhinol. Laryngol.* 87: 797–803.
SUMMITT, J., AND J. REIMERS 1971. Noise: a hazard to divers and hyperbaric chamber personnel. *Aerosp. Med.* 42: 1173–1177.
SUNDMAKER, W. 1973. Vestibular function, In: *Special Summary Program, Predictive Studies III,* edited by C. Lambertsen. Philadelphia: Univ. of Pennsylvania.
TAYLOR, G. D. 1959. The otolaryngologic aspects of skin and scuba diving. *Laryngoscope* 69: 809–858.
TEED, R. W. 1944. Factors producing obstruction of the auditory tube in submarine personnel. *U.S. Nav. Med. Bull.* 44: 293–306.
TERRY, L., AND W. DENNISON 1966. Vertigo amongst divers. *U.S. Nav. Submar. Med. Cent. Spec. Rep.* No. 66-2.
THOMAS, W., J. SUMMITT, AND J. FARMER 1974. Human auditory thresholds during deep saturation helium-oxygen dives. *J. Acoust. Soc. Am.* 55: 810–813.
TJERNSTROM, O. 1973. On alternobaric vertigo: experimental studies. *Forsvarsmedicin* 9: 410–415.
VOROSMARTI, J., AND J. BRADLEY 1970. Alternobaric vertigo in military divers. *Mil. Med.* 135: 182–185.
WRIGHT, B., AND H. BOYD 1945. Aerosinusitis. *Arch.Otolaryngol.* 41: 193–203.

E. Blast

The term *blast* has been used to identify the intense sound wave emanating from a detonated explosive. Bebb (1953) says of underwater blast, "The energy of detonation of an explosive charge is distributed between several phases of the explosion, namely (a) the initial shock wave, (b) the velocity imparted to the water arising from the pressure of the steep-fronted shock wave, (c) the pulses produced by successive collapses of the bubble, (d) the turbulence and thrusting action of the mass motion of the surrounding water."

Blast injury denotes the biophysical and pathophysiological events and the clinical syndrome and pathologico-anatomical changes caused by exposure of a living body to the shock wave generated by the detonation of a high explosive. In air, primary blast injury is the damage inflicted by the primary shock wave itself, secondary injury is caused by the flying debris scattered by the blast, and tertiary injury occurs if the victim is thrown and injured by collision with a stationary object.

Several other terms have been used, particularly for air blast: reflex paralysis, vent du boulet, air concussion, shell shock, blast chest, blast concussion, and wind of shot. This last term reflects the popular belief that a dead soldier without discernible marks on his body was killed by the "breath of the cannonball," the supposition being that the rapid rush of air accompanying the missile was in some way deadly. In all likelihood, the death was caused by fragments hitting a vital area.

Much of the information about underwater blast comes from studies of wartime activities and from present-day U.S. Navy activities of Underwater Demolition Teams (UDT), Explosive Ordinance Disposal (EOD) units, and Sea Air-Land (SEAL) assault divers. The first published report of underwater blast injury was in a paper by Atkins (1940) discussing casualties from the Dunkirk evacuation. This study was a detailed report on 35 casualties treated at a U.K. Naval Hospital, and it gave a rather complete picture of the type and degree of damage to those men surviving long enough to reach a hospital—in this case several days after exposure to an underwater explosion of unknown size while the men were swimming on the surface. All aspects of these cases were subsequently covered: general discussion of injuries (McMullin 1943, Palma and Uldall 1943); surgical report (Pugh 1943); roentgen findings (Gates 1943); pathology (Ecklund 1943); and neurological observations (Hamlin 1943).

The U.S. Navy initiated intensive study of blast injury early in 1942. An early report by Corey (1946) and a later review by Wolf (1970) describe most of what is known about the medical aspects of blast. There is also an extensive review of the literature on blast by C. J. Clemedson (1956).

However, blast is not past history, for explosives are used now both in mining and salvage operations by civilian divers and in demolition, sheet-metal cutting, cable cutting, and making holes in metal. The explosive charges involved in these operations are much smaller than the depth charges dropped on submarines during the war, but they are large enough to require care in handling. Minor explosions have caused personal injury during underwater electric cutting and welding.

1. Physical Aspects

The underwater explosion produces a shock wave that travels outward in all directions from the detonating charge at sonic speed. The nature of the underwater explosion is complex; the interested reader is referred to Hoff and Greenbaum (1943, 1954), Greenbaum and Hoff (1966), and Shilling et al. (1976). However, an understanding of the physical phenomena involved in blast injury is necessary for the clinician to interpret the clinical manifestations.

The intensity of the shock wave and the pressure waves that follow depends on several factors:

1. The size of the explosive charge and the type of explosive utilized. Some explosives produce a high-order, short-duration explosion, resulting in a high-level pressure wave of short duration, while other explosives produce lower-order explosions that result in less intense but longer-duration shock and pressure waves, which do more damage at a longer range.

2. The character of the bottom. A soft bottom may tend to dampen the shock wave; a hard bottom may amplify the effect. The contour of the bottom is also important, since rock strata, ridges, and other topographical features may affect the direction of the shock and pressure waves and produce secondary reflecting waves.

3. The depth of the water. If the explosive is detonated at depth near the bottom, the pressure waves are attenuated by passing through the water to the surface, but an explosion near the surface is not so affected.

4. The distance of the diver from the explosion. In general, the farther away, the greater the attenuation, and thus the greater the diver's safety.

5. The degree of submersion of the diver. A fully submerged diver receives the total effect. It has been experimentally proved that the air-containing parts of the body (sinuses, middle ear, lungs, and intestines) are the most vulnerable to blast injury. If the head and upper body are out of the water, the effect of the shock and subsequent pressure waves will be minimal on the ears and sinuses and somewhat less severe on the lungs. A diver floating on his back on the surface has the greatest unaided protection from blast, and floating on an air cushion or wearing protective clothing or equipment affords the maximum protection to the diver in the water.

A 600-lb charge of TNT detonated underwater at a distance of 50 ft exerts a pressure on the diver of 2180 psi and would certainly be fatal. A pressure wave of 500 psi is sufficient to cause serious and even fatal injury under certain conditions. Ten divers who were experimentally exposed on 46 occasions to calculated underwater explosion pressures of from 4.5 to 55.4 psi of body surface sustained no injuries whatever (Corey 1946). It is considered wise to limit a diver's exposure to pressure to less than 50 or 60 psi or, if at all possible, to remove the diver from the water for the time of the explosion.

An explosion in air has effects that are quite different from an explosion in water. In air much of the damage is due to the fragmentation of the charge container and to foreign bodies and gravel drawn into the explosive wave. Also, in air explosions much of the pressure wave is reflected at the body surface, since this represents a surface of contact between media of different densities.

Since most of the body tissues have a density similar to that of water, in an underwater blast the individual molecules are displaced only a little, except in air- or gas-containing parts of the body, such as the lungs, the sinuses, and the intestines.

2. Clinical Aspects and Pathology

According to Wolf (1970), clinical aspects of underwater blast are derived from animal experiments and from the study of case reports of men in the water after their ships have been attacked. The studies involving men do not, in general, give any idea of the magnitude of the explosion or of the position of the victim relative to the charge. If the victim was swimming on the surface, the primary injury would be to the lungs and the secondary injury would be to the air-filled viscera. Organs not filled with air are seldom injured. Occasionally central nervous system lesions are produced, probably secondary to blood shifts or to air emboli. Also, the middle ear and the sinuses may be involved, but these effects are not life threatening.

1. Effect on the lungs and thoracic cavity. The most prominent feature of severe blast injury is massive lung hemorrhage, which is due to rupture of the alveolar walls (Clemedson 1956). This tearing, shredding, or rupture results from pressure differences between the lungs and the pleural space and is caused by different accelerations of the structural thoracic elements (Clemedson and Granstom 1950). Rupture of the boundaries between alveolar spaces and alveolar capillaries has been demonstrated to lead to arterial air embolism (Benzinger 1951). This type of pulmonary damage is associated with respiratory difficulty, usually slow and shallow breathing accompanied by pain in the chest (Barrow and Rhoads 1944). In severe lung damage with massive hemorrhage the airways may be blocked, and suffocation may result. In most cases, however, lung damage is not sufficient to be the direct cause of death; death is usually due to circulatory failure, air embolism, or complications such as bronchopneumonia (Clemedson 1956). When death occurs shortly after the time of injury, air embolism should be considered as the cause (Benzinger 1951). At autopsy in these cases, air is usually found in the coronary arteries and in the left side of the brain. In some cases the basal brain blood vessels may be virtually filled with air. (See Chapter XV, "Diving Accident Investigation.")

2. As would be expected, severe lung damage has an effect on heart action, circulation, and the nervous system. The effect on the heart, as shown in animal experiments, is an instantaneous and sometimes severe bradycardia. Animal research has also shown that the first postdetonation heartbeat may not occur for 30 sec or more, an effect that has been attributed to vagal nerve reflexes elicited in the damaged lungs (Benzinger 1950; Clemedson 1949).

3. The effect on the circulation is due to the anatomical and pathological changes in the lungs that cause a contraction or obstruction of the pulmonary capillary bed. This results in an increase in pulmonary arterial resistance, which causes, in turn, a drop in aortic and systemic arterial pressure (Clemedson 1956).

4. The effect on the nervous system may not be directly related to lung damage, but neurological involvement has been described both clinically and experimentally. Abnormalities in consciousness, varying from mild delirium to coma, have been reported. Severe headache is common, and pain has been reported in the chest, testicles, and legs, as well as in the abdomen.

5. The effect on the abdomen and air-filled viscera is common and serious. The reason for the vulnerability of the abdominal viscera to blast injury is probably that they normally contain gas and have relatively nonmuscular walls (Wolf 1970). That gas in the intestine is an essential precondition for blast damage was well demonstrated by Graves et al. (1943). These workers removed four short segments of rabbit intestine and ligated them at both ends. One section was completely collapsed, one filled with saline solution, one filled with air, and one with air and saline solution. The collapsed segment and the one filled with saline solution remained intact when exposed to an underwater blast, while the two that had air in them ruptured. The damage from blast is therefore usually found in the gastrointestinal tract, and there is notable absence of injury to the liver, spleen, kidneys, or bladder (Hoff and Greenbaum 1943). In a series of 20 patients

requiring surgery the most consistent findings were retroperitoneal and subserosal hemorrhage. The cecum was perforated in nine patients, the ileum in seven, and there were multiple perforations in four patients. Most perforations occur within one or two days but some are delayed by as much as a week, probably because of secondary infections or ulceration.

In a review of 80 patients who did not require surgery, abdominal pain was the most common symptom, lasting from a few days to months, in some few cases. Melena was present in 82% of these patients and persisted for up to 4 months. Hemoptysis occurred in 20% of the patients and hematemesis in 14%. Radiological studies usually did not reveal abnormalities, and sigmoidoscopy rarely revealed even areas of petechial hemorrhages in the rectum or sigmoid colon.

3. Treatment

Even though the person exposed to an underwater blast may be asymptomatic immediately after the injury, he should be admitted to hospital for observation in case complications develop. There are usually no external signs of injury (e.g., bruising, lacerations) despite internal damage. Until the full extent of the damage is determined, the patient should be maintained on intravenous fluids and nothing should be given by mouth.

Oxygen administration has been unreservedly recommended for the treatment of blast injury to the lungs, but great care must be taken not to further damage the lungs. A monoplace chamber, if available, may be the best way for administering the oxygen.

Appropriate examinations and tests for lungs and abdominal damage should be made and may include complete and differential blood count; x-ray photographs of the chest, including PA views in full expansion, and a plane and upright radiograph of the abdomen (Wolf 1970). When there are signs of peritonitis—i.e., rebound tenderness, rigidity, or decreased bowel sounds—a decision must be reached regarding surgical intervention. Unfortunately, these signs may not be due to perforation of the bowel but to hemorrhagic lesions throughout the bowel affecting the peritoneal cavity. Bleeding from the rectum is common but is not itself an indication for surgery. There must be a reasonable presumption of gastrointestinal perforation before surgical exploration.

4. Prevention and Protective Measures

The NOAA Diving Manual (Miller 1979) presents a detailed discussion of safety measures to be followed in the handling of explosives, and a diver who is involved in a project that includes the use of underwater explosives should study this section to become aware of the general safety precautions.

The most important and probably the only sure way to avoid injury from blast is to be out of the water at the time of the underwater explosion. If that is not possible, the swimmer or diver should attempt to reach the surface and get as much of the body out of the water as possible, taking advantage of anything that he can climb on or use for floatation. If the diver must remain in the water, he should swim or float face up so as to put the thicker tissues of the back between the vulnerable abdominal organs and the shock wave.

In response to a U.S. Navy request, the Navy Science Assistance Program (Christian and Gaspin 1974) completed a detailed study of explosives in deep open water and presented a series of charts that depict the safe zone (safe standoff curves) for a swimmer in relation to weight of explosive charge and distance of the swimmer from the point of detonation. These standoff curves can be used with confidence provided that the particular charge and swimmer configuration described on the curves are observed carefully.

Various types of protective clothing have been suggested for the diver who must remain in the water during a detonation (Medical Research Council 1945; Committee on Amphibious Operations 1952, U.S. Navy 1978), but most of them are bulky and seriously restrict movement and should therefore be considered only when there is no alternative. The ordinary wet or dry suit confers little protection.

Underwater blast is an important problem for all underwater workers, and this hazard has increased in recent years with the greater use of divers in handling both underwater demolition and other work involving explosives.

CHARLES W. SHILLING

References

ATKINS, H. J. B. 1940. Lessons from Dover. *Guy's Hosp. Gax.* 54: 192–195.
BARROW, D. W., AND H. Y. RHOADS 1944. Blast concussion injury. *JAMA* 125: 900–902.
BEBB, A. H. 1953. Underwater blast. Report prepared for the Underwater Blast Subcommittee. London: Medical Research Council, Royal Naval Personnel Research Committee.
BENZINGER, T. 1950. In: *German Aviation Medicine, World War II*. Washington, DC: U.S. Govt. Printing Office, Vol. II, p. 1225.
BENZINGER, T. 1951. Causes of death from blast. *Am. J. Physiol.* 167: 767.
CHRISTIAN, E. A., AND J. B. GASPIN 1974. Swimmer safe standoffs from underwater explosions. Navy Science Assistance Program (NSAP) Project Number PHP-11-73. *U.S. Nav. Ord. Lab. Rep.* NOLX-80.
CLEMEDSON, C. J. 1949. An experimental study on air blast injuries. *Acta Physiol. Scand. Suppl.* 61: 1–220.
CLEMDSON, C. J. 1956. Blast injury. *Physiol. Rev.* 36: 336–354.
CLEMDSON, C. J., AND S. A. GRANSTOM 1950. Studies of the genesis of "rib marking" in lung blast injury. *Acta Physiol. Scand.* 21: 131–144.
COMMITTEE ON AMPHIBIOUS OPERATIONS 1952. Effects of underwater blast. In: *Panel on Underwater Swimmers*, edited by R. Revelle. Washington, DC: Natl. Acad. Sci./Natl. Res. Council.
COREY, E. L. 1946. Medical aspects of blast. *U.S. Nav. Med. Bull.* 46: 623–652.
ECKLUND, A. M. 1943. The pathology of immersion blast injuries. *U.S. Nav. Med. Bull.* 41: 19–26.
GATES, R. 1943. Roentgen findings in immersion blast injury. *U.S. Nav. Med. Bull.* 41: 12–19.
GREAVES, F. C., R. H. DRAEGER, O. A. BRINES, J. S. SHAVER, AND E. L. COREY 1943. An experimental study of underwater concussion. *U.S. Nav. Med. Bull.* 41: 339–352.
GREENBAUM, L. J., AND E. B. C. HOFF 1966. *A Bibliographic Sourcebook of Compressed Air, Diving and Submarine Medicine*. Washinton, DC: Department of the Navy, vol. III.
HAMLIN, H. 1943. Neurological observations on immersion blast injuries. *U.S. Nav. Med. Bull.* 41: 26–31.
HOFF, E. B. C., AND L. J. GREENBAUM 1943. *A Bibliographical Sourcebook of Compressed Air, Diving and Submarine Medicine*. Washington, DC: Department of the Navy, vol. I.
HOFF, E. B. C., AND L. J. GREENBAUM 1954. *A Bibliographic Sourcebook of Compressed Air, Diving and Submarine Medicine*. Washington, DC: Department of the Navy, vol. II.

McMullin, J. J. A. 1943. Foreword to symposium on immersion blast injuries. *U.S. Nav. Med. Bull.* 41: 1–2.
Medical Research Council 1945. Protection of divers against underwater explosions. Rep. RNP 47/374, UWB 1. London: Royal Naval Personnel Research Committee.
Miller, J. W. (editor) 1979. *NOAA Diving Manual. Diving for Science and Technology.* Washington, DC: U.S. Dept. of Commerce, p. 1–15, p. 4–38.
Palma, J., and J. J. Udall 1943. Immersion blast injuries. *U.S. Nav. Med. Bull.* 41: 3–8.
Pugh, H. L. 1943. Surgical report on immersion blast injuries. *U.S. Nav. Med. Bull.* 41: 9–12.
Shilling, C. W., M. F. Werts, and N. R. Schandelmeier 1976. *The Underwater Handbook: A Guide to Physiology and Performance for the Engineer.* New York: Plenum Press, p. 637–646.
U.S. Navy 1978. *U.S. Navy Diving Manual* (Change 2). Washington, DC: U.S. Department of the Navy. (NAVSEA 0994-001-9010.)
Wolf, N. M. 1970. Underwater blast injury: A review of the literature. *U.S. Nav. Submar. Med. Res. Lab. Rep.* SMRL 646.

F. Dangerous Marine Life

Any marine organism that produces human injury or illness may be classified as a form of dangerous marine life, whether the role of the organism is active or passive.

1. Infections from Marine Microorganisms

Dangerous marine microorganisms include primarily the bacteria (Kriss 1963; MacLeod 1965; Oppenheimer 1963; Rheinheimer 1974; Sieburth 1971; Zobell and Upham 1944), fungi, viruses, and protozoa. At present the oceans may be considered to represent dilute solutions of bacteria (Table IX-3), fungi, and viruses that are known or potential human pathogens. The overall objectives for all human afflictions from marine microorganisms are the same: (1) recognize the clinical condition; (2) culture the organism; (3) provide antimicrobial therapy. Cultures, as well as special histological stains (e.g., Gram, acid-fast bacilli, silver), may be helpful when evaluating biopsy or excised specimens.

Marine bacterial flora are of considerable importance when assessing near-drownings, marine trauma (e.g., coral cuts, puncture wounds, fish bites), infection of preexisting surgical incisions, and bacterial food poisoning. *Clostridium perfringens, C. tetani,* and *C. botulinum* are to be specifically ruled out in association with several of these.

a. Infections Associated with Near-Drowning

In near-drowning, infections of the respiratory tract and ears and any traumatic wounds on the body can result from marine bacteria particularly. Pneumonias, aspiration pneumonias, lung abscesses, and pulmonary empyemas can complicate the near-drowning event (Fuller 1963; Hughes et al. 1978; McDanal et al. 1977; Modell 1978; Redding et al. 1970; Rosenthal et al. 1975). Primary inoculation of the pulmonary tract with sea water bacteria, including *Pseudomonas putrifaciens* and *Vibrio parahemolyticus,* can occur. After a thorough initial examination, the ears of convalescent near-drowning

Table IX-3
Representative Marine Bacteria Known to Be Human Pathogens

Acinetobacter lwoffi	*Mycobacterium marinum*
Actinomyces species	*Neisseria catarrhalis*
Aerobacter aerogenes	*Proteus mirabilis*
Aeromonas hydrophila	*Proteus vulgaris*
Aeromonas sobria	*Pseudomonas aeruginosa*
Alcaligenes faecalis	*Pseudomonas putrefaciens*
Bacillus cereus (formerly *Bacillus limosus*)	*Pseudomonas* species
Bacillus subtilis	*Salmonella* species
Bacteriodes fragilis	*Salmonella enteriditis*
Clostridium botulinum	*Serratia* species
Edwardsiella tarda	*Staphylococcus aureus*
Enterobacter aerogenes	*Staphylococcus citreus*
Enterobacter species	*Staphylococcus epidermidis* (formerly
Enterococcus species	*Staphylococcus albus*)
Erysipelothrix species	*Streptococcus* species
Escherichia coli	*Streptococcus faecalis*
Flavobacterium species	*Vibrio alginolyticus*
Klebsiella pneumoniae	*Vibrio cholera*
Micrococcus sedentarius	*Vibrio parahemolyticus*
Micrococcus tegragenus	*Vibrio* species (unclassified)

victims should be periodically checked to exclude otitis. It is presently recommended that prophylactic antibiotics not be given to near-drowners (Hoff 1973; Modell 1978; Modell et al. 1976), but rather that definitive antimicrobial therapy based on cultural and sensitivity results be provided; however, in some cases definitive antibiotic therapy may be started once a culture has been obtained. In addition, it is recommended that steroids not be administered for aspiration of gastric contents (Chapman et al. 1974; Downs et al. 1974).

b. Tetanus

Clostridium tetani, the bacterium responsible for producing human tetanus, has been cultured from the marine environment (Shewan 1938), one human case being possibly attributed to a natural sponge implant (Taylor 1953). For marine wounds, thorough wound cleansing is necessary in order to reduce wound *C. tetani* appreciably, and wound follow-up is needed to ensure that wound anaerobiosis does not develop. The American College of Surgeons (1972) tetanus prophylaxis guidelines are now standard. Penicillin is the antibiotic of choice (Burke 1974) in human tetanus victims not allergic to pencillin.

c. Gas Gangrene

Many clostridia can produce gas gangrene; however, *Clostridium perfringens* and *C. tetani* are the major producers. *C. perfringens* (formerly *C. welchii*) gas gangrene is treatable with hyperbaric oxygenation (HBO), as well as with intravenous fluids and antibiotics (e.g., penicillin).

d. *Mycobacterium marinum* Infections

Mycobacterium marinum (Fisher 1978; Loria 1976; Myrvik et al. 1974; Schaefer and Davis 1961) is an acid-fast bacillus that produces cutaneous granulomas; it is related to *M. tuberculosis*. The cutaneous lesions produced are verrucous scaly nodular or ulcerated granulomas. The primary therapeutic modalities include heat, surgical excision, and antimicrobials. Although *M. marinum* is remarkably sensitive to heat (optimal temperature for growth is 30°C, with reduced growth at 33°C), heat sources at 37°C–50°C may be only variably effective, and scalds and burns may occur if care is not taken. Local surgical excision of one or more lesions may be complicated by subsequent local recurrence. *M. marinum* is generally sensitive to cycloserine, ethionamide, ethambutol, trimethoprim-sulfamethoxazole (Bactrim,® Septra®) and minocycline (Fisher 1978; Knox et al. 1961; Schaefer and Davis 1961). Minocycline has been effective in some instances where combinations have failed. Adult antibiotic therapies for *M. marinum* infections include the following: (1) minocycline hydrochloride (100 mg per os b.i.d., minimum of 10 days); (2) triple therapy—ethionamide (250 mg per os t.i.d.), ethambutol (1000–1200 mg per os daily), and cycloserine (250 mg per os b.i.d.); (3) trimethoprim-sulfamethoxazole (Bactrim,® Septra®) (2 tablets b.i.d., minimum of 10 days). *M. marinum* infections are usually contracted from marine waters, swimming pool waters, fish bites, dolphin bites, puncture wounds from fish fins, general marine trauma, and aquarium maintenance, as well as from handling fish (e.g., cleaning fish).

e. Erysipelothrix Infections

The many names of erysipelothrix infections (Grieco and Sheldon 1970) include fish-handlers' disease and erysipeloid of Rosenbach. Most commonly *Erysipelothrix rhusiopathiae* and *E. insidiosa* are involved. The infection begins with the infection of an open wound or an infection of a wound sustained on fish, crayfish, crabs, coral, fish teeth, fish fins, and marine mammal carcasses. Within 1 to 5 days the small infected wound develops rapid spreading erythema, itching, swelling, and severe pain. Systemic manifestations can occur. The cutaneous lesions are generally sharply demarcated and develop a central clearing. The erysipelothrix are usually quite sensitive to penicillin.

f. Marine Vibrio Infections

Marine vibrio infections (Barker 1974; English and Lindberg 1977; Fernandez and Pankey 1975; Rubin and Tilton 1975) are usually due to *Vibrio parahemolyticus, V. alginolyticus,* and lactose-positive (L+) vibrios. *V. parahemolyticus* and lactose-positive vibrios also cause a postingestion gastroenteritis. Vibrios require special media for culture growth, frequently TCBS (tellurite-citrate-bile salt-sucrose). All three groups of these organisms are generally sensitive to tetracycline, chloramphenicol, and gentamycin.

g. Coral Trauma Infections

Brushing against corals can produce abrasions, contusions, scrapes, gouges, and lacerations that frequently become severely infected. After a few days untreated coral cuts may progress to abscess, cellulitis, granulomas, foreign body granulomas, lymphedema, lymphadenitis, erysipelas, vesicles, bullae, pustules, gangrene, osteomyelitis, or sepsis. Fistulas and draining sinuses that exude pus can develop. Microorganisms involve coral trauma, although more research is needed in this area in order to determine the complete infectious organism spectrum. There is no evidence that corals grow in human tissues, although the foreign body granuloma does increase in size. The coral wound may be cleansed by the following five-step procedure: (1) thorough normal saline irrigation; (2) hydrogen peroxide flush; (3) normal saline flush; (4) povidone-iodine wash; (5) thorough normal saline irrigation. Removal of all foreign bodies and all devitalized tissues is mandatory. Prophylactic antibiotic recommendations depend on suitable prospective clinical studies, although in wound follow-up care the wound can be cultured when purulent, and then antibiotics can be started.

h. Marine Wounds

Wounds sustained in the marine environment are similar to terrestrial wounds in that the wound must be thoroughly cleansed, all devitalized tissues debrided, and all foreign bodies removed.

i. Marine Fungal Infections

One of the most common marine fungal infections is athlete's foot, or tinea pedis, attributable to the fungi *Trichophyton mentagrophytes*, *T. rubrum*, or *Epidermophyton floccosum*. The source is usually showers, shower houses, and boat decks. Depigmented skin lesions also occur in sunbathers; these may be attributed to *Malassezia furfur*.

j. Schistosome Cercarial Dermatitis

Marine schistosomes were identified as a source of human dermatitis when snails infected with schistosomes were recovered from the tidal pools of the same beach used by shell collectors who developed typical pedal schistosome lesions (Chu 1952, 1958; Fisher and Orris 1973). The persons were infected when they entered into the seawater medium of the schistosome at the point in its life cycle between the birds and the snails. The clinical manifestations of the infection include cutaneous prickling sensations, papules, wheals, and a hemorrhagic rash. The infection site usually becomes excoriated secondary to scratching. Treatment includes external application of isopropyl alcohol and calamine lotion and in severe cases the administration of antihistamines or corticosteroids, or both. Dimethyl phthalate (Edmonds et al. 1976) is reportedly an effective schistosome cercarial repellent.

k. Marine Viral Infections

The most important marine viral infections are the hepatitis A, hepatitis B, and hepatitis non-A, non-B viral infections. Serological tests are available for providing a precise diagnosis of the hepatitis virus after the initial liver profile data have been obtained. Corticosteroids are of no benefit in hepatitis A, and hepatitis immune serum gamma globulin also is not beneficial in hepatitis A patients. In hepatitis B, immune serum gamma globulin is of no benefit to the hepatitis patient but is useful for contacts. The isolation in hepatitis A is extensive for the victim's waste products, bedding, and clothing, whereas the hepatitis B victim isolation is largely confined to blood and needles, for example.

2. Poisonous and Venomous Marine Organisms

There are more than 1000 marine vertebrate species that are venomous or poisonous (Edmonds 1978), as well as hundreds of venomous or poisonous marine invertebrates. In this section a brief description is made of certain of these organisms, together with the clinical manifestations to be expected and the treatment of the victim.

a. Blue-Green Algae

Microcoleus lyngbyaceus (Arnold et al. 1959; Banner 1959; Grauer and Arnold 1961; Sims 1981), formerly *Lyngbya majuscula,* although a member of the blue-green algae, is actually a dark olive drab, finely filamentous hairlike alga that elaborates more than two toxins (lyngbatoxin A and debromoaplysiatoxin) when the alga is trapped between the bathing suit and skin of swimmers—hence the name "seaweed dermatitis." Itching, burning, and escharotic lesions can result. The treatment consists of soap and warm water scrubs, particularly if used within 3 hr of exposure.

b. *Gymnodinium breve* (Red Tide)

The dinoflagellate *Gymnodinium breve* (now *Ptychodiscus breve*) (Galtsoff 1948; Hayes and Austin 1951; Hughes and Merson 1976; Music et al. 1973), well known for producing a "red tide," also produces conjunctivitis, rhinitis, bronchitis, and respiratory distress in persons vicinal to beaches where there are offshore red tides and combined water and wind conditions that aerosolize the *G. breve*. The treatment is to move the victim away from the *G. breve* aerosol; oxygen may be required in some cases.

c. Dogger Bank Itch

Dogger Bank itch, a North Sea malady, has been attributed to the filamentous dinoflagellate diatom *Fragilaria striatula* (a plant), as well as to the seaweedlike marine animal colony *Alcyondium hirsutum,* the sea chervil.

d. Green Algae (Phylum Chlorophyta)

In the Philippines the popular edible deep-water algae of the *Caulerpa* species (e.g., *C. racemosa;* see Doty and Aguilar-Santos 1966) becomes toxic in the rainy months; chewing of the raw dried caulerpa algae produces numbness of the extremities, difficult breathing, and ataxia that takes hours to wear off.

e. Brown Algae (Phylum Phaeophyta)

The brown algae include the giant kelp of the Pacific; however, more divers have drowned from entanglement than have ever manifested toxicity from ingestion.

f. Sponges

Of more than 4000 species of sponges worldwide, at least 13 species have been reported toxic to human beings (Halstead 1978; Sims and Irei 1979; Yaffee 1970; Yaffee and Stargardter 1963). All toxic sponges have a microabrading glasslike spicule as well as one or more toxins.

The acute manifestations of human sponge poisoning include local prickling, burning, and itching sensations, followed by pain, erythema, and edema. Vesicles and pustules may appear later, with eczematous desquamation with or without exfoliation developing days to months after the incident. Erythema multiforme and anaphylactoid reactions are rare.

The treatment consists of sponge spicule removal by use of cellophane tape, dilute vinegar soaks (5% acid strengh or less, t.i.d.–q.i.d., for 5–30 min each time). After the exfoliative desquamation the insult is usually over.

g. Nematocyst Envenomizations

A considerable number of coelenterates, or cnidarians, cause human envenomization by using microscopic stinging organelles, the nematocysts (Burnett 1971a, 1971b; Lane 1974). These cnidarians include the sea anemones, marine hydroids, jellyfish, Portuguese man-of-war, stinging fire corals, and stinging true corals. All these coelenterates have nematocysts that have a microscopic thread conveying the multicomponent venom. The severity of the sting varies with the species of the offending coelenterate and the susceptibility of the host. Anaphylaxis is the most serious problem for most of these stings, whereas for the sting of the sea wasps, along with anaphylaxis sudden death can occur from the negative cardiac inotropic component of the venom (Baxter and Marr 1969; Crone and Keen 1971; Endean and Noble 1971).

The nematocyst envenomizations require the management of the most serious problems first (e.g., anaphylaxis, sea wasp antivenin for life-threatening sea wasp stings) as well as removal of the offending tentacles. The tentacles from jellyfish and Portuguese man-of-war can be removed (1) by liberally pouring vinegar onto the tentacles and sting sites, (2) by sprinkling abundant amounts of unseasoned papain meat tenderizers (Arnold 1971) on the tentacles and onto the wounds, and (3) by removing the partially inactivated tentacles with wire pliers or surgical clamps. In anaphylaxis intravenous, intracardiac, or endotracheally nebulized epinephrine can be used (0.01–0.015 mg/kg epinephrine in a total vol of 5–10 ml of sterile water), as well as corticosteroids, and H_1-blocker antihistamines (e.g., diphenhydramine) (Roberts et al. 1979a, 1979b).

Minor coelenterate stings consisting of local wheal and flare, local erythema, and urticaria can usually be managed with the vinegar and meat-tenderizer therapy, antihistamines (e.g., diphenhydramine or hydroxyzine), or subcutaneous racemic epinephrine. A tapering dose of oral corticosteroids can be given for mild focal inflammation; however, prolonged steroid therapy is to be avoided.

h. Spine Puncture Envenomizations

Spine puncture envenomizations can be inflicted by cone shells, crown of thorns starfish, scorpion fish and catfish, stingrays, stonefish, surgeonfish, urchins, weevers, and sea worms.

Cone shells (Hinegardner 1958; Kohn 1958) have a radular tooth in the proboscis of the cone that injects venom into the tissues. The primary clinical manifestations include excruciating pain (which often radiates), wound ischemic changes, and paresthesias. Neurological manifestations and cardiovascular developments may occur. Cone shell venom is a poorly heat labile toxin, so primary therapy is directed toward the relief of pain and decontamination of the wound. A local anesthetic (without epinephrine) is injected into the incised wound, and if the pain is severe, a naloxone-reversible analgesic is given intravenously. Then the wounded part is placed in water as hot (e.g., 45°C–50°C) as the victim can tolerate without scalding, replenishing the hot water as necessary.

Crown of thorns starfish (Furlong and Phil 1970), or *Acanthaster planci*, is a dark red-green-brown starfish with 5 to 21 arms that are studded with elongated sharp venomous spines resembling thorns. Impalement by the spines produces a pink- or red-stained wound that is exceedingly painful. The acute wound may be rinsed with isopropyl alcohol or vinegar and then immersed in nonscalding hot water (45°C–50°C). The puncture wound should be thoroughly evaluated to exclude the possibility of a foreign body, such as a spine tip.

Catfish and scorpion fish (Wiener 1958) have venomous dorsal fin spines and pectoral fin spines, the scorpionfish also having venomous pelvic and anal fin spines. These venomous spines have pain-producing heat-labile toxins, so the primary therapy is directed at pain relief. A local anesthetic (without epinephrine) is injected into the wound, and naloxone-reversible systemic opiates are given intravenously as needed. Then the wound site is immersed in hot water (45°C–50°C) without scalding; with massage, free bleeding from the puncture wound site is promoted. The immersion may require as much as 90 min, with hot water replenishment as needed. Subsequent wound debridement may be necessary to remove all devitalized tissues. A venoconstriction band may be helpful if placed proximal to the wound, as able.

Stingrays (Cross 1976; Russell et al. 1958) and some species of manta rays have one to five cartilaginous serrated spins in the proximal half of the tail, which lashes out with an impaling action. The associated venom is only mildly heat labile. The puncture wound produced may be an irregular laceration and is very painful, pain radiation being frequent. The initial therapy consists of prompt, thorough, local anesthetic (without epinephrine) and infiltration of the wound, followed by systemic (i.m. or i.v.) naloxone-reversible opiate analgesia (Mullanney 1970). The wounded area is then placed in 45°C–50°C hot water, without scalding, with massage to promote controlled free bleeding. The hot water treatment may require up to 90 min of immersion, with hot water replenishment throughout. Again, a venoconstriction band may be helpful if placed proximal to the wound, as able. Subsequent wound repair and debridement may be necessary. In adults 50 mg of an antihistamine (diphenhydramine or hydroxyzine) should be given intramuscularly, with a prescription for oral antihistamines and oral analgesics. A 40-mg tapering dose of methyl prednisolone sodium succinate should be given and the steroid tapered over the next 5 days. Antitetanus prophylaxis should be provided (Mullanney 1970).

Stonefish (Wiener 1958, 1959) are related to the scorpion fish and have venomous dorsal, pectoral, anal, and pelvic fin spines; they are confined to the Pacific and Indian Oceans. Stonefish produce one of the most severe of all envenomizations; the puncture wound is painful and fatalities have resulted. The therapy consists of a local anesthetic injection into the wound, systemic (i.m. or i.v.) naloxone-reversible analgesics, the hot water therapy (immerse affected area in 40°C–50°C hot water, without scalding, and use massage to promote free bleeding from the wound), and in some cases, utilization of the stonefish antivenin (Commonwealth Serum Laboratories, 45 Poplar Road, Parkville, Victoria, Australia, 3052, telephone 389-1911, telegraphic code Serums Melbourne, Telex AA 32789).

Surgeonfish and tangs represent some of the most beautiful fish in the oceans; however, a number of these fish have a switchbladelike venomous spine in the tail. The wounds inflicted are usually either puncture wounds or lacerations, and the venom preliminarily appears to be heat labile. Therapy consists of infiltration of the wound with a local anesthetic (without epinephrine), systemic (i.v. or i.m.) naloxone-reversible analgesics as needed, and the 40°C–50°C hot water therapy. Wound debridement, wound repair, and antitetanus prophylaxis are usually indicated.

Sea urchins (Baden and Burnett 1977; Feigen and Hadji 1974; O'Neal et al. 1964; Rocha and Fraga 1962) have a rigid globoid body that is studded with rigid spines or small jawlike pedicellariae. Painful human injury is the result of rigid spine impalement or pedicellarial "bites." The thick calcified spines produce puncture wounds, and all of the spine must be removed from this nonvenomous wound. The thin spines in some species are venomous, however, and require brief nonscalding hot water therapy at 45°C–50°C (e.g., 5–15 min) until pain is relieved; the sliver spines may be left in if they cannot be removed with a thumb forceps (they will usually be absorbed in 1–4 weeks).

Weevers (Russell and Emery 1960) are highly venomous eastern Atlantic fish whose dorsal fin and opercular fin spines are highly venomous. Spine puncture envenomizations by this fish provide fully florid manifestations of the envenomizations. The management is as with the stingray, with intravenous calcium gluconate being used for paresthesias.

Sea worms have anticoagulant biting jaws (marine leeches) or body bristles called setae. The wounds are painful, erythematous, swollen, and itchy. The treatment consists of removal of the setae with cellophane tape and subsequent local application of isopropyl alcohol or dilute ammonia.

i. Venomous Octopus Bites

Several species of generally small octupuses confer a lethal bite (Gage and Dulhunty 1973; Shemack et al. 1978a, 1978b; Sutherland and Lane 1969; Trethewie 1978) on human beings. The nipping bite produces a painful, erythematous, edematous and bloody wound. The onset of central nervous system manifestations such as dysphonia, dysphagia, paralysis, and coma develops within a few hours. Treatment consists of putting the victim at absolute rest, application of ligature if possible, and removal of venom by incision (do not suck the wound). The remainder of care is supportive, including a respirator as needed.

j. Sea Snake Envenomizations

Sea snakes (Campbell 1975; Reid 1956; Tu 1977) are marine serpents that are noted for their paddle-shaped tails, multiplicity of fangs, relatively painless chewing bite, and remarkably lethal venom. Sea snake venoms have multiple components, many of which are toxic peptides or proteins. The bite may present with from 2 to 20 little dots, and the bite rapidly becomes painless. The victim experiences a lucid period lasting 5 min to several hours before the onset of anxiety, apprehension, or euphoria. The major venom factors are neuromuscular blockers, hypotensive agents, and muscle necroticants. Myoglobinuria, hemoglobinuria, and ptosis are not uncommon. The therapy consists of restraining the victim from movement, application of a venom-confining tourniquet, wound cleansing, administration of sea snake antivenin (if indicated), antitetanus immunization updating, and supportive care.

3. Human Toxic Ingestions

A number of marine organisms when consumed are capable of producing significant human illness beyond the more common bacterial food poisoning and seafood allergies. Fish poisoning refers to the ingestion of a fish that produces human illness in the absence of bacterial food poisoning or allergy. The most common types of fish poisoning include the following: scombroid poisoning, ciguatera poisoning, tetrodotoxication (puffer poisoning).

a. Scombroid Poisoning

Scombroid poisoning (Ferencik 1970; Foo 1975, 1976; Geiger 1955; Kim 1979; Kimata 1961; Ramros 1974; Uragoda 1978; Uragoda and Kottegoda 1977) is caused by the toxic red flesh of scombroids and nonscombroids, numbering at least 18 different species of fish. Tuna, mackerel, sardines, and mahimahi dolphin fish are the most commonly involved. The amino acid histidine in the red fish flesh is decarboxylated into the active histamine by fish flesh bacterial proliferation in the absence of suitable refrigeration. This can be detected by analysis of fish flesh or human blood for histamine or by obtaining urinary histamine metabolites, or by blood procedures. The clinical manifestations are those of a histamine overdose (erythema, flushing), and the treatment consists primarily of antihistamines (e.g., diphenhydramine or hydroxyzine) and gastrointestinal purges, as well as administration of epinephrine or steroids in selected cases.

b. Ciguatera Poisoning

Human ciguatera (Bagnis 1968, 1973; Bagnis et al. 1979; Chungue and Bagnis 1977; Hokama et al. 1977; Hughes and Merson 1976; Miyahara et al. 1979; Rayner 1972; Rayner and Szekerczes 1973; Russell 1975; Scheuer et al. 1967; Yasumoto et al. 1976) poisoning involves more than 500 ordinarily edible reef fish such as the snappers (e.g., red snapper), grouper, sea bass, sea perch, flounder, rock cod, barracuda, parrot fish, and bonito. Numerous toxins are present in ciguatera, particularly ciguatoxin and maitotoxin. Ciguatoxin is produced by *Gambierdiscus toxicus* (Bagnis et al. 1980), a dinoflagellate, which gets passed along the food chain to affect the reef fish. Bagnis et al. (1979) have reviewed the human clinical manifestations of ciguatera poisoning in 3009 cases and have found them to consist primarily of nausea, diarrhea, and paresthesias (although there are more than 150 individual signs and symptoms of ciguatera poisoning).

Itching and the temperature reversal phenomenon (cold objects feel hot to touch, hot objects feel cold) do not usually develop until 2–5 days postingestion, in some cases. The treatment given is highly dependent on the severity of manifestions. In the severe bradycardic-hypotensive (i.e., cardiovascular) form of ciguatera fish poisoning the management consists of intravenous atropine, intravenous dopamine infusion, and intravenous calcium gluconate (J. K. Sims, S. Y. Matsumoto, and S. J. Wallach, unpublished observations). Minor cases can be managed with thorough gastrointestinal purging, progressive liquid diet free of fish and shellfish, megavitamins, and acetaminophen for pain or headache. Dietary fish should continue to be avoided until the patient has been completely symptom free for at least 3–6 months.

c. Puffer Poisoning

Tetrodotoxication (Agner et al. 1978; Fujii et al. 1967; Henderson et al. 1978; Narahashi 1972; Rump and Rabsztyn 1977; Torda et al. 1973) occurs from puffer poisoning. It should be noted that there are many species of puffer, and in some areas the fish is a delicacy, whereas in others it is avoided entirely. In Japan the mortality in 6380 cases over 78 well-monitored years was 59%. The primary clinical manifestations consist of: oropharyngeal paresthesias, hypersalivation, diaphoresis, hypotension, severe hyperemesis, weakness, and dyspnea. Clinical management consists of the provision of oxygen, normal saline infusion for volume, atropine for bradycardia, and nasogastric tube placement. All other care is supportive.

4. Marine Trauma

Marine trauma is unique in the sense of the traumatic events transpiring in a fluid medium of seawater. Marine trauma associated with envenomization by a venomous marine organism is usually an insignificant wound compared to the manifestations of the envenomization. Closed marine trauma is rarely produced by marine life. Most marine trauma is open, such that seawater bacteria, sand, silt, shell fragments, coral fragments, rock fragments, and other seawater debris enter the wound.

The initial management of all acute open marine trauma is the format of "*A*irway, *B*reathing, *C*irculation, *D*econtamination." The standard hemorrhage control matters may be used in open acute marine wounds: direct pressure, pressure bandages, tourniquet, two to four large-bore intravenous infusions of normal saline (or lactated Ringer's), and use of the MAST garment (medical antishock trouser). The administration of a single massive intravenous dose of corticosteroids (e.g., dexamethasone 1 mg/kg i.v., or methyl prednisolone 30 mg/kg i.v. slowly over 15–30 min of infusion time) may be helpful in the management of shock.

Decontamination of open marine wounds involves first ruling out envenomization. The second phase involves the removal of all foreign bodies (e.g., stingray spines) after thorough assessment and using soft-tissue density x-ray techniques for localization. Sand, shell fragments, rocks, coral fragments, shark teeth, and stingray spines can all be assessed by using this x-ray technique. Wound decontamination also involves sufficient wound cleansing to render the wound reasonably sterile.

Wound closure depends on the assessment of the cleanliness of the wound. A clean wound may be sutured primarily if all foreign bodies have been removed and if the wound is adjudged sterile. Unless there is objection, this wound can also be skin grafted primarily. If there are doubts about wound cleanliness, the wound can be closed by second intention or left to granulate in by third intention. At present, every effort should be made to thoroughly cleanse the wound at the onset.

5. Conclusion

There are many organisms that constitute dangerous marine life. Much more remains to be learned regarding these organisms and particularly regarding the therapeutics of treating injuries inflicted by them.

JOEL KEVIN SIMS

References

AGNEW, W. S., S. R. LEVINSON, J. S. BRABSON, ET AL. 1978. Purification of the tetrodotoxin-binding component associated with the voltage-sensitive sodium channel from *Electrophorus electricus* electroplax membranes. *Proc. Natl. Acad. Sci. USA* 75: 2606–2610.
AMERICAN COLLEGE OF SURGEONS 1972. A guide to prophylaxis against tetanus in wound management. *Bull. Am. Coll. Surg.* 57: 32–33.
ARNOLD, H. L., JR. 1971. Portuguese man-of-war ("bluebottle") stings: treatment with papain. *Straub Clin. Proc.* 37: 30–33.
ARNOLD, H. L., JR., F. H. GRAUER, AND G. W. T. C. CHU 1959. Seaweed dermatitis apparently caused by a marine alga—preliminary report (November 25, 1958). *Proc. Hawaii Acad. Sci.* 34: 18–19.
BADEN, H. P., AND J. W. BURNETT 1977. Injuries from sea urchins. *South. Med. J.* 70: 459–460.
BAGNIS, R. 1968. Clinical aspects of Ciguatera (fish poisoning) in French Polynesia. *Hawaii Med. J.* 28: 25–28.
BAGNIS, R. 1973. *Fish Poisoning in the South Pacific.* Sydney, Australia: South Pacific Commission Publ. Bureau.
BAGNIS, R., S. CHANTEAU, E. CHUNGUE, ET AL. 1980. Origins of ciguatera fish poisoning: a new dinoflagellate *Gambierdiscus toxicus* Adachi and Fukuyo, definitively involved as a causal agent. *Toxicon* 18: 199–208.
BAGNIS, R., T. KUBERSKI, AND S. LAUGIER 1979. Clinical observations on 3009 cases of ciguatera (fish poisoning) in the South Pacific. *Am. J. Trop. Med. Hyg.* 28: 1067–1073.
BANNER, A. H. 1959. A dermatitis-producing alga in Hawaii—preliminary report. *Hawaii Med. J.* 19: 35–36.
BARKER, W. H., JR. 1974. *Vibrio parahyemolyticus* outbreaks in the United States. *Lancet* 1: 551–554.
BAXTER, E. H., AND A. G. M. MARR 1969. Sea wasp (*Chironex fleckeri*) venom: lethal, haemolytic, and dermonecrotic properties. *Toxicon* 7: 195–210.
BURKE, J. F. 1974. Sepsis following trauma: prevention and control. In: *Trauma Management,* by E. F. Case, J. F. Burke, and R. J. Boyd. Chicago: Year Book Medical Publ., p. 943–955.
BURNETT, J. W. 1971a. An electron microscopic study of two nematocysts in the tentacle of *Cyanea capillata*. *Chesapeake Sci.* 12: 67–71.
BURNETT, J. W. 1971b. An ultrastructural study of the nematocysts of the polyp of *Chrysaora quinquecirrha*. *Chesapeake Sci.* 12: 225–230.

CAMPBELL, C. H. 1975. The effects of snake venoms and their neurotoxins on the nervous system of man and animals. In: *Topics on Tropical Neurology*, edited by R. W. Hornabrook. Philadelphia: F. A. Davis Co., p. 259–292.

CHAPMAN, R. L., JR., J. B. DOWNS, I. HOOD, AND J. H. MODELL 1974. The ineffectiveness of steroid therapy in treating aspiration of hydrochloric acid. *Arch. Surg.* 108: 858–861.

CHU, G. W. T. C. 1952. First report of the presence of a dermatitis-producing marine larval schistosome in Hawaii. *Science* 155: 151–153.

CHU, G. W. T. C. 1958. Pacific area distribution of fresh-water and marine cercaria dermatitis. *Pac. Sci.* 12: 299–312.

CHUNGUE, E., AND R. BAGNIS 1977. Isolation of two toxins from the parrot-fish *Scarus gibbus*. *Toxicon* 15: 89–93.

CRONE, H. D., AND T. E. B. KEEN 1971. Further studies on the biochemistry of the toxins from the sea wasp *Chironex fleckeri*. *Toxicon* 9: 145–151.

CROSS, T. B. 1976. An unusual stingray injury—the skindiver at risk. *Med. J. Aust.* 2: 947–948.

DOTY, M. S., AND G. AGUILAR-SANTOS 1966. Caulerpicin, a toxic constituent of *Caulerpa*. *Nature (Lond.)* 211: 990.

DOWNS, J. B., R. L. CHAPMAN, JR., J. H. MODELL, AND I. HOOD 1974. An evaluation of steroid therapy in apiration pneumonitis. *Anesthesiology* 40: 129–135.

EDMONDS, C. 1978. *Dangerous Marine Animals of the Indo-Pacific Region*. Newport, Australia: Weidnel Publications. Introduction.

EDMONDS, C., C. LOWRY, AND J. PENNEFATHER 1976. *Diving and Subaquatic Medicine*. Mosman, Australia: Diving Medical Centre, p. 229–241.

ENDEAN, R., AND M. NOBLE 1971. Toxic material from the tentacle of the cubomedusan *Chironex fleckeri*. *Toxicon* 9: 255–264.

ENGLISH, V. L., AND R. B. LINDBERG 1977. Isolation of *Vibrio anginolyticus* from wounds and blood of a burn victim. *Am. J. Med. Technol.* 43: 989–993.

FEIGEN, G. A., AND L. HADJI 1974. Modes of action and identities of protein constituents in sea urchin toxin. In: *Bioactive Compounds of the Sea*, edited by H. J. Humm and C. E. Lane. New York: Marcel Dekker, p. 37–97.

FERNANDEZ, C. R., AND G. A. PANKEY 1975. Tissue invasion by unnamed marine vibrios. *JAMA* 233: 1173–1176.

FERENCIK, M. 1970. Formation of histamine during bacterial decarboxylation of histidine in the flesh of some marine fishes. *J. Hyg. Epidemiol. Microbiol. Immunol. (Prague)* 14: 52–60.

FISHER, A. A. 1978. *Atlas of Aquatic Dermatology*. New York: Grune and Stratton, p. 90–92.

FISHER, A. A., AND W. L. ORRIS 1973. Aquatic contact dermatitis. In: *Contact Dermatitis*, by A. A. Fisher. Philadelphia: Lea and Febiger, p. 327–351.

FOO, L. Y. 1975. Scombroid-type poisoning induced by the ingestion of smoked Kahawai. *N. Engl. J. Med.* 81: 476–477.

FOO, L. Y. 1976. Scombroid poisoning. Isolation and identification of "saurine." *J. Sci. Food Agric.* 27: 807–810.

FUJII, M., K. HARADA, AND M. MATSUDA 1967. Counteraction of the effects of puffer poison by cysteine. *Agric. Bull. Saga Univ.* 24: 1–9.

FULLER, R. H. 1963. Drowning and post immersion syndrome—a clinicopathologic study. *Mil. Med.* 128: 22–36.

FURLONG, M., AND V. PHIL 1970. *Starfish*. Edmonds, WA: Ellison Industries, p. 76–77.

GAGE, P. W., AND A. F. DULHUNTY 1973. Effects of toxin from the blue-ringed octopus (*Hapalochlaena maculosa*). In: *Marine Pharmacognosy*, edited by D. F. Martin and G. M. Padilla. New York: Academic Press, p. 85–106.

GALTSOFF, P. S. 1948. Red tide. Progress report on the investigations of the cause of mortality of fish along the west coast of Florida. *U.S. Fish Wildl. Serv. Spec. Rep.* 46.

GEIGER, E. 1955. Role of histamine in poisoning with spoiled fish. *Science* 121: 865–866.

GRAUER, F. H., AND H. L. ARNOLD, JR. 1961. Seaweed dermatitis. *Arch. Dermatol.* 84: 720–730.

GRIECO, M. H., AND C. SHELDON 1970. *Erysipelothrix rhusiopathiae*. *Ann. NY Acad. Sci.* 174: 523–532.

HALSTEAD, B. W. 1978. *Poisonous and Venomous Marine Animals of the World*. Princeton, N.J.: Darwin Press, p. 79–85.

HAYES, H. L., AND T. S. AUSTIN 1951. The distribution of discolored seawater. *Tex. J. Sci.* 3: 530–541.
HELFRICH, P. 1963. Fish poisoning in Hawaii. *Hawaii Med. J.* 22: 361–372.
HENDERSON, R., J. M. RITCHIE, AND G. R. STRICHARTZ 1974. Evidence that tetrodotoxin and saxitoxin act as a metal cation binding site in the sodium channels of nerve membrane. *Proc. Natl. Acad. Sci. USA* 71: 3936–3940.
HINEGARDNER, R. T. 1958. The venom apparatus of the cone shell. *Hawaii Med. J.* 17: 533–563.
HOFF, B. H. 1973. Multisystem failure: a review with special reference to drowning. *Crit. Care Med.* 7: 310–320.
HOKAMA, Y., A. H. BANNER, AND D. B. BOYLAN 1977. A radioimmunoassay for the detection of ciguatoxin. *Toxicon* 15: 317–325.
HUGHES, J. M., D. G. HOLLIS, E. T. GANGAROSA, ET AL. 1978. Non-cholera vibrio infections in the United States—clinical, epidemiologic, and laboratory features. *Ann. Intern. Med.* 88: 602–606.
HUGHES, J. M., AND M. H. MERSON 1976. Current concepts: fish and shellfish poisoning. *N. Engl. J. Med.* 295: 1117–1120.
KIM, R. 1979. Flushing syndrome due to mahi-mahi (scombroid fish) poisoning. *Arch. Dermatol.* 115: 963–965.
KIMATA, M. 1961. This histamine problem. In: *Fish as Food,* edited by G. Borgstrom. New York: Academic Press, p. 329–352.
KNOX, J. M., S. G. GEVER, R. G. FREEMAN, ET AL. 1961. Atypical acid-fast organism of the skin. *Arch. Dermatol.* 84: 386.
KOHN, A. J. 1958. Cone shell stings. *Hawaii Med. J.* 17: 528–532.
KRISS, A. E. 1963. *Marine Microbiology (Deep Sea).* London: Oliver and Boyd.
LANE, C. E. 1974. Nematocyst toxins of coelenterates. In: *Bioactive Compounds from the Sea,* by H. J. Humm and C. E. Lane. New York: Marcel Dekker, p. 123–137.
LORIA, P. R. 1976. Minocycline hydrochloride treatment for atypical acid-fast infection. *Arch. Dermatol.* 112: 517–519.
MCDANAL, C. E., M. D. ROSARIO, J. O. MCDANAL, ET AL. 1977. Near-drowning from ding-sting surf boarding: a case report. *JAMA* 238: 398.
MACLEOD, R. A. 1965. The question of the existence of specific marine bacteria. *Bacteriol. Rev.* 29: 9–23.
MIYAHARA, J. T., C. K. AKAU, AND T. YASUMOTO 1979. Effects of ciguatoxin and maitotoxin on the isolated guinea pig atria. *Res. Comm. Chem. Pathol. Pharmacol.* 25: 177–180.
MODELL, J. H. 1978. Biology of drowning. *Ann. Rev. Med.* 29: 1–8.
MODELL, J. H., S. A. GRAVES, AND A KETOVER 1976. Clinical course of 91 consecutive near-drowning victims. *Chest* 70: 231–238.
MULLANNEY, P. J. 1970. Treatment of sting ray wounds. *Clin. Toxicol.* 3: 613–615.
MUSIC, S. I., J. T. HOWELL, AND C. L. BRUMBACK 1973. Red tide—its public health implications. *J. Fla. Med. Assoc.* 60: 27–29.
MYRVIK, Q. N., N. N. PEARSALL, AND R. S. WEISER 1974. *Fundamentals of Medical Bacteriology and Mycology.* Philadelphia: Lea and Febiger, p. 358.
NARAHASHI, T. 1972. Mechanism of action of tetrodotoxin and saxitoxin on excitable membranes. *Fed. Proc.* 31: 1124–1132.
O'NEAL, R. L., B. W. HALSTEAD, AND L. D. HOWARD, JR. 1964. Injury to human tissues from sea urchin spines. *Calif. Med.* 101: 199–202.
OPPENHEIMER, C. H. 1963. *Symposium on Marine Microbiology.* Springfield, IL: Charles C Thomas.
RAMRAS, D. G. 1974. Scombroid poisoning from mahi-mahi. *West J. Med.* 121: 415–416.
RAYNER, M. D. 1972. Mode of action of ciguatoxin. *Fed. Proc.* 31: 1139–1145.
RAYNER, M. D., AND J. SZEKERCZES 1973. Ciguatoxin: effect on the sodium-potassium activated adenosine triphosphatase of human erythrocyte ghosts. *Toxicol. Appl. Pharmacol.* 24: 489–496.
REDDING, J. S., R. W. YAKAITIS, AND C. H. KING 1970. Problems in the management of drowning victims. *Md. State Med. J.* 19: 58–61.
REID, H. A. 1956. See snake bites. *Br. Med. J.* 2: 73–85.
RHEINHEIMER, G. 1974. *Aquatic Microbiology.* New York: John Wiley and Sons.
ROBERTS, J. R., M. I. GREENBERG, AND S. I. BASKIN 1979a. Endotracheal epinephrine in cardiorespiratory collapse. *J. Am. Coll. Emergency Physicians* 8: 515–519.

ROBERTS, J. R., M. I. GREENBERG, M. A. KNAUB, ET AL. 1979b. Blood levels following intravenous and endotracheal epinephrine administration. *J. Am. Coll. Emergency Physicians* 8: 53–56.

ROCHA, G., AND S. FRAGA 1962. Sea urchin granuloma of the skin. *Arch. Dermatol.* 85: 146–148.

ROSENTHAL, S. L., J. H. ZUGER, AND E. APOLLO 1975. Respiratory colonization with *Pseudomonas putrifaciens* after near-drowning in salt water. *Am. J. Clin. Pathol.* 64: 382–384.

RUBIN, S. J., AND R. C. TILTON 1975. Isolation of *Vibrio alginolyticus* from wound infections. *J. Clin. Microbiol.* 2: 556–558.

RUMP, S., AND T. RABSZTYN 1977. Effects of some veratrum-like agents on the muscular blocking action of tetrodotoxin. *Toxicon* 15: 521–528.

RUSSELL, F. E. 1975. Ciguatera fish poisoning: a report of 35 cases. *Toxicon* 13: 383–385.

RUSSELL, F. E., AND J. A. EMERY 1960. Venom of the weevers *Trachinus draco* and *Trachinus vipera*. *Ann. NY Acad. Sci.* 90: 805–819.

RUSSELL, F. E., T. C. PANOS, L. W. KANG, AND A. M. WARNER 1958. Studies on the mechanism of death from stingray venom: a report of two fatal cases. *Am. J. Med. Sci.* 235: 566–584.

SCHAEFER, W. B., AND C. L. DAVIS 1961. A bacteriologic and histopathologic study of skin granuloma due to *Mycobacterium balnei*. *Am. Rev. Respir. Dis.* 84: 837–844.

SCHEUER, P. J., W. TAKAHASHI, J. TSUTSUMI, ET AL. 1967. Ciguatoxin: isolation and chemical nature. *Science* 155: 1267–1268.

SHEUMACK, D. D., M. E. H. HOWDEN, I. SPENCE, ET AL. 1978a. Tetrodotoxin in the blue-ringed octopus. *Med. J. Aust.* 1: 160–161.

SHEUMACK, D. D., M. E. H. HOWDEN, I. SPENCE, ET AL. 1978b. Maculotoxin: a neurotoxin from the venom glands of the octopus *Hapalochlaena maculosa* identified as tetrodotoxin. *Science* 199: 188–189.

SHEWAN, J. M. 1938. The strict anaerobes in the slime and intestines of the haddock (*Gadus aeglefinus*). *J. Bacteriol.* 35: 397–405.

SIEBURTH, J. M. 1971. Distribution and activity of oceanic bacteria. *Deep Sea Res. Oceanogr. Abstr.* 18: 1111–1121.

SIMS, J. K., AND M. Y. IREI 1979. Human Hawaiian marine sponge poisoning—case report, literature review, and treatment recommendations for *Tedania ignis* dermatitis. *Hawaii Med. J.* 38: 263–270.

SIMS, J. K., AND ZANDEE VAN RILLAND 1981. Escharotic stomatitis caused by the "stinging seaweed" *Microcoleus lyngbyaccus* (formerly *Lyngbya majuscula*). Case report and literature review. *Hawaii Med. J.* 40: 243–248.

SOLOMON, A. E., AND R. B. STOUGHTON 1978. Dermatitis from purified sea algae toxin (debromoplysiatoxin). *Arch. Dermatol.* 114: 1333–1335.

SUTHERLAND, S. K., AND W. R. LANE 1969. Toxins and mode of envenomation of the common ringed or blue-ringed octopus. *Med. J. Aust.* 1: 893–898.

TAYLOR L. 1958. Tetanus from a marine sponge. *J. Laryngol. Otol.* 72: 762.

TORDA, T. A., E. SINCLAIR, AND D. B. ULYATT 1973. Pufferfish (tetrodotoxin) poisoning—clinical record and suggested management. *Med. J. Aust.* 1: 599–602.

TRETHEWIE, E. R. 1978. Tetrodotoxin in the blue-ringed octopus. *Med. J. Aust.* 1: 506.

TU, A. T. 1977. *Venoms: Chemistry and Molecular Biology*. New York: John Wiley and Sons, p. 151–177.

URAGODA, C. G. 1978. Histamine poisoning in tuberculosis patients on ingestion of tropical fish. *J. Trop. Med. Hyg.* 81: 243–245.

URAGODA, C. G., AND S. R. KOTTEGODA 1977. Adverse reactions to isoniazid on ingestion of fish with a high histamine content. *Tubercle* 58: 83–89.

WIENER, S. 1958. Stonefish sting and its treatment. *Med. J. Aust.* 45: 218–222.

WIENER, S. 1959. The production and assay of stonefish antivene. *Med. J. Aust.* 2: 715–179.

YAFFEE, H. S., AND F. STARGARDTER 1963. Erythema multiforma from *Tedania ignis*. *Arch. Dermatol.* 87: 601–603.

YAFFEE, H. S. 1970. Irritation from red sponge. *N. Engl. J. Med.* 282: 51.

YASUMOTO, T., R. BAGNIS, AND J. P. VERNOUX 1976. Toxicity of the surgeon-fishes—II. Properties of the principal water-soluble toxin. *Bull. Jpn. Soc. Sci. Fish.* 42: 359–365.

ZOBELL, C. E., AND H. C. UPHAM 1944. A list of marine bacteria including descriptions of sixty new species. *Bull. Scripps. Inst. Oceanogr. Univ. Calif.* 5: 239–292.

G. *Spontaneous Pneumothorax*

One of the more difficult problems that I have found in diving medicine is convincing the diver who has suffered a spontaneous pneumothorax that there are significant risks involved in continued diving. Similarly, the prospective diver with this history always finds it hard to understand why diving might be problematic. Part of the problem is that these are usually fit, young individuals who have a keen desire to dive. Another problem is that there are limited data on which to base advice. Very few cases of spontaneous pneumothorax are known to have occurred at depth, and no experimental studies specifically addressing this issue have been published. Thus, one's admonitions to such a diver must be based largely on theoretical eventualities and statistical data on the natural history of this problem in nondiving activities.

Spontaneous pneumothorax (SPTX) was recognized as early as the 17th century, but Laennec (1819) first described its possible relationship to emphysema and bleb formation in 1819. Since then a considerable literature has accumulated on the subject, although there continue to be few reliable figures on the overall incidence of SPTX. The best figures for the United States come from Olmstead County, Minnesota, where there was found to be an age-adjusted incidence of primary spontaneous pneumothorax of 7.4 per 100,000 per year among males and 1.2 per 100,000 per year for females (Melton et al. 1979). The higher incidence in males has been well established.

Spontaneous pneumothorax can be categorized as either primary or secondary. Primary SPTX occurs almost exclusively in young people who have no demonstrable lung disease. Typically these are tall, thin, athletic individuals, and it is in this group that most of the afflicted divers fall. Conversely, secondary SPTX affects individuals who have an underlying pulmonary disease (see Table IX-4); these are usually older persons having chronic lung disease, and there is less relationship to body habitus in these cases (Melton et al. 1981).

Table IX-4
Lung Disease Associated with Secondary Spontaneous Pneumothorax

Emphysema
Chronic bronchitis
Bronchiectasis
Tuberculosis
Pneumoconiosis (silicosis, Shaver's disease)
Eosinophilic granuloma
Sarcoidosis
Idiopathic pulmonary hemosiderosis
Carcinoma (primary or metastatic)
Chronic pulmonary fibrosis
Pulmonary alveolar proteinosis
Familial fibrocystic pulmonary dysplasia
Asthma
Lung abscess
Necrotizing pneumonia (e.g., Staph, *Klebsiella*)
Lung infarct

It is now generally accepted that primary spontaneous pneumothorax results from rupture of subpleural blebs or bullae. This most often accurs at the lung apices where the mechanical stresses within the lungs are greatest (West 1972). Whether these blebs are congenital or postinflammatory or are due to other causes has been much debated; however, recent data strongly suggest a congenital etiology for at least some types of these bullae. Electron microscopic evaluation of surgically resected subpleural bullae from documented cases of SPTX demonstrated marked absence of pleural mesothelial cells in some of these bullae (the Reid type I bullae) and abnormalities in the underlying collagen basal structure (Ohata and Suzuki 1980). These findings also support the idea that air may leak through the walls of such bullae into the pleural space (i.e., cause a pneumothorax) at raised intrapulmonary pressures. How great these pressures have to be is not known.

Although it was formerly believed that SPTX was more likely to occur during vigorous exercise, several studies have found no such relationship, and it is now generally agreed that exercise per se has no significant pathophysiological role. Not known, however, is what effect repeated baric stresses have on these subpleural blebs.

Spontaneous pneumothorax usually occurs unilaterally, affecting each side about equally, although some studies have shown a slight left-sided predomonance. Rarely (1%–2% of cases), simultaneous bilateral pneumothoraxes may occur. The main problem for divers is that once a spontaneous pneumothorax occurs there is a significant chance that it will happen again. Although this may not be a major problem on land, SPTX that occurs at depth is likely to become a fatal tension pneumothorax during ascent.

Reported recurrence rates for spontaneous pneumothorax have ranged from 12 to 52% (Cliff 1957; Cran and Rumball 1967; Ferguson et al. 1981; Gobbel et al. 1963; Lenox-Smith 1962; Lichter and Gwynne 1971), with an average of 20%–30%. If a second SPTX occurs, however, the risk of yet another recurrence increases sizably. After a second recurrence the chance of a further recurrence rises to more than 80%. Furthermore, the recurrence may be contralateral to the originally affected lung. (This further supports a congenital etiology.) The eventual development of bilateral spontaneous pneumothoraxes has been reported in 10%–40% of cases (Cliff 1957; Cran and Rumball 1967; Gobbel et al. 1963; Lenox-Smith 1962; Lichter and Gwynne 1971), also with an average of 20%–30%.

Most recurrences (80%–90%) happen within the first 2 to 3 years after the initial episode (Cliff 1957; Ohata and Suzuki 1980), but documented recurrences after more than 20 years also have been reported (Myers 1954).

Spontaneous pneumothorax probably occurs more often than realized. Many mild cases may not be diagnosed because they produce relatively minor symptoms of pleurisy or chest pain that never come to medical attention or, if they do, are not evaluated with a chest radiograph. Indeed, small pneumothoraxes are a well-known finding in chest x-ray screening programs of asymptomatic persons. Thus, the reported recurrence rates probably underestimate the actual risk.

Screening for the causative subpleural blebs in cases of primary SPTX has been generally unproductive. Chest radiographs have been reported as normal in 50%–77% of documented cases (Cliff 1957; Cran and Rumball 1967; Gobbel et al. 1963; Lenox-Smith 1962). Radioisotopic ventilation-perfusion scans may demonstrate large bullae but have a low sensitivity for the small lesions that are associated with spontaneous pneumothorax. Currently, the most sensitive method of detecting parenchymal bullae is by computerized tomography (CT), although its sensitivity for blebs less than 1 cm in size is less than satisfactory. A normal chest CT certainly does not exclude such blebs. So, at this time, there is no way of reliably screening someone for the presence of bullous changes that might increase the chance of recurrent spontaneous pneumothorax.

If the lung collapse causes significant symptoms or affects more than about 15% of the lung, the preferred treatment for pneumothorax, whether spontaneous or otherwise, is needle aspiration or closed-chest tube thoracostomy. The treatment of choice for recurrent SPTX (i.e., after the pneumothorax is evacuated) is more controversial. Numerous surgical procedures have been advocated for this problem, most of which involve bleb excision combined with some form of pleural scarification or pleurectomy. Recently, simple blebectomy alone has been advocated (Ferguson et al. 1981). Each of the various procedures has ardent supporters who claim complete success in preventing recurrences on the operated side. Unfortunately, follow-up is limited to a few years, at the longest, in most series, and not all investigators report the same degree of success with the same procedure. In addition, unless the procedure has been bilateral there is still a risk of recurrence on the contralateral side.

Clearly, the issue of diving after suffering a spontaneous pneumothorax is not a simple matter. I believe, though, that all authorities would agree that diving is absolutely contraindicated for at least 3 years after a spontaneous pneumothorax. If there has been no recurrence in that time the issue becomes less clear-cut. Even though the chance of a recurrence is much less likely if it has not happened within 3 years, there still remains a small but definite increased risk, which carries with it the likelihood of a catastrophic outcome if it occurs while diving. Whether blebectomy, with or without pleurodesis, will completely prevent recurrences is not entirely clear, either, and even if it did, it would at best be quite radical to recommend that a sport diver have bilateral thoracotomies just to be able to dive. It is conceivable that in some commercial situations this might be a consideration. For such persons, as well as for the very rare sport diver who has already had bilateral corrective procedures,the advice must be individualized and based on the understanding that none of the currently recommended surgical procedures offer absolute protection against recurrent pneumothorax.

Unfortunately, therefore, a history of spontaneous pneumothorax is a contraindication to diving in all but exceptional situations.

KENNETH W. KIZER

References

CLIFF, J. M. 1957. Spontaneous pneumothorax in the Royal Navy. *Proc. R. Soc. Med.* 50: 517–526.
CRAN, I. R., AND C. A. RUMBALL 1967. Survey of spontaneous pneumothoraces in the Royal Air Force. *Thorax* 22: 462–465.
FERGUSON, L. J., C. W. IMRIE, AND J. HUTCHISON 1981. Excision of bullae without pleurectomy in patients with spontaneous pneumothorax. *Br. J. Surg.* 68: 214–216.
GOBBEL, W. G., W. G. RHEA, A. NELSON, ET AL. 1963. Spontaneous pneumothorax. *J. Thorac. Cardiovasc. Surg.* 46: 331–345.

LAENNEC, R. T. H. 1819. *De l'Auscultation mediate, ou traité du diagnostic des maladies des poumons et du coeur.* Paris: Brosson et Chaudé, vol. 1.

LENOX-SMITH, I. 1962. Spontaneous pneumothorax—a study of ninety-four cases. *Br. J. Dis. Chest* 56: 1–10.

LICHTER, I., AND J. F. GWYNNE 1971. Spontaneous pneumothorax in young subjects. *Thorax* 26: 409–417.

MELTON, L. J., N. G. G. HEPPER, AND K. P. OFFORD 1979. Incidence of spontaneous pneumothorax in Olmstead County, Minnesota: 1950 to 1974. *Am. Rev. Respir. Dis.* 120: 1379–1382.

MELTON, L. J., N. G. G. HEPPER, AND K. P. OFFORD 1981. Influence of height on the risk of spontaneous pneumothorax. *Mayo Clin. Proc.* 56: 678–682.

MYERS, J. A. 1954. Simple spontaneous pneumothorax. *Dis. Chest* 26: 420–429.

OHATA, M., AND H. SUZUKI 1980. Pathogenesis of spontaneous pneumothorax, *Chest* 77: 771–776.

WEST, J. B. 1972. Factors affecting localization of disease in the lung. *Thorax* 10: 510.

X

Emergency Treatment While under Pressure

A. *Use of Drugs and Related Substances under Diving Conditions*

The ingestion, inhalation, or injection of either physician-prescribed or over-the-counter substances prior to entering a hyperbaric environment may result in an untoward (adverse or hazardous) reaction. Drug-induced physiological and psychological responses are often altered in the undersea environment. The known and recognized metabolic and excretion patterns of pharmacologically active substances may be significantly and pathologically altered once the diver becomes pressurized. An understanding of the types of changes that occur, the implications of these changes, and the relationships between and among drugs, the environment, and the diver are critical if therapeutic accidents are to be avoided.

Hyperbaric environments may affect the manner in which a drug is psychologically and physiologically dealt with by the mind and body. Specific concerns include the following:

1. The hyperbaric environment may directly affect the manner in which the drug is absorbed, metabolized, and excreted.

2. The perceived effects of the drug or drugs may be altered by direct effects of the hyperbaric environment. The physical effects of the increased density of the gases, the relative temperature of the water or other environment (e.g., divers may work inside ship's fuel tanks, where they are surrounded by diesel fuel), and the degree of exertion all contribute to altered mental and physical states.

3. The indirect effects of a hyperbaric experience include the effects of heavy exercise, which can result in dehydration, mild acidosis, and excessive fatigue. The normal physiological responses of the body's organs may be stressed to such an extent that normal absorption, metabolism, and excretion patterns are altered. These altered responses may adversely affect the manner in which a therapeutic substance is dealt with by the body.

4. Acceptable side effects, like drowsiness from antihistamines, may be tolerated on the surface; in the hyperbaric environment, however, the side effects may become unac-

ceptable, leading in some cases to serious morbidity or even death. Impairment of cognitive functions, neuromuscular strength and coordination, or integration of thought and action can have catastrophic results in either the aqueous or gaseous hyperbaric environment.

This section reviews the physiological and psychological alterations of commonly used prescription and over-the-counter medications in the hyperbaric environment as well as drug-to-drug interactions. This entire discussion is placed in a historical perspective of research activities undertaken to explore the unique effect the hyperbaric environment has on the normal physical and mental processes. General comments concerning the use and prescription of drugs, the physical conditions that require medication, and the classes of drugs that should be used (with caution) in the hyperbaric environment are reviewed.

1. *Physiological Background*

The hyperbaric environment presents four sets of conditions that affect drug absorption, metabolism, and excretion: (1) Direct effects of pressure. (2) Interactions of pressure and breathing gas. (3) Physical and emotional state of the diver. (4) The underwater environment (e.g., cold black water with strong currents).

These conditions are dynamic states that will alter the psychological and physical performance of the diver and these sets of conditions are constantly changing. The limits of human performance and function may be gradually overreached without the knowledge of the diver, or the limits may be exceeded abruptly and calamitously. It is the rate of adverse impact of these sets of conditions that assists in predicting whether the end result will be minor or morbid.

Therefore, it is important to review the effects of each of these sets of conditions in order to appreciate the relative role of each in predicting the effectiveness and safety of pharmacologically active substances consumed prior to entering (or in some cases while actually in) a hyperbaric environment. These variables may be grouped into three categories, although there are interactions among and between any and all of these variables throughout the hyperbaric or diving exposure.

a. Direct Effects of Pressure

Dramatic changes in biological functioning occur at high hydrostatic pressures (in excess of 100 ATA); cell structure is changed, membrane permeability is altered, muscle can become rigid and stiff (Fenn 1969). In the 50–150 ATA range a complex of neurological changes occur; this complex of changes has been referred to as the *high pressure nervous syndrome* (HPNS). Brauer (1975) describes the characteristic HPNS as beginning with motor disturbances (tremors of the extremities), followed by a second stage of isolated myoclonic jerking, usually in the facial areas and upper extremities, increasing in severity until the final stage of generalized clonic or tonic-clonic seizures, which may prove fatal to the victim. These symptoms begin to appear around 800–1000 fsw (245–305 msw) and become more pronounced as pressure increases. At pressures less than 800 fsw the changes become more subtle, and since these effects are often not anticipated, these subtle changes are potentially quite hazardous.

b. Interactions of Pressure and Gas

Increased partial pressures of nitrogen (P_{N_2}), oxygen (P_{O_2}), and carbon dioxide (P_{CO_2}) may have detrimental effects on the diver. Nitrogen narcosis and carbon dioxide retention are the most prevalent detrimental effects on the sport diver breathing compressed air, and these gases could certainly interact with drug effects. Drugs acting on the central nervous system would probably interact directly with the narcotic effects of high P_{N_2} levels. High P_{O_2} and P_{CO_2} levels may cause indirect interactions by changing pharmacokinetic processes (e.g., metabolism). Experiments at the Naval Medical Research Institute have shown a variety of drug-pressure-gas interactions at relatively shallow depths (200 fsw) in subjects breathing compressed air (Walsh 1974). (See Section B of this chapter, *Anesthesia for Emergency Surgery under High Pressure*.)

c. Physical and Emotional State of Diver

The physiological state of the diver is dependent on the interplay of a variety of physical, mental, and environmental factors. Figure X-1 illustrates the types of interactions

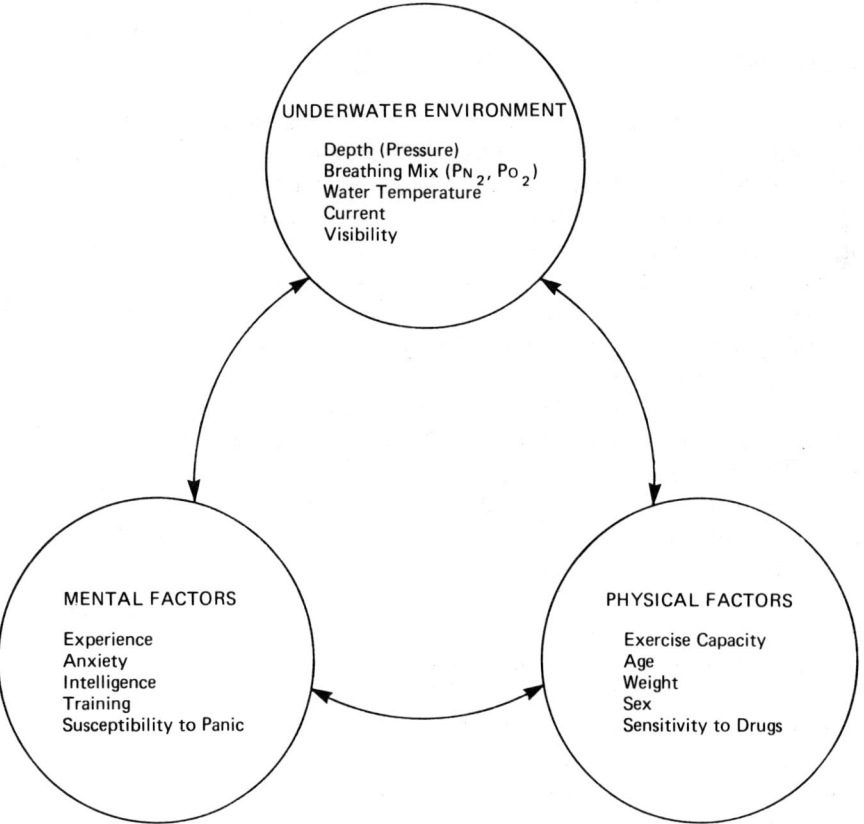

Figure X-1. Interacting variables that may affect drug disposition in a diver.

that may be possible. Each cluster may interact both within its own categories as well as with one or more categories from the other clusters. Even in this simple figure it is readily visible that the types and numbers of different possible combinations are quite large. The relative contribution of any single element is often difficult to determine.

The importance of these factors on the absorption, distribution, metabolism, and excretion of exogenous and endogenous substances is a complex and not well-understood phenomenon. The pharmacokinetics of a drug consumed prior to the initiation of a dive may be modified by the physical and mental state of the diver and the actual parameters of the dive.

Any drug that affects exercise tolerance (e.g., autonomic blocking agents) may be troublesome. Drugs that increase central nervous system (CNS) activity may create high levels of anxiety in response to new diving situations and may exacerbate hyperventilation and panic in response to physical exertion. These effects will also vary with the diver's level of experience and emotional stability. It is quite common for a given pharmacologic agent, in the same dose and route of administration, to have different physiological and psychological effects on the same individual at different moments and in different circumstances. Additional variables associated with the hyperbaric environment create a situation that produces drug effects that are even less predictable.

d. Known Interactions of Drugs with Environment

The basic understanding of the hyperbaric environment has been developed from sound research using animal models under well-controlled conditions in dry hyperbaric facilities. Studies at the cellular level have been conducted in these animal models, one drug or variable at a time often being tested in genetically similar rodents and mammals. The basic finding of these studies indicates that any drug that acts on the neuromuscular junction has the potential for interacting with pressure. Even though sport divers generally stay relatively close to the surface, they can still be vulnerable. Kendig (1979) indicates that "where junctional transmission has already been depressed by drugs, disease, or abnormal metabolic state, pressure may tip the balance toward transmission failure."

Studies in the area of hyperbaric anesthesia have contributed significantly to our knowledge of hyperbaric drug interactions. Detailed description of this work is discussed in section B of this chapter on hyperbaric anesthesia. Behavioral evaluations have provided an integrated appreciation of the overall effects of drugs. Behavior is the output of the functional integrity of the central nervous system; it encompasses sensory, motor, and cognitive factors. In general, the behavioral studies, evaluating human as well as animal subjects, have shown that the nature of the behavioral action of a drug in diving conditions is not predictable from its behavioral action under normobaric conditions. In addition, the drug-induced changes that have been observed are not always in accord with what would be expected by our current understanding of hyperbaric phenomena (Thomas and Walsh 1978; Walsh 1976; Walsh and Burch 1979).

A comprehension of the effects of a specific class of drugs under controlled circumstances ultimately provides the clinician with a basis for making sound judgment on the appropriateness of recommending a drug. This becomes especially important for those drugs that can be demonstrated to have a different range of actions in the normobaric and hyperbaric environments. A substantive body of knowledge indicates that drugs have different effects in the hyperbaric environment. These unanticipated effects have been noted in depths of less than 3 ATA (66 fsw or 20 msw). There remains a great deal that is unknown about the interactions between drug and host environment and among the various organ systems of the body during the conduct of actual diving operations; this unknown quantity produces a number of variables that exceed those currently under investigation in research settings.

In summary, the prescribing physician and the self-medicating diver are thus left with the basic dilemma of determining whether or not the risks of using a therapeutic agent, or other substance in question, outweigh the potential therapeutic benefits.

2. Clinical Applications

A relative-risk approach is taken in reviewing the various classes of drugs that may be taken prior to, or even during, a hyperbaric experience. Scientifically controlled human studies, those investigating the drug-pressure-diver effects and drug-drug-pressure-diver effects, have not been conducted for the great majority of therapeutic and nontherapeutic agents commonly used by divers. Thus the information offered here is a clinical summation of a number of hyperbaric physicians and experts in the field. These comments are made with an awareness of a very limited amount of hard data to support specific recommendations; therefore, general information is presented with the philosophy that to err on the conservative side is a reasonable approach to this problem. Additional clinical knowledge may permit, and in some instances require, a physician or other trained professional to act in a manner differently from that indicated. All contingencies cannot be dealt with in this text. The final arbiter is the clinician and his or her understanding of the clinical situation.

Not all classes of drugs are presented here. It should be noted that nontherapeutic substances are also presented and discussed. Substance abuse, be it alcohol, marijuana, or cocaine, to name a few, is a universal problem that transcends social class, age, sex, and race. In addition, these substances may interact with a number of therapeutic agents. For the purpose of this discussion drugs are presented by their principal site of action or use. The following classifications are discussed: central nervous system agents, including stimulants and depressants; cardiovascular agents; respiratory agents; otorhinolaryngeal agents; antiallergenics; antibiotics; and abused psychoactive agents.

a. Drugs Acting on Central Nervous System

Central nervous system (CNS) agents comprise the most widely used group of pharmacologically active agents. Drugs affecting the CNS can be grossly divided into two categories—stimulants and depressants. Drugs that stimulate the CNS are widely used to increase alertness, improve performance, inhibit fatigue; they may also be used as antidepressants and appetite suppressants. However, their common concomitant effects may be harmful to a diver, for they produce anxiety, euphoria, dizziness, increased rates of total body metabolism through both oxygen and glucose consumption, and increased respiratory and cardiovascular function. Depressants of the central nervous system are used to produce sedation, antiemesis, and a decrease in actual or potential allergic responses. Fatigue, drowsiness, and muscular weakness commonly occur as a function of therapy that uses depressant-type drugs. General information regarding CNS drugs is summarized in Table X-1.

450 Chapter X

Table X-1
Drugs Affecting the Central Nervous System

Subclass	Clinical effects	Examples	Comments
Analgesics and antipyretics	Mild analgesia Anti-inflammatory Reduces fever	Aspirin, acetaminophen, indomethacin, propoxyphene	Aspirin and acetaminophen have been shown to be relatively safe for use in hyperbaric conditions (Walsh and Burch 1979). Narcotic-related analgesics (codeine, propoxyphene) have untoward effects (nausea, dizziness) that could be a problem for a diver.
Hypnotics and sedatives	Depress CNS Induce sleep	Barbiturates, methaqualone, chloral hydrate	Safe diving requires an alert, responsive individual; therefore these drug are contraindicated for divers.
Antianxiety minor tranquilizers	Relieve anxiety Depress CNS (depression is dose dependent)	Benzodiazepines: Chlordiazepoxide Diazepam Others: Meprobamate Hydroxyzine	Generally these drugs cause drowsiness, lethargy, ataxia, and confusion. Hypotension and syncope may also occur. These adverse effects could be fatal in the water. A person who requires tranquilizers for anxiety probably shouldn't be diving.
Antipsychotic major tranquilizers	Relieve anxiety and thought disturbances	Phenothiazines: Chlorpromazine Promazine Butyrophenones: Haloperidol	These drugs produce significant biological changes. Side effects that would endanger a diver include sedation, hypothermia, hypotension, reduction of seizure threshold, cardiac arrythmias. These drugs should be an absolute contraindication for diving.

Antidepressants	Psychostimulant CNS-stimulant Anticholinergic	Tricyclic antidepressants: Amitriptyline Desipramine Monoamine-oxidase inhibitors: Phenylzin Tranylcypromine	Tricyclics cause dry mouth, blurred vision, tachycardia, and cardiac arrythmias. MAO inhibitors have been shown to interact synergistically with high nitrogen pressures (Thomas and Walsh 1978).
CNS stimulants and anorexiants	Increase alertness, inhibit fatigue, suppress appetite, elevate mood	Amphetamines	Dizziness, excessive sweating, euphoria, anxiety, and panic. Amphetamines interact synergistically with increased pressures of air as shallow as 50 fsw and further disrupt behavior (Walsh 1974; Thomas 1973). These drugs contraindicate diving.
Antiemetics	Relieve nausea and vomiting	Phenothiazines Anticholinergics Sedatives Antihistamines	For motion sickness the antihistamines are the only acceptable drugs for divers. Dimenhydrinate and diphenhydramine have been evaluated in U.S. Navy divers and shown to be relatively safe for use (Walsh and Burch, 1979), although drowsiness may cause decreased cognitive abilities.

b. Cardiovascular Agents

Cardiovascular agents affect the heart muscle and its nerves and blood vessels and are generally prescribed to supplement the normal performance of the heart. Implicit then is that the heart cannot function well without them. While some exercise is often a significant component of the treatment of heart disease, it is strongly recommended that heart patients requiring medication not dive. Exercise on land can be controlled; this is not necessarily the case for a diver who finds himself in a heavy current, or in extremely cold water. The use of antihypertensive agents is also a contraindication to diving, for these agents reduce exercise tolerance and therefore place the diver at increased risk for overexertion and possible myocardial ischemia. Clearly, assessment on a case-by-case basis is necessary to determine whether a given patient, using these medications, is fit to dive. Careful examination, with relevant laboratory and radiographic studies including stress electrocardiography, should be carried out to assist the clinician in arriving at a reasonable clinical opinion. The drugs presented in Table X-2 have substantive capability to have impact on the cardiovascular system. If a diver requires more than a single one of these drugs to lead a reasonably normal life, then care should be taken in assessing whether or not the individual should be permitted to dive. The drug-to-drug interactions in the hyperbaric environment are not well known or understood, and extreme care is therefore required.

c. Respiratory Agents

Respiratory agents affect the gas exchange and blood flow in the upper airways and lungs. Those individuals requiring bronchodilators for treatment of their chronic asthma, chronic bronchitis (even if it is secondary to chronic use of tobacco products), or other obstructive airway or lung disorders should not be permitted to dive; they have a predisposition to lung rupture and resultant emboli.

A wide variety of prescription and over-the-counter oral decongestants are available and frequently used by both sport and commercial divers. Though these drugs appear to be reasonably safe on the surface, those that have an antihistaminic component will produce decreased alertness, and fatigue and drowsiness. It might be that these drugs will have a greater effect on the central nervous system in the presence of fatigue, use of alcohol or marijuana, and increased nitrogen pressure (at depth). Oral decongestants, having only epinephrine analogues, are preferred for long-term usage to nasal decongestants. In general, nasal sprays and drops have a reduced effect after repeated use, and a rebound phenomenon that occurs after peak effect is reached may produce reverse ear squeeze during ascent.

The drugs presented in Table X-3 are the more commonly used respiratory drugs. This list is not all-inclusive. Some of these drugs also may have an effect on the cardiovascular system, stressing it to a harmful degree in individuals with a history of angina, previous infarction, or arrhythmia.

d. Otorhinolaryngeal Agents

Otorhinolaryngeal agents affect the ears, nose, and throat. Many of these agents are also used as bronchodilators. Though aural and otopharyngeal preparations are thought to

Table X-2
Drugs Affecting the Cardiovascular System

Subclass	Clinical effects	Examples	Comments
Adrenergic blocking agents	Alpha blockers: produce peripheral vasodilation Use in Reynaud's disease	Alpha: Tolazoline Phentolamine	Tachycardia, nausea, hypotension could cause hypothermia in water when cold stressed.
	Beta blockers: reduce sympathetic activity of heart (decrease HR, myocardial contractility, cardiac output).	Beta: Propranolol	Fatigue, lethargy, severely limits exercise tolerance. Bronchospasm may predispose to air embolism. These drugs indicate conditions that are absolute contraindications for diving.
Antihypertensives	Reduce blood pressure	Thiazide diuretics Methyldopa Clonidine Hydralazine Reserpine Guanethidine Propranolol	Most antihypertensive medications have multiple side effects and reduced exercise tolerance; these medications indicate more than minor cardiovascular disease. Only thiazide diuretics are deemed reasonably safe for divers, provided potassium depletion is monitored.
Coronary vasodilators	To relieve acute angina Management of angina	Amyl nitrite Nitroglycerine	Dizziness, weakness, flushing face. The conditions requiring these drugs contraindicate diving.
Drugs for miscellaneous cardiac disorders	Cardiac glycosides: to control atrial flutter, fibrillation and paroxysmal atrial tachycardia	Propranolol Digitalis	Combination of cardiac disorder presented and adverse side effects of these drugs contraindicate diving.
	Procainamide: for premature ventricular contraction, paroxysmal atrial tachycardia, and ventricular tachycardia	Procainamide	
	Quinidine: prevent aberrant cardiac rhythms	Quinidine	

Table X-3
Drugs Affecting the Respiratory System

Subclass	Clinical effects	Examples	Comments
Bronchodilators	To relieve bronchospasm in: chronic bronchitis, bronchial asthma, emphysema	Isoproterenol, Theophylline, Aminophylline, Epinephrine	Sympathomimetic effects, nervousness, tachycardia. Requirement for these drugs indicates excessive bronchial congestion. Because of the dangers of the expanding lung in decompression, lung obstructions could cause catastrophic results. The requirement of these drugs contraindicates diving.
Decongestants	Provide symptomatic relief of a variety of respiratory conditions	Oral: Pseudoephedrine (Sudafed), Phenylephrine, Promethazine (Phenergan)	In general the side effects of the oral decongestant group are minimal, and if the drug is well tolerated on the surface, it should be relatively safe in the water. The primary disadvantages are the sedative (CNS depressant) effects, which in some individuals are significant. (See Table X-1 for phenothiazine derivatives.)
	Nasal decongestants are generally sympathetic amines	Nasal: Ephedrine, Oxymetazoline, Xylometazoline	The nasal decongestant group has only mild side effects; however, the disadvantages are that with repeated applications, symptomatic relief is short acting and rebound congestion is often significant, which could easily result in reverse squeeze for the diver on surfacing.
Cough remedies Expectorants Mucolytics	Depress medullary cough center. Increase and liquify secretions, loosen sputum	Codeine, Dextromethorphan	Sedative properties of codeine and its drying action on the respiratory tract mucosa would not be helpful to diver. Dextromethorphan has no sedative/analgesic effects, but the requirement of cough suppressants/expectorant/mucolytics contraindicates diving.
Antihistamines	Action is to block the effects of histamine	Chlorpheniramine, Triprolidine, Cyclizine, Meclizine, Diphenhydramine	Most significant side effects for diver are nausea, decreased alertness muscular weakness, drowsiness, impaired ability to concentrate.

be nontoxic and nonsensitizing in the hyperbaric environment, they cannot be used with impunity. Caution should be used because of individual sensitivity to products containing antibiotics. It should be stressed that careful physical examinations and appropriate studies are required for individuals who have required these agents on a routine basis prior to hyperbaric exposures. The symptomatic treatment of apparently minor difficulties does not resolve the underlying pathological etiologies. Ear, nose, and throat agents are presented in Table X-4.

e. Antiallergenic Agents

Antiallergenic agents affect the immune and autonomic systems. Antihistamines are prescribed to minimize the body's response to a noxious agent, while allergy densensitization injections attempt to adapt the body to these noxious agents. Toxic and unpredictable reactions to allergy shots require careful monitoring in the postinjection period. Therefore, divers requiring allergy shots should remain out of the water, and with companions, for at least 4–6 hr after receiving a desensitization injection. (See Table X-5.)

f. Antibiotics

Antibiotics affect the toxic agents causing infection, although they are also used prophylactically. Use of antibiotics is not an absolute contraindication to being exposed to a hyperbaric environment; nevertheless, after an antibiotic is administered for the first dose, regardless of previous exposure to the antibiotic, the diver should not enter the hyperbaric environment for 4–6 hr to ensure that an allergic response will not develop while the diver is under pressure. A number of conditions that usually require antibiotics are absolute contraindications to being exposed to a hyperbaric environment. Active tuberculosis, or any other active pneumonic process with the potential for causing damage to the alveolar walls, will place the individual at risk for emboli. Individuals receiving antituberculous agents prophylactically (conversion of tine test with negative chest roentgenogram) may experience side effects of the central nervous system that include dizziness, disorientation, mental confusion, paresthesias of hands and feet, and a lowered convulsion threshold. If any of these symptoms are experienced, without exposure to a hyperbaric environment, it is recommended that these individuals not be permitted to dive, because if they dive and subsequently become symptomatic, the true cause of the symptoms will be difficult to determine.

Topical antifungals are essentially nontoxic and nonsensitizing. When sensitization does occur it usually occurs as a local reaction. The administration of anthelmintics is a contraindication to diving, for these drugs often produce side effects and adverse reactions that may be confused with the signs and symptoms of decompression sickness.

Table X-6 indicates the more commonly used antibiotics and their most commonly reported side effects. This list would be prohibitively extensive if all antibiotics and all their reported side effects were presented. It would be a part of prudent care to first determine why the antibiotic was required and then assess whether the underlying condition, per se, should be the basis for temporarily restricting the diver's access to the hyperbaric environment.

Table X-4
Drugs Used for Ear, Nose, and Throat

Subclass	Clinical effects	Examples	Comments
Local reactants on nose	Nasal decongestant sprays	Oxymetazoline (Afrin) Xylometazoline (Neo-Synephrine)	Sympathomimetic amines should not be used for prolonged periods, as tolerance develops; rebound symptoms may be especially hazardous to divers. (Also see Respiratory Drug section.)
Oropharyngeal preparations	To relieve: oral and throat infection; gingivitis, dental stomatitis	Betadine gargle Chloraseptic (Phenol) Nystatin Orabase	Generally thought to be nontoxic and nonsensitizing.
Aural preparations	To relieve or prevent ear infections To soften wax	Mostly antibiotic/steroid combinations	Minimal adverse reactions; caution needed for sensitivity to antibiotics.

Table X-5
Drugs Used for Allergic Disorders

Subclass	Clinical effects	Examples	Comments
Antiallergic	H_1 or H_2 receptor blockers	Generally antihistamines and phenothiazines Diphenhydramine Chlorpheniramine Diphenylpyraline Promethazine Cimetidine	Preparations containing antihistamines may cause drowsiness and lack of alertness and may have synergistic effects with other CNS depressants. Phenothiazine derivatives have significant CNS, cardiovascular, and respiratory effects that would contraindicate diving.
Desensitizing preparations	Hyposenitization Immunotherapy	Allergens	Because of the possibility of adverse reactions it is recommended that divers allow 4–6 hr to elapse between allergy shots and diving.

Table X-6
Drugs Used for Infections or Infestations

Subclass	Clinical effects	Examples	Comments
Antibiotics	Antibiotics work through interference with cell wall synthesis, cell membrane permeability, molecular mechanisms	Tetracyclines Penicillins Sulfonamides Cephalosporins Aminoglycosides	Antibiotics produce a wide variety of side effects and their interaction with hyperbaric conditions is unknown. Antimicrobial agents are often overused. If strong clinical evidence requires the use of antibiotic therapy, then careful scrutiny of the infectious condition should be made to determine the individual's physical fitness for diving.
Antituberculous drugs	Antimicrobial	Isoniazid (INH) Ethambutol Rifampin	Decreases in visual acuity most prevalent, although a variety of CNS side effects are included: mental confusion, dizziness, and disorientation; numbness, parasthesia of the feet and/or hands; memory impairment; muscular weakness.
Antifungals		a. Miconazole b. Griseofulvin c. Amphotericin d. Nystatin e. Tolnaftate	(a,b,c) Adverse reaction is most commonly hypersensitivity, although occasionally CNS side effects have been reported. (d,e) Essentially nontoxic, nonsensitizing.
Anthelmintics	Piperazine produces a paralysis of ascaris muscle with expulsion of the worms by intestinal peristalsis	Piperazine (Antepar)	Significant side effects including vertigo, parasthesia, weakness, convulsion, blurred vision, lack of alertness.
	Vermox exerts anthelmintic effect by blocking glucose uptake of susceptible helminths	Mebendazole (Vermox)	Some abdominal pain and diarrhea. These drugs contraindicate diving.

Table X-7
Physiological Contraindications to Diving

Absolute contraindications	Relative contraindications
1. History of spontaneous pneumothorax	1. Severe hay fever or allergy causing blockage of middle ear
2. History of epileptic seizures or syncopal attacks	2. Upper or lower respiratory infection; chest congestion
3. Lung cysts and/or air-trapping lesions visible on radiograph	3. Alcohol intoxication
4. Active asthma	
5. Insulin-dependent diabetes	
6. Drug addiction	

[a]Adapted from Kindwall (1976).

g. Abused Psychoative Agents

Both cognitive and motor performance can be impaired by the abuse of psychoactive agents. Alcohol and marijuana (and other cannabis products) are the most commonly abused central nervous system depressants in the world today. It is apparent that their use is additive and in some cases (e.g., with concurrent administration of barbiturates) can potentiate other central nervous system depressants. These drugs can impair judgment and can thus permit the diver to become involved in physically and mentally dangerous activities.

Cocaine is currently the most commonly abused central nervous system stimulant. Its relatively short action belies its dangerousness to the diver. The hypermetabolic state that occurs during the use of cocaine (it is rarely used alone and is often used with alcohol or marijuana) may place the diver at risk to subsequent fatigue, mental depression, acidosis, and an inability to respond promptly to life-threatening emergencies.

3. Conclusions

The use of prescribed and over-the-counter medications in a hyperbaric environment is a complex issue. There are no simple answers to the questions of which drugs are best for which conditions in a hyperbaric environment. Individual variability, concurrent medical and physical conditions, and the mental and physical requirements of the hyperbaric exposure must all be taken into account prior to the use of any pharmacologically active agent. Consideration must be given to the following elements before the exposure to the hyperbaric environment is permitted:

1. Will the drug interfere with cognitive processes?
2. Will the drug interfere with physical performance?
3. Will the drug impair exercise tolerance?
4. Will the side effects of the drug increase to an unacceptable level the associated risks of diving?
5. Are any of the known or anticipated side effects absolute or relative contraindications to exposure to the hyperbaric environment?
6. What is the half-life of the drug, and what is a reasonable period of time before or after its use that the diver should not be exposed to a hyperbaric environment?

7. Does the drug produce rebound phenomena?

8. Why are the drugs being used initially, and are the underlying conditions relative or absolute contraindications to exposure to the hyperbaric environment?

The clinician has the responsibility to explain the nature of his or her treatment to the diver. The diver has the responsibility to indicate to the treating clinician that an exposure to a hyperbaric environment is anticipated. Divers should be discouraged from using any medications prior to an exposure to a hyperbaric environment. Sharing of medications among divers should also be discouraged. Exposure to a hyperbaric environment is not a good opportunity for either a clinician or diver to determine whether a drug will be satisfactory for a given diver, despite the close monitoring of the subject throughout a test dive.

Diving, as either a sport or an occupation, requires a great deal of self-reliance and common sense. Conservative and safe practices are required for the well-being and survival of the diver. Abstinence from diving may be the most conservative approach for an individual requiring systemic medication. Drugs may permit divers to go diving, but drugs do not permit divers to dive safely.

J. MICHAEL WALSH
HAROLD M. GINZBURG

References

BRAUER, R. W. 1975. The high pressure nervous syndrome: animals. In: *The Physiology and Medicine of Diving and Compressed Air Work* (2nd ed.), edited by P. B. Bennett and D. H. Elliott. Baltimore: Williams and Wilkins, p. 231–247.

FENN, W. O. 1969. The physiological effects of hydrostatic pressures. In: *The Physiology and Medicine of Diving and Compressed Air Work*, edited by P. B. Bennett and D. H. Elliott. Baltimore: Williams and Wilkins, p. 36–57.

KENDIG, J. J. 1980. Interactions between hyperbaric pressure and drugs on excitable cells (nerve and muscle). In: *Interaction of Drugs in the Hyperbaric Environment*, edited by J. M. Walsh. Bethesda, MD: Undersea Medical Society, p. 3–10. (Undersea Med. Soc. Workshop, Bethesda, MD, 1979.)

KINDWALL, E. P. 1976. Medical examination of the diver. In: *Diving Medicine*, edited by R. H. Strauss. New York: Grune and Stratton, p. 341–347.

MARTYS, C. R. 1979. Adverse reactions to drugs in general practice. *Br. Med. J.* 2: 1194–1197.

NICODEMUS, H. F. 1980. Anesthesia under high pressure. In: *Interaction of Drugs in the Hyperbaric Environment*, edited by J. M. Walsh. Bethesda, MD: Undersea Medical Society, p. 61–68. (Undersea Med. Soc. Workshop, Bethesda, MD, 1979.)

THOMAS, J. R., AND J. M. WALSH 1978. Behavioral evaluation of pharmacological agents under hyperbaric air and helium oxygen. In: *Underwater Physiology VI. Proceedings of the Sixth Symposium on Underwater Physiology, 1978*, edited by C. W. Shilling and M. B. Beckett. Bethesda, MD: Fed. Am. Soc. Exp. Biol., p. 69–77.

WALSH, J. M. 1974. Amphetamine effects on timing behavior in rats under hyperbaric conditions. *Aerosp. Med.* 45: 721–726.

WALSH, J. M. 1976. Drugs and diving. In: *Diving Medicine*, edited by R. H. Strauss. New York: Grune and Stratton, p. 197–209.

WALSH, J. M., AND L. S. BURCH 1979. The acute effects of commonly used drugs on human performance in hyperbaric air. *Undersea Biomed. Res.* 6(Suppl):49.

B. Anesthesia for Emergency Surgery under High Pressure

The physician involved with the delivery of medical care to divers must familiarize himself with the compression facilities near the location of his practice. A contingency plan for handling medical emergencies under hyperbaric conditions must include knowledge of the following: size of the chamber and available work space; kind of bed or table in the chamber and its limitation for changing positions; lighting; engineering facilities to assist in setting up such things as a system for gas delivery to the patient, suctions, and monitoring systems; locks for entrance of personnel and supplies; and, not the least, information about the available trained help. These are the same facts that a surgical team needs should the physician require the services of one. The plan must also include a list of available drugs and portable equipment (see Tables X-8). Although most diving facilities stock their own emergency drugs and instrument packs, there is no uniformity, so one cannot always depend on the emergency stock. Adequate preparation is the single most important factor that determines the outcome of a surgical emergency, assuming that anesthesia and surgical skills are available.

The purpose of this chapter is to provide some guidelines in the emergency anesthesia care for the surgical patient while under high pressure. It is hoped that this chapter will help the physician-practitioner of diving medicine to formulate a plan of approach when confronted with a surgical emergency. The plan must be applicable at all depths and at all inspired gas mixtures.

Much of the information about drugs commonly used during anesthesia and about the technical skills necessary for safe practice of anesthesia is well described in standard textbooks of anesthesiology. Two such books that should be part of the physician's library are Dripps et al. (1977) and Moore (1975). It is further recommended that the physician obtain the manual dexterity required in the conduct of anesthesia from practical courses at an anesthesia clinic. Most training centers would welcome such preceptorships by physicians and paramedics.

With increasing use of the saturation dive at ever-increasing depths and its mandatory long decompression time, physicians may find themselves dealing with common surgical emergencies such as appendicitis, bleeding or perforated ulcers, torsion of the testicle, incarcerated hernia, and traumatic injuries to various parts of the body that require immediate surgical intervention.

To meet the increasing demands on his expertise, a practitioner of high pressure medicine must also be familiar with resuscitation, care of the unconscious patient, and the use of hypnotic sedative drugs, muscle relaxants, and some regional anesthetic blocks. While staying on the surface the physician may be expected to direct resuscitation or a minor anesthetic and surgical procedure in an underwater habitat by means of an electronic audiovisual communication system, usually with considerable voice distortion. At depth he may have to administer anesthesia and perform surgical procedures as well as provide postoperative care of a patient recovering from anesthesia.

Most of the anesthetic problems during surgery in a hyperbaric chamber at less than 6 ATA pressure have been previously addressed (McDowal 1964; Pittinger 1966; Severinghaus 1966; Smith et al. 1964; Spence and Smith 1964). The present state of technology easily overcomes many of the problems presented in these references, which are unfortunately based on actual hyperbaric operating room facilities and may not apply in the realistic industrial setting of a saturation dive. Nonetheless, pharmacologic problems remain because of the general lack of information regarding the dose response to drugs when administered to patients while under increased pressure. There is also a paucity of pharmacologic data from animal models closely resembling man.

When confronted with a surgical emergency, the choice is between (1) general anesthesia, i.e., total loss of the patient's consciousness during the entire operative procedure and (2) local anesthesia with or without sedation, i.e., pain relief in a conscious patient who is able to cooperate with the physician during surgery. The ill-defined state between local and general anesthesia, when the patient is unable to cooperate and is neither awake nor asleep, should be avoided. Short-acting general anesthetics should be chosen, especially when decompression is anticipated. Wakefulness is an important sign to be monitored during decompression. When the sensorium is depressed, signs of gas embolism or decompression sickness may be masked or modified by the interaction of pressure, anesthetic, and the gas mixture employed. A delay in the definitive therapy may cause injury or death.

1. Protection of the Airway

Whatever technique is chosen, the anesthetist must have the ability to control the airway adequately. For our use adequate control of the airway may be defined as the set of conditions that allows unobstructed ventilation and removal of secretion, prevents pulmonary aspiration of solid and liquid particles, and enables positive pressure artificial respiration to be administered when necessary. Examples are: an endotracheal tube securely taped in place and connected to a breathing system; a watertight tube cuff that prevents gastric contents from getting into the tracheobronchial tree and allows positive pressure ventilation without too much leak; and a good suction apparatus to guarantee an adequately controlled airway. An overview of tracheal intubation is presented below. Most standard textbooks of anesthesiology have vivid descriptions of tracheal intubation and its indications. Some practice is required to gain these skills.

In most cases, awake intubation is the safest course of action to take. With little practice, blind nasal intubation is the easiest and least traumatic approach and also requires the least equipment. In the uncooperative patient, manual restraints by assistants may be required together with slow, deliberate titration of intravenous sedative, but only to the point when struggling ceases, and certainly not to apnea. In case the breathing stops, artificial respiration by manual compression of the chest allows some tidal exchange, which will serve as a guide to nasotracheal intubation and permit a limited time to perform the necessary steps.

The common misconception that local or spinal anesthesia will do away with the need to control the airway could not be further from the truth. Local or spinal anesthesia may merely put off emergency tracheal intubation, so that when the need arises intubation becomes more difficult and the time available so short that it often leads to avoidable complications such as broken teeth, lacerations in the mouth and lips, aspiration pneumonia, hypoxemic cardiac arrest, and death.

In the course of an inadequate local or spinal anesthesia, when the patient is unable to cooperate, the operative field becomes unsuitable for the completion of the operation.

Table X-8
Suggested Basic Equipment for Anesthesia/Surgery at High Pressure

Equipment	Strength	Size or unit	Quantity
Supplies for airway and positive pressure ventilation (see Fig. X-2)			
Clear plastic masks		Large	1
		Medium	1
Oral airway		Large	1
		Medium	1
Nasal airway		8.5 mm i.d.	1
		7.5 mm i.d.	1
Endotracheal tubes		7.5 mm i.d., uncut	2
Laryngoscope, handle, and extra batteries			
Laryngoscope blades with extra light bulbs		#2 straight blade,	1
		#3 curved blade	1
Suction catheters		14 French	4
		Yankauer	2
Suction apparatus (foot operated)			
Stylet			1
Ophthalamic ointment		Tube	1
Lubricant jelly with or without anesthetic drug		Tube	1
Tracheostomy tube, disposable, with cuff		7.5 mm i.d.	1
		8.5 mm i.d.	1
Nasogastric tube, sump		18 French	2
Monitoring equipment			
Stethoscope			
Esophageal stethoscope			1
Blood pressure cuff and dial			
Stick-on EKG electrode and leads			
CVP manometers			2
Urinary catheters (Foley) and collecting bag		Packs	2
Urine pH test tape			
Dextrostix			
Fluids and administration and procedural supplies			
Dextrose in water	5%	1000-ml plastic bags	4
Ringer's lactate solution	5%	1000-ml plastic bags	4
NaCl solution	0.9%	1000-ml plastic bags	2
Human albumin solution	25%	100-ml	2
Blood recipient sets			3
Macrodrip i.v. infusion sets			6
Microdrip i.v. infusion sets			2
Intravenous extension sets			6
Three-way stopcocks			6
Plastic venous cannulas		14 gauge	12
Plastic venous cannulas		16 gauge	12
Plastic venous cannulas		18 gauge	6
Central venous catheters		14 gauge, 12 in.	4
Central venous catheters		14 gauge, 24 in.	2

Table X-8 Continued

Equipment	Strength	Size of unit	Quantity
Syringes		2 ml	10
		5 ml	10
		10 ml	6
		30 ml	6
		50 ml	3
Needles		18 gauge	20
		20 gauge	20
		22 gauge	20
		25 gauge	20
Spinal needles		22 gauge	3
		25 gauge	3
Intravenous infusion filters			2
Spinal trays, prepacked			2
Tetracaine	2%	Ampules	3
Dextrose in water	10%	5-ml ampules	3
Epidural trays, with catheter,			2
extra catheters in separate packages			2
Epidural lidocaine	1.5% with 1:200,000 parts epinephrine		4
Miscellaneous			
Tapes			
Betadine swabs			
Betadine ointment			
Tourniquets for starting i.v.			

The physician has no other recourse but to resort to general anesthesia. At this gray area of partial anesthesia, many a well-trained anesthetist has wished he had no ears (noise from the patient and the surgeon distracts his attention) but instead had another pair of hands to help in the control of the patient's movements, in the control of the airway, and in the conversion to general anesthesia.

Under hyperbaric conditions, physicians should reserve local or spinal anesthesia for operative procedures that can be completed within the duration of the block or within the range of safe blood level of local anesthetic drug. Local anesthesia for exploratory procedures should be avoided because of the uncertainty of its extent and duration. When toxicity of local anesthetic manifests as convulsion, the airway must be controlled immediately in all patients, especially those with food in the stomach. Intubation under this condition requires a high level of skill.

With a secured, adequately controlled airway, positive pressure ventilation of the patient may be delegated to the less skilled assistant while the physician proceeds with the surgical intervention. A self-inflating resuscitator bag is needed to ventilate the patient's lungs with the existing gas mixture inside the chamber. To maintain humidity and integrity of the tracheal mucosa, 1–2 ml (cc) saline should be instilled into the endotracheal tube every 30 min. If the engineers could set up a flowmeter, the same gas mixture might

464   Chapter X

be led into an anesthesia breathing bag equipped with a nonrebreathing Ruben valve. (See Figure X-2.)

It has been suggested earlier that the physician acquire the skill of tracheal intubation in an operating room setting, with an anesthetized patient, and under the supervision of an anesthetist. The reason for this is to familiarize the physician with the technique under the best of conditions. The patient's position in relation to the laryngoscopist is very important and easily managed in an operating room; in a hyperbaric chamber the table height may not be adjustable. Emergency tracheal intubation while a patient lies on the floor projects an image of a physician on his knees, trying as best he can to relate his position with that of the patient within the limited work space of the chamber. This clearly is not the time a physician should ever attempt direct visual tracheal intubation.

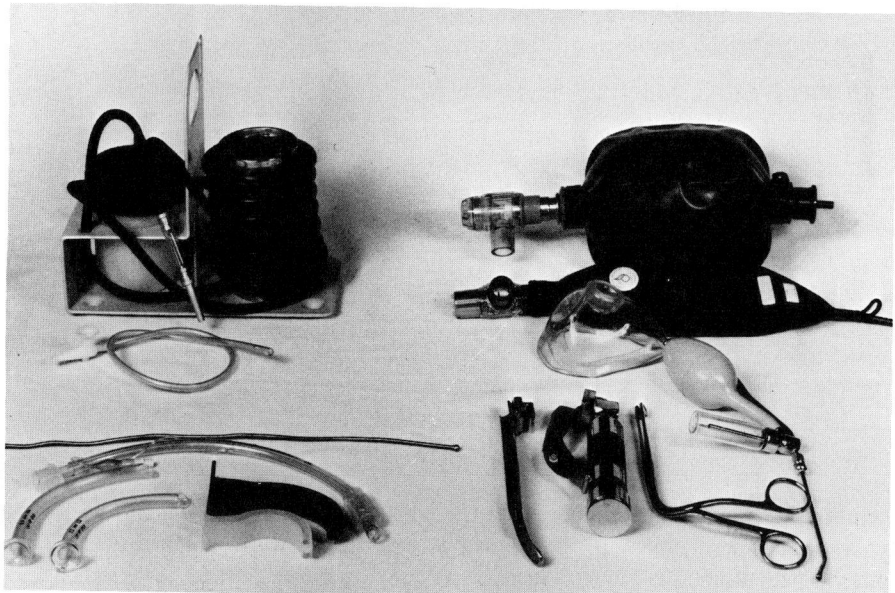

Figure X-2. Basic equipment for airway management. *Top right*, artificial respiration group: self-inflating bag (AMBU); 2-liter anesthesia breathing bag with Ruben valve; clear plastic mask. *Bottom right*, instrumentation group: sprayer; Magill forceps; laryngoscope with curved blade; straight blade. *Bottom left*, airway group: two sizes oral airways; two sizes nasal airways; 7.5-mm i.d. endotracheal tube; stylet. *Top left*, suction group: foot-operated suction; suction catheter.

a. Direct Visual Tracheal Intubation

Direct visualization of the glottis requires a laryngoscope; this is in contrast to indirect visualization, which requires a laryngeal mirror. The technique of direct visual intubation is the same whether the patient is anesthetized or awake; however, the awake patient needs more emotional preparation. It is of utmost importance that rapport and confidence develop between the patient and the physician. The patient must realize that the contemplated procedure is the only safe option he has under the circumstances, and that the physician's approach to the surgical problem offers the highest probability of survival. A note about this transaction should be entered in the patient's record.

If the patient had not fasted and will not allow awake intubation, the last resort is to give an antacid, insert the largest nasogastric tube available, and lavage the stomach till the return is clear. This maneuver does not always remove large food particles but will decrease the volume and acidity of the gastric contents and lessen the morbidity should aspiration take place. The physician may then proceed with direct visual intubation under general anesthesia. An assistant should apply pressure on the cricoid cartilage to prevent regurgitation of the remaining gastric contents during intubation. Unless the physician is certain that he can manually ventilate the patient, using a mask and quick intubation of the trachea, no muscle relaxant should be used. The use of a rapid sequence of induction, then muscle relaxant, then intubation should also be discouraged. This approach should be reserved for physicians with wide experience in anesthesia care.

The physician should stay at the patient's head during laryngoscopy. A 3-in. (7.5-cm) pillow may improve visualization of the glottis. For awake intubation, topical anesthesia of the tongue and pharynx obtained with nebulized 2%–4% lidocaine stops most of the gagging and eases the insertion of the blade. To preserve the cough reflex, in case the patient aspirates, the tracheal mucosa is not anesthetized. The patient is instructed to open the mouth wide or, better yet, to slide the lower jaw anteriorly so as to provide a wide space for insertion of the blade. The blade is held with the left hand and introduced on the right side of the tongue until the epiglottis is visible. Cooperation is better obtained if the patient's attention is directed to his breathing and he is given vocal assurance that he is doing what is required of him. Voice contact with the patient, a most important part of the technique, should not be lost, as this reinforces his confidence and desire to cooperate.

The tip of a curved blade rests on the valecula, whereas the tip of a straight blade is advanced about 2 cm farther in to pick up the epiglottis. A forward and upward lift at a 45° angle raises the mandible and head, exposing the glottis. The wrist of the instrument hand should be held firmly without a prying motion to avoid using the upper incisors as fulcrum for the blade. Several layers of adhesive taped on the part of the blade that touches the teeth, but not obstructing the view, afford added protection to the teeth. (The fragments from a broken tooth must be found, and those that got into the trachea must be removed at any cost, for it acts as foreign body and can cause lung abscess.) Gentle extension of the neck or depression of the thyroid cartilage may improve the view of the glottis. As the laryngoscope supports the entire head, gentle pressure on the occiput may further extend the head to improve the exposure. After several attempts, both the physician and the patient become more familiar with the technique. The endotracheal tube (cuff pretested, 7.5 mm i.d. is adequate for most adults) is inserted on the right side of the mouth without obstructing the view of the glottis. If the curvature of the tube is not correct a stylet will help keep the shape. The tube is inserted until the cuff barely disappears into the trachea. The cuff should be filled with water or saline until it is airtight to assure positive pressure ventilation (Ross et al. 1977).

Similar steps are followed for intubation under anesthesia. Because an anesthetized patient cannot swallow, secretion in the pharynx could be more troublesome. Aspiration of acidic gastric contents could trigger bronchospasm and cyanosis in the patient (Mendelson's syndrome).

b. Blind Nasotracheal Intubation

A pillow should be used to support the patient's head in a sniffing position (as in smelling flowers). The wider naris should be chosen and the nasal mucosa shrunk with phenylephrine or ephedrine, or cocaine if available. Cotton applicators or a nebulizer may be used to apply topical anesthesia on the nasal mucosa, concentrating on the area of the inferior turbinate and floor of the nasal cavity. The surface anesthesia should also include the pharynx, an unnecessary step if the patient is under general anesthesia. A well-lubricated 7.5-mm (i.d.) tube (uncut; cuff pretested for integrity) is inserted directly posteriorly, close to the floor of the nasal cavity, with the bevel preferably sliding on the nasal septum. There is a distinct give as the tip of the tube passes through the posterior naris. When the tube is turned so that the convexity is directed cephalad, the tip then goes in a caudad direction. The breath sound heard through the external end of the tube is loudest as the tube nears the glottis. For alignment of the tube with the glottis, the shaft of the tube is twisted to the right or to the left, increasing or decreasing its curvature; or by observing the bulge on the neck created by the tip of the tube, the physician can manually move the larynx from side to side (Bennett et al. 1978). A short, gentle stabbing motion generally gets the tip past the glottis. Tracheal intubation is indicated by a good airflow through the tube, coughing, and inability to vocalize.

Direct visual nasotracheal intubation requires laryngoscopy similar to oral intubation. Once in the hypopharynx, the tip of the tube is guided as in blind nasal intubation, or with a Magill forceps. The endotracheal tube is taped securely. Extubation is described in the outline for general anesthesia at the end of this chapter.

The complications of intubation of the trachea are laryngospasm if the intubation fails, bronchospasm, mucosal bleeding, and dislodgement of the tube. Laryngospasm is frequent and predisposes to cyanosis and cardiac arrhythmia, although fatalities are rare. To break laryngospasm without using muscle relaxants, the mask is held tightly over the face so that there is no gas leak around the mask, and the breathing bag is gently squeezed to apply progressively firmer pressure on the glottis. A high-pitched sound with each respiration indicates that air is flowing into the lungs. The maneuver generally doesn't fail, but many choose to break laryngospasm with a small dose (5–10 mg i.v.) of succinylcholine. Because the oxygen in the breathing mixture is only a third of an atmosphere, it may take longer for cyanosis to disappear even after the laryngospasm is broken.

2. *Regional Anesthesia*

A large number of major surgical procedures are performed under regional or under field block anesthesia. A successful case of major bowel resection has been reported (Carter and Goldsmith 1970), performed under local field block and sedation while in a hyperbaric chamber with limited space and help. The objection to the use of local anesthesia is the unpredictability that the operation can be completed without having to resort to general anesthesia as well as the need for airway control.

Nearly all surgical procedures in the extremities would involve traumatic injuries ranging from lacerations to fractures with or without nerve or vascular involvement. Most of these operations could be performed with the use of regional anesthetic techniques—spinal anesthesia or a conduction block of a major plexus of nerves. Some of these techniques may be modified so that the anesthetic drug can be applied continuously for long periods. For operative procedures in the lower abdomen and lower extremities, spinal anesthesia is a well-proved, safe, and simple method of pain relief that has the added advantage of total muscle relaxation. These methods are discussed to provide the physician enough information on their use; for more detail, however, Moore's book (1975) is invaluable.

Several authors (Kendig and Cohen 1977; Roth et al. 1976) have reported that pressure reverses nerve conduction block induced with either local or general anesthesia, but whether or not local anesthesia will work is not the concern here. We are assured that local anesthesia is effective under high pressure inasmuch as all clinical methods of bathing the nerves in local anesthetic solution use a concentration high enough to overcome the effect of pressure, to the extent that the anesthetic procedure itself constitutes a gross overdose of anesthetic drug. Of greater interest to the anesthetist is the influence of pressure on the duration of effect. Nicodemus and colleagues (1981) have shown that the duration of tetracaine spinal blocks at pressures as high as 32 ATA lasts as long as those in 1 ATA. The data suggest that blood flow and the subsequent washout of local anesthesia is not or is little affected by the pressure. Unfortunately, the method they reported involved induction of spinal block at 1 ATA and cannot give information on the onset (uptake) if the block had been administered under pressure.

a. Toxicity of Local Anesthetics

Available information indicates that the effect of pressure on the toxicity of drugs constitutes a minor problem (Small 1970). R.E. Herold and H.F. Nicodemus (unpublished data) found that hyperbaric air or oxygen increased the dose of lidocaine needed to induce convulsion in guinea pigs. They concluded that the safe limits of the surface doses of lidocaine are just as safe to use under as much pressure as 6 ATA air. Krenis et al. (1971) presented data that subhypnotic doses of lidocaine and cocaine protected against the central nervous system toxicity of high pressure oxygen. Pretreatment with subhypnotic doses of diazepam nearly doubles the amount of local anesthetic necessary to induce convulsion in cats (de Jong and Heavner 1972). Herold and Nicodemus (unpublished data) failed to show alterations in the anticonvulsant property of diazepam in guinea pigs when challenged with convulsive doses of lidocaine in 3 ATA oxygen or 6 ATA air. Nevertheless, caution should be exercised when diazepam, local anesthesia, and a high partial pressure of nitrogen are combined, because a far greater depression may occur and be misinterpreted as arising from other causes. Furthermore, the increased dose requirement for both local anesthetic drug and partial pressure of oxygen necessary to induce convulsion does not guarantee that the high pressure of oxygen will not cause cellular damage.

Inasmuch as there is little known about the changes in toxicity of drugs when administered under high pressure, the manifestations of toxicity of local anesthetic drugs in 1 ATA also apply under pressure. Toxicity is related to blood level and the speed with which blood level is attained. Some factors that determine the peak level and the rate of rise (Moore 1975) are: (1) intravascular injection; (2) use of too high a concentration;

(3) use of excessive volume; and (4) injection into a highly vascular area. Prevention of toxicity includes (1) use of the least effective concentration to accomplish the block; (2) use of epinephrine-containing solution to delay absorption (except for digital blocks); (3) repeated aspiration for blood during induction of the block; and (4) careful attention to the total dose of local anesthetic. Pretreatment with subhypnotic doses of diazepam will not prevent other signs of toxicity but may prevent or soften the convulsion.

Central nervous system toxicity is related not only to the total dose or intravenous injection but also to the speed with which a convulsive level is reached. In many deaths from dental anesthesia intra-arterial injection of a small amount of local anesthetic led to an overflow into the carotid artery and then to the cerebral circulation, resulting in convulsion (Aldrete et al. 1978). Aspiration for blood before injection should lessen this possibility. Convulsion from central nervous system toxicity to local anesthetics need not be a fearsome complication were it not for the possibility of airway obstruction and aspiration of vomitus or secretion. Although the individual convulsive dose for lidocaine is not known, central nervous system toxicity may be anticipated if the total dose approaches 6 mg/kg body wt. The initial symptoms in human beings consist of lightheadedness and dizziness followed by auditory and visual disturbances such as tinnitus and difficulty in focusing. Drowsiness, disorientation, and temporary loss of consciousness may also occur. Immediate precursors of convulsion are slurred speech, muscle twitching, and tremors of the face and extremities.

Even small doses of either thiopental or diazepam may prevent, shorten, or soften an oncoming convulsion. Discretion at this point is most difficult. The depressant effect of the anticonvulsant potentiates that response to the systemic effect of the local anesthetic: when superimposed on a postictal state the result can be cessation of respiration. In addition, cardiovascular collapse can occur from toxicity of local anesthetics.

Toxicities of other local anesthetic drugs are similar to those of lidocaine. Lidocaine is singled out because it is a drug with many uses other than local anesthesia and because it is one of the most widely studied local anesthetics.

b. Techniques

(i) Spinal Anesthesia. CAUTION: Spinal anesthesia must not be administered if there are symptoms of spinal cord decompression sickness, nor should the patient be decompressed if there is residual spinal block.

Detailed description for administration appears in the recommended textbooks. Spinal anesthesia as discussed here includes pain relief obtained from epidural or subarachnoid application of drugs on the nerves that form the cauda equina. For epidural application of drugs, lumbar and caudal (though the sacral hiatus) methods are popular. Insertion of a fine catheter into the epidural space makes it possible to continuously apply the drug on the spinal nerves. Hypotension may complicate any of the methods of spinal anesthesia. The cause of the fall in blood pressure is sympathetic block occurring during the first 5 min. The most rapid onset is seen in subarachnoid block, a much slower one in epidural block, although the level of hypotension may be the same. Prevention and treatment of hypotension, regardless of the initiating block, are the same. Less frequent and less severe hypotension occurs in the patient preloaded with 0.5–1.0 liter of intravenous fluid before the block is instituted. Rapid fluid infusion, and if necessary, intravenous injection of a vasopressor (ephedrine, 25 mg), generally corrects the hypotension. Repeated injection of vasopressor is seldom required. Elevation of both legs above the level of the body is also a rapid method of infusing about 500 ml of blood into the general circulation and may rapidly reverse the hypotension. For the healthy patient on diving status the only contraindications to spinal anesthesia are minor ones, the most serious of which is hypovolemia as a result of the trauma. The initial therapy consists of fluid replacement, and if the blood volume appears adequate (normal heart rate and no hypotension when the patient sits up), spinal anesthesia may be instituted. Without therapy the sympathetic block could precipitate dangerously severe hypotension and cardiovascular collapse.

Subarachnoid block. As applied to healthy divers, subarachnoid block (SAB) is simple and safe. After the patient is preloaded with intravenous fluid, spinal tap is performed in any of the lumbar spaces but preferably below the first lumbar intervertebral space. A line drawn between the iliac crests passes through the fourth lumbar intervertebral space. Proper positioning of the patient, i.e., having the patient roll up into a ball, widens the spaces. The simplest instruction is for the patient to try to touch his symphysis pubis with his chin. The lumbar puncture may be performed with the patient on his side or sitting up. With 0.2 ml (cc) epinephrine added to the spinal drug the usual duration of the block is 3–4 hr. The doses and the expected level of block as well as the corresponding landmarks are shown in Figure X-3. Strict attention must be paid to asepsis and antisepsis without allowing any of the antiseptic to get into the spinal canal through a contaminated needle.

Because the specific gravity of the spinal drug mixed with an equal volume of 10% dextrose in water is heavier than that of the cerebrospinal fluid (CSF), the drug flows

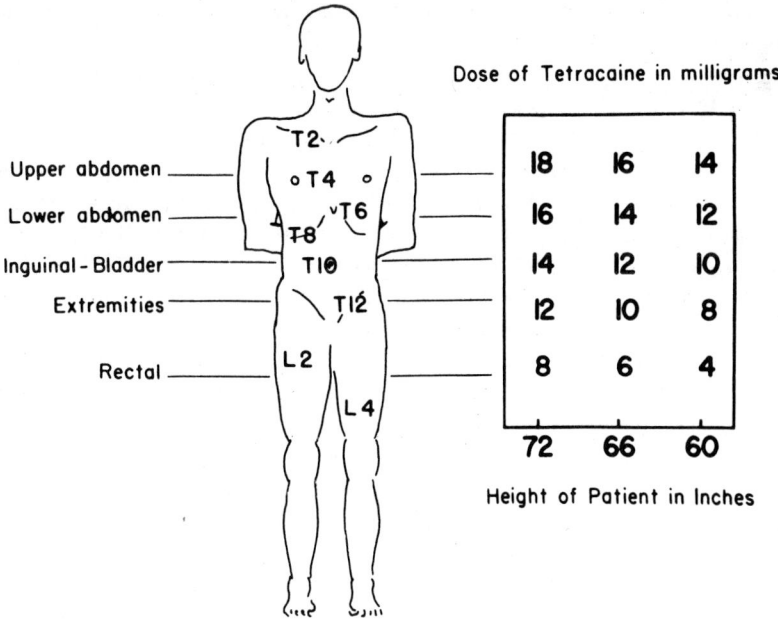

Figure X-3. Approximate sensory levels of anesthesia required for operative site indicated. [From Dripps et al. (1977), with permission.]

"downhill." It is possible to extend the level of the block to a higher thoracic segment during the first 10 min by simply putting the patient in Trendelenberg's position. Once the drug is fixed on the nerves its level cannot be changed with any predictability. Response to pin prick determines the segmental level of sensory block. The physician who rarely administers spinal anesthesia should not allow the level to go higher than T4 or T2 lest it cause respiratory difficulty. Should the block rise to the cervical segments, the patient becomes dyspneic and unable to feel his own breathing. Breathing can be assisted manually with a self-inflating or anesthesia breathing bag and mask. If all respiratory effort disappears, then the block is total and the patient will require control of the airway and artificial respiration until the block recedes to the thoracic segments. It is safer to intubate the patient and complete the operation as in general anesthesia. When food in the stomach is suspected, the patient must be intubated immediately, because coughing is ineffective with high spinal block even without phrenic nerve anesthesia. Once the airway is adequately controlled, ventilation may be delegated to an assistant.

High spinal block often includes the cardiac accelerator nerve and may result in bradycardia in the presence of hypotension. Small, repeated intravenous doses of ephedrine (5–10 mg) or atropine (0.2 mg) generally stabilize the patient's heart rate.

Many physically fit patients with high spinal anesthesia complain of nausea and vomiting. These symptoms may be a prelude to hypotension and may respond well to ephedrine. Occasionally the patient does not become hypotensive, yet nausea may persist. The mechanism is not clear; however, the unopposed vagus nerve may be the reason for the persistent nausea. Small intravenous doses of atropine may help; otherwise verbal assurance is all that may be required. A small amount of vomitus with few or no food particles is reassuring to the physician should he need to proceed or supplement with general anesthesia; it means an empty stomach, and anesthesia may be maintained with bag and mask.

Lumbar epidural block. The indications and procedure for lumbar epidural block are similar to those for SAB except for the insertion of a larger needle—beyond the ligamentum flavum but not puncturing the dura mater. The larger needle allows insertion of the catheter for a continuous or intermittent injection of drug into the epidural space. The catheter and needles needed for the procedure can be obtained prepackaged together with the drugs. The distinct advantage of epidural block over SAB is the absence of postlumbar puncture headache if there has been no dural puncture. Nevertheless, there is no guarantee against this complication even if no CSF is obtained, for the dura mater may be entered during or even after placement of the catheter.

To locate the epidural space, the 17-gauge epidural needle is inserted slowly while a 10-ml (cc) syringe with 2–3 ml saline (no air) is attached to the hub of the needle. The needle is advanced slowly while gentle finger pressure is applied to the plunger. As the needle pierces the ligamentum flavum, the physician feels a sudden loss of resistance to the injection of saline. Under hyperbaric conditions no gas is injected into the epidural space. With saline injection, it may be difficult to distinguish CSF leak (a possible result of subarachnoid placement of the needle) from the backflow of saline. Subarachnoid placement is determined with 2 ml of the anesthetic solution injected through the needle. If the placement is epidural, no block is descernible; however, if it is subarachnoid, a rapid onset and wider distribution of block is obtained.

Kermorgant (1978) believes that it is advantageous to insert a catheter into the epidural space even if a single dose is adequate for the contemplated procedure. He mentions that the catheter will allow egress of gas from the epidural space should the patient undergo decompression. The catheter is advanced 2–3 cm beyond the tip of the needle (there are marks on the catheter); as the needle is withdrawn, the catheter is held with the other hand so as not to change its position. After the catheter is well taped to the back of the patient a test dose of 2–3 ml of the epinephrine-containing solution is again administered, to determine if the catheter remained epidural. Subarachnoid placement is indicated by rapid onset and wider block, whereas intravascular injection may manifest as tachycardia. Inadvertent subarchnoid placement of the catheter may be utilized for continuous SAB with titration of the doses of spinal drug; otherwise the epidural tap should be repeated at another space.

Two milliliters (cc) of anesthetic solution for each spinal segment, or about 20 ml of 1.5% lidocaine with 1:200,000 parts epinephrine, usually suffices for most abdominal procedures and will last about 2.5 hr. Specially prepared solutions without preservative are available in ampules or in vials specifically labeled for epidural use. A 3% solution of 2-chloroprocaine hydrochloride produces faster onset of anesthesia, although it has a shorter duration. Pseudocholinesterase hydrolyzes chloroprocaine so that systemic toxicity is virtually unknown.

The need to reinject anesthesia is determined by the sensory level of the block or by the patient discomfort. Although bacterial filters are often used with the catheter, strict aseptic technique should be followed. The catheter is first aspirated for blood or CSF. If CSF is obtained in the middle of an operation the catheter must be pulled out about 1 cm or until CSF can no longer be aspirated. The test dose is then repeated. If adequate anesthesia occurs with the test dose there is a very good chance that the catheter is still subarachnoid. Use of the catheter may be continued for continuous SAB. On the other hand, if blood is aspirated, the catheter must be withdrawn until blood can no longer be aspirated. A repeat test dose will produce tachycardia (from epinephrine) if the catheter is still intravascular; otherwise the maintenance dose of 10–15 ml of the anesthetic solution is injected. Bleeding in the epidural space is rarely symptomatic, probably because most bleeding is venous and tamponades itself before any pressure can cause nerve damage. Injection of epinephrine-containing solution also helps in making the hole in the vessel wall smaller.

Complications and treatment. With the loss of CSF through the hole in the dura, CSF pressure falls, causing traction on the pain-sensitive structures as the brain settles on the floor of the cranial cavity. Some of the cranial nerves are stretched, causing auditory and visual symptoms along with headache, which is postural in nature—less when the patient is lying down and worse in the head-up position. The incidence, duration, and severity are directly related to the size of the dural hole, so that with a 24-gauge needle there is an incidence of 6% in the general population; with 17-gauge, about 18%. The incidence is higher yet if lumbar puncture was performed for perinatal analgesia.

Treatment of this headache consists of keeping the patient flat in bed to diminish the CSF leak; use of analgesics; attempting to increase CSF pressure by increasing fluid intake; or by tight abdominal binders to dilate the epidural veins (Dripps 1977; Gromley 1960). Enlarged veins in the epidural space decrease the size of the spinal dural tube. Because the rent on the dura created by a large needle may persist for days, the headache may be incapacitating to the patient. The treatment consists of a repeat epidural tap and injection of 20 ml saline into the epidural space. The volume of the injectate makes the dural tube smaller, thereby increasing the CSF pressure and relieving the headache. Some patients, however, require a repeat epidural saline injection. In these cases, after the epidural needle is placed, 10–20 ml of the patient's blood is drawn aseptically from an arm vein and injected epidurally, usually with immediate and lasting relief (Di Giovanni et al. 1972, Glass and Kennedy 1972). The clot that forms patches the dural rent, and the volume tamponades the dural tube, increasing CSF pressure. Very rarely is a repeat blood patch required.

Headache after lumbar puncture has been reported days after the patch, when the patient traveled by air and became decompressed to 10,000 feet above sea level (Mulroy 1979, Vacanti 1972). Similar headaches could occur during decompression from high pressure air.

(ii) Brachial Plexus Blocks. According to an unsigned article in a symposium edited by Carron (1980), for most operations in the upper extremities conduction block on the brachial plexus provides adequate anesthesia to the entire arm and, in some cases, the shoulder. There are several approaches, two of which have the least possibility of serious complications (Moore 1975).

Axillary block. With the patient supine, the arm is abducted to 90°. The forearm is flexed and rotated so that the dorsum of the hand touches the table. The axillary artery is palpated at the apex of the axilla. At this point a 1.0-in. (25-mm) 22-gauge needle is inserted tangential to the artery until a "click" is felt as the needle penetrates the fascial sheath (Fig. X-4). After aspiration for blood, 40 ml of 1.5% lidocaine with 1:200,000 parts epinephrine is deposited. Periodic aspiration makes certain that the injection is not intravascular. If a vessel is punctured, the needle is simply withdrawn until blood can no longer be aspirated, and the drug is injected. Paresthesia may be elicited as the needle touches a nerve; if paresthesia is persistent, the needle is withdrawn and reinserted before injection of the drug. Because the fascial compartment envelops the axillary artery and the nerves, perivascular injection such as described allows spread of local anesthesia to involve the entire brachial plexus. A good block may last up to 3 hr.

Inadvertent phrenic nerve block, vagus nerve or recurrent laryngeal nerve block, and stellate ganglion block are virtually impossible with an axillary approach. Pressure applied on the punctured vessel avoids hematoma formation, but even if it forms it has little clinical significance. Malignancies or lymphadenopathy from active infection in the arm would contraindicate axillary block.

Interscalene brachial plexus block. The fascia that envelops the brachial plexus may be entered high in the neck closer to the origin of the nerves (Winnie 1970). The supine patient, arms at side, rotates the head away from the side of the block. As the patient lifts the head, the clavicular head of the sternomastoid muscle becomes prominent. Starting from the lateral border of the sternomastoid, a finger is rolled across the belly of the anterior scalene muscle to the groove between the anterior and middle scalene muscles. This point corresponds to the tubercle of Chassaignac, which is frequently palpable. A 1.5-in. (30-mm) 22-gauge needle is inserted perpendicular to the skin in a mesiad, caudad, and downward (toward the table) direction until paresthesia is obtained (Figure X-5). The paresthesia should be transient before 20–30 ml of 1.5% lidocaine with 1:200,000 parts epinephrine is injected. Periodic aspiration for blood is needed to avoid intravascular injection.

The technique is indicated when the patient cannot abduct the arm or under conditions where the axillary approach is contraindicated. The anesthesia is adequate for shoulder manipulation and certain operations in the shoulder. Pneumothorax is virtually nonex-

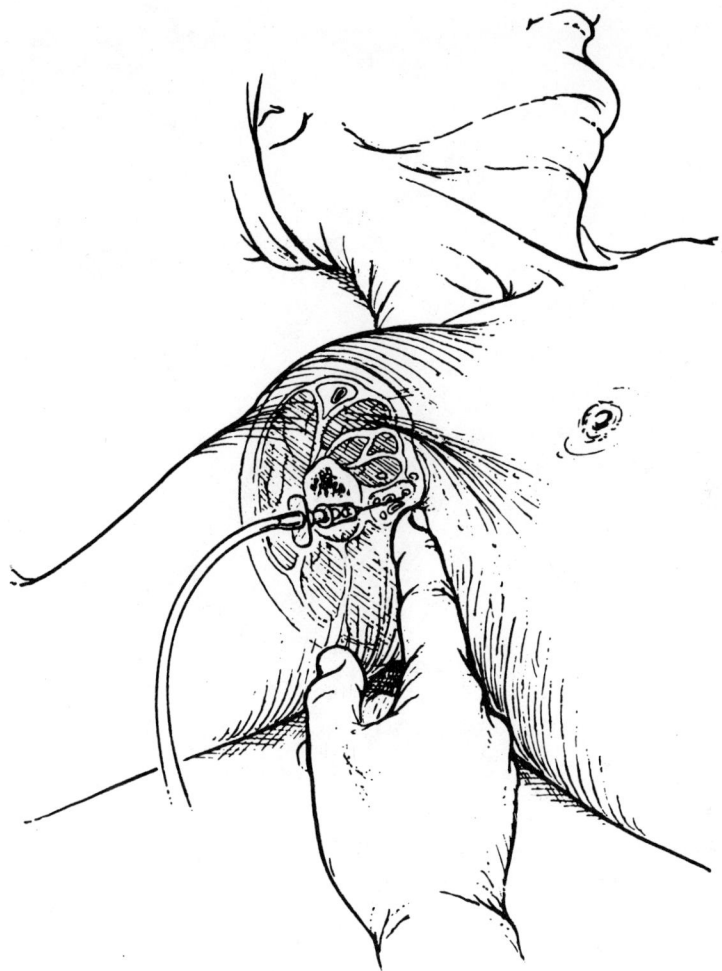

Figure X-4. Schematic diagram of needle placement for axillary block, perivascular approach. Position of the needle is more stable with use of intravenous extension tube. [From Winnie (1970), with permission.]

istent, although stellate ganglion block and phrenic nerve blocks are frequent. Very rarely subarachnoid injection occurs, in which case the treatment is that of total spinal anesthesia, i.e., intubation and manual artificial ventilation of the patient until the block recedes.

With the use of a 20-gauge needle–plastic cannula combination (e.g., Venocath) during the plexus block, the catheter may be left in place for intermittent reinjection, thereby prolonging the block indefinitely. The procedure as such has a high failure rate, however.

(iii) Intercostal Nerve Blocks. Intercostal blocks provide pain relief for multiple rib fractures and many intra-abdominal operations, including hernia. The segmental distribution on the abdomen was described in connection with spinal anesthesia (Figure X-3). The ribs may be counted from the 12th rib along the posterior axillary line upward or downward from the sternal angle of Louis (2nd rib). For wide or total abdominal wall anesthesia, bilateral lower six intercostal block may be performed. Unless pain relief is also required in the back, the block may be done along the midaxillary line.

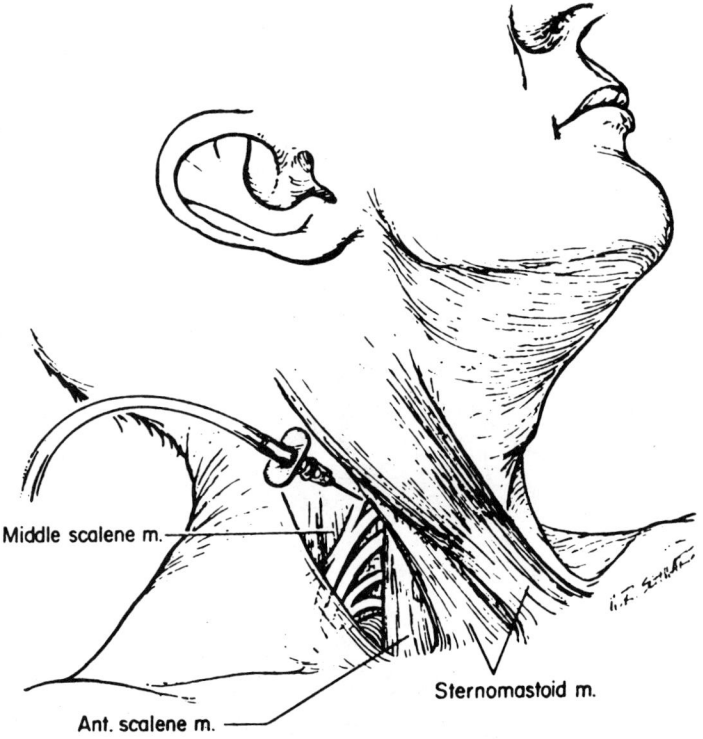

Figure X-5. Schematic diagram of interscalene block. [From Winnie (1970), with permission.]

Although the technique is very useful there is great danger of pneumothorax, which is highest when performed by physicians less familiar with the block. When pneumothorax occurs under the hyperbaric condition the symptoms are those found in 1 ATA; it could, however, become much worse and under tension when the patient undergoes decompression. Of course, the treatment is thoracostomy with underwater seal or Heimlich valve.

The ribs must be mapped out and all the segments to be blocked must be marked. A 22-gauge, 1-in. (25-mm) needle attached to a 10-ml syringe is inserted tangential to the rib and at a small angle so that the syringe practically touches the next lower rib. The lower border of the rib is hit, then the needle is slowly "walked" until it barely misses the lower border of the rib. The needle is advanced about 0.5 cm while hugging the inferior border of the rib with care to not enter the thoracic cavity. Aspiration for blood follows, then injection of 2–3 ml of 1.5% lidocaine with epinephrine. This procedure is repeated with each intercostal nerve. The area of anesthesia is mapped out; partially anesthestized areas are reblocked. Breath sound must be checked before and after the block. With any sign of dyspnea, the possibility of pneumothorax must be considered. When in doubt, the chest must be needled for presence of air and a thoracostomy tube inserted if necessary.

Depending on the number of nerves blocked, the incidence of central nervous system toxicity is high with intercostal blocks because of the wide area of absorption and the vascularity of the chest wall (Moore et al. 1976).

(iv) Other Regional Blocks. The physician caring for traumatic injuries should be familiar with the blocks for small areas of the body such as wrist, ankle, face, and scalp. Area blocks such as these are simpler to perform than infiltration field block. They are more effective and less painful, especially if the operative site is inflamed. These blocks may be studied from the recommended textbooks.

(v) Intravenous Regional Anesthesia (Bier block). Total anesthesia is obtained when local anesthetic solution is injected intravenously into an extremity isolated from the general circulation with a tourniquet (D'Amato and Wielding 1969; Moore 1975). This method is applicable in both the lower and upper extremities and is most conveniently effective for operations in the leg or foot and in the forearm. The requirements are simple and include dilute local anesthetic without epinephrine, 50 ml and 100 ml for upper and lower extremities, respectively; a double tourniquet or two pneumatic tourniquets, and a regulator or reducing valve that can apply constant pressure to the tourniquets to as much as 500 mmHg above the ambient pressure.

Technique. The pneumatic tourniquets are applied side by side on the extremity. An intravenous catheter (18-gauge) is secured in one of the veins distal to the tourniquets. The extremity is exsanguinated with Esmarch's bandage. If the appendage is painful and cannot be moved, Esmarch's bandage is optional. An alternate method that may be used is to apply pressure to occlude the major arterial supply proximal to the tourniquets and elevate the extremity to drain out venous blood. The proximal tourniquet is inflated to 250 mmHg and to 450 mmHg for the upper and lower extremities, respectively. Injection of the local anesthetic (lidocaine 0.25%–0.5%) intravenously into the isolated extremity produces complete anesthesia in 10 min. Anesthesia remains as long as the tourniquet remains inflated. Sensation returns in minutes after deflation and blood flow has been reestablished.

Because the proximal tourniquet is on an unanesthetized segment, pressure from the tourniquet will soon become unbearable. For relief the distal tourniquet on the anesthetized segment is inflated and then the proximal one is deflated.

To prevent a high peak level of local anesthesia at the end of the operation the tourniquet is deflated in stages. A quick deflation, followed by reinflation, flushes out a fraction of the local anesthetic into the systemic circulation. Two to three minutes should be allowed for redistribution before totally deflating the tourniquets. The redistribution avoids a high peak in the plasma level and central nervous system complications. Pretreatment with diazepam (5 mg i.v.) also prevents convulsion from a sudden high blood level of the drug. An alternative method is to allow arterial flow into the extremity while the venous flow is still occluded. Blood (50–100 ml) may then be drawn out of the still-isolated extremity. When the tourniquet is finally released, the total systemic dose will be much less. With use of an indwelling catheter anesthesia may be reinduced with a repeat dose after the tourniquet has been reinflated as previously described. The regulator requires reasonable accuracy; too much pressure may cause pressure damage to the nerves.

3. *General Anesthesia*

General anesthesia is indicated for all operations that cannot be safely performed under regional anesthesia. With reasonable care, general anesthesia is safer than regional or local anesthesia and is certainly more convenient for the patient. The preparation and the equipment required are similar for both regional and general anesthesia. If the physician's task is to be both surgeon and anesthetist, he should opt for general anesthesia whenever practicable. Once the patient is intubated and the breathing is controlled by an assistant, the physician can then proceed with the operation.

a. Inhalation Agents

At pressures higher than 6 ATA, inhalation anesthesia becomes less desirable or impossible. Some of the reasons mentioned by McCracken and colleagues (1979) are: (1) the desire to not contaminate the enclosed atmosphere with anesthetic gases; (2) the difficulty of using flowmeters in a high-density atmosphere of the chamber where flow settings are inaccurate and would require difficult monitoring of the vapor concentration for each chamber pressure setting; (3) the need for a monitoring system for assurance that the patient is normoxic; and (4) the unpredictability of anesthetic dose required to induce and maintain anesthesia under pressure. Flammability, however, is no longer an issue, because of newer nonflammable agents (Baker and Unsworth 1978).

Even if proper calibrations for flowmeters and vaporizers are obtained at an operational depth, and even if contamination of the atmosphere is prevented with proper and efficient scavenging systems, the reluctance to use inhalation anesthetics under high pressure will still exist. Wisely (1976) suggested that inhalation anesthesia is "out of the question" at about 20 ATA. He further suggested the use of intravenous agents, like alfaxalone (Althesin)—a drug mixture whose potency is known to be reduced at high pressure (Bailey et al. 1977).

As mentioned already, one reason for the reluctance to use gaseous anesthetics is the absence of information on dose response of these agents. Anesthesia can be obtained by simply increasing the inspired concentration that might be needed under pressure. It is not known, however, if there is a parallel increase in the tolerance of other organ systems to the agent. For example, the increased alveolar concentration of halothane required to abolish response to painful stimulation under pressure may be devastating to the cardiovascular system, just as methoxyflurane is damaging to the kidneys, making either agent unsafe for hyperbaric use. Furthermore, pressure antagonism and therefore dose requirement is nonlinear, at least for some anesthetic agents (Smith et al. 1979). Unless the physician has had extensive experience at 1 ATA in monitoring the depth of anesthesia and the corresponding cardiovascular responses, it would be safest to stay away from potent inhalation agents.

If this section appears to condemn inhalation methods, it is because of the lack of information for guidance in its safe usage at greater than 3 ATA (Ross et al. 1977).

b. Intravenous Anesthesia

Intravenous general anesthesia is likely to be the choice under hyperbaric conditions despite the known interaction between pressure and anesthesia (Halsey et al. 1978). Pressure is known to increase the requirement for anesthetic and shorten the duration of sleep induced with a wide variety of unrelated compounds (Bailey et al. 1977; McCracken et al. 1979; Nicodemus et al. 1980; Tobey et al. 1978). Furthermore, most of these compounds interact with the gases used during the compression. For example, 3 ATA oxygen increases the dose requirement for induction of sleep with diazepam but shortens the duration by 50%. In 6 ATA air the partial pressure of nitrogen is very likely the reason for the diminished requirement for diazepam. The shortened duration of effect in 6 ATA is not a pressure effect but probably a function of the small dose. Less time is required to remove the small amount of diazepam from its site or sites of action (Nicodemus et al. 1980).

(i) Balanced Anesthesia. Balanced anesthesia is a method of intravenous general anesthesia now used in most clinics for a wide variety of surgical procedures, from intracranial to open heart surgery. In this technique a drug is administered for a specific indication: narcotics to provide pain relief, barbiturates to provide loss of consciousness, and muscle relaxants to provide varying degrees of muscle paralysis. Induction of sleep is accomplished with any of the ultrashort-acting barbiturates, e.g., thiopental. Unrelated drugs may be substituted to achieve similar effects; e.g., diazepam, a benzodiazepine derivative, may be substituted for a barbiturate. In fact diazepam, singly or in combination with ketamine or with a narcotic, is widely used and could be expected to gain prominence under hyperbaric conditions. Diazepam offers some degree of amnesia and it softens the hallucinogenic effect of ketamine (Burnap 1974). The combination has little circulatory depressant effect; in some instances it even supports a borderline cardiovascular state. Induction of anesthesia with ketamine is recommended when hypovolemia is suspected in a patient, because it sustains the blood pressure. Diazepam is a popular induction agent for coronary artery bypass procedures where cardiac venticular function is questionable, and it may be adapted for all indications for intravenous general anesthesia.

Pain relief. Narcotics, singly (Stanley et al. 1979) or in combination with a neuroleptic drug (Innovar), have proved adequate as primary anesthetic agents. The long duration of action of the neuroleptic drug, however, precludes its use for hyperbaric work; because pressure also antagonizes morphine analgesia (Tofano and DeBoer 1976), a larger dose would be required. In patients allergic to morphine, more severe reactions and hypotension from the released histamine can be expected. Instead of morphine, fentanyl, a short-acting synthetic narcotic with less histamine-releasing property, would seem more logical to use for most anesthesia and pain relief under hyperbaric conditions. In case of untoward effect, the time it takes for the effect to disappear would be much shorter than with morphine. Alfaxalone may be substituted for narcotic, although its short duration of action would require frequent administration, a very troublesome problem if the anesthetist is also the surgeon. The control of depth of this anesthetic is most difficult, especially in the paralyzed patient.

In most cases of untoward reactions, such as hypotension or marked respiratory depression or prolonged narcosis, can a specific antagonist be used? Physostigmine salicylate reverses the effects of diazepam and other sedatives (Biduwai et al. 1979; Rosenberg 1974). Can one expect similar results at high ambient pressure? No a priori reason exists for antagonists to be ineffective; however, the dose requirement may be different from that recommended for 1 ATA. Among the antagonists that should be of interest to the physician providing anesthesia and pain relief under pressure are nalorphine and naloxone. Nalorphine has its own depressant effect if morphine is not present, whereas naloxone has virtually no effect of its own in the absence of narcotics. The efficacy of these drugs under pressure needs proper documentation in a patient who has received narcotics and who otherwise would need ventilatory support. Mechanical ventilation in a hyperbaric chamber is not easy, even to those familiar with it at surface conditions. The narcotic effect may outlast the effect of the antagonist so as to require reintubation or a repeat dose of the antagonist. It is better to err on keeping the airway in place for a longer time than to err on extubation that is too early.

The list of recommended drugs (Table X-9) includes a large amount of plain lidocaine because of its analgesic properties. When combined with other drugs (e.g., thiopental, diazepam), lidocaine may be used as an intravenous general anesthetic (Bartlett and Hutaserani 1961; Phillips et al. 1960; Steinhaus and Gaskin 1964; Steinhaus and Howland 1958). Systemic lidocaine is also a good cough suppressant, and when given 1–2 min before extubation it prevents laryngospasm. With the use of intravenous lidocaine, ventilation must be ascertained before extubation.

Muscle relaxants. Muscle relaxation is necessary for adequate surgical exposure. It should be noted that the information on neuromuscular function and the effects of muscle relaxants thereof were reported mostly from works on isolated nerve-muscle preparations and do not shed light on the duration of effect (Gountis-Bonikos et al. 1977; Kendig and Cohen 1976). The degree of myoneural block can only be inferred from these studies. The contribution of dilution of the drug with extracellular fluid, protein binding, and the effect of blood flow awaits confirmation in a patient who has been under pressure for some time. L. E. McCracken has data (unpublished) on the use of succinylcholine in intact guinea pigs at 31 ATA helium and oxygen. Like others (Gountis-Bonikos et al. 1977), he noted increased height of twitch tension. In addition his study revealed that the duration of paralysis is not different from that of surface control, a further indication that at high pressures there is an intact and functional pseudocholinesterase system. Note that this enzyme also hydrolyzes some of the local anesthetics.

For a procedure of short duration a depolarizing block with succinylcholine (1 mg/ml i.v. drip), titrated to the point where the patient can still initiate ventilation, should prove adequate. For longer procedures nondepolarizing blocks with either curare or pancuronium bromide is the choice. Curare, with its mild ganglionic blocking effect and its ability to release histamine, may worsen a borderline cardiovascular state. In this case pancuronium bromide is the choice, as it is not known to cause hypotension. On the other hand it can cause tachycardia and should not be used if tachycardia is not desirable.

Redistribution and metabolism or pharmacologic reversal with cholinesterase inhibitors terminate the muscle paralysis. Even with an overdose of succinylcholine in a patient with an adequate level of pseudocholinesterase in the plasma, muscle function should return within an hour. When pharmacologic reversal of a nondepolarizing block is desirable, neostigmine (a cholinesterase inhibitor) is an effective antagonist, but it should be given only after a dose of atropine. There is meager information about the ability of atropine to block the muscarinic effect of neostigmine under pressure. If uninhibited, the muscarinic effects are bradycardia, bronchoconstriction, and bronchorrhea. It also increases intestinal motility, which together with the gas contents of the bowel constitutes an important consideration during decompression.

The interaction between muscle relaxants and antibiotics with or without such other factors as low serum calcium, electrolyte imbalance, and narcotics can lead to difficult pharmacologic reversal and prolonged muscle paralysis. This interaction is difficult enough to unravel at 1 ATA and is totally undocumented under high pressure. Dripps et al.

Table X-9
Anesthetic and Other Drugs to Have on Hand for Emergency Medical and Surgical Procedures

Substance	Quantity	Strength	Unit	Unit dose	Use
Aminophylline (bronchodilator)	4	250 mg	Ampule	5–6 mg/kg initially; then 0.5 mg/kg/hr	Administer by i.v. infusion; monitor EKG; see package insert.
Atropine (for bradycardia)	4	1 mg	Prepacked syringe	0.4–1.0 mg	Administer i.m. or i.v.
Calcium chloride	4	1 g	Prepacked syringe	1 g	Administer i.v. slowly.
2-Chloroprocaine hydrochloride, epidural	3	3%		1.5–2.0 ml per segment to be blocked	
Dexamethasone (steroid)	4	4 mg/ml	5-ml vial	4–8 mg	Administer i.m. or i.v.
Diazepam	6	10 mg	Prepacked syringe	5–10 mg	Administer i.v. as sedative, more if sleep is to be induced. Potentiates narcotics and depressant effect of local anesthetics. Watch ventilation.
Digoxin	4	0.5 mg	Ampule	0.5 mg initially; then 0.25 mg. 1.2 mg	Administer i.m. or i.v. initially; then i.m. or i.v. every 4–6 hr. Digitalizing dose.
Diphenhydramine hydrochloride (antihistamine)	4	50 mg	Prepacked syringe	50 mg	Administer i.m. or i.v.
Dopamine	4	200 mg	Ampule	8–12 µg/kg per hr	Administer by i.v. infusion only; monitor BP and urine output; see package insert.
Edrophonium	4	10 mg	Ampule	10 mg	Administer i.m. or i.v. for reversal of muscle relaxant or conversion of atrial tachycardia; have atropine ready; see package insert.
Ephedrine	4	25 mg	Ampule	10–25 mg More	Administer i.v. or i.m. for hypotension. Administer for asthma.
Epinephrine	4	1 mg	Ampule	0.25–0.5 ml	Administer i.m for anaphylaxis.
Fentanyl	20	0.5 mg/ml	5-ml ampule	0.05 mg/kg	Administer as sole anesthetic with or without muscle relaxant.

(Continued)

Table X-9 Continued

Substance	Quantity	Strength	Unit	Unit dose	Use
Fentanyl (*cont.*)				Considerably less	If used with other anesthetic.
				0.1 mg equipotent with 10 mg morphine	Administer for pain, but relief will last only 0.5–1.0 hr; chest wall spasm if given rapidly i.v.; patient may need mechanical ventilation.
Furosemide (diuretic)	4	20 mg	Ampule	20–40 mg	Administer i.m. or i.v.
Heparin	2	10 ml	Multidose vials	10,000 U initially; then 5000 U	Administer i.v. intermittently; then every 4–6 hr.
				20,000–40,000 U/day	Administer by i.v. infusion, continuously.
				5000 U	Minidose, every 8–12 hr.
Hydralazine (lowers BP)	4	20 mg	Ampule	20–40 mg	Administer i.v. or i.m.; monitor BP.
Hydrocortisone 21-sodium succinate	2	250 mg	Prepacked vial	100–250 mg	Administer by i.v. infusion.
				Larger dose	Administer for pharmacologic effect.
Isoproterenol	4	1 μg	Ampule	0.5–5.0 μg/min	Administer by i.v. infusion; monitor BP and heart rate.
Lidocaine hydrochloride (antiarrhythmic)	4	100 mg	Prepacked syringe	100 mg initially then 1–2 mg/min	Administer i.v. Then continuous i.v. infusion; monitor EKG.
Lidocaine hydrochloride, plain	6	2%	20-ml vial	6 mg/kg total dosage	Administer for local anesthesia: CNS toxicity more likely at total dosage; add epinephrine to desired concentration; dilute with sterile water as necessary for Bier block.
Lidocaine hydrochloride, plain	6	1%	50-ml vial		
Mannitol (diuretic)	4	12.5 g	Ampule	1–2 ampules	Administer as 25% solution i.v.
Morphine	10	15 mg	Prepacked syringe	1 mg/kg	Administer this amount i.v. as sole anesthetic.
				Less	Administer i.v. if combined with other anesthetic; use artificial ventilation and/or reversal with naloxone.
Naloxone (antinarcotic)	6	0.4 mg	Ampule	5–15 mg	Administer i.v. or i.m. for pain relief.
Neostigmine	3	10 mg	Vial	0.4 mg	Administer i.m. or i.v.; repeat p.r.n.
				5 mg	Administer i.v.; combine with 1.2 mg atropine for reversal of pavulon or curare; evaluate effect after each i.v. dose

Emergency Treatment While under Pressure 481

Drug				
Nitroglycerin (lowers BP)	1	0.6 mg	100-tablet vial	1 tablet	Administer sublingually p.r.n. for angina.
				12 mg/250 ml	Administer as i.v. infusion to desired effect; use i.v. millipore filter; dosage rate, 0.3–4.5 μg/kg/min.
Pancuronium bromide	2	10 mg	Multidose vial	5–7 mg	Administer i.v. as muscle relaxant; ventilate patient.
Phenylephrine hydrochloride (elevates BP)	2	10 mg	Ampule	5–10 mg/liter fluid 0.25%	Titrate to desired effect; monitor BP. Use as nasal drops as anticongestant.
Phenytoin	6	250 mg	Ampule	150 mg	Administer i.v. slowly for status epilepticus, not to exceed 50 mg/min.
				100–200 mg	Administer i.m. or i.v. 4 hr before surgery if prophylactic; see package insert.
Potassium chloride	6	20 meq	Ampule	20 meq/liter	Administer by infusion as required.
Procainamide hydrochloride (antiarrhythmic)	2	1 g	Multidose ampule	100 mg	Administer i.m. or as infusion of 25–50 mg/min.
Prochlorperazine	4	10 mg	Ampule	10 mg	Administer i.m. or i.v.
Propranolol (antiarrhythmic; causes bronchospasm)	4	1 mg	Ampule	1–2 mg	Administer by slow i.v.; monitor BP and heart rate.
Sodium bicarbonate	6	44 meq	Prepacked syringe		Administer i.v. a total dose of 1/3 body wt. in kg × base deficit. Check arterial pH.
Sodium chloride	25	0.9%	Ampule	5 ml	
Sodium nitroferricyanide	2	50 mg	Multidose ampule	0.5–10.0 μg/kg/min	Administer by i.v. infusion; monitor BP; watch for tachyphylaxis and acidosis with large doses; see package insert.
Succinylcholine	2	200 mg	Vial	50–100 mg	Administer i.v. for muscle paralysis, relaxation. By infusion 1 mg/ml in 500 ml saline. Ventilate patient. For longer duration of muscle paralysis, use pancuronium bromide or curare.
Thiopental	3	500 mg	Package with diluent	2–4 mg/kg	Administer i.v. for induction of sleep or rapid treatment of convulsion.

(1977) covered some of the differential diagnoses, which really are not immediately essential as long as the patient receives adequate ventilation. More work on the efficacy of antibiotics similar to that reported by Argamaso and Wiseman (1967) is needed to provide the physician a choice of antibiotics that do not interact with the muscle relaxants. Among the antibiotics, the following have muscle-blocking property that can act synergistically with neuromuscular blockers: streptomycin, neomycin, polymyxin A and B, gentamycin, colistin, and lincomycin. Other drugs that may increase neuromuscular blocks are ganglionic blocking drugs, cholinesterase inhibitors, local anesthetics, and antiarrhythmic drugs such as quinidine, procainamide hydrochloride, and phenytoin.

Parenthetically, Bennett and co-workers (1974) abolished most of the tremors in high pressure nervous syndrome (HPNS) by adding nitrogen to the inspired gas. Those tremors that occurred with purposeful movement nevertheless persisted and were troublesome. Because pressure is known to increase twitch tension height (Gountis-Bonikos et al. 1977), it is not illogical to expect jerky movement during exposure to high pressure. Inasmuch as muscle contraction is initiated with a train of nerve impulses (tetanus), this jerky movement is reminiscent of the post-tetanic facilitation seen in partially curarized muscles. Kendig and her associates (1978), however, have reported that repetitive impulse generation in the nerve terminal may be the basis for the hyperactivity in HPNS. The physician who has to descend to the operational depth of a dive may have to take time or be incapacitated by HPNS.

(ii) Catecholamines, Adrenergic Blockers, Vasodilators. The close relationship among catecholamines, adrenergic blockers, and vasodilators has necessitated the grouping of these drugs for discussion. The most consistent effect of high pressure on the cardiovascular system is bradycardia. Evans' section on cardiac effects in Chapter III of this book reviews the literature and enumerates several causes of bradycardia. Among them are: (1) direct effect of pressure; (2) effect of high partial pressure of oxygen; (3) effect of gases other than oxygen; (4) reduced beta adrenergic stimulation; and (5) increased parasympathetic activity. The effect of pressure on cardiac output is inconclusive.

How does one relate the physiological effect of pressure on the cardiovascular system in an anesthetized patient? Under high pressure the stress of infection has been shown to increase the amount of circulating catecholamines (Won and Ross 1975). Although high sympathetic tone may be expected (Hammond and Akers 1974), the response of the target organs to the catecholamines is further modified by the presence of anesthesia. Evans and Greenbaum (1970) reported that pressor response to epinephrine is unaltered in cats at 200 ATA. Inasmuch as adrenergic response is either alpha (represented by vasoconstriction) or beta (represented by increased heart rate and vasodilation), there is a need for better characterization of the autonomic response of the anesthetized patient when under increased pressure. These responses would vary, depending on the drug or combinations of drugs that are used for anesthesia.

One of the hallmarks of balanced anesthesia is an intact and sensitive sympathetic nervous system able to respond to the surgical stimulation. If peripheral resistance becomes unduly high because of intense vasoconstriction during anesthesia, the strain on the myocardium may precipitate acute heart failure. In this situation vasodilators are indicated. The cardiovascular dose responses to ganglionic blockers and to the more specific alpha or beta blockers are largely undocumented at high pressure. Moreover, information on the efficacy of two locally acting vasodilators, nitroglycerin and sodium nitroprusside, is not available to help ensure their safe and rational use while under high pressure. Other antihypertensive drugs also deserve documentation.

Should acute heart failure develop, rotation of tourniquets to decrease venous return, diuretics, and digitalization are accepted therapy. In the presence of factors such as anesthesia, electrolyte imbalance, loss of potassium due to pressure diuresis, altered catecholamine response, altered response to calcium, and altered membrane physiology, rapid digitalization is a perfect setup for ventricular dysrhythmia or even ventricular fibrillation. To say that electrical defibrillation is difficult in a hyperbaric chamber is an understatement and extreme care must be exercised in using cardiac glycosides.

The key to the use of the drugs under this grouping is adequate monitoring. Technically the problems of electrocardiography, continuous blood pressure measurement, or even cardiac output determination are surmountable. What may be required, though, is a reinterpretation of some of the changes in the vital signs of a patient exposed to hyperbaric conditions (Gutsche et al. 1966). For example, a patient may show electrocardiographic signs of cardiac strain, increased blood pressure, and rapid heart rate in the presence of blood loss. Traditionally, hematocrit, cardiac output, and peripheral resistance are the determinants of oxygen delivery to the tissues. In a critical care situation at 1 ATA, a given set of values may determine the need for more red blood cells or, if the hematocrit is normal, more fluids to improve blood flow. When the patient is under pressure, oxygen delivery could be improved, or at least brought to near normal values regardless of hematocrit, by simply increasing the inspired oxygen concentration. The increased amount of dissolved oxygen may be enough to meet the basal requirement, but increased dissolved oxygen (as opposed to oxyhemoglobin) may cause greater cellular damage. More information is needed in this area for more logical conclusions and actions. To be complete, the algorithm must also include the appropriate fluid—whether crystalloids, colloids, or a mixture of both plus red blood cells.

Monitoring should include urine output. Balanced anesthesia that includes narcotics could change the antidiuretic hormone output. It is known, however, that pressure reverses the antidiuretic effect of morphine (Tofano and DeBoer 1976). To be sure, urine output must be measured together with urine pH. A question to be asked is: Do pressure and exposure to different gases alter the response to test tapes for determination of urine pH?

(iii) Nonpharmacologic methods of pain relief. Other modes of pain relief that have been introduced include electronarcosis, transcutaneous electrical stimulation of nerves, acupuncture, and hypnosis. Biofeedbacks have also been tried. The efficacy of all these should be tested under high pressure. Electronarcosis does not require uptake, distribution, and metabolism; neither will it contaminate the atmosphere in the chamber. Electronarcosis therefore appears ideal for hyperbaric use.

c. Suggested Course of Action for General Anesthesia under High Pressure

I. Consider awake tracheal intubation in all patients after topical anesthesia (two alternatives).
   A. Awake blind nasal intubation.
   B. Awake direct visual, oral, or nasal intubation.

II. When airway is secured, administer drug intravenously.
   A. Narcotic. (Sole anesthetic with or without relaxant; smaller doses if combined with other agents; artificial respiration needed. Shorter acting drugs are recommended.)
      1. Fentanyl, .05 mg/kg, administered slowly to avoid chest wall spasm; muscle relaxant may be required.
      2. Morphine, 1 mg/kg, if fentanyl is unavailable.
   B. Hypnotic sedative.
      1. Thiopental, 2–4 mg/kg.
      2. Diazepam. 10–20 mg.
      3. Other drugs, optional:
         a. Ketamine, 1–2 mg/kg; preferred when adequacy of blood volume is questionable.
         b. Lidocaine, 5–10 mg/kg initial dose.
III. Monitor depth of anesthesia after induction.
   A. Monitor blood pressure and pulse rate every 5–10 min.
   B. Manual ventilation:
      1. Self-inflating bag.
      2. Anesthesia breathing bag with Ruben valve if gas mixture can be delivered to the patient.
IV. Administer muscle relaxants to improve surgical exposure and to lessen requirement for intravenous anesthetics.
   A. Pancuronium bromide, 5 mg initially, titrated intravenously to near apnea.
      1. 1–2 mg maintenance dose every 45–60 min.
   B. Other relaxants, optional:
      1. Curare 0.5–0.6 mg/kg; 0.15 mg/kg maintenance dose every 30–45 min.
V. Maintain anesthesia.
   A. Signs of light anesthesia indicating need for more drugs:
      1. Sweating.
      2. Lacrimation.
      3. Movements, facial grimace, opening of the eyes.
      4. Increased blood pressure and pulse rate.
      5. Increased frequency and depth of breathing.
   B. Maintenance doses—generally 25% of initial induction doses (good practice to administer fractions of narcotic, hypnotic sedative, and relaxants to deepen anesthesia).
   C. With increase in time less of the drug required to maintain anesthesia.
   D. 1–2 ml normal saline solution instilled into endotracheal tube every 30 min for humidity.
VI. End of operation.
   A. Breathing should be present—steps to take if breathing is shallow:
      1. Reverse relaxants with atropine (1.5 mg) and neostigmine (5 mg) in one syringe, divided into two doses.
      2. Reverse narcotic with naloxone if ventilation is still inadequate or if patient fails to awaken after reversal of relaxant (0.4 mg i.v. × 2 p.r.n.).
      3. Reverse diazepam with physostigmine (1–2 mg i.v.)—rarely necessary.

B. Extubation, only under these conditions:
1. Patient is wide awake and struggles to remove endotracheal tube.
2. Patient breathes spontaneously and can hold head off the table for 5 sec or more.
3. Patient coughs when endotracheal tube is moved.
C. Physician may opt for keeping endotracheal tube longer.
VII. Recovery—(applicable to either general or regional anesthesia).
A. Check for bleeding at operative site.
B. Check for wakefulness, orientation, ability to follow simple commands.
C. Check for adequacy of respiration; more reversal p.r.n.
D. Watch for vomiting and aspiration.
E. If patient is restless, consider the following:
1. Full bladder: catheterize once.
2. Pain: treat with half recommended dose of narcotic, i.v.; titrate dose to desired effect.
3. Emergence delirium (rare with balanced anesthesia); treat with small doses of narcotic or diazepam i.v.
F. Assess urine output for adequacy of fluid therapy and replacement. Urine output should be 0.5–1.0 ml/kg/hr.
G. Assess adequacy of blood volume; monitor blood pressure and pulse.

Caution: Do not decompress if patient is not fully conscious or has residual regional block.

Preparation of this section was supported in part by Research and Development Command Task Number M0095PN001 and M0099PN001.

HONORATO F. NICODEMUS

References

ALDRETE, J. A., F. ROMO-SALAS, R. WILSON. AND R. RUTHERFORD 1978. Reverse arterial blood flow as a pathway for central nervous system toxic response following injection of local anesthestics. *Anesth. Analg. Cleve.* 57: 428–433.

ARGAMASO, R. V., AND G. M. WISEMAN 1967. The use of combined hyperbaric oxygen and polymixin B in the treatment of pseudomonas infection in mice. *Plast. Reconstr. Surg.* 1: 81–86.

BAILEY, C. P., C. J. GREEN, M. J. HALSEY. AND B. WARDLEY-SMITH 1977. High pressure and intravenous anesthesia in rats. *J. Appl. Physiol.: Respir. Environ. Exercise Physiol.* 43: 183–188.

BAKER, A. B., AND I. P. UNSWORTH 1978. No ignition risk with hyperbaric enflurane. *Anesth. Inst. Care* 6: 157–159.

BARTLETT, E. E., AND O. HUTASERANI 1961. Xylocaine for the relief of postoperative pain. *Anesth. Analg. Cleve.* 40: 296–304.

BENNETT, E. J., E. M. GRUNDY. AND K. P. PATEL 1978. Visual signs in blind nasal intubation. *Anesthesiol. Rev.* 5: 18–20.

BENNETT, P. B., G. D. BLENKARN, J. ROBY. AND D. YOUNGBLOOD 1974. Suppression of high pressure nervous syndrome in human deep dives with He-N$_2$O. *Undersea Biomed. Res.* 1: 221–236.

BIDUWAI, A. V., T. H. STANLEY, C. ROGERS. AND E. K. RIET 1979. Reversal of diazepam-induced post anesthetic somnolence with physostigmine. *Anesthesiology* 51: 256–259.

BURNAP, R. W. Ketamine/diazepam solution as general anesthetic. 1974. In: *European Congress of Anesthesiology, 4th, Madrid, 1974*, p. 177.

CARRON, H. (editor). 1980. Regional anesthesia for upper extremity surgery symposium. *Regional Anesth.* 5: 2–12.

CARTER, L. H., AND G. A. GOLDSMITH 1970. The ordeal of Donald Boone. *Nutr. Today* 5: 1–9.

D'AMATO, H., AND S. WIELDLING (editors). 1969. Intravenous Regional Anesthesia, An International Conference. *Acta Anaesth. Scand. Suppl.* 36.

DEJONG, R. H., AND J. E. HEAVNER 1972. Local anesthetic seizure prevention—diazepam vs. pentobarbital. *Anesthesiology* 36: 449–457.

DIGIOVANNI, A. J., M. W. GALBERT. AND W. M. WAHLE 1972. Epidural injection of autologous blood for post lumbar-puncture headache. *Anesth. Analg. Cleve.* 51: 226.

DRIPPS, R. D., J. E. ECKENHOFF. AND L. D. VANDAM 1977. *Introduction to Anesthesia: Principles of Safe Practice* (5th ed.) Philadelphia: Saunders.

EVANS, D. E., AND L. J. GREENBAUM, JR. 1970. Pressor response to epinephrine in hyperbaric atmosphere. *Aerosp. Med.* 41: 738–740.

GLASS, P. M., AND W. F. KENNEDY, JR. 1972. Headache following subarachnoid puncture: Treatment with epidural blood patch. *JAMA* 219: 203–205.

GOUNTIS-BONIKOS, C., J. J. KENDIG, AND E. N. COHEN 1977. The actions of neuromuscular relaxants at hyperbaric pressures. *Anesthesiology* 47: 11–15.

GROMLEY, J. B. 1960. Treatment of postspinal headache. *Anesthesiology* 21: 565–566.

GUTSCHE, B. B., J. R. HARP. AND C. R. STEPHEN 1966. Physiologic response of anesthetized dog to oxygen at 5 ATA. *Anesthesiology* 27: 615–623.

HALSEY, M. J., B. WARDLEY-SMITH, AND C. J. GREEN 1978. Pressure reversal of general anesthesia—a multisite expansion hypothesis. *Br. J. Anaesth.* 50: 1091–1097.

HAMMOND, R. E., AND T. K. AKERS 1974. The effect of hyperbaria on neuroeffector drugs in the isolated heart. In: *Aerospace Medical Association Annual Scientific Meeting, Washington, D.C., 1974.* Preprints, p. 205–206.

KENDIG, J. J. 1980. Interactions between hyperbaric pressure and drugs on excitable cells (nerve and muscle). In: *Interaction of Drugs in the Hyperbaric Environment*, edited by J. M. Walsh. Bethesda, MD: Undersea Med. Soc., p. 3–10. (Undersea Med. Soc. Workshop, Bethesda, MD, 1979.)

KENDIG, J. J., AND E. N. COHEN 1976. Neuromuscular function at hyperbaric pressures: pressure-anesthetic interaction. *Am. J. Physiol.* 230: 1244–1249.

KENDIG, J. J., AND E. N. COHEN 1977. Pressure antagonism to nerve conduction block by anesthetic agents. *Anesthesiology* 47: 6–10.

KENDIG, J. J., T. M. SCHNEIDER. AND E. N. COHEN 1978. Repetitive impulses in nerves: a possible basis for HPNS. In: *Programs and Abstracts, Undersea Medical Society, Inc., Annual Scientific Meeting, 1978. Undersea Biomed. Res.* 5 (Suppl.): 49.

KERMORGANT, Y. 1978. Anaesthesia in a hyperbaric atmosphere. In: *Congress of the European Undersea Biomedical Society on Medical Aspect of Diving Accidents, 1978*, p. 96–113.

KRENIS L. J., P. L. LIU. AND S. H. NGAI 1971. The effect of local anesthetics on the central nervous system toxicity of hyperbaric oxygen. *Neuropharmacology* 10: 637–641.

MCCRACKEN, L. E., H. F. NICODEMUS, R. E. TOBEY, AND R. C. BAILEY 1979. Ketamine and thiopental sleep responses in hyperbaric helium oxygen in guinea pigs. *Undersea Biomed. Res.* 6: 329–338.

MCDOWAL, D. G. 1964. Anaesthesia in a pressure chamber. *Anaesthesia* 19: 321–336.

MOORE, D. C. 1975. *Regional Block* (4th ed.). Springfield, IL: Thomas.

MOORE, D. C., L. E. MATHER, P. O. BRIDENBAUGH, L. D. BRIDENBAUGH, R. I. BALFOUR, D. F. LYONS. AND W. G. HORTON 1976. Arterial and venous plasma levels of bupivacaine following epidural and intercostal nerve blocks. *Anesthesiology* 45: 40–45.

MULROY, M. F. 1979. Spinal headache and air travel. *Anesthesiology* 51: 379.

NICODEMUS, H. F., R. C. BAILEY, J. P. SUMME, AND H. MCELROY 1980. Dose-responses of guinea pigs to diazepam at recompression depths. *Undersea Biomed. Res.* 7: 1–9.

NICODEMUS, H. F., H. MCELROY. AND R. LEVY 1981. The efficacy of spinal anesthesia at high pressure. In: *Underwater Physiology VII. Proceedings of the Seventh Symposium on Underwater Physiology*, edited by A. J. Bachrach and M. M. Matzen. Bethesda, MD: Undersea Med. Soc, p. 853–856.

PHILLIPS, O. C., A. T. NELSON, W. B. LYONS, T. D. GRAFF, L. C. HARRIS, AND T. M. FRAZIER 1960. Intravenous lidocaine as an adjunct to general anesthesia. *Anesth. Analg. Cleve.* 39: 317–322.
PITTINGER, C. 1966. Problems of anesthesia in hyperbaric atmosphere. *J. Am. Assoc. Nurse Anesthetists* 34: 321–325.
ROSENBERG, H. 1974. Physostigmine reversal of sedative drugs. *JAMA* 229: 1168–1170.
ROSS, J. A. S., H. J. MANSON, A. SHEARER, AND C. R. DUNDAS 1977. Some aspects of anesthesia in high pressure environments. In: *Proceedings International Congress on Hyperbaric Medicine, 6th, Aberdeen, Scotland, 1977*, p. 449–452.
ROTH, S. H., R. A. SMITH, AND N. D. M. PATOU 1976. Pressure antagonism of anaesthetic-induced conduction failure in frog peripheral nerve. *Br. J. Anaesth.* 48: 621–628.
SEVERINGHAUS, J. W. 1966. Anesthesia and related drug effects. In: *Fundamentals of Hyperbaric Medicine*. Washington, DC: Natl. Acad. Sci./Natl. Res. Council, p. 115–127.
SMALL, A. 1970. The effects of hyperbaric helium-oxygen on acute toxicity of several drugs. *Toxicol. Appl. Pharmacol.* 17: 250–261.
SMITH, R. A., M. SMITH, E. I. EGER II, M. J. HALSEY, AND P. M. WINTER 1979. Nonlinear antagonism of anesthesia in mice by pressure. *Anesth. Analg. Cleve.* 58: 19–22.
SMITH, R. M., D. CROCKER, AND J. G. ADAMS 1964. Anesthetic management of patients during surgery under hyperbaric oxygenation. *Anesth. Analg. Cleve.* 43: 766–776.
SPENCE, A. A., AND G. SMITH 1964. Problems associated with the use of anesthetic and related equipment in a hyperbaric environment. *Int. Anesthesiol. Clin.* 12: 165–179.
STANLEY, T. H., L. BERMAN, O. GREEN, D. H. ROBERTSON, AND M. ROIZEN 1979. Fentanyl-oxygen anesthesia for coronary artery surgery: plasma catecholamine and cortisol response. *Anesthesiology* (Suppl) 51: S139.
STEINHAUS, J. E., AND L. GASKIN 1964. A study of intravenous lidocaine as suppressant to cough reflex. *Anesthesiology* 24: 296–304.
STEINHAUS, J. E., AND D. E. HOWLAND 1958. Intravenously administered lidocaine as a supplement to N_2O thiobarbiturate anesthesia. *Anesth. Analg. Cleve.* 37: 30–46.
TOBEY, R. E., L. E. MCCRACKEN, A. SMALL AND L. D. HOMER 1978. Effect of hyperbaric helium on anesthetic action of thiopental. In: *Underwater Physiology VI. Proceedings of the Sixth Symposium on Underwater Physiology, Bethesda, MD, 1978*, edited by C. W. Shilling and M. W. Beckett. Bethesda, MD: Fed. Am. Soc. for Exp. Biol., p. 267–272.
TOFANO, M. E., AND B. DEBOER 1976. Effects of hyperbaria upon morphine antidiuresis and analgesia in rats. *Aviat. Space Environ. Med.* 47: 26–28.
VACANTI, J. J. 1972. Post-spinal headache in air travel. *Anesthesiology* 37: 358–359.
WINNIE, A. P. 1970. Interscalene brachial plexus block. *Anesth. Analg. Cleve.* 49: 455–466.
WISELEY, I. C. F. 1976. High pressure medicine. *Br. Med. J.* 1: 340.
WON, W. D., AND H. C. ROSS 1975. Catecholamines and phagocyte response in infected mice exposed to hyperbaric helium-oxygen atmosphere. *Aviat. Space Environ. Med.* 46: 191–193.

XI

Physical and Psychological Examination for Diving

A. *Physical Standards For Diving*

1. *Background*

The preceding chapters have contained accounts of a variety of physiological, psychological, and pathological stresses that are imposed on an individual who enters the underwater hyperbaric environment. When a man places himself underwater he is at a great disadvantage with regard to his ability to propel himself through the dense medium and to protect himself against excessive heat loss, both activities requiring high energy expenditure. He must breathe gases of increased density in or through appliances to maintain adequate gas exchange of oxygen, carbon dioxide, and inert gases, utilizing a cardiorespiratory system that has been altered as a result of exposure to the direct effects of pressure. He must be able to adequately accommodate changes in gas volume and pressure in his anatomical and pseudoanatomical spaces to prevent morbid changes. Lastly, he must function within narrowly defined limits imposed by the indirect effects of pressure, i.e., the effects of the partial pressure of gases, which cause toxic, narcotic, stimulatory, and gas solubility alterations to bodily functions.

Because of these obligatory stresses of underwater exposure, an individual must possess certain physical and physiological attributes and must be devoid of certain limitations or conditions in order to function safely in this unique environment. The physical requirements and limitations fall into two major categories. The first are those that concern everyone exposed to pressure, no matter if one is dry, wet, in a deep-sea rig, in a caisson, or enjoying a "wall-dive" at a Caribbean dive resort. The second major category that defines limitations or influences requirements is the type of diving in which an individual intends to engage. The author suggests the following types of diving are decreasingly stringent in physical requirements though not necessarily in potential risk: (a) military diving;

(b) commercial diving; (c) scientific and technical diving; (d) semiprofessional diving; and (e) recreational (sport) diving.

a. Military Diving

Divers of the uniformed service initially must meet stringent physical standards for enlisted service and even more stringent standards for officer status. Additional restrictions and standards are then applied for diving status and are typified by U.S. Navy standards (U.S. Navy 1980). These strict standards are necessary, since military diving may be under combat conditions and may be performed in arduous, dangerous situations such as salvage in the open sea, disposal of explosive ordnance, clandestine operations, or the extremely urgent nature of rescue and assistance in escape from a sunken submarine. Military divers in performance of their duties may use compressed air or semiclosed or closed-circuit mixed-gas scuba; closed-circuit oxygen apparatus; deep-sea gear, with both air and helium-oxygen mixtures supplied; or advanced bell and saturation systems. Military divers have no choice about whether they perform their duties or not, as is the case of a commercial diver who can simply quit, or the recreational diver who can dive when and where he pleases. Therefore, excellent physical fitness among these individuals must be assured without question.

b. Commercial Diving

Commercial diving activities range from shallow work (underwater construction, cleaning ship hulls of marine growth, marine salvage, etc.) to the deep diving in support of offshore petroleum and gas exploration and production. Offshore petroleum exploration and production diving poses the greatest area of risk. Many deep-diving operations are carried out hundreds of miles from shore and are lacking in medical and support facilities. Inclement weather may hamper medical attention or evacuation of a casualty. One estimate gives the annual fatality rate of offshore employment, other than diving, at 22 fatalities per 10,000 persons per year and that of offshore diving, for the year 1974, at 111 fatalities per 10,000 persons per year. This is contrasted to the general construction industry and mining industry—approximately 2.6 fatalities per year per 10,000 persons engaged. These figures come primarily from experience in the North Sea oil fields and from the Gulf of Mexico oil fields (Grorud and Bøl 1976). In these geographical areas there is reasonable governmental oversight to assure the most reasonable adherence to prudent safety precautions and safe diving techniques. In more remote areas, however, and particularly in those around the underdeveloped countries, conditions are considerably worse.

Selection criteria for employment in commercial diving are strict, not only because of the hazardous and heavy labor conditions involved, but because the risk of litigation for injuries incurred during work or for aggravated injury is extremely high for the employer and third-party insurers. "Zero defect" is the dictum for selection of commercial divers. Not only does an employer face potential disability liability for work-related injury under the normal applications of Workmen's Compensation procedures, but he faces essentially unlimited financial liability with the application of the Jones Act, a federal law passed to protect U.S. merchant seamen on the high seas. Legal precedent has placed commercial divers under the provisions of this law (*United States Code*). As a result, commercial diving firms in the United States are extremely selective, in terms of physical standards, in screening potential employees. Commercial divers may utilize the entire spectrum of diving modes—from compressed air scuba to deep saturation mixed gas. They may be expected to go from one type of diving to another and from employer to employer, for a variety of reasons. When passed "fit," a diver is physically qualified for all types of diving unless a specific limitation has been imposed (Linaweaver 1977).

The Federal Occupational Safety and Health Administration (OSHA), the U.S. Coast Guard, and state occupational safety and health organizations (e.g., CALOSHA) all require commercial divers to have annual physical examinations and reexamination after an illness or injury of more than 72 hr or after an episode of unconsciousness relating to diving activity (OSHA and USCG 1977). Although the tests and examinations required are explicit, the standards set by these regulatory agencies are vague concerning the criteria for fitness, thus leaving the responsibility for selection to the employer and the examining physician.

c. Scientific and Technical Diving

Those individuals who use diving as a tool or mode to practice their primary scientific or technical skill in the marine environment are usually associated with universities or other laboratories, and they enjoy universally an excellent safety record. Their activities are generally in shallow water, and they work under strict rules and regulations established by their local diving regulatory body, such as a university diving safety board. Most scientific divers are required to have annual physical examinations that are quite comprehensive. Their diving mode is primarily shallow air, but many use techniques of mixed gas and even bottom habitat saturation.

d. Semiprofessional Diving

So-called semiprofessional divers are self-employed divers such as the divers for California abalone and sea urchin, the operators of dive shops and dive-boat enterprises, and those part-time marine handymen who clean boat bottoms and change the propellers. This group has no standards with regard to physical requirements or training, and they are not under any regulatory control. In California this group does not enjoy a favorable safety record.

e. Recreational Diving

The group of recreational or sport divers is the largest of those engaged in underwater activity; they number internationally in the millions. Most have had good basic training supervised by the recognized training agencies such as the YMCA, National Association of Underwater Instructors (NAUI), the Professional Association of Diving Instructors (PADI), and others. Most of those so trained have not had physical examinations, although most have answered a health questionnaire. Positive answers on these questionnaires require an individual to have clearance by a physician before training. This questionnaire is used primarily as legal protection for the dive shop operator, instructor, or sponsoring training agency, and true physical evaluations are recommended but not required. Each agency has an appropriate medical form such as that of NAUI (Appendix A) when an examination is required. The dropout rate after initial amateur sport training is high in spite of the considerable investment in equipment and training courses. The exact population at risk and their frequency of diving is essentially unknown. Treatment statistics, however, do indicate a much higher incidence of serious conditions than one sees among the professional or military divers (see Tables XI-1 and XI-2). Numerous factors influence these data and further elaboration is not undertaken here.

Table XI-1
Typical Types of Diving Accidents Treated

Treatment facility	Type I DCS, %	Type II DCS, %	Air embolism, %
University of Southern California, Catalina Island	13	54	33
Pearl Harbor, Hawaii, civilian facility	48	52	a
Grand Cayman, Dutch West Indies	19	38	45
U.S. Navy, military facility	89	11	a

[a] Not recorded.

Table XI-2
Summary of Number of All Underwater Fatalities, by Year, 1970–[a]76

Purpose of underwater activity	Fatalities													
	1970		1971		1972		1973		1974		1975		1976	
	M[a]	F[a]	M	F	M	F	M	F	M	F	M	F	M	F
Nonprofessional underwater	99	11	104	8	107	12	118	7	129	15	123	8	137	10
Professional, scuba diving	3	0	2	0	2	0	0	0	6	0	4	0	6	0
Professional[b] surface-supplied air or mixed gas	6	0	2	0	2	0	4	0	8	0	8	0	7	0
On duty military	0	0	0	0	0	0	0	0	2	0	1	0	1	0
Skindiving	18	1	17	0	15	1	22	0	25	2	16	1	11	3
Totals, M + F	138		133		139		151		187		161		175	

[a] M, Male, F, Female. [b] Includes one nonprofessional hose diver.   [From NOAA (1976).]

2. Physical Evaluation of Divers

Physical examination of divers requires of the physican a knowledge of the physiology of diving and a fundamental understanding of the type of work in which the individual diver will be engaged. The examiner must be an astute clinician to elicit a careful history and perform an equally careful physical examination to detect disqualifying or potentially hazardous conditions. He must be consistent in his application of his findings and clinical judgment concerning the certification or disqualification of divers. The physician must consider himself a member of a team responsible for the health and safety of divers: this may require, besides his clinical efforts, active participation in research and other aspects of preventive medicine.

A careful history, as in any physical examination, is of upmost importance. There is little disagreement among experts that specific conditions would automatically disqualify a potential diving candidate, whether for recreational or commercial endeavors, and these are discussed under the anatomical and organ system parts of the physical examination.

The physical examination should be conducted with the thought in mind to detect signs of absolute or relative or temporary disqualifying conditions. The requirement for laboratory studies and ancillary studies is an area for controversy and further discussion. Lastly, the physician has a distinct responsibility to the diver, as a patient, in terms of preventive medicine. He should look carefully for the telltale signs of excessive smoking, which can only be injurious to the individual—nicotine-stained fingers, chronic hyperemic pharynx, chronic cigarette cough. He should look also for telltale signs of substance abuse— tremor, alcohol odor on the breath. Poor muscle tone, lack of conditioning, and obesity and other evidences of dietary indiscretion should be a stimulus to the physician to advise his diver-patient in constructive fitness programs.

The diver candidate that you, the physician-reader, will most often encounter is the sport or recreational diver. Remember, sport diving is for *fun*, and any condition present that could hurt the diver or result in injury to his buddy diver should be considered disqualifying. The buddy-diver system is the universally recognized practice of pairing scuba divers for mutual safety and implies that each of the pair is fully capable of providing effective aid to the other in any emergency. Or you may be called upon to determine the fitness of a commercial diver, especially if you indicate an interest in providing such a service to the industry. There is a good chance you might be asked to examine a candidate for one of the many schools that train commercial divers. For this reason, commercial standards in some detail, as well as general standards, are presented in this chapter. An individual can spend as much as $4000 or invest two years of time in studying to become a commercial diver. He should know, at the outset, his employability chances from the physical point of view.

In considering the specifics of the physical examinations and selection criteria for diving, I have sought advice and comments from a heterogenous group of diving medical experts[1] to make the opinion stated herein as universally acceptable as possible.

---

[1] I wish to express my sincere gratitude to these experts in the field of undersea medicine for the input of their knowledge, experience, and forthright opinion on physical standards for diving: Capt. Robert C. Bornmann, MC, USN, Washington, DC: undersea medicine; Capt. Mark E. Bradley, MC, USN, Bethesda, MD: occupational medicine; Col. Jefferson C. Davis, MC, USAF, San Antonio, TX: aerospace medicine; Christopher Dueker, M.D., Palo Alto, CA: anesthesiology; David Elliott, M.B., D. Phil., M.R.C.P., London, England: consultant undersea activities; Hugh D. Greer III, M.D., Santa Barbara, CA: neurology; Eric P. Kindwall, M.D., Milwaukee, WI: hyperbaric medicine; Barry S. Kronman, M.D., Melbourne, FL, otorhinolaryngology; John Paul Jones, Jr., M.D., Lakeport, CA: orthopedic surgery; Rev. Edward H. Lanphier, M.D., Madison, WI: physiologist; LCDR Tom S. Neuman, MC, USN, San Diego, CA: internal/pulmonary medicine; Lawrence W. Raymond, M.D., Orange, NJ: internal medicine; Capt. Lewis H. Seaton, MC, USN, Groton, CT: ophthalmology; Michael B. Strauss, M.D., Long Beach, CA: orthopedic surgery; Capt. James Vorosmarti, MC, USN, Bethesda, MD: occupational medicine; Robert D. Workman, M.D., Picayune, MS: physician.

a. Age

It is difficult to set a minimum age for diving: individual variation in development, strength, maturity, and intelligence is too wide. From a practical standpoint, several of the established training agencies will train 12-year-olds in the company of a responsible family adult 18 years or older. Such training leads to a *junior diver* certification. The normal minimal age for *basic* certification training is 15 years. By practice 18 years is the accepted minimum age for commercial diving in the United States, and it is the age mandated by regulation in the United Kingdom and other jurisdictions. At the other end of the age scale, to begin a commercial diving career after the age of 30 is a doubtful venture and should be discouraged because of the reluctance of commercial diving companies to hire these older individuals; but there is really no age limit for sport diving. Careful attention to neuromuscular, pulmonary, and cardiovascular condition of the diver is recommended for both commercial and sport divers. Susceptibility to diving accidents, such as an increased incidence of decompression sickness, has been documented for increasing age. The U.S. Navy permits only supervisory activity for divers older than 45. For sport divers and scientific divers, physiological age is more important than chronological age.

b. Sex

Sex, per se, should not affect an individual's selection for any type of diving. I refer the reader to the part of Chapter III concerning women in diving activities, particularly diving and pregnancy.

c. Body Build

Obesity represents a hazard to divers because of the effect of inert gas exchange and its relationship to decompression sickness and it also is a reflection of general physical fitness. A value of more than 20% over ideal weight (with body build and age being considered) should at least temporarily disqualify commercial, scientific, and military divers. Sport divers should be discouraged from diving until they fall within acceptable levels, but there is no way to enforce such recommendations. With average skin-fold thickness measurements from the midtriceps, subscapular, and sacroiliac areas, the estimate of percentage of total body fat can be obtained from several nomograms. Total body fat of less than 25% is desirable.

d. Nervous System

Sudden loss of motor control, sensory neural failure, and loss of consciousness are unacceptable occurrences in any diving situation. The risk of drowning and the likelihood that pulmonary overpressurization accidents will occur as a result of nervous system failure in the diving situation make the neurological history and careful neurologic examination of divers paramount in importance. The following conditions are considered totally unacceptable for diving:

- A seizure disorder, excepting childhood febrile convulsions, whether controlled by medications or not

- Neurosyphilis, brain or spinal cord tumors, or demylinating disease
- Head trauma with unconsciousness for longer than 24 hr, depressed skull fracture, brain laceration, intracranial hemorrhage, severe brain contusion, or persistent neurological or electroencephalographic abnormalities
- Narcolepsy, catelepsy, and similar states
- Unexplained loss of consciousness
- Central nervous system (including spinal cord) paralysis secondary to diving, if residua exist

For brain trauma of lesser degrees than listed, careful consideration is warranted prior to allowing an individual to dive, with close consultation between the neurosurgeon, neurologist, and diving physician over a sufficient period posttrauma to assure no sequelae. The presence of a normal neurological examination and electroencephalogram is also a requisite.

The examiner should perform and document in detail the result of the neurological examination. Reflexes including deep tendon reflexes and superficial abdominal and cremasteric reflexes must be tested, and the presence or absence of abnormal reflexes should be elicited and documented. Motor strength and cutaneous, vibratory, and position sense must be described. Documentation is extremely important. The postdive evaluation of a diving accident may reveal changes from the base-line data indicating a serious condition that might otherwise go unrecognized and thus untreated.

Migraine can be quite disabling and, if occurring during or following a dive, may be confused with central nervous system decompression sickness. It should be disqualifying for commercial and military diving; sport diving may be permitted on a case-by-case basis, again in close consultation between the examiner and neurological physician.

Psychosis or severe psychoneurosis is usually listed as cause for rejection. However, unless the examiner personally knows the candidate or the history, or unless bizarre behavior becomes manifest during the examination, the chances of detecting these disqualifying conditions are slim.

e. Ear, Nose, Throat

The anatomical and functional interrelationship between the ear structures, conducting airways of the nose, pharnyx, and air spaces of the head makes the otorhinolaryngologic evaluation extremely important in assessing a candidate's ability to dive.

Chronic inability to equalize pressure in the middle ear and sinus spaces or a history of recurrent infections of these spaces, or both, render the candidate unsuitable for diving. Morbidity involving these organs represents the most common presenting complaints among all divers. Most of the morbidity is minor, consisting of various degrees of squeeze or overpressurization. However, serious disabling conditions attributable to barotrauma can occur that may result in deafness or acute disability involving the equilibrium. The examiner must look closely for patent nasal pharyngeal airways and note the presence of obstructive polyps or turbinates, purulent discharge, or the telltale inflammatory mucosa of the "nose-drop habitué." Most important, the individual must prove his ability to move the tympanic membrane during a Valsalva maneuver.

Chronic perforations of the tympanum are disqualifying for all forms of diving. Cold water entering the middle ear through a perforation can cause vertigo, nausea, vomiting, and disorientation, and the entrance of bacteria or other foreign material creates the potential for middle ear infection. Temporary perforation or a history of ear surgery must be evaluated on an individual basis.

The great majority of traumatic diving-related ruptures of the tympanum result in minimal hearing loss and vertigo and will heal spontaneously in 1 to 4 weeks. Diving should be prohibited for 4 to 6 weeks following clinical healing. The lack of spontaneous healing usually indicates complicating eustachian dysfunction or middle ear disease. A tympanoplasty repairs the hole in the drum, and if the complicating factor is temporary, the repaired tympanum should withstand normal stresses of diving. If that factor was permanent or recurrent, the repair may fail at some variable time in the future. Once a tympanoplasty fails in a diving (or flying) situation, the sport diver should be advised against further diving, and commercial or scientific and technical divers should be disqualified. Successful stapes mobilization need not be disqualifying, but stapedectomy with wire or plastic prothesis insertion should disqualify for all types of diving. This is due to the possibility that pressure changes could force the prothesis through the oval window and cause a fistula. Ménière's disease, as contrasted to simple, acute self-limited labyrinthitis, should be disqualifying for diving. Electronystagmography may be useful in doubtful cases.

The decision to permit an individual to resume diving activities after surgical repair of round window fistula caused by barotrauma, which is now more often recognized as a diving accident (Freeman 1978), is still a matter of controversy. Wiesskopf (1978) reported a 20% failure rate of surgical repairs of round window fistulas. The unusually high frequency of refistulization, as compared with a low rate of occurrence of fistulas following stapedectomy, implies that abnormal pressure relationships are present and that ambient pressure changes should be avoided. Electronystagmography, tympanometry, and audiometry should be done prior to consideration of requalification following the repair of a round window fistula. In this regard, initial and annual audiograms are required of all commercial divers, and some companies require base-line electronystagmograms on preplacement physical examinations.

There are no prescribed standards for hearing acuity. For commercial diving, unilateral deafness (defined as an average of 80-dB loss at 500, 1000, and 2000 Hz), or an average 40-dB bilateral loss in the speech range (250–3000 Hz) should probably disqualify. In the case of commercial divers, annual audiometry is required by OSHA regulations. Because of gas flow characteristics, many hyperbaric chambers and diving helmets have noise levels in the decibel range that can produce occupational hearing loss (Summitt and Reimers 1971).

Chronic or recurrent external otitis may prove temporarily disabling for diving and should disqualify saturation divers. External otitis is a common disorder during saturation dives, even among divers without predisposition to the condition. Exostoses of the external auditory canal are commonly seen among aquatic-oriented males. They may become so large as to cause obstruction of the canal, causing conductive hearing loss and predisposing to external otitis. Surgical correction is recommended, and when severe the condition may be considered temporarily disqualifying for all commercial divers (DiBartolomeo 1979).

The ability to equalize pressure in sinuses is difficult to determine clinically, and for military, commercial, and scientific and technical divers, a pressure test should be required. The sport diver will probably eliminate himself because of repeated barotrauma, and the cost of a pretraining pressure test at a hyperbaric facility could be avoided.

Examination of the oropharnyx should reveal good oral hygiene, the absence of extensive dental caries or significant gingival disease. Improperly filled teeth may be the cause of dysbaric odontalgia, which can only be determined by the application of pressure; if present, reconstruction of the suspect restoration is required. The candidate should demonstrate the ability to securely hold a mouthpiece. Dental protheses that could obstruct the diver's airway should not be considered disqualifying for any type of diving, but the protheses should not be worn during diving. A commercial diver may be temporarily disqualified until his oral hygiene is corrected, since very often he must work in locations where dental care either is not available or is substandard. The development of an acute periapical abscess or a toothache in a saturated diver has obvious consequences. To abort a commercial saturation dive for such causes would be an embarrassing economic faux pas.

f. Eyes

Active disease of the eyes and adnexae should bar from all types of diving because pressure changes and physical contact with water may aggravate the underlying condition. Visual standards are quite specific for military divers and for scientific divers under the jurisdiction of NOAA (NOAA 1975, U.S. Navy 1980). There are no standards for the commercial divers in the United States. Commercial divers under the jurisdiction of the United Kingdom and Norway require as a minimum acceptable standard for uncorrected distant vision 6/36 for o.d. and o.s. and 6/24 for o.u. This corresponds to 20/120 and 20/80 Snellen, respectively. For near vision, Jaeger 16 for each eye separately and Jaeger 15 for both eyes together, corresponding to 20/100 and 20/90, respectively, are required. A more reasonable approach would be to consider binocular visual efficiency (BVE) as a limiting criterion at 80% efficiency. Table XI-3 illustrates and describes how to derive the BVE percentage rating (U.S. Navy 1980).

Thus, a diver could have congenitally or developmentally poor vision in one eye, e.g., caused by amblyopia, with vision measured at 20/200, but with 20/20 in his good eye he would have a BVE at 80%. It is believed that such use of the BVE would be a much more practical way to judge the commercial diver's visual ability. The examining physician should know at the time he is conducting the examination what visual tasks any diver is expected to perform. Visual acuity requirements for the sport diver should be quite lenient. Basically, the visually deficient sport diver should have sufficient acuity with or without corrective lenses (should he lose them under water) to be able to surface and maintain visual contact with his buddy, see his dive boat, or find the beach from which he started his dive.

Color vision tests should be performed using standard techniques such as the pseudoisochromatic plate test available in several forms or the Farnsworth New London Navy lantern test. Color-deficient divers should not needlessly be disqualified unless they are required to perform tasks that involve color-coded electrical or compressed gas circuits. In questionable cases testing for demonstrated ability should be performed, in which the

Table XI-3
Binocular Visual Efficiency Computation[a]

Left eye	Right eye							
	20/20	20/30	20/40	20/50	20/70	20/100	20/200	20/400
20/20	100	98	96	94	91	87	80	76
20/30	98	92	90	88	85	81	74	69
20/40	96	90	84	82	79	75	68	64
20/50	94	88	82	77	73	70	62	58
20/70	91	85	79	73	64	60	53	49
20/100	87	81	75	70	60	49	42	38
20/200	80	74	68	62	53	42	20	16
20/400	76	69	64	58	49	38	16	3

[a]Instructions: Using the corrected Snellen vision in the right eye, find the appropriate vertical column and come down to the horizontal line that corresponds to the corrected vision in the left eye. The number where these columns meet is the corrected binocular visual efficiency expressed in percentage.

subject is shown samples of work requiring color discrimination and his abilities recorded. The Federal Aviation Administration (1970) uses this technique to certify color-deficient pilots.

g. Respiratory System

Diving, by its very nature, involves breathing gases that are under increased pressure and therefore are increased in density; this increases the work of breathing because of the increase in airway resistance, which is a function of gas density, cross-sectional area of the airway, and length of the airway. During inspiration, air flow is dependent on muscular work. During expiration, air flow is due primarily to the passive recoil of the lungs, is essentially independent of effort, and is dependent on airway flow capacity. Thus, any condition that affects gas flow (e.g., changes in the power of respiratory muscles, elastic properties of the lung, or the condition of the airway) can limit ventilation capacity, and this in turn limits a diver's effort potential.

Immersion in water has a definite effect on the airways by means of hydrostatic compression of the thorax and alteration of lung volume (Minh et al. 1977). In immersion, the diaphragmatic contraction is greater but the tidal volume is decreased, implying a stiffening of the lung. The result is that to maintain normal ventilation more work is required (Minh et al. 1978). Roentgenographic studies have been made of changes in the thoracic shape, and tantalum bronchographic studies have been performed that dramatically show the effects on the airways of the lungs, including marked decrease in diameter and length in the airways simply due to passive, hydrostatic effects. There is some evidence of early airway closure in the small airways, simply due to immersion (Dahlback and Lundgren 1972). With increasing depth the work of breathing increases in these attenuated airways by the addition of increasing density and possible viscosity of the respired gases (Wood 1963, Anthonisen et al. 1971). Anyone with limited ventilatory capacity on the surface is further restricted under pressure, and breathing through a diving appliance further restricts the diver.

Avoidance of pulmonary overpressurization is a primary concern of all engaged in diving, and especially of those responsible for selection of diving candidates, because of the potential seriousness of the triad of pathological conditions resulting (Linaweaver 1963). The triad consists of pneumothorax, mediastinal emphyema, and traumatic arterial gas embolism, the last-named being the most serious of the triad. In traumatic arterial gas embolism the dissection of gas into the left heart and then directly out into the arterial circulation, and usually to the central nervous system or the systematic arteries (including the coronaries), causes immediate obstruction of blood flow. Survival times of tissues beyond this obstruction have a finite limit, roughly 4–10 min. Immediate recompression therapy of air embolism casualties is indicated.

Any condition that can result in air trapping is contraindicated in diving of *all types*. It should be clear from the discussion so far that the most careful appraisal of the pulmonary system—historically, physically, roentgenographically, and by special testing—is indicated in the evaluation of a diver. In the history, general information should be obtained regarding, for example, smoking habits, occupational exposure, presence of dyspnea, cough, quantity and characteristics of sputum, pulmonary or bronchial infections.

Inquiry should be made regarding the history of the following specific conditions that may be absolute or relative contraindications to diving.

- Spontaneous pneumothorax
- Pneumothorax due to trauma
- Pneumothorax, subcutaneous or mediastinal emphysema, or arterial air embolism due to pulmonary overpressurization incidents
- Thoracotomy
- Established diagnosis of chronic pulmonary disease, whether obstructive, restrictive, neoplastic, or suppurative
- Asthma

(i) Pulmonary Disorders. Spontaneous pneumothorax is an absolute contraindication for all forms of diving. There is a high incidence of recurrence, as high as 44% (O'Hara 1978), in the same lung as well as the contralateral lung. Lung collapse, which can occur under pressure with expansion of the trapped extrapulmonary gas volumes upon surfacing, is an extremely hazardous situation. Pneumothorax caused by trauma (e.g., rib fractures, penetrating chest wounds, concussive injuries such as blast effect) also fall into the category of absolute contraindication for all types of diving. The injury results in damaged lung tissue which, although clinically healed, leaves scars, pleural adhesions, and other structural distortion predisposing to entrapment of air and the possibility of pulmonary overpressurization incidents. In the case of overpressurization accidents, many experts believe that further diving is contraindicated. Others, including myself, are of the opinion that if the individual "deserved" the accident (e.g., by breathholding during ascent, or by uncontrolled rapid ascent such as has occurred with accidental inflation of a bouyancy compensator), his return to diving activity should be on a case basis. If normal results are obtained from chest roentgenography, pulmonary function studies including xenon ventilation studies with washout, and monitored exposure to pressure under controlled conditions in a chamber, an individual can reasonably safely resume diving. Similar reasoning can be applied to the postthoracotomy diver. The training candidate or preemployment commercial diving applicant should not be qualified after thoracotomy. However, the experienced diver might be considered on a case basis, depending on why the procedure was done, how the procedure was done, by whom the procedure was done, and the result—using the same criteria described under accidents from overpressurization.

Most commercial firms would not accept such a diver, and the United Kingdom and Norway regulations forbid diving after thoracotomy. For example, an internationally known self-employed underwater photographer began to develop mediastinal and subcutaneous emphysema after each dive. He consulted a thoracic surgeon familiar with diving physiology. Use of the xenon ventilation-washout technique in the clinical workup revealed an area of gas trapping in the lingula. Thoracotomy with excision of the affected segment was performed with careful attention to surgical technique. Postthoracotomy evaluations with repeated xenon testing and hyperbaric pressures testing were normal, and the diver is again practicing his occupation. If large amounts of lung tissue are removed, such as a lobe, requalification should not be considered, since the remaining lung tissue overexpands to compensate for the lost lung volume and reduces the safety margin for overpressurization accidents. In summary, the presence of the chronic pulmonary conditions listed here are contraindicated for diving because of decreased pulmonary reserve and the increased risk of air trapping.

(ii) Asthma. Because of conflicting opinions among experts regarding the asthmatic individual and diving, the problem of asthma is presented in somewhat greater detail. One definition of asthma is as follows: "Bronchial asthma is a type of pulmonary incompetency due to constriction of the bronchi and edema of the bronchial mucosa, caused by the response of a susceptible bronchial tree to specific, allergic and/or nonspecific, irritative stimuli" (Sherman 1963). Today there is no doubt that allergy is an important factor in those patients whose asthma attacks are elicited by exposure to antigenic substances such as pollens, spores, or animal hairs or dander (allergens). This type of asthma is often called *extrinsic asthma* and is common among young and otherwise healthy people. In many patients with asthma, however, an association of symptoms with allergen exposure cannot be demonstrated; such patients who suffer from this condition are often classified as having *intrinsic asthma* (Bouhuys 1974). In asthma, airway resistance, mainly reflecting large airway diameter, is increased and maximum expiratory flows, which reflect small airway diameter, are decreased. Thus, both large and small airways appear to be affected; however, it is probable that small airway obstruction predominates. In a recent study from the University of California, San Diego, Wagner et al. (1978) measured the ventilation/perfusion relationship in asymptomatic asthma patients. Their study showed that in some of the asymptomatic asthmatic patients, as many as one-half of the lung units lay behind completely closed airways and had very low ventilation/perfusion ratios ($\dot{V}_A/\dot{Q}$) as a result of collateral ventilation. They demonstrated that even though standard pulmonary ventilatory function studies may appear grossly normal (because measurements are being made predominately of the large airways, or 80% of the ducting system), small airways may be closed. In a diving situation, respiring with closed airways cannot be tolerated. The possibility exists of developing acute, symptomatic, or asymptomatic bronchospasm in presensitized or predisposed airways by a variety of stimuli, including specific allergens, infection, chemicals, or physical stimuli, such as temperature changes or an aerosolized spray of water from a regulator. Psychophysiological effects affecting the vagus and other portions of the autonomic nervous system can cause bronchospasm (Horton et al. 1978). Hypocapnia caused by the hyperpnea of exercise can cause bronchoconstriction and could be compounded by the hyperventilation of the panicking diver (Zeballos et al. 1978). Airway muscle hypertrophy and increased responsiveness exists in these typical individuals, and, indeed, an increase in tone of airway muscle causing

airway constriction and development of asthma can occur whether the individual is aware of it or not. In the condition of acute asthma vital capacity decreases, even in the presence of a normal or increased total lung capacity, because of increase in residual volume. At residual volume, we can assume that the small airways are virtually closed, their flow resistance approaching infinity. The individual is then forced to breathe at an increased functional residual capacity (FRC), closer and closer to the total lung capacity (TLC). This causes dyspnea. Not only overpressurization but also overexpansion of the lung is a requisite for overpressurization accidents. The asthmatic, breathing at an elevated FRC near total lung volume (VL_{tot}), has already lost the margin of safety before overexpansion occurs. These factors result in increased susceptibility to overpressurization and the development of the triad of pathological conditions previously mentioned.

I don't think there is any informed physician who would say that an active asthmatic should dive. But should the individual who "grew out" of his asthma be allowed to dive? Based on experience, my answer is No, unless the individual is equipped to carry his own recompression chamber wherever he goes. The individual who has not had an asthmatic attack since he was 12 will, frequently, wheeze during forced expiration and not be aware of it. Pulmonary function studies on asthmatics will show decrease in the expiratory phase of the flow-volume curve and, in particular, the maximal midexpiratory flow (FEF_{25-75}), will be diminished (Weng and Levison 1969). To repeat the test with bronchodilators may prove fallacious, for many of the smaller airways (diameters of 2 mm), which have few muscle fibers, may not respond to the bronchodilators. It is always tempting to give in to the usually young, bright, eager, enthusiastic individuals, but the risk is too great. Once an asthmatic, always an asthmatic. If the diagnosis of asthma is in doubt or if the patient is asymptomatic, a positive histamine or methacholine test (or both) substantiates its existence. In asthmatics, hyperreactivity to methacholine persists for years, even in the absence of active asthma. In proper hands this test is a safe diagnostic tool (Townley et al. 1971).

(iii) Chest Examination. In examining the chest, the examiner should be looking for evidence of the conditions already described as well as a general assessment of the health and function of the pulmonary system. Several specific items should be looked for during inspection. During inspiration, is there equal expansion bilaterally or intercostal or lower rib retraction? Are accessory muscles of respiration being used? Are there surgical scars to suggest thoracotomy, placement of chest tubes, or penetrating wounds of the chest? The expansion of the chest should be measured with a measuring tape at the nipple level and the descent of the diaphragms should be percussed and the result documented. On auscultation, the usual signs of bronchial or parenchymal disease should be listened for specifically over each major lobe area during forced expiration for evidence of bronchoconstriction; the expiratory effort should be timed. If these observations are normal, then one can be almost certain that the examinee can safely dive. Why only almost? Because the presence of disqualifying lesions such as pulmonary cysts, bullae, atelectasis, parenchymal and pleural abnormalities, and solid lesions such as tumors and granulomata cannot be detected by physical examination. These lesions can only be detected by chest roentgenograph. Military, commercial, and most scientific or technical divers are required to have 14 × 17 posterior-anterior and lateral chest roentgenography initially. The frequency for follow-up chest x-ray examination varies widely, depending on the diving regulations that apply to the particular diver: ordinary military divers, triennially; satu-

ration and experimental military divers, annually; Occupational Safety and Health Administration (OSHA), initially only; California OSHA (CALOSHA), biennially; United Kingdom and Norway, annually; most companies belonging to the Association of Diving Contractors, annually. Sport divers should have a posterior-anterior (PA) and lateral x-ray examination initially, but it is not required by most training agencies. I will not certify any diver as being fit unless the examinee has had a normal 14 × 17 PA chest roentgenograph within a year, interpreted either personally or by a radiologist who understands the physical requirements for diving.

The need for pulmonary function tests is at the discretion of the examining physician for commercial divers under United States jurisdiction. It is recommended, and is required by the United Kingdom and Norway that at each examination a forced vital capacity (FVC) and a 1-sec forced expired volume ($FEV_{1.0}$) be measured. A value of less than 80% of the predicted FVC or a ratio of the actual $FEV_{1.0}$/FVC of less than 70% should disqualify. Other special tests such as xenon studies and methacholine challenge have previously been discussed. If arterial blood gas analysis is considered necessary by the physician, then the diver's fitness is suspect at the outset.

h. Cardiovascular System

Ordinary diving activities are strenuous, requiring high oxygen consumption and therefore high cardiac output. Emergency situations may stress the cardiac capacity to the limit. Any chronic heart disease, regardless of the underlying abnormalities (congenital, valvular, hypertensive, conductive, arteriosclerotic) that limit cardiac output, should be considered disqualifying. The physician must determine whether the presence of abnormalities are hemodynamically significant. Heart murmurs may be innocent or abnormal. Arrhythmias may be functional or clinically significant. If the arrhythmia worsens with exercise or is associated with preexcitation (Wolff-Parkinson-White syndrome) or midsystolic click (mitral valve syndrome), the diver should be disqualified. Septal defects that are clinically insignificant may become very important in the diving situation. Neuman et al. (1980) studied sheep exposed to pressures with an exposure time and decompression profile known to preclude clinical decompression sickness. In the studies, bubble formation was confirmed by Doppler bubble detection, and a rise in pulmonary arterial resistance and pulmonary arterial pressure and a decrease in wedge pressure (left atrial pressure) were found. These findings suggest that a right-to-left shunt through a septal defect or patent foramen ovale is possible during decompression and could lead to potential systemic bubble emboli. Since approximately 20% of the population have asymptomatic and undiagnosable (short of autopsy) patent foramen ovale, this postulate might explain the unexpected and unusual cases of decompression sickness of the upper central nervous system, e.g., scintillating scotomata, tunnel vision, or auditory and vestibular decompression sickness.

There are no universally recognized acceptable upper limits for blood pressure. The U.S. Navy limit for divers is 145 mmHg systolic and 90 mmHg diastolic without medication. The United Kingdom and Norway mandate 144 mm/90 mm without therapy for commercial divers. It is reasonable to find physically fit scientific or technical and recreation divers with blood pressures up to 150 mm/90 mm even when diuretic therapy is required to maintain this level. The addition of other medications usually indicates more severe hypertension; their use pharmacologically alters the autonomic nervous system function (and response to stress), and diving is not recommended.

Arteriosclerotic cardiovascular disease of any degree is disqualifying for military and commercial divers. The presence of exertional angina or history of myocardial infarction or coronary bypass surgery should render all other divers unfit. The latter condition carries two strikes against the diver—the disease itself and the condition of being postthoracotomy, which usually requires insertion of a chest tube and other violations of the chest wall and pleurae. Special consideration in the case of the noncommercial diver can be argued where the cardiac status has normalized after myocardial infarction. That is to say, if exercise tolerance is normal, and if electrocardiographic and coronary angiographic tests (and special studies such as isotopic myocardial imaging under stress) indicate adequate circulation and no significant myocardial injury, a noncommercial diver could be permitted to dive. However, he should be informed that he is statistically at greater risk for recurrent disease.

Arteriosclerotic peripheral and cerebral vascular disease is rare in the military and commercial age group but is disqualifying if present. These conditions should be looked for in the older, noncommercial diver, the degree of impairment assessed, and a recommendation for diving derived on an individual basis.

Venous varicosities or hemorrhoids should not restrict diving activities unless of a severe nature; clinical judgment is indicated.

The blood is considered as part of the cardiovascular system, and any condition that alters oxygen delivery capacity, carbon dioxide transport, and normal buffering capacity should eliminate a candidate. Chronic anemia, 2, 3- diphosphoglycerate deficiency, hemoglobinopathies (especially sickle-cell disease) are disqualifying for all types of diving. In the latter condition, the hemoglobin crystallizes under conditions of decreased oxygen tension—acidosis or statis—predisposing to sludging of the blood, thrombosis and infarction, and even aseptic bone necrosis. For this reason, a sickle-cell test is required by most diving companies on preemployment physical examinations. Coagulopathies are also disqualifying for obvious reasons. All military and commercial and most scientific and technical divers are required to have initial and periodic hemoglobin, hematocrit, and white cell count determinations.

i. Alimentary System

Common sense about the alimentary system should prevail in determining fitness. The active enteropathies such as Crohn's disease and ulcerative colitis makes those individuals unfit for diving because of stress and changes in bowel gas volumes that accompany pressure changes, and these individuals are usually debilitated to some degree. Active peptic ulcer disease should disqualify the professional diver who might have to work overseas, offshore, or in a saturation or deep-diving mode requiring long decompression. The risk of hemorrhage, perforation, or obstruction warrants such disqualification. A diver can be requalified after he demonstrates healing of the ulcer and that he does not require an elaborate medical regimen to remain asymptomatic. Clinical judgment must prevail in considering the fitness of sport, harbor-type commercial divers, and scientific or technical divers, since they usually are proximate to medical care should a problem arise. A history of diverticulitis should be considered in a similar manner.

Hernias that might incarcerate should be repaired prior to allowing an individual to be exposed to pressure changes. Pancreatitis is disqualifying for professional diving because of the underlying precipitating causes as well as its relationship to aseptic bone necrosis. Multiple abdominal surgical procedures should disqualify the military and commercial diver because of the high risk that mechanical bowel obstruction from postsurgical adhesions could occur with pressure changes. I was personally involved with such a case in a saturation diver who, fortunately, was only at 40 ft during the decompression phase of a heliox saturation dive when he developed a mechanical bowel obstruction. His decompression was hastened by oxygen breathing, and he was successfully transferred to a hospital for definitive treatment before any morbidity occurred. What if he had been at 500 ft?

j. Musculoskeletal System

The musculoskeletal system provides an individual with mechanical support, protection, prehension, dexterity, locomotion, flexibility, strength, and durability. The system consists of muscles, connective tissue, cartilage, bone, and attendant nerves and blood vessels. A diver requires all of these functions and components to be intact in order to function effectively and safely under water.

Each tissue described reacts differently to injury. Muscles and connective tissue structures—including ligaments, tendons, and fascia—respond to injury by forming scar tissue; scar tissue cannot contract or stretch and is relatively avascular. Cartilage covers joint surfaces and has no direct blood supply; when damaged, cartilage is replaced by scar and leaves the underlying bone of the joint uncovered and subject to arthritic changes. Bone when injured can heal, reforming living bone, and bone rebuilds in response to stress. Bone healing depends to a great extent on viable surrounding soft tissue to provide blood supply, oxygen, and nutrients. Nonunion of bone fractures can occur if concurrent damage to soft tissue at or near the fracture site is extensive or results in excessive scar tissue with attendant decrease in blood supply. An intact blood supply is essential for adequate decompression of any tissue, and scar formation can alter inert gas exchange dynamics. There is no clear evidence that the presence of malunion, nonunion, or extensive injury to bone or soft tissue with scarring predisposes to decompression sickness per se. However, my experience suggests that a bend tends to localize at the site of previous trauma and, especially, at the site of a previous bend.

There are no universally accepted criteria for determining fitness for diving from an orthopedic point of view. As with other systems, consideration must be given to whether the diver will be in a decompression situation that uses mixed gases as opposed to shallow sport or professional diving with air, and any condition that significantly compromises blood supply to the musculoskeletal system should render a diver unfit.

Neuromuscular and muscular disease, such as a muscular dystrophy, myotonia, amyotonia, myasthenia gravis, polymyositis, and related diseases, are absolutely disqualifying for all types of diving. Many of the progressive connective tissue diseases fall into this category also. The presence of unstable major joints subject to dislocation or subluxation, which might occur under water, would be extremely hazardous to the diver.

The presence of a nonunion or pseudoarthrosis and the presence of fixation devices for long bone fractures are contraindicating for commercial or any decompression diving. Their presence indicates that the injury was of such significance that normal healing was not possible or that surgery was required to achieve healing. Sport diving, with these conditions, may be possible with advice from an orthopedist.

Most authorities agree that the presence of dysbaric osteonecrosis in the juxta-articular location should disqualify all divers, even sport divers, who would dive deeper than 30 ft (9 m). Currently, there is controversy whether individuals with shaft osteonecrosis should also be found unfit. Further decompression diving is not recommended if the shaft lesion developed in the absence of precipitating causes, such as omitted decompression, untreated decompression sickness, or alcoholism, suggesting an individual predisposition to osteonecrosis.

Back surgery for removal of a herniated disc or fusion of a spine precludes further commercial diving because of the associated extraordinary disability and the vulnerability of the diving employer under the current legal climate. In view of the recent work on the etiology of spinal cord decompression sickness by Hallenbeck and Sokoloff (1978), decompression diving may be contraindicated following disk injuries or back surgery due to alteration of the epidural vertebral-venous system. Because of the extreme liability for back injuries, many U.S.-based diving contractors require preemployment lumbosacral spine x-ray pictures. These radiographs are interpreted and classified according to a protocol of *unknown origin* ranging from Classes I–V (see Appendix B). Classes I and II are employable. Class III is employable at the discretion of the examining physician. Classes IV and V are employed by "special approval of the management," which in the real world is never forthcoming. This practice is the source of much controversy. Several ad hoc meetings of knowledgeable persons in the fields of radiology, orthopedics and diving medicine have been held to deliberate the problems (Daugherty 1979). The results of most of these meetings have been to deplore this automatic disqualification without benefit of clinical evaluation. However, the practice continues. Other industries have questioned the rationale of preemployment back x-ray pictures because no correlation was found in the incidence of back problems and the presence of abnormal x-ray studies. When back injuries do occur, however, those with abnormal studies have longer and more costly disabilities. Whether one agrees with the practice or not, many major companies that hire divers do follow the protocol (probably at the insistence of third-party insurers). Therefore, the candidate for a commercial diving training program should be advised to have the back radiograph to determine his employability before starting the application procedure.

The loss of a major extremity renders an individual unfit for military and commercial diving, although there have been some notable exceptions in the past. The amputee diver, particularly if fitted with an appropriate prosthesis, may be able to perform his duties in a satisfactory manner. Offshore diving, and the requirement for transfer at sea from small boats and helicopters, and very hazardous heavy industrial activities aboard an offshore platform—all put the amputee at considerable disadvantage in a very unsafe environment. The sport diving amputee should dive in accordance with his limitations that only he can define.

k. Skin

Skin infections are very common among commercial divers who must stay for long periods of time in chambers with high humidity and relative lack of sanitary conditions, as well as among those commercial divers who work in polluted waters. A commercial diving candidate with active skin diseases, such as impetigo, extensive furunculosis, and other forms of pyoderma, must be treated before being found fit. The presence of widespread or severe atopic skin conditions also should be considered disqualifying. The presence of surface-dwelling parasites such as scabies or head, body, or pubic lice should be carefully looked for and treated.

l. Metabolic Disorders

Any significant metabolic disorder involving the pituitary, adrenal, or thyroid gland precludes an individual from commercial diving. Diabetes is disqualifying unless controlled by diet alone. Most experts consider the requirement for oral hypoglycemics or insulin to control diabetes to be highly dangerous for diving.

m. Genitourinary Disorders

Chronic renal disease or a history of multiple renal calculi disqualifies the commercial diver, while other urinary tract diseases or conditions must be considered on a case basis, as is the fitness of a scientific or sport diver.

3. *Special Studies Required for Divers*

Besides the history and physical examination, OSHA requires the following laboratory or special testing for commercial divers: initial only 14 × 17 PA chest radiograph; initial standard 12-lead electrocardiogram; initial and annual audiogram to American National Standards Institute (ANSI) standards; initial tests of visual acuity and color vision; initial and annual hematocrit, hemoglobin, white blood count, and routine urinalysis. Bone and joint radiographs are required initially and triennially for those commercial divers engaged in dives outside the no-decompression depth-time limits. The use of the protocol established by the British Medical Research Council Decompression Sickness Registry is required (Appendix C). Many diving contractors have additional requirements: an initial electroencephalogram and electronystagmogram; initial and annual pulmonary function tests (usually FVC and $FEV_{1.0}$); stress electrocardiography initially and reexamination after reaching a certain age level, usually age 30. Many of the diving contractors are requiring the use of chemistry panels, particularly to look for evidence of alcoholic hepatitis and stress indicators such as cholesterol and uric acid levels. Recently, they have also been insisting on a urinalysis for chromatographic drug screening for evidence of drug abuse.

4. *Physical Fitness to Dive*

In the preceding paragraphs much emphasis was placed on conditions that would render a diver fit or unfit to perform the activities for which he was being examined. In assessing an individual's fitness to dive, in addition to screening the above-described liabilities or attributes that pertain to safe diving, assessment should be made of physical qualities of strength and endurance as well as emotional qualities of maturity, risk acceptance, motivation, and stability. Physical strength and endurance can be qualitatively derived in the physician's office. Cardiac response to exercise can be quantitatively obtained through use of a variety of equipment and following several equally valid protocols and these results can be used as an estimate of cardiovascular fitness (Hellerstein 1979a, 1979b). The more subtle emotional factors and transient physical conditions, such as intercurrent infection, fatigue, hangover, minor trauma, must be assessed immediately predive. A diver's fitness must go beyond the initial or annual vist to the physician; it must be continued as an on-the-spot assessment of the individual by the dive master, scuba instructor, offshore rig supervisor, or paramedic—to ensure safe diving among all types of divers (Miles 1977). The need for continuing physical fitness should be emphasized to all who dive, and the physician should be prepared to render specific recommendations on how to achieve this goal. Some diving companies have their own medical examination forms. Most have standardized their forms based on those published by the Underwater Engineering Group of the Construction Industry Research and Information Association of the United Kingdom. (See Appendix D.)

A diver who intends to dive in an area under the jurisdiction of the United Kingdom must have his examination performed by a "doctor approved to issue certificates of medical fitness." Approval of the physician is granted by the Secretary of State, after consultation with the Director of Medical Services at the Office of the Health and Safety Executive, London. A similar approval is required in Norway to certify divers under that jurisdiction. Original forms of fitness must be issued to the diver; photostatic copies are not recognized (Appendix E). The commercial diver who presents himself for examination is required to have his current diving logbook bearing his picture and signature to identify himself to the examiner. (Apparently, use of ringers in examinations has been a problem in the past.)

In conclusion, the physician who undertakes the responsibility of examining divers must have a thorough knowledge of the physiological and psychological stresses involved in underwater activities. The type of diving the examinee is intending to perform must be known by the physician, for the risks, standards, and legal requirements vary with the type of diving. Lastly, the safety of the diver and his codivers is paramount in arriving at the decision of fitness.

PAUL G. LINAWEAVER

APPENDIX A

NATIONAL ASSOCIATION OF UNDERWATER INSTRUCTORS
POST OFFICE BOX 630, COLTON, CALIFORNIA 92324
MEDICAL FORM

Please print or type

NAME_____ AGE_____ SEX_____

ADDRESS_____ CITY_____ ZIP_____

OCCUPATION_____ HOME PHONE_____

HEIGHT_____ inches   WEIGHT_____ POUNDS

To The Physician:

This person is an applicant for training in diving with self-contained underwater breathing apparatus (SCUBA). This is an activity which puts unusual stress on the individual in several ways. Your opinion of the applicant's medical fitness is desired. Scuba diving requires heavy exertion. The diver must be free of cardiovascular and respiratory diseases. An absolute requirement is the ability of the middle ear and sinuses to equalize pressure. Any condition that risks the loss of consciousness should disqualify the applicant.

You will note that the medical examination form presents three (3) alternative choices under IMPRESSION. If you conclude that diving is not in the individual's best interest, please discuss your opinion with the person. If he/she persists in desiring to dive, and if definite threat to life and health is NOT involved, CONDITIONAL APPROVAL may be indicated. This will be considered with the understanding that the applicant has been told why you do not consider him/her fully qualified and that the individual accepts the responsibility for going ahead with the program.

References of possible value to the physician conducting medical examinations for scuba diving:

*Athletic Institute, Human Performance and Scuba Diving, 1970.
*CNCA, New Science of Skin and Scuba Diving, 1974.
*Dueker, Medical Aspects of Sport Diving, 1970
Miles, Underwater Medicine, 1969
USGPO, U.S. Navy Diving Manual, 1973.

*Available from NAUI

If there are any questions, please contact:

Instructor name, address, phone

Physician's Notes (see reverse side for medical history): ....

PLEASE RETURN THIS FORM TO THE APPLICANT

IMPRESSION: _____ 1. APPROVAL (I find no defects which I consider incompatible with diving.)

_____ 2. CONDITIONAL APPROVAL (I do not consider diving in this person's best interest but find no defects which present marked risk. I have discussed my impression with the patient.) Reason for conditional approval_____

_____ 3. DISAPPROVAL (This applicant has defects which in my opinion clearly would constitute unacceptable hazards to health and safety in diving.)

Date_____ Signature_____, M.D.

Address_____ Phone_____

Physical and Psychological Examination

NATIONAL ASSOCIATION OF UNDERWATER INSTRUCTORS
POST OFFICE BOX 630, COLTON, CALIFORNIA 92324

MEDICAL HISTORY FORM

Before your medical examination by the physician, this entire side and the top of the reverse side are to be completed. Be prepared to discuss any abnormalities or problems with your physician.

Check the appropriate blank if you have ever had any of the following apply to you, and explain under remarks, indicating the number.

.... 1. Previous diving experience	.... 15. Sinus trouble	.... 29. Tuberculosis
.... 2. Participate in active sports	.... 16. Motion sickness	.... 30. Respiratory problems
.... 3. Electrocardiogram	.... 17. Claustrophobia	.... 31. Persistent cough
.... 4. Mental or emotional problems	.... 18. Nervous breakdown	.... 32. Breathing difficulty
.... 5. Operation or illness	.... 19. Glasses or contacts	.... 33. Smoke
.... 6. Hospitalized	.... 20. Hearing difficulty	.... 34. Diabetes
.... 7. Serious injury	.... 21. Alcoholic beverages	.... 35. Chest pain
.... 8. Physical handicap	.... 22. Dental plates	.... 36. Use of street drugs
.... 9. Regular medication	.... 23. Trouble equalizing pressure	.... 37. Over 40 years old
.... 10. Allergies, including drugs	.... 24. Dizziness or fainting	.... 38. Pregnant
.... 11. Frequent colds or sore throat	.... 25. Epilepsy	.... 39. Using tranquilizers
.... 12. Severe or frequent headaches	.... 26. Heart trouble	.... 40. Bronchitis
.... 13. Rejected from any activity for medical reasons	.... 27. Ear trouble	.... 41. High blood pressure
.... 14. Hay fever	.... 28. Asthma	.... 42. Any medical problem not listed

PRINT OR TYPE REMARKS: ....

....

....

....

Date of chest x-ray ....

IF STUDENT IS A MINOR, BOTH PARENTS OR GUARDIANS MUST SIGN THIS FORM.

Date of previous medical examination ....

_____   _____
Parent/Guardian Signature   Date

_____   _____   _____   _____
Student Signature   Date   Parent/Guardian Signature   Date

Legal Name (for certification or records) ....

Nickname (for informal course use) ....

Home Address .... City .... State .... Zip ....

Birthdate .... Age .... Sex .... Home Phone ....

Occupation .... Company ....

Course applied for: .... City ....

In case of emergency, contact:

Name .... Relationship .... Phone ....

Doctor .... Day Phone .... Night Phone ....

Medical Insurance Co. .... Policy No. .... Phone ....

How did you learn of this course? ....

1/76

APPENDIX B

CURRENT LUMBOSACRAL SPINE X-RAY PROTOCOL
PRE-EMPLOYMENT LOWER BACK X-RAY

Class I and Class II applicants are eligible for employment. Class III applicants are eligible for employment at the discretion of the examining physician, with a negative history of back complaints or injury.
Class IV and Class V cannot be employed without special approval of the Management.

1. NORMAL SPINE—No abnormality—Class I

2. ARTHRITIS
    A. Osteoarthritis
        1. Single Spicule 2 mm. or less—Class II
        2. Multiple spicules 2 mm. or less—Class III
        3. Any spicule 3 mm. or more—Class V
        4. Hip or Hips any degree or type—Class V
    B. Rheumatoid arthritis, any degree—Class V
    C. Degenerative arthritis or destructive arthritis, any degree—Class V

3. ARTICULAR FACETS
    A. Ununited without arthritic changes—Class IV
    B. Ununited with arthritic changes—Class V
    C. Facets in different planes (AP) but clear on obliques—Class II
    D. Articular spaces obliterated on obliques—Class III
    E. Rudimentary or infantile facets—Class IV
    F. Marked difference in size of corresponding facets—Class IV
    G. Fracture old or recent—Class V

4. BONE DISEASE
    A. Any evidence of inflammatory or granulomatous disease—Class V
    B. Osteoporosis—Class V
    C. Osteosclerosis
        1. Single island, 10 mm. or less in diameter—Class II
        2. Multiple islands or generalized disease—Class V
    D. Pagets Disease—Class V

5. CURVATURE—Abnormal spinal
    A. Scoliosis
        1. With no associated pathology
            a. 10 mm. or less deviation from mid-sacral line—Class I
            b. 10 mm. to 20 mm. deviation from mid-sacral line—Class I
            c. More than 20 mm. deviation from mid-sacral line—Class V
        2. Any associated with rotation or arthritic changes—Class V
    B. Absence of normal lumbar curve—Class V
    C. Kyphosis any degree—Class V

6. FOREIGN BODIES
   A. Any, without special approval of the Management—Class V
   B. Opaque medication in soft tissues, without special approval of the Management—Class IV

7. FRACTURES
   A. Transverse Processes or Ribs
      1. Single ununited—Class III
      2. Multiple ununited, all on one side—Class IV
      3. Multiple ununited, bilateral—Class V
   B. Vertebral Body
      1. Questionable or definite, old or recent—Class V
   C. Any of pelvis, hips or otherwise unlisted—Class V

8. INTERSPACE CHANGES (measure at mid-portion of intervertebral space)
   A. Lumbo-sacral (compared with first normal interspace above)
      1. Narrowing up to 50%—Class III
      2. Narrowing 50% or more—Class V
   B. Any narrowing above the lumbo-sacral space—Class V
   C. Widening of the space or cupping of the vertebrae—Class IV
   D. Suggestive or definite evidence of pathological disc—Class V

9. LUMBO-SACRAL ANGLE (measured by Ferguson's method)
   A. 45 to 60 degrees—Class III
   B. 60 degrees or over—Class IV

10. NEOPLASMS
    A. Any evidence of primary or metastatic bone or soft tissue including osteochondroma, cysts, hemangioma, etc.—Class V

11. OPAQUE MEDIA IN VERTEBRAL CANAL–Class V

12. PELVIS AND HIPS
    A. Legg-Perthes—Class V
    B. Slipped epiphysis—Class V
    C. Evidence of fracture—Class V
    D. Deformity of pelvis or hip—Class V
    E. Any abnormality of sacro-iliac, unilateral or bilateral—Class V

13. SOFT TISSUE SHADOWS
    A. Definite evidence of abnormal or enlarged abdominal organs—Class V
    B. Calculic biliary, renal, ureteral, prostatic, pancreatic—Class V
    C. Calcification of pancreas, adrenals, spleen, aorta, or other vessels—Class V
    D. Calcified mesenteric node, without special approval of the Management—Class V

14. SPINA BIFIDA
    A. First sacral only—Class II

B. Last lumbar only—Class III
C. First sacral and last lumbar—Class III
D. Multiple sacral segments—Class III
E. Any single vertebra cephalad to the last lumbar—Class IV
F. Multiple vertebrae cephalad to the last lumbar—Class V

15. SPINOUS PROCESSES
    A. Evidence of fracture or other abnormality—Class V

16. SPONDYLOLISTHESIS
    A. Any degree, any level—Class V

17. SPONDYLOLYSIS (defect of pars interarticularis or isthmus)
    A. Unilateral or bilateral, any level—Class V

18. SURGERY (any evidence of)
    A. Myelogram—Class V
    B. Previous surgery, back, pelvis or hips—Class V

19. TRANSVERSE PROCESSES
    A. Ununited first lumbar or lumbar rib—Class II
    B. Sacralization or lumbarization
       1. Bilateral complete (no anomalous joint)—Class II
       2. Unilateral complete (no anomalous joint)—Class III
       3. Incomplete with anomalous joint (unilateral or bilateral)—Class V
    C. Fusion or anomalous articulation above lumbo-sacral—Class V
    D. Fracture—see paragraph 7

20. VERTEBRAL BODIES
    A. Butterfly vertebra—Class V
    B. Cupping of bodies (due to enlarged disc or notocordal rest)—Class IV
    C. Fusion of vertebral bodies—Class V
    D. Hemi-vertebrae or other such abnormalities—Class V
    E. Persistant vertebral body epiphysis—Class IV
    F. Schmorl's nodules
       1. Less than three, all less than 3 mm. deep—Class II
       2. Three or more, all less than 3 mm. deep—Class IV
       3. Any 3 mm. or more deep—Class IV
       4. Three or more, and 3 mm. or more deep—Class V
    G. Unusual number, 4 or 6 normal lumbar vertebrae—Class II
    H. Vertebral epiphysitis (Schuireman's Disease)—Class V

NOTE: When two or more separate pathological conditions exist in the same individual he should be put in one class below the maximal he would occupy with a single defect. These changes apply to ALL THORACIC as well as lumbar vertebrae that can be visualized.

APPENDIX C

SANTA BARBARA MEDICAL FOUNDATION CLINIC
Commercial Diving Physical Examination
PROTOCOL FOR RADIOGRAPHIC EXAMINATION FOR DYSBARIC OSTEONECROSIS OF COMMERCIAL DIVERS
STANDARD OSHA

(Based on British Medical Research Council—Decompression Sickness Panel Standards).

The examination must include independent views of the head and proximal shaft of the humerus and femur and lateral views of each knee, including two-thirds of the femur shaft and one-third of the tibia shaft. While other views may be included if suspicion of clinical involvement is present, they are not included in the standard survey views.

I. The following factors are standard on each view:

Moving Bucky grid (employing 1:16 ratio grid if available)
10 × 12 cassettes
Par Speed Screens
40 inch distance (variable with equipment available)
One view per film
Gonadal shielding, ¼ inch lead or equivalent

II. The following independent views comprise a routine ten film survey:

Right shoulder and left shoulder joint with humeral shaft
    Grashey position internal rotation
    Grashey position external rotation
Right hip and left hip joint with femoral shaft
    Antero-posterior projection
    Frog-leg lateral
Right and left knee
    Lateral projection

III. The following positioning descriptions must be employed in obtaining the aforementioned views:

a) *Shoulder*—The patient is placed in a supine position with the trunk rotated at an angle approximately 45 degrees to bring the shoulder to be radiographed in contact with the table. This arm is straight and follows the trunk. Center 1 inch below the coracoid process of the scapula. Angle the tube head 5 degrees caudally (toward feet). Cone to show as much humerus as possible bringing in the lateral diaphragm to show only the head and shaft of the humerus. This positioning should show a clear joint space and the acromion should not overlap the head of the humerus.

With the patient positioned as above, and without moving body position, the two required views are accomplished as follows:

Internal Rotation—Palm down with the hand flat against the table
External Rotation—Palm up with the hand flat against the table

b) *Hip. Antero-posterior* positioning. The patient is placed in a supine position with the feet 90 degrees to the table top. The edge of the Gonad shield should be as near the femoral head as possible but not obscuring the femoral head. Center the cone over the head of the femur, that is 1 inch below the mid-point of a line joining the anterior superior iliac spine and the upper border of the pubic symphysis.

Frog-leg lateral—The patient is placed in a supine osition on the table with the foot of the side for examination level with the opposite knee. The flexed knee is elevated about 10 degrees and supported. Gonadal shielding and centering are the same as in the hip antero-posterior view.

c) *Knee. Lateral Projection*. The patient is placed in a supine position on the table and rotated to bring the outside of the knee to be examined in contact with the table and the leg straight. The opposite leg is rotated anteriorly to the knee being examined to result in the pelvis being perpendicular to the table. Center at the level of the upper border of the patella. The field should include the lower $\frac{2}{3}$ of the femur and the upper $\frac{1}{3}$ of the tibia and fibula.

GONAD SHIELDING MUST BE EMPLOYED IN ALL VIEWS. Forego the survey if shielding is not available. Immediate notices will be forwarded to facilities that do not employ gonadal shielding.

The radiographs in this survey must be of a high standard and must show good trabecular detail. A radiologist review and reading at the time of survey is requested unless a radiologist is not available to the facility. Probably the greatest error lies in underpenetration of the radiographs resulting in inadequate trabecular detail in which small dense areas near the joint surfaces will not be identified. Other difficulties in interpretation arise from malformation of the shoulder joint resulting in the superior border of the greater tuberosity appearing as a dense layer which could be misinterpreted as osteonecrosis.

APPENDIX D

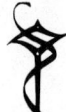

SANTA BARBARA MEDICAL FOUNDATION CLINIC

Medical examination of commercial divers

Section 1 To be completed by the diver   Cross out YES or NO whichever is incorrect

NAME: Surname _____ Forenames _____   Office use ▢▢▢▢▢▢
ADDRESS: _____   Date of birth ▢▢▢▢▢▢

Where were you brought up? _____   NHS _____
NAME AND ADDRESS OF YOUR OWN DOCTOR _____
_____   NI _____

Have you filled in one of these forms before? Yes / No
If Yes to above say when? _____ and where? _____
Can you swim? Yes / No   Are you afraid of heights, confined spaces or darkness? Yes / No If 'Yes' which? _____
Where did you do your basic diver training? _____
In what year was this? _____
Who is your present employer? _____

What is the maximum depth to which you have dived? _____ metres
How long at that depth? _____ days _____ hours _____ mins
What is the duration of your longest dive? _____ days _____ hours _____ mins
What is the maximum depth of your longest dive? _____ metres
How many times have you dived deeper than 152m (500 ft) _____
How many times have you dived deeper than 50m (165 ft) _____
How many saturation dives have you done? _____
How many hours have you spent at saturation? _____
How many bends have you had? Type I _____ Type II _____
Have you been involved in a diving accident since your last examination? Yes/No

3. Have you had any of the following:

Tuberculosis	Yes / No	Poor circulation	Yes / No	Bowel trouble	Yes / No	Other Fevers	Yes / No
Pneumonia	Yes / No	Sinusitis	Yes / No	Piles	Yes / No	Kidney or bladder trouble	Yes / No
Bronchitis	Yes / No	Ear trouble	Yes / No	Giddiness	Yes / No	Diabetes or sugar in urine	Yes / No
Collapsed lung or pneumothorax	Yes / No	Rheumatic Fever	Yes / No	Nervous breakdown	Yes / No	Operations or anaesthetics	Yes / No
Asthma	Yes / No	Heart disease	Yes / No	Fits or blackouts	Yes / No	Concussion	Yes / No
Hay Fever	Yes / No	High blood pressure	Yes / No	Recurrent headaches	Yes / No	Serious injury	Yes / No
Spitting of blood	Yes / No	Indigestion	Yes / No	Motion sickness	Yes / No		
Nose bleed	Yes / No	Ulcers	Yes / No	Tropical diseases	Yes / No		

Have you been treated by a doctor during the past year? Yes / No   If yes, why? _____
Are you taking any drugs, injections, medicines or tablets now? _____

4. Dates of last inoculations and x-rays:

For Typhoid/TAB _____ Tetanus _____ BCG _____ Smallpox _____ Polio _____ Cholera _____ Typhus _____
Yellow Fever _____   Other injections _____
Bone & joint X-rays _____   Where taken _____
Chest X-ray _____   Where taken _____
Other X-rays _____   Where taken _____

I declare that the answers given above are true to the best of my belief, and I give permission for the result of this examination to be disclosed to other doctors who examine me and to my Employer.

Signed _____   Date _____

5. Doctor's comments:

FORM NO. 395   White - Employer / White - Chart / Pink - Diver / Yellow - Overseas Regulatory Authority

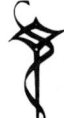

SANTA BARBARA MEDICAL FOUNDATION CLINIC
Medical examination of commercial divers

Section 2 To be completed by the doctor   Cross out YES or NO whichever is incorrect

Surname 8 _____ Forenames 6 _____ 7 _____ 16 DOB ☐☐☐☐ Computer No. 1 (Office Use) ☐☐☐☐

SEX: Male/Female 22 ☐   Height 23 ☐☐ Metres   Weight 26 ☐☐☐.☐ kg

EAM normal? R. Yes / No L. Yes / No	Any sinus abnormality? R. Yes / No L. Yes / No	Audiometry normal? R. Yes / No	**ENT normal?** 49 Yes / No
Ear drums normal? R. Yes / No L. Yes / No	URT Infection R. Yes / No L. Yes / No		
Eustachian tubes patent? R. Yes / No L. Yes / No	Nasal airways normal? R. Yes / No L. Yes / No L. Yes / No		

Are teeth and gums in good condition? Yes / No   Any dentures? Yes / No   FEV₁ _____   FVC _____ 30
Lungs normal? Yes / No   Current CXR normal? Yes / No   FEV₁/FVC _____ %

Respiratory system normal? 50 Yes / No

Apex beat in normal position? Yes / No   32 syst   35 diast   37
Heart sounds normal? Yes / No   Blood pressure ☐☐ ☐☐   Heart rate (beats per minute) ☐☐
Heart murmurs? Yes / No
Peripheral circulation normal? Yes / No   Sickle cell trait? Yes / No   PCV? 39 ☐☐
Varicose veins? Yes / No   ECG Normal? Yes / No

Cardiovascular system normal? 51 Yes / No

Is abdominal palpation normal? Yes / No   Hernia? Yes / No   Skinfold 41   43
Skin rashes, infections or infestations? Yes / No   L.Biceps ☐☐   L.Triceps ☐☐
Lymphatic glands normal? Yes / No   45   47
External piles? Yes / No   L.Subscapular ☐☐   L.Sacro-Iliac ☐☐
Genito urinary system normal? Yes / No

Alimentary system normal? 52 Yes / No
Skin normal? 53 Yes / No

Limbs normal? Yes / No   Spine normal? Yes / No   Current joint x-rays normal? Yes / No

Limbs & bones normal? 54 Yes / No

Are the cranial nerves normal: Are reflexes normal:
I Yes / No   V Yes / No   IX Yes / No   Rt. Tri. Yes / No | AJ Yes / No   Lt. Tri. Yes / No | AJ Yes / No
II Yes / No VI Yes / No X Yes / No   Bi. Yes / No | Abdo Yes / No   Bi. Yes / No | Abdo Yes / No
III Yes / No VII Yes / No XI Yes / No   Sup. Yes / No | Plantar Yes / No Sup. Yes / No | Plantar Yes / No
IV Yes / No VIII Yes / No XII Yes / No   KJ Yes / No   KJ Yes / No

Nervous system normal? 55 Yes / No

Power and tone of limbs normal and equal? Yes / No   Proprioception normal? Yes / No   Cerebellar function normal? Yes / No
Normal sensation to: Pinprick? Yes / No   Light touch? Yes / No   Temperature? Yes / No
Vestibular function normal? Yes / No   Rombergism? Yes / No

Vision without glasses: R. 6/ ___ L. 6/ ___   Vision with glasses: R. 6/ ___ L. 6/ ___
Visual fields normal? R. Yes / No L. Yes / No   Colour vision normal? Yes / No   Fundi normal? R. Yes / No L. Yes / No

Eyes normal? 56 Yes / No

Normal exercise tolerance test? Yes / No   General appearance

ETT normal? 57 Yes / No

Urine: Identifying features, scars, tatoos, etc.
Albumin? Yes / No   Sugar? Yes / No
Blood? Yes / No   Ketones? Yes / No

Urine normal? 58 Yes / No

Comments on any abnormalities mentioned above:

Fit? 59 Yes / No

In your opinion:
1. Is the candidate free from physical defect and disease? Yes / No   2. Has he the physique for prolonged exertion? Yes / No
3. Is he fit to dive without limitation? (If no, specify) Yes / No   4. Is he fit for service in a tropical climate? Yes / No

66
Signature of medical examiner _____ Qualifications _____ Date 60 ☐☐ ☐☐ ☐☐
                                                                                           day month year
Address Calle Real at San Marcos Pass Road   P.O. Box 1200 Santa Barbara CA 93102

FORM NO. 396   White - Employer / White - Chart / Pink - Diver / Yellow - Overseas Regulatory Authority

APPENDIX E

THE OFFSHORE INSTALLATIONS (DIVING OPERATIONS) REGULATIONS 1974
THE MERCHANT SHIPPING (DIVING OPERATIONS) REGULATION 1975
THE SUBMARINE PIPE-LINES (DIVING OPERATIONS) REGULATIONS 1976

Certificate of Medical Fitness to Dive issued by a Doctor approved by the Secretary of State

(1) Insert full name of diver in block capitals

1 IT IS HEREBY CERTIFIED that[1]

_____

(2) Insert private address of diver in block capitals

of [2] _____

_____

(3) Insert day, month, and year

(hereinafter called 'the diver') whose date of birth is[3]

_____ 19 _____

has been medically examined by me and that he is fit to dive.

(4) See note 1(a) overleaf

2. This certificate is issued subject to the conditions(s) that[4] (a) the diver shall not dive to a depth greater than _____ metres;

_____

_____

_____

and in accordance with the relevant provisions of the Regulations is not valid for diving operations as defined in those Regulations other than diving operations in which those conditions are satisfied.

(5) See notes 1(b) and 2(b) overleaf

3 The diver should be medically examined within a period of _____ months from the date of this certificate[5]

(6) Not more than seven days after date of examination

Date of issue[6] _____ 19 _____

Signature of approved doctor

_____

(7) Block capitals

Full name of approved doctor[7]

_____

Address of approved doctor[7]

_____

NOTES

1 FOR THE ATTENTION OF THE APPROVED DOCTOR:

(a) The certificate may be issued subject to such conditions as you consider necessary to the safety and health of the diver. Delete and initial the condition set out in paragraph 2 if it is unnecessary, and/or insert any other condition necessary to his safety and health.

(b) The Regulations forbid a diver to be employed or to take part as a diver in diving operations unless not more than 12 months beforehand a certificate has been issued by an approved doctor that the diver is fit to dive, but a certificate may state that the diver should be medically examined within a shorter period. If you consider that the diver should be reexamined within less than 12 months state the shorter period in paragraph 3. The diver is then forbidden to dive after that period unless a fresh certificate is issued by an approved doctor that the diver is fit to dive. If you consider that no such stipulation is necessary delete paragraph 3 and initial the deletion.

2 FOR THE ATTENTION OF THE DIVER AND THE EMPLOYER OF DIVERS:

(a) This certificate must be given to the employer of the divers (as defined in the Regulations)

(b) The diver must not be employed or take part as a diver in diving operations (as defined in the Regulations) after 12 months from the date of this certificate, or if a shorter period is stated in paragraph 3 of this certificate after that period, unless a fresh certificate that the diver is fit to dive is issued by an approved doctor before he is again employed or takes part as a diver in diving operations.

(c) If conditions are specified in paragraph 2 of the certificate, it is not valid for diving operations other than diving operations in which these conditions are satisfied.

(d) If by reason of illness or physical injury the diver is unable for a continuous period exceeding 7 days to work underwater as a diver, this certificate shall cease to be valid.

(e) The diver should obtain the certificate from the employer of divers when the diver leaves his employment or when the diver ceases to take part as a diver in diving operations with which the employer of divers is concerned, as the case may be.

NOTE: The statutory provisions relating to the above are contained in:

Regulation 12 of the Offshore Installations (Diving Operations) Regulations 1974

Regulation 12 of the Merchant Shipping (Diving Operations) Regulations 1975

Regulation 12 of the Submarine Pipe-lines (Diving Operations) Regulations 1976

References

ANTHONISEN, N. R., M. E. BRADLEY, J. VOROSMARTI. AND P. G. LINAWEAVER 1971. Mechanics of breathing with helium-oxygen and neon-oxygen mixtures in deep saturation diving. In: *Underwater Physiology IV. Proceedings of the Fourth Symposium on Underwater Physiology*, edited by C. J. Lambertsen. New York: Academic Press, p. 339–345.
BOND, M. B. 1964. Low back X-rays. Criteria for their use in placement examinations in industry. *J. Occup. Med.* 6: 373–380.
BOUHUYS, AREND 1974. *Breathing: Physiology, Environment and Lung Disease*. New York: Grune and Stratton.
DAHLBACK, G. O., AND C. E. G. LUNDGREN 1972. Pulmonary air-trapping induced by water immersion. *Aerosp. Med.* 43: 768–774.
DAUGHERTY, C. G. 1979. Report of Ad Hoc Committee on low back X-rays (in the diving industry). New Orleans, LA.
DIBARTOLOMEO, JOSEPH R. 1979. Exostoses of the external auditory canal. *Ann. Otol. Rhinol. Laryngol.* 88: Suppl. 61.
FEDERAL AVIATION ADMINISTRATION 1970. *Guide for Aviation Medical Examiners*. Washington, DC: Federal Aviation Administration.
FREEMAN, PETER 1978. Rupture of the round window membrane. *Otolaryngol. Clin. N. Am.* 11: 81–93.
GRORUD, H. F., AND C. BÖL 1976. Hazards of offshore operations and control. In: *Automation in Offshore Oil Field Operations*, edited by F. L. Galtung et al. New York: Elsevier-North Holland.
HALLENBECK, J. M., AND L. SOKOLOFF, 1978. Blood flow studies during spinal-cord damaging decompression sickness in dogs. In: *Underwater Physiology VI. Proceedings of the Sixth Symposium on Underwater Physiology*, edited by C. W. Shilling, and M. W. Beckett. Bethesda, MD: Fed. Am. Soc. Exp. Biol., p. 579-585.
HELLERSTEIN, HERMAN K. 1979a. Specifications for exercise testing equipment. *Circulation* 59: 849A—854A.
HELLERSTEIN, HERMAN K. 1979b. Standards for adult exercise testing laboratories. *Circulation* 59: 421A–430A.
HORTON, D. J., W. L. SUNDA, R. D. KINSMAN, J. SOUHRADA. AND S. L. SPECTOR 1978. Bronchoconstrictive suggestions in asthma: a role for airways hyperreactivity and emotions. *Am. Rev. Respir. Dis.* 117: 1029–1038.
LINAWEAVER, P. G. 1963. Injuries to the chest caused by pressure changes, compression and decompression. *Am. J. Surg.* 105: 514–521.
LINAWEAVER, P. G. 1977. Physical examination requirements for commercial divers. *J. Occup. Med.* 19: 817–818.
MILES, S. 1977. Fitness to dive. In: *Proceedings of the Sixth International Congress on Hyperbaric Medicine*. Aberdeen, Scotland: Aberdeen Univ. Press, p. 415–418.
MINH, VU-DINH, G. F. DOLAN, P. G. LINAWEAVER, P. J. FRIEDMAN, R. G. KONOPKA. AND B. B. BRACH 1977. Diaphragmatic function during immersion. *J. Appl. Physiol.: Respir. Environ. Exercise Physiol.* 43: 297–301.
MINH, VU-DINH, G. F. DOLAN, D. D. NAM, P. G. LINAWEAVER. AND C. HARVEY 1978. Immersion vs. pressure-breathing and diaphragmatic function in the upright position. *Respir. Physiol.* 36: 36–49.
NATIONAL OCEANIC AND ATMOSPHERIC ADMINISTRATION 1975. *NOAA Diving Manual*. Washington, DC: U.S. Dept. of Commerce.
NATIONAL OCEANIC AND ATMOSPHERIC ADMINISTRATION 1976. *U.S. Underwater Diving Fatality Statistics*. Washington, DC: U.S. Department of Commerce.
NEUMAN, TOM, R. SPRAGUE, P. WAGNER. AND K. M. MOSER 1980. Cardiopulmonary consequence of decompression. *Respir. Physiol.* 41: 143–153.
O'HARA, VINCENT S. 1978. Spontaneous pneumothorax. *Mil. Med.* 143: 32–35.
OSHA and USCG 1977. Commercial diving operations, medical requirements, *Fed. Regist.* 42(141); Article 1910.41.
SHERMAN, WM. B. 1963. Asthma. In: *Textbook of Medicine* (11th ed.), edited by P. B. Beeson and W. McDermott. Philadelphia: W. Saunders.
SOMERS, LEE H. 1978. *Research Diver's Manual*. Ann Arbor: Univ. of Michigan Press.
SUMMITT, J. K., AND S. D. REIMERS 1971. Noise: a hazard to divers and hyperbaric personnel. *Aerosp. Med.* 42: 1173–1177.

TOWNLEY, R. G., V. Y. RYO, AND B. KANG 1971. Bronchial sensitivity to methacholine in asthmatic subjects free of symptoms from one to twenty-one years. *J. Allergy Clin. Immunol.* 47: 91–92.
United States Code 1964. Vol. 46, Sect. 688.
U.S. NAVY 1980. Physical examinations. In: *Manual of the Medical Department.* Washington, DC: U.S. Department of the Navy, chap. 15 (NAVMED P-117).
WAGNER, P. D., D. R. DANTZKER, V. E. JACOBONI, W. C. TOLMIN, AND J. B. WEST 1978. Ventilation-perfusion inequality in asymptomatic asthma. *Am. Rev. Respir. Dis.* 118: 511–536.
WEISSKOPF, ALEX, J. T. MURPHY, AND M. M. MERZENICK 1978. Genesis of the round window rupture syndrome: some experimental observations. *Laryngoscope* 88: 389–397.
WENG, T. R., AND N. LEVISON 1969. Pulmonary function in children with asthma at acute attack and symptom-free status. *Am. Rev. Respir. Dis.* 99: 719–728.
WOOD, W. B. 1963. Ventilatory dynamics under hyperbaric states. In: *Proceedings of the Second Symposium on Underwater Physiology*, edited by C. J. Lambertsen and L. J. Greenbaum. Washington, DC: Natl. Acad. Sci./Natl. Res. Council, p. 108–123 (Publ. 1181).
ZEBALLOS, R. J., R. SHTURMAN-ELLSTEIN, J. F. MCNALLY, JR., J. E. HIRSCH, AND J. F. SOUHRADA 1978. The role of hyperventilation in exercise-induced bronchoconstriction. *Am. Rev. Respir. Dis.* 118: 877–884.

Pertinent References Not Cited but Recommended for Review by the Reader

COX, ROBIN D. F. The medical examination of commercial divers. *Practitioner* 212: 861–866, 1974.
DUEKER, CHRISTOPHER W. *Medical Aspects of Sport Diving.* Cranbury, NJ: A. S. Barnes, 1969.
KINDWALL, ERIC P. Medical aspects of commercial diving and compressed air work. In: *Occupational Medicine: Principles and Practical Applications*, edited by C. Zenz. Chicago: Year Book Med. Publ., 1975, p. 361–421.
KINDWALL, ERIC P. Medical examination of the diver. In: *Diving Medicine*, by R. H. Strauss. New York: Grune and Stratton, 1976, p. 341–347.
STRAUSS, RICHARD H. State of the art: diving medicine. *Am. Rev. Respir. Dis.* 119: 1001–1023, 1979.
WALDER, D. N. The prevention of decompression sickness. In: *The Physiology and Medicine of Diving and Compressed Air Work* (2nd ed.), edited by P. B. Bennett and D. H. Elliott. Baltimore: Williams and Wilkins, 1975, p. 456–470.

B. *Psychological Standards for Diving*

A review of the available literature on diver selection and evaluation suggests that most of the problems associated with adjusting to underwater life could be resolved easily if divers had the intellect of a Nobel laureate, the courage of a gladiator, the perseverance of a missionary, the social adaptiveness of a politician, and the humility of a monk—in short, those who are most suited to work at watery depths should be able to walk on the surface as well.

In a discussion of submariner and diver selection written in 1945, Dr. Albert Behnke made several keen observations that would be true as well for many divers today, especially saturation divers. Personnel should not be selected "who are temperamentally unfit for close association and the type of teamwork that requires judgment and insight" (Behnke 1945). Research conducted nearly 25 years later will show that possession of interpersonal skills—referred to as *social adjustment, socialization,* or *sociability*—may well prove to be the most important characteristic that differentiates overall success among divers.

Behnke was adamant in stating that evaluations involving detection of abnormal personality traits in normal clinical settings would prove fruitless in diver selection. This has indeed been the case, as demonstrated by several investigators (Radloff and Helmreich 1968, Biersner and Cameron 1970, Weybrew 1974). This later work showed that the interaction between normal personality traits (as defined by demographic information) and diving stress would be most predictive of performance effectiveness, much as Behnke suspected in 1945. Research by Biersner and Ryman (1974a) found that divers did not differ from a matched nondiver control group in the prevalence of either neuroses or psychoses. These findings should not, however, deter the examining physician from denying admission or qualification to prospective (or active) divers who demonstrate abnormal behavior or perceptions; such cases should be referred to mental health professionals for more extensive evaluation. In the case of those who have a past history of psychosis or neurosis, referral to a mental health professional is recommended in order to ensure the total absence of disorder and the return of normal, healthy coping skills. Previous work cited above only indicates that psychopathology is likely to be a rare occurrence among divers and diver candidates and that the limited clinical and evaluating resources normally available would be better dedicated to other types of problems and to screening methodologies.

1. Recent Selection and Evaluation Research

For the purposes of this discussion the term *diver* is defined primarily as one who derives a major portion of income and livelihood from working at atmospheric pressures of more than 1 ATA and who is engaged in the following diving activities: commercial diving (e.g., construction, engineering, inspections) and in diving for research and noncombatant military support (e.g., ship salvage and husbandry, search and rescue). This definition excludes sports divers and submersible systems operators, including those who operate 1-ATA armored diving suits such as the JIM system, as well as Underwater Demolition Teams (UDT) and Explosive Ordnance Disposal (EOD) groups. Emphasis is on military research in diver selection, especially that research involving Divers First and Second Class[2] and saturation divers, because such research has dominated the research literature on selection and evaluation. Research on civilian divers, both scientific and commercial, is cited as appropriate.

a. Mechanical and Arithmetic Aptitudes

Inasmuch as diver training courses usually have substantial reading and computational requirements, aptitude tests that measure verbal intelligence and mechanical and mathematical aptitudes have been found useful in predicting diver training performance. These measures, however, have not been used to evaluate performance under operational diving conditions. In the first research involving selection for Diver First Class (DFC) training, Wise (1963) found that three of the Navy Basic Test Battery (BTB) measures (Mechanical, Arithmetic, and General Classification tests) correlated significantly with the final grade

---

[2] Divers First Class in the U.S. Navy have been trained for both air and mixed gas (helium-oxygen) diving and are permitted to dive to depths greater than 200 fsw. Divers Second Class are trained for air diving only and are normally restricted to depths of 200 fsw or less.

earned by 137 candidates in the course. A combination of the Mechanical and Arithmetic tests best predicted this criterion (R = 0.43). If a combined score of 80 on the two tests was used to select candidates, the attrition rate would have been lowered from 20% to 8%, with a false negative rate of only 3% (i.e., rejecting only 3% of applicants who would have succeeded). This standard, however, was not adopted by the U.S. Navy. Instead, a combined score of 105 on the Mechanical and Arithmetic tests was used. Berghage (1972) later found that a combination of the General Classification and Arithmetic tests was the best predictor (R = −0.29) of pass-fail performance among 464 DFC candidates. Berghage stated, however, that insufficient criterion variance (R^2 = 0.09) was accounted for by these measures for them to be of any practical use for selection purposes. Berghage further stated that the existing Navy aptitude selection standards for diver training were too stringent. On the sample of divers used for the Berghage analysis, combined Arithmetic and Mechanical test scores of 105 would have resulted in an unacceptably high false negative error rate—i.e., had this standard been used, 113 candidates who passed the course would have been denied training.

The importance of mechanical and arithmetic aptitudes in diving may also account for the relationship found by Ross (1968) between scientific background and success in a university diver training course. Science majors were found to volunteer more often for diving training and had nearly twice the success rate as those with academic backgrounds in the social sciences and arts. The success of science majors could be related to their greater mechanical or arithmetic aptitudes as well as to greater motivation (scientists have more to gain from diving than social science majors), the planning and organizational abilities that they may bring to diving situations, a higher level of risk-taking, and interpersonal skills. The exact factors involved in this relationship cannot be determined from these findings.

Convincing evidence that tests of mechanical aptitude, spatial perception, and verbal intelligence contribute significantly to the prediction of training performance in a civilian course in deep diving was found by Moray et al. (1979). Among 154 candidates the Bennett Mechanical Comprehension test (a written test of mechanical aptitude), the Raven Progressive Matrices (tests assessing spatial perception and nonverbal intelligence), and the Cattell Culture Fair test (a measure of nonverbal intelligence) were found to correlate most highly with grades on theoretical or purely academic subject matter, and to a lesser extent, with overall course grades. Interestingly, a test in which the candidates were required to attach nuts and bolts of various sizes to a small work bench as fast as possible (the Bennett Hand Tool Dexterity test) was not predictive of either total course grades or practical grades. This unexpected finding may indicate that the course did not involve performance of this type, that such performance was not important in grade determinations, or that the candidates were so efficient at performing this task that most of the scores clustered together (i.e., little variance existed among the candidates).

Biersner and Ryman (1974a) found that Navy aptitude test scores could be used to reduce the neuropsychiatric rate among a variety of diver classification groups. If a combined Mechanical and Arithmetic score of 80 had been used to select divers, about 5% of the psychiatric casualties would have been eliminated, against a loss of about 2% of the normal divers. If a combined score of 105 had been used, subsequent incidence of psychiatric casualties would have been reduced about 50%; 28% of the normal divers, however, would have been lost. While this false negative rate is too high for practical use, the data do nonetheless indicate that divers with low aptitudes are often placed in difficult situations with which they cannot cope, the result being situational maladjustment and acting-out behavior, and subsequent hospitalization.

b. Age

Another important variable in predicting diver training success is age. Researchers with both the French and Dutch navies (Mensh 1970, Vroegop 1973) have found that older candidates have a higher rate of training success than younger candidates. The French data, however, indicate that a curvilinear relationship exists between age and training success; divers less than 20 and more than 28 years old do more poorly than those who are between 20 and 28. Biersner et al. (1978) found that experienced U.S. Navy divers who volunteered for diver training during the first 4-year enlistment period made more dives and deeper dives (as reported on OPNAV Form 9940/1) than those who were trained in the second enlistment period. The young diver group also experienced more diving accidents than the older group, probably because they dove more frequently and to deeper depths than the older group. More importantly, the younger group appears to leave diving much earlier than the older group, perhaps because of the greater diving risks they take. These data indicate that if younger divers are selected, they may assume more risks than older divers, but they may also have to be replaced sooner.

c. Demographic Factors, Medical History, Social Adjustment

In the U.S. Navy, deep sea divers must first successfully complete scuba training, the most common type of diving under operational conditions (Biersner 1975a). In predicting performance during this phase of diver training, a number of measures have been found to be related to pass-fail (Biersner and Ryman 1974b). Demographic and medical history information are particularly useful in predicting pass-fail performance during scuba training. Among the demographic variables, education and order of birth in the family were found to be related positively to training success (the more educated and the more senior in birth, the higher the likelihood of success). Medical history items involving visual and psychological problems were found to correlate negatively with success. Attitude scales that measured "Training Concern" and "Leadership" were also correlated with the criterion. The combined correlation of these demographic, health, and attitude scales with pass-fail was 0.45.

The findings just discussed emphasize several important features about divers and diver training. First, social adjustment and maturity are important in diver training success. Education, for example, may be more significant as an indicator of perseverance, motivation for achievement, and social conformity or adjustment than as an indicator of intelligence or acquired skills. High school graduation is an indication of willingness to conform to prescribed conventions, largely dictated by adults, in order to obtain a socially important goal. Birth order is also a measure of social conformity—those children most senior in birth order typically acquire goals and direction from adult authority (i.e., parents), whereas the more junior children are more responsive to peers (i.e., other children in the family). Responses to the Leadership scale provided evidence that motivation for achievement, status, and dominance among peers was important to training success. The combination of the above characteristics—perseverance, achievement, satisfactory relationships with authorities and subordinates, and social dominance—would be beneficial to success in many training situations. Of these, adequate relationships to authorities and to subordinates may be the most important factor because of the decisive position that instructors have in determining course outcomes. Instructors are likely to prefer those who demonstrate strong motivation to succeed in the face of difficulty, as well as those who show proper deference to authority (i.e., the instructors). Social adjustment and deference to authority are, therefore, important dimensions to evaluate in determining whether prospective candidates will succeed in diver training.

Mechanical aptitudes and manual dexterity do not appear to be predictive of diver training performance if training success is estimated by experienced diving supervisors. Baddeley et al. (1978) have found that a number of tests—including the Bennett Mechanical Comprehension Test and the Bennett Hand Tool Dexterity Test, as well as the Raven Standard Progressive Matrices and the 16 Personality Factors (16 PF) Test—were not related significantly to commercial diver training success. These authors state that the failure of these measures to correlate with interview scores (the criterion of success) "was expected, and is supported by a huge volume of research showing that the function of the interviews is not to measure abilities." While not stated directly, the purpose of interviews would appear to be to subjectively determine the interpersonal dynamics and perseverance of the candidates. None of these predictor measures, including the 16 PF, was designed to assess these characteristics. Personality tests such as the 16 PF are usually designed to measure only extremes in personality characteristics, not variations of personality characteristics within the normal range. This shortcoming has resulted in the failure of personality tests to account for significant variations in diver performance (see below). As part of the same research, Baddeley and associates (1978) asked experienced divers to define the characteristics of effective divers. Of the 13 characteristics mentioned, at least nine had some relationship to social adjustment, maturity and perseverance. These characteristics were, in order of frequency: "sense of humor," "staying power," "experience," "ability to switch off to others' foibles," "reliable," "doesn't talk diving socially," "sociable and mixes will," "not only in for the money," and "will ask if he doesn't know." Other characteristics were: "thorough knowledge of and concern for gear," "level-headed, with a healthy respect for fear," "common sense" and "native cunning," and "capacity for drink" (which may have social implications as well).

The above findings indicate that social adjustment characteristics may be as important to operational effectiveness as to training success and should be evaluated in determining the suitability of a candidate for operational diving. Some caution must, however, be exercised in determining operational suitability. If the criterion of suitability is the adequacy with which the candidate performs typical tasks under water, then tests of mechanical aptitude, spatial perception, and general intelligence are appropriate, provided the divers are to be judged eventually only on this type of performance. If, however, the criterion of effectiveness is much broader, involving such factors as motivation, job satisfaction, and interpersonal relationships, then evaluation should include measures of social effectiveness, maturity, and perseverance.

In the preceding paragraph, mention was made of problems associated with using personality tests for predicting training or operational performance. These problems are associated with the purpose of many of these tests—identifying and diagnosing psychopathology. This purpose necessitates that documentation of extremes of personality, which by definition are rare occurrences. In addition, while Biersner and Ryman (1974a) showed that the psychiatric incidence rate for Navy divers (17 per 1000) was more than twice the rate for a comparison group of Navy personnel matched for age and pay grade (about 8 per 1000), this rate nonetheless compares favorably with the national rate for young adult males of 18 per 1000 (Tansey et al. 1979). Tests designed for detecting psychopathology, therefore, are of little use under these low-incidence conditions because the variability of the criterion (i.e., psychopathology) is too low to be predictable.

The test most often used for determining psychopathology is the Minnesota Multiphasic Personality Inventory (MMPI). Biersner and Cameron (1970) found that only one of the 14 MMPI scales differed significantly between experienced U.S. Navy Divers First Class and male Navy enlisted personnel matched for age and pay grade. The significant difference obtained for the single scale was attributed to chance. Both groups (divers and matched controls) were well within the normal range of scores on each of the 14 scales. These findings were essentially replicated by Weybrew (1974), who found that a mixed group of Navy divers (consisting mostly of Divers First and Second Class) differed from Navy enlisted male submariners on 4 of the 14 scales. Only 2 of these scales, however, documented personality traits directly. The scores of the divers on these 2 scales were more normal than the scores of the submariners. In addition, Radloff and Helmreich (1968), in conducting psychological research during SEALAB II, found that only one personality scale among the 70 that were used correlated significantly with a composite criterion of adjustment and performance. This single significant case was attributed to chance. Ross (1968) also found that personality tests (the Maudsley Personality Inventory and the Pensacola Z Scale) were not especially useful in discriminating between candidates who passed a university diving course and those who failed.

The Edwards Personal Preference Schedule (EPPS), a personality test used typically to differentiate psychological characteristics among normal (as opposed to psychopathological) populations, has been found to discriminate between U.S. Navy divers and a Navy comparison group matched for age and rank (Biersner and Cameron 1970). Responses to the EPPS showed that divers were significantly less self-reflective, affiliative, and nurturing, were more aggressive, and demonstrated a higher need for variety than the comparison group. These results provided evidence that divers are motivated toward tasks and objects and prefer to ignore or avoid interpersonal responsibilities and social interactions. Using a projective personality test, Biersner and associates (1974) substantiated previous EPPS data showing that divers preferred to interact more with objects than with people.

A modified version of the MMPI (reduced from 566 to 26 items) that emphasized social adjustment characteristics was found to discriminate between candidates who passed and those who failed a basic deep sea diving course offered by the Royal Canadian Navy (Johnson 1961). If Canadian divers who had MMPI scores (on the shortened form) of 12 or more had not been admitted into the course, then 60% of those who eventually failed the course would have been eliminated, while 23% of those who later passed would also have been denied training.

The importance of social dynamics to performance effectiveness under operational diving conditions was substantiated in the research of Radloff and Helmreich (1968). These researchers found that among divers participating in SEALAB II, those who interacted most frequently with other divers in the habitat also spent longer periods diving and made more diving sorties than those who remained socially isolated. These data were later replicated during TEKTITE II (Helmreich 1971). Among the civilian scientists and engineers participating as divers on TEKTITE II, those who interacted extensively with the other participants completed more marine science tasks than those who remained socially inactive. In addition, teams led by scientists were found to complete more tasks than teams led by engineers, perhaps because the scientists had a vested interest in accomplishing the tasks or because they were more active interpersonally than engineers. Marine science accomplishments were also related significantly to intelligence, school performance, parental employment and discipline, and early work responsibilities and financial independence, among other factors. A personality measure (the Allport-Vernon-Lindzey Study of Values) did not correlate significantly with this criterion of task performance.

One feature should be noted about the research just described: The demographic (predictor) variables appear to represent subtle, complex social dynamics involving competition with peers (i.e., school performance), relationships with authority (i.e., parental affection and punishment), and achievement motivation (i.e., early work and financial responsibilities). As such, these findings are consistent with the interpretation that established patterns of interpersonal effectiveness are critical determinants of success in diving situations.

While some caution should be exercised in accepting the above findings because of the small sample sizes (about 40), the data were replicated on a different but still small ($n = 38$) sample of candidates for Navy Diver Second Class training (Helmreich 1971, Radloff 1971). In this case the performance criterion was success or failure in the course. Again, demographic factors that included parental discipline, birth order, a history of delinquency, and paternal education were found to be associated with the pass-fail criterion.

Evidence showing that demographic factors could be used to indicate major socialization traits related to diver performance was also found by Biersner (1973). Experienced Navy Divers First Class were found to have a significantly higher incidence of pre-Navy delinquency, including arrests, traffic tickets, truancy, and running away from home, than other enlisted personnel matched for age, pay grade, and rating. These findings indicate that U.S. Navy divers can be described as being socially independent and having mild difficulty in conforming to accepted standards of social conduct. These findings should not, however, be taken to imply that U.S. Navy divers are antisocial or psychopathic. Previous research (Biersner et al. 1979) demonstrated that the minority of divers who are high in antisocial traits perform ineffectively in several categories of diving activity.

Some of the findings so far described appear at first to be equivocal in that social adjustment and coping skills appear to be necessary for success in diver training, yet divers who are successful under operational conditions (by virtue of experience) appear to have at least mild problems interacting effectively with others. The two conditions, however, are not necessarily contradictory. Most of the demographic and some of the personality data show that successful divers are autonomous, self-sufficient, and task-motivated individuals with little empathy or emotional responsiveness to others, especially peers and subordinates, who may be regarded as objects to be used in goal attainment. Divers are also motivated for achievement and recognition by authority (i.e., instructors and supervisors). They actively seek to exercise control over the environment, instead of passively responding to the environment or leaving future events to chance. This trait is referred to as *field independence*, and experienced divers have been shown to score high on measures of this trait (Biersner (1975b). Witkin et al. (1977) have shown that those who score high in measures of field independence have been found to enter occupations and professions in which the tasks can be readily structured and organized, such as engineering and science (and now, diving).

In addition to showing field independence, those who perceive that they are competent in controlling events would most likely (1) score high on measures of Training Confidence and Leadership and low on measures of Training Concern; (2) be praised and rewarded—not criticized and punished—by parents; and (3) experience educational success as well as success in attaining early employment and financial independence. Medical history, too, may be a subtle indicator of the extent to which they perceive the diving environment to be controllable. Do they overcome stress and avoid or deny accidents and illnesses, or do they succumb to stress and become the victims of events and conditions that they perceive as uncontrollable and unpredictable? The data described above have shown that these competency factors are important predictors of diver success in a variety of training and operational situations. The findings of Baddeley et al. (1978) showed that effective divers were described by diving supervisors as being "level headed" and "jacks of all trades," possessing "common sense," "knowledge of gear," "respect for fear," and "native cunning," as well as demonstrating skill in planning and organizing dives. These findings provide credence to my earlier interpretations that successful divers can rapidly and thoroughly assess the requirements (and risks) of a diving situation and can effectively structure (or plan) the situation so that performance is as efficient as possible and risks are minimal. In short, successful divers impose structure and control on risky situations, thereby reducing risk and concomitant anxiety.

The research findings described so far provide evidence that the typical U.S. Navy diver (and the commercial diver as well) is socially rigid (i.e., defers to authority but is domineering to peers and subordinates), is skilled at determining factors related to harmful or fatal outcomes (i.e., can assess risks), and can assume risks that can be calculated and controlled (i.e., knows that while the outcomes may be harmful or fatal, such outcomes are largely avoidable and occur only if correct procedures or equipment are not used).

Future diving, which will probably involve more saturation diving than is done now, will most likely require that divers be exposed to hyperbaric conditions for longer periods than is currently the case. Under these conditions, risk-taking, social autonomy, and poor interactions with peers and subordinates will become a serious liability to safety and operational effectiveness. A recent saturation dive conducted for research purposes noted that social stress was high throughout the dive and may have impaired performance (O'Reilly 1977). The recommendation of that author was that "judicious selection of team members should be accomplished to minimize the effects of environmental stressors and reduce the disruptive influence of maladaptive individuals." A similar recommendation was made by Aquadro (1965) in discussing diver selection. Aquadro stated: "The compatability and continued effectiveness of the worker as a member of a group or crew is often as important as his individual capabilities. Cohesion of the group, particularly for prolonged periods in restricted quarters, is of considerable importance in effective team performance and successful accomplishment of its mission." While little research has been done on selection of personnel for saturation diving, the findings described above for SEALAB II (Radloff and Helmreich 1968) and TEKTITE II (Helmreich 1971) were obtained from saturation divers. These data would appear to substantiate the importance of social characteristics and dynamics to performance effectiveness under saturation diving conditions. In addition, Biersner et al. (1976) showed that those who volunteered for saturation diving could be differentiated from Divers First Class just by using occupational information that is readily available from OPNAV Form 9940/1 or from official personnel records. Saturation diving candidates were found to make deeper dives as well as more semiclosed-circuit scuba dives, complete more diving courses to enhance their qualifications, and to make more cold water dives than the Diver First Class group. Divers First Class, however, had more special qualifications such as UDT or EOD training than the saturation diving candidates. These findings provide evidence that those who enroll in saturation diving training assume more risks and achieve more professional recognition than peers who remain Divers First Class. Such an interpretation is consistent with the above discussion indicating that effective divers are motivated for achievement and demonstrate (through prior accomplishments and performance) that they perceive the environment to be amenable to organization and control.

2. *Summary and Conclusions*

The research discussed in this section indicates that the selection and evaluation of divers is a complex process. Whether selection and evaluation procedures should be implemented is largely dependent on the size of the available personnel pool and the magnitude of false positive and false negative errors. If attrition is high and the selection pool is small, psychological selection and evaluation will be of little practical use. If the pool exceeds the number of operational or training vacancies by at least 25%–50%, then implementation of some selection techniques may be useful in avoidance of unnecessary attrition, thereby enhancing training or operational effectiveness. The measures to be used in the selection and evaluation process may vary substantially with the availability of competent professionals, time, and testing facilities. The measures that are administered, however, should be of demonstrated reliability and validity. In addition, the research described shows that effective performance, whether in training or in operational diving, involves a wide variety of psychological dimensions. The selection and evaluation process should, therefore, include a number of measures to assess these psychological dimensions.

Several tests and measures, demonstrated through research to predict training or operational performance among divers, can be recommended for selection and evaluation purposes. Selection and evaluation of personnel for more global types of criterion behavior (such as frequency of performing tasks, supervisor ratings, total course grades or grades in the theoretical or academic portion of a course, and pass-fail performance) appear to rely on measures of arithmetic and mechanical aptitudes (e.g., the Navy Basic Test Battery), perceptual style (e.g., field independence or dependence), and interpersonal effectiveness and social adjustment. Mechanical and arithmetic aptitudes are significant predictors of training success among deep diving candidates because these aptitudes are involved in calculating decompression schedules, fabricating structural parts, and so forth. The higher the score, the more likely the candidate is to succeed. Field independence or dependence can be measured by use of several instruments (e.g., the Hidden Patterns Test, the Rod and Frame Test, the Embedded Figure Test). These tests appear to assess the extent to which the respondent actively structures a situation and determines interactions among situational components. Successful divers should be field independent. Another measure, the Internality-Externality Text, assesses a similar psychological dimension but has not been used to predict diver performance. The assumption would be, however, that successful divers would have low scores, indicating a disposition toward internality.

Interpersonal effectiveness and social adjustment can be assessed from use of demographic questionnaires. These questionnaires should ask about previous disciplinary problems, with those candidates found to have a history of disciplinary actions being least likely to succeed. Also useful are items regarding pride in school performance, parental interactions, and early work history. Those candidates with more schooling (and more achievements in school) and positive and rewarding interactions with parents, and those who assumed work responsibilities as teenagers, are predicted to do well in diver training and as operational divers.

Age is also a significant predictor of diver performance. The relationship of age to diving performance, however, is not linear but is instead curvilinear. Younger personnel (17–19 years old) and older personnel (more than 24 years old) were not as successful or effective as those in the intermediate age group. This finding has been demonstrated across different types of diving classifications and for divers and diving candidates from several different countries. An explanation of this finding is not readily apparent, although the unrealistic expectations of younger personnel and the availability of other employment opportunities for older age groups may be involved.

Attitudes have also been shown to be important predictors of training success for deep diving personnel. Particularly useful in predicting training outcomes were attitudes toward expected training success (Training Confidence) and the assumption of major responsibilities within groups (Leadership). Higher scores have been associated with training success. Attitudes about being injured or harmed during training (Training Concern) have been found to be important predictors of pass-fail performance, the lower scores being associated with successful training outcomes. These three attitudes appear to describe an important dimension in diver effectiveness—the skill to assess true risks in a situation and to perceive as controllable a potentially harmful situation.

Personality tests, especially those designed to diagnose psychopathology, have not been particularly useful in differentiating diver performance under either operational or training conditions. The only measure of this type that may prove useful for this purpose is the Edwards Personal Preference Schedule. Experienced divers were found to be low on scales that assessed nurturance, affiliation, and self-reflection and high on scales that measured the need for change and aggression. Presumably, these traits would be characteristic of those who would succeed in diver training and who would be operationally effective as well.

While research is worthwhile in identifying tests and measures that are predictive of diver performance, the final judgment of probable effectiveness is that of the physician. Interviews and the impressions formed from interactions with the diving candidate should provide a major source of information from which to make this judgment. If these impressions are integrated with objective test results, this judgment is likely to be more valid than using either source of information alone.

ROBERT J. BIERSNER

References

AQUADRO, C. F. 1965. Examination and selection of personnel for work in underwater environment. *J. Occup. Med.* 7: 619–625.

BADDELEY, A. D., D. GODDEN, N. P. MORAY, H. E. ROSS, AND N. E. SYNODINOS 1978. Selection of diving trainees. Final Report. London: Training Services Agency.

BEHNKE, A. R. 1945. Psychological and psychiatric reactions in diving and submarine warfare. *Am. J. Psychiatry* 101: 720–725.

BERGHAGE, T. E. 1972. The use of standard Navy classification test scores for the selection of Diver First Class candidates. Rep. 20–72. Washington, DC: U.S. Navy Experimental Diving Unit.

BIERSNER, R. J. 1973. Social development of Navy divers. *Aerosp. Med.* 44: 761–763.

BIERSNER, R. J. 1975a. Factors in 171 Navy diving decompression accidents occurring between 1960–1969. *Aviat. Space Environ. Med.* 46: 1069–1073.

BIERSNER, R. J. 1975b. Sustained performance in training for military swimmer/diver operations. In: *Proceedings of the American Psychological Association, Chicago.*

BIERSNER, R. J. AND B. J. CAMERON 1970. Betting preferences and personality characteristics of Navy divers. *Aerosp. Med.* 41: 1289–1291.

BIERSNER, R. J., M. L. DEMBERT, AND M. D. BROWNING 1978. The aging diver: Do the older become bolder? *Faceplate* 9: 19–21.

BIERSNER, R. J., M. L. DEMBERT, AND M. D. BROWNING 1979. The anti-social diver: performance, medical, and emotional consequences. *Mil. Med.* 144: 445–448.

BIERSNER, R. J., D. EDWARDS, AND L. W. BAILEY 1974. Effects of N_2O on responses of divers to personality tests. *Percept. Mot. Skills* 38: 1091–1097.

BIERSNER, R. J., D. A. HALL, AND P. G. LINAWEAVER 1976. Occupational differences between conventional and saturation divers. *Aviat. Space Environ. Med.* 47: 29–32.

BIERSNER, R. J., AND D. H. RYMAN 1974a. Psychiatric incidence among military drivers. *Mil. Med.* 139: 633–635.

BIERSNER, R. J., AND D. H. RYMAN 1974b. Prediction of SCUBA training performance. *J. Appl. Psychol.* 59: 519–521.

HELMREICH, R. 1971. Human reactions to psychological stress. Technical Report No. 14. Austin, TX: University of Texas.

JOHNSON, J. A. 1961. Selection of men in the Esquimaux port division for clearance diver (ship). Tech. Rep. No. PC 61–3. Ottawa, Ont.: Department of National Defence (Navy).

MENSH, I. N. 1970. La plongée et les plongeurs. *ONR Eur. Sci. Notes* 24: 1–4.

MORAY, N., H. ROSS, AND N. SYNODINOS 1979. Test battery for the selection of trainee divers. Final Report. Stirling, England: Stirling University.

O'REILLEY, J. P. 1977. Hana Kai: a 17-day dry saturation dive at 18.6 ATA. VI: Cognitive performance reaction time, and personality changes. *Undersea Biomed. Res.* 4: 297–305.

RADLOFF, R. 1971. Life history and success in diving school. Rep. M4306.03-1010. Bethesda, MD: Naval Medical Research Institute.

RADLOFF, R., AND R. HELMRIECH 1968. *Groups Under Stress: Psychological Research in SEALAB II.* New York: Appleton-Century-Crofts.

ROSS, H. E. 1968. Personality of student divers. *Underwater Assoc. Rep.* 1968: 59–62.

TANSEY, W. A., J. M. WILSON, AND K. E. SCHAEFER 1979. Analysis of health data from 10 years of Polaris submarine patrols. *Undersea Biomed. Res.* 6: Suppl., S217–S246.

VROEGOP, P. 1973. Psychodiagnostic selection of divers: study review, 1972. Hilversum, Netherlands: Hilversum Diving Medical Center. (NAVSHIPS transl. 1416.)

WEYBREW, B. B. 1974. Shallow habitat air dive (SHAD-I): psychological screening of divers as subjects for long duration saturation experimentation. *US Nav. Submar. Med. Res. Lab. Rep.* 776.

WISE, D. A. 1963. Aptitude selection standards for the U.S. Navy's first class diving course. Res. Rep. 3–63. Washington, DC: U.S. Navy Experimental Diving Unit.

WITKIN, H. A., C. A. MOORE, P. K. OLTMAN, D. R. GOODENOUGH, F. FRIEDMAN, D. R. OWEN, AND E. RASKIN 1977. Role of the field-dependent and field-independent cognitive styles in academic evolution: a longitudinal study. *J. Educ. Psychol.* 69: 197–211.

XII

Stress Physiology and Behavior Underwater

A. Introduction

In this chapter we consider an important biomedical area—that of stress underwater—beginning with a discussion of the general nature of stress; factors that contribute toward stress problems in diving; the effects of variables such as cold, exercise, and fatigue (particularly as they relate to cardiovascular problems and performance); diving accidents; and, as an ultimate potential event to which all these factors contribute, the problem of diver panic, which is implicated in many if not most of the fatalities among recreational divers.

B. Concept of Stress

Stress is one of those words of wide usage and unclear definition. In everyday usage it has taken on an almost exclusively negative connotation, and courses in "stress management" as a way of life (or frequently billed as a way of saving one's life) are gaining in popularity. Perhaps part of the origin of this approach comes from engineering, where stress is viewed as a force impacting on an object or element, such as concrete, and resulting in changes in the shape or form of that object. In any case, stress is a complex and involved concept and one that is central to experiences such as diving where physical and psychological forces and pressures do indeed impact on the individual.

Stress is always viewed as some sort of induced imbalance, and our current conceptualization of stress derives in large measure from the homeostatic theory of Bernard (1856) for whom balance—"the constancy of the internal milieux"—was central to physiological function. Homeostasis is the restoration to balance of imbalance induced by stressors, internal or external, and is basic not only to Claude Bernard's approach but to that of Cannon (1939) and, more recently, to that of Selye (1971).

Four aspects of stress need discussion (Bachrach, 1981). First, stress is complex. Response to stress is highly individual in nature, the same stressor differentially effecting varied responses among individuals, so that some people may actually demonstrate an improvement in performance under conditions of stress, whereas others respond negatively with a diminution of performance; still others show no reaction and may be considered "immune" (Appley and Trumbull 1967). The individual nature of a stress response demonstrating a behavior few individuals could engage in is illustrated in Figure XII-1.

A second attribute of stress is that it is to a large degree culturally determined. In our society, for example, boredom or ennui is considered stressful, an attitude that is not in evidence in many other cultures. Leisure activity in our culture is in many ways different from that in other cultures, in that leisure is almost always equated with activity. Even our colloquialisms demonstrate an inability to cope effectively with nonactivity—for example, the phrase *killing time* is unique to western culture.

A third characteristic of stress is related to cultural determination; stress is largely learned. Interpreting an event as a stressor is largely a matter of learning, of conditioning. Certain phobias represent this conditioning in some measure. If you were to ask a group of people how many were afraid of snakes you would, in all likelihood, get a high number of positive responses. If you were to then ask the same group how many of those with a fear of snakes had actually had a direct, threatening experience with a snake, the chances are the number would be zero. Modeling of phobic responses by parents or peers is a major means by which stressors become interpreted as aversive.

Finally, an important characteristic of stress is that it is not necessarily a negative experience. Earlier, I mentioned that stress has taken on an almost inevitably negative connotation, but two factors suggest this is not necessarily so. First, a response to external stress can be a form of mobilization for action: for example, a tournament swimmer is expected to peak heart rates of around 185 beats/min just before entering the water, an imbalance that is not negative. The second factor deals with thrill seeking (in an extreme form) or certainly a sought imbalance for the apparent pleasure of stimulation and restoration. The human animal is unique in the animal kingdom in that it will ride a roller coaster.

In the area of recreation, it is strongly suggested that the human is going to be increasingly a thrill seeker. This thought comes from a recent extensive study of trends relevant to consumer marketing (*Yankelovich Monitor* 1979, p. 56). One trend was identified as "flirtation with danger," an eagerness to enter into high-risk activities such as high-speed auto racing, hang gliding, skydiving, and scuba diving, all sports that apparently satisfy a number of varied motives. In this interesting study one identified motive for entering into high-risk sports activity was excitement. A related motive had a "self-worth" component, which involved a firm belief that mastering dangerous activities can make one a much better person and that "'driving yourself to the brink' is a path to better self-understanding." Another thrill-seeking activity that may have other types of risk but, nevertheless, is included in the flirtation-with-danger complex is that of shoplifting, an apparently exciting, unlawful activity among classes of people who do not really need the item thus acquired.

A detailed discussion of risk taking appears in Zuckerman (1979).

Risk taking is not necessarily to be equated with suicidal behavior. In the German diving magazine *Tauchen* a recent article (Fritz 1979) asked the question in its title "Sind Taucher selbsmörder?" ["Are divers suicidal?"], a question prompted by the large number of diving fatalities in German waters.

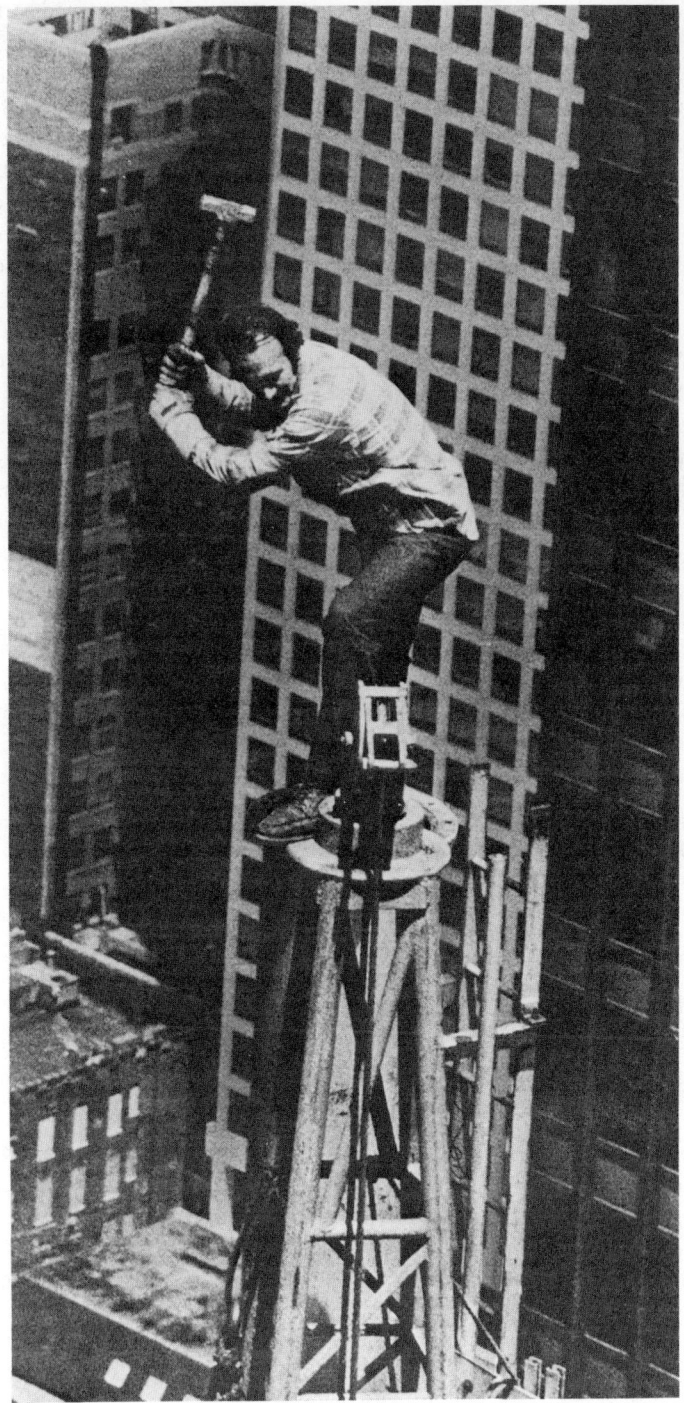

Figure XII-1. Individual nature of a stress response. (*Chicago Tribune* photo.)

To define risk taking as suicidal we should use the criterion proposed by Durkheim in his classic essay on suicide (1951): if an individual enters a high-risk behavior and believes there is a chance that he or she will emerge alive, then this is not suicidal; the behavior can be termed suicidal only if there is a belief that there is no chance whatever of survival. In this chapter I have used the term *risk taking* to indicate that there is hazard involved in such recreational activities as scuba diving and hang gliding but that it is not likely that such risk taking is a self-destructive behavior. Even though an individual goes into a sought-for imbalance for the excitement, in my opinion there is a fundamental belief that control is not lost. The individual going on a roller coaster believes that the engineering of the device is sound, that safety measures have been observed, and that the titillation of the ride will be, nonetheless, a safe stress. The individual who scuba dives or skydives believes that he or she has control over the equipment and the use of it in that unique environment and, moreover, that the equipment used has been designed for safe and efficient use. Blau (1980) in an article on diving makes the interesting observation that "risk-taking occurs when a diver does not follow the rules." Blau's observation is a cogent one, although my personal belief, as I have noted, is that entering an environment such as the ocean, where demands are greater and different from land requirements, incurs some hazard and, therefore, some risk. Blau goes on to explain his comment by stating that a properly trained diver may still make decisions that are incompatible with good training and practice, such as diving when tired or diving in strange waters, presumably without proper planning. To be sure, a diver who had driven 5 hr to get to a dive site only to find the waters inhospitable may be unwilling to give up completely and return home without at least giving it a try—a practice probably contrary to good sense. I would not disagree with Blau's definition of risk taking; my only modification would be that diving always entails some degree of risk, by the very nature of the activity; the risk is made more severe by poor diving practice.

C. Stress in Diving

1. Training to Alleviate Stress

a. Organized Training Programs

Diving in the United States has become a popular sport. As Egstrom (1982) observes, "Organized diving instruction appears to have had its beginings with the scientific diving training program at Scripps Institute of Oceanography in 1953." This was followed quickly by the first public scuba program offered by the Los Angeles County Department of Parks and Recreation. Shortly thereafter the YMCA and the Council for National Cooperation in Aquatics began developing materials for training. Egstrom notes that the assumption strongly held in these early programs was that the scuba trainee was strong in watermanship—the ability to swim and perform in water. This assumption has evolved over the years to a different view that assumes minimal watermanship skills. Egstrom makes the cogent observation that most courses enable individuals to dive within their own limitations rather than meet a rigorous standard of performance. He also states that "the development of equipment which makes diving 'easier' has tended to place an emphasis upon reliance upon the equipment rather than upon personal fitness and watermanship skills" (Egstrom 1982). Early divers such as Guy Gilpatric were called *gogglers* because goggles were the prime piece of equipment they wore (their primitive equipment made excellent water skills imperative). Contrast these early divers with the current divers who may not worry about knowing proper weighting techniques because the buoyancy compensators they wear can always be inflated for buoyancy control; thus they can rely on equipment rather than on personal skill.

It is perhaps ironic that the diminished emphasis on personal skill in the diver has coincided with the growing view of the diver in the United States that Egstrom (1982) describes as "fully certified and more or less independent in contrast to other countries where 'club' activity is generally supervised and additional training becomes an accepted goal." The British Sub-Aqua Club, for example, has four classes of divers with continual training requirements and experience. The highest rank, First Class Diver, requires passage through many and varied skill and training experiences along with a minimum of 100 dives. Unsupervised divers in the United States, once certified, are rarely challenged regarding maintenance of learned skills, nor are they required to continue training. This, I believe, is an inadequacy in our training programs and a serious source of potential danger to divers under stress.

Another problem I see is that most training courses do not have controlled training for emergency. The loss of a mask underwater is, or should be, at most a marked inconvenience but not a reason for panic, for an individual can do very well without a mask. Learning to do without a mask in a training situation in a pool, so that the event, if it occurs, will not be a novel and disrupting experience, strikes me as a logical part of training. Training for similar emergencies, such as buoyant ascents, should also be considered. Situation-dependent training is all-important: the stimulus conditions and performance requirements differ in varying situations, so a diver who is comfortable in an open-sea situation should not automatically be assumed to be equally competent in kelp beds or caves. Training in such specialties as cave diving should do much to minimize the effects of stress.

b. Physician's Role in Training

Part of the purpose of this book is clarification of the role of the physician in the training of divers—in particular, the medical screening needed for individuals who wish to enter a course of training. Elsewhere in this book medical examinations are more carefully considered (see Chapter XI). From my viewpoint as a stress psychophysiologist, I would hope that the diving physical would be thorough and the physician alert to potential problems, not only the usual pulmonary and cardiovascular factors but others such as, for want of a better word, "personality types." For example, the macho, Type A, aggressive person may well have labile hypertension; such individuals are described by Bove (1977) as "presumably . . . showing manifestations of sympathetic activity induced by emotional factors." It is possible that labile hypertension may not be detected during normal screening.

In the United States medical screening is minimal and repeat physicals are ususally not required; this is, again, in contrast to other countries. For example, in Canada the

Ontario Underwater Council requires a medical examination on entry and, to maintain certification, an annual physical for divers over 40. The British Sub-Aqua Club requires an entry medical examination; this must be repeated every 5 years until age 50 and then every 3 years to maintain diving certification. The physician's role in screening is crucial and needs further reinforcement, particularly in the United States.

2. Diver Motivation—A Stress Factor?

The motives that lead people to become divers are obviously varied and individual, but it is probable the excitement and adventure, as the market research people suggest, play an important role. Certainly appreciation of beauty and the opportunity to see things unlike the land motivate the diver, and the satisfaction of accomplishment—of having met a challenge—is very real. These are positive motivations, but one of the major sources of stress and resulting problems in diving is the macho motivation, i.e., the individual who is not competing with himself to develop greater skills or take better underwater photographs but is aggressively competitive with others. The greatest marine hazard is the person who says he or she "can dive deeper on less air" than you. This type of performance places the macho diver at risk, along with his or her diving partners. Earlier I mentioned that labile hypertension might be one of the physical signs physicians should look for in physical examinations for diving and that Type A aggressive behavior was also an important psychological sign. This behavior clearly relates to a potential hazard in diving, that of sudden death, which will be discussed in more detail later. For the moment it underscores the problems inherent in macho motivation, as noted by Engel (1978) in discussing vasodepressor (vasovagal) syncope, which he states, "occurs in our machismo culture more commonly among men than women, especially in settings in which the man feels the ambience to be one of strong social disapproval of any display of weakness" (Engel 1978). This is indeed a potentially dangerous motivation, for the likelihood of serious consequences is created by the probability that an individual will get into trouble by entering a situation in which he or she is not comfortable or one in which there is a lack of the needed skills. "Loss of face," the fear of looking foolish in front of one's peers, is a source of problems if it leads an individual to go beyond his or her realistic limits of performance. Of course, we all have our own little devices—many divers have found a "sinus block" can keep them from diving when they really don't want to!

Another positive motivation for divers is the social interaction provided by the clubs that are active in all regional areas. Identification with groups is an important part of diving, and the pleasures of diving appear close to the pleasures of sharing experiences and reliving them in a social situation. One reason why underwater photography has burgeoned as a hobby is the increased ability to share a diving experience long after it has happened. An outward symptom of diving as a social enterprise is evidenced in the number of patches worn by diving enthusiasts on their jackets, dive bags, et cetera. Reg Vallintine, Director of the London Underwater Centre, described such decorated diving enthusiasts as being afflicted with "emblemism." The proper channeling of social interaction over and above the pleasures of sharing an experience can well be the use of peers as support in proper dive planning and execution for safe, enjoyable diving.

3. Physical and Physiological Stress Factors

a. Fatigue

Contributing to the stress that impacts on a diver are physical and physiological factors that act as additional stressors. The underwater environment itself, the drag of equipment, and exercise all lead to a primary stressor—fatigue.

The medium of the water itself is a stressor in that a human is not proficient in moving through water. From an engineering standpoint, as Kidd (1969) observed, the efficiency of propulsion achieved, expressed as a function of fuel consumed, is very uneconomical. Kidd further noted that an Olympic-class swimmer, swimming without an aid, can achieve an efficiency of slightly better than 2%; with fins efficiency rises to 6%–8%; with fins and scuba efficiency drops to 2%–4%. Egstrom (1981) observed that the additional draping of equipment over the diver's body continues to increase the drag. Starting, let us say, with a basic wet suit, the mask, fins, weight belt, tanks, buoyancy compensator, regulator, goody bag (to mention the major pieces of equipment, to which may be added camera gear) all create projections from what may have started out to be a streamlined profile. In 1969, before the larger buoyancy compensators came into use, Kidd estimated the addition of scuba gear increased the drag on a submerged diver by about 30% (Kidd 1969). Thus, it is patent that swimming is hard work and that the addition of gear to permit submergence for periods of time increases the level of effort.

Equipment can be a problem in other ways as well. Egstrom (1970) measured heart rates during normal dressing for a dive and found that, in midsummer, a diver donning equipment that included a 45-lb tank, 10–20 lb of lead, and wearing a wet suit ¼ in. thick peaked heart rates in excess of 160 beats/min, a measure of a heavy work load. The wet suit was also evaluated by Egstrom (1981) in his analysis of equipment; he found that divers who weight themselves for shallow diving and then dive deeper encounter problems with compression of wet suits; these problems result in overweighting, an event that has led to casualties in California waters. Most divers are overweighted at the beginning of a dive. Earlier I noted the reliance on equipment rather than on personal skill; this is illustrated in the use of buoyancy compensators in some situations rather than the exercise of care in selecting the proper weights. Overweighting requires even greater effort and exercise and creates additional problems. A recent accident leading to a fatality in Canada resulted in part from a diver who weighted himself for salt water, as was his custom, but dived to 80 ft in fresh water and was thus greatly overweighted.

Exercise, in short, is a function of a number of variables: physical condition; the medium in which the effort is expended (difficult because water is a viscous medium), the nature of the environment with respect to cold, which further taxes performance; and the equipment, which, while aiding the diver to remain in the environment and perform therein, also taxes strength and stamina. All of these factors contribute to the stress of fatigue.

As a function of increased effort in moving through the water the possibility of fatigue is markedly increased, both in the level of fatigue and the time of onset. On land, a fatigued individual who is exercising can stop to rest, a feat much more difficult to achieve under water. The cost of exercise, coupled with such factors as cold and progressive hypothermia as the course of the dive continues, markedly exacerbates fatigue. Cold, as we shall see, affects performance and judgment and makes fatigue potentially even more hazardous. In addition, fatigue can contribute in the susceptible individual to cardiac arrhythmias, another topic to be considered as a stress response in diving.

In summary, the water environment provides a medium that requires effort for divers whose propulsion efficiency is severely reduced; in most waters of the world an environment of cold further affects divers, placing them under additional stress.

b. Cold

Cold is considered to be the major stressor in the diving environment. In this section I focus on the effects of cold as a stress factor, particularly as it relates to performance and the cardiovascular factors that contribute to a stress response. Cold, as stress, when coupled with other stress factors can be a potentially serious hazard for divers. More detailed information about physiological response to hypothermia appears in Chapter III in this volume.

To refer to the ocean as a heat sink is something of a cliché; however, according to the second law of thermodynamics, heat transfers from the warmer medium to the cooler, and because virtually all of the waters of the world are cooler than the human entering therein, the waters form a heat sink. Heat loss in water is 25 times that in air. The progressive drain on the human caused by heat exchange even in relatively warm waters has led authorities such as Egstrom (1976) to recommend use of a protective wet suit everywhere, including the tropics.

There is, of course, no constant and invariant transfer of heat. Differences in body habitus, posture, and a host of personal elements contribute to heat exchange. Mechanisms of heat loss vary, and factors such as the activity in which the individual is engaged play important roles in the degree of heat transfer. Heat loss normally occurs by radiation, conduction, convection, and evaporation. Egstrom (1977) has observed that heat loss from radiation and convection, as well as from evaporation, is minimal in a diver: in deep diving respiratory heat exchange is the primary source of heat loss. This is a function of the breathing mix: helium creates more heat loss than air. Heat loss is also a function of depth, with loss through skin conduction primarily occurring during dives shallower than 130 ft.

Flynn et al. (1981) state that "during water immersion heat is lost from the body through the respiratory tract and by convective conductance from the skin. Cutaneous evaporation and radiation play no role." The respiratory heat loss comes from breathing dry, cold air from a tank or surface supply, which the diver breathes, heats, moistens, and expires. Thus, evaporation occurs when the air comes in contact with moist lung tissue. Webb and Annis (1966) demonstrated that divers breathing air at 1 atm lost approximately 10% of their metabolic heat through respiration. This loss is further exacerbated when the diver breathes a mixture of helium and oxygen under pressure. Helium, which causes heat loss at a rate seven times that of air, was breathed by divers at 7 ATA, with a resulting 28% metabolic heat loss through respiration (Webb and Annis 1966). Helium provides another difficulty: a layer of heliox next to the skin provides far less insulation than does a layer of air. Thermal physiologists have recommended that heliox be heated when divers are scheduled for depths approaching 600 fsw (183 msw). Nonetheless, respiratory heat loss remains a significant problem in helium-oxygen diving.

(i) Hypothermia. Much of the interest in hypothermia has centered around immersion hypothermia, particularly accidental immersion such as is encountered in boating accidents and shipwrecks. The first real recognition of hypothermia as a source of fatalities in shipwrecks appears to have been an article by Molnar (1946) in which hypothermia and survival

were discussed. Before this time deaths in wrecks such as the *Titanic* were almost inevitably attributed to drowning, with no implication of the effects of cold water. Recent experiments and analyses of immersion hypothermia include reports by Bangs (1980), Collis (1976), Cooper (1976), Golden (1972), Harnett and Bijlani (1979), Hayward and Steinman (1975), Keatinge (1969), MacInnis (1979), and Webb (1974). These reports of accidental immersions and subsequent hypothermia are, for the most part, concerned with individuals who are not protected by clothing designed to minimize the effects of cold water. Divers normally wear wet suits or dry suits. In commercial and military salvage diving, suits are heated with hot water. Wet suits, the most frequently used form of protection, offer limited protection against cold—limited by pressure (below shallow depths their effectiveness is markedly reduced) and also limited by time (the longer the exposure the greater the heat loss that will occur). Bayne (see Flynn et al. 1981), in an experiment conducted with working Navy divers, found "drops in rectal temperatures up to 3.6°F in a 30-min scuba dive performed at 30 fsw with a complete 3/8" wet suit." The dive was accomplished in the Anacostia River (Washington, D.C.) in February in water temperatures ranging from 0°C to 4°C.

The problem of slow cooling, or progressive hypothermia, has been recognized as an operational problem by Hayward and Keatinge (1979), who described progressive or "silent" hypothermia as a possible cause of diving accidents in commercial diving. They commented on the cases of loss of consciousness reported by Childs and Norman (1978) in the North Sea and suggested that the probable cause of this loss of consciousness was progressive hypothermia. Webb (1974) observes that there is no significant body of either physiological or performance data on cold that has been drawn from open-sea diving experience. As he notes, "it is possible to say that divers routinely get cold" and that they may self-select their occupation on the basis of greater tolerance to cold. Webb also believes it is reasonable to assume that cold is a "seriously limiting factor in many diving operations and . . . that occasionally hypothermia, with its insidious onset, has caused fatal diving accidents." He does caution, however, that the very routine nature of cold exposure associated with diving operations may make cold acceptable to a point where its "potential for harm [is] discounted" (p. 1).

Bradley (1981) reported on diving accidents among commercial divers and stated that in 11% of the fatalities cold was implicated as a contributing or causative factor. What makes progressive hypothermia a problem is the apparent inability of the diver to detect the changes that occur with time; hence the term "silent" hypothermia. In a discussion of temperature perception Garrard et al. (1981) observed that there have been both pictorial and anecdotal accounts of divers who were scalded in their hot water suits without any apparent recognition of the temperature change. A similar problem in temperature perception was reported by Keatinge, et al. (1980), who found in a series of saturation dives to 427–476 ft (130–145 m) in the North Sea that divers suffered hypothermia without any definite sensation of cold. The risks of undetected hypothermia, these authors suggest, can be a mental confusion, loss of consciousness, and death. The signs of hypothermia from a performance standpoint can be confusion and a loss of judgment; Hayward and Keatinge (1979) describe this phenomenon as "unexplained confusion and bad judgment leading to diving accidents." This description agrees with the findings of Bradley's (1981) study of diving accidents, which has reported that 15% of the North Sea fatalities were attributed to poor judgment on the part of the diver, probably an effect of cold. Part of this problem in judgment may be what Childs (1978) described as performance degradation and discomfort resulting from cold, which rendered the diver less aware of possible threats to safety. As he states, "Loss of manual dexterity due to cold accounts for the greater part of performance decrement, but with falling core temperature, attention narrowing may further impair performance to the point where safety is threatened" (Childs 1978, p. 17).

Childs (1978) further observes that "distraction due to discomfort may cause the diver to ignore threats to his safety underwater and finally, realizing he is in danger, he may be in further difficulty because of loss of power and dexterity in his hands." In the initial period of the dive, distraction owing to exposure to cold is common (Vaughan 1977), with tasks such as reaction time and target detection time degraded early in the dive. In another study, Vaughan (1975) studied trained Navy operators in two-man wet submersibles in the cold (6°C) waters of Puget Sound. Despite protective equipment it was found that the divers lost a large amount of heat over the time in the water, with concurrent degradation of performance. Errors in maintaining correct headings increased and task concentration was degraded. Davis and colleagues (1975) found a distraction effect in cold water (5°C) with degradation of capability for simple arithmetic, logical reasoning, word recall, word recognition, and manual dexterity. Egstrom et al. (1972) found vigilance and reasoning ability in a 30-min exposure in 40°F (4°C) water were not significantly affected, although memory function was. These authors also found the motivation of the diver to be a critical factor in resisting potential degradation.

Results have not been entirely consistent from study to study, probably a result of task and subject variability (Bachrach 1975); there is a general view, however, that cold water degrades performance and that progressive hypothermia can impair performance such as judgment to a point where the diver is at hazard.

For the commercial diver this risk is inherent in cold exposure and pressure. For the sport diver, probably less adequately protected by a wet suit, the problem of progressive hypothermia that can degrade performance becomes more of a problem of coping with potential emergencies than the loss of consciousness or other risks experienced by the commercial diver. In both circumstances heat loss is a stress response that is dangerous.

(ii) Cardiovascular effects of cold. So far I have briefly discussed changes in the performance of the diver associated with exposure to cold, changes that can adversely affect ability to complete a task or even to recognize potential threats to safety owing to loss of judgment. A major effect of cold exposure is the marked set of physiological changes that occur immediately upon immersion. The best known of these cold effects is the *diving reflex*, a reflex vagal response leading to bradycardia (Angell James and Daly 1972). Immersion in water can produce bradycardia, although Hurwitz and Furedy (1979) have suggested that the combination of water immersion and breath holding produces the greater heart response. In their study they compared the effects of three groups of conditions: (1) face immersion and breath holding, (2) face immersion and breathing through snorkel, and (3) breath holding only. Group 1—facial immersion and breath holding—produced the greatest effect, with no return to base-line heart rate until the end of the 40-sec exposure. Similar results were reported by Bruce and Speck (1979), who found that facial cooling by wetting combined with apneic immersion precipitated the diving reflex. Moreover, lowered water temperatures markedly increased the effects.

The interaction of swallowing and bradycardia has been reported by Huang and Peng (1981), who found that swallowing during face immersion appeared to inhibit bradycardia in almost half of their subjects; inspiratory effort also attenuated bradycardia in some cases. This finding is similar to that of Gandevia et al. (1978) who found that bradycardia was reduced with an inspiratory effort against a closed glottis. Huang and Peng (1981) also reported that although inspiratory efforts and swallowing could modify bradycardia, they had no effect on vasoconstriction as measured by a finger plethysmograph. Space does not permit a detailed analysis of or speculation about the complexities of the diving reflex, but the interaction of facial sensation, respiratory functions, and temperature within a neural framework remains an important research area. Findings such as those suggested by Abrahamsson and Jansson (1973) in their report on reflex vagal inhibition of esophageal motility are of value to the diving physician (see also Sessle and Storey 1972; White and McRitchie 1973).

Further complexities derive from the large number of stimuli impinging on a diver, which range from the wet and cold stimulation of the water to the possible impact of equipment and physiological events associated with diving. Many investigators (cf. Bove et al. 1973; Dejours 1965) have reported that hypoxia and hypercapnia cause bradycardia and vasoconstriction by the stimulation of chemoreceptors during apnea. Bove et al. (1973) suggested that the bradycardia resulting from the diving reflex may be a significant factor in underwater blackout; they believe unconsciousness may occur in individuals who are more prone to blackout owing to a higher tolerance of hypoxia and hypercapnia. In analyzing underwater loss of consciousness, Craig (1961) suggested the "hyperventilation preceding breath-holding and exercise may delay the sensation of the urge to breathe."

Shepherd and Vanhoutte (1979) have stated that "during a dive the sensory endings of the trigeminal nerve are activated first," an event that initiates the trigeminal reflex, which in turn causes a cessation of respiration and eliminates the lung inflation reflex. The vagal efferent to the sinus and atrioventricular nodes is activated, thus effecting bradycardia. In this stimulation of the trigeminal nerve by face immersion (leading to apnea and vagal-induced bradycardia) we can only speculate on elements of the trigeminal nerve that relate to diving equipment. For example, face masks and regulators may have yet-undemonstrated stimulating effects on branches of the trigeminal nerve, particularly on the maxillary and mandibular division (see Figure XII-2), with cutaneous stimulation from the pressure exerted on these areas. Andersen (1966) demonstrated that the diving reflex depended on the integrity of the ophthalmic branch of the trigeminal nerve. For those interested, related work may be found in Griffin and Harris (1975). It is patent that other neural interactions are involved, certainly the vestibular effects (see for example, Akert and Gernandt 1962) and the glossopharyngeal nerve, but space does not allow for a consideration of these exquisite complexities.

This brief excursion into the neural aspects of the diving reflex is intended to highlight the importance of facial immersion and interactions with breathing patterns in the dive reflex. The diving reflex has been documented in a number of diving animals (Andersen 1966; Scholander 1961–1962) and has been called the *oxygen conserving reflex* because the slowing of the heart and lowered oxygen consumption permit longer breath-hold dives. What is important for us to consider in this discussion is the temperature-dependent nature of the reflex—assuming the high frequency, if not universality, of the dive reflex in human divers. Hong (1976) observes, "Regardless of whether one is engaged in actual breath-hold diving or breath-hold face immersion, the degree of bradycardia increases with the decrease in water temperature," a finding consonant with that noted earlier by Bruce and Speck (1979). Cutaneous cold receptors, Hong indicates, "play a very important role in the development of diving bradycardia."

Cold water was implicated in diving bradycardia in a study by Hughes and associates

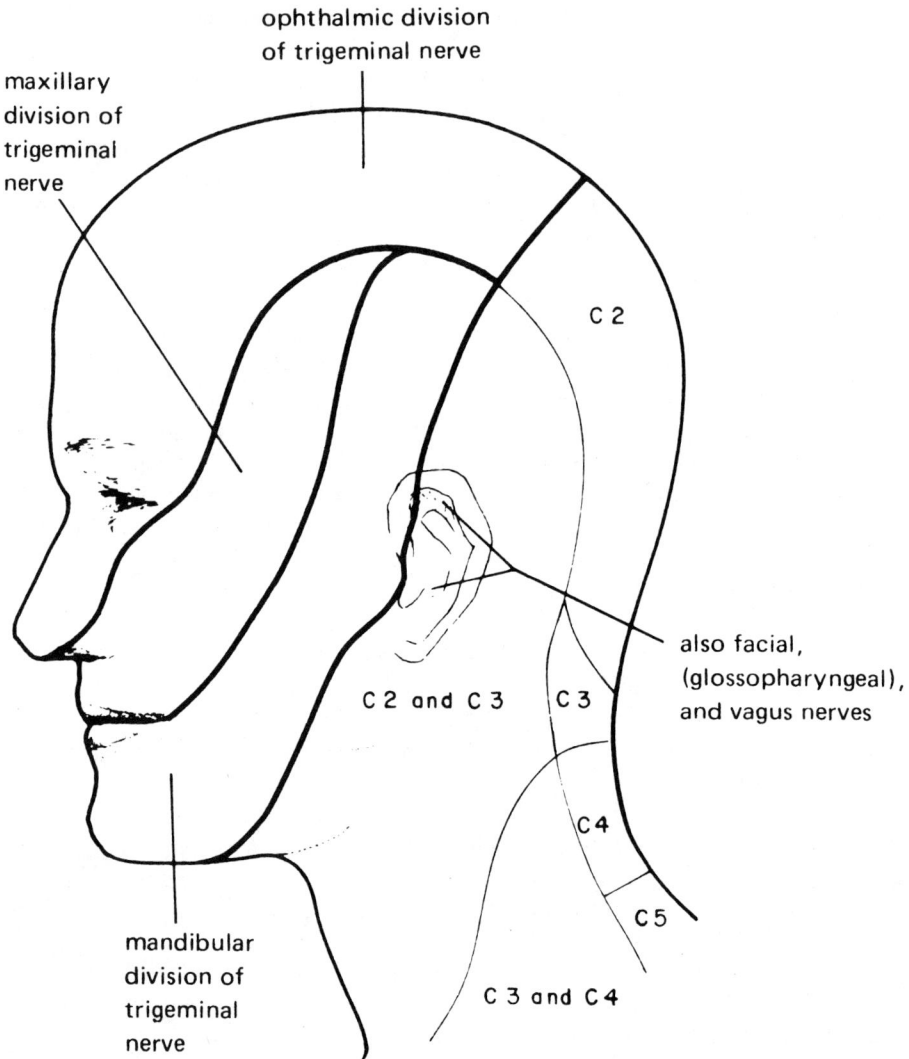

Figure XII-2. Cutaneous innervation of the head and neck. From Barr (1979).

(1978); these investigators consider emotional stress a contributing factor and state that bradycardia "is susceptible to complex central modulation." Central nervous system modulation was also implicated by Wolf (1967), who reported a series of experiments in which subjects were directed to immerse their faces in water; the predictable heart slowing followed. However, Wolf stated, "when the subjects were distracted . . . or harassed in any way, the reflex bradycardia often failed to occur, despite the fact that the face was underwater."

Wolf (1967) also observed that heart slowing began in some subjects "immediately after the order to immerse was given and before the face reached the water." He considered this finding demonstrated that the reflex occurred "in anticipation of immersion." These reports strongly support a higher nervous system component in the reflex.

c. Cardiovascular Disorders and Sudden Death

In recent years a particular cardiovascular problem in divers has received attention—the problem of sudden death. Case histories and studies of drowning, sudden cardiac death, and cardiovascular reflexes underwater were analyzed by Eldridge (1979a, 1979b). She reported, "A substantial number of sport scuba diving fatalities in cold water have been middle-aged males who suddenly and unexplainably lost consciousness." The number of deaths in the past 2 years in California waters has been around 10—all males between the ages 35 and 55. Eldridge reported that the victims were unresponsive to mouth-to-mouth resuscitation and that the timing of the deaths suggested cardiac arrhythmia and arrest as the underlying cause of the fatality. Diving partners in general reported the victims to be "calm" with no overt signs of panic or struggle; reports of being "tired" were frequent among the victims before sinking. Most of the victims in Eldridge's study had previous cardiovascular problems such as hypertension or a history of arrhythmias. Autopsy showed significant coronary artery stenosis in others. Unfortunately, in recording these diving fatalities the cause of death was invariably listed as "drowning," which, as we see in a later discussion of diving accidents, is the last event in a series of events associated with the fatality.

A crucial finding in Eldridge's survey was the inevitability of cold water as the site of the fatality. We have seen that bradycardia is affected by lowered water temperatures. Marked cardiovascular responses are associated with cold. Cold water is a potent stimulus and, in view of the autopsy data on the diving fatalities, Eldridge suggests that divers with functional or anatomical cardiovascular problems may be especially vulnerable to disruptions in heart rhythms elicited by cold water. Minor cardiac irregularities that physicians detect on physical examination may cause problems in susceptible individuals diving in cold water.

This preliminary survey offers much in the way of speculation. Arrhythmias evoked by cold, fatigue, exercise, and related events in diving are normal. An oversimplified view of these arrhythmias is to consider stress and balance; we have seen in the earlier discussion of the nature of stress that body imbalance and restoration of balance (homeostasis) is a normal event and that, indeed, deliberate invocation of imbalance is engendered in the search for thrills. Here, the interaction of two divisions of the autonomic nervous system, the sympathetic and the parasympathetic, is germane. Bradycardia, an oxygen-conserving reflex, is evoked by trigeminal stimulation of vagal efferents to the sinus and atrioventricular nodes. As Wolf observes, the dive reflex is "a good example of the simultaneous activation of both cholinergic and adrenergic elements," with "apnea, bradycardia, peripheral and visceral vasoconstriction, often elevation of systemic arterial pressure and a shift by the tissues to anaerobic metabolism" (1969, p. 32).

Hypothermia, especially in a susceptible individual, is a major cause of disorganized rhythm. Changes in heart rhythm as a result of stress such as cold are normal, and restoration of rhythm after cardiac arrhythmias are induced is usual in the normal individual. But as Childs (1978) notes, a falling core temperature in an immersed individual may result in death, "usually in a cardiac arrhythmia."

Childs states, "The possibility exists that maximal thermal shivering may require an increase in cardiac output that can only just be met by a fit myocardium; if further stresses are applied, for example, by frantic swimming efforts, or if the myocardium is unfit for any reason, high output cardiac failure may follow" (1978, p. 6). Animal research such as that reported by Auld (1978) supports such a hypothesis. Auld found that cold exposure caused an increase in oxygen uptake (resulting from the increased oxygen requirements of maximal shivering) of three times that of normal as well as a similar threefold increase in cardiac output in dogs. Like exercise, the ability to handle thermal stress can be improved with physical conditioning.

4. Cardiovascular Effects of Stress: Emotional Factors

The layman and the poet have always fully believed that the heart is the seat of emotion and is acutely sensitive to passions of a positive and negative nature. Shakespeare relates emotion to fatigue, monitored by the heart:

> A merry heart goes all the day,
> Your sad tires in a mile.
> —Shakespeare, *The Winter's Tale*

And Coleridge relates a negative emotion, fear, to a life-threatening condition:

> Fear at my heart, as at a cup,
> My life-blood seem'd to sip.
> —Coleridge, *The Ancient Mariner*

The scientist has evidence that such stress factors as fatigue (which can evoke cardiac arrhythmias) and fear can produce marked cardiovascular effects. Earlier I talked about Type A behavior, a cluster of behavioral characteristics described by Friedman and Rosenman (1974) as a coronary-prone pattern. According to Friedman and Rosenman, the Type A individual (probably male) demonstrates a complex of actions and emotions while struggling incessantly against opposing forces for the purpose of achieving as much as possible in the least amount of time.

Documentation for this behavior pattern has come from other investigators. Glass et al. (1980), for example, refer to studies in which Type A individuals worked on a treadmill, at a level closer to their limits of endurance, at the same time admitting to less fatigue. A double-blind study conducted by Rosenman et al. (1964) analyzed 3000 men between the ages of 39 and 59, judging exactly half of them to be Type A on the basis of structured interviews. A follow-up study (Rosenman et al.1975) accomplished almost 9 years later showed that the Type A group had an incidence of coronary heart disease of twice the rate of the non-Type A (Type B). Moreover, traditional risk factors such as cigarette smoking and hypercholesterolemia did not account for the differential rate, which suggests, as Glass and associates (1980) note, that the behavior pattern of Type A does not appear to exert pathogenic influence through other coronary risk factors and that this behavior pattern appears to be related to clinical manifestations of coronary heart disease as well as to the underlying atherosclerotic disease process. The latter suggestion finds some support in a study by Blumenthal et al. (1978) that used techniques of coronary arteriography, in which it was found that a significantly greater degree of coronary occlusion occurred in patients classified as having Type A behavior patterns.

Obviously no simple relationship between behavior and coronary-prone patterns can be drawn. How much the life style contributes to a behavior pattern and how much of the life style is created by other factors of a physical or social nature is difficult to determine. Nevertheless, there is strong evidence that the emotional nature of the individual contributes markedly to cardiovascular disorders. Earlier I cited Engel as noting that the macho individual in our culture who is unable to display weakness appears to have a higher incidence of vasodepressor (vasovagal) syncope. Engel (1978) further comments that "the need to exaggerate bravery, strength, aggressiveness, and other culturally defined attributes of manliness and to deny, minimize, or at least not acknowledge fear, coupled with a shame for failure to live up to such standards, constitute the classic psychologic preconditions for vasodepressor syncope" (p. 404).

Given the high percentage of cardiovascular disorders found in Eldridge's study (1979a, 1979b) of sudden cardiac death among male middle-aged divers, discussed previously, we can only speculate about the psychological profile of victims in this group of fatalities: Did they have a modicum of machismo that related to a Type A unwillingness to limit activity? We can only speculate regarding the physiological events as well. If, indeed, these cases of sudden cardiac death in the water involved a predisposition to cardiovascular disorder, and if the physical event leading to death was a vasovagal syncope, it is useful to look briefly at Engel's concept of the psychological factors in vasodepressor syncope, which, as he noted, is almost invariably a function of male machismo. The predominance of males in these accounts as well as the Type A behavior patterns described by Rosenman and Friedman (1974) are, in themselves, of interest, especially when correlated with the data from the cave diving fatality analysis of Desautels and Poulton (1980) (discussed later in this chapter) in which 205 of 207 cave fatalities were male. Surely, the ratio of males to females participating in diving is not that overwhelming.

Engel (1978) noted that the initial circulatory changes in vasovagal syncope are an increase in heart rate and blood pressure (diastolic more than systolic) as well as an increase in systemic resistance and cardiac output (largely autonomic nervous system activity). These responses are similar to the sympathetic activation reported by Bove (1977) in a study in which anxiety was experimentally induced in animals and physiological events were carefully recorded. Bove stated that the anxiety-induced animals showed alterations in circulation typical of sympathetic activation, including tachycardia, elevated blood pressure, increased cardiac output, increased coronary blood flow, tachypnea, and elevated levels of free fatty acids and glucose in the blood. Fain and Czech (1975) demonstrated that, under conditions of stress, corticosteroids increase the sugars available in the blood stream and inhibit the transport of glucose into fat cells, thereby raising the level of release of free fatty acids—findings consonant with Bove's.

The catecholamines under stress are a subject so complex that the brief compass of this chapter does not permit any but the most shallow note. One such observation is that rises in blood pressures, elevated heart rates, and initiation of cardiac arrhythmias, among cardiovascular problems, are a function of sympathetic nervous system activity, which engenders discharge of catecholamines such as epinephrine and norepinephrine (Eliot 1979). Glass et al. (1980) reported on research that showed higher urinary norepinephrine rates among Type A men during the work day; Rosenman and Friedman (1974) found higher plasma norepinephrine rates during conditions of stress; still another study showed greater elevations in plasma epinephrine in Type A men exposed to a hostile competition. Glass and associates (1980) found that active coping with a stressor heightened catecholamine activity; Engel (1970) stated that the rise and fall of catecholamines and related shifts between sympathetic and parasympathetic activation under stress may be an important mechanism underlying sudden death. Lown et al. (1980) have presented evidence that sympathetic-adrenergic mechanisms are implicated in the susceptibility to ventricular fibrillation resulting from psychological stress such as anxiety; they sum up their report by observing, "psychophysiological factors can no longer be ignored if the trigger mechanisms for the sporadically occurring ventricular arrhythmias are to be comprehended" (p. 1333).

To be sure, the links between emotional stress and cardiovascular disorders are not clearly delineated. That emotional stress plays some role seems not to be in much doubt, but what the role may be is still a matter of discussion. A U.S. Public Health Service (1972) report on hardening of the arteries states that emotional or prolonged stress and strain may contribute to heart attacks. The report adds that many medical persons believe the role of pressure becomes critical only after a hardening of the arteries has created a setting for an attack.

An important consideration in conducting the physical examination for diving, in any case, should be a sensitivity to personality factors that may render an already susceptible individual further liable to stressors such as cold, fatigue, and exercise associated with diving, as well as add to the potential for excitement and fear-inducing stimuli.

A final note: explicit in the characterization of the macho (Type A) individual is the marked need of such a person to be in control of a situation; this is associated with a low ability to tolerate frustration and opposition. Glass (1977) has noted that Type A individuals work hard initially to assert and maintain control over events that may be uncontrollable; however, continued lack of control leads to a sense of failure and frustration and, as Glass observes, Type A persons are believed to give up efforts at control more quickly than their Type B counterparts, who apparently react with less intensity and a higher tolerance for frustration. This is an interesting hypothesis illuminated by an observation of Wolf (1969) dealing with regulatory inhibition of autonomic nervous system—sympathetic and parasympathetic—activity: "Regulatory inhibition appears to be enhanced in situations that tend to concentrate attention on purposeful action and to be diminished in situations that are interpreted as overwhelming and without hope, such as situations of total social exclusion, of hopeless dejection, or of sudden fear. Under such circumstances, the loss of regulatory inhibition may provide a mechanism of death" (p. 34). The reader interested in such a hypothesis may well turn to writers such as Cannon (1942) on voodoo death and to Richter (1957).

Control and the loss of control as psychophysiological factors are further explored in a later section dealing with the ultimate in loss of control—diver panic.

D. Diving Accidents

In the course of these discussions on stress responses in diving there have been passing references to diving accidents, including the effects of hypothermia and cardiovascular changes. The concatenation of stressors to which the diver is subjected markedly affects his or her performance; this effect may have minimal negative results unless an unforeseen event exacerbates the stress. Such an unforeseen event is referred to as an "accident." As a prelude to discussing diving accidents, I discuss hazards and accidents, putting emphasis on the methodology of accident research.

1. Hazards and Accidents

Much has been written about diving accidents in commercial diving (Bradley 1981) and in recreational diving (McAniff 1980). These reports illustrate the difficulties inherent in accident reporting: the problems in obtaining accurate accounts of each incident and sufficient detail to be able to examine possible causative factors. Blau (1980), citing various reports, points out that diving is unusual in that there are relatively few minor accidents in comparison to reported fatalities. Part of this, of course, is the problem of gathering accurate data regarding incidents even in cases of fatalities, as we see later on, and it is almost certain that minor mishaps go unreported. Nonetheless, the ratio of mishaps to fatalities is unusual, but perhaps not unexpected. An incident in water does not allow for the recovery that a mishap on land might permit. Blau compares skateboarding with diving in noting that in the former the National Safety Council statistics revealed that in 1976 there were 27,000 hospitalizations resulting from skateboarding, and 9 fatalities.

Accident reporting in itself is a methodology not entirely agreed upon; various approaches are suggested by Blackman (1975), Licht (1975), Manning (1974), Missirtlu and Foy (1978), Pezoldt (1977), and Yanowitch (1975). What is usually called an accident in many circumstances is the final event resulting from a sequence of events. In some situations the word *accident* is used synonymously with the word *casualty*. In a like manner, *drowning* is frequently given as the cause of death in a diving accident, when drowning is actually the last event in a series. It is my belief that a more fruitful approach to assessing diving accidents is the accident methodology proposed by Licht (1975), who defined an accident as an unforeseen event that is sudden, unplanned, and has a potential for producing injury or damage. The key to the methodology is the aspect of control.

Licht (1975) explains, "As long as the situation is under control, an accident by definition cannot occur" (p. 532). The accident occurs at the moment control is lost: what happens thereafter constitutes the *consequences* of the accident; the accident itself is the event that caused the individual to lose control. For example, an accident occurs when a car skids out of control on an icy patch of road. The responses that take place to restore control may determine the consequences of the accident. The driver either does or does not regain control. This sequence may be diagrammed as follows:

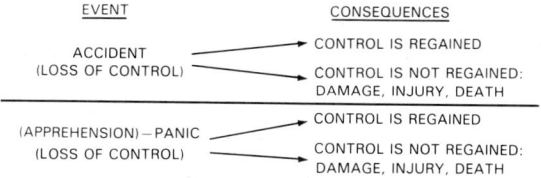

Because an accident is an unforeseen event, Licht (1975) suggests that the term *accident prevention* is at best meaningless and that the emphasis should be on *accident mitigation*, which would reduce the potential for damage from consequences attendant upon an accident. A hard hat, he noted, does not prevent accidents, but it might mitigate the consequences. When such a methodology is used, the concentration shifts from the final event, usually called the accident, to the first event, in which control was lost. In addition, evaluating mitigation as the important element leads to several behaviors. For example, the emphasis on preparation is strengthened: training is underscored, and training for emergency response takes on more importance. The assessment of individual capabilities for emergency response also takes on greater emphasis. If one assumes an accident to be a sudden, unforeseen event with a potential for harm, then preparation for restoration of control—an evaluation of the environmental conditions and the individual characteristics—can be better approached. With regard to an individual who is performing, Waller (1977) has described an accident as the "moment at which task demand exceeds the performance" of the individual or the group. The individual (or group) must have certain capabilities to respond so that the loss of control can be corrected. Waller (1977) suggests four such crucial capabilities:

1. The knowledge that "one has about one's self in relation to different aspects of the environment." This is knowledge that depends on capabilities such as education, training, basic intelligence, and experience as well as culturally determined beliefs and attitudes.

2. The ability to "receive information about the environment through inherent senses." These include perception through sight, touch, and hearing.

3. "The ability to make rapid judgments about one's self in relation to the environment as a result of the combination of the information received through the senses and knowledge applied in interpreting such information."

4. "The capability to act in response to judgments that suggest danger may exist" (p. 34).

From Licht's comments and those of Waller we may observe that accident mitigation is required to restore control lost as a result of an accident. The individual must have the ability to obtain and receive information about the environment and his or her situation accurately, be able to process the information in a timely manner, and react with an appropriate and effective response. *Timely* and *rapid* have appeared as adjectives describing the event and the response. It is precisely the suddenness of the accident that creates the greatest problem. Dean and Thatcher (1975), in their analysis of human factors in aircraft accidents, list *rapidity of events* as the first of several factors leading to loss of control by pilots in an accident; other factors constitute related problems: departures from preplanned parameters (the unforeseen event), time-sharing (several events occurring at once), concentration of attention (an effort rendered more difficult by the time-sharing of events), and, finally, later realization or delayed reaction (a production problem in information processing and response).

The environmental aspects to be assessed in accident mitigation may be concentrated in an evaluation of the potential for hazard in the particular environment. In comparing ocean performance with that on land we have seen that, for example, fatigue can be handled more successfully on land because there is greater opportunity for resting. By inspection, the ocean environment suggests an infinitely greater hazard cluster than land. Kates (1970) has proposed a model for discussing hazards; he limns two types of hazards: (1) Intensive hazards, which are "characteristically small in area extent, intense in impact, of brief duration, sudden onset, and poor predictability" (p. 405). These characteristics appear to fit well with our definition of an accident. (2) Pervasive hazards, which are, by contrast with intensive hazards, "widespread in extent, have a diffuse impact, a long duration, gradual onset, [and are] . . . predicted more accurately" (p. 405).

In the ocean environment the likelihood of the appearance of hazards is high. Pervasive hazards such as storm systems, which are predictable to a large degree, are not as much a problem for the diver as intensive hazards such as sudden changes in sea states, the appearance of marine hazards, equipment malfunction, and similar limited intensive hazards that can be associated with the loss of control represented by an accident.

2. Diving Hazards and Accidents

At best, it is difficult to estimate what percentage of United States divers is represented in the worldwide number of fatal diving accidents because there are no hard data regarding the numbers of active divers. We do have hard data on the numbers of divers trained by certifying training agencies such as the National Association of Underwater Instructors and the Professional Association of Diving Instructors. These agencies and the others actively engaged in instruction certify approximately 250,000 scuba divers a year. How many of these quarter of a million divers go on to active participation in recreational diving can only be guessed; attrition is estimated to be high. (By active participation I mean, as a rough criterion, getting one's head wet at least three times a year; this is probably a stringent requirement.) Many professionals in diving would guess that there are perhaps close to 2 million reasonably active scuba divers in the United States. If that were so, less than 200 fatalities would not appear to be high. Compared to other active sports such as skiing the ratio is high, but, of course, the possibilities of regaining control or, at most, breaking a limb and therefore recovering from a skiing accident are higher than in the diving environment, where errors or loss of control lead to more drastic consequences. An article in a medical journal some years ago referred to "the ballistics of skiing" in which an object moving at a certain momentum impacts another stationary object with measurable force (and predictable consequences). No such ballistics can be applied under water.

With regard to commercial diving fatalities, again accurate statistics are difficult to obtain. And, once again, the estimated number of accidents in which divers have lost control is much higher than the actual number of reported casualties, injuries, or deaths. Bradley (1981) reports on an estimated 905 commercial divers working in the Gulf of Mexico, and statistics indicate that the total fatalities from 1968 to 1975 would yield an average of 2.49 deaths per 1000 working divers per year. In the British sector of the North Sea a somewhat higher rate prevails; from 1971 to 1978 a fatality rate of 4.82 per 1000 per year was found. Commercial diver fatalities occurred at depths that ranged from 0 to 340 fsw (104 msw) in the Gulf of Mexico (the mean depth at which there was a fatality was 136 fsw, or 41 msw). In the North Sea the mean depth of fatalities was 223 fsw (68 msw), with a range of 0–500 fsw (0–152 msw). Virtually all of these dive operations were associated with oil exploration, recovery, maintenance, and inspection.

Comparing commercial diving casualties with military diving casualties is not a reasonable enterprise for a major reason: most Navy diving operations are at relatively shallow depths. Berghage and associates (1975) analyzed a total of 127,103 U.S. Navy dives logged from January 1972 through December 1973. These authors found that 99% of the dives were accomplished in less than 200 fsw (61 msw), with a mean of 47 fsw (14 msw), and an average time on bottom of 31 min. In addition, the majority of dives were done in waters in which the temperature exceeded 50°F (10°C) and the surface temperature was rarely below 55°F (13°C). Similar data, with the exception that water temperatures were slightly higher, were obtained for commercial divers operating in the Gulf of Mexico. Statistics from such dives are not comparable to those for North Sea commercial dives, where waters are much colder, the length of operational dives much longer, and the depths of work much deeper.

The depth of a dive determines the breathing gas used. In dives deeper than 190 fsw (58 msw) compressed air is replaced by a mixture of helium and oxygen, a mixture that allows for less pulmonary stress and attendant problems of oxygen toxicity. Thus most of the U.S. Navy dives must have been on air. In the North Sea 63% of the fatal accidents occurred with a breathing mix of helium and oxygen; in the Gulf of Mexico, 67% of the fatal accidents occurred while the diver was breathing compressed air (Bradley 1981).

Accidents with a negative consequence to recreational divers have become a source of great interest and concern not only in the United States but also in other parts of the world. For example, in recent years accident reports have appeared from Israel (Melamed and Ohry 1980) and New Zealand (Lewis 1979) and from Great Britain through a series of reports from the British Sub-Aqua Club Diving Officers' Conference (Skuse 1980). These reports, and similar ones, have analyzed diving incidents and accidents leading to injury, casualty, or fatality, in an attempt to detail conditions and causes. The statistics vary from study to study. In Israel, Melamed and Ohry (1980) estimated an increased activity among Red Sea and Mediterranean divers from 500 in 1971 to more than 7000 divers in 1977. The diving accident data accumulated during the years 1974–1978 showed a total of 130 diving incidents leading to injury or physical damage. In New Zealand, Lewis (1979) reported fatalities as a consequence of diving accidents, showing a total of 28 deaths between 1971 and 1973, of which 21 were scuba divers and 5 were skin divers. The British experience reported by Skuse (1980) showed a total of 360 diving incidents, of which 38 resulted in a fatality during the years 1978–1980. In all of these reports from foreign diving experiences the number of incidents at relatively shallow depths is striking. In the Israeli data, for example, almost a third of the incidents involved depths of less than 30 m; the British data showed that, for the years 1979 and 1980, 84 out of 137 divers were at less than 98 ft (30 m) when an incident occurred, and another 52 divers were on the surface. In New Zealand, Lewis (1979) reported, "Two-thirds of the scuba deaths occurred in water less than 15 m deep, 5 of these on the surface." The inference from these and related data is that the divers may not have been down deep enough or long enough, in most cases, to have suffered from problems of decompression.

There are no clear statistics regarding the number of accidents or incidents in diving (nor in any other risk recreation)—if we adhere to our definition of an accident as an unforeseen event in which control is lost and either regained or not regained. The number of near misses or unreported incidents can be only roughly estimated. What are generally referred to as accident statistics, as we have seen, are usually casualty statistics or injury statistics reflecting a loss of control leading to damage or death.

Two basic problems continue to haunt the reporter of accident statistics in diving: First, there is no clear denominator, i.e., what is the ratio of incidents to exposures? How many incidents or accidents occurred during how many dives? Second, many of the reported incidents are anecdotal in nature and therefore lack clearness and objectivity. Myers (1979) reported on recompression procedures in a resort community, the Cayman Islands. In comments during the Undersea Medical Society Workshop at which his paper was presented, Myers stated that there were, in 1 year, 8 divers that were treated in a chamber out of as many as 250,000 dives. He indicated that the denominator was derived from interviews with all of the dive-shop owners: he simply asked for the total number of tank fills they had accomplished during the year; the assumption that one tank fill equaled one dive gave him his denominator. This technique has merit, although there are some problems associated with it—largely, to touch on a sensitive point, because tank fills are commercial interactions in which cash changes hands and taxable income might have to be declared!

McAniff (1980) reported diving accident statistics in the United States through the data center at the University of Rhode Island. (See Chapter XV, "Diving Accident Investigation.") Although this center is working closely with diving agencies and groups, McAniff acknowledges that for the 1977–1978 fatality data, 65% of the 1977 data and 72% of the 1978 data came from press clippings. With all due respect to newspaper reporting, information reported in the press is not always complete or accurate. McAniff also indicates that the accuracy of reporting from a presumably more responsible quarter, the medical examiners, leaves something to be desired. McAniff (1980) made a colorful comment regarding the medicolegal system in the United States in saying that it "ranges from extremely talented forensic pathologists with excellent facilities and well-trained staffs to small towns with only a local politico who simply looks at a body and determines that it is dead" (p. 1).

Allowing for the problems of possibly inaccurate reporting, I believe the reports from the University of Rhode Island provide valuable information to the diving scientist and physician. McAniff's 1980 report covers the years 1970–1978 and presents an analysis of diving fatalities. A brief review of the salient data from this report is useful in assessing underwater problems. The data for fatalities to skin divers and nonprofessional scuba divers for the years 1970–1978 are in Table XII-1.

Table XII-1
Fatalities to Skin Divers and
Nonprofessional Scuba Divers in the
United States, 1970–1978[a]

	Skin divers		Nonprofessional scuba divers	
Year	Male	Female	Male	Female
1970	18	1	99	11
1971	17	0	104	8
1972	15	1	107	12
1973	22	0	118	7
1974	25	2	129	15
1975	16	1	123	8
1976	11	3	137	10
1977	18	1	98	4
1978	13	3	95	21

[a]Data from McAniff (1980).

A 25% decrease in the number of fatalities from the high levels of 1975–1976 is important, in part reflecting the dramatic drop in cave diving fatalities (mostly in Florida) from a total of 66 for the years 1974–1976 to a total of 20 for 1977–1978.

California and Florida have always had the highest diving fatality rates, undoubtedly because of higher numbers of dive exposures. Saltwater fatalities, also a reflection of frequency, represented 60% of the totals in McAniff's report. The fatalities in fresh water were mostly in lakes and ponds, those from cave diving being close behind in numbers. Why fatalities from cave diving have decreased so dramatically is a source of conjecture. McAniff suggests that there is greater private control of caves than before and that local regulations have been effective. Some of the more dangerous caves have been sealed off. In another analysis of diving fatalities Desautels and Poulton (1980) reported on 207 deaths (205 male, 2 female) in 138 incidents associated with cave diving from 1960 to 1979; the age range was from 15 to 50 yr (mean age, 23 yr) and only 50% of the fatality victims held a valid basic scuba certification at the time of death. Fewer than 15% of these divers were experienced in cave diving and only 5% had been certified by the National Association of Cave Divers (see Chapter I footnote). Divers' bodies were found between 10 and 1000 ft within the caves (mean distance 290 ft or 88 m from the entrance) at depths ranging from 25 to 290 ft (mean depth 80 ft or 24 m). These authors observed that nearly 75% of the divers who died were equipped inadequately. The lesson from this study is clear: diver error in judgment, planning, training, and technique all contributed to fatalities. Another factor related to training and screening is important here: diving in each different type of area requires a specialized skill. The diver who is trained and comfortable in an open-sea situation may not be equally prepared to enter a kelp bed or a cave.

In McAniff's study there are other interesting data: the most frequent diving platform for fatalities was shore, beach, or pier (e.g., in 1978, 61 out of a total of 116 fatalities), and the second most frequent platform was private recreational vessels (in 1978, 26 out of 116); diving charter boats had a lower incidence of fatalities (in 1978, 14 out of 116). These figures correlate with the higher number of fatalities occurring in heavy surf and current; moreover, they suggest that private recreational vessels do not have the control or precautions exercised in professionally chartered dive boats. Experience, as noted in the Desautels and Poulton (1980) data on cave-diving, was also a crucial factor in McAniff's report. Almost half of the 1978 fatalities occurred in a first open-water dive or in a dive soon after training; some of the divers who died had some experience, few had considerable experience.

The various reports on diving fatalities clearly point out the roles of human performance and human error in the accidents and their consequences. Poorly equipped and inexperienced divers—those who may not have adequate training and who do not plan well for a dive—place themselves (and their diving partners) at risk. Equipment failure in diving fatalities does not appear to be a contributing factor. In San Diego a committee examined every piece of gear used by divers who died; they uncovered no significant problems in function. McAniff reports only one documented failure in well-maintained equipment in approximately 1100 cases in 9 years; obtaining the equipment after a fatality is, however, often a problem.

The phrase "well-maintained" is another key phrase here. As Egstrom (1982) observes, much of the equipment in use by divers is not given sufficiently careful routine maintenance. Another observation from the same paper is germane. In a study of regulators, Egstrom found that almost all the regulators on the market allowed comfortable inhalation and exhalation at 6 breaths/min. Normal breathing rates are closer to 15 breaths/

min, but even these higher breathing rates create no problem for comfortable divers unless tank pressures fall to levels of 300 psi, where, at depth, some difficulty may occur. These findings assume a comfortable diver breathing easily and with regularity. The problem with regulators becomes acute at low tank pressure when a diver, who is perhaps apprehensive and fatigued, breathes at rates of 25 to 30 breaths/min—a hyperpnea probably associated with growing apprehension that can lead to possible panic. Thus, equipment may be functional within normal limits of performance but may become stressed as the diver becomes stressed. Because I believe panic to be the single most important factor in diving fatalities and negative consequences of accidents, the next section deals in detail with diver panic.

E. *Diver Panic*

>. . . and panic, panic was the biggest danger, enemy, the only danger there was in diving.
>—James Jones, *Go to the Widow Maker*

In previous discussions panic has been alluded to in a number of comments. Most diving investigators believe that panic is the cause of eventual fatalities in many if not most of the recreational diving accidents in the United States (and probably elsewhere, for that matter). The topic of panic has been explored, with information drawn from observed incidents of panic as well as the general stress literature (Bachrach 1970, 1973, 1979, 1980, 1981; Bachrach and Egstrom 1977; Bevan 1973; Blau 1980; Curley 1978; Egstrom and Bachrach 1971). A definition of panic that has emerged from such studies is: "a strong, fearful perception by an individual that he is out of control, that he is not capable of coping with the situation in which he finds himself, leading to behaviors that not only do not solve the problem posed by the danger but actually may work directly against such solution" (Bachrach 1970).

The key phrase is *out of control*; it is related to the discussion on accident methodology in which we defined an accident as an unforeseen event in which control is lost, either to be regained (with no negative consequences) or not regained (with damage, injury, or death). The discussions that have preceded this consideration of panic have prepared the groundwork for a detailed analysis of the events in a panic reaction. Figure XII-3 presents a diagram of the interaction among various events. Having entered the water dressed in equipment that in itself is stressful, the diver is subjected to two additional stressors—cold and exercise. All three contribute to fatigue. As the course of the dive continues, the initial response to cold may become a progressive and silent hypothermia in which the diver is not aware of changes in the ability to make judgments and changes in other cognitive performance demonstrated to be degraded by cold. In addition, cold and fatigue begin to degrade the strength, dexterity, and stamina of the diver so that there is not only a lowered ability to cope with problems in a cognitive manner but also a diminished physical competence. The effects of cold, exercise, and fatigue may also engender physiological reactions such as induced cardiac irregularities and arrhythmias, which, as has been discussed, in the susceptible individual might lead to the serious consequences of ventricular fibrillation and sudden cardiac death. This cardiac event is a rare one, but the reduction of physical and psychological competence in the diver under these stress conditons is not infrequent.

Also occurring during the course of the dive is the gradual reduction of the finite air supply the diver carries in the scuba bottle. As the title of Figure XII-3 states, these are the major predisposing factors in a panic reaction. The diver has diminished physical and behavioral ability to cope; this diminution is accompanied by physiological changes, and the lessened supply of vital air may require extra breathing effort because of lowered tank pressures. The last column in Figure XII-3 is titled "Unforeseen Events: Accident." Here the diver, already subjected to stress, encounters an event that was not planned: it may be a change in sea state with increased wave action, it may be the appearance of a shark, or it may be an equipment malfunction. The result of this unforeseen event—diving accident—is crucial; what the diver does in response to the accident will, as seen in the discussion of accidents, determine the consequences of the accident. It would be expected that the well-trained, experienced diver who has encountered difficulties in past dives would immediately take action to cope in the most efficient manner possible. But what creates the problem and potential casualty is the inability to cope. The definition of panic offered earlier in this discussion emphasized that the individual in a panic reaction not only perceives that he or she is not in control of the situation but may actually engage in behaviors that further contribute to the danger. This is seen, for example, in stereotypy of responding in which the individual engages in responses that do not work but, perhaps, have worked in the past; thus the individual is engaged in what amounts to almost superstitious response. An example of such a situation is the continued and aggressive

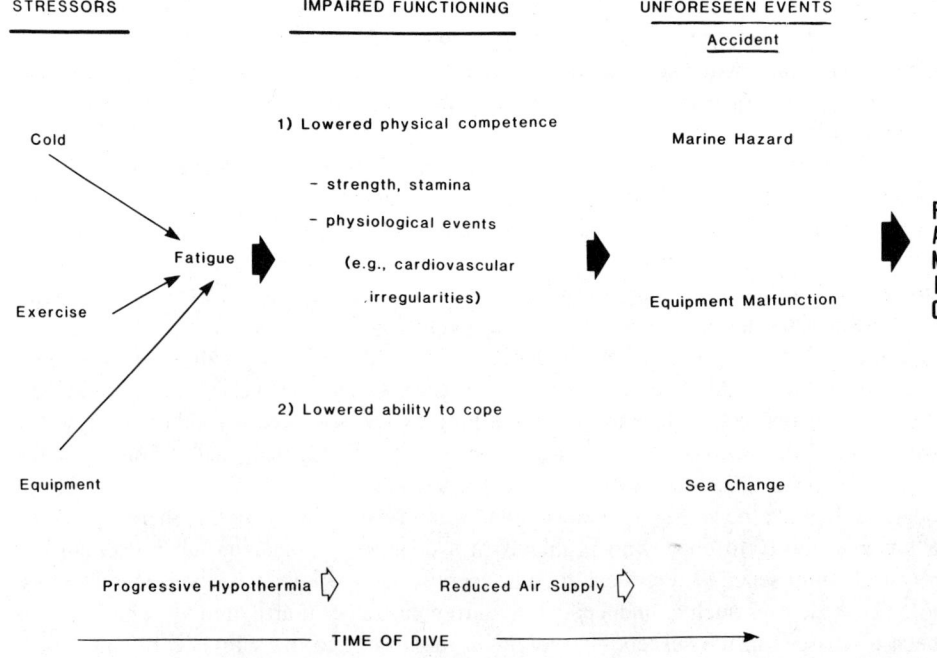

Figure XII-3. Major predisposing factors in a panic reaction.

pulling of the reserve J-valve despite the fact that it had already been tripped accidentally, perhaps on kelp. Continuing to pull the reserve is indeed a stereotyped response, one that had been reinforced in the past but is not currently successful. Thus, not only does it fail to work but it prevents the individual from attempting responses that might help to solve the danger situation.

Part of this stereotype of responding is a function of what has been referred to as a *narrowed perception* in divers under stress. Weltman and Egstrom (1966) conducted experiments on perceptual narrowing in novice divers, followed by Baddeley (1972), who observed "one way in which danger effects performance is through its influence on the subject's breadth of attention." Narrowing of perception and attention is not only in terms of visual fields, although Weltman and Egstrom have demonstrated that a literal narrowing of perception can occur. What is more important to our discussion is the narrowing of perception in terms of perceiving courses of action to be taken to extricate oneself from the danger situation. This, again, is the lowered ability to cope—which places the individual at greater hazard. Narrow attention under stress has been a source of interest to behaviorists for many years, beginning in particular with the classic work of Callaway and Dembo (1958), in which neurochemical and neurophysiological elements in narrowed attention were explored. These investigators hypothesized that narrowed attention was a psychological phenomenon that accompanies a specific physiological change, a *central sympathomimetic activity* as a stress response. Callaway and Dembo (1958) were able to induce narrowing of perception in human subjects through administration of epinephrine, methamphetamine, and amyl nitrite. The interaction of behavioral and physiological events undoubtedly is critical in the reduced ability to cope.

1. Helplessness and Anxiety

a. Behavioral Reactions

Earlier in a discussion of sudden death it was noted that theorists such as Wolf (1969), drawing in large measure on researchers such as Richter (1957) and Cannon (1939, 1942)—the latter in particular with regard to voodoo or hexed death—speculate that sense of helplessness in the face of stress can contribute to marked physiological changes. We continually are drawn to compare the restoration of control on a land situation with restoration of control in open water. Individuals faced with loss of control and the necessity to regain it stand an infinitely better chance of restoration on land, where they are not also battling a surging, somewhat weightless environment while encumbered with gear and probably in a condition of hypothermia. The sense of helplessness that occurs when control is lost and panic begins is central to anxiety. Mandler (1979) has discussed the unavailability of appropriate responses or action alternatives in coping with stress; he considers this helplessness in the face of the environment to be the essential psychological basis of the subjective reactions classified as anxiety.

In another related approach to anxiety (Bachrach 1980a) I have invoked the paradigm of Schoenfeld (1950) in which the temporal nature of anxiety is defined:

$$S_1 \text{-----} R_{T_{(av)}} \text{----} S_2$$

in which S_1 is the warning stimulus that signals the oncoming presentation of the noxious stimulus (S_2), creating the condition where the individual engages in a response to avoid or postpone the onset of the aversive, noxious stimulus. This avoidance response ($R_{T(av)}$ either can be a coping response in which the individual takes action to cope with the warning stimulus or can be a response of avoidance in which certain neurotic components come into play, such as phobic responses that avoid but never solve previously interpreted aversive stimulus conditions (Lief 1955). Superstitious responses occur with greater frequency under conditions of uncertainty (Bachrach 1962, 1980b; Malinowski 1925). The time course presumes that the individual will, in some manner, cope with the onset of the aversive event following the warning stimulus. As we have seen, a major characteristic of accidents is their rapid onset, which allows little time to assess action alternatives for coping with the incident, a circumstance especially serious under stress conditions in which rapid control is essential, as in aircraft accidents and, of course, open-water accidents. This inability to cope effectively is the main reason that training should develop an overlearned emergency response in divers so that no cognitive complexities are required and coping becomes virtually automatic.

So far attention has been directed to the behavioral events that are associated with the onset of an accident in which panic is a consequence, concentrating on the behavior of the panicked individual in a potentially uncontrolled situation. How this individual is perceived by others in the water is, understandably, largely anecdotal, relying on descriptions of the event by observers. As mentioned earlier in the sudden cardiac death cases discussed by Eldridge (1979a), the victims were usually described by their diving partners as "calm" and frequently as "tired." In the panic situation a different behavioral constellation appears. Figure XII-4 is an artist's conception drawn from observers' descriptions. It depicts the diver in panic—in a vertical posture, head held out of the water,

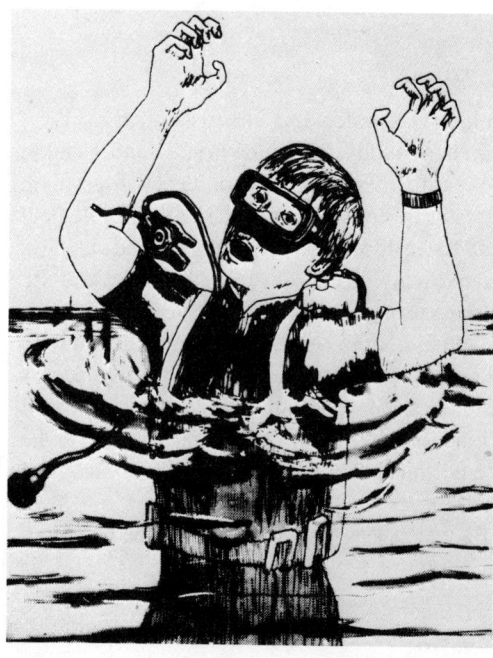

Figure XII-4. Artist's conception of a diver in panic.

quiet, hands clawing the air, mouthpiece out of the mouth, and buoyancy compensator unfilled. Bevan (1973) also indicated that wide eyes, easily seen through the mask, are a sign of panic. Obviously, this is not a universal picture of panic but is sufficiently frequent to present a general view. The head weighs about 17 lb; holding the head high therefore demands work effort. The head normally rests on a fulcrum forward of the neck, so holding it high and back is work that can only be performed for periods of less than 60 sec without fatigue. Clawing the air places more strain in holding the body erect and unrelaxed; this strain is exacerbated by the probable lack of buoyancy ordinarily expected from the buoyancy compensator, which is designed to assist in emergencies but is probably not inflated by the panicked diver. It is obvious that the actions described further contribute to the problem. The "quiet" description so often found may relate to the psychological response of *freezing* under stress or, again a speculation, perhaps air is at a premium and breathing is also difficult, rendering even a call for aid a problem.

Apprehension, which is also observable by others, is not uncommon among divers. All divers have, at one time or another, had a sense of being apprehensive about a dive. During the period in which some apprehension may occur there is time to plan courses of action to damp out apprehension and prepare for coping, before the situation has gone out of control (Bachrach and Egstrom 1977). Signs of potential panic are also observable, and primary among these is *agitation*, which may be noted in two major signs.

(i) Changes in Respiration. In all stress situations, on land or underwater, changes in breathing patterns appear to be the first (or at least an early) sign of apprehension and impending panic. The comfortable diver's breathing is smooth, regular, and relatively slow. The apprehensive individual's breathing pattern changes to rapid breathing that is, for the most part, irregular. The term *hyperventilation* is usually used to describe such breathing, but properly speaking, the term hyperventilation would define an excessive ventilatory exchange in which a small increase in partial pressure of oxygen in arterial blood (Pa_{O_2}) occurs accompanied by a marked decrease in Pa_{CO_2}. The term is not synonymous with tachypnea or hyperpnea, although it is frequently used in this manner in the literature. (Rapid breathing is tachypnea; increased ventilation with normal blood-gas levels of oxygen and carbon dioxide is hyperpnea.) For example, Childs and Norman (1978) in their analysis of commercial diving accidents observe: "The commonest problems associated with all incidents were related to breathing and included breathlessness, hyperventilation, and difficulty in breathing. Hyperventilation pronounced enough to be noticed over the communications systems is the most accurate indicator at present available of a potentially dangerous situation" (p. 128). This observation is important and reinforces the concept that breathing irregularity is a crucial and reliable indicator of impending problems under stress, but as I have noted, it is not entirely accurate, inasmuch as hyperventilation (or hypoventilation) can only be determined by *measuring* blood gas levels of oxygen and carbon dioxide. Listening to the breathing over the communications system is an observed event just as watching a fellow diver change breathing rate in the water is an observed event.

Consideration is given to the *Physiological Events in Panic* in the next part of this chapter. At the moment I wish to emphasize the importance of observable changes in breathing patterns as a first sign of agitation.

(ii) Changes in Swimming Movements. A second sign of agitation is the change in swimming movements from smooth and regular to irregular. Bevan (1973) has stated

that "a diver on the verge of panic tends to bring his knees forward and fin like a novice, with small, jerking strokes, starting from the knees instead of the thighs" (p. 312).

Thus, breathing and movement changes can be observed by alert diving partners, in time, it is hoped, to assist the potentially panicked diver to take corrective action.

(iii) Changes in Orientation of Diver. Still another sign that may be observed is orientation of the diver. The comfortable diver is usually oriented toward buddies or partner or toward the bottom, where he or she is observing, or oriented straight ahead. The apprehensive diver is oriented toward the surface, presumably where safety lies in the presence of the diving boat and natural air. Again, this is speculation regarding motive, but the observation of such behaviors is clear and frequent.

(iv) Overattention to Equipment. Checking of equipment is a normal part of a dive—checking to see how much air remains in the tanks, for example—but overchecking of equipment suggests a condition of apprehension (Bachrach and Egstrom 1977).

(v) Other Signs of Apprehension. Signs of apprehension can be observed before the divers enter the water—for example, on the dive boat going to the dive site. Remarks about sharks and other dangers and "gallows humor" about terrible things that can happen are not infrequent and can, indeed, be a sort of safety valve to relieve tension. Too much or too intense gallows humor can be an indicator of marked apprehension (as can profound silence) and should be noted by the sensitive divemaster (Bachrach 1970).

2. *Physiological Events in Panic*

Accompanying the psychological responses in a panic reaction, and further exacerbating them, are physiological changes that occur. To start, let us look again at breathing patterns.

Observing the regularity or irregularity of breathing rate and depth by auditory or visual cues is, as we have seen, possible. The physiological consequences of these changes in breathing pattern can only be inferred if measurement of blood gases is not possible, as is certainly the situation underwater. Most of the research in hyperventilation (and other areas in respiratory physiology) stems from studies of subjects breathing air at surface pressure, from clinical studies, and from anesthesiology reports. In air on the surface breathing resistance is minimal, but add equipment that restricts breathing (mask, snorkel, regulator) and immerse the subject in water, and the breathing resistance increases markedly. The effects of pressure and gas density have been well documented in research, but the work was done under simulated conditions in hyperbaric chambers. Actually, there is not clear documented evidence of precisely whether hyperventilation occurs as a possible consequence of marked changes in breathing patterns in water at depth. It may be useful to consider the consequences of both hyperventilation and hypoventilation as we know them from research accomplished on the surface and extrapolate some possible events underwater.

a. Hyperventilation

Hyperventilation is noted by Missri and Alexander (1978) to be "commonest in visibly anxious persons and is often precipitated by obvious stress" (p. 2093). Johnson

(1967), in a comprehensive review of the physiology of hyperventilation, discussed changes in acid-base balance along with many other changes cited in the literature, including a shift in body electrolytes, alterations in heat and water exchange, changes in ventilatory mechanics and the intrapulmonary distribution of blood and gas, changes in blood gas and circulation, as well as neuromuscular irritability and impairment of psychomotor performance.

For our purposes, a few of these changes related to the diver can be discussed. Heat and water exchange, as we have seen, is a potential problem in hypothermia, in which air is moistened and heated by the respiratory process, then expired. Warming and moistening the inspired air obviously serves a critical function in that "it protects the alveolar membrane from thermal injury." Hyperventilation effects greater total loss of heat and water (Johnson 1967, p. 78–79), thus contributing to the hypothermia. Overbreathing also contributes greatly to fatigue and exhaustion, further placing the diver at hazard. Increases in the amount of expired CO_2 with concomitant fall in Pa_{CO_2} elevates the blood pH and results in acute respiratory alkalosis. With regard to cardiovascular effects, a reduction of Pa_{CO_2} can occcasion severe vasoconstriction of the cerebral arteries and the possibility of cerebral anoxia (Missri and Alexander 1978). Johnson (1967) observes, "Whether due to impaired perfusion or acid-base disturbances of the brain many of the manifestations of the hyperventilation syndrome are considered to be evidences of impaired central nervous system respiration" (p. 91). He also cites the work of Brown (1953), in which hypocapnia appeared to cause marked deterioration in tests of psychomotor performance.

These potential central nervous system changes that are likely to affect judgment and problem solving, creating further problems for the diver, are among the more serious consequences of cerebral effects of hyperventilation. Neuromuscular irritability, as manifest by numbness and tingling, may accompany these changes (Brown 1953).

The relationship between hyperventilation and anxiety states is well documented, each seeming to contribute to and exacerbate the other. As Missri and Alexander (1978) noted, many of their patients have reported that their awareness of a rapid, forceful heartbeat has caused them to hyperventilate, and the rapid heartbeat, a sinus tachycardia, is often the result of an anxiety attack. Given all these complex physiological events that can occur as a function of hyperventilation, it is important once again to note that the events are disproportionately magnified in an underwater situation where control is less likely to be exercised.

As I have noted, these effects of hyperventilation have been well documented in a surface situation but are speculative when extrapolated to a diving condition. Moreover, the probability of a diver hyperventilating underwater is questionable. The increased gas density will produce increased airway resistance, which is added to the increased airway resistance caused by immersion, and, as noted, the equipment creates further resistance. The usual result of the confluence of these factors that increase breathing resistance is to make the diver hypoventilate rather than hyperventilate. Thus, the one time that a diver might hyperventilate is on the surface and, as I have described, panicked divers often are observed on the surface, flailing about, with mouthpieces spit out. Under these circumstances it is possible that the tachypnea observed, also reported in panicked divers, many engender hyperventilation and induce some of the physiological consequences I have discussed.

b. Hypoventilation

That hypoventilation occurs at depth underwater is very probable. The anxious diver, exhibiting tachypnea, may have breathing rates that approach 25–30 breaths per min. These rates are, of course, fatiguing and will put a strain on the regulator at low tank pressures; as Egstrom (1982) has suggested, such a situation produces a sensation of inadequate air supply or "air hunger," which will in turn further contribute to the sense of panic and a loss of control. The breathing resistance would render such a tachypnea difficult to sustain.

There is unequivocal evidence that loaded respiration increases resistance to airflow. In the event that hypoventilation results from severely decreased air flow the physiological consequences will be marked. Inadequate ventilatory exchange will increase the concentration of carbon dioxide in the body. Just as hyperventilation and resulting hypocapnia can induce central nervous system changes leading to impaired psychomotor performance, so can an increase in carbon dioxide evoke deterioration of cognitive capabilities such as judgment. Although there is an abiding controversy regarding nitrogen narcosis and its etiology, the role of carbon dioxide retention in increasing the impairment associated with narcosis underwater remains an area of speculation (Bennett 1966); a possible synergistic effect of nitrogen and carbon dioxide under pressure is hypothesized. If this were indeed true, the judgment and problem-solving capability of a diver under stress could be further impaired.

F. Concluding Remarks

These discussions have moved from a definition of stress to a consideration of that very special stress condition, the underwater environment, in which a diver experiences physical, physiological, and behavioral events that can produce serious problems. The obvious pleasures of diving have not been sufficiently considered, to be sure, but the role of the biomedical specialist is not as crucial when problems do not arise. So concentration has rested on those circumstances where there is a need to understand the importance of effective medical screening in reducing risks in divers, to recognize how critical adequate training is in preparing a diver for the emergency that may arise, to recognize the effects of cold, fatigue, and exercise on the physiological state of the diver. The general model described is the impact of such factors as cold, exercise, and fatigue on the diver during the course of an underwater exposure, particularly when the most effective physical and psychological competence is needed, as in the case of an accident, an unforeseen event in which control is lost. The physician who is well acquainted with the stresses of the underwater environment and the physical and physiological demands on the diver entering therein can perform an invaluable service to the diving community in screening, in training, and in contributions to the theory and practice of diving.

I wish to express my profound thanks to Mrs. Mary Margaret Matzen, Mrs. Doris N. Auer, and Miss Regina E. Hunt for their splendid editorial help and to Dr. Fred Bove for his critical comments on the manuscript.

ARTHUR J. BACHRACH

References

ABRAHAMSSON, H., AND G. JANSSON 1973. Reflex vagal inhibition of esophageal motility. *Acta Physiol. Scand.* 89: 600–602.
AKERT, M. D., AND B. E. GERNANDT 1962. Neurophysiological study of vestibular and limbic influences upon vagal outflow. *Electroencephalogr. Clin. Neurophysiol.* 14: 904–914.
ANDERSEN, H. T. 1966. Physiological adaptations in diving vertebrates. *Physiol. Rev.* 46: 212–243.
ANGELL JAMES, J. E., AND M. DEB. DALY 1972. Some mechanisms involved in the cardiovascular adaptations to diving. In: *The Effects of Pressure on Organisms*, edited by M. A. Sleigh and A. G. Macdonald. New York: Academic Press, p. 313–339.
APPLEY, M. D., AND R. TRUMBULL 1967. *Psychological Stress.* New York: Appleton-Century-Crofts.
AULD, C. D. 1978. Cited in Childs, C. M. 1978. Loss of consciousness in divers—a survey and review. In *[Proceedings] Medical Aspects of Diving Accidents Congress, Luxembourg/Kirshberg, 12–13 October 1978*, p. 3–23.
BACHRACH, A. J. 1962. An experimental approach to superstitious behavior. *J. Am. Folklore* 75: 1–9.
BACHRACH, A. J. 1970. Diving behavior. In: *Human Performance in Scuba Diving. Proceedings of the Symposium on Underwater Physiology, Scripps Institution of Oceanography, La Jolla, California, April 1970.* Chicago: Athletic Institute, p. 119–139.
BACHRACH, A. J. 1973. Never mind the diver's mind. *Skin Diver* 22: 30–33.
BACHRACH, A. J. 1975. Underwater performance. In: *The Physiology and Medicine of Diving and Compressed Air Work* (2nd ed.), edited by P. B. Bennett and D. H. Elliott. London: Baillière, Tindall, p. 183–196.
BACHRACH, A. J. 1979. Diving stress. *Undersea J.* 12: 14–15.
BACHRACH, A. J. 1980a. Learning theory. In: *Comprehensive Textbook of Psychiatry* (3rd ed.), edited by H. I. Kaplan, A. M. Freedman, and B. J. Sadock. Baltimore: Williams and Wilkins, vol. 1, p. 378–392.
BACHRACH, A. J. 1980b. *Psychological Research* (4th ed.). New York: Random House.
BACHRACH, A. J. 1980c. Stress in sport diving. In: *Man and the Sea*, edited by J. K. Adams, R. F. Leahy, P. R. Lynch, and R. L. Miller. Philadelphia: Ctr. Marine Studies, Temple Univ., p. 11–15.
BACHRACH, A. J., AND G. H. EGSTROM 1977. Apprehension and panic. In: *British Sub-Aqua Club Manual.* London: British Sub-Aqua Club, p. 40–45.
BADDELEY, A. D. 1972. Selective attention and performance in dangerous environments. *Br. J. Psychol.* 63: 537–546.
BANGS, C. C. 1980. Immersion hypothermia. *Emergency* Jan: 43–45.
BARR, M. L. 1979. *The Human Nervous System* (3rd ed.). New York: Harper and Row, p. 105.
BENNETT, P. B. 1966. *The Aetiology of Compressed Air Intoxication and Inert Gas Narcosis.* London: Pergamon Press.
BERGHAGE, T. E., P. A. ROHRBAUGH, A. J. BACHRACH, AND F. W. ARMSTRONG 1975. Navy diving: who's doing it and under what conditions? Bethesda, MD: Naval Medical Research Institute.
BERNARD, C. 1856. *Leçons de physiologie expérimentale à appliquée à la médecine. Cours du semestre d'été.* Paris: Baillière, vol. II, pp. 49–52.
BEVAN, J. 1973. Diver panic—and how to beat it. *Triton* 18: 311–312.
BLACKMAN, A. C. 1975. What really causes accidents. *Int. J. Occup. Health Saf.* 44: 30–32.
BLAU, T. H. 1980. The lure of the deep: scuba diving as a high-risk sport. In: *The Many Faces of Indirect Self Destructive Behavior*, edited by N. L. Farberow. New York: McGraw-Hill, p. 410–427.
BLUMENTHAL, J. A., R. WILLIAMS, Y. KONG, S. M. SCHANBERG, AND L. W. THOMPSON 1978. Type A behavior and angiographically documented coronary disease. *Circulation* 58: 634–639.
BOVE, A. A. 1977. The cardiovascular response to stress. *Psychosomatics* 18: 13–17.
BOVE, A. A., A. L. PIERCE, F. BARRERA, A. AMSBAUGH, AND P. R. LYNCH 1973. Diving bradycardia as a factor in underwater blackout. *Aerosp. Med.* 44: 245–248.
BRADLEY, M. E. 1981. An epidemiological study of fatal diving accidents in two commercial diving populations. In: *Underwater Physiology VII. Proceedings of the Seventh Symposium on Underwater Physiology*, edited by A. J. Bachrach and M. M. Matzen. p. 869–876. Bethesda, MD, Undersea Medical Society.
BROWN, E. B. 1953. Physiological effects of hyperventilation. *Physiol. Rev.* 33: 445.
BRUCE, D. S., AND D. F. SPECK 1979. Human simulated diving experiments. *Physiologist* 22: 39–40.
CALLAWAY, E., AND D. DEMBO 1958. Narrowed attention: a psychological phenomenon that accompanies a certain physiological change. *AMA Arch. Neurol. Psychiatry* 79: 74–90.

CANNON, W. B. 1939. *The Wisdom of the Body.* New York: Norton.
CANNON, W. B. 1942. "Voodoo" death. *Am. Anthropol.* 44: 169–181.
CHILDS, C. M. 1978. Loss of consciousness in divers—a survey and review. In: *[Proceedings] Medical Aspects of Diving Accidents Congress, Luxembourg/Kirshberg, 12–13 October 1978,* p. 3–23.
CHILDS, C. M., AND J. N. NORMAN 1978. Unexplained loss of consciousness in divers. *Med. Aeronaut. Spat. Med. Sub. Hyp.* 17: 127–128.
COLLIS, M. L. 1976. Survival behavior in cold water immersion. In: *Proceedings, The Cold Water Symposium.* Toronto: Royal Life Saving Soc., p. 25–27.
COOPER, K. E. 1976. Hypothermia. In: *Diving Medicine,* edited by R. H. Strauss. New York: Grune and Stratton, p. 211–226.
CRAIG, A. B. 1961. Underwater swimming and loss of consciousness. *JAMA* 176: 255–258.
CURLEY, M. D. 1978. Psychological stress in diving. *Faceplate* 9: 11–13.
DAVIS, F. M., A. D. BADDELEY, AND T. R. HANCOCK 1975. Diver performance: the effect of cold. *Undersea Biomed. Res.* 2: 195–213.
DEAN, P. J., AND R. F. THATCHER 1975. Analysis of human factors in aircraft accidents. *Aviat. Space Environ. Med.* 46: 1260–1262.
DEJOURS, P. 1965. Hazards of hypoxia during diving. In: *Physiology of Breath-Hold Diving and the Ama of Japan,* edited by H. Rahn and T. Yokayama. Washington, DC: Natl. Acad. Sci./Natl. Res. Council, p. 183–193.
DESAUTELS, D. A., AND T. J. POULTON 1980. Cave-diving fatalities: twenty years experience (Abstract). Annual Scientific Meeting, Gulf Coast Chapter, Undersea Medical Society, March 1980.
DURKHEIM, E. 1951. *Suicide,* transl. by J. A. Spaulding and G. Simpson. Glencoe, IL: Free Press, Book I. (1st ed. 1897.)
EGSTROM, G. H. 1970. Effect of equipment on diving performance. In: *Human Performance and Scuba Diving. Proceedings of the Symposium on Underwater Physiology, Scripps Institution of Oceanography, La Jolla, California, April 1970.* Chicago: Athletic Inst., p. 5–16.
EGSTROM, G. H. 1976. Diving equipment. In: *Diving Medicine,* edited by R. H. Strauss. New York: Grune and Stratton, p. 23–34.
EGSTROM, G. H. 1977. Thermal regulation in man. In: *Thermal Problems in Diving,* edited by G. H. Egstrom. Wilmington, CA: Commercial Diving Ctr., p. 3–16.
EGSTROM, G. H. 1981. Human engineering of scuba diving equipment. In: Program, Underwater Canada '81, Toronto, Canada, March 28, 1981.
EGSTROM, G. H. 1982. SCUBA-diving practice and equipment. In: *The Physiology and Medicine of Diving and Compressed Air Work* (3rd ed.), edited by P. B. Bennett and D. H. Elliott. London: Ballière, Tindall 31–45.
EGSTROM, G. H., AND A. J. BACHRACH 1971. Diver panic. *Skin Diver* 20: 36ff.
EGSTROM, G. H., G. WELTMAN, A. D. BADDELEY, W. J. CUCCARO, AND M. A. WILLIS 1972. Underwater work performance and work tolerance. Rep. UCLA-ENG-7243. Los Angeles: Univ. of California Sch. Eng. Appl. Sci., p. 63.
ELDRIDGE, L. 1979a. Cardiovascular problems in scuba diving. In: *Proceedings of the 11th International Conference on Underwater Education, Houston, Texas, October 11–14, 1979.* Colton, CA: Natl. Assoc. Underwater Instructors, p. 105–118.
ELDRIDGE, L. 1979b. Sudden unexplained death syndrome in cold water scuba diving. In Program and Abstracts, Undersea Medical Society, Inc., Annual Scientific Meeting. *Undersea Biomed. Res.* 6: Suppl., 41.
ELIOT, R. S. 1979. *Stress and the Major Cardiovascular Disorders.* New York: Futura.
ENGEL, G. L. 1970. Sudden death and the "medical model" in psychiatry. *Can. Psychiatr. Assoc. J.* 15: 527–538.
ENGEL, G. L. 1978. Psychological stress, vasodepressor (vasovagal) syncope, and sudden death. *Ann. Intern. Med.* 89: 403–412.
FAIN, J. N., AND M. P. CZECH 1975. Glucocorticoid effects in lipid mobilization and adipose tissue metabolism. In: *Handbook of Physiology. Ednocrinology. Adrenal Gland,* edited by J. Blaschko, G. Sayers, and A. D. Smith. Washington, DC: Am. Physiol. Soc., sect. 7, vol. 6, p. 169–178.
FLYNN, E. T., P. W. CATRON, AND G. BAYNE 1981. Immersion hypothermia and thermal protective garments for divers. Lesson 40. In: *Diving Medical Officer Student Guide.* Memphis, TN: Naval Technical Training Command.

FRIEDMAN, M., AND R. H. ROSENMAN 1974. *Type A Behavior and Your Heart*. New York: Knopf.
FRITZ, M. 1979. Sind Taucher selbsmörder? [Are divers suicidal?] *Tauchen* 2: 24–25.
GANDEVIA, S. C., D. I. MCCLOSKY, AND E. K. POTTER 1978. Inhibition of baroreceptor and chemoreceptor reflexes on heart rate by afferent from the lungs. *J. Physiol. (Lond.)* 276: 369–381.
GARRARD, M. P., P. A. HAYES, R. F. CARLYLE, AND M. J. STOCK 1981. Metabolic and thermal status of divers during simulated dives to 55 bars. In: *Underwater Physiology VII. Proceedings of the Seventh Symposium on Underwater Physiology,* edited by A. J. Bachrach and M. M. Matzen. Bethesda, MD: Undersea Medical Society, p. 517–538.
GLASS, D. C. 1977. *Behavior Patterns, Stress, and Coronary Disease*. Hilldale, NJ: Erlbaum.
GLASS, D. C., A. B. CONTRADA, AND A. B. SNOW 1980. Stress, type A behavior and coronary disease. *Weekly Psychology Update* 1(1): 2–7. Princeton, NJ: Biomedia, Inc.
GOLDEN, F. ST. C. 1972. Accidental hypothermia. *J. R. Nav. Med. Serv.* 58: 196–206.
GRIFFIN, C. J., AND R. HARRIS 1975. The regulatory influences of the trigeminal system. *Monogr. Oral Sci.* 4: 65–86.
HARNETT, R. M., AND M. G. BIJLANI 1979. The involvement of cold water in recreational boating accidents. Final Report, Contract DOT-C672074-A. Washington, DC: U.S. Dept. of Transportation.
HAYWARD, J. S., AND A. M. STEINMAN 1975. Accidental hypothermia: an experimental study of rewarming. *Aviat. Space Environ. Med.* 46: 1236–1240.
HAYWARD, M. G., AND W. R. KEATINGE 1979. Progressive symptomless hypothermia in water: possible cause of diving accidents. *Br. Med. J.* 5 May 1979: 1182.
HONG, S. K. 1976. The physiology of breath-hold diving. In: *Diving Medicine,* edited by R. H. Strauss. New York: Grune and Stratton, p. 269–286.
HUANG, T. F., AND C. T. PENG 1981. The influence of the inspiratory effort and swallowing on the cardiovascular response to simulated diving and breath-holding. In: *Underwater Physiology VII. Proceedings of the Seventh Symposium on Underwater Physiology,* edited by A. J. Bachrach and M. M. Matzen. Bethesda, MD: Undersea Medical Society, p. 267–271.
HUGHES, T., J. G. CARTER, AND S. WOLF 1978. Changes in cardiac rate, rhythm and conduction in man during the dive reflex (Abstract). *Clin. Res.* 26: 548A.
HURWITZ, B., AND J. J. FUREDY 1979. The human dive reflex: an experimental, topographical and physiological analysis (Abstract). *Psychophysiology* 16: 192–193.
JOHNSON, C. 1967. The physiology of hyperventilation. In: *Hyperventilation and Hysteria,* edited by T. P. Lowy. Springfield, IL: Charles C Thomas, p. 34–104.
JONES, J. 1968. *Go to the Widow Maker*. New York: Dell Publ.
KATES, R. W. 1970. Experiencing the environment as hazard. In: *Environmental Psychology: Man and His Physical Setting,* edited by H. M. Proshansky, W. H. Ittelson, and L. G. Rivlin. New York: Holt, Rinehart and Winston, p. 401–418.
KEATINGE, W. R. 1969. *Survival in Cold Water*. Oxford: Blackwell Scientific Publ.
KEATINGE, W. R., M. G. HAYWARD, AND N. M. MCIVER 1980. Hypothermia during saturation diving in the North Sea. *Br. Med. J.* 280: 6210.
KIDD, D. J. 1969. Underwater activities—physiology. In: *Conference on Man in Cold Water*. Ottawa: Canadian Society of Oceanology.
LEWIS, P. R. F. 1979. Skin diving fatalities in New Zealand. *New Zealand Med. J.* 1979: 472–475.
LICHT, K. F. 1975. Safety and accidents—a brief conceptual point of view. *J. School Health* 45: 530–534.
LIEF, H. I. 1955. Sensory association in the selection of phobic objects. *Psychiatry (Wash. DC)* 18: 331.
LOWN, B., R. A. DESILVA, P. REICH, AND B. J. MURAWSKI 1980. Psychophysiological factors in sudden cardiac death. *Am. J. Psychiatry* 137: 1325–1335.
MCANIFF, J. J. 1980. U.S. underwater diving fatality statistics 1970–1978. Rep. No. URI-SSR-80-13. Kingston: Univ. of Rhode Island. (Rep. NOAA Grant No. 4-3-158-31.)
MACINNIS, J. 1979. The icy facts on how cold water kills. *Quest Magazine*. June.
MALINOWSKI, B. 1925. Magic, science and religion. In: *Science, Religion and Reality,* edited by J. Needham. New York: Macmillan.
MANDLER, G. 1979. Thought processes, consciousness and stress. In: *Human Stress and Cognition: An Information-Processing Approach,* edited by V. Hamilton and D. M. Warburton. New York: Wiley, p. 179–201.
MANNING, D. P. 1974. An accident model. *Occup. Health Saf.* Jan.: 14–15.

MELAMED, Y., AND A. OHRY 1980. the treatment and the neurological aspects of diving accidents in Israel. *Paraplegia* 18: 127–132.

MISSIRTLU, C., AND B. FOY 1978. Underwater accident statistics: a Bayesian approach. In: *Proceedings of European Undersea Biomedical Society and Medical Committee of the European Diving Technology Committee Congress on Medical Aspects of Diving Accidents.* October 1978.

MISSRI, J. C., AND S. ALEXANDER 1978. Hyperventilation syndrome: a brief review. *JAMA* 240: 2093–2096.

MOLNAR, G. W. 1946. Survival of hypothermia by men immersed in the ocean. *JAMA* 131: 1046–1050.

MYERS, D. 1979. Cayman Island divers recompression chamber. In: *Therapy of Serious Decompression Sickness and Arterial Gas Embolism.* Bethesda, MD: Undersea Medical Society, p. 71–73. (Workshop.)

PEZOLDT, V. J. (editor) 1977. *Rare Event/Accident Research Methodology.* Washington, DC: National Bureau of Standards, Sp. Publ. 482.

RICHTER, C. P. 1957. On the phenomenon of sudden death in animals and man. *Psychosomatic Med.* 19: 191–198.

ROSENMAN, R. H., AND M. FRIEDMAN 1974. Neurogenic factors in pathogensis of coronary heart disease. *Med. Clin. N. Am.* 58: 269–279.

ROSENMAN, R. H., M. FRIEDMAN, R. STRAUS, M. WURM, R. KOSITCHEK, W. HAHN, AND N. T. WERTHESSEN 1964. A predictive study of coronary heart disease: the Western collaborative group study. *JAMA* 189: 15–22.

ROSENMAN, R. H., C. D. JENKINS, R. J. BRAND, M. FRIEDMAN, R. STRAUSS, AND M. WURM 1975. Coronary heart disease in the Western collaborative group study: final followup experience of 8½ years. *JAMA* 233: 872–877.

SCHOENFELD, W. N. 1950. An experimental approach to anxiety, escape and avoidance. In: *Anxiety,* edited by P. J. Hoch and J. Zubin. New York: Grune and Stratton.

SCHOLANDER, P. 1961–1962. Physiological adaptations to diving in animals and man. *Harvey Lect.* 57: 93–110.

SELYE, H. 1971. The evolution of the stress concept—stress and cardiovascular disease. In: *Society, Stress, and Disease—The Psychosocial Environment and Psychosomatic Diseases,* edited by L. Levi. London: Oxford Univ. Press, p. 299–311; 453–457.

SESSLE, B. J., AND A. T. STOREY 1972. Periodontal and facial influences of the laryngeal input to the brain stem of the cat. *Arch. Oral Biol.* 17: 1583–1595.

SHEPHERD, J. T., AND P. M. VANHOUTTE 1979. *The Human Cardiovascular System: Facts and Concepts.* New York: Raven.

SKUSE, G. 1980. Report of the Diving Incidents Panel, Diving Officer's Conference. London: British Sub-Aqua Club.

U.S. PUBLIC HEALTH SERVICE 1972. *Hardening of the Arteries.* Washington, DC: Department of Health, Education and Welfare. (DHEW Publ. 73-431.)

VAUGHAN, W. S. 1975. Diver temperature and performance changes during long-duration, cold water exposures. *Undersea Biomed. Res.* 2: 75–88.

VAUGHAN, W. S. 1977. Distraction effect of cold water on performance of higher-order tasks. *Undersea Biomed. Res.* 4: 103–116.

WALLER, J. A. 1977. Epidemiologic approaches to injury research. In: *Rare Event/Accident Research Methodology,* edited by V. J. Pezoldt. Washington, DC: National Bureau of Standards (Sp. Publ. 482.)

WEBB, P. (Chairman) 1974. *Thermal Problems in Diving.* Bethesda, MD: Undersea Medical Society (6th Workshop).

WEBB, P. 1982. Current concepts of metabolism and thermal physiology. In: *Underwater Physiology VII. Proceedings of the Seventh Symposium on Underwater Physiology,* edited by A. J. Bachrach and M. M. Matzen. Bethesda, MD: Undersea Medical Society, p. 493–502.

WEBB, P., AND J. F. ANNIS 1966. Respiratory heat loss with high density gas mixtures. Final Rep. Contract NONR 4965(00). Washington, DC: Office of Naval Research.

WELTMAN, G., AND G. H. EGSTROM 1966. Perceptual narrowing in novice divers. *Human Factors* 8: 499.

WHITE, S. W., AND R. J. MCRITCHIE 1973. Nasopharyngeal reflexes: integrative analysis of evoked respiratory and cardiovascular effects. *Aust. J. Exp. Biol. Med. Sci.* 51: 17–31.

WOLF, S. 1967. The bradycardia of the dive reflex—a possible mechanism of sudden death. *Cond. Reflex* 1967: 88–95.

WOLF, S. 1969. Central autonomic influences on cardiac rate and rhythm. *Mod. Concepts Cardiovasc. Dis.* 38: 29–34.

YANKELOVICH MONITOR 1979. Trend No. 44, Flirtation With Danger. New York: Yankelovich, Skelly and White, Inc.

YANOWITCH, R. E. 1975. Medical and psychiatric aspects of accident investigation. *Aviat. Space Environ. Med.* Oct.: 1254–1256.

ZUCKERMAN, M. 1979. *Sensation Seeking: Beyond the Optimal Levels of Arousal*. Hillsdale, NJ: Erlbaum.

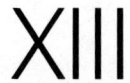

Safety Considerations

A. Introduction

Because preventive medicine is one of the most important aspects of the practice of medicine, this chapter has particular significance in a book designed for the clinician. If the diver-physician is not interested in safe practices, then to whom can we look for help in cutting down the deplorable number of accidents and deaths among divers?

A major step in the direction of diving safety among sport divers was the production of the excellent booklet put out by the National YMCA Center for Underwater Activities. This work, titled "SLAM" (Scuba Lifesaving and Accident Management), is a document that should be read by all who are interested in making sport diving safer (Doubt 1979). This YMCA report was organized as "SLAM through CARE [Cognizance, Assessment, Rescue, Evacuation]."

"Cognizance on the part of an individual trained in Scuba Lifesaving and Accident Management refers to the ability of that individual to detect signs in a diver or in a diving situation which identify or predict the possibility of a diving accident" (Doubt 1979). The report points out that the signs exhibited by the potential scuba victim are often quite subtle and then lists signs that the physician is more likely to notice than the untrained individual— signs of anxiety, distress or illness and many other signs indicating that the diver needs help.

"Assessment is a continuous evaluation of all the variable factors that can have an effect on a lifesaving situation" (Doubt 1979). The sections of the report on victim condition, environment, and apparatus are certainly areas of which the diver-physician should continuously be aware. The rescue and evacuation sections are less directly related to the physician's experience and interest but are areas that need consideration.

Figure XIII-1 presents graphically the accidents, illnesses, hazards, and environmental difficulties that might occur under different exposures to different divers (center). The diver has been carefully selected and trained and is in a satisfactory predive condition, yet his sensory and physiological reactions are altered in the underwater environment (circle 1); he encounters unexpected physiological and psychological problems (circle 2) that may develop insidiously to a danger point before he is even aware of any problem. The outer

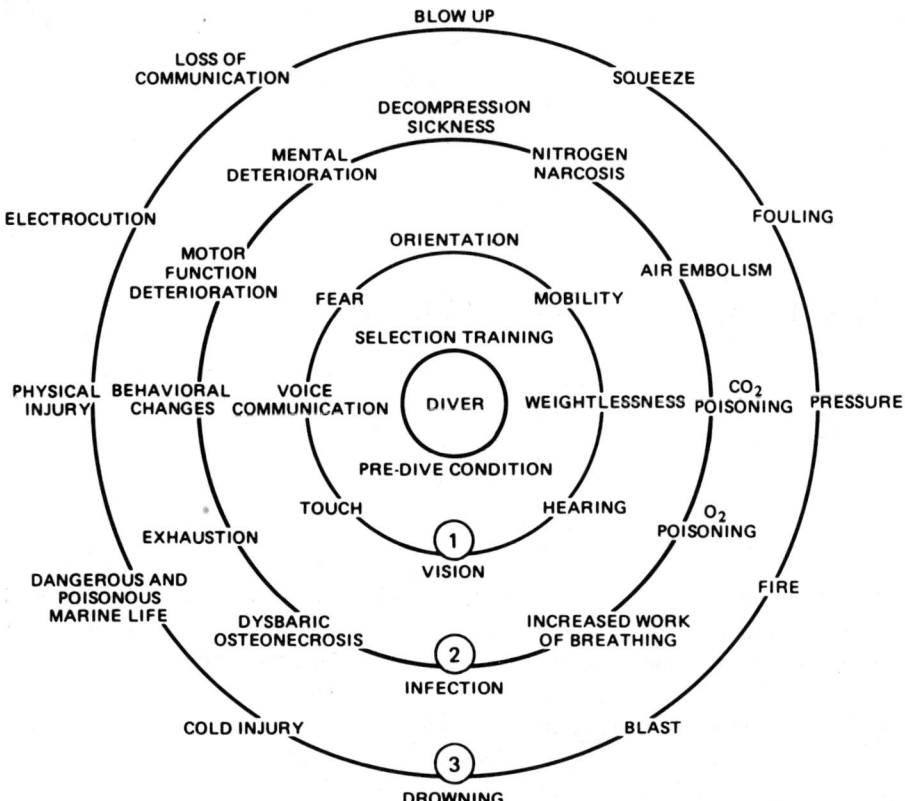

Figure XIII-1. Organization and planning. Accidents, illnesses, hazards, and environmental difficulties affecting performance. *Center:* The diver, selected, trained, in good condition. *Circle 1:* The immediate circle of sensory awareness. *Circle 2:* Physiological and psychological problems inherent in underwater work. *Circle 3:* Possible environmental accidents. [From Shilling et al. (1976).]

circle (circle 3) shows possible environmental accidents. The elements of all three circles are interrelated, and a relationship exists between cause and effect in some cases.

It is to be hoped that the physician brings to the various safety considerations presented in this chapter a thorough grounding in emergency medical care to be related to diving medicine, for the civilian diving physician has a great responsibility to the entire nonmilitary diving community—university research divers and commercial divers, as well as sport divers.

B. The Diver

It is assumed that each diver has previously had a complete physical and psychological examination and has been adequately trained, but it is the task of the physician to check on this prior to a diving operation in which he is involved. To cope with a stressful situation, both physical well-being and emotional stability are important, and if the planned dive is considered to be either particularly difficult or hazardous, great care must be exercised to ensure that the diver is ready.

The following list of basic diving principles as presented in Dueker (1978) will, if adhered to, greatly reduce the chances of getting into trouble:

1. Do not dive when feeling ill.
2. Do not dive when under the influence of alcohol or debilitating drugs.
3. Have medications evaluated before use when diving.
4. Maintain proper diving fitness.
5. Do not dive alone.
6. Dive only with adequate, well-maintained equipment.
7. Evaluate conditions before diving: storms, currents, surf, condition of the sea, and possible entanglements.
8. Remember that specialty diving requires specialty training.

1. Selection of the Diver

a. Physicial Examination

If the diver has a record of a formal physical examination all that is necessary is a check on the items mentioned below under *Predive Condition*. If there has been no recent examination, the physician should conduct one in accordance with the rules as set forth in Chapter XI of this book. If there is any doubt about the quality of the previous physical examination it would be well to consider the limitations set forth by Mecklenburg (1972); Major contraindications to diving are: epilepsy, diabetes, inability to equalize pressure in middle ears and sinuses, alcohol or drug addiction and mental retardation. Other contraindications to be evaluated are: overweight, poor physical condition, high blood pressure, perforated ear drums, sinus problems, claustrophobia, asthma, emphysema, myocardial infarction, and cardiac defects. Obviously individuals with conditions listed in the second group will require medical judgment on the severity and careful evaluation of each individual problem. (See also Section A of Chapter XI in this volume.)

b. Psychological Evaluation

Usually psychological evaluation is considered to be a part of the original physical examination. But it is well for the physician to check on the individual diver's reaction to the planned dive of the day. Is there fear or apprehension? Does the diver seem nervous or distraught?

c. Diving History Evaluation

Diving history evaluation is concerned with the time interval since the last dive and with elicitation of information on any difficulties experienced during previous dives.

2. Training

Training is probably the single most important element in the prevention of diving accidents. In a study of 38 skilled scuba divers, J. D. Taylor (1959) found that "in the opinion of the divers, the greatest hazards to life resulting from diving are man-made: namely, panic, ignorance, foolhardiness, other careless divers, poor training, air embolism and bends." It is plain that all but the last two are directly related to training and the last two may be indirectly related.

A person must not be allowed to dive unless a certificate or other evidence is presented attesting to proper training.

3. Predive Condition

Regardless of the past record of the diver, it is imperative that his condition be checked just prior to the proposed dive. Several of the following items are covered in more detail elsewhere in this volume but are mentioned here because they must be part of the check list.

a. Age

For the original qualifying examination age is more important than it is for the predive check, but it is generally agreed that persons over 45 should not be called upon for strenuous and deep-dive missions.

b. Drugs

In general, drugs include chemical substances taken with the intent of helping the individual (medicines), and those that are taken for recreation (alcohol, tobacco, or illicit drugs). In diving we may add two more categories: drugs used to make diving possible or more enjoyable (decongestants used to help clear the ears and sinuses), and drugs used to prevent or to treat diving maladies (drugs used to prevent inert gas narcosis, oxygen toxicity, and decompression sickness). It is well to realize that although some drugs have been considered worthy of inclusion in the last-mentioned group, none have been proved efficacious.

It has been found by the work of Walsh (1976; see also Section A of Chapter X of this volume) at the U.S. Navy Medical Research Institute that under pressure some drugs are potentiated, some antagonized, and some yield opposite effects from those observed in normal atmospheric environments. He has pointed out that the only conclusions possible at present are: to avoid all drugs while diving; if diving under medication is absolutely essential, it must be understood that the most harmless of drugs may become behaviorally toxic and that extreme caution must be exercised. According to Summers (1972), with use of marijuana in warm water "the diver may become ultrarelaxed, sleepy, unaware, lazy, and his work ability may be reduced significantly." Groner-Strauss and Strauss (1976) have given the following advice: "For the sports diver there is probably no place for drugs in diving today. If medications are necessary in order for a diver to dive, activity should be postponed until the underlying condition has resolved." Nemiroff (1977) has pointed out that drugs, including alcohol, depress the level of consciousness and act synergistically with nitrogen to cause narcosis; he has strongly advised that divers with a history of chronic use of drugs—even drugs such as insulin or thyroid taken for medical purposes—should not be certified to dive. This is particularly true for commercial divers.

Not only should alcohol and other drug abuse be probed for by the examining physician but it is well for him to find out what drugs are being taken for disease conditions. For, as pointed out by Dueker (1978): "A diver taking penicillin for pneumonia, for example, should not dive because of the danger of pneumonia, not because of the penicillin."

The British Sub-Aqua Club Medical Committee (Kaifman 1976) has taken a very strict stand on drugs and diving by pointing out that "if a candidate has been using psychotropic drugs, including tranquilizers, sedatives and hypnotics, he should not dive for at least three months after cessation of therapy, without the consent of the Medical Referee."

Drugs and the diver is covered in more detail in Chapter X, "Emergency Treatment While under Pressure," but the problem is included here to call attention to the need for a careful evaluation of the diver—whether sport, research, or commercial. In summary, it is wise to allow only drugs prescribed by a physician who knows that the individual is diving; it is also wiser to cancel a dive than to hide a problem with drugs.

c. Alcohol

Divers, like other people, use alcohol to "feel good" and "relax" without realizing that even relatively small amounts can produce significant, temporary adverse effects on the mental processes, motor coordination, physical stamina, and tolerance to cold. Alcohol consumption can also add to the effects of fatigue, seasickness, and nitrogen narcosis.

The effect of hyperbaric air alone and in combination with alcohol, 2 ml/kg, on standing steadiness at 1, 4, and 6 ATA was studied in eight divers (Jennings et al. 1977). Body sway was measured with eyes open and with eyes closed. It was concluded that "there was a clear synergistic relationship between alcohol and pressure. It was proposed that alcohol and pressure may interact to seriously disturb the processing of visual information."

All selection criteria lists have recommended turning down the chronic alcoholic for diving. But none of them describe the reason as picturesquely as King (1970): "Chronic alcoholism also disqualifies a man from working in compressed air. One of the workers' terms for neurological bends is 'the staggers.' When 'the staggers' are 80 proof in origin, diagnosis and treatment become inordinately complex." Dawson (1972) quoted Lloyd's of London as decreeing: "Care should be taken to avoid absolutely the use of alcoholics or psychiatric patients in diving."

The physician should carefully check and insist on 24 hr of elapsed time between heavy drinking and diving. Any individual should not dive for at least 4 hr after drinking any alcoholic beverage, and, of course, a chronic alcoholic should never be allowed to dive.

d. Cigarettes

Many divers smoke, but as pointed out by Dueker (1978) "this does not prove its advisability." The evidence is solid that smoking causes lung damage and no one will argue that lung damage is desirable, particularly for a diver. Smokers have trouble eliminating their respiratory tract secretions, and the accumulations of these secretions can make equalizing pressure in ears and sinuses difficult. Most importantly, the type of damage—emphysema, bronchitis, and the bronchoconstriction that smoking may induce—may be conducive to air trapping and embolism. There is also evidence that heavy smoking causes damage to the heart and blood vessels; in diving there is enough strain on a normal heart.

A diver or a tunnel worker should not smoke. And a long-time heavy smoker should be warned against undertaking any arduous underwater task.

e. Diet

For the normal, healthy diver, evidence points to the desirability of a low-fat but otherwise standard diet. Some points are mentioned here for the check-off. Diving should not be undertaken until 2 hr after the last meal. No alcoholic beverages should be consumed. No carbonated beverages should be used because of their gas content.

Lack of food has been incriminated in fainting and collapse. Some people faint easily, but fainting is much more likely to happen among those who "take a last meal between 6 and 7 p.m. in the evening and are content with a cup of tea and a cigarette for breakfast. Forenoon diving with such a routine is not recommended" (Miles 1969).

f. Obesity

The evidence is incontrovertible—a fat rat is more susceptible to decompression sickness than a lean one. In studying decompression sickness in rats Philp (1967) demonstrated that "body fat causes an increase in the incidence." Gowdey and Philp (1965) found that both the incidence and severity of decompression sickness were related to the amount of body fat regardless of the age of the animal. "Fat rats were more susceptible and very lean rats more resistant to bends than normal rats following prolonged compression, even when the lean ones were in a poor nutritional condition."

Apparently the only situation in which a layer of fat is advantageous is in temperature control while swimming in cold water. Pugh (1965) reported: "Experiments showed that while a fat channel swimmer maintained body temperature after several hours of swimming in water at 15.8°C, a thin swimmer lost 2.9° of heat after 30 minutes and was unable to continue." In writing about the Korean ama, Rennie (1965) said: "Cold tolerance is generally related to the thickness of the subcutaneous layer of fat. Women have a greater body insulation than men because of the greater thickness of their subcutaneous layer of fat."

Some authorities say that for regular underwater activity the weight of the individual should not be more than 10% greater than that given in the standard table. Even though the diver reports with a valid certificate, it is the physician's duty to point out to the obese individual that the extra fat is an additional hazard in diving.

g. Fatigue

Fatigue is closely related to a number of aspects of diving and hyperbaric activity and thus is mentioned in several other sections of this *Guide*; it is treated here in some detail because it is a major hazard to safe diving and thus directly related to safety considerations. Overexertion, fatigue, exhaustion, respiratory embarrassment, panic, and resultant accident is the repeated sequence of events leading to a fatality.

One study (Webster 1966) considered physical exhaustion as probably leading to the cause of death in more than half the diver fatalities. Sawyer (1972) listed "fatigue and exhaustion" as the primary factor leading to injury of scuba divers. An analysis of accidents in the San Diego area (R. H. Strauss 1976) led to the conclusion that most accidents are the result of human error, and perhaps the result of exhaustion, fatigue, and panic. Strauss stated that less than adequate physical condition "can lead to a loss of control which seems to be implicated in most sports-diving accidents." The U.S. Navy (1970) agreed that "a man who neglects his physical condition may discover that what was once a normal work rate now tires him very quickly."

Physical fitness was also stressed by Bray (1979), who pointed out that the sport diver often underestimates the work load associated with the following: donning the equipment; entering the water; pressure of the wet suit on the chest and the resistance of the regulator, causing increased work of breathing; and cold stress of the water. "Underestimation of these environmental stresses brings on fatigue, which is frequently a contributing cause of diving accidents. Psychologic stress added to fatigue often results in panic and tragedy."

The need for a careful predive check is clear. The U.S. Navy (1978 Change 2) expresses it this way: Medical personnel assigned to a diving unit should take an active interest in the day-to-day condition of each diver, and the diving supervisor must verify the fitness of each diver immediately before a dive. Signs of any irregularity, such as cough, nasal congestion, apparent fatigue, emotional stress, skin or ear infection, intoxication or any indication of the use of narcotics or other dangerous drugs, should put a man on the sick list until the problem is corrected.

Physiological fatigue is a common experience and the respiratory response to overexertion is seldom a problem on the surface, where shortness of breath passes rapidly once the work is slowed or stopped. However, under water, especially at increased depths, the situation may become serious. Breathing resistance, both in the diver's own airways and particularly in self-contained diving equipment, makes the work of breathing difficult and, coupled with anxiety, may lead to an accident. The symptoms of overexertion and exhaustion, as listed by the *U.S. Navy Diving Manual* are: extreme fatigue, increasing weakness, labored breathing, and anxiety and tendency toward panic. Behnke (1970) has prepared a check-off list of danger signs and symptoms, which is presented in Table XIII-1.

Subjective signs of fatigue were studied in professional divers during a very deep saturation dive at 40 ATA (Janus III, at Comex). Seki and Hugon (1975) reported that "subjective symptoms were related to alertness and physical fatigue; symptoms were most marked during compression and saturation, and were reduced during decompression; fatigue symptoms were similar morning and evening; and fatigue symptoms differ markedly from one subject to another."

However, it is well to bear in mind, as pointed out by Sayers (1942), that psychological and environmental factors are more important causes of fatigue than are physiological factors. In writing of panic Dueker (1978) points out that the "physically comfortable diver is less likely to be fearful. When he can enter the surf and swim without fatigue, the ocean seems a pleasant place. But the cold, exhausted, and seasick diver finds even small problems frightening."

Table XIII-1
Manifestations of Acute and Chronic Fatigue: Impairments That Preclude an Individual on any Given Day From Diving: A Checkoff List for the Supervisor Responsible[a]

Intellectual functions	Impairment Referable to Somatic Systems			Affective behavior
	System or region	Overt	Covert	
Difficulty in thinking and in concentration, impaired memory, insight, and judgment	Cephalic	Drowsiness	Heavy head, headache	Anxiety, tension, irritability, exaggerated fears
Fixation of ideas	Respiratory	Shortness of breath; shallow, rapid breathing	Feeling of suffocation	Depression, lethargy
	Vasomotor	Sweating, pallor, rapid pulse	Weakness	
	Cardiac	Decreased ability to work; rise in diastolic blood pressure	Precordial distress	Euphoria, excitement, hilarity, pugnacity
	Gastric	—	Loss of appetite; distress, nausea	
	Intestinal	Diarrhea	Cramps	
	Neuromuscular	Impaired coordination; tremors, speech disorders	Fatigue	

[a] Axiom: The actions of the emotionally aroused individual are unpredictable. From Behnke (1970) with permission of the Athletic Institute.

In considering psychological fatigue it should be remembered that motivation and job satisfaction are especially significant aspects of physically and psychologically demanding, hazardous occupations such as deep-sea diving.

Behnke (1975) has referenced the work of VanDerAue et al. (1951) in showing that fatigue is related to inadequate decompression. In submarine escape training during the course of successive exposure to 100 ft (4 ATA) followed by a 30-sec ascent to the surface, the first ascent may be symptom free, the second followed by delayed fatigue, and the third may be followed by frank bends. "The gradation of reactions varies from no symptoms, to fatigue, itch, fatigue and itch, and mild decompression sickness" (Behnke 1975, p. 412).

Dewey (1962) has pointed out that one of the prominent symptoms of decompression sickness is fatigue, and "a plea is made for heightened alertness not only to the rising incidence of this entity but most especially to the fact that it constitutes a true medical emergency, requiring expeditious management if lasting impairment is to be avoided."

A diver who is accustomed to being cold seems to know when to stop before he becomes seriously fatigued. That is, he will stop when he becomes unable to carry out the tasks he has been assigned. Fatigue is very likely related to being cold. "The old hands at diving have probably learned, like the Korean ama, just when to stop. Perhaps they have experienced the insidious effects of developing hypothermia, and have nearly had serious accidents," according to Paul Webb (1975, p. 296). He goes on to say, "The reverse is likely to be true: that those men who ignore these symptoms do not become old hands in the underwater world."

Vaughan and Strauss (1975) cited distraction, fatigue, and motivational factors as potential sources, other than body cooling, of individual differences in perceptual and cognitive tasks.

To prevent the chain of events leading to accident the diver should follow these precepts: know his own limits and stay within them; discontinue the dive if it exceeds his powers; use good gear in good condition; concentrate on training and experience to help eliminate panic; use weights and line when working in strong current; stop to rest and ventilate before becoming overfatigued; and wear adequate cold-water protection.

The *U.S. Navy Diving Manual* (1978) says that the fatigued diver should stop and rest if possible; inform buddy or tender; terminate dive if resting fails to help; and surface when practical, observing proper rate of ascent and decompression stops if required. His buddy should render all possible assistance, particularly in getting him to the surface. The surface personnel should give help in getting the diver aboard and should provide rest, warmth, nourishment, and treatment as needed.

J. B. MacInnis (1975, p. 31) summarizes it very well: "Every successful ocean dive depends upon the skills and experience of the operating personnel. Early attention must therefore be given to the number of men required, their qualifications and responsibilities, and their physical and mental condition. Diving accident studies show that the latter is the one most often ignored, and that fatigue is its commonest element."

h. Physical Condition

Since there is general agreement that exercise, properly conducted, helps develop physical fitness, and since physical fitness is required for diving, it follows that divers should have a physical fitness exercise program. According to Bray (1979) physical fitness for the sport, research, and commercial diver is most important if he is to keep out of trouble. There are three major components of an exercise program to promote fitness: stretching, strengthening exercises, and cardiovascular-respiratory conditioning such as jogging or swimming.

The *U.S. Navy Diving Manual* (1978) advises that before a man can even begin training as a diver, he must meet the specific physical requirements for divers as set forth by the Bureau of Medicine and Surgery. "Once qualified, it is his own responsibility to keep in good health and in top physical condition." But the *Manual* goes on to require medical personnel to take an active interest in the day-to-day condition of each diver.

Exercise is definitely related to the problems of decompression from a dive and to the possibility of developing decompression sickness. It is well known and accepted that gas uptake in body tissues during exercise is far greater than during rest, because of increased cardiac action. It follows that heavy exercise or work while under pressure will lead to earlier and more complete saturation of the body tissues.

On land, at sea level, the limiting factor on the amount of work that can be performed is considered to be the cardiovascular system, whereas at depth under the water the limiting factor probably is the respiratory system. Because of the density of the breathing gas and the resistance of the breathing equipment the amount of breathing gas reaching the alveoli may be insufficient to clear out the carbon dioxide being produced, and heavy exercise under these conditions may lead to carbon dioxide buildup.

Strauss (1974) evaluates rebreathing equipment and says that "with strenuous exercise, there is an increased oxygen requirement which may be in excess of that supplied by the flow rate for the particular gas mixture chosen. With increased oxygen consumption, there is also an increased carbon dioxide production, which places an added load on the absorbent system. Thus the dangers of both hypoxis and carbon dioxide toxicity are increased."

i. Emotional Stability

Everyone knows that panic is not an appropriate response to an emergency situation; and as every physician knows, it is most difficult to handle. Yet both Bachrach (1973) and Strauss (1976) report that panic is a most important cause of serious and often fatal diving accidents.

One of the major problems is that panic occurring underwater leads to an attempt to get to the surface (and safety), and this often leads to a rapid breath-hold ascent and thus to air embolism and death. Hanson and Young (1975) say: "In the underwater environment panic can lead to a fatality from a simple problem which should have been overcome."

An important point is that although the stable or normal individual is usually able to handle stress because of a compensatory reserve, everyone has a breaking point. Also it is well to bear in mind that panic is not limited to the diver but may be exhibited by the personnel at the surface as well. The diving physician must be constantly aware of possibility of emotional instability in any member of the team.

All agree that training is the most important single method of preventing panic. Egstrom and Bachrach (1971) spoke of "overlearning" both diving techniques and the use of diving equipment so that action underwater becomes as automatic as walking on the ground. In another paper Bachrach (1973) stressed that it is extremely important for a working diver to master a task so completely that he can perform it automatically.

Prevention of panic, according to Strauss (1976), is adequate training, good physical condition, and (most importantly) the acquisition of as much information as possible about the dive to be undertaken, the equipment needed, and the possible problems; thus apprehension is reduced by information gathering. He pointed out that apprehension is normal for an unknown situation like cave diving or diving in kelp, but it can be reduced by getting as much information as possible ahead of time.

The best protection against panic according to Hanson and Young (1975) is correct training to give those involved in diving operations confidence in themselves and in the other members of the team. Although panic is most common in the inexperienced diver, it can occur in anyone, no matter what his experience, if the emotional trauma is great enough.

Smith (1975) lists as probable causes of "stress-induced behavioral dysfunction": cold, exertion, physical threat, task loading, time pressure, ego threat, or a combination of any of these. He lists the symptoms to be on the lookout for: behavioral narrowing, increased heart rate, hyperventilation, breathing in very short breaths, muscular tension, human error, the "wild-eyed look," and finally the culminating symptom—panic.

The problem of emotional instability is mentioned here because it is so important for the physician in determining the predive condition; for details please read Chapter XII, "Stress Physiology and Behavior Underwater."

j. Infections

Diving-related infections are discussed in Chapter IX, "Diagnosis and Treatment of Other Diving-Related Conditions." Here are treated only those conditions that should be considered during the predive physical check.

Upper respiratory infections such as colds, sore throat, and sinusitis are important to consider because pressure equalization may be difficult or impossible, and diving may lead to barotrauma, vertigo, or disorientation if in the water. Chest colds and bronchitis add other complications. For example, holding the mouthpiece in place while coughing is quite impossible. In addition a lower respiratory infection can lead to the forming of mucus; this would cause trapping of alveolar air, which in turn can lead to rupture of the alveolae and air embolism. Except in a real emergency a diver must not be permitted to go in the water with a fever and other signs of respiratory infection.

The most common complaint concerns ear problems. Otitis externa is frequently associated with swimming and diving and is the most pressing problem in habitat living. The external ear canal must be kept dry, so diving should be discontinued as long as the condition is present.

Aerotitis media (middle ear squeeze) in diving is usually caused by blockage of the eustachian tube, causing a failure in equalizing the pressure in the middle ear. Nature satisfies the relative vacuum by filling the middle ear with fluid and blood. Obviously, until the condition is cleared, a ruling of "no diving" is indicated.

Skin disease, whether acute or chronic, must be carefully evaluated, since it may be infective or offensive to others if clothing has to be shared. In some cases the condition may be exacerbated by diving, particularly saturation diving or habitat dwelling.

Either in a habitat or in a chamber with a water-filled compartment the occupants are found to be more than usually prone to infection. J. N. Miller (1975) reports that "fungal infections of the skin and infections of the external ear are common." This is especially true in tropical waters. In a study of habitat living Gulyar and associates (1974) found that most body functions are normal. "However, resistance to infection decreased and certain infections (pustular and fungal, upper respiratory tract, etc.) appeared." Oser (1972) reported a similar experience in the German habitat HELGOLAND.

k. Previous Diving History

There probably is no occupation or sport in which the medical history of the participant is more important than in diving. The medical history of the diver is crucial, and a history of appropriate training is also important. Both are considered in Chapter XI.

In the predive check-off the history of the immediately preceding dive or dives is the variable to be weighed. A dive that is less than 12 hr after a previous dive is considered to be a repetitive dive. The proper decompression schedule of the standard air table cannot be selected on the basis of the repetitive dive alone but must be calculated on the basis of the repetitive dive, the surface interval, and the previous dive. The detailed method of calculation can be found both in the *NOAA Diving Manual* (Miller 1979) and in the

U.S. Navy Diving Manual (1978). Additional treatment of the subject is also found in Chapter IV of this guide.

Another reason for checking on the history of recent dives is to determine if the diver has had any problems. If, for example, he has had a serious case of decompression sickness it is important to determine how soon diving can be resumed, or if it should be resumed at all.

C. The Dive

1. Organization and Planning

The most important point in planning is for a knowledgeable person to be in charge. This is true whether the dive be military, commercial, scientific, or just for sport. Regardless of how much fun diving may be, it is well to remember that all diving is associated with hazards not encountered on dry land, and someone must therefore be responsible for the well-being and safety of the divers. This person is often the medical member of the team or group.

No matter what type of diving is contemplated, one must not forget that bottom time is always at a premium, and planning should aim not only at assuring greater safety but also at greater efficiency while on the bottom.

The following eight steps in planning of diving operations are listed in the *U.S. Navy Diving Manual* (1978):

1. Define objectives.
2. Collect and analyze data.
3. Establish operational tasks.
4. Select diving technique.
5. Select equipment and supplies.
6. Select and assemble the diving team.
7. Make final preparations and check all safety precautions.
8. Start operation.

Adequate planning will assure the diver that proper equipment is available, with backup spares, and that he can count on proper assistance from a buddy or from the surface crew.

2. General Safety Precautions

This entire chapter deals with safety considerations for various environmental conditions and for different types of diving. A general checklist that applies to the planning for most diving activities would include the following:

>Where is the nearest recompression chamber?
>How can transportation to the chamber be obtained?

Where is the closest medical assistance? (You may be the one.)
If an accident occurs, do you have in mind the best method of handling all contingencies?
Have possibly interested parties been notified of the planned dive?
Has a competent person been designated to be in charge?
Is the available equipment adequate for the task to be undertaken?
Have environmental conditions been taken into account: weather, sea state, depth, type of bottom?
If the dive is to be of a length or to a depth requiring decompression, are appropriate tables available?
If the dive is for pleasure:
   Have buddies been chosen?
   Have they agreed on what they wish to do?
If the dive is to accomplish work:
   Has the total operation been carefully planned?
   Have the divers been briefed on the work?
   Is all the necessary equipment available?

3. *Personnel: Qualified, Trained, Ready to Dive*

It is important to be certain that all divers have been properly selected and adequately trained, and that they are presently in condition to dive (see the Section B.3., *Predive Condition*, in this chapter). In addition, it is important to check for the following:

- Are the divers qualified for the depth of the dive anticipated, and are they experienced in the type of work contemplated?
- Are the divers familiar with the equipment planned for use?

4. *Natural Hazards: Environmental Conditions*

Natural hazards are always present when terrestrial man attempts to become an aquatic animal. But additional hazards may be present due to atmospheric or weather conditions; storms, high wind, snow, and cold expose the diver, his tender, and his equipment to disruption, delays, and danger (*U.S. Navy Diving Manual* 1978).

As stated earlier, extremes of temperature are usually more of a problem for the surface crew than for the divers, so that sunburn, windburn, frostbite, and heat exhaustion must be guarded against.

The surface of the body of water adds problems that can cause delays or disruption: seasickness; water entry and exit; handling of heavy equipment in rough seas; maintaining diving location in tides and currents; and the presence of ice and various natural obstacles such as kelp, oil spills, or other contaminants. Wave action can affect everything from the stability of the mooring to the vulnerability of the crew and divers to seasickness and accident.

There are also hazards under the water and on the bottom: exposure to low temperatures; dangerous marine life; tides and currents; limited visibility; obstructions and other dangerous bottom conditions (e.g., mud, drop-offs, sewer outfalls). The type of bottom will affect the mobility of the diver and, particularly if it is mud bottom, his ability to see. Visibility is usually not adversely affected by other types of bottom: rock, coral, gravel, shell, or sand. An environmental checklist modified from the *U.S. Navy Diving Manual* calls attention to all these details (Table XIII-2).

Although natural hazards are important, the most important underwater consideration is that the dive and the decompression be in accordance with standard tables for the depth and time of the dive.

Table XIII-2
Environmental Checklist

SURFACE

Atmosphere:	**Sea Surface:**
Visibility _____	Sea State _____
Sun _____	Wave Action:
Moon _____	Height _____
Temperature (air) _____	Length _____
Humidity _____	Direction _____
Barometer _____	Current:
Precip. _____	Direction _____
Cloud Descrip. _____	Velocity _____
% Cover _____	Type _____
Wind Direction _____	Surf. Visibility _____
Force (knots) _____	Surf. Wat. Temp. _____
Other: _____	Local Characteristics: _____

SUBSEA

Underwater and Bottom:	**Visibility:**
Depth _____	Underwater—
Wat. Temp.	_____ ft at _____ depth
_____ depth _____	_____ ft at _____ depth
_____ depth _____	_____ ft at _____ depth
_____ depth _____	Bottom:
_____ bottom _____	_____ ft at _____ depth
Thermoclines _____	Bottom:
_____	Type: _____
Current:	
Direction _____	Obstructions: _____
Source _____	_____
Velocity _____	_____
Pattern _____	_____
Tides:	Marine Life: _____
S High Water _____ time	_____
S Low Water _____ time	_____
Ebb dir. _____ vel. _____	
Flood dir. _____ vel. _____	Other Data: _____
	_____
	_____

Adopted from U.S. Navy Diving Manual.

5. On-Site Hazards

The *U.S. Navy Diving Manual* (1978) lists six on-site hazards to diving: local marine traffic; high-powered active sonar; other conflicting naval operations; conflicting commercial operations; radiation exposure due to radioactive contamination; and pollution.

a. Traffic

Local marine traffic is indeed a hazard, for (as pointed out elsewhere) divers have been killed by the propellers of boats or ships passing through the area. (See *Diving Operations,* later in this chapter.) In a similar way other conflicting operations may lead to confusion. For instance, two different groups working on the same wreck without proper coordination could lead to difficulty.

b. Sonar

Sonar is an acronym derived from the expression *Sound Navigation and Ranging* and is used to indicate either the method or the equipment for using underwater sound techniques to detect the presence, location, or nature of objects in the sea. Sound is the result of vibrations transmitted to the ear through some form of matter. It is transmitted through water as a series of pressure waves; high-intensity sound is transmitted by correspondingly high intensity of pressure waves.

The low-intensity sonars, such as depth finders and fish finders, do not produce pressure waves of an intensity dangerous to divers, but antisubmarine sonars cause the diver to become disoriented, and this is a most serious problem. Thus it is prudent to suspend diving operations if a high-powered sonar transponder is being operated in the area.

c. Radioactive Contamination

Radioactive contamination is considered to be deposition of radioactive material in any place where radiation from it may harm persons, spoil experiments, or render products or equipment unsuitable or unsafe for some specific use. The *U.S. Navy Radiological Control Manual* (1970) lists safe levels of tolerance to radioactive material.

The chance that the ordinary scuba diver will encounter any significant radioactive contamination is almost nonexistent. The commercial diver, however, may be asked to dive in slightly radioactive water—for example, the coolant water for a nuclear reactor. This can be accomplished by wearing a complete and body-covering dry suit and carefully scrubbing the suit before removing it. This will prevent any significant radiation from reaching either the diver or the tenders.

6. Object Hazards

The *U.S. Navy Diving Manual* (1978) lists the following hazards from objects: entrapment, entanglement; toxic pollution; explosives or other ordnance; and shifting or "working" of an object. Under that heading other texts (Miller 1979; Shilling et al. 1976) also discuss these hazards. Explosives and the resultant blast are covered in Chapter IX of this guide; fouling and pollution are discussed here.

a. Fouling

The diver, supplied from the surface with lifeline and air hose, is more likely to become fouled than the scuba diver, but the scuba diver may become entangled with various underwater obstructions from kelp to a wrecked ship. Both divers may be caught by cave-in of a tunnel or by the shifting of a heavy object that blocks the route of exit from a wreck. Fouling does occur, and divers should be reminded of that possibility when diving under conditions likely to contribute to it.

The diver wearing self-contained equipment is in the most danger, since his air supply is limited and he has no other communication with the surface. His best assets in such a situation are calmness and common sense, his buddy diver, and his knife. Immediate struggling to free himself will often lead to a worsened situation. With care it is usually possible to work free, especially if the buddy is there to help.

Whether a diver emerges safely from fouling depends very much on his own actions even though the help of another diver is often required to free him. For either type of diver the action recommended by the Navy (1978) is as follows:

- Remain calm; think.
- Describe situation to tender or call buddy's attention to situation.
- Carefully and systematically attempt to determine cause of fouling and to clear self. Use knife cautiously to avoid cutting airhose or breathing apparatus.
- In fouling with self-contained apparatus, regard ditching diving gear and free ascent as a last resort, but prepare to do this in case it proves necessary.
- If efforts to clear prove futile, be quiet and wait for air.
- Remember that frantic, ill-planned efforts usually not only fail but make the situation worse. Futile struggling and panic can result in death from exhaustion.

In most cases fouling can be prevented by using proper precautions and studying the situation beforehand. But it is important to have a buddy if scuba diving and a tender and reserve diver on the surface if diving with surface-supplied equipment.

b. Pollution

Pollution of the air supply and pollution of the water may both affect the diver.

Air pollution is one of the most likely types for the diver to encounter. The gas mixture may be wrong, with too little or too much oxygen; the carbon dioxide may become too high because of faulty absorption; and carbon monoxide may be contaminating the breathing air. This may occur when the air intake for the compressor is located where it draws air from the engine exhaust.

Water pollution may be thermal, chemical, radioactive, or microbial. Thermal pollution may be great enough to cause a shift in the fauna and flora of the area, but it seldom changes enough to cause any problem for the diver. Chemical pollution may be encountered as a result of accidental spills or illegal dumping of chemical material. A dive must be accomplished with the same precautions already pointed out for radioactive pollution. Nuclear radiation (discussed under *On-Site Hazards*) may be encountered as a result of accident, proximity to weapons or propulsion systems during salvage, or, occasionally, in the natural state.

The *U.S. Navy Diving Manual* (1978) points out that a diver working near sewer outlets or industrial discharges may be exposed to the hazards of disease or chemical poisoning. Oil leaking from underwater wellheads or damaged fuel tanks can cause fouling of equipment and seriously impede a diver's movements. Toxic materials or volatile fuels leaking from barges or tanks can irritate the skin and corrode equipment. When using scuba a diver may inadvertently take polluting materials into his mouth, posing both physiological and psychological problems. As in radioactive water, in planning for operations in water known to be polluted, full protective clothing and appropriate preventive medical procedures must be provided.

7. Special Situations

No general presentation of operational safety considerations can hope to cover all types of diving. Construction Industry Research and Information Association (CIRIA 1972) lists the following as requiring special plans and special arrangements:

- Diving in shark-infested waters
- Diving in wrecks
- Diving on or near ship's bottom
- Diving in the vicinity of a ship's propellers
- Diving in locks, basins, and culverts
- Diving to place underwater explosives
- Diving in sewers and in natural and artificial underground waters
- Diving from drilling rigs or other high platforms
- Diving from a pipe-laying vessel
- Diving from a basket slung from a crane
- Diving from a diving bell operated from a crane
- Divers operating a wet submersible

8. Recompression Chamber

Recompression chambers are discussed in some detail in Chapter I, "The Diving Environment," and Chapter XIV, "Equipment and Procedures." Here it is important to stress that before any dive is undertaken the location of the nearest recompression chamber must be known to all personnel—Where is it located? What is the best means of getting there? Is it covered 24 hr a day?

It is best, as the U.S. Navy requires, to have a chamber immediately available, but for sport scuba diving this is often not possible.

Once again, since the average diver seldom thinks of safety or possible emergencies, it is up to the physician diver to have the facts.

9. Equipment, Regular and Emergency

The physician safety officer should check to determine the following:

- Does everyone have appropriate diving equipment for the type of dive being undertaken?
- Is there spare equipment available in case of need?
- Has the equipment been tested to see that it is in working order?
- Does every diver have an adequate supply of compressed gas?

This last is particularly crucial when cave diving, for coming to the surface for air in a water-filled cave is dangerous.

Detailed information on various types of equipment is presented in Chapter I, "The Diving Environment," and Chapter XIV, "Equipment and Procedures."

10. Orientation

Both postural and geographic orientation are adversely affected by the underwater environment, which reduces both visual and kinesthetic cues. Orientation to gravitational vertical may be lost to the extent that the diver may literally not know "which end is up." Some details of this problem are presented in Chapter XII, "Stress Psychology and Behavior Underwater," but here attention is called to this additional hazard to safe diving in order to alert the physician to the problem.

11. Diving Operations

Safety during diving operations is largely a matter of careful planning and then adherence to detail. Most of the following considerations apply to any type of diving, but there are some differences between scuba and surface-supplied diving that are noted whenever indicated. Certain of the following items are presented in depth, since they are not considered elsewhere in this guide. Further detail on any point is available in the diving manuals of the U.S. Navy (1978) and of NOAA [see Miller (1979)] and the CIRIA 1972 publication.

a. Diving Platform

Entry into the water may be made from a dock, a seawall, or from the open beach, but it is generally from a boat. If from a boat it is important that the boat be positioned in the most advantageous position for the underwater activity contemplated and that the boat be moored so that it will not shift.

b. Warning Signals

Divers are killed every year by being struck by motor boats cruising into the diving sites. If there is any chance at all that boats not related to the dive are moving in the area, it is necessary to display the appropriate diving flags, which are shown in Figure XIII-2.

A float supporting the diver's flag should be used when diving from the beach or when operating from a boat. The float may be a simple buoy, and flag, or it may be as large as a small raft. The float most frequently used is an automobile inner tube with the center lined with net. The float should be brightly colored and have the diving flag

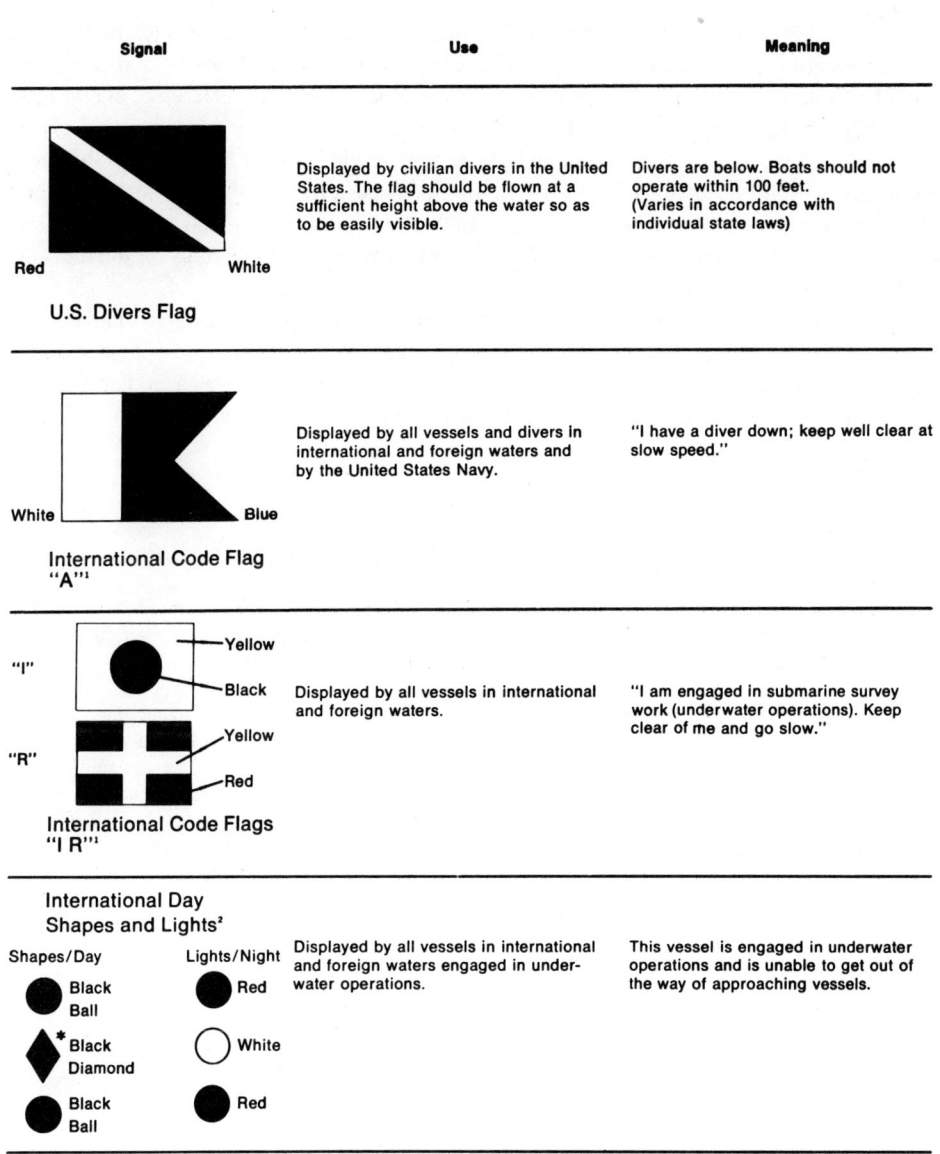

[1] U.S. Navy, *International Code of Signals*, United States Edition, 1969.
[2] U.S. Coast Guard, *Navigation Rules: International—Inland*, May 1, 1977.

Figure XIII-2. Signal flags, shapes, and lights. [From NOAA Diving Manual (Miller 1979).]

attached on the staff. A line attached to the float will allow the diver to keep the float with him, and a small anchor, hook, or snap at the end of the line will enable him to hold it on the bottom while he is working.

Figure XIII-2 and its legend explain the international diving flags and their meanings.

c. Line Signals

With surface-supplied equipment line signals may be used as a backup to voice communication or as a primary means of communication. Line signals can also be used by divers using self-contained equipment to communicate with the surface or, in restricted visibility, with another diver. A line-pull signal consists of one or a series of sharp, distinct pulls on the line, strong enough to be felt by the diver or the tender. Obviously there must be no slack in the line if a signal is to be felt. A failure to answer signals may mean too much slack but it may also mean that the line is fouled or that the diver is in trouble. The same type of signals can be given by light flashes, taps on the air tank, and even by hand squeeze.

The actual signals vary between different nations and even in different parts of the United States, so it is wise to review and agree upon the signals for use in the diving being contemplated. The line signals used by the U.S. Navy are given in Table XIII-3 and are suggested as the standard basis to which may be added signals for special work being contemplated.

Table XIII-3
Line-Pull Signals[a]

From tender to diver	Special signals from diver
1 Pull "Are you all right?"	1-2-3 Pulls "Send me a square mark"
When diver is descending, one pull means "stop"	5 Pulls "Send me a line"
2 Pulls "Going down"	2-1-2 Pulls "Send me a slate"
During ascent, 2 pulls mean "you have come up too far, go back down until we stop you"	*Searching signals—without circling line*
3 Pulls "Stand by to come up"	7 Pulls "Go on (or off) searching signals"
4 Pulls "Come up"	1 Pull "Stop and search where you are."
2-1 Pulls "I understand," or "answer the telephone"	2 Pulls "Move directly away from tender if given slack; move toward the tender if strain is taken on the life line"
From diver to tender	3 Pulls "Go to your right"
1 Pull "I am all right" or "I am on the bottom"	4 Pulls "Go to your left"
2 Pulls "Lower" or "give me slack"	
3 Pulls "Take up my slack"	*Searching signals—with circling line*
4 Pulls "Haul me up"	7 Pulls Same
2-1 Pulls "I understand" or "answer the telephone"	1 Pull Same
3-2 Pulls "More air"	2 Pulls "Move away from the weight"
4-3 Pulls "Less air"	3 Pulls "Face the weight and go right"
	4 Pulls "Face the weight and go left"

Emergency Signals
2-2-2 Pulls   "I am fouled and need the assistance of another diver"
3-3-3 Pulls   "I am fouled but can clear myself"
4-4-4 Pulls   "Haul me up immediately"
All signals will be answered as given—except for emergency signal 4-4-4

[a] From *U.S. Navy Diving Manual* (Change 2).

d. Hand Signals

Hand signals may be the only method of communication in certain situations underwater, and it is important that everyone understand what signals are to be used and their meaning. Those shown in Figure XIII-3 are worth adopting.

e. Descent

(i) Air. If diving in a surface-supplied diving dress, it is important to continue to adjust the air during descent so that breathing is easy and so that pressure inside the suit is maintained to prevent body squeeze.

(ii) Rate. The rate of descent is governed by such factors as the diver's ability to clear the ears; environmental factors such as currents and reduced visibility; and the need to approach the bottom with caution. The maximum rate of descent, under any conditions, is 75 ft/min.

(iii) Line. The surface-supplied diver is connected to the surface by his umbilical, which carries his air hose, a communication cable, and usually a lifeline. The scuba diver often operates without a lifeline attachment to the surface. In all cases it is advisable to have a descending line attached to a weight on the bottom or to some stationary object on the bottom. When using a descending line the diver can control his descent by locking his legs around a line and holding on with one hand while the other hand is free to adjust his air flow or buoyancy, if necessary. A descending line is mandatory for cave diving, under-ice diving, or in a strong current. The most commonly used type of line is made of nylon, dacron, or polypropylene. The descending line should normally be attached directly to a weight on the bottom or to some stationary object, and an additional line (a distance line) may be attached at the sea bed to assist the diver in a search pattern when he is on the bottom. If decompression is contemplated or required, the descending line, which then becomes the ascending line, should have markers every 10 ft (3 m) from the surface so that decompression stops can be accurately determined.

f. Fouling

Every effort should be made to anticipate difficulty and to prevent fouling. For example, for exploration or work inside a wreck a fellow diver should tend the distance line at the point of entry of the diver working inside. (See subsection on *Object Hazards* in this chapter.)

g. Explosives

If explosives are being used precautions must be taken so that all divers are out of the water when detonation occurs. (See section *Blast* in Chapter IX.)

h. Electric Power

If electric power is being used for underwater cutting or welding it is important that the diver be properly dressed and grounded and insulated from any possible source of electric current. (See section *Electrical Safety*, later in this chapter.)

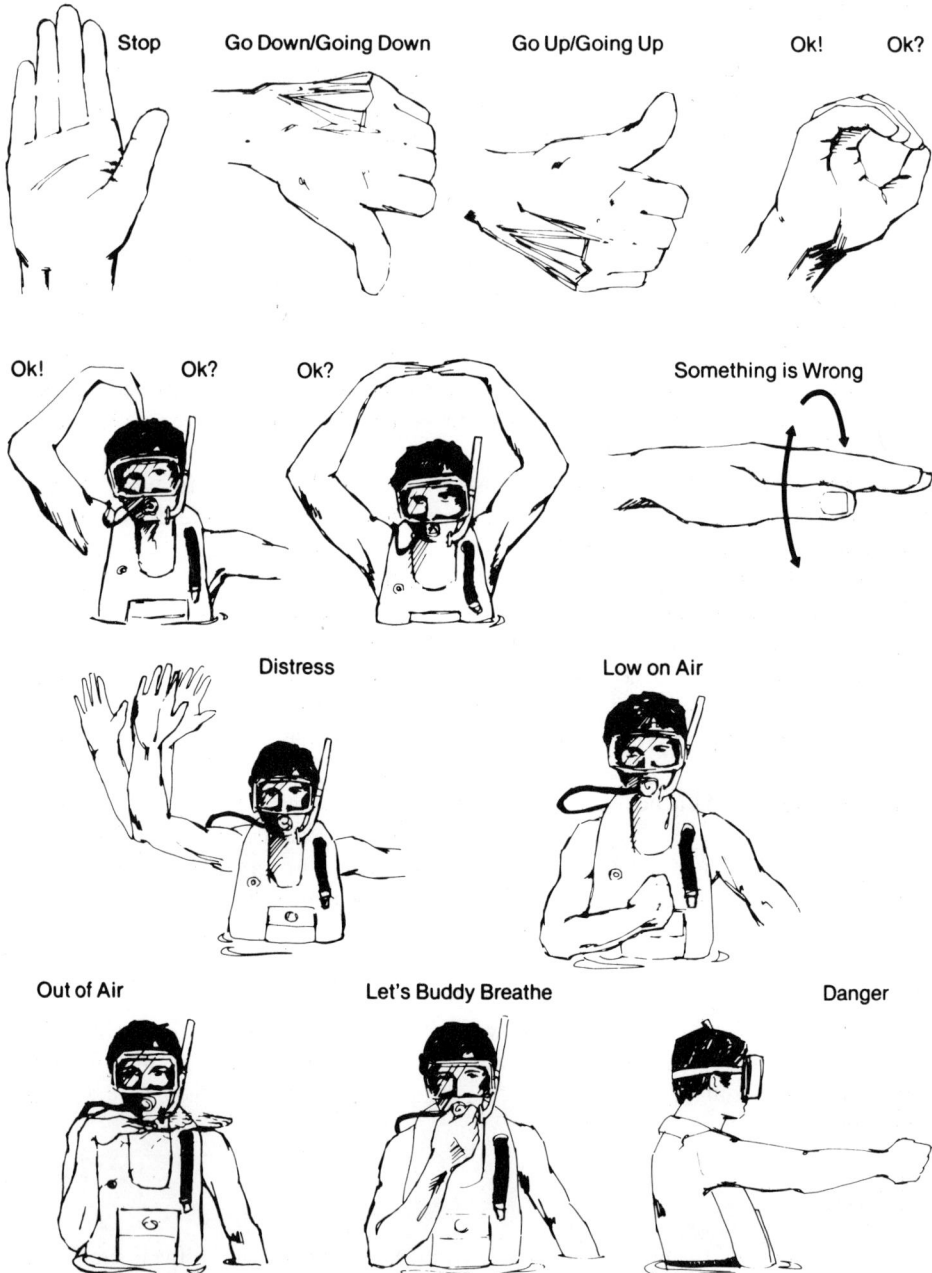

Figure XIII-3. Hand signals. *1.* Hand raised, fingers pointed up, palm to receiver, like a policeman's Halt! sign. Meaning: STOP. *2.* Thumb extended downward from clenched fist. Meaning: GO DOWN, or GOING DOWN. *3.* Thumb extended upward from clenched fist. Meaning: GO UP or GOING UP. *4.* Thumb and forefinger making a circle with three remaining fingers extended, if possible. Meaning: OK! or OK? *5.* Two arms extended overhead with fingertips touching above head to make a large O-shape. Meaning: OK! or OK? *6.* Hand flat, fingers together, palm down, thumb sticking out, then hand rocking back and forth on axis of

i. Shark Defense

The diver's problem with dangerous marine life is covered in Chapter IX. Here we present three operational devices used to protect against sharks. The simplest (and probably the oldest) antishark device is a 3- to 4-ft-long wooden club with a short nail on one end; the slab is counterweighted for effective underwater handling. The device is commonly called a "shark billy" and is used to fend off the shark or strike it, preferably on the nose.

If the shark must be killed there is a device called the "bang stick," a short pole at the end of which is a chamber that holds a shotgun shell. It can be shot at the shark or set to fire upon being pushed against the body of the shark. Another device available commercially is the "shark dart." This consists of a hollow stainless steel needle 5 in. long that is connected to a small CO_2 cartridge. The dart is thrust through the abdominal wall and releases enough gas to force the shark to the surface.

j. Decompression

If the contemplated dive is at a sufficient depth or the time on bottom is long enough to require decompression it is important that appropriate arrangements be made ahead of time. The descending (ascending) line should have markers at 10-ft (3-m) intervals from the surface, and the applicable decompression tables must be at hand. Details of decompression are discussed in Chapter IV, "Decompression Theory," and elsewhere in this book.

D. *Diving at Altitudes above Sea Level*

When diving in mountain lakes or at high altitudes the normal sea level decompression schedules must be adjusted to compensate for atmospheric pressure and density of water at the dive site. Extensive research was conducted by Boni et al. (1976) on decompression after diving in Swiss mountain lakes. They pointed out that "the major factor that causes a decompression accident is the ratio of nitrogen pressure in the tissue to ambient pressure; therefore, for the same depth and the same bottom time but for a lower ambient pressure, longer decompression times are necessary."

According to CIRIA (1972), the adjustments should be as follows:

1. Dives at altitudes of less than 100 m (about 300 ft): no adjustment is required.

2. Dives between altitudes of 100 m and 300 m (about 300 to 1000 ft): add one-fourth of the depth to give the comparable depth of the dive.

3. Dives between altitudes of 300 and 2000 m (about 1000 to 6500 ft): add one-third of the depth to give the comparable depth of the dive.

---

forearm. Meaning: SOMETHING IS WRONG. 7. Hand waving over head (may also thrash hand on water). Meaning: DISTRESS. 8. Fist pounding on chest. Meaning: LOW ON AIR (quantity has been agreed on in advance). 9. Hand slashing or chopping throat. Meaning: OUT OF AIR. *10*. Fingers pointing to mouth. Meaning: LET'S BUDDY BREATHE. *11*. Clenched fist on arm extended in direction of danger. Meaning: DANGER. [Adapted from *NOAA Diving Manual* (Miller 1979).]

4. Dives between altitudes of 2000 and 3000 m (about 6500 to 10,000 ft): add one-half of the depth to give the comparable depth of the dive.

For example, a dive to a depth of 24 m at an altitude of 1000 m should be treated as a dive to a depth of 32 m.

As pointed out by Miller (1979, p. 9–18), an important factor to consider when diving at altitudes above sea level is the effect the increased elevation will have on the various types of depth gauges. "Neither oil-filled nor capillary depth gauges will provide accurate depth indication when used at altitude. Oil-filled depth gauges are designed to read zero feet at 1 ATA. At reduced atmospheric pressure, the gauge will read less than zero . . . and consequently in the water the gauge will always give a reading that is shallower than the actual depth. . . . Due to the reduced density of the air trapped in the capillary gauge, less water pressure is required at altitude than at sea level to compress the air to a given volume. As a result, the capillary gauge will always indicate a depth greater than the actual depth."

We are reminded by Dueker (1978) that "upon arriving at a mountain lake, the diver has excess nitrogen remaining from his life at sea level. . . . At least twelve hours should pass before diving so that the first dive is not a repetitive one."

E. Flying after Diving

In keeping with the times, many scuba divers fly to and from their diving sites. In the usual small private plane there is no pressurization, and even in a commercial pressurized-cabin aircraft there is some additional decrease in ambient pressure, since the cabin atmosphere in most modern pressurized aircraft is usually maintained at an altitude of 8000 ft or 2450 m (0.74 atm; see Edel et al. 1969). See Table XIII-4 for both altitude and underwater pressure equivalents.

Following a dive or exposure to increased pressure in a chamber, the elimination of inert gas from body tissues continues for a period of 24 or more hr before complete equilibrium with ambient, or surface, inert gas (nitrogen) is complete. Thus, if the flight occurs shortly after surfacing from a dive the change in pressure may be sufficient to precipitate decompression sickness, even though the dive itself was conducted in accordance with the U.S. Navy decompression tables.

Because of the growing rate of sport, commercial, research, and military diving, Strauss (1974) urges that not only the divers themselves but air crews and physicians be made aware of the signs, symptoms, and primary care of this condition.

The first authenticated case to be published (Miner 1961) was of some air crew members who had been diving both morning and afternoon and then developed decompression sickness on their return international flight that evening. Since that time both animal and human experiments have demonstrated the hazards of flying after diving.

To more clearly define the problem, an experimental program was initiated at the Naval Medical Research Institute (Furry et al. 1966); large dogs were exposed to pressure and then decompressed to determine a "no-bends" threshold. Then they were subjected to an altitude exposure of 10,000 ft (3000 m, 10.11 psia) after surface decompression intervals of 1, 3, 6, and 12 hr. After the 1-hr surface interval 92.9% developed de-

XIII-4
Comparison of Altitudes and Air Pressure
at Various Pressures of Seawater

Altitude or depth		Pressure	
ft	m	ATA	psi
30,000	9150	0.30	4.41
20,000	6100	0.46	6.76
10,000	3050	0.68	10.11
8,000	2440	0.74	10.92
5,000	1525	0.83	12.20
4,000	1220	0.86	12.69
3,000	915	0.90	13.17
2,000	610	0.93	13.66
1,000	305	0.96	14.17
Sea level	—	1.00	14.70
−100	−30.5	4.00	58.80
−250	−76.3	8.55	125.88
−500	−152.5	16.15	237.41
−1,000	−305.	31.30	460.11

compression sickness; after 3 hr, 61.5%; after 6 hr 27.8%; but after 12 hr none exhibited signs of decompression sickness at altitude.

More recently Balldin (1978) used Doppler ultrasound in human subjects to detect intracardial gas bubbles, and symptoms of decompression sickness were noted at simulated altitude of 9000 m within 12, 18, and 24 hr after exposure to 15 or 39 m of simulated water depth, not allowing for stage decompression. Bubbles and symptoms appeared within 17 min even after a 24-hr period; for prolonged flights it appears that an even longer surface decompression period is necessary.

From work with both animals and humans, Furry et al. (1966) recommended a sound and accepted set of guidelines: "All personnel who have engaged in compressed-air diving to depths of 25 feet of water or its equivalent should not fly in other than pressurized commercial aircraft or in a cabin altitude greater than 8,000 feet or its equivalent within 12 hours following termination of a compressed-air exposure." Further work with human volunteers (Edel et al. 1969) confirmed this, but they added that "Divers who make dives beyond the 'no-decompression' limits should allow a surface interval of 24 hours before decompression to a commercial aircraft's cabin altitude pressure if they are to avoid the risk of bends." The French (Lavernhe 1970) agree with this dictum but add that any diver showing symptoms of decompression sickness should observe a minimum period of 24 hr after symptoms clear before boarding an aircraft. The CIRIA group (1972) consider it inadvisable to fly above 600 m (approximately 2000 ft) in any aircraft within 24 hr of completion of a dive.

If it becomes necessary to fly immediately after diving, as in the case of injury requiring treatment not available at the dive site, the *NOAA Diving Manual* (Miller 1979) recommends that "the diver should be transported at a low altitude by helicopter or aircraft, or in a pressurized aircraft which does not exceed a cabin atmosphere of 800 feet of altitude." In addition the diver should breathe oxygen during the flight.

F. Fire Safety

Even though you may consider that the operation of the recompression chamber is not your province, it is well to remember that the physician is expected to be safety conscious at all times. In this case we must consider the fire hazard of an oxygen-enriched atmosphere. This is especially important in a recompression chamber, for compressed air at a pressure equivalent of 200 fsw has an oxygen partial pressure of 1.5 atm; at 300 fsw, 2 atm. When the subject is breathing 100% oxygen either during decompression or in treatment, the partial pressure of oxygen in the chamber may rise rapidly.

Added to the ordinary risk associated with fire is the impracticality of escape because of the physiological danger of a sudden decrease in pressure; in most situations escape is impossible in time to save the lives of those in the chamber. Although fires in pressure chambers have been rare, there have been fatal fires in a Navy chamber, in an Air Force chamber, in a NASA space capsule, and in commercial diving operations.

The reader is encouraged to read carefully the treatment of this subject in Chapter XIV, "Equipment and Procedures," for full details.

G. Electrical Safety

Electricity is used extensively by the diver in the conduct of underwater activity: electric lighting, electric heating, power for tools, and power for movement of all types of underwater vehicles. Yet electricity is one of the many potentially dangerous agents with which the diver must contend. Of particular importance is the intimate coupling between the diver and the water in which he is immersed; because of the high conductivity of seawater, even low voltages can cause large currents to flow through the body.

Although management of electric power is an engineering problem, electric power can be made intrinsically safe if it is designed to comply with one or more of the following: voltage or current limitation and high frequency if AC is used, low-wattage circuits, earth screen, double insulation, continual monitoring, or circuits with automatic cutoff.

There are numerous sources of possible electric shock in a diving operation: power for the vehicle in which the diver may be riding, power tools, electric light, electric welding, and even the electrically heated diving suit.

The use of electricity over hot water to heat the diver has many advantages and an all-out effort is being made to make this type of heating safe (Taylor 1979).

For the purpose of this section it is sufficient to recognize that if electric power is being used for any purpose during the dive, the system must be inspected beforehand by a qualified person to make certain that it has been made as safe as possible.

H. Blast

Blast is mentioned here to call attention to the serious danger of blasting associated in any way with either swimming on the surface or diving beneath the water while blasting operations are being conducted in the vicinity of the dive.

I. Drowning

Drowning is an important problem, for in the United States there are 7000 to 8000 drowning deaths each year, and many studies indicate drowning as the single most frequent cause of death in young adults. It is well to remember that if a person dies in the water and no other cause of death is immediately apparent, then drowning is the coroner's report. However, the U.S. Navy (1970) reported that drowning is the most frequent cause of death in self-contained diving equipment. But drowning is extremely unlikely in diving operations from a surface-supplied, deep-sea, hard-hat rig. It can occur, however, if the diver gets in an upside-down position with the spitcock open or the chin button depressed. Such an occurrence has been unofficially reported in North Sea oil exploration—the diver became fouled and tried to blow himself loose.

Numerous opportunities for accidents can occur to a diver using self-contained equipment: loss or flooding of mask or mouthpiece; exhaustion of the gas supply; failure or improper functioning of the gear; surface exposure in rough water; and almost any mishap that is followed by panic and failure to follow emergency procedures.

For the breath-hold diver or skin diver or swimmer the most likely cause of drowning is blackout (see *Breath-Hold Diving* in Chapter III for details of blackout), and, of course, any condition leading to exhaustion or panic can lead to drowning. The U.S. Navy in its 1970 *Diving Manual* reported that the most common cause of drowning is physical exhaustion resulting from swimming after surfacing.

The physiology and the treatment of the nearly drowned person are presented in Chapter VIII, but here the emphasis is on prevention. Both the *U.S. Navy Diving Manual* (1970, 1978) and the *NOAA Diving Manual* (Miller 1979) list training as the most important single asset in the prevention of drowning. A recent NOAA-supported UMS Workshop (UMS 1979) concluded that emergency ascent training was important in preparing the diver for any emergency that might arise. Other elements of prevention of mishaps are: proper equipment in good working condition; diver adequately trained in operation of equipment to be used; use of life jacket with scuba; lifeline with lightweight outfit; proper planning and preparation for the dive; buddy system for scuba and skin diving; tenders trained to handle emergencies in other forms of diving; appropriate boats, floats, diving flags; and readiness to go to the aid of a diver in distress.

The basic diving principles suggested in Dueker (1978) and listed in section *The Diver*, in this chapter, will, if adhered to, greatly reduce the chance of drowning. These principles are just as applicable in preventing accidents of any type.

J. Hazards of Marine Life

Of the myriad life forms that live in the oceans most are completely innocuous, some are potentially hazardous to divers, and a few are life threatening. This problem is treated in detail in a section in Chapter IX, but it is mentioned here to remind the physician to inquire about the conditions in the area in which diving is planned. The most complete treatise on this subject is the three-volume set by Halstead (1965), but both the *U.S. Navy Diving Manual* (1970, 1978) and the *NOAA Diving Manual* (Miller 1979) carry all the information needed by the average diver.

K. *Escape and Rescue*

1. *Submarines*

a. Escape

Military submarine activity is, in general, not considered in this guide, but the following material dealing with escape and rescue is considered to be so closely related to similar problems encountered in civilian underwater submersibles and habitats that a short review is presented.

A more detailed review of this entire subject is found in two bibliographies produced by the Defense Documentation Center (DDC 1968); although specifically related to military submarines, they give material on deep-submergence vessels, search techniques, escape and rescue, and passive and active communication to and from the distressed craft. Much of this may have application to habitats and various types of deep-submergence vessels.

Submarine disasters have occurred in every one of the world's major navies. In only a few of the shallow-water sinkings have any of the men escaped. The first recorded escape was from a German submarine in 1851 in Kiel Harbor in 60 ft of water. Wilhelm Brauer, trapped with a number of men, realized that the only hope of opening the hatches was to raise the internal pressure by flooding. Flooding allowed the hatches to burst open and some of the men shot to the surface (Miles 1969).

It is well to remember that a hatch cannot be opened unless the pressure is equalized on both sides; at a depth of only 100 ft (a little over 4 ATA) the pressure would be 14,130 lb or a little over 7 tons (45 psi on a 20-in.-diam hatch), assuming atmospheric pressure inside the submarine.

The first escape in the British Navy occurred in 1916 after H.M. Submarine E-41 collided with another submarine and went to the bottom in 30 ft of water. Stoker Petty Officer Brown found himself alone behind the watertight bulkhead in the engine room. He began to flood the compartment so as to equalize pressure and enable him to open the hatch. The hatch popped open and a bubble of air was released, and then the hatch slammed shut. This was repeated several times until the air in the engine room was almost exhausted, when the hatch remained open, allowing Brown to escape.

Because of obvious need for the men to be able to breathe during flooding and during the actual escape, there was early development of escape equipment. The German Navy developed the Draeger breathing apparatus; the U.S. Navy the submarine escape apparatus (Momsen lung); and the British the Davis submarine escape apparatus (DSEA). These were self contained but were all rather complicated, and since all that was really needed was a space in which to breathe, it was logical that the "hooded" systems were developed. The U.S. Navy has the Steinke hood, and the British have a hooded system combined with an exposure suit. There has been ample demonstration that the hoods and the various escape configurations will work. Escape from a disabled submarine is fraught with a number of problems, however. To more thoroughly understand them a workshop was held at the U.S. Navy Submarine Medical Research Laboratory in 1972 (Gell and Parker 1974); seven countries were represented, and many aspects of marine escape were considered: doctrine and training; decompression predictions; high pressure nervous syndrome; contaminated atmosphere; ear, nose, and throat considerations; free ascent; thermal problems; human factors; and escape techniques and devices.

Because of these and other problems, individual escape is limited in the British Navy to depths not in excess of 600 ft (Elliott 1971) and this only for individual tower escapes, where pressurization time is 20 sec, bottom time 1.5 sec, and the original pressure in the submarine is not more than 2 ATA. In the U.S. Navy group escape is possible for shallower depths (100 ft and less) by using the Steinke hood.

b. Rescue

The U.S. Navy has always stressed rescue from the outside; the use of the McCann rescue chamber to remove 33 men from the U.S.S. *Squalus* on the bottom at 240 ft is the classic and only example of a mass rescue.

However, since the diving bell can only be used at depths at which a diver can function in fastening the down-haul cable to the hatch ring, the U.S. Navy has developed the deep submarine rescue vehicle (DSRV); this device can operate at great depths, mate with the submarine hatch, and bring to the surface 24 men at a trip.

2. Submersibles and Habitats

A *submersible* is any of the four general types of vehicle for underwater operation: *dry* refers to a submersible in which the occupants are maintained in a dry environment at near atmospheric conditions; *wet* is a free-flooding submersible in which the occupants are exposed to the ambient environment; *self-propelled* is a submersible operating under its own power; and *lock-out* is a submersible that has a compartment maintained at 1-atm pressure for the pilot and observer and a compartment that can be pressurized to ambient pressure so that the diver can enter and exit (lock out) to perform underwater work.

The *habitat*, on the other hand, is a seafloor structure, either movable or fixed, in which divers can live for extended periods and from which they can make excursions. Habitats are of many types and sizes and many are used for marine biological observations and research.

A *bell* is defined as a tethered underwater support platform, providing life-support services and used to transport divers. A bell may be closed or pressurized, may be open to the water, and may be used as a personnel transfer capsule, an observation chamber, or a submersible decompression chamber.

From the standpoint of escape and rescue all have one thing in common—it is most difficult if not impossible to escape, and rescue is extremely difficult. The Johnson SEA-LINK tragedy in 1973 certainly demonstrated the need for developing a capability for escape or rescue. The U.S. Navy Submarine Development Group One developed an airborne system that included a diving bell, recompression chamber, air compressor, mixed gas supply, scuba and hard hat gear, and support equipment and tools (Pfeiffer 1974).

What is needed is a means of transferring the diver saturated at even a shallow depth (e.g., 60 ft) from the underwater vehicle or habitat to the surface in a transfer capsule that can be mated to the deck decompression chamber so that the diver, still under pressure, can move into a more comfortable place for the duration of the long decompression. Although this is done routinely in the commercial diving industry, many of the research, observation, and exploration rigs used by research and sport divers are not so safety oriented; however, in detailed discussion of diving bell escape systems at a recent conference, there was agreement that a great deal of safety progress had been made (Nuytten 1974). But the scientific and sport diving communities must take steps to make submersible and habitat activities as safe as they now are in the commercial community.

L. Ice Diving

There is no question that very cold conditions affect diving operations, but such conditions do not necessarily prevent diving. Since it is impossible to change the elements of the polar world, it is wise for the diver to learn to work with and not against the elements if survival and accomplishment of the objective are to be realized. The additional problems encountered as a result of diving in extreme cold may be overcome by proper use of special clothing, diving equipment, and support equipment, and by carefully following support and safety measures.

Much of the research accomplished in this specialized field has been conducted by the U.S. Navy or with Navy support. A series of manuals by Jenkins (1973, 1974, 1976) have reported work under the auspices of the Naval Coastal Systems Laboratory, and they constitute a most valuable source of information.

Diving under the ice is not just a stunt, for both the U.S. and Canadian Navy divers have logged many hours of work in such tasks as assisting in the DEW line construction, changing propellers, clearing underwater obstructions, laying pipeline; inspecting hulls, recovering crashed and submerged aircraft, and engaging in routine search and salvage.

The environmental characteristics of polar diving (and to a lesser extent lake diving) that complicate diving operations include such conditions as extreme and rapid temperature changes; wind, snow, and ice storms; flooding and freezing around the entry hole; alternate thawing and freezing; and the variable characteristics of the ice cover.

Careful planning for ice diving is even more important than for any other type of diving activity. Shelter should be provided over the ice hole for the tenders and for the necessary equipment: proper clothing for protection at the surface and for the underwater activity is mandatory. Transportation and communications present special problems that must be solved; detailed planning for emergency situations is of prime importance.

Falling overboard in polar water or falling through the ice hole is a life-threatening situation because survival time is only a few minutes in near-freezing water. An individual should not attempt to swim unless forced to by lack of life jacket or because there is no chance of rescue by other people. Nor should one attempt to keep warm by exercising while floating in the life jacket; exercise will have the reverse effect. Those on the surface should stay clear of the entry holes unless they are needed to assist the diver, for the ice is usually slick around the perimeter of the holes.

A breathing system failure may occur because of freezing of the respirator. In such event the diver should switch to the backup system, should notify his partner or tender, and should exit to the surface. If the diving suit floods, the diver should surface immediately, since the extreme chilling effect of near-freezing water will put the diver in thermal stress within a few minutes.

If an uncontrolled ascent results from a suit blowup or a lost weight belt, the diver should use this procedure: exhale during ascent; relax against the ice; if suit blowup occurs, purge the exhaust valve; signal the tender to haul in the tether; and wait for assistance from buddy diver or tender. In the event the diver becomes lost under the ice the procedure should be to notify the tender or buddy if possible and make an initial search for the entry hole. If the hole cannot be found, the diver should ascend to the overhead ice cover, maintain positive buoyancy, relax as much as possible (to conserve air), and wait for assistance.

Ice diving requires not only careful planning but the use of common sense. Those who try to outlast and outperform other divers by the use of brute force are a threat not only to themselves but to the entire mission. Necessary risks are bad enough, and dares should neither be offered nor taken. Success depends on planning, attention to detail, and hard work—not on heroics.

CHARLES W. SHILLING

References

BACHRACH, A. J. 1973. Panic. In: *Oceans 2000. Third World Congress of Underwater Activities*. London: British Sub-Aqua Club, p. 29–31.

BARNARD, E. E. P., W. J. EATON, AND R. E. SNOW 1971. Experiments in submarine escape. Rapid compression of men to 625 feet (191 meters). Alverstoke, Engl.: R. Nav. Physiol. Lab. Rep. 10-71.

BALLDIN, U. I. 1978. Intracardial gas bubbles and decompression sickness while flying at 9,000 m within 12–24 h of diving. *Aviat. Space Environ. Med.* 49: 1314–1318.

BEHNKE, A. R., JR. 1970. Reaction 1 [to paper on Diving Behavior]. In: *Human Performance and Scuba Diving. Proceedings of the Symposium on Underwater Physiology, Scripps Institute of Oceanography, La Jolla, CA, Apr. 1970*. Chicago: The Athletic Institute, p. 139–143.

BEHNKE, A. R. 1975. Early quantitative studies of gas dynamics in decompression. In: *The Physiology and Medicine of Diving and Compressed Air Work*, (2nd ed.), edited by P. B. Bennett and D. H. Elliott. London: Ballière, Tindall, p. 392–416. (Baltimore: Williams and Wilkins.)

BEHNKE, A. R. JR., AND T. L. WILLMON 1941. Cutaneous diffusion of helium in relation to peripheral blood flow and absorption of atmospheric nitrogen through the skin. *Am. J. Physiol.* 131: 627–632.

BENNETT, P. B., AND D. H. ELLIOTT 1975. *The Physiology and Medicine of Diving and Compressed-Air Work* (2nd ed.). London: Ballière, Tindall. (Baltimore: Williams and Wilkins.)

BONI, M., R. SCHIBLI, P. NUSSBERGER, AND A. A. BUHLMANN 1976. Diving at diminished atmospheric pressure: air decompression tables for different altitudes. *Undersea Biomed. Res.* 3: 189–204.

BROUHA, L. 1943. The step test: A simple method of measuring physical fitness for muscular work in young men. *Res. Q. Am. Assoc. Health Phys. Educ.* 14: 31–35.

BROWN, C. V. 1976. Drugs and diving. *NAUI News*: 2–3; Mar. 1976 and 12–13; Apr. 1976.

CIRIA UNDERWATER ENGINEERING GROUP 1972. *The Principles of Safe Diving Practice*. London: Construction Industry Research and Information Association.

DAWSON, J. 1972. Safety in the sixth continent. *Mar. Technol. Soc. J.* 6: 28–31. (Professional Diving Safety. Second Annual Symposium of Marine Technology Society, New Orleans, Nov. 1971.)

DEFENSE DOCUMENTATION CENTER 1968a. A DDC bibliography on submarine escape and rescue. Washington, DC: Def. Doc. Cent. Rep. DDC-TAS 6801, vol. 1, Aug. 1968 (AD 838,825).

DEFENSE DOCUMENTATION CENTER 1968b. A DDC bibliography on submarine escape and rescue. Washington, DC: Def. Doc. Cent. Rep. DDC-TAS 68-26, vol. 2, Aug. 1968 (AD 838,665).

DEWEY, A. W., JR. 1962. Decompression sickness. An emergency recreational hazard. *N. Engl. J. Med.* 267: 759-765, 812-819.
DOUBT, T. 1979. The YMCA diving medic program—a first. *Accent Lines* 8(2):10.
DUEKER, C. W. 1978. *Scuba Diving Safety.* Mountain View, CA: World Publications.
EDEL, P. G., J. J. CARROLL, R. W. HONAKER. AND E. L. BECKMAN 1969. Interval at sea-level pressure required to prevent decompression sickness in humans who fly in commercial aircraft after diving. *Aerosp. Med.* 10: 1105-1110.
EGSTROM, G. H., AND A. J. BACHRACH 1971. Diver Panic. *Skin Diver* 20: 36-39.
ELLIOTT, D. H. 1971. Submarine escape from 600 ft. using rapid compression and buoyant ascent. In: *1971 Offshore Technology Conference, Apr. 1971, Houston, TX. Preprints.* Published by the Conference, vol. 2, p. 191-194.
FURRY, D. E., E. REEVES. AND E. BECKMAN 1966. Relationship of scuba diving to the development of aviators' decompression sickness. NUMRI Res. Rep. 5 on MF 011.99-1001. U.S. Navy Underseas Med. Res. Inst. (*Aerosp. Med.* 38: 825-828.)
GELL, C. F., AND J. W. PARKER (editors) 1974. International workshop on escape and survival. U.S. Nav. Submar. Med. Res. Lab. Rep. (NSMRL 794, Oct. 15, 1974.)
GOWDEY, C. W., AND R. B. PHILP 1965. Etiology and treatment of experimental decompression sickness with special references to body lipid. *Mil. Med.* 130: 648-652.
GRONER-STRAUSS, W., AND M. B. STRAUSS 1976. Divers face special peril in use/abuse of drugs. *Physician Sports Med.* 4: 30-36.
GULYAR, S. A., YU. M. BARATE. AND YU. N. KUKLEVICH 1974. Basic principles of human adaptation to the conditions of shallow-depth underwater laboratories. *Usp. Fiziol. Nauk* 5: 82-101.
HALL, D. A., AND J. K. SUMMITT 1970. Simulated deep submarine escape from 495 feet of sea water. U.S. Nav. Submar. Med. Cent. Rep. (SMRL 617, Mar. 18, 1970.)
HALSTEAD, B. 1965-70. *Poisonous and Venomous Marine Animals.* Washington, DC: U.S. Govt. Printing Office, vol. 1, 1965; vol. 2, 1967; vol. 3, 1970.
HANSON, R. DE G., AND J. M. YOUNG 1975. Diving accidents. In: *The Physiology and Medicine of Diving and Compressed Air Work* (2nd ed.), edited by P. B. Bennett and D. H. Elliott. London: Ballière, Tindall, p. 545-556. (Baltimore: Williams and Wilkins.)
JENKINS, W. T. 1973. *A Summary of Diving Techniques Used in Polar Regions. A Preliminary Manual.* Panama City, FL: Naval Coastal System Lab.
JENKINS, W. T. 1974. *A Guide to Polar Diving.* Panama City, FL: Naval Coastal System Lab.
JENKINS, W. T. 1976. *A Guide to Polar Diving.* Panama City, FL: Naval Coastal System Lab.
JENNINGS, R. D., W. JONES, J. ADOLFSON, L. GOLDBERG. AND C. M. HESSER 1977. Changes in man's standing steadiness in the presence of alcohol and hyperbaric air. *Undersea Biomed. Res.* 4:A16. (Abstracts of papers presented at Undersea Medical Society Annual Scientific Meeting, May 13-16, 1977, Toronto, Canada.)
KAIFMAN, M. S. 1976. Drugs and diving. *Triton* 21: 168-169.
KING, W. One clinic's criteria for employment in a compressed air environment. 1970. *J. Occup. Med.* 12: 113-116.
LAVERNHE, J. 1970. Plongées sous-marine et voyage aerien. *Presse Med.* 78: 1449.
MACINNIS, J. B. 1975. Open-sea diving techniques. In: *The Physiology and Medicine of Diving and Compressed Air Work* (2nd ed.), edited by P. B. Bennett and D. H. Elliott. London: Ballière, Tindall, p. 20-33. (Baltimore: Williams and Wilkins.)
MARRIOTT, J. 1969. Submarine search and rescue. *Underwater Sci. Technol. J.* 1: 140-145.
MECKLENBURG, R. L. 1972. To dive or not to dive. *Del. Med. J.* 44: 91-92.
MILES, S. 1969. *Underwater Medicine* (3rd ed.). Philadelphia: Lippincott.
MILLER, J. N. 1975. Life support systems. In: *The Physiology and Medicine of Diving and Compressed-Air Work* (2nd ed.), edited by Bennett, P. B., and D. H. Elliott. London: Baillière, Tindall, and Cox. (Baltimore: Williams and Wilkins.)
MILLER, J. W. 1979. *The NOAA Diving Manual. Diving for Science and Technology.* Washington, DC: Natl. Oceanic and Atmospheric Admin., U.S. Dept. of Commerce.
MINER, A. D. 1961. Scuba hazards to air crew. *Business Pilots Safety Bulletin 61-204.* New York: Flight Safety Foundation.

NEMIROFF, M. J. 1977. Drugs and divers—Case report and comments. *SPUMS J./Newsletter* 17–18; Jan./Mar. 1977.

NUYTTEN, P. 1974. Diving bell escape systems: Some observations and test results. In: *1974 Offshore Technology Conference, May 1974, Houston, TX: Preprints*. Published by the Conference, vol. 1, p. 313–318.

OSER, H. 1972. Medizinische Erfahrungen beim Einsatz des Unterwasserlaboratoriums 'Helgoland' in Herbst 1971. DFVLR-Nachrichten, Aug. 1972, p. 307–308.

PARKER, J. W., AND D. A. HALL 1970. Experimental training for open-sea submarine escape. U.S. Nav. Submar. Med. Cent. Rep. (SMRL 622, Mar. 30, 1970.)

PARKER, J. W., D. A. HALL, AND J. J. MELLON 1970. Open sea, surface evaluation of submarine escape and immersion equipment. U.S. Nav. Submar. Med. Cent. Rep. (SMRL 614, Feb. 20, 1970.)

PFEIFFER, R. 1974. Fly-away diving system near. *Faceplate* 5: 10–11.

PHILP, R. B. 1967. Decompression sickness in experimental animals. In: *Underwater Physiology. Proceedings of the Third Symposium on Underwater Physiology, March 1966, Washington, DC.*, edited by C. J. Lambertsen. Baltimore: Williams and Wilkins, p. 412–424.

PUGH, L. G. C. E. 1965. Temperature regulation in swimmers. In: Rahn, H., and T. Yokoyama (editors). *Physiology of Breath-Hold Diving and the Ama of Japan*, edited by H. Rahn and T. Yokoyama. Washington, DC: Natl. Acad. Sci./Natl. Res. Council, p. 325–348.

RENNIE, D. W. 1965. Thermal insulation of Korean diving women and nondivers in water. In: Rahn, H., and T. Yokoyama (editors). *Physiology of Breath-Hold Diving and the Ama of Japan*. Washington, DC: Natl. Acad. Sci./Natl. Res. Council, p. 315–324.

SAWYER, R. N. 1972. Some aspects of scuba in college health. *J. Am. Coll. Health Assoc.* 20: 323–327.

SAYERS, R. R. 1942. Major studies in fatigue. *War Med. Chicago* 2: 786–823.

SEKI, K., AND M. HUGON 1975. Fatigue subjective et dégradation de performance en environnement hyperbare à saturation. (Subjective fatigue and deterioration of performance in a saturated hyperbaric environment.) *Trav. Hum.* 38: 368–369.

SHILLING, C. W. 1964. *Atomic Energy Encyclopedia in the Life Sciences*. Philadelphia: Saunders.

SHILLING, C. W., M. WERTS, AND N. SCHANDELMEIER (editors) 1976. *The Underwater Handbook. A Guide to Physiology and Performance for the Engineer*. New York: Plenum.

SMITH, R. W. 1975. Application of a medical model to psychopathology in diving. In: *Proceedings of the Sixth International Conference on Underwater Education, Oct. 1974, San Diego, CA*. Natl. Assoc. Underwater Instructors, p. 377–385.

STRAUSS R. H. (editor). 1976. *Diving Medicine*. New York: Grune and Stratton.

STRAUSS, S. 1974. Decompression sickness due to altitude exposure following compressed air diving: a review. New London, Groton, CT: U.S. Nav. Undersea Med. Inst. Thesis.

SUMMERS, L. H. 1972. Research divers manual. Ann Arbor, MI: Univ. of Michigan. (Sea Grant Tech. Rep. 16, MICHU-SG-71-212 A, Aug. 1972.)

TAYLOR, J. D. 1959. The otolaryngologic aspects of skin and scuba diving. *Laryngoscope* 69: 809–858.

TAYLOR, W. F. 1979. Electric heating of divers. In: *International Diving Symposium '79, Association of Diving Contractors, New Orleans, LA, Feb. 1979*, p. 57–62.

UNDERSEA MEDICAL SOCIETY 1979. *Emergency Ascent Training*. Bethesda, MD: Undersea Med. Soc. (Workshop, Bethesda, MD, Dec. 1977.)

U.S. NAVY 1970. *U.S. Navy Radiological Control Manual*. Washington, DC: U.S. Navy Dept. (NAVSEA 0389-LP-015-3000.)

U.S. NAVY 1970. *U.S. Navy Diving Manual*. Washington, DC: U.S. Navy Dept. (NAVSHIPS 0994-001-9010.)

U.S. NAVY 1978. *U.S. Navy Diving Manual (Change 2)*. (NAVSEA 0994-001-9010.)

VANDERAUE, O. E., O. E. KELLER, E. S. BRITTON, G. BARRON, H. D. GILLIAM, AND R. J. JONES. 1951. Calculation and testing of decompression tables for air dives employing the procedure of surface decompression and the use of oxygen. Res. Rep. I. Washington, DC: U.S. Navy Exp. Diving Unit.

VAUGHN, W. S., JR., AND M. B. STRAUSS 1975. Exploratory analysis of predictors of diver performance decrement during 3-hour cold-water exposures. Tech. Rep. on Contract N00014-72-C-0309. Landover, MD: Oceanautics, Inc.

WALSH, J. M. 1976. Drugs and diving. In: *Diving Medicine*, edited by R. H. Strauss. New York: Grune and Stratton, 1976, p. 197–209.

WALKER, D. 1976. Provisional report on diving-related deaths in 1975 (Stickybeak Project). *SPUMS J./ Newsletter* 19–25; Apr.–June.
WEBB, P. 1975. Cold Exposure. In: *The Physiology and Medicine of Diving and Compressed Air Work* (2nd ed.), edited by P. B. Bennett and D. H. Elliott. London: Ballière, Tindall, p. 285–306. (Baltimore: Williams and Wilkins.)
WEBSTER, D. P. 1966. Skin and scuba fatalities in the U.S. In: *U.S. Public Health Rep. 81*. Washington, DC: U.S. Govt. Printing Office, p. 703–711.
WIDMANN, B. 1976. The early warning signs of diving accidents. In: *Proceedings of the Seventh International Conference on Underwater Education, Sept. 1975, Miami Beach*. Natl. Assoc. Underwater Instructors, p. 448–455.

XIV

Equipment and Procedures

A. *Treatment Chambers*

1. *Multiplace Chambers*

a. Introduction

For at least three centuries hyperbaric chambers have been used for a variety of scientific and medical applications. British physician H. Henshaw is credited with being the first to use a hyperbaric chamber for medical treatment (Simpson 1857). In 1664 he published an essay in which he proposed to use an airtight room (domicilium) constructed of masonry where the sick person could remain while the surrounding air was compressed or rarified. He used an organ bellows to compress and rarify air ". . . to help digestion, to promote insensible respiration, to facilitate breathing and expectoration, and consequently, of excellent use for the prevention of most afflictions of the lung." With the advent of the air pump in 1650, Otto van Guerick provided the instrument with which early "pneumatic chemists" and physicians could begin to define the hyperbaric environment. In his studies of pressure-volume relationships, Sir Robert Boyle experimented extensively with laboratory animals, and, in 1670, observed bubbles in living tissue as a result of pressure changes on the eye of a viper. Diving bell operations to 60 ft, for up to 90 min, were conducted by Edmund Halley in 1690, and by 1716 he had published *The Art of Living Underwater*. However, it was not until the advent of the air compressor in 1790 that a large chamber could be pressurized for extended durations, thus making compressed air chambers practical.

In the early 1800s at least 50 hyperbaric chamber facilities were constructed throughout Europe, and "compressed air baths" came into vogue. These early compressed air chambers were used to treat a variety of respiratory, cardiovascular, and surgical problems. Little was known about "compressed air illness," or decompression sickness, at that time. In 1879 a French physician, J. A. Fontaine, described his mobile, 10-person hyperbaric chamber: "With this chamber one can do surgery in hospitals, sanitaria, and private homes." Monsieur Pean, a well-known French surgeon, performed 27 operations in the Fontaine chamber in three months and planned a large hyperbaric surgical amphitheater that would hold 300 people. An unfortunate hyperbaric chamber accident that resulted in Fontaine's death made him the first martyr in hyperbaric medicine and prevented construction of the amphitheater (Jacobson et al. 1965). Apparently this accident also seriously impeded the progress of other therapeutic hyperbaric chambers in Europe, for a short time later an English physician, C. T. Williams (1885), wrote in the *British Medical Journal*: "The use of atmospheric air . . . is one of the most important advances in modern medicine . . . [and] we are astonished that in England, this method of treatment has been so little used."

In reviewing the history of compressed air chambers, one finds that safety factors developed for caisson and diving activities provided important preliminary guidelines for establishing safe hyperbaric chamber environments.

b. Contributions of Caisson Work

In 1839, a French engineer, M. Triger (1841), successfully employed the technique of using air pressure to keep water out of mine shafts—the *caisson*. Using a pressurized iron tube 3 ft in diameter, he was able to reach a deep vein of coal in the valley of the Loire, through 62 ft of quicksand. In 1841 he wrote that coal miners suffered cramps and muscle pains after leaving the caisson, but appeared to get better upon returning to work in the caisson. This strange, new disease was first scientifically described in 1854 by two French physicians, B. Pol and T. J. J. Watelle, who presented a complete discussion with many case histories. By 1850 use of compressed air in mining had become well established, and it was being used for pier building in England. By 1868 caissons were being used for pier and bridge abutment construction across the Mississippi River, and by 1879 the procedure was used for tunnel construction under the Hudson River.

Serious study of the hazards of caisson operations was initiated following the 1854 mining caisson explosion that caused the death of 6 workers (Goodman 1961). The first known fatality from decompression sickness in the United States occurred in 1870 during construction of the Mississippi River bridge caisson (St. Louis Bridge). Decompression sickness was common among workers in the St. Louis Bridge and Brooklyn Bridge caissons during the 1870s. A St. Louis physician, A. Jaminet (1871), wrote of his own caisson disease episode after exposure in the St. Louis Bridge caisson. He described his treatment with Old Jamaica rum (a popular, all-purpose remedy of the time). Jaminet's article on the St. Louis Bridge tunnel work reported 119 cases of caisson disease, 52 developing permanent paralysis and 14 dying, for a 12% mortality rate.

During construction of the Brooklyn Bridge, Dr. A. H. Smith (1873), the surgeon of the New York Bridge Company, described caisson disease as a disease depending on increased atmospheric pressure but always developing after removal of the pressure. He proposed to have a special iron treatment lock (9 ft × 3.5 ft) built, in which workers stricken with caisson disease would be recompressed to a pressure equal to that at which they had been working previously, followed by several hours of decompression to the surface. In 1873 his printed rules (Smith 1873) for caisson workers on the Brooklyn Bridge project at pressures greater than 24 psig were as follows:

1st   Never enter the caisson with an empty stomach.

2nd   Use as far as possible a meat diet, and take warm coffee freely.

3rd	Always put on extra clothing on coming out and avoid exposure to cold.
4th	Exercise as little as may be during the first hour after coming out, and lie down if possible.
5th	Use intoxicating liquors sparingly; better not at all.
6th	Take at least eight hours sleep every night.
7th	See that the bowels are open every day.
8th	Never enter the caisson if at all sick.
9th	Report at once all cases of illness, even if they occur after going home.

In spite of 4-hr work cycles (2 per day) and medical examinations to eliminate "heart and lung diseases and those enfeebled by age or intemperance," 110 cases of caisson disease were reported, 3 of which were fatal.

When French physiologist Paul Bert formulated the bubble theory of compressed air illness in his 1878 classic work *Barometric Pressure*, he provided convincing evidence for using a recompression chamber to treat caisson disease. In 1879 when the Hudson River tunnel project began, compulsory medical exams were required on the 14,300 workmen. Despite these medical clearances there were 1575 cases of decompression sickness and three deaths (Goodman 1961). A recompression chamber was installed at the Hudson River tunnel at Jersey City in 1889, in which Sir Ernest W. Moir was able to effectively treat patients suffering from decompression sickness.

In order to protect caisson workers, the State of New York adopted a legislative bill for prevention of compressed air illness in 1909. New York subsequently established the first state code regulating work in compressed air in 1910. This was followed by New Jersey (1914) and Pennsylvania (1917) bills. The documents were prepared by the American Association for Labor Legislation. The 1921 Public Service Commission analysis of tunnel morbidity reported 680 cases of decompression sickness in 1,361,461 decompressions (Penzias and Goodman 1973). By 1939 safety codes for work in compressed air had been adopted by eight states. These codes specified the hours of work at specific depths, the decompression rules, a period of observation following decompression, and the number of air chambers that had to be used in a tunnel (Hoff 1948). Later safety codes developed for caisson workers were to have a profound influence on recompression chamber equipment and use. Much that had been learned about the medical management of caisson disease thus created a safer environment for occupants of recompression chambers. Conversely, acceptable equipment (such as wood deck flooring and electric motors) and customs (such as smoking) in the moist, compressed-air environment of the caissons would later prove to be fatal in the dry, oxygen-enriched environment of recompression chambers.

c. Contributions of Diving

When Augustus Siebe introduced his original brass-helmeted, leather diving suit in 1819 it became practical for divers to work with surface-supplied air at depths up to 100 ft (30.5 m) for extended periods of time. William H. James' design of a self-contained diving outfit in 1825 provided the diver with a portable air supply and the freedom to dive without a surface air supply. Slow, continuous descents and ascents at rates of about 5 ft/min were a common practice.

Exhaustion and decompression sickness were common among these early divers, particularly whenever they performed work at depths greater than 70 ft (21 m). A French physician, L. R. de Mericourt (1869), published the first comprehensive medical report on diver's decompression sickness. It was not until 1882 that U.S. Navy divers received instruction in diving procedures at the U.S. Naval Torpedo Station, Newport, Rhode Island (Penzias and Goodman 1973). Although graduates of the Seaman Gunners School were qualified to dive only to 60 ft of seawater (fsw) or 18 m (msw), they were employed for several salvage and construction projects, and for ship repairs.

In 1905 the British admirably acknowledged the need for improved safety in diving, and appointed a deep-diving committee to investigate the hazards of compressed air diving. A member of the committee, British physiologist J. S. Haldane, and his colleagues (Boycott et al. 1908) made two significant contributions to diving safety: First, he demonstrated that the amount of air pumped to a diver must increase in proportion to the increase in pressure. Second, he derived a rational basis for computing decompression schedules, and recommended the "stage decompression" method for safe ascent to the surface. The admiralty adopted Haldane's recommendation in 1907 and set the limit on diving operations at 210 ft (64 m).

In December 1912, U.S. Navy Warrent Gunner George T. Stillson was granted permission by the Bureau of Construction and Repair to test the practicality of the stage decompression method for U.S. Navy divers. For this purpose, his group was established as the U.S. Navy Experimental Diving Station at the New York Naval Shipyard in Brooklyn. Extensive tests were conducted in the "diving tanks" at the factory of A. Schrader's Son, Inc., in Brooklyn. Sea tests were conducted from the deck of the U.S.S. *Walke* in Long Island Sound at depths as great as 274 ft or 84 m (Penzias and Goodman 1973). These successful tests quadrupled the maximum diving depths for U.S. Navy divers. This was fortunate, because the rapidly expanding U.S. submarine fleet was plagued with a series of accidents, collisions, and mishaps over the next two decades. These submarine disasters drew heavily on the U.S. Navy diving capability for rescue and salvage (U.S. Navy 1978).

In 1924, the U.S. Navy Diving School was established at Newport, Rhode Island, and the first *U.S. Navy Diving Manual* was published. The manual specified the requirement for compression chambers to support deep-diving operations: "In all cases of deep-diving operations, a compression chamber of some sort is essential, as without the compression chamber there is no efficient method of treating caisson disease other than to send the diver down again to the proper depth of decompression." By 1924 rigid physical standards and frequent reexaminations were required for deep-sea divers in the U.S. Navy. Furthermore, divers were automatically disqualified when becoming 40 years old (Shilling 1938). Surface decompression was first used by the U.S. Navy in salvage operations for the submarine *S-51* in 1925. Surface decompression became routine by the 1930s, and the U.S. Navy entered the recompression chamber business. Later, the breathing of oxygen or oxygen mixtures during treatment decompression was recommended by A. R. Behnke and L. A. Shaw (1937). Research and treatment profiles using oxygen advanced more rapidly than the supporting chamber safety program, and a series of accidents occurred, principally due to fire in the oxygen-enriched atmosphere. One example was a 1939 shipboard chamber interior that was ignited by a chamber attendant's cigar when he opened the door to the oxygen-enriched environment. The four occupants had been oxygen decompressing by mask, causing exhalation gases to accumulate within the chamber. The chamber had been pressurized with air from an oil-lubricated compressor. Fortunately, the four occupants survived (A. R. Behnke, personal communication).

In order to facilitate realistic escape training for all submarine personnel, large training tanks were constructed at the New London and Pearl Harbor submarine bases 1930–1932. The 138-ft high steel cylinders provided a 100-ft vertical column of water with submarine escape locks providing entry points at 18-, 50-, and 100-ft depths (Figure XIV-1). Trainees were provided "vigorous training in submarine escape" under condi-

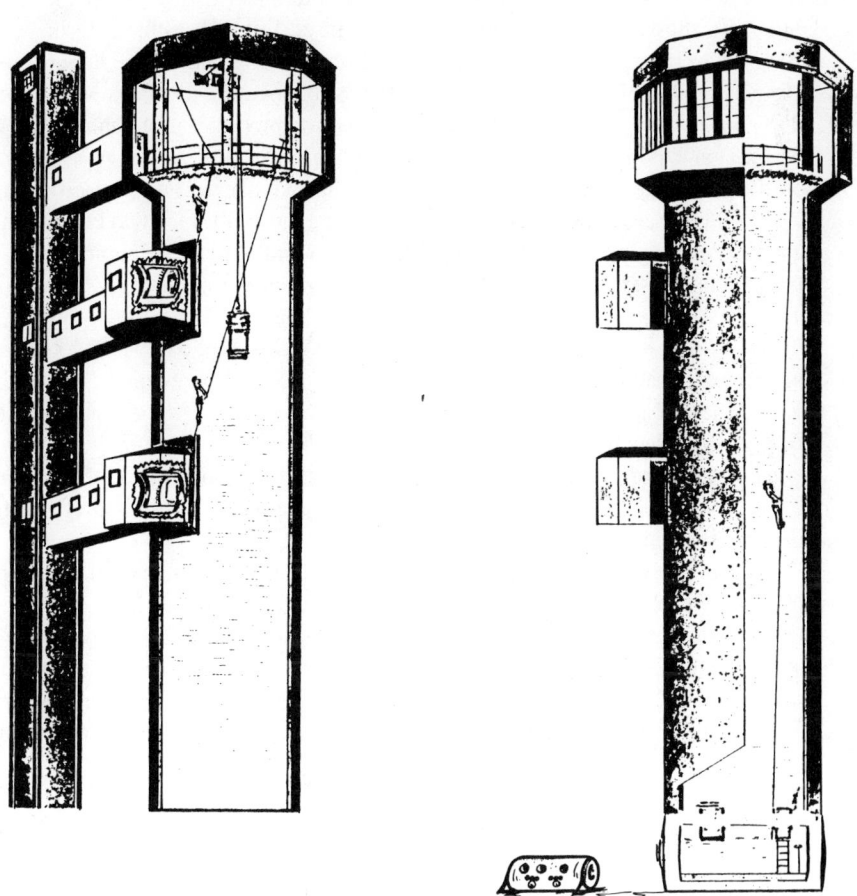

Figure XIV-1. Submarine Escape Training Tank, U.S. Navy Submarine Center, New London, CT, in 1953. This submarine escape training tank was constructed at a cost of $120,000 and completed in August 1930. It has an overall height of 138.5 ft and contains a vertical column of water 100 ft high and 18 ft in diameter. Submarine escape locks are located at depths from the top of the tank at 18 ft, 50 ft, and 100 ft. Before surfacing, the trainee must perform a controlled breathing exercise, enter the tank through a submarine lock, and continuously exhale during ascent. While equalizing lung pressure with decreasing external pressure, the trainee may surface at rates up to 375 ft/min.

tions identical to those existing in similar depths at sea. In the first 15 years of operation approximately 83,000 submarine trainees received this valuable training in the New London tank alone. Recompression chambers were positioned at the training tanks for treatment of air embolism among trainees and decompression sickness in rare occasion among instructors. According to Submarine Medicine Practices instructions written in 1956 (U.S. Navy 1956b), attendance of a medical officer was required at training exercises, but his capacity was "... advisory rather than authoritative. During normal tank operation his attention is devoted to prevention of casualties; any violation of safety measures or other undue hazards should be brought tactfully to the attention of the tank officer who is present in order for the situation to be remedied. In medical emergencies the doctor takes charge of his patient." During the 27-year period 1930–1957, 62 accidents occurred, 17 of which occurred during recompression treatment (Moses 1964).

To cope with the severe mental impairments caused by air breathing during deep diving, testing and research on helium-oxygen mixtures were initiated at the U.S. Bureau of Mines Experimental Station in Pittsburgh, Pennsylvania. By 1927 the need for a centralized diving-related research and testing effort prompted the establishment of the Naval Experimental Diving Unit (NEDU) at the U.S. Naval Gun Factory (Washington, D.C.) Soon afterward, the Navy School of Diving and Salvage was also reactivated at the Washington Navy Yard. The facilities installed during the 1930s included two pressure tanks capable of working pressures of 350 psi (788 fsw) and adjoining double-lock, 200 psi (450 fsw) recompression chamber. The NEDU recompression chambers were also equipped for altitude experimental work (U.S. Navy 1956a).

In the mid 1930s, three U.S. Navy physicians, C. W. Shilling, A. R. Behnke, and O. E. VanDerAue, became the first medical staff at the Navy Experimental Diving Unit (Carter 1977). Their monumental compression chamber research efforts resulted in the institution of surface decompression for divers in shipboard decompression chambers, the installation of air conditioning systems in submarines, the establishment of maximum safe limits for oxygen breathing at depth, and the establishment of safe use of helium-oxygen mixtures for deep-sea diving.

By 1939 chamber dives had been made to 500 ft using helium-oxygen breathing, and at-sea testing was ready to start, when the submarine *Squalus*, with a 50-man crew, sank in 243 ft (74 m) of water near Portsmouth, New Hampshire. All the 33 crew members who survived the initial sinking were rescued by a "rescue chamber"—a specially equipped diving bell designed by Commander Allen R. McCann. Combining helium-oxygen diving and surface decompression using oxygen, salvage divers were also able to raise the *Squalus* (Carter 1977).

By the early 1950s rapid advancement in helium-oxygen diving technology necessitated the construction of recompression chambers with increased depth capability and improved built-in breathing systems. From oxygen toxicity studies came the establishment of oxygen-breathing limits for working scuba divers. In 1958 unmanned testing in the chambers became possible through the introduction of a breathing machine that simulated the gas flow requirements of the diver.

Although F. L. Keays (Keays 1909) had reported 3692 cases of decompression sickness in 1909 and had insisted that recompression was the treatment of choice for decompression sickness, there was no accepted recompression schedule until 1924, when the first standard recompression treatment procedure was published in the *U.S. Navy*

Diving Manual. Unfortunately, the Navy's air decompression procedure resulted in recurrence of symptoms in more than 50% of the individuals treated (VanDerAue et al. 1945). Research conducted by A. R. Behnke and L. A. Shaw (1937) resulted in an oxygen treatment table recognized by the U.S. Navy Bureau of Medicine and Surgery in 1937. However, the early oxygen treatment schedules provided little change in the symptom recurrence rate. In 1945 investigators at the Naval Medical Research Institute reported the results of a series of tests to formulate comprehensive tables for treatment of decompression sickness and air embolism. Results of these studies provided the treatment tables (Tables I–IV) used by the U.S. Navy until 1965. Because of a low success rate for the more severe cases of decompression sickness, M. W. Goodman and R. D. Workman (1965) developed the Oxygen Treatment Tables 5, 5A, 6, and 6A, which are now considered the standard for treating decompression sickness and air embolism.

Perhaps one of the most revolutionary developments in diving technology was the postwar modification of scuba. The Aqua-lung by J. Y. Cousteau, and E. Gagnan and C. J. Lambertsen's Amphibious Respiratory Units were routinely used during World War II in prediving operations such as reconnaissance and demolition of underwater obstacles (U.S. Navy 1978). Scuba-related equipment developed in the 1950s became available to the public, and the publication of the U.S. Navy Standard Air Decompression Tables in 1959 (U.S. Navy 1959) met a ready commercial market as sport scuba diving became one of the nation's fastest growing sports. Then hyperbaric chambers took on a new challenge: treatment of sport diving casualties. In a 10-year (1956–1965) statistical summary of U.S. Navy diving accidents, T. E. Berghage (1966) reported that the Navy Experimental Diving Unit received 78 diving accident reports per year. In the medical management of decompression sickness (51.2%) and overpressure of the lungs (9.6%), he estimated that 4600 man-hours were spent each year to treat U.S. Navy divers with recompression and another 3800 man-hours were spent annually for recompression treatment of civilians and other military personnel.

The feasibility of saturation diving techniques was proved in the 1960s by the separate efforts of three individuals: Jacques Yves Cousteau, Edwin A. Link, and Captain George F. Bond. By 1969, submerged "sea lab" habitats had enabled humans to remain in the sea at depths exceeding 205 ft (63 m) for periods as long as 30 days (U.S. Navy 1978). This led to the development of the deep-diving systems of the 1970s, which provided a method for maintaining the saturated divers under pressure in a dry environment. Furthermore, development of the U.S. Navy Unlimited Duration Excursion Tables enhanced the vertical mobility of saturation divers (U.S. Navy 1977).

The 1975 relocation of the Navy Experimental Diving Unit to the world's largest hyperbaric complex in Panama City, Florida, provides researchers with immense new capability for research in its ocean-simulating facility at depths up to 2250 ft or 686 m (Carter 1977).

d. Contributions of Aviation

As early as 1917 Yandell Henderson predicted the possibility of decompression sickness in aviators. In the 1930s, when balloon and aircraft altitude records were set at altitudes above 50,000 ft (15,250 m), altitude decompression sickness became a common occurrence. Prior to 1959, among the 743 serious (Type II) cases of this disorder, at least

18 aviators died from altitude decompression sickness (Davis et al, 1977). Meanwhile, the medical community argued about its etiology and management and used a variety of descriptive or made-up words to describe the disorder. Although A. R. Behnke treated an altitude decompression sickness case in 1941, it was not until the 1959 case described by A. M. Donnell and C. P. Norton (1960) that compression therapy became the recognized treatment of choice for altitude decompression sickness. Dramatic successes in the hyperbaric chamber treatment of military aviators suffering altitude decompression sickness between 1959 and 1963 led to the establishment of a formal Hyperbaric Medicine Program in the U.S. Air Force.

In the early 1960s, the U.S. Air Force School of Aerospace Medicine installed a sophisticated hypo-hyperbaric chamber at Brooks Air Force Base, Texas, for conducting animal studies to elucidate mechanisms and treatment methods for altitude decompression sickness. Studies demonstrated the bubble etiology of altitude decompression sickness as seen in divers, and confirmed the effectiveness of compression to greater than sea level pressure for those cases that persisted after return to ground level. In 1965 the U.S. Air Force, under the guidance of Colonel J. C. Davis, initiated a program to install hyperbaric chambers at strategic locations in the United States and abroad to treat altitude decompression sickness. The early staff of physicians and technicians were trained in the U.S. Navy's formal courses.

The Air Force purchased eight standard Navy double-lock recompression chambers and located them to augment existing Navy and civilian hyperbaric chambers. In 10 years, more than 145 cases of altitude decompression sickness were treated (Davis et al. 1977). Since the institution of this program there have been no fatalities due to altitude decompression sickness and, with the exception of one small but permanent scotoma, all patients treated have fully recovered. Refinements in the oxygen-breathing/air-breathing periods for the treatment tables were instituted at the U.S. Air Force Hyperbaric Center, and were recognized by the U.S. Navy in the 1978 *U.S. Navy Diving Manual*. Modern systems and methods of transportation via air evacuation from remote diving areas to recompression chambers have been a spin-off of this program.

e. Contributions of Clinical Chambers

Meanwhile, other important clinical applications for hyperbaric oxygenation were being considered. In 1955, W. H. Brummelkamp, J. Hoendijk, and I. Boerema (1961) at the University of Amsterdam Medical School used hyperbaric oxygenation (HBO) to treat anaerobic infections and perform open-heart surgery. In 1960, when I. Boerema and his associates (1960) published the classic "Life Without Blood" documenting his research involving removal of erythrocytes from pigs with no ill effects during hyperbaric oxygen exposures, the medical community developed new enthusiasm for hyperbaric oxygen therapy. When the concept of performing open-heart surgery in room-size hyperbaric chambers was introduced, several large facilities were installed in U.S. civilian medical centers. Early use of these chambers for vascular surgery was generally disappointing and they are now rarely used for this purpose. During the 1960s monoplace chambers using 100% oxygen were introduced to apply HBO during radiation therapy for cancer. This application of HBO also was disappointing. On the other hand, at the first and second international conferences on hyperbaric medicine (Amsterdam, 1963;

Glasgow, 1964) good results were reported in the treatment of clostridial myonecrosis (gas gangrene) (Brummelkamp et al. 1961) and carbon monoxide poisoning (Douglas et al. 1964).

In 1965 U.S. Air Force hyperbaric medicine teams began accepting life- or limb-saving cases of gas gangrene and carbon monoxide poisoning, with excellent results in cases referred promptly upon diagnosis (Davis et al. 1973).

By the early 1970s there were reports of success in clinical series using HBO in chronic refractory osteomyelitis (Depenbusch 1972), maxillofacial osteoradionecrosis (Mainous and Boyne 1974), osteogenesis enhancement of bone grafts (Mainous et al. 1973), preservation of failing skin grafts (Perrins 1970), and promotion of granulation and epithelial coverage of chronic, nonhealing wounds in soft tissue (Niinikoski 1969). Laboratory animal studies by T. K. Hunt and M. P. Pai (1972) indicated increased fibroblastic activity when oxygen tension of ischemic, hypoxic wounds was elevated toward normal. S. A. Ketchum and associates (1970) demonstrated extensive capillary proliferation by Day 18 in experimental burn wounds of rats, after daily HBO treatments. G. D. Winter and D. J. D. Perrins (1970) reported an HBO dose-response in the epithelization of experimental wounds in pigs. It appeared from many similar studies that wound healing was enhanced with intermittent HBO.

As a result of these studies, in 1974 the Air Force Surgeon General established a hyperbaric center at the U.S. Air Force School of Aerospace Medicine, Brooks Air Force Base, Texas, for a comprehensive evaluation of this clinical modality. By September 1979, more than 1000 patients had been treated with HBO with an 80% success rate. Perhaps the most important contribution to hyperbaric chamber safety in recent years was the 1977 publication of *Hyperbaric Oxygen Therapy* by J. C. Davis and T. K. Hunt. This textbook, published by the Undersea Medical Society, summarizes the modern practice of hyperbaric medicine and current safety practices (Davis and Hunt 1977).

f. Development of Safety Codes

Advancements in hyperbaric oxygen therapy brought a new dimension to medicine. It also carried new safety considerations. The medical condition of each patient demanded a variety of medical support equipment and services inside the chamber: i.e., equipment for electrocardiography, defibrillation, suction, blood gas analysis, and other supportive equipment. The literature contained warnings and concern about general safety features in design and operation of clinical chambers (Boerema 1965; Brown and Smith 1965; Meijne 1973). New potential dangers included communications, fire potential, mechanical injury, oxygen toxicity, and decompression methods. The warnings were not unfounded, as three fatal fires occurred in rapid succession: in 1965, a fatal fire at the Naval Experimental Diving Unit; in 1965, a fatal fire in the 100% oxygen altitude chamber at Brooks Air Force Base, Texas; and in 1967, the fatal fire in the 100% oxygen Apollo Command Module. Extensive studies were made into the causes and circumstances of catastrophic accidents in both altitude and diving chambers. One report discussed 11 fires in chambers (7 in hyperbaric chambers) with enriched oxygen atmospheres, most of which had been ignited by an electrical source (Alger and Nichols 1971). Safety of the patients and personnel suddenly became a prime consideration in chamber design and operation. In an attempt to establish firm safety guidelines, particularly concerning fire safety, a number of safety codes were wisely developed for hyperbaric chambers. In 1968, the U.S. Navy initiated a system certification program to certify hyperbaric chambers and diver equipment used by Navy personnel (U.S. Navy 1973). Other organizations also developed safety codes for hyperbaric facilities: Compressed Gas Association (1966), National Fire Protection Association (1970), U.S. Department of Labor, Occupational Safety and Health Administration (1977), and others. Application of these codes unquestionably reduced risk to persons using the chambers. In some areas, however, particularly in fire safety, some of the codes became so restrictive as to be unrealistic, making compliance virtually impossible, until their revision in the 1980s. The ever-increasing use of deep-diving systems in support of offshore oil exploration and underwater pipelines resulted in international concern for the safety of divers and in special safety legislation for those hyperbaric facilities. The Department of Labor OSHA standards (1977) developed for these chambers reflect the U.S. Government's concern over the safety aspects of the chamber.

Design and construction criteria for pressure vessels have existed for many years. Construction in accordance with American Society of Mechanical Engineers (ASME) codes has proved to be a satisfactory approach to practical, safe hyperbaric chambers. And more recently, ASME codes were expanded to include design and construction of pressure vessels for human occupancy (ASME 1977). For the most part, hyperbaric chambers constructed in the United States today follow the stringent structural safety guidelines of the ASME codes. But the operational safety aspect of the chamber is delegated to the physician and his staff who operate it.

As the use of hyperbaric chambers becomes more diversified in the treatment of deep-diving casualties and a larger list develops for clinical applications of hyperbaric oxygen treatment, it becomes imperative that the physician understand basic principles for safe chamber operations. Figures XIV-2 to XIV-4 show exterior and interior views of a hyperbaric treatment chamber.

g. Principles of Safe Treatment Chamber Operations

To safely utilize the treatment chamber, the physician must understand the engineering design and adhere to prescribed operating procedures. Specifically, these safety principles must be considered: (1) Structural integrity of the pressure boundary, (2) Safety in handling gas, (3) Electrical safety, (4) Fire safety, (5) Operational safety, (6) Chamber crew qualification. Although there have been hundreds of thousands of safe, manned dives, a few accidents have occurred when safe practices were disregarded (Sheffield and Heimbach 1981).

(i).Structural Integrity of the Pressure Boundary. The hyperbaric chamber must be carefully engineered, and then tested to ensure structural integrity of the pressure vessel prior to its use as a treatment chamber (Sheffield, Davis, and Cutrona 1977). Failure of the pressure vessel would result in rapid decompression of its occupants, and, depending on the rate of decompression, severe injuries such as pneumothorax, air embolism, or decompression sickness could occur.

> *Case 1.* A 60-yr-old patient with advanced bladder cancer was in his second week of daily treatments in a study to combine use of hyperbaric oxygen at 3 ATA with 200 rads daily from a cobalt-60 unit. The patient was

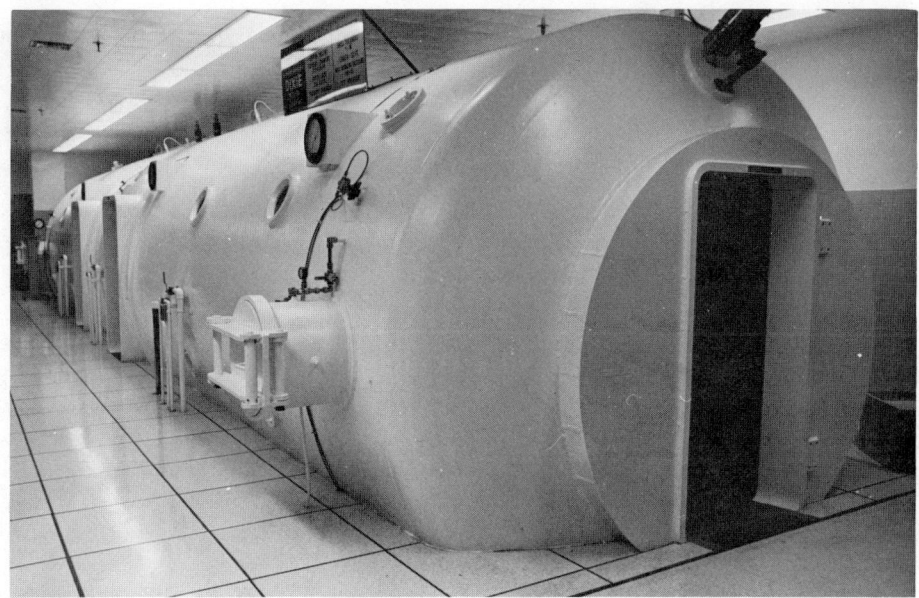

Figure XIV-2. Exterior of a multiplace hyperbaric treatment chamber. (Photo Maryland Institute for Environmental Medical Services.)

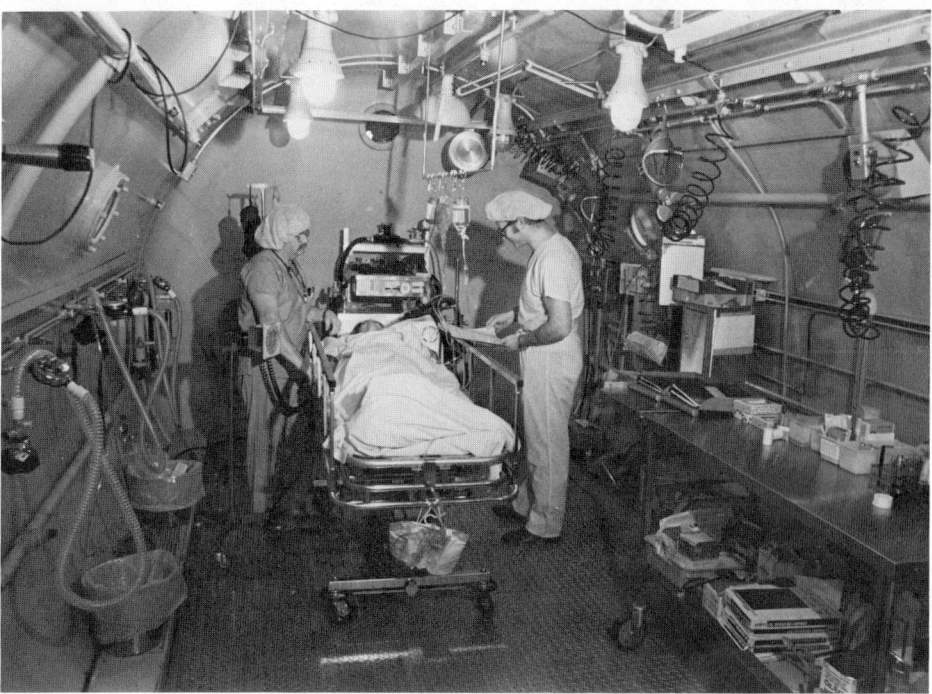

Figure XIV-3. Interior of a multiplace hyperbaric treatment chamber being used for treatment. (Photo Maryland Institute for Environmental Medical Services.)

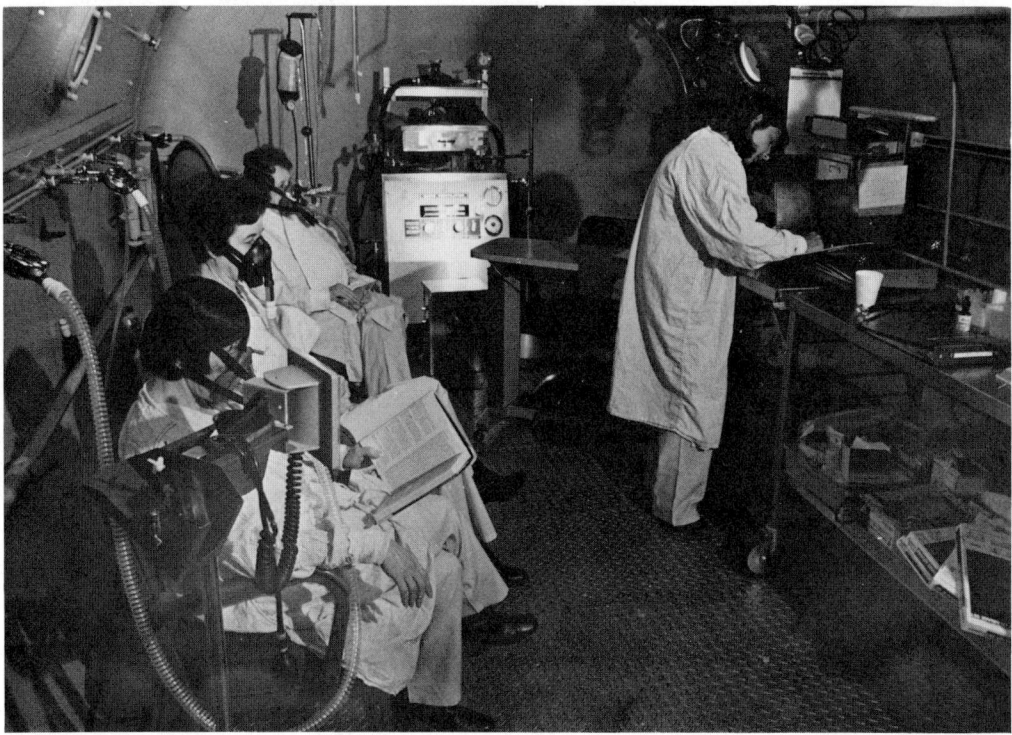

Figure XIV-4. Interior of same multiplace chamber as in Figure XIV-3, this time being used for simultaneous treatment of three seated patients. (Photo Maryland Institute for Environmental Medical Services.)

pressurized in a monoplace plastic chamber to 3 ATA on 100% oxygen. At 29 min into the treatment cycle the plastic portion of the chamber spontaneously ruptured, resulting in explosive decompression of the patient to the surface. Large chunks of plastic were propelled with projectile velocity around the cobalt unit room. The radiation technician, who was standing some distance away, incurred lacerations over the forehead. The research director, who was bending over the chamber at the time of explosion, received the full force of the exploding plastic on his mandible and was thrown back across the room. His injuries included multiple mandibular fractures, lumbar and left shoulder injuries, and extensive facial lacerations. The patient suffered a bilateral hemopneumothorax that was relieved by chest tube. The patient was able to reinitiate radiation therapy in 10 days (Tobin 1971).

Pressure integrity is not assured forever when a newly installed chamber passes the hydrostatic and pneumatic pressure tests. However, periodic inspection and specific maintenance procedures can virtually assure it. Periodic inspection for corrosion and surface cracks should be made, particularly around welds. The chamber must be kept clean and dry. Viewport seals and door gaskets should be cleaned and inspected regularly. Viewports should be protected from thermal stress and mechanical damage. As a safety precaution, metal disks or "port plugs" are maintained in some chambers and can be used by the inside occupant to cover a damaged viewport for immediate recompression. Heat from high-intensity lights is known to have caused rupture of a glass viewport in one instance.

Case 2. A new surgical procedure in a pressurized animal chamber was being televised. Under the extreme heat of high-intensity television lights, the viewport failed. (Failure of the glass was caused by a temperature differential from the cold air on the interior during decompression and heat on the exterior from the television lights.) Fortunately, no one was injured, but there was considerble damage to the wall adjacent to the chamber (Sheffield and Heimback 1981).

Pressure integrity of both the piping and pressurized support equipment is important. One technician was severely injured by the explosion of an oxygen cylinder he was filling.

Case 3. Violating established safety procedures, a technician charged a low pressure (450 psi) oxygen cylinder from a high pressure source without using a pressure gauge. During this process, the technician held the low pressure cylinder between his legs, planning to charge the cylinder until it was warm to touch. The resulting explosion caused severe lacerations and trauma to the technician's thighs and genitalia. Calculations revealed that the low pressure cylinder had been charged to about 850 psi when it exploded.

(ii.) Safety in Handling Gas. Chamber Air. The chamber can be pressurized by one of three methods: compressed gas provided directly from a compressor; compressed gas stored in an accumulator; or mixed oxygen and nitrogen from a cryogenic hyperbaric gas system. Monoplace chambers are usually pressurized with pure oxygen from an accumulator source. Multiplace chambers are usually pressurized with compressed air, and occupants receive special gases via a mask or head tent delivery system. An accumulator is usually used to store the air prior to chamber pressurization. Compressor air should be checked for possible contaminants at intervals not to exceed 6 months, but preferably every month. Carbon monoxide, oil mist, and occasional solvents are typical contaminants. Oil-lubricated compressors require high-quality filtration systems and strict filter maintenance to ensure delivery of air uncontaminated by oil and carbon monoxide. They also require continuous monitoring for contaminants (carbon monoxide, carbon dioxide, and hydrocarbons). Maximum levels for contaminants are shown in Table XIV-1. Standards of air purity established by the U.S. Navy Bureau of Medicine and Surgery

TABLE XIV-1

Maximum Levels for Contaminants in Hyperbaric Chamber Air[a]

Oxygen concentration	20% to 22% by volume
Carbon dioxide	0.05% by volume (500 ppm)
Carbon monoxide	0.001% by volume (10 ppm)
Gaseous hydrocarbons (e.g., methane, ethane)	0.0025% by volume (25 ppm)
Halogenated solvent	0.00002% by volume (0.2 ppm)
Oil and particulate matter	0.005 mg/liter, wgt/vol
Total water	0.3 mg/liter, wgt/vol
Odor	None

[a] Adapted from Hamilton and Sheffield 1977.

(U.S. Navy 1978) for scuba operations are slightly more liberal for carbon dioxide (1000 ppm) and carbon monoxide (20 ppm).

When air samples show contamination by oil and particulate matter, the air flasks and accumulator should be cleaned with an alkaline-type cleaner (such as lye), rinsed with clean, hot water (100°C), and air dried. The source of carbon monoxide in the air system is usually through the intake of contaminated air, but it can also be a product formed by "flashing" of an overheated, oil-lubricated compressor. When carbon monoxide is detected in the compressed gas, the source must be found and eliminated. Intake pollution can be controlled with suitable absorbers. However, the best practice is to avoid placing the compressor intake near areas where atmospheric pollution occurs, such as sewage manholes or engine exhausts, or where toxic or noxious gases are released into the atmosphere.

> *Case 4.* A treatment dive was terminated when the high pressure, oil-lubricated compressor failed. It was noticed to be spraying oil through the pop-off valve. Gas analysis of air pumped in the backup air flasks immediately prior to compressor failure indicated the presence of 14% carbon monoxide.

Oxygen Delivery and Control. The breathing gas system in a chamber is the life-support system for chamber occupants. It provides the patient and inside medical attendants with oxygen, compressed air, or mixed gases via mask or head tent. Because of the shallow depths used in therapeutic chambers, mixed gases are usually restricted to: heliox (a mixture of 80% helium and 20% oxygen), which is sometimes used to prevent nitrogen narcosis in dives to pressures greater than 4 ATA; and nitrox (a mixture of 50% nitrogen and 50% oxygen), which is sometimes used as a treatment gas at pressures of 4–6 ATA.

One must always ensure that the gas in the cylinder is consistent with the label on the bottle and never assume that the vendor has delivered the gas shown on the label.

> *Case 5.* Gas analysis before a treatment dive revealed 80% oxygen in the 100% oxygen line. Treatment was delayed until an alternate oxygen source could be obtained. Investigation revealed that the vendor had mistakenly recharged the hospital liquid oxygen ball with liquid nitrogen.

A breathing gas system is essential for therapeutic multiplace chambers, since they are pressurized with compressed air. The system is usually used only for oxygen delivery to patients during therapy and to attendants during oxygen decompression schedules. However, it also serves as an emergency breathing gas system in the rare event that contamination of chamber air is suspected. A properly fitted anesthesia or aviator's mask will deliver essentially 100% oxygen to the patient, whereas other hospital masks will deliver only about 40%–80% oxygen (Sheffield, Stork, and Morgan 1977). Pure oxygen breathing should never be used at pressures greater than 3 ATA because of toxic effects on the central nervous system. In any case, the life-support system should be equipped with an overboard dump capability to exhaust exhaled gases outside the chamber.

Ventilation Requirements. The buildup of carbon dioxide from individuals enclosed in the chamber demands that the carbon dioxide be removed. This can be accomplished by venting the chamber with fresh air or by scrubbing the carbon dioxide with an absorber such as Sodasorb or lithium hydroxide. Limits established by the *U.S. Navy Diving Manual* (1978) allow an effective (surface equivalent) carbon dioxide concentration of not more than 1.5%. To keep the concentration at a safe level, the chamber can be continuously vented at a rate of 4 ft^3/min (1.22 m^3/min) per occupant. If this well-established ventilation procedure is used to control chamber carbon dioxide levels, continuous carbon dioxide monitoring of therapeutic hyperbaric chambers is unnecessary.

Whenever 100% oxygen is breathed by chamber occupants there is a potential for increased oxygen concentration inside the chamber, and continuous monitoring is required. Venting requirements are minimized by using a mask overboard dump system. The *U.S. Navy Diving Manual* (1978) allows a true oxygen percentage (at any pressure) of not more than 29%, but others recommend a more conservative value of 23% (Hamilton and Sheffield 1977). Venting of the chamber should be accomplished at a rate to keep the oxygen concentration within an acceptable range as shown by the oxygen monitor.

One must not forget that the hyperbaric chamber is a sealed environment. As persons inside the chamber consume oxygen in an unvented chamber, the potential for hypoxia exists. The time required to consume the oxygen inside the chamber will vary with the size of the chamber and number of occupants. Hypoxia can be insidious and deadly, particularly when the chamber is accidentally diluted with inert gas. Dizziness occurs when oxygen concentration drops below 10% at 1 ATA, and unconsciousness and death occur at levels below 5% at 1 ATA.

Hypoxia is not a constant threat in large therapeutic chambers, because of the large chamber volume and because the oxygen concentration is usually elevated. However, the chamber team must understand the danger, and provide an adequate oxygen exchange schedule, especially when special gas mixes are used.

> *Case 6.* A research chamber was decompressed to atmospheric pressure while the gas inside the hyperbaric chamber contained an oxygen content of only 5%. Upon surfacing, the four divers inside were found by the outside crew to be dozing peacefully. Upon exposure to atmospheric air, they recovered from the hypoxic episode with no ill effects (Sheffield and Heimbach 1981).

(iii.) Electrical Safety. Electrical components are important considerations in chamber safety because of the potential shock hazard and the potential ignition source for a chamber fire. Conductive surgical shoes are recommended for chamber occupants (Sheffield, Davis, Bell, and Gallagher 1977). All electrical components should share a common ground, and ultraisolation transformers should be used on all instruments with leads passing into the chamber. Power wiring should not share penetrations or be bundled with physiological leads (Hamilton et al. 1970). If power is supplied to equipment inside the chamber, it should be isolated and have a ground-fault interrupter to shut off the electric power supply to the chamber should there be any abnormal fluctuation in current. Temporary electrical appliances should be avoided whenever possible, since these devices have been the principle ignition source in chamber fires. In Alger and Nichol's (1971) survey of 11 hypobaric and hyperbaric chamber fires, 10 were ignited by an electrical source in the presence of increased oxygen concentration.

> *Case 7.* "Fire! Turn off the electricity!" was the cry from inside the chamber. Within 10 sec the chamber was engulfed in flames. The fire started in the polyvinyl insulation of an extension cord that provided temporary power to a fluorescent lamp and camera assembly. In the 75%–80% oxygen, 2-ATA environment, flames rapidly spread to papers on the floor. In the absence of a fire suppression system, two physicians and two patients perished while trying to stamp out the fire with their feet (Alger and Nichols 1971).

(iv) Fire Safety. Fire prevention is a primary safety concern because of the special considerations of the hyperbaric environment: increased flammability in oxygen-enriched environments, the problems of extinguishment and escape, and the rapid rise in chamber pressure that accompanies the temperature change. The fatal hyperbaric chamber fires to date were caused by a combination of factors: elevated oxygen concentration, abundance of burnables, inadequate extinguishments, and faulty electricial components (Alger and Nichols 1971, Dorr 1971). Three components must be present in order to produce a fire: burnable materials, oxygen concentration greater than 6%, and an ignition source. Vigilance and constant monitoring of these factors will essentially eliminate the danger of fire.

Materials. Burnable materials should be restricted to the bare essentials. Those required for patient therapy (such as medical supplies, tissues, towels) should be stored in flameproof or metal boxes when not in actual use. Volatile, flammable liquids such as ether and alcohol should not be used. Oil, grease, and other hydrocarbon contaminants must be excluded from the chamber, because fire or explosion can spontaneously occur in the presence of oxygen (Hamilton and Sheffield 1977).

> *Case 8.* An inside occupant of a diving chamber called over the intercom, "We have got a fire in here!" Two outside observers noted a flame coming from the carbon dioxide scrubber. Immediately thereafter, a flash fire engulfed the entire compartment. Before the occupants could attempt firefighting with the bucket of water, they were incapacitated. The pressure surged from 91 fsw to 260 fsw, corresponding to a temperature rise to approximately 427°C. Primary cause of the fire was determined to be an overheated scrubber motor, causing spontaneous ignition of the cellulose filter element within the carbon dioxide scrubber. The filter element had been previously impregnated with a kerosenelike liquid, and mistakenly installed inside the chamber. Oxygen concentration was 28% and there was an abundance of burnables present. Two casualties resulted from toxic fumes and heat (Alger and Nichols 1971).

Whenever possible, chamber clothing, mattresses, pillows, sheets, and blankets should be made of flame-retardant materials such as Teflon®, fiberglass (Beta cloth®), polybenzimidazole (PBI), or Durette Gold® (Hamilton and Sheffield 1977). Some clothing materials that do not burn at atmospheric air (such as Nomex®) will, however, burn in enriched oxygen atmospheres.

> *Case 9.* Despite established safety procedures, a student performed welding operations in a chamber pressurized to 190 fsw while wearing synthetic polyester street clothing. (The established fire safety procedure required the diver to wear a swim suit and, if possible, to stand waist deep in water during the welding procedure). Sparks from welding ignited the diver's clothing, causing fatal burns. The only items consumed by the fire were the diver's clothing (Sheffield and Heimbach 1981).

Oxygen Concentration. Except for saturation dives where occupants may require oxygen concentration of less than 6%, the majority of chamber operations involve a fire risk. Whenever 100% oxygen is breathed by chamber occupants, there is a potential for increased oxygen concentration. Although burning rates and ease of ignition are only slightly increased in compressed air, they increase twofold in oxygen-enriched pressurized environments. Thus, oxygen concentrations should be continuously monitored and maintained at levels below 23%. Oxygen concentration can be controlled by purging (see Glossary), but a mask overboard dump system that exhausts exhaled gases outside the chamber is a more efficient method.

Case 10. A monoplace chamber was pressurized with 100% oxygen to treat an infant. After completion of the treatment, the chamber was opened and the infant removed. As the attendant left the room carrying the infant, the mattress was observed to spontaneously ignite. Combustion of the oxygen-saturated mattress was attributed to a static charge in the Fiberglas mattress tray that was caused by defective grounding (Sheffield and Heimbach 1981).

Ignition Sources. Potential ignition sources must be excluded from the chamber. Matches, cigarette lighters, static sparks, temporary electrical cords, and volatile substances constitute a hazard. Under no circumstances should grease or oil lubricants be used on any chamber component. Static sparks are minimized by avoiding the use of plastics, by avoiding the use of switches and unplugging of cords, and by maintaining the chamber humidity above 50%.

Case 11. During oxygen decompression at 30 fsw, a diver draped his cotton dungaree shirt around the incandescent light bulb to cut down the amount of light. After approximately 30 min, the shirt ignited and fire consumed the chamber contents. The diver had time to shut off his oxygen breathing valve but could not use the bucket of water in the chamber before he was overcome by toxic fumes and heat (Alger and Nichols 1971).

Extinguishment and Escape. Many test fires have shown that time is available for fire extinguishment and escape. A manually operated, water deluge system is the best method of extinguishment. The nozzles must be designed and arranged to give full chamber coverage to all treatment depths. A hand-held hose should also be provided in each compartment. Water pressure in the water deluge system should be maintained at 40 psig greater than the internal chamber pressure. Activation of the fire suppression system should deactivate the interior chamber power supply. Automatic activation is not recommended due to the possibility of accidental deluge of patients undergoing treatment (Hamilton and Sheffield 1977). It is essential to have a plan for fire extinguishment and escape via the lock compartment and to practice the plan periodically.

Case 12. A ventilating fan began sparking, and ignited the wood grating in the floor of a shipboard recompression chamber that was pressurized to 2.3 ATA (40 fsw). The chamber was decompressed to the surface. Two occupants perished, but one survived (Alger and Nichols 1971).

(v) Operational Safety. Clearly defined supervision is imperative for chamber safety. The supervisor must ensure that the crew is trained and motivated and that the chamber equipment is working properly. Repairs and maintenance must be performed regularly and recorded in an equipment log. A complete operations manual and written emergency procedures must be readily available at the chamber. Emergency procedures should be regularly practiced so that every crew member is proficient in all duty positions. Emergency decompression procedures should be established prior to any treatment dive. Finally, the supervisor must ensure that every team member is aware of any condition or circumstances that could cause harm to chamber occupants or the crew.

Case 13. A 35-year-old male patient undergoing hyperbaric oxygen treatment in a monoplace chamber experienced an oxygen seizure after 28 min of exposure to 100% oxygen. Following standard procedures, the patient was brought immediately to the surface. On removal from the chamber, the patient continued to experience Jacksonian seizures. One minute later, the patient's breathing and heart action ceased and he became flaccid. Cardiopulmonary resuscitation was unsuccessful and recompression was not attempted. Autopsy findings confirmed the diagnosis of fatal cerebral gas embolism (Bond 1977).

Case 14. A professional deep-sea diver had completed a working dive 50 miles at sea and ascended to the surface in a diving bell, still pressurized to 190 fsw (58 msw). Upon reaching the surface, the diving bell was swung aboard a barge and married to a large decompression chamber. Having completed his work period, the diver sought the "instinctual comforts of dry clothes and a bowel movement." While he sat on the toilet, a worker outside, unaware of the diver's presence, vented the valve of the disposal system at the precise moment that the diver flushed the toilet. In response to the 90-psi pressure differential, the diver's buttocks formed a seal on the seat and he was suddenly eviscerated into the toilet bowl. He was able to break the seal and, with the help of another diver, move to a bunk, where heroic surgery was later performed at a pressure equal to 190 fsw, followed by a 3-day decompression to the surface. The patient survived (Carter and Goldsmith 1970).

(vi) Chamber Crew Qualification. Safe chamber operations require knowledgeable physicians and operators who meet high qualification standards. Like any other medical equipment, the hyperbaric chamber should be operated only by fully qualified personnel. Inside medical attendants should be trained in chamber operating procedures as well as the medical aspects of diving. No matter how intrinsically safe the chamber may be, lack of crew proficiency can result in serious danger to inside occupants and operating personnel.

Case 15. The 22 March 1976 *Medical World News* carried an account of a hyperbaric chamber disaster in Germany that resulted in five deaths. According to the article, "There were 20 patients with a variety of heart, lung, rheumatic and stroke illnesses in the chamber when one . . . complained of trouble breathing. To bring him out for treatment, the pressure was reduced quickly—apparently much too quickly." According to the article, two patients died at the clinic later that evening and, "within the next two days three more patients . . . died in local hospitals; air embolism caused all five deaths. . . . It was not clear who was actually in charge when the mishap occurred." (Sheffield and Heimbach 1981.)

The medical aspects of this accident are discussed by Richter and Loblich (1978). The message from this accident is quite clear: Safe hyperbaric chamber operations demand a full-time, experienced, and supervised crew who understand all aspects of decompression procedures and chamber safety.

h. Summary

The physician must bear the ultimate moral and legal responsibility for both patient care in the hyperbaric facility and safety of equipment. Provision of this safety is normally beyond the expertise, time, and energy of the physician in charge of the hyperbaric facility. He must, then, assemble a team of experts on whom he can rely to install the equipment and to assist him in operating the facility. The hyperbaric chamber is safe when the engineering design concepts and operating procedures are fully understood and adhered to, and a trained, experienced crew operates the chamber.

PAUL J. SHEFFIELD

References

ALGER, R. S., AND J. R. NICHOLS 1971. Survey of fires in hypobaric and hyperbaric chambers. Silver Spring, MD: Naval Ordnance Lab. (NOLTR 71-128).
AMERICAN SOCIETY OF MECHANICAL ENGINEERS 1977. *ANSI/ASME Safety Standard for Pressure Vessels for Human Occupancy*. New York: American Society of Mechanical Engineers. (PVHO-1.)
BEHNKE, A. R., AND L. A. SHAW 1937. The use of oxygen in the treatment of compressed-air illness. *U.S. Nav. Med. Bull.* 35: 1–12.
BERGHAGE, T. E. 1966. Summary statistics: U.S. Navy diving accidents. Res. Rep. 1-66. Washington, DC: U.S. Navy Experimental Diving Unit.
BERT, PAUL 1878. *Barometric Pressure:* Researches in Experimental Physiology, transl. by M. A. Hitchcock and F. A. Hitchcock. Columbus, OH: College Book Co., 1943. Republ. Bethesda MD: Undersea Medical Society, 1978.
BOEREMA, I. 1965. The large chamber. In: *Hyperbaric Oxygenation Symposium. Ann. N.Y. Acad. Sci.* 117: 883–887.
BOEREMA, I., N. G. MEIJNE, W. W. BRUMMELKAMP, S. BROWN, M. H. MENSCH, F. KAMERMANS, M. STERNHAUF, AND W. VAN ALDEREN 1960. Life without blood: a study of the influence of high atmospheric pressure and hypothermia and dilution of blood. *J. Cardiovasc. Surg.* 1: 133.
BOND, G. F. 1977. Arterial gas embolism. In: *Hyperbaric Oxygen Therapy,* edited by J. C. Davis and T. K. Hunt. Bethesda, MD: Undersea Medical Society, p. 141–152.
BOYCOTT, A. E., G. C. C. DAMANT, AND J. S. HALDANE 1908. The prevention of compressed air illness. *J. Hyg.* 8: 342–443.
BROWN, I. W., JR., AND W. W. SMITH 1965. General safety features in chamber design and operation. In: *Hyperbaric Oxygenation Symposium. Ann. N.Y. Acad. Sci.* 117: 801–813.
BRUMMELKAMP, W. H., J. HOENDIJK, AND I. BOEREMA 1961. Treatment of anaerobic infections (clostridial myositis) by drenching the tissues with oxygen under high atmospheric pressure. *Surgery* 49: 299–302.
CARTER, L. H., AND G. A. GOLDSMITH 1970. The ordeal of Donald Boone. *Nutr. Today* 5: 2–9.
CARTER, R. C. 1977. Pioneering inner space: The Navy Experimental Diving Unit's first 50 years. Rep. 1-77. Panama City, FL: Navy Experimental Diving Unit.
COMPRESSED GAS ASSOCIATION 1966. Standard for hyperbaric facilities intended for use in medical application. New York: Compressed Gas Assoc. (Pamphlet P-2.3T).
DAVIS, J. C., J. M. DUNN, C. O. HAGOOD, AND B. E. BASSETT 1973. Hyperbaric medicine in the U.S. Air Force. *JAMA* 224: 205–209.
DAVIS, J. C., AND T. K. HUNT 1977. *Hyperbaric Oxygen Therapy*. Bethesda: Undersea Medical Society.
DAVIS, J. C., P. J. SHEFFIELD, L. SCHUKNECHT, R. D. HEIMBACH, J. M. DUNN, G. DOUGLAS, AND G. K. ANDERSON 1977. Altitude decompression sickness: hyperbaric therapy results in 145 cases. *Aviat. Space Environ. Med.* 48: 722–730.
DEPENBUSCH, R. L., R. E. THOMPSON, AND G. B. HART 1972. Use of hyperbaric oxygen in the treatment of refractory osteomyelitis: a preliminary report. *J. Trauma* 12: 807–812.
DONNELL, A. M., JR., AND C. P. NORTON 1960. Successful use of the recompression chamber in severe decompression sickness with neurocirculatory collapse. *Aerosp. Med.* 32: 1004–1008.
DORR, V. A. 1971. *Compendium of Hyperbaric Fire Safety Research*. Washington, DC: U.S. Navy Office of Naval Research (AD 720353).

DOUGLAS, T. A., D. D. LAWSON, I. MCA. LEDINGHAM, J. N. NORMAN, G. R. SHARP, AND G. SMITH 1964. Carbon monoxide poisoning. In: *First International Congress on the Clinical Application of Hyperbaric Oxygen,* edited by I. Boerema, W. H. Brummelkamp, and N. G. Meijne. New York: Elsevier, p.161–167.

FONTAINE, J. A. 1879. Effets physiologiques et applications therapeutiques de l'air comprimé. Paris: Germer-Baillière.

GOODMAN, M. W. 1961. The syndrome of decompression sickness in historical perspective. Rep. 368, Vol. 22. Washington, DC: U.S. Navy Medical Research Laboratory.

GOODMAN, M. W., AND R. D. WORKMAN 1965. Oxygen breathing approach of treatment of decompression sickness in divers and aviators. Res. Rep. 5-65. Washington, DC: U.S. Navy Bureau of Ships. (Project SF 01106-05, Task 11513-2.)

HAMILTON, R. W., JR., T. D. LANGLEY, AND V. A. DORR 1970. Safe instrumentation for physiological research in the hyperbaric environment. *Trans. N.Y. Acad. Sci.* 32: 458–470.

HAMILTON, R. W., JR., AND P. J. SHEFFIELD 1977. Hyperbaric chamber safety. In: *Hyperbaric Oxygen Therapy,* edited by J. C. Davis and T. K. Hunt. Bethesda, MD: Undersea Medical Society, p. 47–60.

HENDERSON, Y. 1917. Effects of altitude on aviators. *Aviation* 2: 145–147.

HOFF, E. C. 1948. Bibliographical source book of compressed air diving and submarine medicine. Washington, DC: U.S. Navy Bureau of Medicine and Surgery, Vol. 1. (NAVMED 1191).

HUNT, T. K., AND M. P. PAI 1972. The effect of varying ambient oxygen tensions on wound metabolism and collagen synthesis. *Surg. Gynecol. Obstet.* 135: 561–567.

JACOBSON, J. H., II, J. H. C. MORSCH, AND L. RENDELL-BAKER 1965. The historical perspective of hyperbaric therapy. In: *Hyperbaric Oxygenation Symposium. Ann. N.Y. Acad. Sci.* 117: 651–670.

JAMINET, A. 1871. Physical effects of compressed air . . . . St. Louis: R. and T. A. Ennis.

KEAYS, F. L. 1909. Compressed-air illness with a report of 2,692 cases. *Publ. Cornell Univ. Med. Coll.* 2: 1–55.

KETCHUM, S. A., A. N. THOMAS, AND A. D. HALL 1970. Angiographic studies of the effects of hyperbaric oxygen or burn wound revascularization. In: *Proceedings of the Fourth International Conference on Hyperbaric Medicine,* edited by J. Wade and T. Iwa. Baltimore: Williams and Wilkins, p. 388–394.

MAINOUS, E. G., AND P. J. BOYNE 1974. Hyperbaric oxygen in total rehabilitation of patients with mandibular osteoradionecrosis. *Int. J. Oral Surg.* 3: 297–301.

MAINOUS, E. G., P. J. BOYNE, G. B. HART, AND B. C. TERRY 1973. Restoration of resected mandible by grafting with combination of mandible homograft and autogenous iliac marrow and post-operative treatment with hyperbaric oxygenation. *J Oral Surg.* 35: 13–20.

MEIJNE, N. G. 1973. Hyperbaric oxygen, increased pressure and the activities in this field in Boerema's department in the period 1956–1972. *Arch. Chir. Neerl.* 25: 195–213.

MERICOURT, LE ROY DE 1869. Hygiène des pêcheurs d'èponges. *Ann. Hyg. Publ. Med. Leg. Paris* 31: 274–286.

MOSES, H. 1964. Casualties in individual submarine escape. Rep. 438. Groton CT: U.S. Navy Submarine Center.

NATIONAL FIRE PROTECTION ASSOCIATION 1970. Standard for hyperbaric facilities. Boston: National Fire Protection Association. (NFPA 56D 1970.)

NIINIKOSKI, J. 1969. Effect of oxygen supply on wound healing and formation of experimental granulation tissue. *Acta. Physiol. Scand. Suppl.* 334: 1–72.

PENZIAS, W., AND M. W. GOODMAN 1973. *Man Beneath the Sea.* New York: Wiley Inforscience, p. 17–37.

PERRINS, D. J. D. 1970. The influence of hyperbaric oxygen on the survival of split skin grafts. In: *Proceedings of the Fourth International Congress on Hyperbaric Medicine,* edited by J. Wada and T. Iwa. Baltimore: Williams and Wilkins, p. 369–376.

POL, B. AND T. J. J. WATELLE 1854. Memoire sur les effects de la compression de l'air. *Ann. Hyg. Publ. Med. Leg. Paris* 1: 241–279.

RICHTER, K., AND H. J. LÖBLICH 1978. Letale Dekompressionskrankheit nach therapeutischer Uberdruckbehandlung. *Z. Rechtsmed.* 81: 45–61.

SHEFFIELD, P. J., J. C. DAVIS, G. C. BELL, AND T. J. GALLAGHER 1977. Hyperbaric chamber clinical support: Multiplace. In: *Hyperbaric Oxygen Therapy,* edited by J. C. Davis and T. K. Hunt. Bethesda, MD: Undersea Medical Society, p. 25–39.

SHEFFIELD, P. J., J. C. DAVIS, AND C. J. CUTRONA 1977. Fabrication and design considerations for a multiplace clinical hyperbaric facility. Brooks AFB, TX: USAF School of Aerospace Medicine. (SAMTR77-7.)

SHEFFIELD, P. J., AND R. D. HEIMBACH 1981. The physician and chamber safety. In: *Hyperbaric and Undersea Medicine,* edited by J. C. Davis. San Antonio: Medical Seminars, Inc., vol. 1(24).

SHEFFIELD, P. J., R. L. STORK, AND T. R. MORGAN 1977. Efficient oxygen mask for patients undergoing hyperbaric oxygen therapy. *Aviat. Space Environ. Med.* 48: 132–137.

SHILLING, C. W. 1938. Compressed air illness. *U.S. Nav. Med. Bull.* 36: 9–17; 233–259.

SIMPSON, A. 1857. Compressed air as a therapeutic agent in the treatment of consumption, asthma, chronic bronchitis, and other diseases. Edinburgh: Sutherland and Knox.

SMITH, A. H. 1873. The effects of high atmospheric pressure including the caisson disease (Prize essay of the Alumni Association of the College of Physicians and Surgeons). Brooklyn, NY: Eagle Print.

TOBIN, D. A. 1971. Explosive decompression in a hyperbaric oxygen chamber. *Am. J. Roentgenol. Radium Ther. Nucl. Med.* 3: 621–624.

TRIGER, M. 1841. Memoire sur un appareil à air comprimé, pour le percement des puits de mines et autres travaux, sous eaux et dans les sables submergés. *C. R. Acad. Sci.* 13: 884.

U.S. DEPARTMENT OF LABOR, OCCUPATIONAL SAFETY AND HEALTH ADMINISTRATION 1977. Commercial diving operations, occupational safety and health requirements. *Fed. Reg.* 42: 37650–37674.

U.S. NAVY 1924. *U.S. Navy Diving Manual.* Washington DC: Department of the Navy.

U.S. NAVY 1956a. History of diving and its development in the U.S. Navy. In: *Submarine Medical Practice.* Washington, DC: U.S. Navy Bureau of Medicine and Surgery, p. 9–14.

U.S. NAVY 1956b. The submarine escape training tank. In: *Submarine Medicine Practice.* Washington, DC: U.S. Navy Bureau of Medicine and Surgery, p. 325–330.

U.S. NAVY 1959. *U.S. Navy Diving Manual. Pt. 1. General Principles of Diving.* Washington, DC: Department of the Navy. (NAVSHIPS 250-538.)

U.S. NAVY 1973. System certification procedures and criteria manual for deep submergence systems. Washington, DC: Department of the Navy. (NAVMAT P-9290.)

U.S. NAVY 1977. *U.S. Navy Diving Manual, Vol. 2, Mixed Gas Diving.* Washington, DC: Department of the Navy. (NAVSEA 0994-LP-001-9020.)

U.S. NAVY 1978. *U.S. Navy Diving Manual.* Washington, DC: Department of the Navy. (NAVSEA 0994-LP-001-9010.)

VANDERAUE, O. E., W. A. WHITE, JR., R. HAYTER, E. S. BRINTON, R. J. KELLAR, AND A. R. BEHNKE 1945. Physiological factors indulging the prevention and treatment of decompression sickness. Project X-443, Rep. No. 1. Bethesda, MD: U.S. Nav. Med. Res. Inst.

WILLIAMS, C. T. 1885. Lectures of the compressed air bath and its uses in the treatment of disease, Lecture I. *Br. Med. J.* 1885: 769–772.

WINTER, G. D., AND D. J. D. PERRINS 1970. Effects of hyperbaric oxygen treatment on epidermal regeneration. In: *Proceedings of the Fourth International Congress on Hyperbaric Medicine,* edited by J. Wada and T. Iwa. Baltimore: Williams and Wilkins, p. 363–368.

2. Monoplace Chambers

a. Introduction

More than 1500 monoplace chambers have been produced and distributed in the past score of years (personal communications from four international firms). With this plethora one would expect several reflections on its use in decompression sickness in the medical literature. Paradoxically, the experience reported is small. Lamy annd Hanquet (1973) note two instances in which a monoplace chamber may be used: "pulmonary overpressure [air embolism, interstitial pulmonary emphysema, etc.] providing the patient evidences no major respiratory or circulatory distress", and second, "the average decompression accident (patient in a satisfactory clinical state) if long distances have to be covered and especially if there are passes to be flown over before arriving at the treatment center." They further note some disadvantages in the use of the chamber, noting they are uncomfortable, may involve a loss of time in transporting, and are difficult to handle due to weight or adaptation to or into a multiplace chamber. There are only two articles (Hart 1974, 1976) reflecting an experience of using the monoplace chamber as a primary treatment device in decompression illness and air embolism, and these are concerned with only 62 patients.

It is noted in Edmonds et al. (1976) that these chambers are to be used only in the most "dire circumstances."

My experience would indicate that the monoplace chamber, by careful adaptation, may be used to treat patients with decompression sickness except for those requiring concurrent surgical procedures.

b. Optimal Monoplace Chamber System

The equipment design of a monoplace chamber must meet the strict codes of fabrication outlined by the American Society of Mechanical Engineers for occupied pressure vessels (ASME 1974a, 1974b). They must be installed, housed, maintained, and operated as specified in the National Fire Protection Association pamphlet regarding human single-occupancy chambers (NFPA 1982).

A properly equipped chamber (Figure XIV-5) should have a heat exchanger to cool or warm the incoming gases for patient comfort. An adjustable flow regulator is preferred to increase or decrease flow of gases across the patient, again for patient comfort. The effluent gases should be exhausted to the exterior of the building in which the chamber is housed.

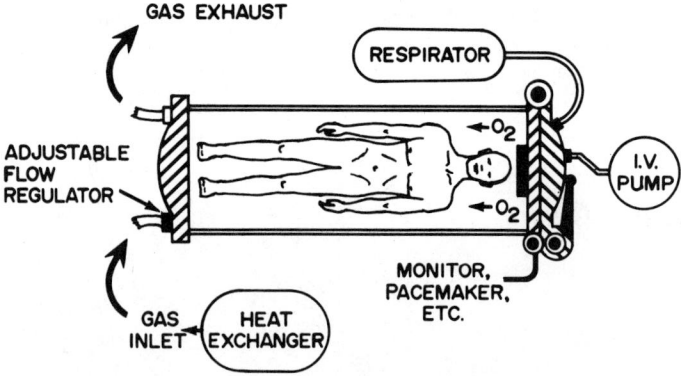

Figure XIV-5. Optimal monoplace chamber system.

Life-support equipment for the monoplace system includes a respirator to support the patient who is apneic or suffering respiratory insufficiency, and a positive displacement pump that may be used to administer intravenous fluids or drugs. A physiological monitor is required for monitoring of blood pressures, temperature, and ECG of the patient. A pacemaker has been required in the past in patients with cardiac dysfunction. These items are "glanded" through the cephalic bulkhead behind the patient's head. A demand valve with mask or mouthpiece is a useful accessory allowing for flexibility in using "air breaks" or other gas mixtures during treatment.

Presently available monoplace chambers are pictured in Figure XIV-6. Chambers with steel hulls have the disadvantage of having only viewports for observation of the patient, whereas the acrylic hulls give excellent patient visibility. Both may be mounted or unmounted, and the mounts may be detachable. The telescoping and collapsible types have an obvious space-saving advantage when not in use; this consideration may or may not outweigh the reported unreliability of these more fragile hulls. Monoplace chambers with working pressures to 7 atm are manufactured; most models, however, use the lower pressure of 3 atm. The heavier chambers weigh approximately 900 lb (410 kg), the lighter approximately 300 lb (135 kg). Accessory gas inlets adaptable to diving tanks are useful in close support of diving activities and further evacuation of the individual to a treatment facility. Transport chambers with interlocking sleeves facilitate the wedding of the monoplace to the multiplace chamber, avoiding the space problems created by placing one inside the other.

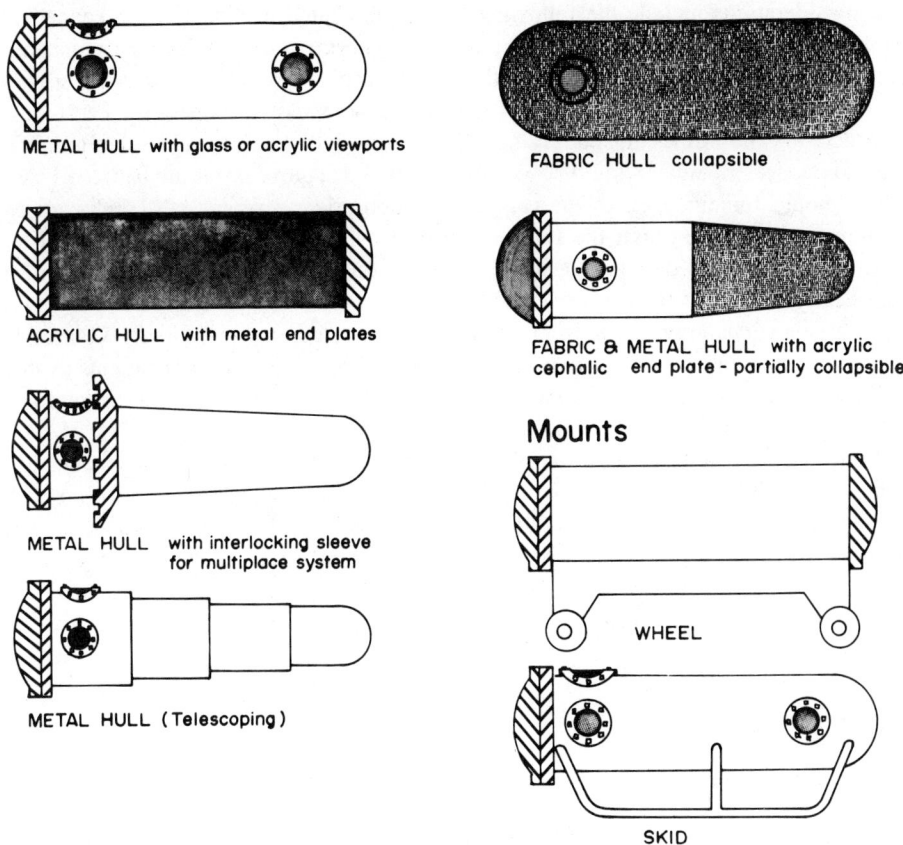

Figure XIV-6. Monoplace hyperbaric chamber systems.

Models are available with recycling capabilities that may be advantageous when gas supplies are expensive. These recycling units may have devices for cooling or warming, or both, that may be used for patient comfort. A humidification device (Ackerman 1967) may be attached to the gas inlet when dryness is a concern. My experience indicates adequate humidification within the chamber is achieved by the patient's evaporative loss and is not required.

An intrinsically safe communication system is essential to proper patient control. It may also be used as a form of entertainment with radio or television programs. A complete supply of drugs and equipment must be at hand for medical emergencies.

c. Application of the Monoplace Chamber

Cotton apparel is preferred, for it does not collect a static charge. Fire safety in this system is assured by absolute exclusion of ignition sources of significant magnitude to cause combustion at 3 ATA oxygen. Greases, oils, and ointments are avoided in order to reduce buildup on surfaces and filters, and gas sources are routinely checked for impurities.

Careful planning must precede insertion of the critically ill patient into the chamber. These considerations include the following: (1) the intubated patient must be connected to the respirator and the air in the cuff replaced with normal saline; (2) where indicated, external pacemaker leads must be passed through the cephalic bulkhead (the pulse energy is insufficient for ignition); (3) ECG, EEG, blood pressure and/or temperature leads must be attached; (4) chest tubes must be drained through a no-return valve such as the Heimlich valve; (5) nasogastric tubes should be to open drainage in a glove or plastic bag; (6) Foley catheter should remain open to drainage in an appropriate receptacle; (7) intravenous lines must be passed through the bulkhead to maintain fluid requirements, administer vasoactive drugs, and sedation as needed; (8) the unconscious or disoriented patient must be physically restrained for his protection.

Emergency decompression is rarely if ever indicated in the properly controlled patient. Three patients have been extracted emergently in a series of 3000 patients treated for all diseases, i.e., gas gangrene, acute burns, cerebral edema, etc. None of the three were under treatment for dysbarism.

Long or short tables may be used as preferred by the supervising physician. My group prefers a short, low-pressure oxygen table with maximum pressure of 3 ATA with extended treatments according to residual, and we find comparable results with the longer, higher-pressure tables if the patient is received within 4 hr of injury. Presently we advise a purge rate of 3 liters/kg body wt for chambers with adjustable control. Pressurization and depressurization is performed commensurate with the patient's ability to equalize his air passages.

d. Maintenance and Safety

A routine inspection by a biomedical engineer is mandatory to safe chamber operation. Damaged equipment must be repaired before further use, and valves, seals, cylinders, and parts should be replaced and cleaned as recommended by the manufacturer. Flammable liquids, oils, and waxes must be excluded from the chamber area. Gas supply alarm systems must be checked routinely and maintained in working condition. Chamber personnel must be trained in safety routines periodically and must practice them regularly. Appropriate fire fighting equipment must be at hand and routinely checked.

e. Conclusion

The monoplace chamber may be used in treatment of dysbarism when applied by trained, experienced personnel. It may not, however, be used in cases where concurrent surgical procedures must be performed.

GEORGE B. HART

References

ACKERMAN, N. B. 1967. Engineering problems in design and utilization of hyperbaric oxygenation equipment. *Am. J. Surg.* 114: 77–86.
AMERICAN SOCIETY OF MECHANICAL ENGINEERS 1974a. *ANSI/ASME Safety Standard for Pressure Vessels for Human Occupancy*. New York: American Society of Mechanical Engineers, PVHO-1.
AMERICAN SOCIETY OF MECHANICAL ENGINEERS 1974b. *ASME Boiler and Pressure Vessel Code, Section VIII, Unfired Pressure Vessels*. New York: American Society of Mechanical Engineers.
EDMONDS, C., C. LOWRY. AND J. PENNEFATHER (editors) 1976. *Diving and Subaquatic Medicine*. Mosman, Australia: Diving Medical Centre, p. 70.
HART, G. B. 1974. Treatment of decompression illness and air embolism with hyperbaric oxygen. *Aerosp. Med.* 45: 1190–1193.
HART, G. B. 1976. Screening test for decompression sickness. *Aviat. Space Environ. Med.* 47: 993–994.
LAMY, M. L., AND M. M. HANQUET 1973. Modern aspects of treatment of decompression sickness. *Acta Anaesthesiol. Belg.* 24: 215–229.
NATIONAL FIRE PROTECTION ASSOCIATION 1982. *Hyperbaric Facilities*. Boston: National Fire Protection Association. (NFPA 56D.)

B. Scuba Diving

1. Introduction

The diving mode most likely to have been used by an accident victim who may require the medical services of readers of this book, particularly nonhyperbaric physicians, is commonly known as *scuba*. Scuba diving—not to be confused with breath-hold or "skin" diving—derives its name from the acronym for the type of breathing equipment the diver uses, i.e., *s*elf-*c*ontained *u*nderwater *b*reathing *a*pparatus. The diver who uses this type of equipment is characterized as free swimming and independent of the surface by virtue of the fact that the source of breathing gas, usually compressed air, is carried in one or more cylinders on the diver's back.

This subchapter is intended to provide the nonhyperbaric physician with some brief background information on the development of scuba, and the scuba diving community. The major portion of this section, however, focuses on specific information about the equipment and procedures commonly used by scuba divers, with particular emphasis on those aspects that may aid in the diagnosis, treatment, and general understanding of dive-related medical problems.

2. Development of Modern Scuba

There is evidence based on the nature of artifacts of civilizations that date from 4500 B.C. to suggest that man has been engaged in breath-hold diving activities since that time. Aristotle, in his fourth century B.C. writings, expressed the idea that man can operate underwater using a submerged source of breathing air. The general history of diving covers an incredible span of time. Both the *U.S. Navy Diving Manual* (1975) and Larson (1959) offer interesting and informative summaries of this history, the latter specifically dealing with self-contained diving.

Modern scuba breathing equipment has developed from the technological innovations of the Frenchmen La Prieur and Fernez, working in the 1920s and 1930s, and the Frenchmen Cousteau and Gagnan, working in the 1940s. La Prieur and Fernez sought to develop an underwater breathing device that would allow a diver longer periods of submerged time than were available to a skin diver, yet would retain the skin diver's underwater swimming mobility. Two devices were eventually designed and built, both of which proved functional but extremely inefficient in terms of air supply duration. Their basic operating principle was that of open-circuit (exhaled into the surrounding water), continuous, low pressure air flow (i.e., free flow), delivered to a mouthpiece or a full face mask from a cylinder of compressed air carried by the diver. The chief differences between the two models were the means by which air was delivered to the diver, and the capacity and number of cylinders carried by the diver. La Prieur's second model reportedly supplied 30 min of air at 23 ft, 20 min at 33 ft, and 10 min at 40 ft. Subsequent further increases in cylinder capacity allowed durations of 25 min at 66 ft. These devices saw very little use in the late 1930s by French diving enthusiasts (Larson 1959).

The major drawback of the La Prieur-Fernez scuba device was the limitation on diving depth and duration imposed by the free flow operating principle. It was Cousteau and Gagnan's adaptation of a demand intake valve (activated by the negative pressure associated with inspiration) to the basic La Prieur-type equipment that was responsible for overcoming this drawback. Fitted with the demand valve, the breathing device delivered air at ambient pressure to the diver only when the diver inhaled, or "demanded," air. Like the La Prieur device, Cousteau's was open-circuit, but because air was only used as the diver's breathing cycle demanded it, both depth and duration capabilities of the diver were greatly extended. This simple modification made scuba equipment commercially feasible and literally paved the way for the dramatic surge in the use of scuba for recreational and occupational purposes.

3. The Scuba Diving Community

Most divers who use scuba are a rather diverse group who dive strictly for recreation. These sport divers participate in such varied underwater activities as wreck diving, underwater photography, tropical fish collecting, spearfishing, underwater archaeology, and just plain underwater sightseeing, to name just a few. Some sport diving enthusiasts seek their underwater thrill in the challenge of diving in submerged caves and springs and in diving under ice. Recreational divers pursue their sport in almost every conceivable body of water—oceans, lakes, rivers, and quarries—and under all kinds of environmental conditions.

While most scuba diving is done for recreation, scuba is also used in the occupational setting. Law enforcement organizations and fire department rescue services use scuba in some situations. Shallow scuba diving is used as a tool by the marine science academic community in many aspects of its research. Certain segments of the commercial fishing industry also make use of scuba. The stereotypical commercial diver, such as one employed by an offshore diving contractor, does not use scuba extensively. However, scuba is frequently used in some types of construction and inspection activities of commercial diving, mostly by smaller diving firms not involved in offshore oil field diving.

The size of the sport diving population is not actually known. The most recent Federal study that deals with the issue estimated that in 1973 there were some 1.9 million individuals in the United States with diving skills, but, of these, only slightly less than 0.5 million were actually practicing the sport (NOAA 1975). There is little doubt, however, that today these numbers have grown considerably.

Most recreational divers have received some basic level of training in the use of scuba from any of several diver training agencies. These organizations all provide several levels of diving skills development and most offer specialty diving courses. These agencies have formed the backbone of and are maintaining a thriving industry based on the public's growing recreational desires. They are constantly working to improve the safety of the sport and the quality of instruction provided by their instructor-affiliates. Consensus standards for training and some procedures have been developed and subsequently endorsed by the American National Standards Institute.

The public's interest in diving as a recreational pursuit has spawned an active and innovative equipment manufacturing industry that is fiercely competitive. The attractions of diving also naturally support a vigorous travel and tourism and charter industry in the Caribbean area, as well as in such states as Florida, California, and Hawaii.

4. Scuba Procedures

Whether recreational or occupational, scuba diving must be recognized as an activity that has its risks. With proper recognition of these risks and a liberal dose of common sense, however, these are usually quite manageable. As a result, scuba diving can be as safe and satisfying as any other physical sport or occupation.

Accident prevention and diving safety are both a state of mind and of practice. Most scuba diving accidents are preventable and most underwater emergency situations can be controlled and resolved before ever reaching accident seriousness. Why then does the medical profession continue to encounter the number of scuba diving accidents that it does?

Four basic tenets of diving safety, if faithfully observed by the diver, can significantly reduce the likelihood of a diving casualty. Briefly, these are: (1) to be in proper physical and mental condition for diving; (2) to be adequately trained for the type of diving anticipated; (3) to be properly equipped for the type of diving anticipated; (4) to practice sound general diving procedures. While accidents have occurred because of failure to observe each of these tenets, the failure to practice sound diving procedures has been the major causal factor of most accidents. A diver can be in excellent physical and mental condition and can be thoroughly trained and properly equipped, but if sound procedures are not followed, all the rest is for naught in preventing an accident.

It is useful to define what is meant by *scuba procedures,* to preclude some common misconceptions that lead to narrow viewpoints. A scuba procedure (or a diving procedure) is that action whose proper and timely execution by the diver provides for maximum safety in the conduct of a dive. Thus, sound scuba procedures include actions to be carried out *prior to* and *following* the submerged period, as well as during it. The remaining discussion of scuba procedures in this subsection deals with those generally applicable to every type of scuba diving activity. Any discussion of specific procedures unique to specialty activities, such as cave diving or diving under ice, is beyond the scope of this chapter.

Perhaps the most serious mistake made by the casual or inexperienced diver is the failure to realize that proper diving procedures for a safe dive begin long before he enters the water. Dive planning is one of the most basic and important procedures with which every diver should concern himself. The planning of a dive is not just a mere statement of intention, such as, "Let's go dive for lobster at Key West." It is a much more serious process. Careful and thorough planning is imperative for safety, for good planning can readily indicate the extant hazards, at which point common sense and mature judgment can suggest the best approach to then minimize the hazard. Planning the dive can also be a social activity that lends as much fun and enjoyment to its participants as the anticipated dive itself! Both the *U.S. Navy Diving Manual* (1975) and the *NOAA Diving Manual* (Miller 1979) provide extensive discussions on all aspects of dive planning. These discussions are easily adaptable to every conceivable type of scuba diving.

The most important element in any dive plan is the clear definition of arrangements for emergency assistance. While they don't actually prevent an accident from occurring, these arrangements are essential in securing *prompt* help for the unfortunate victim, should one occur. As a minimum, these arrangements should include the location, status, and contact procedures for the nearest accessible recompression chamber (not all chambers are available to the public), the location, contact procedures, and response time of the nearest search and rescue unit, first aid treatments for the more serious types of diving accidents (gas embolism, decompression sickness, and drowning), and a sequence of on-scene actions to smoothly effect the evacuation of the victim when help arrives.

Since the more serious diving accidents are life-threatening and require immediate recompression therapy, it should be obvious that time is of the essence in securing professional assistance. Delay in reaching the means of definitive treatment can significantly decrease the chance of a full recovery. A well-thought-out and verified emergency assistance plan is the best assurance of obtaining help in the shortest possible time. It goes without saying that the means of summoning assistance must be immediately available at the scene.

Other elements to be considered in a good dive plan are the general purpose or goal of the dive, the nature of the expected environmental surface and underwater conditions and any known hazards associated with them, the organization and leadership of the dive team and any support people on the surface, the type and amount of diving equipment necessary for the chosen diving platform, the desired depth and duration of the dive as well as any repetitive dive or stage decompression plans, a prearranged set of underwater hand signals and a recall system, and a careful review of possible underwater emergency situations and the best means of responding to each. This last element is particularly important, especially when the dive involves divers of different levels of skill.

The most commonly encountered diving medical emergency seen by the physician is decompression sickness. In its acute form, decompression sickness, or the *bends,* is one of the most serious of all diving accidents. It is also one of the most preventable, as its development usually results from failure to follow acceptable decompression procedures. The decompression procedures in use today are based on a series of schedules designed to afford the diver the most probable combinations of time and depth exposures that will result in safe ascent to the surface. It is acknowledged, however, that there may be variations in individual susceptibilities to decompression sickness and that cases of the sickness may present even after the affected diver has properly followed correct decompression procedures. These variations can be attributed to such stress factors as heavy exercise, poor physical condition, fatigue, anxiety, hypoglycemia, and thermal stress (Kidd and Elliott 1975).

In the United States, the accepted standard of practice for scuba diving decompression procedures is that developed and used by the U.S. Navy. Founded on years of accumulated evidence, the U.S. Navy decompression tables, together with their comprehensive rules for application, represent the best information and procedures currently available. Since all dives require decompression, either direct decompression or stage-to-stage decompression, the Navy tables provide decompression procedures for every combination of depth and bottom time likely to ever be experienced by a scuba diver. Most incidents of scuba diver decompression sickness occur simply because divers fail to understand or use correctly these very straightforward procedures. It is not uncommon for scuba divers to virtually disregard the Navy tables and procedures or to simply divine their own decompression procedures and schedules. Such practice is sheer stupidity on the diver's part.

5. *Basic Scuba Diving Equipment*

Scuba diving, for whatever purpose, requires the use of several essential pieces of equipment. While it is not the purpose of this book to provide a detailed discussion of every aspect of scuba equipment, the physician may find it useful to consider the nature and function of the diver's equipment as an aid in understanding the role that equipment may play as a contributing factor in diving accidents.

While, undeniably, there are equipment-related aspects to many scuba diving accidents, the outright failure of a piece of diving equipment, as a direct cause of an accident, is thankfully not a common occurrence. Equipment that is properly worn and used during the dive, and properly handled and maintained, should rarely cause a diver grief. While it is often easy to blame an accident on "equipment failure," a closer investigation of the circumstances of the accident will usually reveal that some procedural error on the diver's part, misuse of equipment, lack of or improper equipment maintenance, or any combination of these factors, was the true cause of the accident.

The basic pieces of equipment necessary for any type of scuba diving are most easily discussed in six arbitrary but commonly associated groupings.

a. Cylinder Group

The cylinder group consists of the cylinder itself, the cylinder valve, and the harness or backpack in which the cylinder is carried (see Figure XIV-7). The cylinder contains the compressed gas to be used by the divers. This is usually air but may contain another gas mixture in some special circumstances. Scuba cylinders are seamless, weldless, ellipsoid-bottomed pressure vessels designed to safely contain compressed gas at working pressures up to 3000 psig. They are constructed from various alloys of steel or aluminum that are blended to balance maximum strength with malleability (Hall 1976). Cylinders capable of working pressures of 5000 psig are reportedly under development. Scuba cylinders must be manufactured to meet specific federal pressure standards, and must continue to meet these standards throughout their service life. With proper handling, use, and maintenance, they can remain durable and serviceable for extremely long periods of time.

The most significant problem associated with scuba cylinders is corrosion. In comparative tests, Cichy et al. (1978) found that steel cylinders were considerably more susceptible to corrosion than aluminum cylinders. (Upon pressurization, a corrosion-

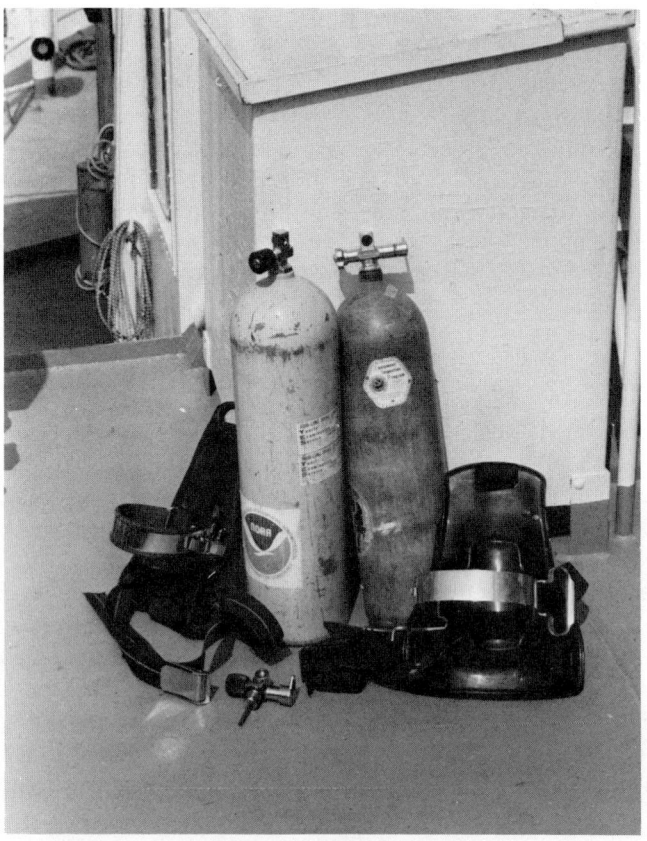

Figure XIV-7. Cylinder group.

weakened cylinder can explode.) Corrosion most commonly occurs after water has been introduced into the cylinder, usually through some action of the diver.

Undetected corrosion, which can progress to serious proportions surprisingly rapidly under some circumstances, can certainly contribute to diving accidents. Flakes of corroded metal that separate from the cylinder wall can block the cylinder valve during a dive, suddenly cutting off the diver's air supply. The possible consequences of this situation are easily imagined.

A different type of corrosion-related problem in scuba cylinders is discussed in Schenck and McAniff (1976). In this case, a diver died from hypoxia less than 5 min into a 12-ft dive in a canal. The accident investigation revealed that the victim had stored a partially charged cylinder for about three months prior to the dive. In that period, internal corrosion apparently chemically consumed some 90% of the oxygen in the cylinder. Analysis of the remaining air in his cylinder showed an oxygen level of only 2%–3% instead of the normal 21%.

Proper internal visual inspection of the cylinder on a regular basis (an annual inspection is common), or at any time water is suspected to have entered (or condensed in) the cylinder, readily detects dangerous corrosion. Subsequent remedial maintenance usually obviates the immediate problem of flaking. The cylinder of the hypoxia victim described had reportedly not been visually inspected in ten years. Hydrostatic testing will also reveal the existence of corrosion so advanced that cylinder wall thickness has been reduced to the point where pressure standards can no longer be met. In the absence of visual inspections, however, the statutory 5-year interval for hydrostatic tests may not, in itself, detect a seriously corroded cylinder before it reaches a dangerous condition.

Scuba cylinders are commercially available in several capacities, with those of 72 and 80 standard cubic feet (scf) being predominant. The capacity of a cylinder is the volume of gas at surface pressure (1 ATA or 14.7 psi) that can be compressed into a cylinder at its rated pressure. (See Table XIV-2.)

The important device that passes high pressure air from the cylinder to the attached regulator's first stage is the cylinder valve. Located in the neck of the cylinder, this valve can be one of two types. A K-valve is a standard on-off valve assembly. A J-valve is also an on-off assembly, but it incorporates a manually actuated air-reserve mechanism. This air-reserve mechanism serves two important purposes: it warns the diver that the air supply is almost exhausted, and it can provide the diver with a quantity of reserve air, sufficient to return to the surface (U.S. Navy 1975).

Table XIV-2

Capacities of Various Size Cylinders at Their Rated Pressures

Cylinder Type	Working Pressure, psig*	Capacity,**
Steel "72"	2475	71.55
Steel "72"	2250	65.05
Aluminum "72"	3000	72.40
Aluminum "80"	3000	79.87

* psig, lb/in.² gauge.
**scf, standard ft³.

The J-valve is a spring-loaded check valve that is preset to close at cylinder pressures of 300–500 psi. While it provides unrestricted air flow at higher cylinder pressures, as the preset pressure is approached, the spring forces a flow check against the valve orifice, restricting air flow and increasing breathing resistance. At the preset pressure the spring totally closes the orifice and stops air flow. To regain air flow of the remaining 300–500 psi in the cylinder the diver must manually override the spring by hand-actuating the reserve lever on the valve, reopening the orifice.

Improper cylinder filling procedures or accidental actuation of the reserve mechanism during the dive can contribute to underwater emergencies that could lead to serious consequences. Divers should not absolutely depend on the availability of reserve air for ascent.

On dives during which a diver does use the reserve air, attention should be paid to the depth from which ascent will be made. The duration of this reserve air supply is a function of depth and the diver's respiratory minute volume (RMV). For example, a diver whose RMV is 1.0 absolute cubic foot per minute (acfm), and who is using a steel 72 cylinder, would only have enough air at 300 psi at 100 fsw for a little more than 2 min. Since ascents should be performed at 60 ft/min this diver should begin ascent immediately when the reserve is actuated, or face a potentially hazardous, out-of-air, emergency swimming ascent whose improper execution might very well result in lung barotrauma.

Another feature of the cylinder valve is its blow-out plug, which is a safety feature designed to prevent dangerously high cylinder pressures. The pressures at which these plugs activate depends on the rated pressure of the cylinder. For cylinders rated for 2250 psi the burst pressure for the plug is 3400 psi, while for 3000 psi cylinders the plug will burst at 3900 psi. It is important that the proper plug be used for each cylinder and that the plug's integrity be established before a cylinder is used. The following incident is illustrative of the consequences of inattention to this detail and it is not hard to conceive of a more grim outcome that what luckily resulted.

A diver placed a fully-charged (2250 psi) set of twin scuba cylinders in the trunk of his car after having gauged their pressure. These cylinders were left in the trunk under a hot July sun for some period of time before the dive. Without rechecking their pressure, the diver donned the cylinders and proceeded to make an 8-ft to 20-ft dive near an old pier. When low on air, the diver attempted to surface but was unable to leave the bottom. He released his weight belt but was still unable to surface. He moved to a nearby piling and pulled himself up the piling to the surface. Even the inflation of his buoyancy vest did not provide sufficient buoyancy to keep him on the surface, but he managed to kick and bob ashore. Upon inspection of his cylinders, it was discovered that one of the blow-out plugs had ruptured; during the dive, the water pressure was sufficient to force water into the cylinder, completely filling it through the ruptured plug (Naval Safety Center 1978). This situation could have easily had much more serious consequences.

The third member of the cylinder group is the harness or backpack. This equipment secures the cylinder and valve to the diver's back through a combination of straps. The cylinder is securely held in the backpack by various styles of clamping bands. The backpack itself is a lightweight frame that is molded to conform to a diver's back and his contours. The shoulder and waist straps are adjustable and usually fitted with quick-release buckles. The diver must exercise care to ensure that these straps do not foul the weight belt or the collar of the buoyancy compensator.

b. Regulator Group

The regulator group consists of the regulator itself and several commonly used pieces of ancillary equipment. The regulator is the single most important piece of diving equipment required by the diver. None of the accessories that can be attached to the regulator are essential for diving; however, when in place and properly used all can add to diver safety.

The purpose of the regulator is simply to reduce the pressure of the air stored in the cylinder to ambient water pressure and deliver it to the diver upon demand. The volume of air that the regulator must deliver to the diver is a function of the diver's depth and his respiratory minute volume. While modern regulators are engineered so that they automatically adjust to changes in depth and respiratory rates, there are upper limits to their abilities to meet unusually high flow requirements. These limitations, often not considered by divers, can be exceeded, with the result that the regulator appears to be failing, and a situation is created where improper diver response could lead to an accident. The importance of an awareness of the limitations of diving equipment is underscored by Egstrom (1976).

Two basic styles of regulators are in use today. The single-hose, two-stage demand regulator (Figure XIV-8 *top*) is in widest use. Indeed, this style dominates the commercial market. The double-hose, two-stage demand regulator (Figure XIV-8 *middle*) which is the style directly descended from the Cousteau-Gagnan device, is still in use, but production is declining. While each style has its own advantages and disadvantages in particular uses, the basic principle of operation is the same. Each style has two pressure reduction stages, a breathing hose, a mouthpiece, and a means of exhausting exhaled air into the surrounding water.

In the first stage of a single-hose regulator, high pressure air from the cylinder passes through a valve assembly that reduces the pressure to 100–130 psi over the ambient pressure at depth. There are three commonly used types of first-stage valves: the standard, the balanced, and the piston types. While different in their specific operations, all are designed to supply a controlled intermediate pressure to the second stage. The reader is referred to the *NOAA Diving Manual* (Miller 1979) for a detailed discussion of these operations.

In the second stage, to which the mouthpiece is connected, intermediate-pressure air passes down the breathing hose to the demand valve. In the second-stage assembly, ambient water pressure is applied to one side of a movable diaphragm, which has a low pressure chamber on its opposite side. This diaphragm makes contact with the demand valve through a mechanical linkage. When no pressure differential exists across the diaphragm, it is centered in the housing and the demand valve is closed. As the diver inhales, the negative pressure of inspiration creates a partial vacuum in the low pressure chamber, drawing the diaphragm inward. This diaphragm movement causes the mechanical linkage to open the demand valve that provides air flow to the diver. The deeper the inspiration, the deeper is the negative pressure gradient across the diaphragm, and the greater the air flow to the diver.

As the diver completes his inspiration, pressure is once again equal across the diaphragm and the demand valve closes with the beginning of exhalation. As the diver exhales, the exhausted air passes through the exhaust check valves and is vented into the

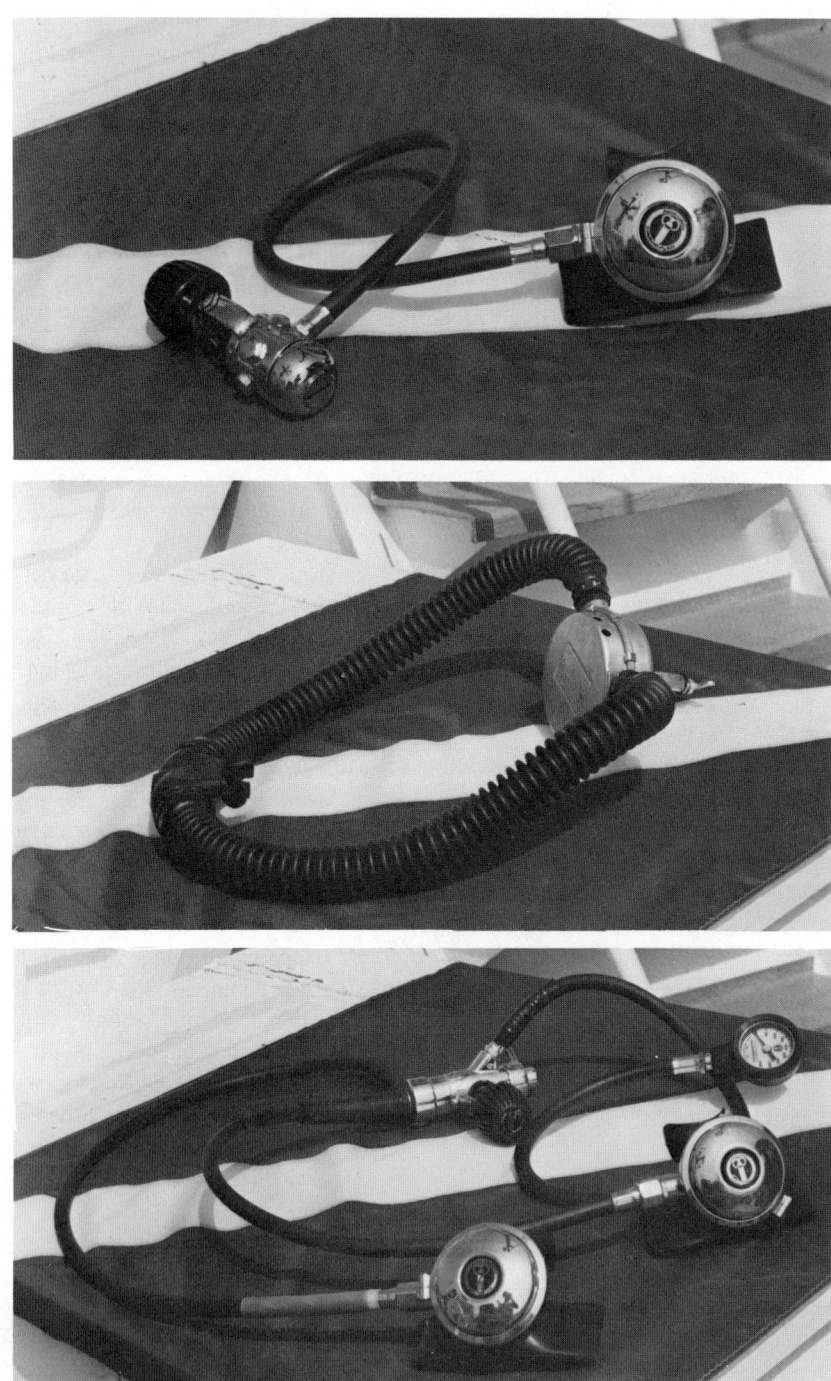

Figure XIV-8. Regulator group. *Top*: Single-hose, two-stage demand regulator. *Middle*: Double-hose, two-stage demand regulator. *Bottom*: Single-hose regulator with submersible pressure gauge and octopus regulator.

surrounding water. Second-stage assemblies are engineered to limit the amount of air rebreathed by reducing dead space to a minimum.

The major advantage of two-stage pressure reduction lies in the fact that the air is supplied at a nearly constant pressure that allows reductions in breathing resistance and in fluctuations in breathing resistance caused by changes in depth or cylinder pressure. Most of the major recent advances in regulator technology have focused on further decreasing the breathing resistance of two-stage regulators to increase the ease of breathing for the diver.

In a program related to its internal Navy mission, the U.S. Navy Experimental Diving Unit (NEDU) conducts comprehensive evaluations of many commercially produced scuba regulators (as well as other types of diving equipment) to determine the suitability of each for Navy diving purposes. These evaluations are based on performance criteria established by Navy operational requirements, and while certainly not conducted for the benefit of the equipment manufacturers, do provide the manufacturing industry with valuable information concerning the performance of their products. Because of their impartiality, these Navy evaluations also benefit the diving public for guidance in making equipment selections; indeed, acceptance of a manufacturer's product by the Navy has become a coveted marketing tool.

The failure of an intact regulator to deliver air at depth would be a most serious matter, one that could easily precipitate a sequence of events resulting in the serious injury, even death, of a diver. It is certainly not unusual for a diver to attribute an underwater emergency to regulator failure. In view of the potential seriousness of such an event, such claims bear careful scrutiny.

In this regard, it is instructive to note two recent findings. First, Egstrom (1976), as a result of extensive functional performance studies of contemporary regulators, has observed that the regulator is a highly reliable instrument whose performance characteristics are predictable. He further observes that it is entirely possible for a poorly trained diver (or any diver for that matter) to place demands upon a regulator that can result in excessive differential pressures and work of breathing. Second, Schenck and McAniff (1978) have not turned up one case, in seven years of investigation and analysis of U.S. diving fatalities, in which the cause of the accident was shown to be the failure of a properly maintained regulator. These findings suggest quite strongly that regulator failure incidents might more properly be incidents where a regulator's performance limits were exceeded by the diver, or where the diver was using a poorly maintained regulator.

While the failure to deliver air because of overbreathing or improper maintenance might not be considered true regulator failure, the failure of a regulator due to a hose rupture certainly is, with the same potentially serious consequences. Failure of the low pressure breathing hose, or either of the other common types of low pressure accessory hoses (the octopus or the power inflator hoses), is usually caused by stress on the crimped metal fittings on either end of the hose. Over time this stress can insidiously weaken the hose fitting connections, or the hose itself, resulting in actual rupture of the hose or explosive separation of the hose from the regulator first stage. Rupture of the hose can deplete the entire air charge of a full cylinder in about 5 min or so. Explosive separation causes immediate loss of air to the diver and is the most serious type of hose failure.

There are three commonly used pieces of accessory equipment often attached to the first stage of single-hose regulators. There are the octopus rig, the submersible pressure gauge, and the power inflator or "whip". A regulator fitted with all three accessories can be seen Figure XIV-8 *bottom*.

The octopus rig is actually an additional regulator second stage on a longer breathing hose that is connected to an available port on the first-stage housing. While it may serve for other functions, the primary purpose of the octopus is to provide a safety device to allow two divers to breathe from the same air supply in situations that would otherwise require the buddy breathing exchange of a mouthpiece during ascent.

While the octopus regulator offers definite advantages for diving safety, there are cautions to observe as well. Care must be taken to protect the octopus from fouling or clogging when not in use, and it must receive the same maintenance as the primary second stage. Divers must also remember that when the octopus is in use, usually following the depletion or loss of one diver's air supply, both divers are now breathing from the same air supply and consuming that supply, which might also be approaching low levels. In addition, the demands placed on the regulator by two divers at one time can exceed the design flow capabilities of the regulator.

The submersible pressure gauge is a safety device that allows the diver to continuously monitor the pressure of the air remaining in the scuba cylinder. It is the only device available that has this capability, and most divers today have incorporated it into their equipment. The gauge consists of a length of high pressure hose attached to the high pressure side of the first stage of the regulator, and a bourdon-type mechanism, within a protected housing, which indicates the pressure remaining. An excellent discussion of the technical details of these instruments can be found in McKenney (1976a). While their safety advantages should be obvious, they are subject to inadvertent abuse if they are not properly secured during a dive. Since they are designed to handle pressures up to 3000 psi, they can be potentially hazardous if the gauge lens has been damaged and then is subjected to high pressure. Blowout of the lens can cause eye damage if a diver does not turn the gauge away from the face when opening the cylinder valve.

The power inflation devices, or whips, are low pressure hoses used to inflate buoyancy devices and variable-volume diving suits from the diver's air supply. These whips are connected to ports on the regulator first stage and to manually activated inlet valves on the vests or suits, via quick-disconnect fittings. The greatest hazard from these whips is hose blowout if the stress of use has weakened the fittings or hose walls. The danger of blowup in a variable volume suit is discussed in another portion of this section on scuba.

c. Masks, Fins, Snorkels

McKenney (1973) describes the mask as "the most important piece of equipment a diver owns. Without a regulator one can still snorkel dive; without fins scuba diving is still possible But a mask provides sight—the one vital sense that's a must to enjoy diving to its fullest." It is doubtful that there is much serious argument over the importance of the mask to diving.

Masks are available in literally dozens of styles, a few of which are represented in Figure XIV-9 top left. Features usually considered in mask selection are size and weight, internal displacement, extent of field of view, efficiency of sealing at the skirt, type of glass used, and the presence or absence of a purge valve. Properly fitting masks rarely

Equipment and Procedures 637

cause a diver any problem if carefully maintained. Diver injuries from the mask are usually confined to squeeze that results from a diver's failure to equalize the pressure in the enclosed air space.

Snorkels (see Figure XIV-9 *bottom*), while not an essential piece of equipment, are commonly used as means of conserving compressed air on the surface while swimming. They are usually a curved piece of plastic or rubber tubing with a 180° bend and a mouthpiece at one end. Tube diameters range from ⅝ in. to ¾ in. and have lengths up to 15 in.

Fins, like masks and snorkels, are available in a variety of styles and sizes. They provide the diver with propulsive force for movement through the water. A common style of fin usually worn with protective suits is seen in Figure XIV-9 *top right*. Selection

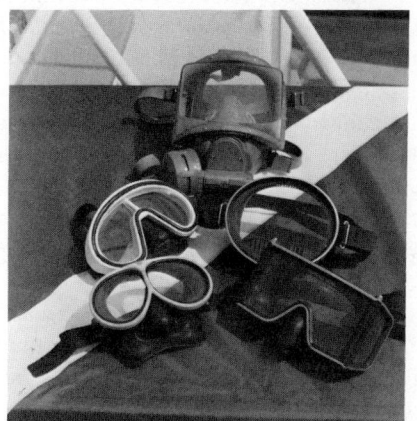
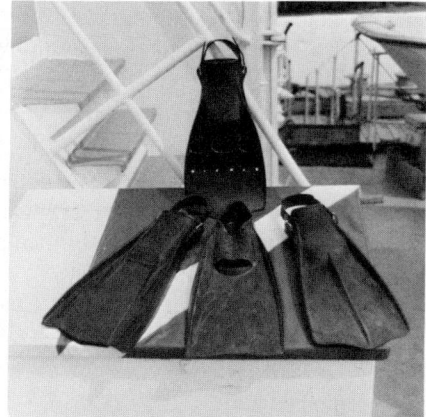
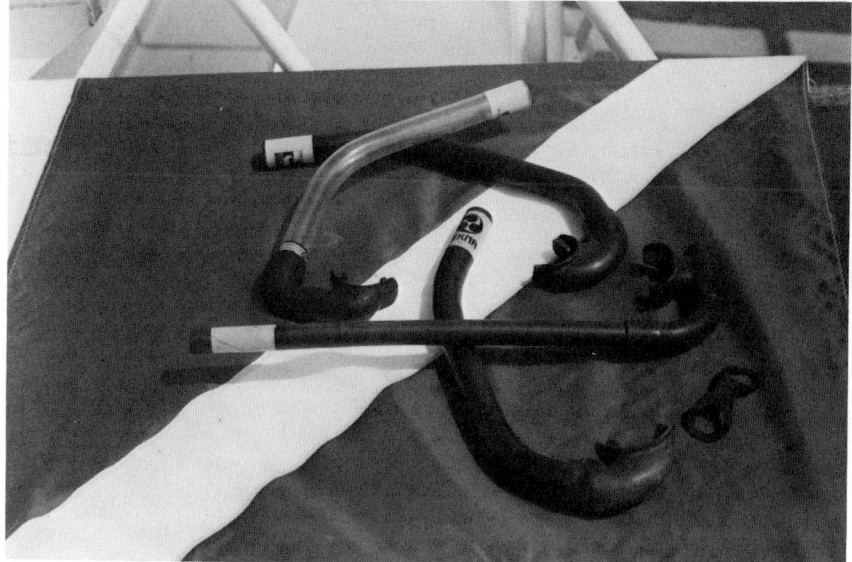

Figure XIV-9. Masks (*top left*), fins (*top right*), and snorkels (*bottom*).

638   Chapter XIV

of fins involves the consideration of characteristics such as shape of the foot pocket; surface area; shape, angle, and degree of stiffness of the blade; and overall weight. Properly fitted and maintained fins, when selected as appropriate for the type of diving anticipated, rarely if ever cause a diver problems. An ill-fitting or otherwise improper fin selection can, however, contribute to early diver fatigue or to painful muscle cramps, either of which can precipitate emergency situations if not recognized and properly handled.

d. Buoyancy Control Group

Safe diving requires the diver to have a working understanding of the effects of buoyancy. Water's buoyant effects on immersed objects are succinctly described in the 1970 *U.S. Navy Diving Manual* as a series of "laws of flotation" derived from Archimedes' principle. The weight systems and the various types of inflatable devices that compose the buoyancy control equipment group are designed to permit adjustment and control of buoyancy by taking advantage of these natural laws.

The manipulative skills involved in properly adjusting and controlling buoyancy are among the most critical to be possessed by the diver. Buoyancy control equipment is more often than not a causal factor in diving accident situations—a sad result of common misunderstanding of its purpose and its proper use.

The diver's buoyant status is established by simply subtracting total individual weight from the weight of water displaced by the individual. Very few people are negatively buoyant by nature, and natural buoyancy varies among individuals mostly because of differences in such physical traits as bone weight, degree of obesity, and lung capacity. External factors such as the buoyancy characteristics of protective sutis and scuba cylinders must also be considered.

To overcome natural and equipment-derived positive buoyancy, a weight system such as the standard weight belt (Figure XIV-10 *top*) is used to achieve a negatively buoyant state. The proper weight to be added is only that amount necessary to become neutral or slightly negatively buoyant at the surface.

The weight belt is by no means the simple piece of gear that it seems. It must hold the proper amount of weight, must be mounted on the waist in a balanced manner that distributes the weight equally, must be worn in such a manner that it can always be jettisoned without fouling on other equipment, and it must incorporate a quick-release buckle operable with a single motion of either hand. Hardy and Sleeper (1976) provide an analysis of weight systems and common problems associated with them. McAniff (1975) recounts a fatal accident case that offers a tragic reminder of the importance of wearing the weight belt and other equipment in such a way as to permit unhindered jettisoning of the weight belt. A diver apparently acted properly in an emergency and ditched the weight belt; the belt, however, became fouled on the diver's knife sheath on the outside of the lower leg. This diver was eventually found, thus fouled, on the bottom and out of air. Another detail frequently overlooked by many divers is the necessity to keep the quick-release buckle in the front. Swimming motions and the compression of the protective suit at depth often cause the position of the buckle to move around the body, making it inaccessible for jettisoning in an emergency.

While the weight systems are used primarily to help produce the proper amount of negative buoyancy, they do not afford the diver an opportunity to vary buoyancy as diving conditions change. Adjustment of buoyancy during a dive is normally accomplished by using an inflatable device generically known as a "personal flotation device." (See Figure XIV-10 *bottom*.) Divers today have a variety of these devices to choose from—each with its own particular advantages and disadvantages. All operate on the same basic principle.

The most common style of personal flotation device in use is typically referred to as a *buoyancy compensator*. This is a horse-collar type of vest that can be inflated by

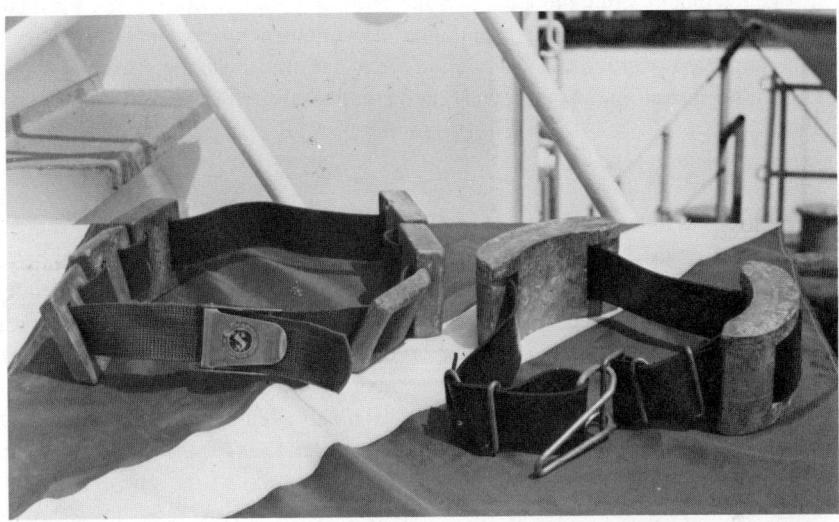

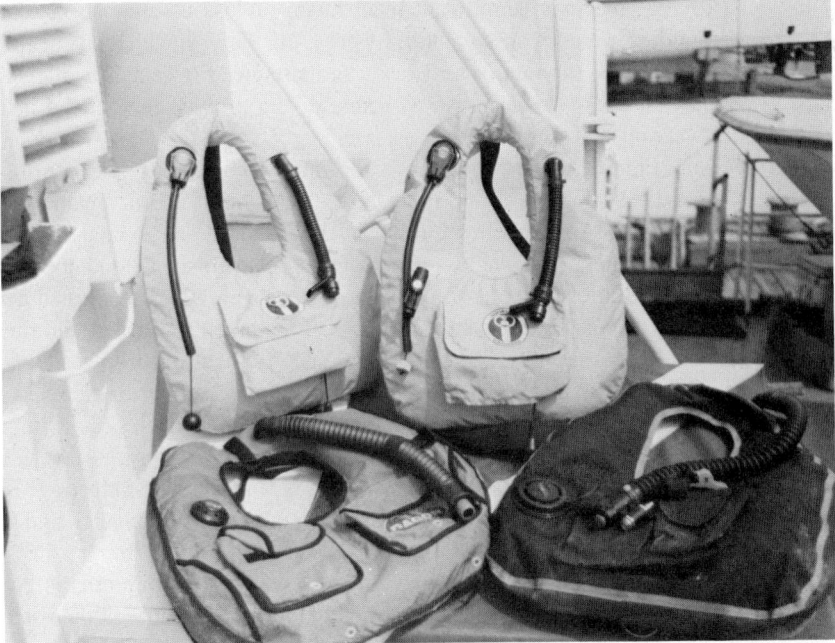

Figure XIV-10. Buoyancy control group. *Top*: Weights and weight belts. *Bottom*: Buoyancy compensators

any combination of the following methods: orally; by a CO_2 cartridge; from an integral compressed air "pony bottle"; and by low pressure inflation via a whip from the scuba cylinder and regulator. Most of these compensators incorporate an overpressure relief valve and will float an unconscious diver in the faceup position on the surface. McKenney (1976a) offers an excellent general description of these devices. Other equipment designs that allow for adjustment and control of buoyancy are discussed in McKenney (1976b) and Tzimoulis (1977). A final device that can be used to control buoyancy is the variable-volume dry suit, which is described in the discussion of the protective clothing group.

Typical accident situations in which the buoyancy equipment has been a factor can usually be described as stemming from improper maintanence, accidental inflation causing sudden unexpected positive buoyancy and ascent, failure to use the device at all when it should have been used in the emergency, and compensating for excessive overweighting.

e. Protective Clothing Group

Heat loss, together with its attendant physiological effects, is one of the more insidious and probably least appreciated problems faced by the diver. Fortunately, heat loss can be one of diving's most manageable problems. The protective clothing equipment group consists of various types of diver dress and accessories to deal with this problem.

The reasons for heat loss in the water environment are physiologically quite complex; they are usually explained in generalities comparing the differences in the thermal conductivity and specific heat of water and air at the same temperature. The details of this heat loss notwithstanding, the most important consideration for the diver is to minimize body heat loss as effectively as possible—for the duration of the immersion and even afterwards.

In scuba diving, the most significant mechanism of loss is conduction across the skin to the surrounding water. Consequently, by covering the skin with a layer of material of high insulative quality, the rate of heat loss can be reduced over reasonable exposure periods. Two diver dress systems in use by scuba divers provide the desired insulating protection: the wet suit and the dry suit.

The wet suit (Figure XIV-11 *top left*) is the most commonly worn form of scuba diving dress, and the "shortie suit" (Figure XIV- 11 *bottom left*) is a variation of it. These suits are fabricated from neoprene rubber. The standard design consists of a layer of closed-cell foamed neoprene enclosed between two layers of smooth neoprene. A popular option is an additional lining of nylon for greater strength. The foamed neoprene layer contains many tiny gas bubbles that are more or less evenly distributed throughout. The entrapped gas has a thermal conductivity and specific heat much lower than water, thus giving the material its insulative property by creating a thermal barrier.

Wet suits are available in thicknesses ranging from ⅛ in. to ½ in. (3–13 mm). The standard suit consists of pants and a jacket. In use, the suit admits a thin layer of water between the insulating layer and the skin. This water is warmed by conduction. Because of a slow circulating flushing action, this water is continuously lost, replaced, and warmed again.

Several factors can influence the effectiveness of wet suits in minimizing heat loss. Effectiveness can be increased by ensuring a proper fit, and also through the use of such accessories as various styles of hoods, vests, gloves, and boots (Figure XIV-11 *bottom right*), which help to reduce the volume of circulating water. The additional protection of hoods, gloves, and boots becomes essential in water temperatures lower than 60°F (NOAA 1975).

An important factor in reducing effectiveness is suit compression, i.e., a reduction in the thickness of the suit material as the depth increases. Suit compression also has a noticeable effect on buoyancy. The wet suit's characteristics that contribute to gradual

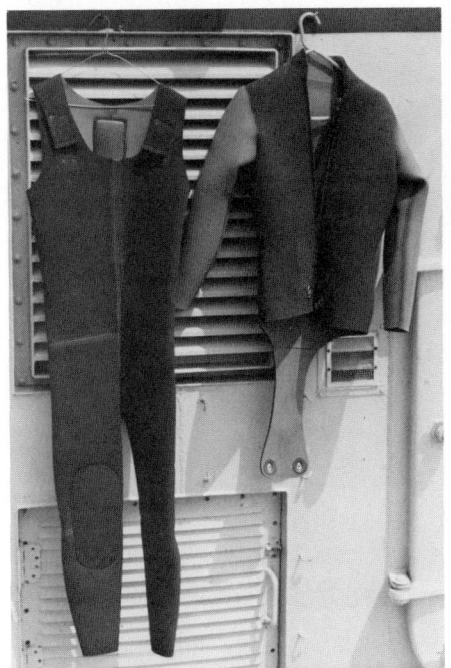
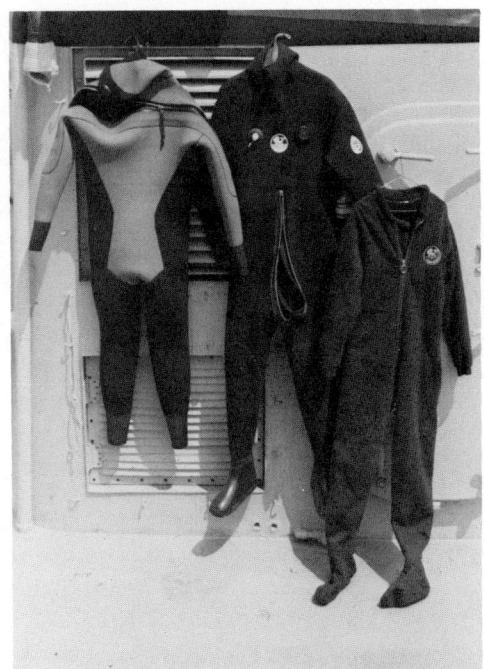
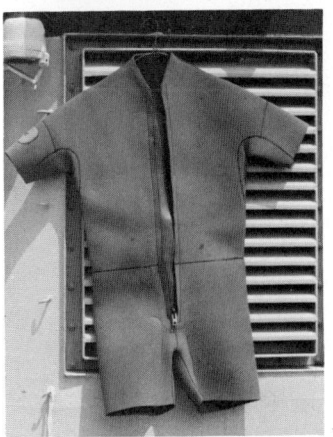
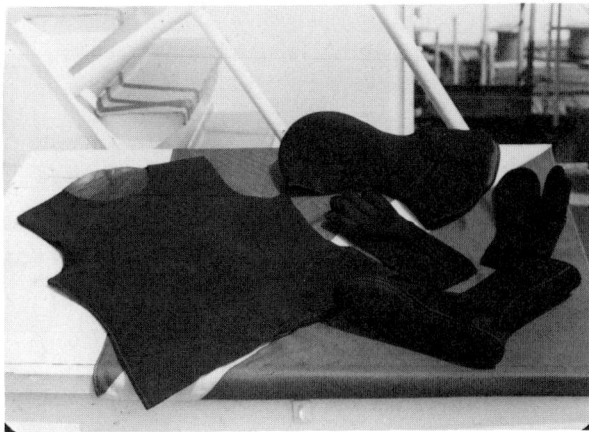

Figure XIV-11. Protective clothing group. *Top left*: "Farmer John" style of wet suit. *Bottom left*: Shortie suit. *Top right*: Variable-volume dry suits. *Bottom right*: Wet suit accessories.

conductive heat loss, suit compression, and buoyancy changes find appreciable relief in the other forms of diver dress—the dry suit.

The dry suit utilizes a layer of trapped air between the diver's skin and the suit fabric as the insulating medium. This air creates an extremely efficient thermal barrier, permitting considerably longer exposure times than is possible with wet suits. In the Arctic, modern dry suits have been used under ice in water at 28.5°F for 2 hr (NOAA 1975).

Unlike the latex rubber dry suits of the 1950s, the modern dry suits are nearly all manufactured of closed-cell foamed neoprene with nylon linings; all are of one-piece construction. Air can be introduced into the suit via an oral inflation hose or a low pressure inflator from the regulator first stage connected to a separate inlet valve. The trapped air can be vented to the surrounding water through the oral inflation hose or through a separate exhaust valve. Boots and hoods may be integral parts of the suit, or they may be donned over watertight seals. Gloves are donned over wrist seals. Entry is easy, by means of various schemes of waterproof zipper placement.

Dry suits, which can be inflated and deflated at will by the diver, are generically termed variable-volume suits (Figure XIV-11 *top right*). These suits permit the diver to offset the noticeable effects of suit compression and buoyancy loss, a disadvantage of wet suits worn without external buoyancy devices. With increasing depth (i.e., increasing pressure), the wet suit material shrinks and compresses against the skin. This action reduces the thermal barrier and the buoyancy provided by the suit material. In the variable-volume dry suit, admitting more air into the suit compensates for the effects of compression and thus maintains the thermal barrier, while the additional air also maintains the suit's buoyancy.

Protective suits are designed to minimize the occurrence of the physiological consequences of heat loss. Usually any diving accident in which the thermal status of the diver was a contributing factor is not the fault of the suit but rather the direct result of the diver having exceeded the design limitations of his suit—either in terms of environmental conditions or of exposure periods.

Dry suits have been involved in accident situations where the immediate cause was a sudden increase in the diver's buoyancy. Because of the greater buoyancy of dry suits inherent in their design and use, a diver must necessarily wear greater amounts of weight. The sudden loss of a heavy weight belt while the suit is inflated or the malfunction of an inlet valve can lead directly, and quickly, to an uncontrolled buoyant ascent, sometimes called a blowup. Such an occurrance, should it befall an inexperienced or ill-trained diver, might well result in some form of extraalveolar air syndrome.

f Instrument Group

Depth gauges and diving watches make up the important instrument group. Their respective purposes should be obvious. Both instruments are usually worn on the same wrist; depth gauges, however, can also be incorporated into equipment "consoles." (Figure XIV-12 *left*). Depth gauges can be of four different types: capillary, bourdon tube, diaphragm, and electronic.

The capillary gauge measures depth by using a simple volumetric principle of physics; this type is most accurate in shallow depths. The bourdon tube and diaphragm types utilize various schemes of mechanically transmitting pressure changes to moving parts.

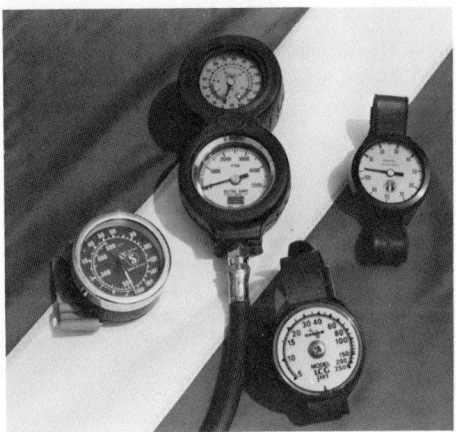 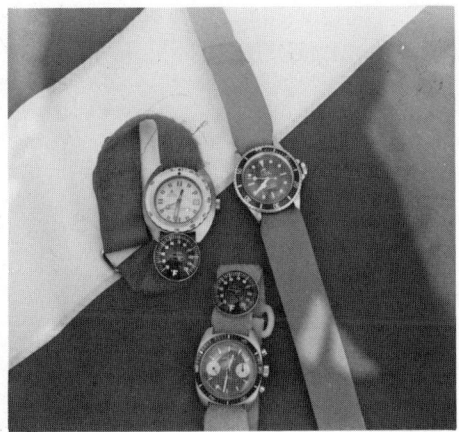

Figure XIV-12. *Left*: Depth gauges, wrist and console styles. *Right*: Diving watches.

They are probably the most common types in use but, because of their delicate internal mechanisms, are also the most sensitive to damage, malfunction, and error. The electronic depth gauge uses a small pressure transducer to electrically measure changes in ambient pressure and converts these changes into an light-emitting diode (LED) display of depth.

Diving watches are waterproof and pressure-proof and are usually equipped with a rotating bezel to directly indicate elapsed bottom time (Figure XIV-12 *right*). Watch faces are normally luminous for readability in reduced visibility. A relatively recent innovation is a pressure-actuated underwater stopwatch.

Decompression sickness (the bends), of all the diving-related medical problems, is the most likely condition the physician will encounter from scuba divers. The information the depth gauge and diving watch provide to the diver are extremely important if the probability of an incident of decompression sickness is to be minimized. Because of the reliance placed upon these instruments, particularly on the depth gauge, an understanding of their design limitations is necessary. Failure to appreciate these limitations is often the contributing factor in inadvertent cases of decompression sickness. Failure to use these instruments at all is an even greater contributing factor to such incidents!

The absolutely accurate scuba depth gauge has yet to be designed. Capillary gauges can be extremely accurate over the shallow depth range of its logarithmically generated scale only if they are carefully maintained. The bourdon tube and diaphragm gauges are limited in their reliability by the accuracy of the movement of their delicate internal mechanisms. Manufacturers' accuracy standards for these types of gauges permit acceptable tolerances in depth indication of various percentages of the full scale over the full scale, or over specific depth increments. Ackerman (1976) presents an excellent discussion on depth gauge accuracy.

6. Conclusion

As market forces continue to generate improvements in equipment design and function, as well as greater variety and increasing sophistication, changes or adjustments in both teaching practices and diving procedures are necessary. This is particularly true where they may relate to the manner in which a diver should conduct himself in an underwater emergency situation. The diver who fails to use his equipment properly, either through lack of training in its correct use or a misunderstanding of its function and limitations, becomes a potential candidate for the physician's services.

DAVID H. PETERSON

References

ACKERMAN, N. 1976. Depth gauges—the inside story on mechanics and accuracy. *Skin Diver* May 1976: 40–46.
CICHY, F. C., H. SCHENCK, AND J. MCANIFF 1978. Corrosion of steel and aluminum scuba tanks. Kingston: Univ. Of Rhode Island, Marine Technical Report 62.
EDMONDS, C. 1976. Barotrauma. In: *Diving Medicine*, edited by R. H. Strauss. New York: Grune and Stratton, p. 49–61.
EGSTROM, G. H. 1976. U.C.L.A.—diving safety research program. In: *Addendum to the Proceedings of the Eighth International Conference on Underwater Education*. National Association of Underwater Instructors, p. 8–11.
HALL, J. 1976. How scuba tanks are made. *Skin Diver* Nov. 1976: 34—38.
HARDY, J., AND J. B. SLEEPER 1976. The last ditch attempt—weight systems. In: *Proceedings of the Eighth International Conference on Underwater Education*. National Association of Underwater Instructors, p. 139–143.
KIDD, D. J., AND D. H. ELLIOTT 1975. Decompression disorders in divers. In: *The Physiology and Medicine of Diving and Compressed Air Work* (2nd ed), edited by P. B. Bennett and D. H. Elliott. Baltimore: Williams and Wilkins Co., p. 471–495.
LARSON, H. E. 1959. *A History of Self-Contained Diving and Underwater Swimming*. Washington, DC: Natl. Acad. Sci./Natl. Res. Coun. (Publ. 469.)
MCKENNEY, J. 1973. Up to our snorkels in masks. *Skin Diver* June 1973: 18–22.
MCKENNEY, J. 1976a. Submersible pressure gauges—what they are and how they work. *Skin Diver* Feb. 1976: 34–36, 71.
MCKENNEY, J. 1976b. The ins and outs of buoyancy compensators. *Skin Diver* April 1976: 42–47, 82–86.
MCKENNEY, J. 1976c. The ups and downs of B/C packs. *Skin Diver* July 1976: 52–57.
MILLER, J. W. (editor). 1979. *NOAA Diving Manual* (2nd ed.). Washington, DC: National Oceanic and Atmospheric Administration, U.S. Dept. of Commerce.
NATIONAL OCEANIC AND ATMOSPHERIC ADMINISTRATION. 1975. An analysis of the civil diving population of the United States. Washington, DC: U.S. Dept. Commerce.
NAVAL SAFETY CENTER. 1978. Diving safety note. Oct. 1978.
SCHENCK, H. V., AND J. J. MCANIFF 1975. *United States Underwater Fatality Statistics—1973*. Rep. No. URI-SSR-75-9. Washington, DC: National Oceanic and Atmospheric Administration, U.S. Dept. of Commerce.
SCHENCK, H. V., AND J. J. MCANIFF 1976. *United States Underwater Fatality Statistics—1974*. Rep. No. URI-SSR-75-10. Washington, DC: National Oceanic and Atmospheric Administration, U.S. Dept. of Commerce.
SCHENCK, H. V., AND J. J. MCANIFF 1978. *United States Underwater Fatality Statistics—1976*. Rep. No. URI-SSR-78-12. Washington, DC: National Oceanic and Atmospheric Administration, U.S. Dept. of Commerce.
SHILLING, C. W., M. F. WERTS, AND N. R. SCHANDELMEIER. 1976. *The Underwater Handbook. A Guide to Physiology and Performance for the Engineer*. New York: Plenum.
TZIMOULIS, P. J. 1977. The calypso compensator. *Skin Diver* Jan.: 52–55, 89.
U.S. NAVY 1970. *The U.S. Navy Diving Manual*. Washington, DC: U.S. Navy Department. (NAVSHIPS 0994-001-9010.)
U.S. NAVY 1975. *The U.S. Navy Diving Manual*. Washington, DC: U.S. Navy Department. (NAVSEA 0994-LP-001-9010.)

C. Surface-Supplied Diving

1. Air Diving

In surface-supplied air diving numerous types of diving equipments and ancillary support equipments are utilized; they vary with diving companies and individual divers. This type of diving is normally limited to 190 ft (58 m) of sea water (fsw or msw) but may be used to a maximum depth of 220 fsw (67 msw) for less than 30 min bottom time.

A basic component of the surface-supplied air diving system is the diving helmet/mask; pictorial representations of these are shown in Figure XIV-13.

All of these helmets/masks should have these features: a ventilation rate capability of 4.5 absolute cubic feet per minute (acfm) at all operating depths, a non-return valve at the attachment point of the diving hose, an exhaust valve, and provision for two-way voice communication between the diver and topside personnel.

In conjunction with the diving helmet/mask, which may be a free flowing or a demand apparatus, is the diver's dress. This dress can vary from a simple wet suit as shown in Figure XIV-14, a variable-volume suit as shown in Figure XIV-15, or a hot water diver heated suit as shown in Figure XIV-16. In addition to the diving dress a suitable weight belt is selected. The diving dress, either active or passive, provides thermal protection to the diver and abrasion protection within the diving environment. A dry suit diving dress must have an independent exhaust valve if it is not directly connected to the exhaust valve of the helmet/mask.

Also worn by the diver is a safety harness that has a positive buckling device and an attachment point for the umbilical. The harness attachment point prevents a strain from being applied to the helmet/mask while a pulling force of the tended umbilical is being distributed over the entire body. A diving umbilical is connected from the diver to the surface and normally contains a diver's air hose, a strong cable (the "strength member"), a communications cable, and some means to determine the diver's depth. The diving hose or umbilical is marked from the diver in 10-ft (3-m) intervals to 100 ft and in 50 ft intervals thereafter. The working pressure of the diving hose equals or exceeds the pressure equivalent of the maximum depth of the dive relative to the supply source, plus 100 psig and a bursting pressure of 4 times its maximum working pressure. Diving umbilicals are so made up that when a surface pulling force is applied to the safety harness attachment point, the full force is carried by the strength member of the umbilical.

A portable or installed diver control console or diving station is located on the surface platform and provides a means for the diving supervisor to monitor the diver. Normally this control station provides the desired air flow and pressure to the diver, a depth gauge or recorder to indicate the diver's depth, a communication system to communicate with the diver, a timekeeping device, and a means of shifting from a primary air supply system to a secondary air supply system should the need arise. The console or control station may also have a diver heating control system should a hot water heating system be put to use.

The primary and secondary air supply system is normally provided by air compressors, air flasks, or a combination of both. Some diving equipments use an emergency diver-carried air supply ("come home bottle") with a sufficient amount of air to enable the diver to return to a safe haven or to the surface. The air systems may be either portable or permanently installed. Compressor intakes must be located well away from areas containing exhaust fumes or internal combustion engines or other hazardous contaminants. A compressor must be equipped with an ASME-coded volume tank that is equipped with a check valve on the inlet side, a pressure gauge, a relief valve, and a drain valve.

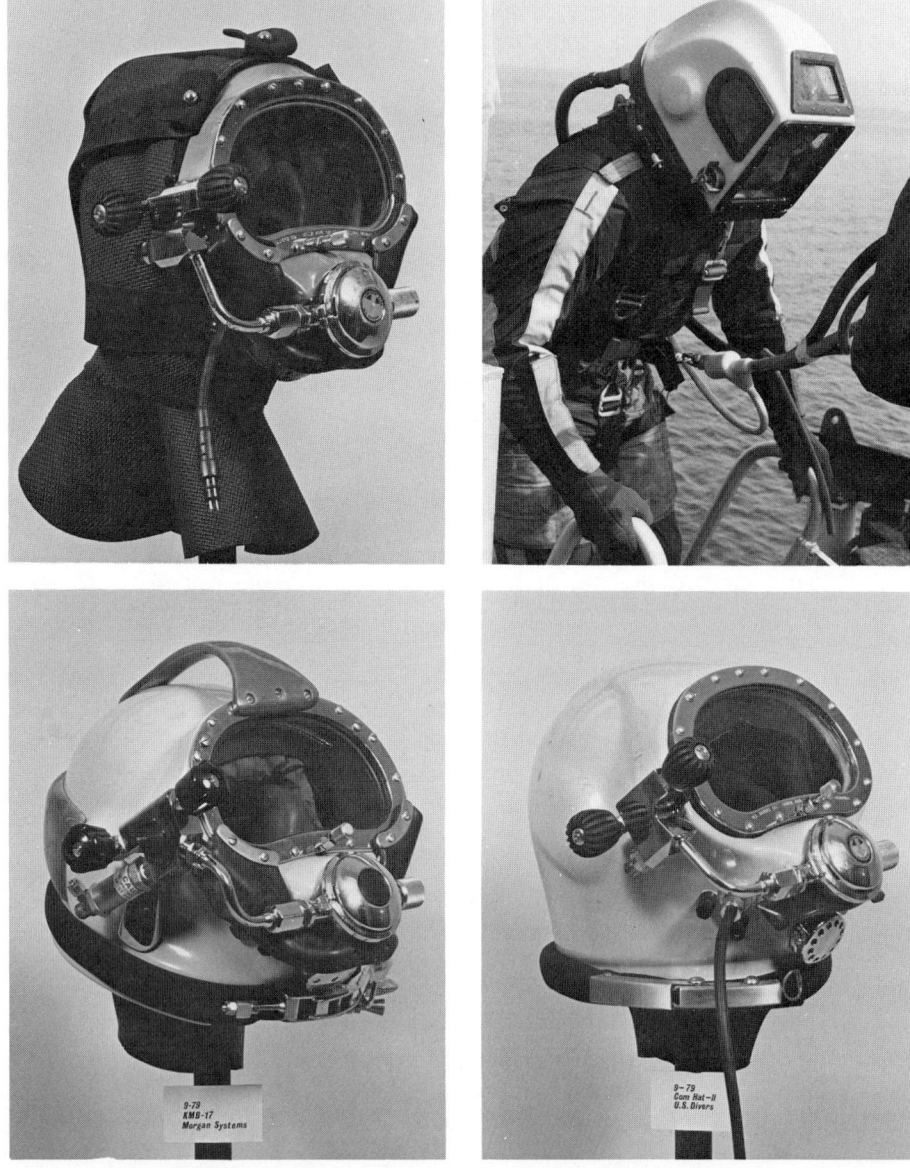

Figure XIV-13. *Top left:* U.S. Navy MK 1 MODO diving mask. *Top right:* U.S. Navy MK 12 deep-sea air helmet. *Bottom left:* Kirby/Morgan KMB-17 helmet. *Bottom right:* U.S. Divers Com-Hat-11.

Outputs of diving compressors must pass through an efficient filtration system that provides air of the purity set forth in Table XIV-1 earlier in this chapter.

The primary breathing supply must be of sufficient capacity to provide adequate air for the diver and the standby diver, and, when required, for open bell and recompression chamber operation. The secondary breathing supply must be of sufficient capacity to provide adequate air for returning the diver to the surface, for the standby diver, and

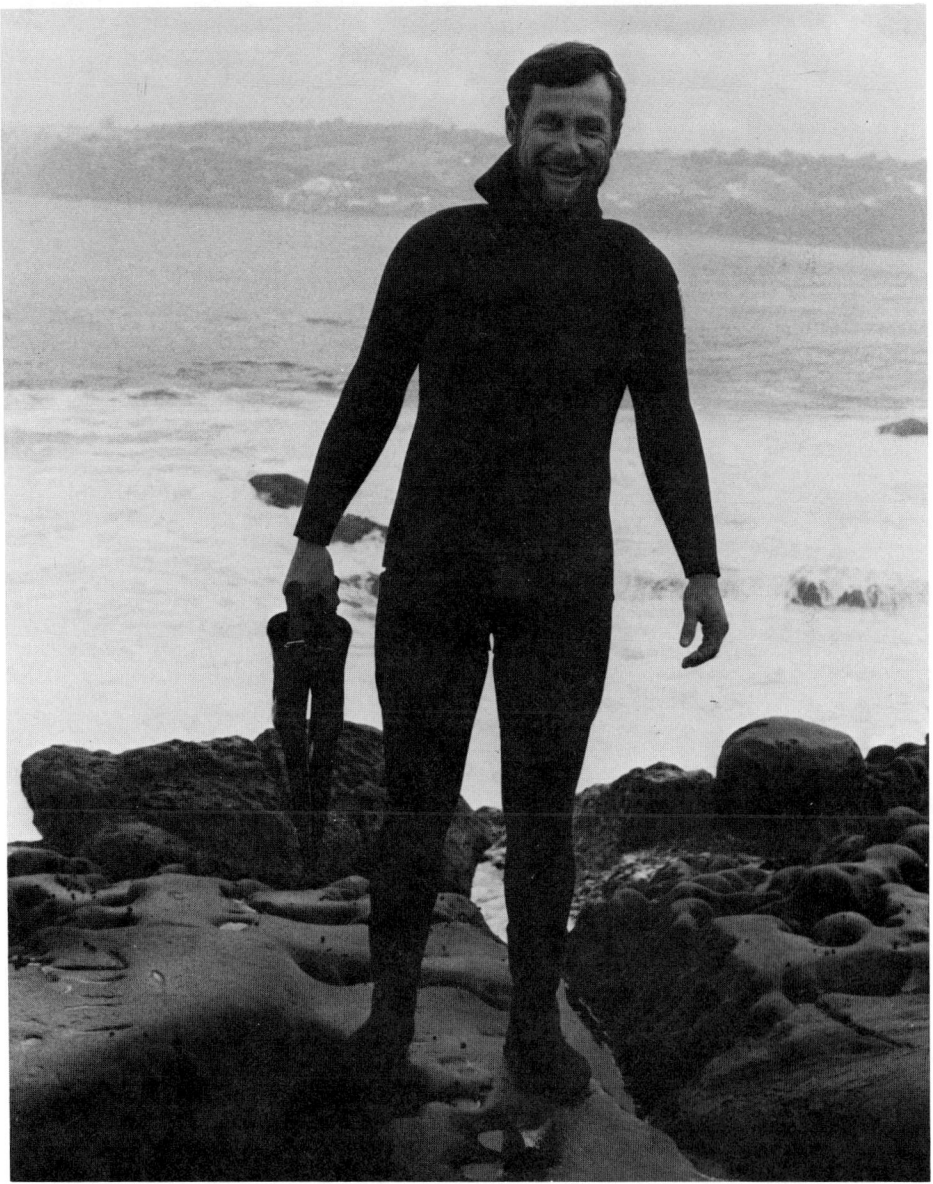

Figure XIV-14. Wet suit with attached hood.

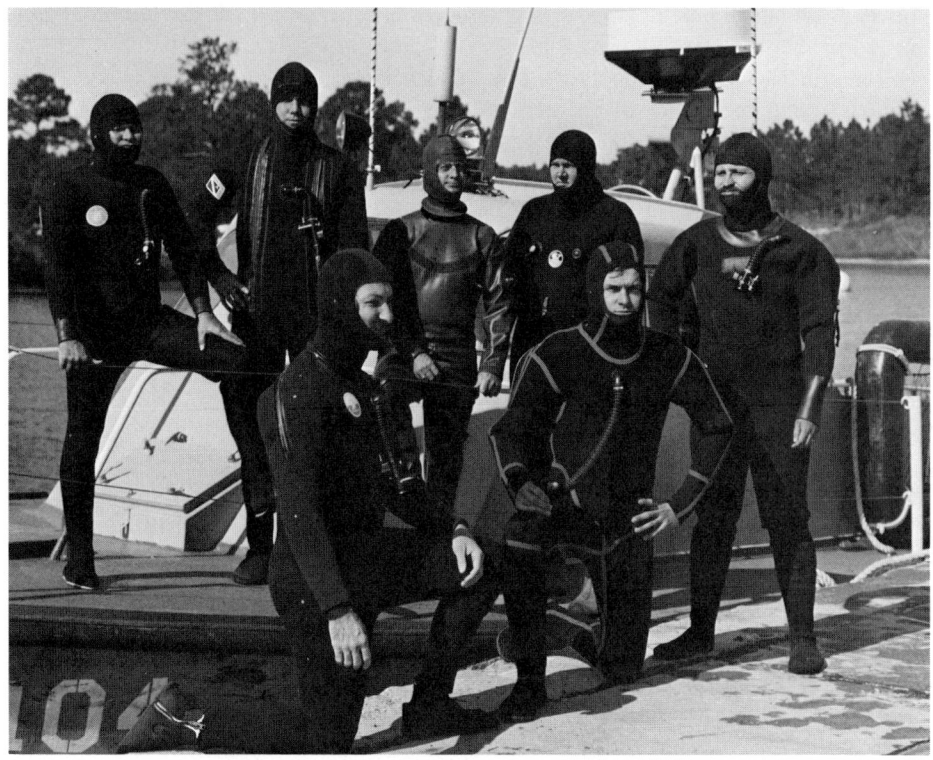

Figure XIV-15. Dry variable-volume diving dresses. (Photo U.S. Navy.)

when required, for returning the open bell to the surface or for supplying the recompression chamber.

An open diving bell may be used in surface-supplied air diving operations; it provides a haven for divers, serves as a diver's stage, and may have additional air sources for diver availability. Figure XIV-17 is representative of one of the numerous types of open bells now in use.

A recompression chamber (pressure vessel for human occupancy, or PVHO) provides a means of treating decompression sickness and for conducting surface decompression dives. Recompression chambers are equipped with means to maintain the atmosphere below a level of 25% oxygen by volume, have a fire extinguishing system, and are ASME-coded. A recompression chamber must be capable of being pressurized to the maximum depth of the dive or to appropriate treatment depth.

The foregoing is not intended to be an optimum or all-inclusive list of surface-supplied air diving equipment; rather, it presents an overview of conventional equipment.

The best diving equipment is only as good as the personnel utilizing it and the procedures they execute. A surface-supported air diving operation varies in complexity from a basic 60-ft (18-m) shallow-water open dive in temperate, clear water to a 190-ft (58-m) dive in cold, turbid water inside a ship's hull. No one set of procedures can encompass all aspects of every dive profile, but a few general procedures are applicable to all diving.

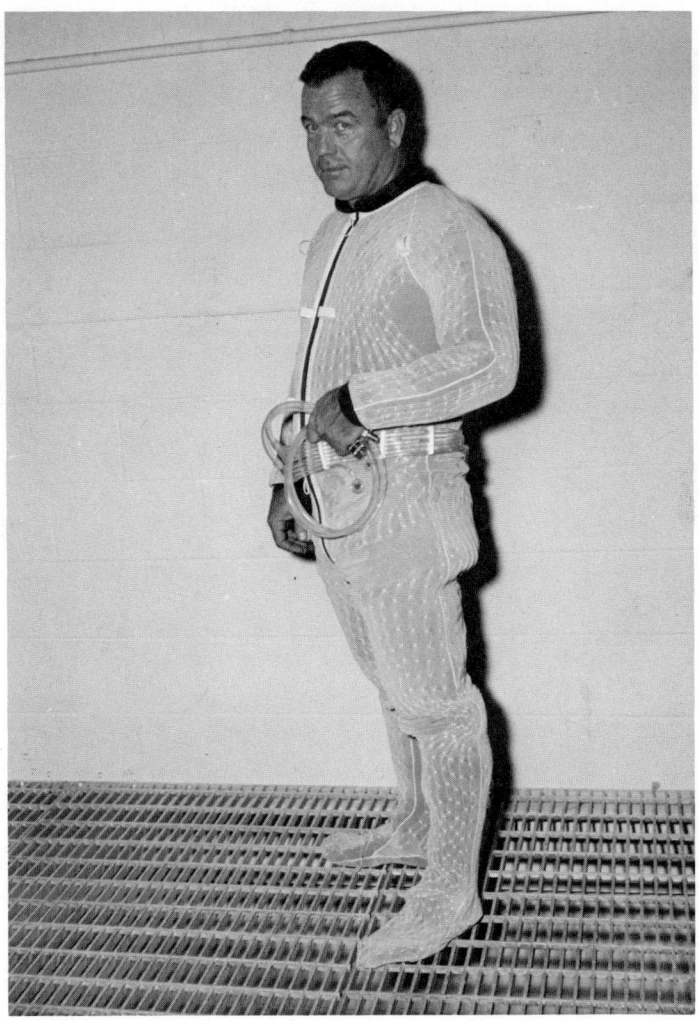

Figure XIV-16. Hot water inner garment tubular suit. (Photo U.S. Navy.)

Any diving task has an objective and, based on that objective, a dive plan is developed to meet that objective in the safest yet cost-effective manner. The dive plan depends on the task at hand and the thoroughness and attention to detail applied to it by the diving supervisor and the divers. The completeness of the dive plan is normally in direct proportion to the success of the dive.

The diving supervisor, by the very title, must be experienced, trained, qualified, and so designated by the diving company. He plans the diving operation, executes it, and is responsible for all aspects of the dive. He must have at his immediate disposal: (1) a company-furnished diving operations manual; (2) written safety procedures and checklists for each item of diving equipment or system; (3) specific emergency procedures and checklists for handling of possible diving casualties; (4) decompression tables; and (5) checklists for diving platform casualties that might impact on the success of the dive.

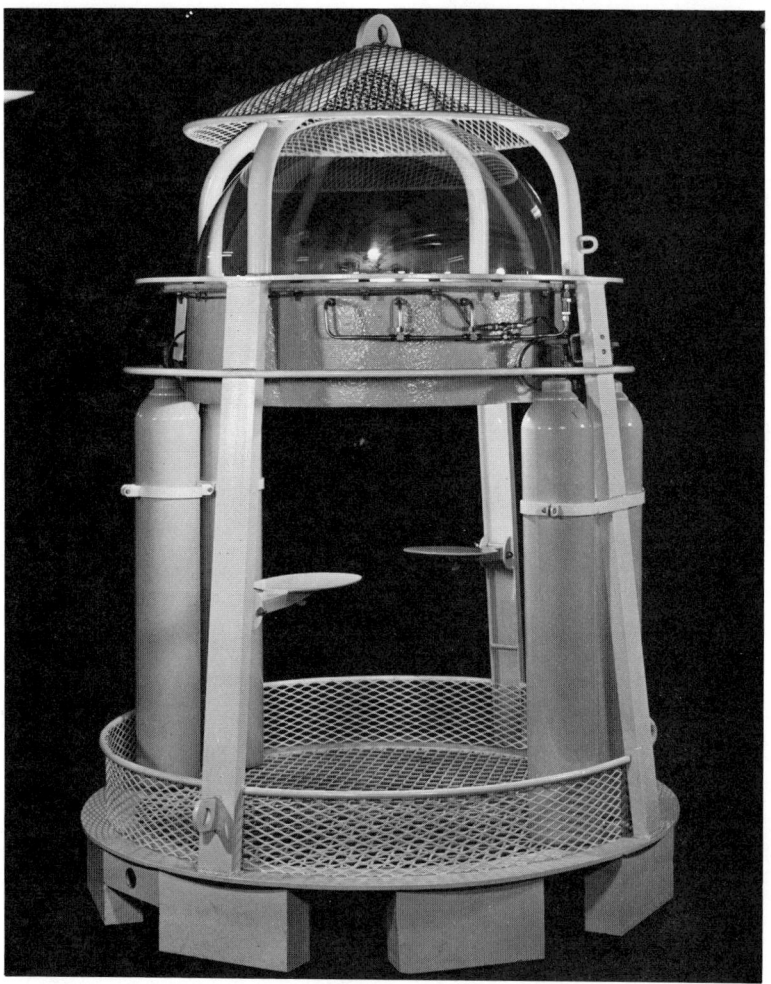

Figure XIV-17. Open diving bell. (Photo courtesy of Nautilus Engineering, Inc.)

It should be noted that the key to effective checklists is that they must be brief enough to be functional, yet detailed enough to ensure an adequate level of safety.

In developing his dive plan, the diving supervisor gives due consideration to many elements: environmental and underwater conditions at the dive site, both present and projected; diving and diving support equipment; manning levels, especially if a diving bell is to be used or if a recompression chamber is required; communications; first aid; air supplies; nearest diving treatment facility; nearest physician trained in diving medicine; diving platform and water interfaces; and decompression schedules to be used, including provision for surface decompression. The dive plan, when complete, is explained to all members of the diving team; they are fully briefed on their individual assignments and are questioned to ensure they fully understand them. The supervisor makes certain that each member of the diving team is physically capable of performing his assigned duties and that he is qualified for the task.

The number of persons engaged in diving operations must be sufficient to conduct and tend the dive but must also be numerous enough to provide backup at full capability in handling emergency or casualty procedures.

The diving equipment is laid out in accordance with the dive plan and is surface tested with the appropriate checklists completed. When the diving supervisor has been assured that all required preparations have been completed and that all systems are properly functioning, he will then commence diving operations. The diver is appropriately tended and the dive plan is executed as scheduled. Discipline on the diving station must always be enforced. The supervisor ensures that depth control is rigidly maintained and that tenders are fully alert. The diver's bottom time is noted to be sure it corresponds to the dive plan, and appropriate decompression schedules are carefully followed. Communications with the diver are frequently made, not only to report job progress but to ascertain the diver's well-being.

An official diving log with appropriate notations about times and facts is kept by assigned personnel, and the dive supervisor ensures that the record of the dive reflects a true documentation of it. In the event that an accident does occur during the span of the dive, then subsequent action is executed in accordance with the emergency and casualty procedures already included in the contingency planning for the dive. The procedures for handling accident victims requiring recompression chamber treatment are discussed in earlier chapters of this book.

Following a dive, a diving supervisor conducts a postdive review to check the physical condition of the diver and review the conduct of the dive to evaluate the possibility of improving future dive plans. If the dive was deeper than 100 fsw (30 msw) or required in-water recompression then the diver must be kept awake and in the vicinity of the recompression chamber for at least 1 hr; if the diving operation is to be terminated the divers must be informed of the potential hazards of flying after diving.

2. Mixed-Gas Diving

As air diving progressed to deeper depths the use of an inert gas with oxygen as a breathing medium was required to eliminate the narcotic effect experienced in utilizing air alone. The U.S. Navy took the lead in this area and commenced modifying open-circuit air systems to accommodate carbon dioxide canisters and develop semiclosed-circuit systems. Semiclosed-circuit systems afforded a means of conserving gas consumption, yet they provided the diver with suitable flows of breathing gas. Commercial endeavors in this area were minimal until offshore oil production moved to deeper waters. The first canisters used carbon dioxide absorbents that were extremely caustic if moisture was introduced into the canister bed; present-day absorbents used in mixed-gas diving systems are much less caustic. Numerous types of mixed-gas diving equipment are used by U.S. diving companies and the U.S. Navy; a sampling is set forth in Figures XIV-18 and XIV-19.

Mixed-gas diving contains the very same principles set forth in Air Diving. With the introduction of helium–oxygen, however, additional areas of concern must be considered by the diver and diving supervisor.

(i) Communications. Helium in the breathing medium produces a Donald Duck quality to the voice, and the diver's voice message is not always easily discernable. The

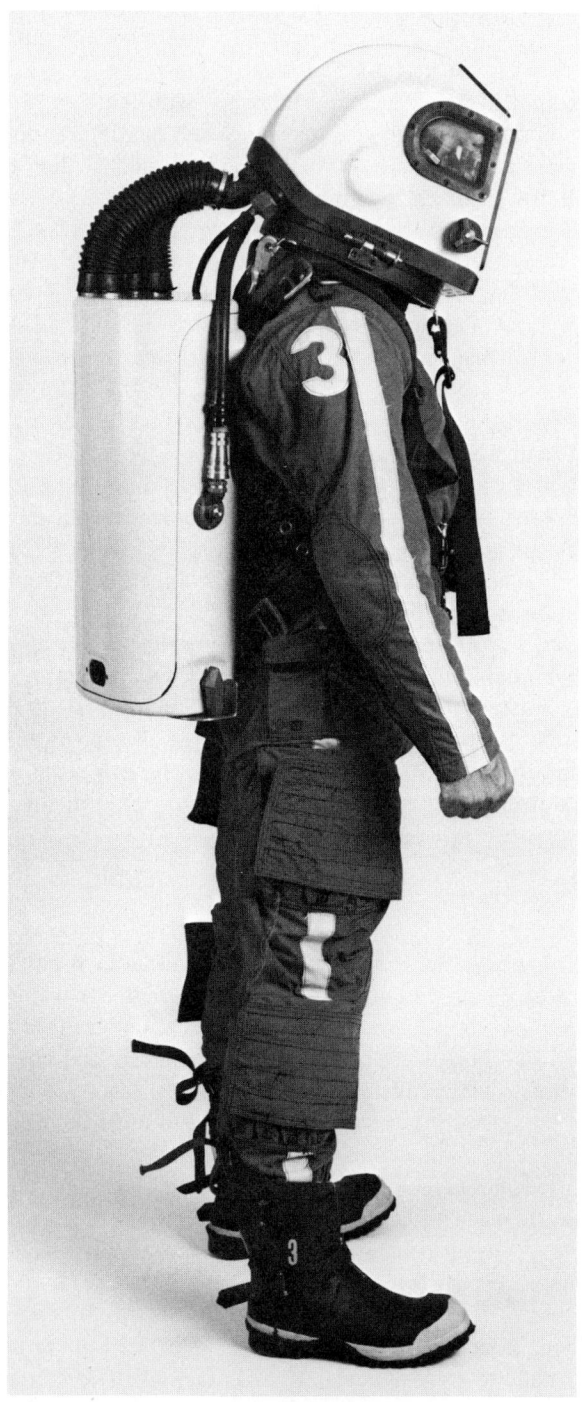

Figure XIV-18. Mixed-gas diving helmet. U.S. Navy MK 12. (Photo U.S. Navy.)

Equipment and Procedures 653

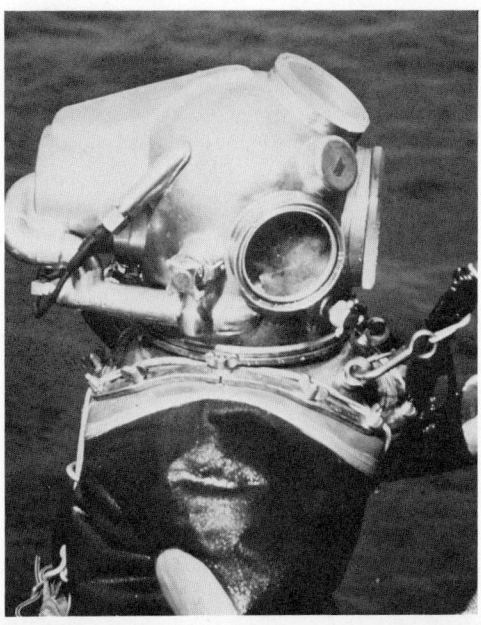

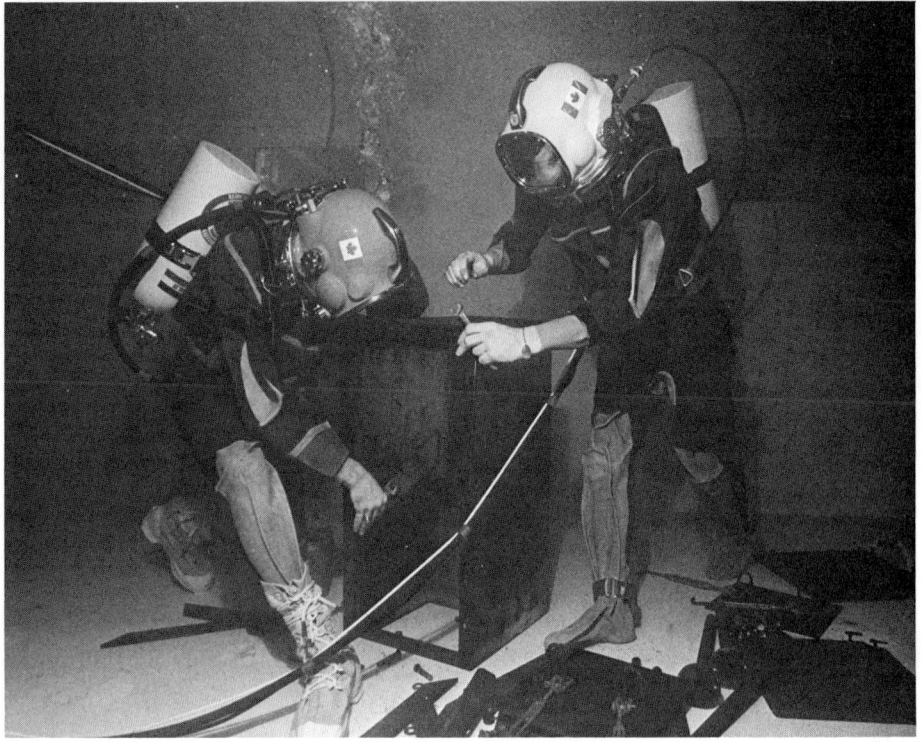

Figure XIV-19. Mixed-gas diving gear. *Top:* recirculating mixed-gas diving gear. *Bottom:* Canadian divers using rat hat.

use of helium speech unscrambler may be necessary to ensure positive communication with the diver.

(ii) System Cleanliness. All diving systems are kept clean, but those systems and piping exposed to oxygen in excess of 40% of the breathing mixture require special oxygen cleaning and maintenance of oxygen cleanliness.

(iii) Thermal Protection. The use of helium in a breathing medium introduces heat loss by the diver not experienced in air diving. The use of additional thermal protection systems are normally required to ensure diver comfort and efficiency. These systems could include inhalation gas heaters.

(iv) Oxygen Toxicity. Decompression schedules call for the use of 100% oxygen in mixed-gas diving decompression either during surface decompression or in a recompression chamber. Accordingly, due attention must be given to careful observation for oxygen toxicity symptoms in the diver who is breathing 100% oxygen.

(v) Gas Stowage. Gas is normally supplied by gas storage racks composed of high pressure gas flasks nested together. Gas may be premixed to the selected percentage or a "mixmaker" device fed by 100% helium and 100% oxygen may be used. It is not meant to imply that all mixed-gas diving is conducted with only helium-oxygen mixtures; some companies use trimixes, some use hydrogen, but the vast majority use helium-oxygen.

(vi) Diver Stage. A diver's stage such as an open diving bell must be provided for all helium/oxygen diving whereby the fully suited diver is lifted out of the water and onto the diving platform.

Mixed-gas diving requires additional operational requirements to ensure safe diving. A recompression chamber must be available for all mixed-gas diving. If dives will be conducted deeper than 200 ft (61 m) or more than 120 min bottom time, an open or closed bell must be used; dives deeper than 300 ft mandatorily require a closed bell. Unless divers are utilizing heavy-duty equipment, a diver-carried emergency mixed-gas supply ("come home bottle") is mandatory. When using heavy-duty equipment, then a standby gas hose, in addition to the gas hose for the standby diver, must be readily available.

The procedures for mixed-gas diving are basically the same as those for air diving; however, dive planning must include the additional areas of concern mentioned. Additional training is required for all divers performing mixed-gas diving, but the principles of safe diving are common to all diving operations.

WALT BERGMAN

D. Deep Diving and Saturation Systems

The preceding section discusses surface-related diving, in which the diver goes to and from the underwater work site from a dive station located at the surface. This section discusses a class of diving in which the diver is primarily based in a deep diving system or pressurized habitat.

Diving bells of one sort or another have been in use for generations. Surface-oriented diving may utilize a "wet" or open bell in which the diver takes his decompression stops during ascent, but the use of this equipment calls for little change in the basic procedures.

During the mid-1960s a new concept of diving came into use in commercial diving. This can be termed *bell diving* or diving with the use of a *deep diving system*. This method protects the diver from exposure to the sea except when he is actually working. Special equipment, gases, and procedures are required. Some of the equipment referred to here is discussed also in Chapter I, under the section of man-made pressure environments.

There are two general categories of bell diving: short-duration or bounce diving, and saturation diving.

1. *Diving with a Deep Diving System: Deep Bounce Diving*

Bell diving is performed using a deep diving system. As a minimum a deep diving system consists of a diving bell, a handling system, and a deck chamber, with the necessary controls and instruments. The diving bell has to be constructed so it can be sealed against both internal and external pressure. A means of handling the bell on deck and lowering it to and recovering it from the seafloor work site is required. The handling system is usually an inverted U-frame with associated winches and pulleys, but the simplest systems handle the bell with a crane or davit. Positive handling, such that the bell never actually swings free, is the safest and most dependable approach.

The bell may or may not be positively buoyant. There is disagreement over which approach is best, but there have been accidents with both approaches, some due to inadvertant surfacing and others due to the bell's being dropped onto the sea floor. In any case there has to be an alternative method of recovering the bell in the event the main lift cable fails, and the bell should be protected against accidental ascent. If a bell is lost on the sea floor the divers should be equipped with survival equipment to ensure an adequate oxygen supply, to remove carbon dioxide, and to provide thermal protection.

The bell should be designed to mate with a deck decompression chamber so that the divers can transfer from the bell to the deck chamber while still under pressure. The deck chamber is normally equipped with bunks, lighting, and control of temperature, oxygen, and carbon dioxide.

The equipment described here as deep diving systems and the saturation diving systems described in the next section both incorporate many of the same characteristics.

The bell is serviced by an umbilical, which carries hoses for gas and hot water and cables for power and communications. Umbilicals may range from 5 to 10 cm in diameter, and while they are usually held together (or bundled) with wraps of duct tape every meter or so, some of the more sophisticated ones may be enclosed in a molded vinyl jacket or woven cover. The umbilical may be stored on a special large-diameter winch (necessarily equipped with slip rings and swivel joints), but many are quite effectively handled manually and coiled in a large basket; this approach eliminates the need for slip rings. The umbilical is generally separate from the strength member, a cable that supports the weight of the bell.

One utility virtually always present in a bell umbilical is a hot water supply hose. Because depths achieved in bell diving lead uniformly to cold water, diver heating is needed. Open-circuit hot water flooded through a diver's suit designed for that purpose is the most popular and most effective means of diver heating. In most deep diving it is also necessary to heat the diver's breathing gas; this is usually also done with hot water.

The procedures used for deep nonsaturation or bounce dives have evolved primarily to support the exploration phase of petroleum production. The diver's job is usually to make a quick repair, turn a valve, attach a cable, or perform a similar job taking from 10 to 30 min. (Longer jobs requiring an hour or more are usually done with saturation procedures, next section). The operational procedures that have been developed are based on this requirement. They are a composite of gas logistics, decompression, life support, and handling.

Two divers (nearly always) enter the diving bell at the surface and seal off the bell, with air at atmospheric pressure inside. The bell is lowered to the work site, still at one atmosphere inside. It may be possible to perform the needed observation or work without having to pressurize a diver, especially if the bell has manipulator arms. Otherwise, when the divers are ready to go to work they pressurize the bell with the appropriate gas mixture until pressure inside the bell equals that outside; the hatch can then be opened and the diver can "lock out" and go to work.

While working he is supplied with breathing gas from the surface via the umbilical. This lockout or bottom gas and the one used to pressurize the bell are chosen to have a proper oxygen level at bottom pressure, usually a partial pressure of 1 to 1.5 b (atm). The highest possible level of oxygen that does not exceed toxicity limits is used, to minimize the decompression obligation and to reduce the diver's chances of becoming hypoxic if something should go wrong. The mixtures normally used are primarily oxygen and helium, with nitrogen included at up to 15%, sometimes more, to improve the diver's voice and in some cases to improve decompression and also to reduce the cost of the helium.

The working diver locks out of the bell to work, and the other diver or bellman helps handle the diver's umbilical and otherwise acts as a tender. The diver's umbilical is perhaps 30 m long and contains his gas, hot water, and communication leads. The bellman is suited up and need only don his helmet or mask in order to go out and rescue the diver should that be necessary. Divers wear a harness, and the umbilical hose is attached to the harness to prevent tension on the hose from pulling off the mask. The bell is equipped with a pulley arrangement so that an unconscious diver could be hoisted into the bell by his harness.

The diver's gas supplied through the bell umbilical is reduced to an appropriate pressure (about 7–10 b) at the bell. Most divers wear a mask or helmet incorporating a demand type of breathing regulator. This is the type most commonly used for surface-supplied diving as well. The diver receives gas when he inhales, and his exhaled gas is normally exhausted into the sea. His mask may be of the "band," type which has a rubber hood attached to the faceplate (with a band), or he may wear a full helmet. In both cases the diver inhales from an oronasal cup or mouthpiece. Extra gas can be directed into the helmet or mask space by a bypass or free flow valve controlled by the diver; it flows down over the faceplate to clear it of moisture and exits near the bottom. The diver wears on his backpack a "bail-out bottle" or emergency tank of gas that will supply his needs for a few minutes should the umbilical supply fail.

When his work is finished, or if his planned time is up, the diver returns to the bell for ascent. The bell internal hatch is sealed, and the bell is hoisted toward the surface. As the bell ascends the divers then bleed the gas out of the bell, reducing the pressure according to the pressure profile called for by the decompression schedule. A change to a higher oxygen mixture or air may be called for, or the divers may breathe special decompression gases by mask.

When the bell reaches the surface the bell and deck chamber are mated. Pressure in the transfer lock of the deck chamber is adjusted to that of the bell (which is appropriate for the decompression profile at that moment) and the divers transfer or lock in to the deck chamber. Often the deck chamber itself is filled with air, and the divers wait until the switch to air is called for by the decompression table before transferring. With the divers now in the deck chamber, decompression is completed by appropriate pressure reductions and gas switches. Generally the divers will breathe pure oxygen for 2 or 3 hr, with periodic breaks. To prevent a buildup of oxygen in the chamber (a serious fire hazard) the masks are equipped with overboard dump capability such that exhaled gas is vented outside the chamber.

2. Saturation and Saturation-Excursion Diving

Diving with a deep diving system may take one of two general forms, depending on the duration of the working time on the bottom and the ensuing decompression. The short ($\frac{1}{2}$–1 hr) bounce dives have been discussed. This section considers the longer dive, generally referred to as saturation diving.

Both equipment and procedures used for saturation diving can be regarded as a special case or subset of diving with a deep diving system; the differences all relate to the duration of the job.

The term *saturation* refers to the diver's inert gas status or decompression obligation. The implication of the term is that his body is saturated with gas at a particular pressure and will not take up any more gas no matter how long he stays at that pressure. Whether or not this reflects the actual biophysical situation is not important; the practical reality is that after a certain duration of exposure the decompression time reaches an upper limit that is not increased with an increasing stay at pressure. Thus saturation diving is free from the worry of racing to meet a decompression-related time limit and also involves much simpler decompression profiles.

A saturation diving system involves the same components as mentioned for a deep diving system: a bell, a handling system, a deck chamber complex, and control and instrumentation equipment. It is usually larger, more complex, and has more capability.

The saturation bell may be big enough for 3 or possibly 4 divers. Strictly speaking, the bell need not be capable of holding external pressure, as the divers are already at pressure when they lock in and the bell is never supposed to have a lower pressure than the surrounding water.

The deck chamber, or more generally the complex of deck chambers, are large enough for comfortable habitability for durations of up to 30 days. The life-support and environmental conditioning equipment are capable of maintaining well-controlled diving conditions for as long as a saturation job lasts; this may be longer than the stay of any one diver. The control system maintains oxygen, carbon dioxide, temperature, and humidity. While the short-duration deep diving system may have only a camp stool or chemical toilet, saturation systems are usually furnished with complete shower and hygienic facilities. Meals are served through a pass-through lock.

An important aspect of running a saturation diving operation is to establish the desired values and tolerance limits for these environmental variables.

While it is not the most difficult to control, oxygen is the most important contributor to the diver's well being. It has both high and low limits. The consideration in saturation diving is to maintain as high an oxygen level as can be tolerated without damage, especially keeping in mind lung toxicity and fire safety. A high value is desired because it increases the safety margin against hypoxia in the event of pressure loss or a disturbance in gas or control. Also, regular normoxic levels (e.g., 0.21 b) have proved to be inadequate at great depths. A good range is 0.4 to 0.45 b (i.e., atm). It is said that values up to 0.5 b can be tolerated indefinitely (Clark and Lambertsen 1971), and up to 0.6 b for a few days without significant risk of lung damage. The matter of what constitutes a proper range for pulmonary oxygen limits is a controversial topic, and it depends on the exposure to oxygen during lockouts for work as well as on the residence exposure.

Carbon dioxide is normally scrubbed from the atmosphere of the saturation chamber continually, and in most cases the level stays so low it hardly need be considered. When the scrubbing systems are noisy or expensive to run, it may make sense to run the scrubbers only enough to keep chamber carbon dioxide below a certain maximum. This value is customarily taken at 0.5% sea level equivalent (5 mb or 3.8 mmHg), but the effects of higher levels (1% or 1.5% equivalent) are promptly reversible without detrimental effect after the brief exposure periods normally involved in saturation dives (Schaefer 1979).

Temperature is an important variable, first because it has to be maintained rather precisely, and also because large deviations can be dangerous (Webb 1977). The helium-oxygen environment of a deep saturation dive has a high thermal conductivity and hence rapid heat exchange with the diver's body. The comfortable zone gets narrower and the comfortable temperature gets warmer as saturation holding depth increases. One is comfortable in air at sea level at 23°C (75°F), but in helium-oxygen at 15 b pressure about 30°C (86°F) is chosen, while at 30 b this goes up to perhaps 32°C (90°F) (Webb 1973). In hyperbaric helium the heat stress of temperatures only slightly higher than these can be considerable, and long exposures to the low end of the comfortable range can lead to significant body hypothermia.

Another thermal factor in saturation diving is that the long work periods in the water afford plenty of time for the diver to become hypothermic if he is not adequately protected. It is especially important for the breathing gas to be warmed. Guidelines for temperatures to be used are given in Figure XIV-20.

Humidity level is not important in an exposure of only a few hours if the temperature is correct, but in an exposure of more than a day or two it should have an average level of no more than 75% relative humidity, and preferably lower, especially if divers are making daily excursions into the water. The problem is with the ears, and with skin in general. Keeping the environment relatively dry is not alone sufficient to prevent and control external ear infections, but control is nearly impossible under high humidity. Ear infections can disable the entire dive team.

Saturation divers perform their work by making excursions into the sea. The saturation depth or pressure may be the same as that of the work site, or divers may go to a different pressure. This involves choice of a breathing mixture appropriate for the depth, and provisions must be made for proper decompression. Transfer to the work site from the deck chamber is made in the bell. The pressure change may be within time limits found to be tolerable for indefinite periods (e.g., U.S. Navy unlimited duration tables)

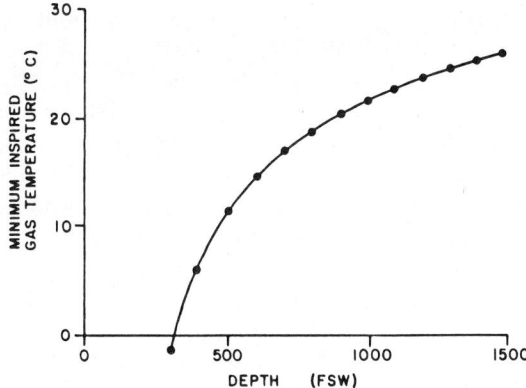

Figure XIV-20. Proposed U.S. Navy minimum inspired helium-oxygen temperatures for saturation depths between 300 and 1500 fsw. [From Piantadosi (1982).]

or may follow procedures involving a timed exposure and controlled return to saturation depth. Even though substantial pressure changes can be managed, saturation at work depth may be the best choice because of the large amounts of gas used in pressurizing and decompressing the bell during excursions.

The discussion thus far has dealt primarily with helium-oxygen (heliox) saturation diving. Another type of saturation diving based on air and nitrogen-oxygen mixtures (sometimes called NOAA OPS diving) has been developed by the National Oceanic and Atmospheric Administration and the U.S. Navy and is gradually being adapted to commercial diving. These procedures are detailed in the *NOAA Diving Manual* (Miller 1979). Air can be used as the gas in the saturation chamber down to depths of about 50 fsw (15 msw), and excursions can be made using air. Saturation can also be with nitrogen–oxygen mixtures having a lower oxygen fraction than air (Miller et al. 1976).

An interesting phenomenon of adaption to narcosis seems to occur when saturation is with air or a nitrox mixture, such that the observed narcosis is reduced approximately by the depth of saturation (Hamilton et al. 1973). This is, a diver saturated at 100 fsw (30 msw) would experience narcosis in a dive to 250 fsw (76 msw) at about the same degree that he would observe on a dive to 150 fsw (46 msw) from the surface. Thus decompression and narcosis are more or less under control, and the limitations to deep diving with air from nitrogen-based saturation becomes one of tolerance of the oxygen level in air.

Recently, development of a new class of diver breathing equipment is dedicated to saturation diving. This is the concept referred to as *push–pull*. The engineering approaches vary somewhat, but the end results are to capture the diver's exhaled gas and return it to the bell or support vessel for reprocessing and reuse. This approach makes no economic sense for half-hour dives, but for long work at great depths, the savings in gas and hence in the cost may be considerable.

Most push-pull systems are adaptations of demand breathing apparatus, with a special valve to collect expired gas yet prevent any possibility that a suction will be applied to the diver's lungs. At least one push–pull design offers something more—essentially a *free flow* system, it reduces the inhalation breathing resistance to much less than that of the demand valve.

An interesting anomaly has developed regarding the status aspects of deep diving. In most diving circles the saturation diver has the highest level of recognition. The amount of work accomplished in this mode and the investment in equipment for saturation diving certainly validate the importance of the concept, but the implication that saturation diving requires the highest level of skill is totally unwarranted. The deep bounce dive is much more demanding. The bounce diver is subjected to rapid pressurization, has to work against the clock, and he and the entire team have to carry out a complex sequence of gas and pressure changes and decompression; all this has to be done correctly and following a tight time schedule. Properly, deep bounce diving should be carried out only by those who have proved themselves through success in saturation operations.

3. Habitat Diving

Another aspect of saturation diving with a slightly different approach is habitat diving. This procedure involves a chamber placed on the sea floor in which the diver or aquanauts live, making excursions for their work. Early habitat programs (Link's Man-in-the-Sea, Sealab, Cousteau) demonstrated the capability of using a helium-oxygen atmosphere, but in recent years habitat atmospheres have been predominantly based on nitrogen or air (TEKTITE, Hydrolab, FISSH).

The techniques for habitat diving have been developed most highly by NOAA and are well described in the *NOAA Diving Manual* (Miller 1979). A detailed account of medical support of the TEKTITE program has been prepared by Beckman (1972).

R. W. HAMILTON

References

BECKMAN, E. L., AND E. M. SMITH 1972. Tektite II: Medical supervision of the scientists in the sea. *Tex. Rep. Biol. Med.* 30: 1–204.

CLARK, J. M., AND C. J. LAMBERTSEN 1971. Pulmonary oxygen toxicity: A review. *Pharmacol. Rev.* 23: 38–133.

HAMILTON, R. W., JR., D. J. KENYON, M. FREITAG, AND H. R. SCHREINER 1973. NOAA OPS I and II: Formulation of excursion procedures for shallow undersea habitats. Tarrytown, NY: Union Carbide Corp. (UCRI-731).

MILLER, J. W. (editor) 1979. *The NOAA Diving Manual* (2nd ed.). Washington, DC: National Oceanic and Atmospheric Administration, U.S. Dept. of Commerce.

MILLER, J. W. (editor), G. M. ADAMS, P. B. BENNETT, R. CLARKE, R. W. HAMILTON, JR., D. J. KENYON, AND R. I. WICKLUND 1976. *Vertical excursions breathing air from nitrogen-oxygen or air saturation exposures.* Rockville, MD: National Oceanic and Atmospheric Administration, U.S. Dept. of Commerce.

PIANTADOSI, C. A. 1982. Respiratory heat loss limits in helium-oxygen saturation diving. Rep. 10-80, rev. 3-82. Panama City, FL: Navy Experimental Diving Unit.

SCHAEFER, K. E. 1979. Physiological stresses related to hypercapnia during patrols on submarines. In: Preventive aspects of submarine medicine, edited by K. E. Schaefer. *Undersea Biomed. Res.* 6 (Suppl).

WEBB, P. 1973. The thermal drain of comfortable hyperbaric environments. *Nav. Res. Rev.* 26: 1–7.

WEBB, P. 1977. Human tolerance to thermal extremes. In: *Thermal Problems in Diving,* edited by G. H. Egstrom. Wilmington, CA: Commercial Diving Center.

XV

Diving Accident Investigation

Underwater swimming using self-contained underwater breathing apparatus (scuba) not only is a popular sport for several million Americans but also has achieved a significant role in military and commercial operations. Accidents are the leading manner of death among Americans of less than 35 years of age, and they rank fourth for deaths in all age groups in the United States. Drowning is the third most common cause of accidental death and more than 8000 deaths by drowning occur annually. Among accidents involving underwater swimmers, drowning is the leading cause of death.

A. Accident Reporting

When an accident occurs, attention is directed to the rescue, resuscitation, transport, and treatment of the victims. If death results from the accident and an autopsy is authorized, attention is often directed to determination of the cause of death, without knowledge of the circumstances of the accident, the equipment used by the diver, and the methods used for resuscitation and treatment of the diving casualty. Thus every accident, whether fatal or nonfatal, is a challenge for the physician to try to elucidate the cause and thus add to the meager knowledge now available for structuring future standards for diving—diver training, standards for physical condition of the diver, modification of equipment, and general management of diving activity.

Unfortunately, investigations of diving accidents are often conducted by inexperienced persons who are unfamiliar with the circumstances, the equipment, the physiology of diving, the significance of pathologic findings, and the necessity for an organized, multidisciplinary approach.

Webster (1966), for example, studied the newspaper accounts of 86 deaths of underwater swimmers and concluded that lack of knowledge concerning the circumstances of these accidents prevented the development of guidelines for improvements of diving safety. Bayliss (1969), Denney and Read (1965), Goldhahn (1977), and Hendry have reported their experiences with scuba diving fatalities in the United States, Australia, and Great Britain.

Knight and Stahl (1976) recommended the preparation of a comprehensive plan to investigate diving accidents in the U.S. Navy and the formation of a multidisciplinary investigative team to include specialists in diving, diving equipment, undersea medicine, and forensic pathology. This approach to the investigation of diving accidents has been used succcessfully in Great Britain and Australia and in Los Angeles in the United States, and it is similar to the investigative methods that have been used for more than 20 years to investigate military and civil aircraft accidents in the United States, Great Britain, and Canada (Mason and Reals 1973; Stevens 1970).

Not until 1981, however, was there a national effort in the United States to develop a repository for such data and to coordinate an organized, uniform method for diving accident investigation that would be consistent with the approach by such groups as the Medical Research Council Decompression Sickness Panel of Great Britain and the Royal Australian Navy School of Underwater Medicine.

In the United States we have DAN, a national Diving Accident Network (in 1983 renamed Divers Alert Network), supported by several federal agencies and assigned to Duke University (Durham, NC) for operation. This consists of a national system of centers organized to handle all emergencies that may arise in diving activity and is, of course, available for the treatment of iatrogenic air embolism. In case of a diving accident, all that need be done is to call the switchboard at Duke University Medical Center (telephone number at time of this printing 919-684-8111) and say "DAN." Referral will then be made to the appropriate one of the seven centers or the closest satellite treatment facility.

Comprehensive reporting of all diving accidents, fatal and nonfatal, is a further function of the Diving Accident Network. The Undersea Medical Society, Inc., studied a number of accident reporting forms while developing in 1979 a standard reporting form they proposed for use by the network. This form constitutes the Appendix to this chapter. It is expected that detailed report forms will help remedy the lack of statistically reliable data on underwater accidents heretofore available. A clearing house for the reporting of fatal accidents has been maintained for a number of years by the National Underwater Accident Center, University of Rhode Island (P.O. Box 68, Kingston, RI 02881). Unfortunately, all fatal accidents have not been faithfully reported, though requested, and nonfatal accidents have not been reported at all.

The reporting and recording of occupational accidents to the commercial diver have become well standardized in many parts of the world, especially in the areas surrounding the North Sea. For the benefit of the commercial diver in the United States, accident reporting is mandated by the Occupational Safety and Health Act of 1970, divers for universities and scientific organizations being covered under the same standard regulations. The U.S. Navy reports analyses of all its diving accidents. There are no regulations, however, to cover the reporting and handling of accidents to sport divers. Fortunately, although during the past 15 years the number of sport scuba divers has increased from approximately one million to more than four million, there has not been a significant increase in scuba diving fatalities, which remain about 100 per year. An organized approach toward training and certification of scuba divers, as well as improved equipment and diving safety, has undoubtedly contributed to the prevention of a greater number of fatal accidents.

B. *Objectives of Diving Accident Investigation*

Whereas accidents in the aquatic environment are often attributed to drowning, or near-drowning, a dynamic interaction that exists between the underwater swimmer and this environment may present unexpected hazards resulting in disability or death. Witnesses to these events are often not available. Investigators have the responsibility to determine the circumstances, to establish the chronological sequence of events, to record their observations accurately, and to provide opinions and recommendations that will lead to the prevention of similar accidents and will contribute to improvement of diving education and safety. The investigation of a diving accident is not a simple matter. If the casualty of the accident has survived, information concerning the circumstances is often available. When death results from the accident, however, delays in recovery, putrefactive changes, postmortem injuries, or artifacts resulting from attempts at resuscitation, recompression, or treatment may obscure the findings. All members of the multidisciplinary investigative team, including the pathologist who will perform the postmortem examination, must have adequate information to guide them in the performance of their respective duties. Otherwise, their conclusions and recommendations will not be meaningful. As recommended by Goldhahn (1977) and Davis (1980), the investigation of diving accidents should include consideration of all factors that may have contributed to the accident:

1. *Human Factors*

- Health of the diver, including evidence of preexisting diseases, prescribed medications, and use of alcohol or illicit drugs.
- Training and experience of the diver.
- Mental status of the diver, possibly contributing to panic, breach of diving safety guidelines, poor judgment, or the manner of death.
- Postmortem findings, including evidence of injury and the results of toxicological studies.

2. *Environmental Factors*

- Plan, location, and depth of the dive.
- Weather and water conditions, including temperatures of the air and water, tides, currents, pollution of the water, and topography of the underwater floor.
- Dangerous or venomous aquatic animals and plants.
- Hazards related to entrapment, fouling, explosion, or electricity.

3. *Equipment Factors*

- Improper use of or failure to use equipment, including snorkel, life vest, knife, mask, watch, immersion suit, weight belt, swim fins, and quick-release straps.
- Malfunction or fouling of equipment, including air hoses, mouthpiece, valves, and regulator.
- Contamination of air supply with carbon monoxide or other toxic gases.
- Absence of residual air in tank, or tank filled with toxic gases instead of air.
- Corrosion of interior of tank with blockage of valves.

4. *Other Factors Bearing on the Accident*

An adequate investigation of a fatal diving accident, including the postmortem examination, should allow the investigators to answer the following questions, which may have importance to the next of kin, the insurance companies of the deceased, the executor and attorney responsible for settlement of the estate, and the litigants involved in civil actions:

- How did the accident occur? What were the circumstances that resulted in the fatal accident?
- Where did the accident occur?
- Did the victim die at the time of the accident, or subsequently as the result of complications during recovery, transport, resuscitation, recompression, or treatment? Was appropriate treatment rendered to the victim?
- Who is the victim of the accident?
- What is the cause of death? What injury or disease, or combination of both, resulted in the fatality?
- What is the mechanism for death? What physiological derangement or biochemical disturbance may be related to the cause of death?
- What is the manner of death? Did the victim die as the result of preexisting natural disease, homicide, suicide, or accident, or in an undetermined manner?
- Were there any contributory causes for death or for disability of the diver during immersion, including preexisting diseases, exposure to cold, entrapment, failure of equipment, fatigue, intoxication by alcohol or drugs, or environmental hazards?
- Did the death occur before or after immersion in water?
- Did any of the injuries occur after the death of the victim?
- Among the human, environmental, and equipment factors considered during the investigation, which factor, or combination of factors, caused the accident?
- Could the accident have been prevented?
- What is recommended to prevent further accidents of this type and to improve the practice of diving safety?

C. Authority for Investigation and Autopsy

Investigation of deaths and the performance of autopsies are based on laws, policies, and regulations. The conduct of an investigation or the performance of an autopsy without appropriate authorization may result in civil litigation or criminal penalties. While the regulations in the United States pertaining to investigations and autopsies are similar among the Armed Forces, there is no uniformity of laws governing the medicolegal investigation of deaths among the states and territories. If there is no statutory authority for medicolegal investigation and autopsy, or if the next of kin refuse to grant permission for autopsy, the investigation of a diving accident fatality is essentially thwarted.

When an accident is reported in a civilian jurisdiction, rescue and law enforcement personnel will respond to the request for assistance. If the victim has survived, or is believed to be alive, the rescue personnel will render appropriate emergency care and will transport the victim to the nearest hospital. The law enforcement personnel will conduct an investigation of the accident to the extent required by the laws of that jurisdiction. If the accident has resulted in death, the medicolegal investigation and perhaps the autopsy become the responsibility of either the coroner or the medical examiner of the state or territory, depending on the type of medicolegal system of the region. In many states with coroner systems, the coroner is neither a physician nor a pathologist, and, in fact, there are often no specific professional qualifications for election to this political office. Medical examiners, however, are appointed as the result of their professional qualifications and experience. The majority of medical examiners are pathologists or forensic pathologists. The monograph by Wecht (1977) is a comprehensive survey of medicolegal autopsy laws, and it contains information such as the statutory authority for autopsies, the circumstances for authorization of a medicolegal autopsy, and the designation of persons who may perform medicolegal autopsies. The U.S. Department of Health, Education and Welfare also published an analysis of laws governing medicolegal death investigations (1978). A comprehensive law for a medicolegal system will require investigation and allow for authorization of autopsy in the following categories of deaths: (1) Violent death by homicide, suicide, or accident. (2) Death under suspicious, unusual, or unnatural circumstances. (3) Sudden, unexpected deaths. (4) Death resulting from occupational diseases and injuries. (5) Death during imprisonment or police custody.

Some jurisdictions, however, have unduly restrictive laws, and death investigations in these medicolegal systems may allow authorization for autopsies only in homicides or suspected homicides.

In the State of Maryland in 1939 when the state legislature enacted the Maryland State Postmortem Examiners Law, the medical examiner system replaced the coroner system. The Office of the Chief Medical Examiner, State of Maryland, serves as an example of an established, well-organized, medicolegal investigative system. The Chief Medical Examiner, a forensic pathologist, is assisted by a staff that includes forensic pathologists, toxicologists, serologists, technologists, investigators, and clerical personnel. Physicians for each county of the State are appointed as deputies to assist the Chief Medical Examiner in investigations of death. The Chief Medical Examiner, as well as the assistant and deputy medical examiners, has the authority to investigate deaths, to take affidavits, and to authorize autopsies when death has resulted from violence, suicide, or casualty; has occurred suddenly to an individual in apparent health or when unattended by a physician; or has occured in any unusual or suspicious manner (Maryland 1979).

The investigation of deaths among active-duty personnel of the Armed Forces is the responsibility of either a military investigative agency, or investigators appointed by the commanding officer, or other fact-finding body, provided the military service has exclusive jurisdiction for the investigation. The various regulations of the three branches of the Armed Forces concerning authorization for autopsy are similar, and the following section pertains to the Navy (U.S. Navy n.d.).

> An autopsy shall be performed on the remains of any person who dies in the military service while serving on active duty or active duty for training, when the commanding officer of his own volition or upon the recommendation of an investigating officer or other fact-finding body or medical officer, deems such procedure necessary to determine the true cause of death, to secure information for the completion of medical records, or to protect the welfare of the military community. When death occurs while serving as an aircrew member of a military aircraft, the medical officer shall recommend to the commanding officer having custody of the remains that an autopsy be performed to determine the cause of death. Under these circumstances, the commanding officer may authorize such an autopsy. The "cause of death" in this connection is interpreted to mean any correlation between pathological evidence and the accident cause factors.

In cases of death of submariners/divers, a copy of the autopsy protocol and the certificate of death shall be forwarded to the Officer-In-Charge, Naval Submarine Medical Research Laboratory, Naval Submarine Medicine Center, Naval Submarine Base, New London, Groton, Connecticut 06340.

. . . [T]he appointed investigating officer, or other fact-finding body, shall provide the medical officer designated to conduct the autopsy with a detailed preliminary report of the circumstances surrounding the death. Upon completion of the autopsy, the medical officer conducting the autopsy shall provide the investigating officer, or other fact-finding body, with a copy of the preliminary autopsy findings as to the cause of death and, when completed, a copy of the final protocol. The investigating officer, or other fact-finding body, shall provide the medical officer with a copy of the final investigation report. Autopsies shall be recorded on Standard Form 503, Autopsy Protocol.

D. *The Autopsy in Diving Accident Investigations*

Although Goldhahn (1977) has stressed the need for more thorough evaluation of deaths of scuba divers, the performance of an autopsy as part of the medical investigation is dependent not only on statutory authority or permission of the next of kin but also on the adequacy and statutory authority of the medicolegal investigative system for the jurisdiction in which the death occurred. The pathologist who performs the autopsy needs to know information not only about the victim, the equipment, and the on-the-scene investigation but also about the methods used for recovery, rescue, resuscitation, recompression, and treatment of the casualty. Without this information the pathologist may be unable to determine the cause, mechanism, and manner of death. Except for certain regions of the United States (e.g., Miami and Los Angeles), few pathologists have had the opportunity to participate in the medical investigation of diving accidents, and there is no central repository for this knowledge and experience. Wright and Tate (1980) believe that forensic pathologists are best qualified to evaluate traumatic deaths of concern to the community. They have also shown that the autopsy, as well as information concerning the medical history, circumstances of death, and the environment in which the death occurred, is required to determine the cause, mechanism, and manner of death. Spitz (1980b) has compared the differences between the objectives of the autopsy performed to evaluate natural death in a hospital and the medicolegal autopsy performed to determine the identity of the victim, the time and place of death, the pathologic conditions or injuries that may have contributed to death, and the relationship of these findings to the cause, mechanism, and manner of death. Lundberg and Voight (1979) found that presumptive diagnoses in sudden, unexpected deaths of adults were often unreliable when compared with the results of postmortem examinations. They concluded that in addition to the usual benefit of the autopsy in determining the cause of death, the autopsy has value for environmental epidemiology as well as for adjudication of insurance and medical negligence claims. Although the number of autopsies performed in hospitals has declined significantly in recent years, Mergner and associates (1980) have used the autopsy, as well as special studies such as immunochemistry, microprobe analysis, electron microscopy, and scanning electron microscopy, to advance medical knowledge, to educate physicians, and to serve as a basis for quality control of the clinical practice of medicine.

E. Medical Investigation of Fatal Diving Accidents

A methodical, multidisciplinary approach is required for investigation of fatal diving accidents. To fulfill the objectives of the investigation, including the postmortem examination, planning and coordination are required, not only to evaluate the human, equipment, and environmental factors that may have contributed to the fatal event but also to determine the jurisdiction, authority, and responsibilities for each member of the investigative team. In many jurisdictions the medicolegal system will serve as the basis for the investigation, but the consultative assistance of diving and equipment specialists may be required. At the onset of the investigation it is important to obtain records and information concerning the victim of the accident and to establish a plan for action, consistent with Table XV-1. The effects of recovery, resuscitation, recompression, and treatment, as well as the effects of putrefaction, often obscure significant pathologic findings and cause difficulty in the interpretation of the findings. It is essential that the pathologist responsible for the postmortem examination have information about the health and diving experience of the victim, the circumstances of accident, the equipment, and the treatment of the victim prior to the autopsy.

Table XV-1.
Medical Investigation of Fatal Diving Accidents

Circumstances of death, including on-the-scene investigation and photographs, interviews of witnesses, evaluation of environmental conditions and hazards, and review of diving safety procedures
Review of methods for recovery, resuscitation, and treatment of the victim
Review of health and dental records, including radiographs
Training and experience of the diver
Examination of diving equipment, clothing, and personal effects
Identification of the diver
Photographs of diver, clothing, equipment, personal effects, and significant pathologic findings, including evidence of injury
Total body radiographs
Established chain-of-custody procedure for physical evidence, including clothing, equipment, personal effects, and specimens for toxicological or other special examinations
Postmortem examination, including evidence of injury and preexisting diseases, microscopic examinations, and toxicological studies
Determination of cause, manner, and mechanism of death
Determination of human, equipment, or environmental factors that contributed to the fatal accident
Recommendations for prevention of similar accidents to improve the practice of diving safety

1. Identification of Victim

The prompt identification of victims of diving accidents is required in order to notify the next of kin, to complete official records such as certificates of death, and to provide information for the settlement of estates and claims resulting from torts. While the personal effects and the equipment of the diver may contribute to the identification of the victim, the effects of decompression and putrefaction usually preclude personal recognition by friends or relatives. Identification is based on comparison of objective scientific data derived from examination of the victim with the available records for the putative person (Fig. XV-1). In the United States, comparison of fingerprints is the most reliable method for identification. Dental records and radiographs, when compared with the results of dental examination and radiographs of the victim, are often helpful if records of fingerprints are not available (Figs. XV-2, XV-3). Other scientific methods for identification include comparisons of exemplar specimens, or available records, with skeletal and anthropometric data, hair, serologic and cytologic studies, and radiographs obtained from postmortem examination of the victim (Stahl 1977, 1980).

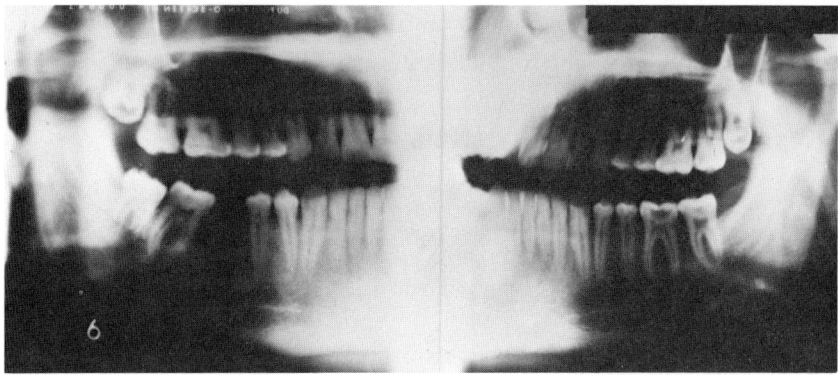

Figure XV-1. Panographic dental radiograph from antemortem dental records of the putative, decomposed victim served as basis for identification of the remains. Teeth of anterior segments are duplicated in this type of radiograph, which was compared with the results of the postmortem dental examination and radiographs. [Armed Forces Institute of Pathology (AFIP) Neg. No. 74-14889-3.]

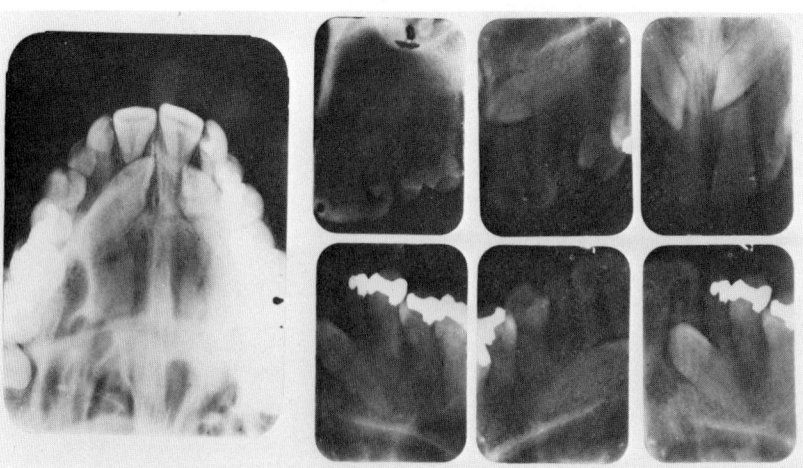

Figure XV-2. Antemortem dental radiographs from burned remains of a victim of homicide show amalgam restorations, retained deciduous teeth, and unerupted permanent cuspids. (AFIP Neg. No. 70-6371.)

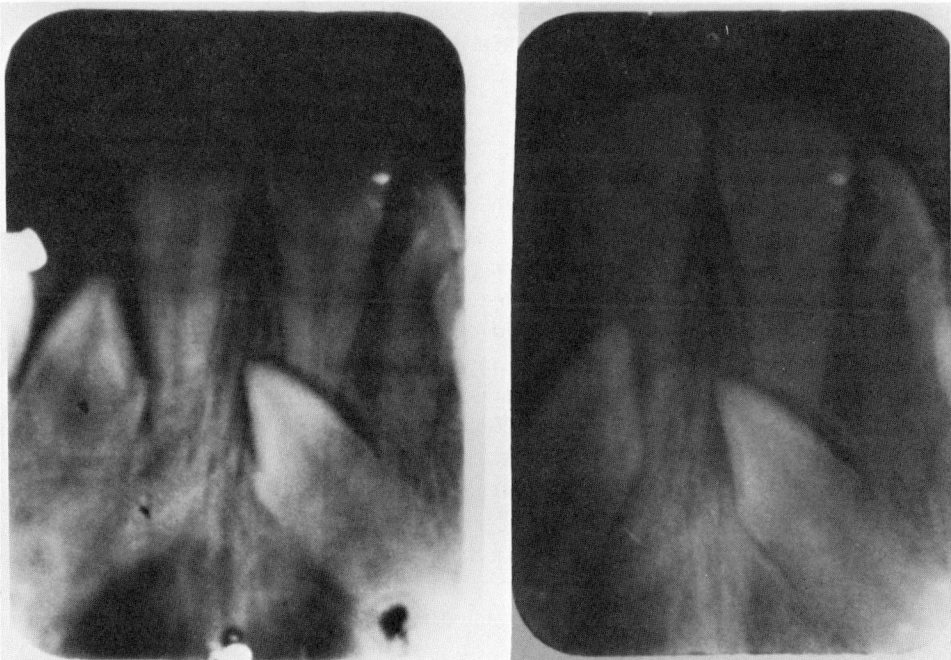

Figure XV-3. Comparison of antemortem (*right*) and postmortem (*left*) dental radiographs show unerupted permanent cuspids that contributed to the identification of the burned body. (AFIP Neg. No. 70-9865-2-A.)

2. Examination of Equipment

The pathologist should examine the clothing and equipment with the consultative assistance of an experienced diver, or diving equipment specialist, to determine the adequacy of the equipment for the dive, the condition of the equipment, and the function of the self-contained underwater breathing apparatus. The examiners need to determine the amount and composition of residual air in the tank and to examine the interior of the tank for corrosion (Temple et al. 1975). Toxicological examination of residual air is required to detect contamination of the air supply by carbon monoxide or other gases.

3. Total Body Radiography of Victim

Whereas dental radiographs are useful to confirm the identity of the victim, total body radiographs contribute not only to identification (when other radiographs are available for comparison) but also to the detection of fractures, foreign bodies, dysbaric osteonecrosis, pneumothorax, and air in vessels, organs, tissues, or body cavities.

4. Photographic Record of Investigation

Color photographs of the on-the-scene investigation, the diver, and the equipment, and of the significant pathologic findings are used to support the procedures for identification and to complement the reports of investigation and autopsy. Each photograph should contain a scale for comparison with the dimension of pathologic findings illustrated.

5. *Postmortem Examination*

The autopsy contributes to the determination of the cause, manner, and mechanism of death, as well as to the determination of relationships among the effects of preexisting diseases, environmental hazards, barotrauma, antemortem and postmortem injuries, intoxication by ethanol or drugs or carbon monoxide, treatment, and artifacts. Drowning, the most common cause for death in diving accidents, is discussed in recent textbooks (Giersten 1977, Spitz 1980a, Stahl 1979), and other causes for death in diving accidents, such as air embolism and decompression sickness, have been presented in a series of accounts of diving fatalities (Bayliss 1969, Denny and Read 1965, Eckert 1977, Edmonds and Thomas 1972b, Goldhahn 1977, Hendry 1977). To provide the distinction among drowning, air embolism, and decompression sickness as causes for death in diving accidents, attention has often been directed to complex autopsy procedures for detection of bubbles in vessels. Ideally, the autopsy should be performed in a chamber at the site and at the ambient pressure where the body is found, but this is impractical and unrealistic. Bubbles result from putrefaction of bodies immersed in water, from the decompressive effervescence in bodies of saturated divers recovered from water, and from recompression treatment of divers who are decompressed after death occurs (Davis 1980, Goldhahn 1977, Hendry 1977). Hanson and Young (1975) have indicated that postmortem gas bubbles in vessels may not have significance in a diver who dies under pressure. The experimental studies by Brown et al. (1978) support the hypothesis that dissolved gas in deceased scuba divers recovered from depths of water will expand during decompression, and that these bubbles are seen as artifacts during autopsy. The significance of intravascular bubbles, therefore, is doubtful when there is lack of correlation with circumstances of death that are consistent with either air embolism or decompression sickness (Brown et al. 1978, Goldhahn 1977, Hendry 1977), or when there is evidence of putrefaction, or when recompression therapy has preceded death. Elaborate autopsy procedures are usually not required, and the techniques recommended by Spitz (1980c) and by Ludwig (1979) are sufficient for most cases.

a. External Examination and Search for Evidence of Injury

After procedures for identification have been completed and total body radiographs and photographs have been obtained, the pathologist conducts a thorough external examination. Since hypothermia (Donahue and Peters 1979; Johnston and Burger 1971; Keatinge 1969) and systemic hyperthermia (Hendry 1977) have resulted in fatal diving accidents, liver and rectal temperatures of the body should be correlated with environmental temperatures of air and water in which the body was found. Evidence of barotrauma of descent—including mask squeeze, immersion suit squeeze, and rupture of tympanic membranes—is detected by careful examination of the skin and eyes as well as by otoscopic examination of the ears (Schulte 1964). The skin is also examined for evidence of antemortem injuries, such as electrothermal burns, lacerations, contusions, abrasions; injuries such as stings, bites, or punctures by marine animals, including sharks, coelenterates, stingrays, sea snakes, venomous fishes, and cone shells (Banner 1977, Edmonds and Thomas 1972a, Strauss and

Orris 1974); and injuries by propeller blades or grappling hooks. Subcutaneous emphysema, bubbles in the conjunctival and retinal vessels detected by opthalmoscopic examination, blotchy discoloration of the tongue (Liebermeister's sign), hemorrhagic froth in the nares and airway, and bite wounds of the lips and tongue from uncontrolled seizures, may each provide clues for barotrauma of ascent, including air embolism. Radiography may offer further evidence of barotrauma of ascent when either pneumothorax or pneumomediastinum or pneumoperitoneum is observed. Rose and Jarczyk (1978) have reported spontaneous pneumoperitoneum in a scuba diver who made an emergency ascent, had symptoms of decompression sickness, and was treated by recompression. Since no abdominal organs were ruptured, the air from ruptured pulmonary alveoli apparently dissected from the retroperitoneum into the peritoneal cavity.

b. Internal Examination and Search for Evidence of Injury

The preferred sequence for the internal examination is head, chest, and cardiopulmonary systems to evaluate the possibility of the extra-alveolar air syndrome, which includes air embolism as well as interstitial pulmonary emphysema, pneumothorax, and pneumomediastinum (Davis 1980). After reflection of the scalp and removal of the calvarium, the basilar artery as well as the circle of Willis and its branches is examined in situ. If bubbles are observed in these arteries, photographs are obtained. The carotid arteries are cut proximal to clamps, and the brain is removed for further external examination and fixation in 10% formalin solution. The dura is stripped from the base of the skull and the petrous portions of the temporal bones are examined for hemorrhage in the region of the middle ear (Fig. XV-4). At one time, hemorrhage in the middle ears was believed pathognomonic of drowning (Mueller 1969), but, more recently, it has also been associated with a variety of hypoxic conditions that include carbon monoxide intoxication, drug intoxication, and head injury. By use of the techniques of Spitz (1980b) and Ludwig (1979) when there is suspicion of pneumothorax, the chest is examined and air is collected for measurement and gas analysis. After the thoracic reflections have been made and the sternum has been removed, the mediastinum, pericardium, and heart are similarly examined for evidence of air embolism. Samples of air are collected and retained for gas analysis. If the circumstances of death and the autopsy findings are consistent with air embolism, analysis of the air samples should indicate a composition of approximately 20% oxygen and 80% nitrogen. Further evidence of air embolism from barotrauma of ascent is provided by pulmonary bullae, hemorrhage, atelectasis, and interstitial emphysema, or by evidence of air trapping by broncholiths or pulmonary scars. The lungs in drowning often show nonspecific pathologic changes (Fig. XV-5). Arterial bubbles may also be observed when the contents of the abdomen are examined. Sections of the heart and brain may reveal hemorrhagic infarcts. Decompression sickness rarely results in death, but when it does, death is often delayed. The pathologic findings are less specific and require careful correlation with the circumstances of death. Ischemic infarcts of the spinal cord and scattered cerebral hemorrhages have been reported (Goldhahn 1977).

The remainder of the autopsy is performed in the usual manner and is directed to detection of preexisting diseases that may have contributed to the fatal accident. When there are radiographic changes in long bones consistent with osteonecrosis, sections of these bones, particularly the humeral and femoral heads, distal femur, and proximal tibia, should be obtained for microscopic examination (Ludwig 1979).

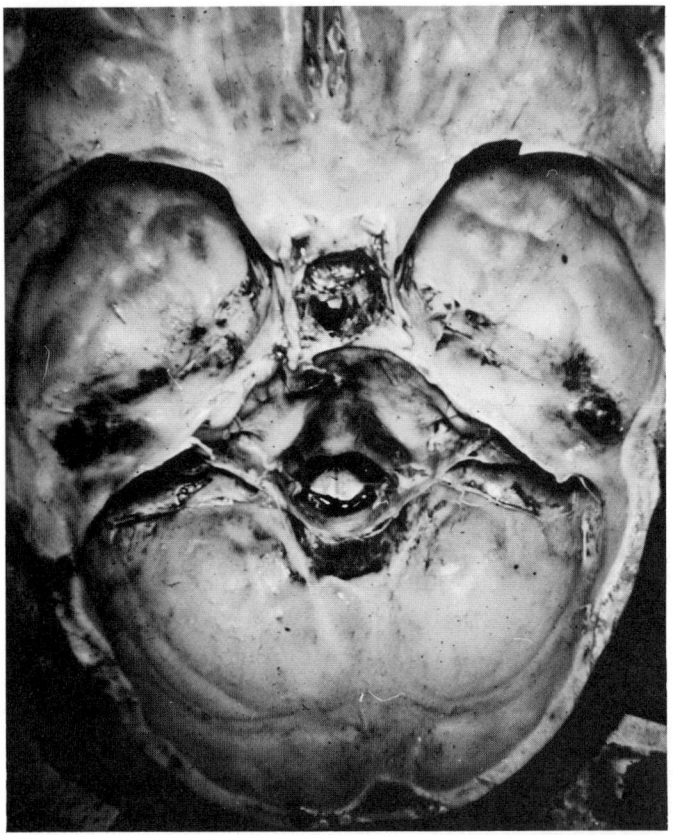

Figure XV-4. After the dura is removed from the base of the skull, the petrous portions of the temporal bones are examined for hemorrhage in the region of the middle ears. (AFIP Neg. No. 64-5204-3.)

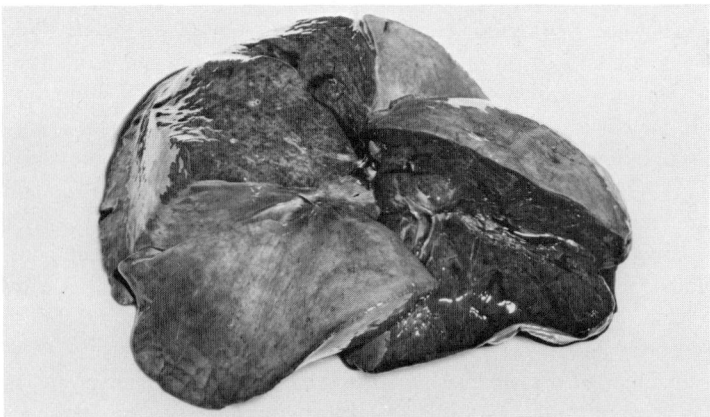

Figure XV-5. Gross photograph of a lung from a victim of drowning. The lung is heavy, edematous, and hemorrhagic, but these pathologic findings are not pathognomonic of drowning. (AFIP Neg. No. 58-12255-A-B.)

c. Microscopic Examination

Microscopic examination will confirm the observations of the gross examination and provide histologic evidence for diagnosis of preexisting diseases. If the victim survived for a period of time after recovery from water, there is often evidence of pneumonia (Figs. XV-6, XV-7) or aspiration of gastric content. Attempts at resuscitation are reflected by pulmonary fat and bone marrow emboli. The presence of diatoms in the lungs may contribute to the diagnosis of drowning, provided similar diatoms are found in the water from which the body was recovered (Fig. XV-8). Occasionally, microscopic sections of skin will reveal nematocysts discharged from coelenterates, such as Portuguese man-of-war and sea wasp, which have incapacitated divers (Figs. XV-9, XV-10).

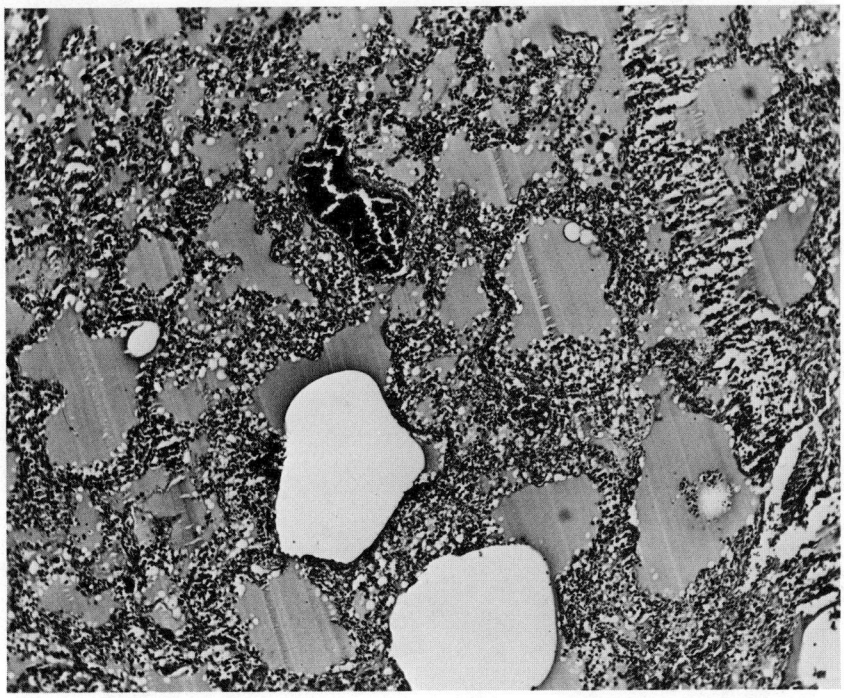

Figure XV-6. After near-drowning, the casualty survived for a brief period and showed clinical signs of the postimmersion syndrome. Histologic sections of the lungs revealed pulmonary edema, congestion, and inflammation. Hematoxylin and eosin stain, ×70. (AFIP Neg. No. 61-5582.)

d. Chemical and Toxicological Examinations

Although the medical literature contains numerous references to chemical tests for the diagnosis of drowning, none of these studies have proved satisfactory. Attempts have also been made to correlate blood gas analyses of the victims of diving accidents with the physiological mechanism for death, but the results of these studies are usually misleading and unrewarding. There is a need, however, to obtain frozen samples of blood and urine, as well as frozen samples of brain, liver, kidney, and bile, for toxicological examinations

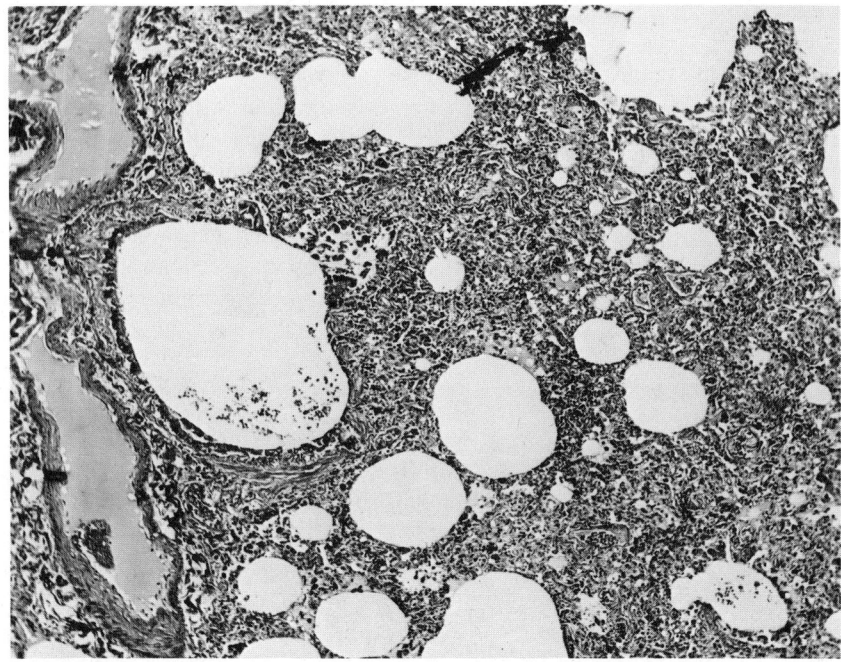

Figure XV-7. Evidence of pneumonia in histologic sections of lungs after the delayed death of a victim of near-drowning. Hematoxylin and eosin stain, ×70 (AFIP Neg. No. 61-5590.)

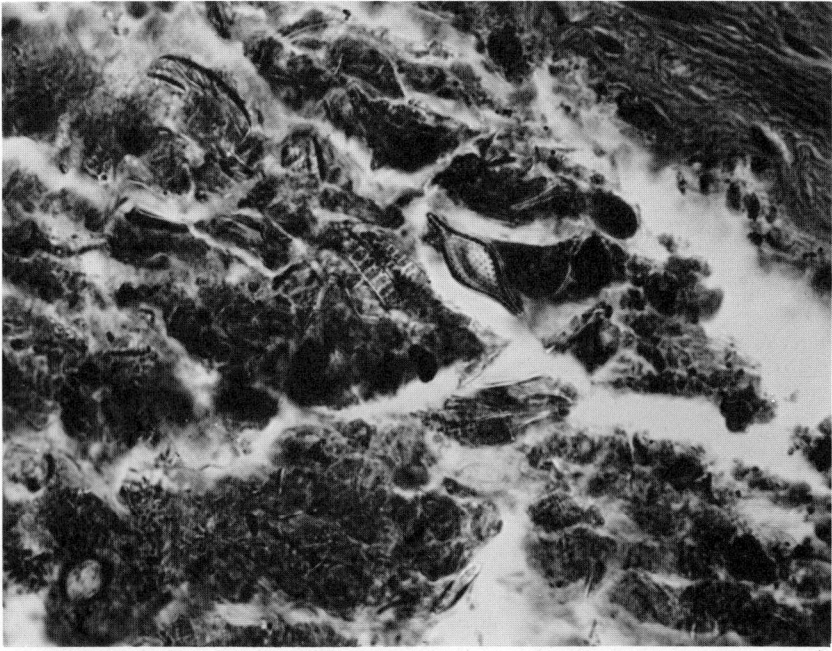

Figure XV-8. Diatoms in histologic sections of lung from a scuba diver who drowned. Hematoxylin and eosin stain, ×600. (AFIP Neg. No. 62-4984.)

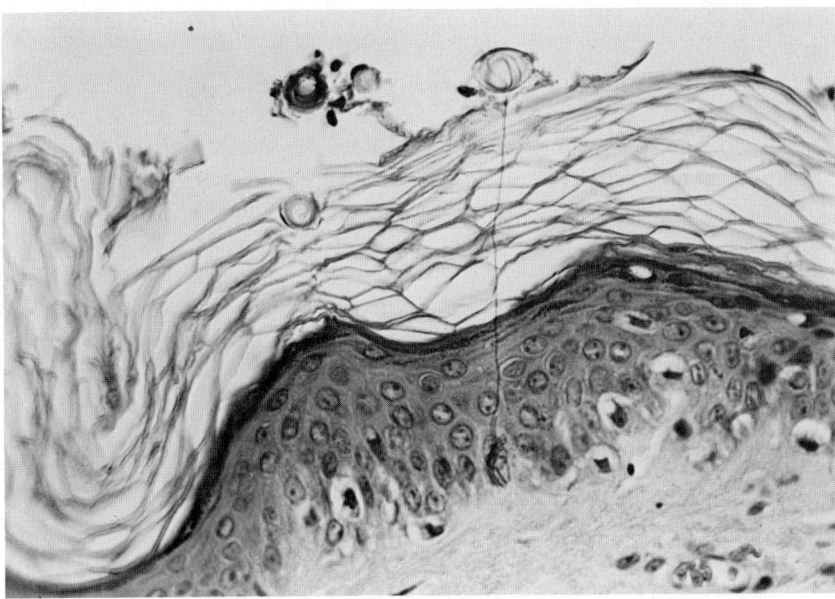

Figure XV-9. Histologic section of skin showing a discharged nematocyst of Portuguese man-of-war on the keratin layer and the penetration of a thread tube to the basal layer of the epidermis. Hematoxylin and eosin stain, ×350 (AFIP Neg. No. 64-6560.)

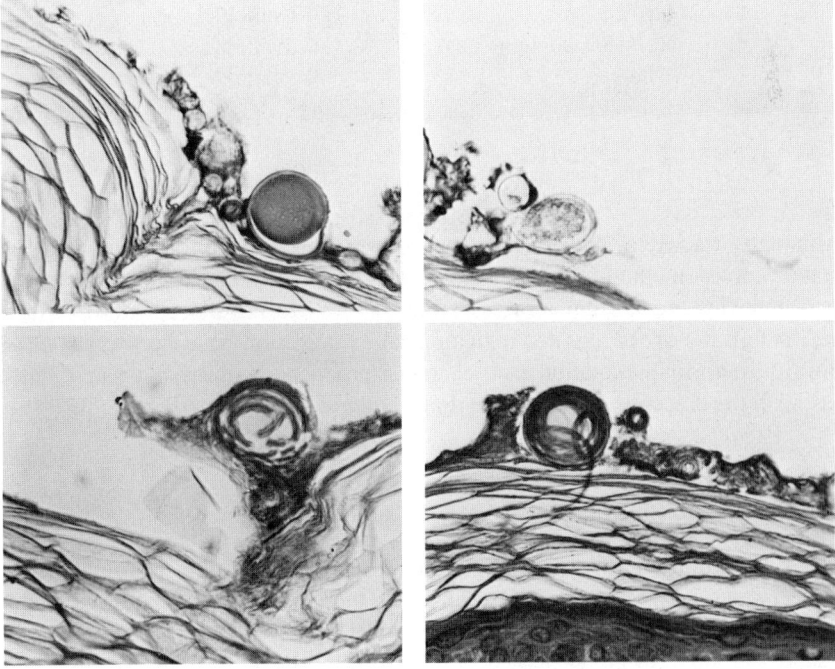

Figure XV-10. Histologic section of skin with coiled and discharged nematocysts of Portuguese man-of-war on the keratin layer. Hematoxylin and eosin stain, ×350 (AFIP Neg. No. 64-7069-B.)

that include tests for ethanol and carbon monoxide and screening studies for acid, basic, and neutral drugs.

The results of the toxicological examinations may enable the pathologist to determine the significance of these studies and to relate them to the medical history, circumstances of death, and pathologic findings of the victim. Underwater swimmers who recognize the potential hazards of proprietary and prescribed medications, alcoholic beverages, and contamination of their air supply by carbon monoxide will not take the risk to jeopardize their personal safety. There are persons, however, who will ingest alcoholic beverages, use medications, or take illicit drugs prior to sport dives. Most clinical laboratories in hospitals do not have the resources for toxicological examinations, but, as described by Garriott (1980), forensic toxicology laboratories are components of a modern medicolegal investigative system. Not all the specimens collected at the time of autopsy may be required, but once the body is released for burial, there is no further opportunity to obtain these specimens.

Physical evidence obtained during the postmortem examination, including specimens for toxicological examination, must be placed in separate, labeled containers, which are accompanied by a recorded chain of custody to assure legal accountability and security for the specimens and to prevent their contamination (Fox and Cunningham 1973, Int. Assoc. Chiefs of Police 1979, U.S. Dept. Justice 1981). The following types and amounts of specimens are suitable for most toxicological examinations, including distribution studies:

Specimen type	Amount
Vitreous humor	all available
Urine	all available
Stomach contents	all available
Bile	all available
Kidney	one
Liver	200 g
Brain	200 g

Although a variety of preservatives have been recommended for toxicological specimens, the simplest method for preservation is freezing. The medical investigators should ensure that bodies are not embalmed, or that tissues are not placed in 10% formalin solution, before the specimens for toxicological examination have been obtained. Embalming fluids, formalin solution, and chemical products of putrefaction may not only interfere with the detection of ethanol or drugs but will also cause considerable difficulty for the toxicologist.

e. Microbiological and Serological Examinations

The blood group and type of the victim are compared with medical records of the putative person to assist with identification. With the onset of putrefaction intravascular dissemination of aerobic and gas-forming anaerobic enteric bacteria cause crepitation in subcutaneous tissues, cystic spaces in organs, and intravascular bubbles. Usually, the effects of putrefaction are readily apparent, but aerobic and anaerobic cultures of blood may be desired for confirmation and to distinguish between air embolism and putrefaction. Either anaerobic bacteriological cultures or gas-liquid chromatography may be used to distinguish between air of the extra-alveolar air syndrome and gases of putrefaction. Ludwig (1979) and Findley (1977), however, have suggested use of the pyrogallol test; pyrogallol, a trihydric phenol, is a white, odorless crystalline power that absorbs oxygen from air readily and turns brown in alkaline solution. Gases of putrefaction, however, will not produce this reaction. Although pyrogallol is available as a chemical reagent, it is rarely used and is probably not available in clinical laboratories of hospitals. It is, therefore, impractical to recommend this test.

F. Summary

The successful investigation of fatal diving accidents requires planning to establish procedures and to coordinate the services of consultants in advance of the incident. A multidisciplinary approach is recommended, and the medicolegal system for the jurisdiction in which the death occurred may serve as the basis for the investigation. The medical history of the victim and the circumstances of death, as well as the examination of equipment and the results of the postmortem examination, are necessary to determine the cause, manner, and mechanism of death, as well as the relationship among the factors that may have contributed to the accident. The information derived from the investigation should be used to comfort the next of kin, to prevent similar accidents, and to improve the practice of diving safety.

CHARLES J. STAHL

APPENDIX

It is apparent that there is a need for a common approach to the investigation of all types of underwater accidents, and the suggestions that follow are considered to be a guide that will lead to a clearer understanding of the problems in need of solution; they should also lead to a more meaningful verdict than the usual coroner's statement: "Death by drowning." What were the events that led up to this final epidosde?

The check list that follows was developed by the Undersea Medical Society for use by the national Diving Accident Network (Divers Alert Network) pending preparation and adoption of a comprehensive underwater accident report form; such a form will be constructed with full consideration of the need for easy scoring and analyzing of the information obtained. It is fully realized that all the blanks cannot be filled in for every accident, but as much information as possible should be supplied—to ensure proper handling of the incident as well as to provide factual data for use in future study of diving accidents. The information considered necessary is merely listed, except for the one page dealing with equipment, where more detail is requested.

A. *Identification of Individual*
   Name_____
   Address_____
   Phone_____
   Next of kin_____
   Age_____
   Sex_____
   Social security number_____
B. *Human Factors*
   (Causal or contributory to the accident)
   1. *Training*
      C-card agency_____
      Date completed_____
      Instructor_____
      Highest credential earned_____
   2. *Experience*
      No experience_____
      Student diver_____
      Certified novice_____
      Occasional diver_____
      Experienced veteran_____
      Professional_____
   3. *Emotional Factors*
      Level of common sense_____
      Judgmental error_____
      Fear, panic_____
      Suicide_____
      Criminal motive_____
   4. *Physiological Factors*
      Level of physical fitness_____
      Illness at time of accident____
      Alcohol consumption_____
      Smoking history_____
      Use of drugs_____
C. *Witnesses*
   1. Buddy_____
   2. Supervisor_____
   3. Instructor_____
   4. Other_____
   5. Address_____
   6. Phone_____
D. *Environment*
   1. Where diving?
      a) Geographic location:
         (1) State_____
         (2) County_____
         (3) Nearest town (Locate on map or chart*)_____
      b) Water:
         (1) Ocean_____
         (2) Lake_____
         (3) River_____
         (4) Quarry_____
         (5) Swimming pool_____
   2. *Diving from*
      a) Shore_____
      b) Dock_____
      c) Pier_____
      d) Boat_____
      e) Rig_____
      f) Cave_____
      g) Kelp_____
      h) Bell—open_____
      i) Bell or habitat saturation_____
   3. *Weather*
      a) Stormy_____
      b) Sea state_____
      c) Rain_____
      d) Fog_____
      e) Clear_____
      f) Snow_____
      g) Air temperature_____
      h) Water temperature_____
      i) Water depth_____
      j) Obtain water sample for salinity, plankton, diatoms._____
E. *Type of Diving*
   1. *Breath-hold (skin)*_____
   2. *Scuba*
      a) Closed circuit (air, mixed-gas?)__
   3. *Tethered*
      a) Surface supplied air?_____
      b) Mixed-gas?_____
F. *Equipment Being Used*
   The accompanying page from the Underwater Accident Report of the National Underwater Accident Data Center, covers the matter of equipment

* *Note:* If at all possible, inspect the site. Obtain statements and complete as many of the questions as possible.

completely and is recommended for use. However, in the examination of equipment the following points are important:

1. Evidence of vomitus in second stage regulator (single-hose or two-hose type).
2. Sample of air from tank for oil vapor, CO, etc. (record amount of pressure gas present in tanks).
3. Technical examination of regulator 'J' valve, pressure gauge, etc. for proper operation. Check weight belt release mechanism.
4. Measure wet suit thickness; examine for defects where water would be in direct contact with skin.

EQUIPMENT DATA

NOTE: *Equipment Brand, Type and Serial Number data need be included only if malfunction or failure was contributory to the incident.*

Equipment Data, Date and Time of Inspection	Brand, Type	Present Before Diving (Yes or No)	Present of Time of Recovery (Yes or No)	Condition	Equipment	Brand, Type, Serial No.	Present Before Diving (Yes or No)	Present at Time of Recovery (Yes or No)	Condition
Diving Suit					Knife (Posit.)				
Hood					Ab Iron				
Boots or Socks					Flashlight				
Gloves or Mits					Depth Gauge				
Mask					Spear Gun				
Snorkel					Compass				
Fins					Regulator				
Weight Belt (lbs.)					Tank				
Buckle					Reserve				
Flotation Device					Watch				
Other Equipment									

Flotation Device: Used _____ (Yes or No)
Tested after event? _____ (Yes or No)
Regulator Tested? _____ (Yes or No)
Results _____

Tank: Air Left _____ MFG _____ Date _____
                (PSIG)
Last Hydro-Test Date _____
Last Visual Inspection Date _____
Internal Condition: Clean _____
  Slight Corrosion _____
  Extensive Corrosion _____

By: _____
        NAME   ADDRESS   PHONE
Special Comments on Equipment _____
Equipment Inspected by: _____
                            NAME   ADDRESS   PHONE
Equipment: Release to/or Held by: _____
                                    NAME   ADDRESS   PHONE

G. *The Dive*
1. *Dives within the last 12 hours including accident dive*

Depth	Time on bottom	Decompression	Surface interval

2. *Activity engaged in at time of accident*
   a. *Commercial Diving*
      (1) Offshore construction_____
      (2) Salvage_____
      (3) Oil and gas exploration_____
      (4) Construction_____
      (5) Salvage_____
      (6) Repair_____
      (7) Fisheries (abalone, sea urchins, black coral, etc.)_____
      _____
      (8) Instructor_____
      (9) In training_____
      (10) Treasure_____
      (11) Archaeological_____
      (12) Photography_____
      (13) Other (specify)_____
   b. *Academic*
      (1) Scientific research_____
      (2) Archaeological_____
   c. *Recreational*
      (1) Instructor_____
      (2) In training_____
      (3) Cave diving_____
      (4) Ice diving_____
      (5) Spear fishing_____
      (6) Photography_____
      (7) Night diving_____
   d. *Government*
      (1) Military_____Service_____
      (2) Civil Service_____
         Agency_____
      (3) Fire department_____
      (4) Police_____
      (5) Rescue unit_____

3. *Diving associates at time of accident*
   a. Diving alone_____
   b. Diving with buddy_____
   c. Buddy distance_____
   d. Diving with group_____
   e. Distance to nearest diver_____

H. *Handling of Emergency*
   1. *Rescue*
      a. Distress signal given_____
         Describe_____
      b. Distance to victim_____yards
      c. Diver free_____, trapped_____
      d. Diver found on surface_____
         submerged_____other_____
      e. Time to reach diver_____minutes
      f. Time to bring diver to surface
         _____minutes
      g. Time to bring diver to shore
         _____minutes
      h. How many involved in rescue attempt?_____
      i. Was safety mat or float used in rescue attempt?_____
      j. Was diver's head above water throughout rescue?_____
   2. *Agency called and responding*
      a. U.S. Coast Guard_____
      b. State Police_____
      c. Local Police_____
      d. Fire Department_____
      e. Other_____
   3. *Transported by*
      a. Coast Guard_____
      b. Police_____
      c. Friend_____

In:
a. Helicopter_____
b. Airplane_____
c. Ambulance_____
d. Car_____
e. Portable pressure chamber_____
4. *First aid administered*
a. At site_____
b. En route_____
c. Hospital emergency room_____
By:
a. Physician_____
b. Emergency Medical Technician_
c. Fellow diver_____
d. Unknown person_____
5. *Condition of the diver*
a. Signs of life prior to resuscitation
   Breathing_____
   Pulse_____
b. Response to resuscitation
   Time elapsed to response_____
6. *Type of first aid given*
a. Mouth-to-mouth resuscitation___
b. External cardiac massage_____
c. Oxygen given_____
d. Mechanical resuscitator_____
e. Any medication given_____
f. Recompression chamber_____
7. *Time elapsed*
a. Surfaced_____
b. First aid started_____
c. Transportation started_____
d. Arrived at definitive pressure chamber care_____

References

BANNER, A. H. 1977. Hazardous marine animals. In: *Forensic Medicine. A Study in Trauma and Environmental Hazards,* edited by C. G. Tedeschi, W. C. Eckert, and L. G. Tedeschi. Philadelphia: W. B. Saunders, vol III, p. 1378–1436.

BAYLISS, G. J. A. 1969. Civilian diving deaths in Australia. *J. Forensic Med.* 16: 39–44.

BROWN, C. D., W. KIME, AND E. L. SHERRER 1978. Postmortem intravascular bubbling: A decompression artifact? *J. Forensic. Sci.* 23: 511–518.

DAVIS, J. H. 1980. Asphyxial deaths. In: *Modern Legal Machine, Psychiatry, and Forensic Science,* edited by W. J. Curran, A. L. McGarry, and C. S. Petty. Philadelphia: F. A. Davis, p. 264–265.

DENNEY, M. K., AND R. C. READ 1965. Scuba-diving deaths in Michigan. *JAMA* 192: 220–222.

DONEHUE, W. C., AND E. L. PETERS 1979. Immersion hypothermia. *U.S. Nav. Med.* 70: 27–28.

ECKERT, W. G. 1977. Injuries from increased atmospheric pressure. In: *Forensic Medicine. A Study in Trauma and Environmental Hazards,* edited by C. G. Tedeschi, W. C. Eckert and L. G. Tedeschi. Philadelphia: W. B. Saunders, vol. I, p. 636–640.

EDMONDS, C., AND R. L. THOMAS 1972a. Medical aspects of diving—Part 2. *Med. J. Aust.* 2: 1256–1260.

EDMONDS, C., AND R. L. THOMAS 1972b. Medical aspects of diving—Parts 3 and 4. *Med. J. Aust.* 2: 1300–1304; 1367–1370.

FINDLEY, T. P. 1977. An autopsy protocol for skin- and scuba-diving deaths. *Am. J. Clin. Pathol.* 67: 440–443.

FOX, R. H., AND C. L. CUNNINGHAM 1973. *Crime Scene Search and Physical Evidence Handbook.* Washington, DC: Law Enforcement Assistant Admin., U.S. Department of Justice, p. 168–173.

GARRIOTT, J. C. 1980. Forensic toxicology: General considerations. In: *Modern Legal Medicine, Psychiatry and Forensic Science,* edited by W. J. Curran, A. L. McGarry, and C. S. Petty. Philadelphia: F. A. Davis, p. 1056–1061.

GIERTSEN, J. C. 1977. Drowning. In: *Forensic Medicine. A Study in Trauma and Environmental Hazards,* edited by C. G. Tedeschi, W. C. Eckert, and L. G. Tedeschi. Philadelphia: W. B. Saunders, vol. III, p. 1317–1333.

GOLDHAHN, R. T. 1977. Scuba deaths: A review and approach for the pathologist. In: *Legal Medicine Annual: 1976,* edited by C. H. Wecht. New York: Appleton-Century-Crofts, p. 109–132.

HANSON, R. G., AND J. M. YOUNG 1975. Diving accidents. In: *The Physiology and Medicine of Diving and Compressed Air Work* (2nd ed.), edited by P. B. Bennett and D. H. Elliott. Baltimore: Williams and Wilkins, p. 554.

HENDRY, W. T. 1977. Autopsy appearances in diving accidents. *Proceedings of the Sixth International Congress on Hyperbaric Medicine.* Aberdeen, Scotland: Aberdeen Univ. Press, p. 364–370.

INTERNATIONAL ASSOCIATION OF CHIEFS OF POLICE 1979. *Guidelines on the Collection and Handling of Physical Evidence.* Gaithersburg, MD: Equipment Technology Center. (Bull. 79-8.)

JOHNSTON, D. G., AND W. D. BURGER 1971. Injury and disease of scuba and skin divers. *Postgrad. Med.* 49: 134–139.

KEATINGE, W. R. 1969. *Survival in Cold Water.* Oxford, England: Blackwell.

KNIGHT, D. R., AND C. J. STAHL 1976. Naval diving accidents: A challenge for thorough investigation. *U.S. Nav. Med.* 67: 30–31.

LUDWIG, J. 1979. *Current Methods of Autopsy Practice* (2nd ed.). Philadelphia: W. B. Saunders, p. 237–239, 363–366.

LUNDBERG, G. D., AND G. E. VOIGT 1979. Reliability of a presumptive diagnosis in sudden, unexpected death in adults. *JAMA* 242: 2328–2330.

MARYLAND, STATE OF. DEPARTMENT OF POST MORTEM EXAMINERS 1979. *Maryland State Post Mortem Examiners Law and Rules and Regulations Governing Medical Examiner Cases.*

MASON, J. K., AND W. J. REALS (editors) 1973. *Aerospace Pathology.* Chicago: College of American Pathologists.

MERGNER, W. J., J. C. SUTHERLAND, W. D. TIGERTT, AND B. F. TRUMP 1980. To answer questions. A review of an autopsy service. *Arch. Pathol. Lab. Med.* 104: 167–170.

MUELLER, W. F. 1969. Pathology of temporal bone hemorrhage in drowning. *J. Forensic Sci.* 14: 327–336.

ROSE, D. M., AND P. A. JARCZYK 1978. Spontaneous pneumoperitoneum after scuba diving. *JAMA* 239: 223.

SCHULTE, J. H. 1964. Diving accidents and treatment methods. *Mil. Med.* 129: 485–489.

SPITZ, W. U. 1980a. Drowning. In: *Medicolegal Investigation of Death. Guidelines for the Applications of Pathology to Crime Investigation, (2nd ed.),* edited by W. U. Spitz and R. S. Fisher. Springfield, IL: Charles C Thomas, p. 351–364.

SPITZ, W. U. 1980b. The medicolegal autopsy. *Hum. Pathol.* 11: 105–112.

SPITZ, W. U. 1980c. Selected procedures at autopsy. In: *Medicolegal Investigation of Death. Guidelines for the Application of Pathology to Crime Investigation, (2nd ed.),* edited by W. U. Spitz and R. F. Fisher. Springfield, IL: Charles C Thomas, p. 590–591.

STAHL, C. J. 1977. Identification. In: *Forensic Pathology: A Handbook for Pathologists,* edited by R. S. Fisher and C. S. Petty. Washington, DC: U.S. Govt. Printing Office, p. 64–71.

STAHL, C. J. 1979. Drowning. In: *Textbook of Medicine* (15th ed.), edited by P. B. Beeson, W. McDermott, and J. B. Wyngaarden. Philadelphia: W. B. Saunders, p. 105–108.

STAHL, C. J. 1980. Identification of human remains. In: *Medicolegal Investigation of Death. Guidelines for the Application of Pathology to Crime Investigation* (2nd ed.), edited by W. U. Spitz and R. S. Fisher. Springfield, IL: Charles C Thomas, p. 39–70.

STEVENS, P. J. 1970. *Fatal Civil Aircraft Accidents. Their Medical and Pathological Investigation.* Bristol, England: John Wright and Sons.

STRAUSS, M. B., AND W. L. ORRIS 1974. Injuries to divers by marine animals: A simplified approach to recognition and management. *Mil. Med.* 139: 129–130.

TEMPLE, J. D., R. T. BOSSHARDT, AND J. H. DAVIS 1975. Scuba tank corrosion as a cause of death. *J. Forensic Sci.* 20: 571–575.

U.S. DEPARTMENT OF HEALTH, EDUCATION AND WELFARE 1978. *Death Investigation: An Analysis of Laws and Policies of the United States, Each State and Jurisdiction (as of January 31, 1977).* Washington, DC: Publ. No. (HSA) 78-5252.

U.S. DEPT. OF JUSTICE, FEDERAL BUREAU OF INVESTIGATION 1981. Washington, DC: *Handbook of Forensic Science.*

U.S. NAVY n.d. *Manual of the Medical Department, U.S. Navy.* Washington, DC: Department of Navy. (NAVMED P-117, Article 17-2.)

WEBSTER, D. P. 1966. Skin and scuba diving fatalities in the United States. *Public Health Rep.* 81: 703–711.

WECHT, C. H. 1977. *The Medicolegal Autopsy Laws of the Fifty States, the District of Columbia, American Samoa, the Canal Zone, Guam, Puerto Rico, and the Virgin Islands* (rev. ed.). Washington, DC: Armed Forces Institute of Pathology.

WRIGHT, R. K., AND L. G. TATE 1980. Forensic pathology. Last stronghold of the autopsy. *Am. J. Forensic Med. Pathol.* 1: 57–60.

Appendixes

A

Glossary of Diving and Hyperbaric Terms

Prepared by the Undersea Medical Society

In 1978 the Undersea Medical Society issued a "Glossary of Diving and Hyperbaric Terms" that was the result of the work of a number of scientists, educators, divers, and international representatives. The background statement for that publication is still pertinent.

> Every speciality has a typical jargon used by the members of the group. In time, the terms become accepted and even begin to appear in dictionaries. In the specialty of hyperbaric and diving activity, the language seemed particularly chaotic. For example, a review of the literature disclosed 48 other terms used to describe the condition we now call dysbaric osteonecrosis; terms ranged from "bone rot" to "osteoarthropathies due to dysbaric aeroembolism."

The glossary was originally designed for the nonphysician. This version includes most of the original as well as many new terms.

The preparation of the original Glossary was supported by The Manned Undersea Science and Technology Program, Office of Ocean Engineering, The National Oceanic and Atmospheric Administration, U.S. Department of Commerce, Washington, D.C.

CHARLES W. SHILLING

ABORT   To terminate dive ahead of schedule or before completion of the task.

ABORT PROFILE   Decompression schedule used to bring a diver safely to the surface when a dive must be aborted.

ABSOLUTE PRESSURE   *See* PRESSURE.

ACOUSTIC BEACON   *See* BEACON.

AEGIR   Underwater habitat developed in Hawaii and used for dives ranging from 100 to 580 feet. It is currently at the Makai Range on Oahu and needs to be refurbished.

AERODONTALGIA *(also* BARODONTALGIA)   Pain in a tooth elicited by changes in ambient pressure.

Appendix A

AEROEMBOLISM   Obsolete term for altitude decompression sickness; also used to mean gas embolism.

AIR COMPRESSOR   *See* COMPRESSOR.

AIR DIVE   Dive in which compressed air is used as the diver's breathing gas. *See also* DIVE.

AIR EMBOLISM   *See* EMBOLISM, AIR OR GAS.

ALTERNOBARIC   Pertaining to changes in pressure.

ALTITUDE CORRECTIONS   Adjustments to decompression schedules necessitated by the reduced barometric pressure prevailing at altitude.

ALTITUDE DIVING   *See* DIVE AT ALTITUDE.

ALVEOLAR VENTILATION   Product of the respiratory frequency and the difference between the expired volume per breath and the dead space.

AMBIENT   Pertaining to the surrounding environment.

AMBIENT PRESSURE   *See* PRESSURE.

ANOXIA   Absence of oxygen. *See also* HYPOXIA.

ANTHROPOMETRY   Measurement of the size and shape of the human body.

APNEA   Cessation of breathing for short periods of time.

ARC SEARCH   *See* SEARCH PATTERN, UNDERWATER.

ARGON   Symbol Ar; atomic number 18; atomic weight 39.944. A colorless, odorless gas that does not react chemically under standard conditions.

ARMORED 1-ATM SUIT   Obsolete term. *See* DIVING SYSTEM.

ARTHRALGIA   Pain in the joints.

   COMPRESSION   Pain in the joints during compression, particularly during rapid compression to pressures greater than 10 atmospheres.

   DECOMPRESSION   Pain in the joints during decompression.

   HYPERBARIC   General term describing either decompression or compression arthralgia; sometimes described by divers as "no joint juice."

ASCENT   Movement in the direction of reduced pressure, whether simulated or due to actual elevation in water or air.

   BUOYANT   Ascent aided by an inflated flotation device.

   EMERGENCY   Unplanned ascent to the surface without stopping at required decompression stops. *See also* BLOWUP.

   EMERGENCY BUOYANT   Rapid ascent to the surface caused by dropping the weight belt and inflating the emergency flotation device; the diver continuously exhales in order to avoid pulmonary barotrauma.

   EMERGENCY CONTROLLED   Ascent to the surface using the breathing apparatus, at a rate that ignores standard ascent rates or decompression stops; ascent rate is *controlled* by the diver (in contrast to uncontrolled, as when a flotation device is used).

EXHALING ("FREE")   Ascent in which diver exhales all the way to the surface without breathing apparatus of any kind.

HOODED   Buoyant ascent during which diver breathes from air-containing hood.

SWIMMING   Controlled ascent with breathing device, but without the aid of a buoyancy device or line.

ASEPTIC BONE NECROSIS   *See* OSTEONECROSIS.

ASPHYXIA   Type of anoxia caused by cessation of effective gas exchange in the lung.

ATMOSPHERES ABSOLUTE   The sum of barometric and hydrostatic pressures.

ATMOSPHERIC PRESSURE   *See* PRESSURE.

ATTENDANT   *See* TENDER.

ATTENDED DIVING *(also* TETHERED DIVING, SURFACE-SUPPORTED DIVING)   Diving with a lifeline and a tender.

BACKPACK   A light frame modeled to conform to the back and hip contours of the diver, used to carry diving equipment.

BAILOUT BOTTLE   Extra bottle of air supply carried in boat.

BARALYME   Carbon dioxide absorbent chemical.

-BARIC   Suffix pertaining to the weight of the atmosphere.

BARODONTALGIA   Pain in teeth associated with changes in barometric pressure.

BAROTRAUMA   Physiological injury caused by pressure changes.

BATHYSCAPH   Navigable submersible ship for deep-sea exploration having a spherical, watertight cabin attached to its underside; example, *Trieste*.

BATHYSCAPHE *(also* BATHYSCAPH, BATHYSCAP, BATHYSPHERE)   Early one-atmosphere vehicles designed for deep ocean exploration.

BATHYSPHERE   Tethered, strongly built diving sphere for deep-sea exploration; example, *Cachalot*.

BEACON   Underwater locating device that emits an acoustic signal.

BÉANCE TUBAIRE VOLONTAIRE (BTV)   Voluntary opening of the eustachian tubes by a maneuver during which the nose, mouth, and glottis are open; the maneuver is performed to equalize pressure.

BELL   Tethered underwater support platform providing life-support services and used to transport divers. *See also* PERSONNEL TRANSFER CAPSULE.

OBSERVATION BELL *(also* OBSERVATION CHAMBER)   Tethered one-atmosphere bell used for search and observation.

BELL, OPEN   Bell open at the bottom and containing a gas pocket in the upper part; used as an elevator or haven.

BELT, WEIGHT   Belt worn by a diver to achieve desired buoyancy.

BENDS   Imprecise term denoting any form of decompression sickness.

BINAURAL INTENSITY DIFFERENCE   Intensity differences at each ear that account for directional hearing.

BINAURAL TIME DIFFERENCE   "Sound shadow effect" that results from one ear being nearer the sound than the other, enabling one to judge direction.

BLOW-OUT PLUG   See PLUG, BLOW-OUT.

BLOWUP   Uncontrolled and rapid diver ascent in a deep-sea dress or variable-volume dry suit.

BODY SQUEEZE   See SQUEEZE.

BOTTOM TIME   Total elapsed time from when the diver leaves the surface in descent to the time (next whole minute) that he or she begins ascent, measured in minutes. (U.S. Navy usage. Other locales may not use descent time.)

BOUNCE DIVE (*also* INTERVENTION DIVE)   Short non-saturation dive beginning and ending at the surface.

BOURDON TUBE   Gauge for measuring pressure, consisting of a coiled sealed tube.

BOYLE'S LAW   See LAWS.

BREATH-HOLD DIVING   See DIVE.

BREATHING APPARATUS   Device for delivering respirable breathing mixture.

BREATHING GAS   See GAS.

BREATHING RESISTANCE   Sum of resistance to flow within the airways and breathing apparatus. *See also* WORK OF BREATHING.

BTV (BÉANCE TUBAIRE VOLONTAIRE)   Method of voluntary opening of the eustachian tubes.

BUBBLE   More or less spherical collection of gas within a liquid. The pressure within such a bubble depends on the surface tension of the liquid, the shape of the bubble, and the external pressure.

SILENT (COVERT) BUBBLES   Gas bubbles that may be detected in the blood vessels or tissues but cause no signs or symptoms of decompression sickness; may be demonstrated by ultrasonic flow techniques such as Doppler.

BUDDY BREATHING   Procedure in which two divers breathe alternately from the same mouthpiece.

BUOYANCY   Upward force exerted by a fluid on an immersed or floating body.

NEGATIVE   State in which the weight of the submerged body is greater than the weight of the displaced liquid, so the body will sink.

NEUTRAL   State in which the weight of the body is equal to the weight of the displaced liquid, so the body will remain suspended in the liquid, buoyed neither upward nor downward.

POSITIVE   State in which the weight of the displaced liquid is greater than the weight of the submerged body, so the body will float or be buoyed upward.

BUOYANCY COMPENSATOR   Device worn and controlled by the diver to regulate his buoyancy.

CAISSON   Watertight pressure chamber used for underwater construction.

CAISSON DISEASE   See DECOMPRESSION SICKNESS.

CARBON DIOXIDE NARCOSIS   The carbon dioxide theory of narcosis suggests that the reduced mental and motor functions observed at depth are the result of retained carbon dioxide rather than the partial pressure of the inert gas.

CAVITATION   Formation of a phase separation (bubbles) due to a localized partial vacuum in a liquid; in the ocean this occurs as the result of the passage through water of a swiftly moving object. In the human body ultrasonic energy may cause cavitation, as it acts to produce substantial but transient reductions in the local fluid pressure; pressure, temperature, and supersaturation have a bearing on the rate of growth of cavitation bubbles.

CHAFING GEAR   Overgarment worn on lower body to protect diving suit.

CHAMBER   Vessel designed to withstand differential pressures.

> ALTITUDE   A chamber whose internal environment simulates the air pressures, humidities, and temperatures encountered at various altitudes.
>
> COMPRESSION   Chamber used for compression.
>
> DECK COMPRESSION, DECOMPRESSION (DDC)   Hyperbaric chamber that is an integral part of a deep diving system and is located on a surface platform from which diving is conducted.
>
> DOUBLE-LOCK   Chamber with two compartments that can be pressurized independently.
>
> HYPERBARIC   Chamber designed to withstand high internal pressures; used in hyperbaric experimentation, diving simulations, and medical treatment.
>
> MONOPLACE   Portable one-person hyperbaric chamber used for therapy in a hospital setting and for transport.
>
> MULTIPLACE   Pressure chamber designed to be used by more than one person at a time; usually a double-lock chamber.
>
> SINGLE-LOCK   Pressure chamber with only one pressurizable compartment.
>
> SUBMERSIBLE DECOMPRESSION (SDC)   Chamber that can be lowered into the water to transport divers between the surface and the work site, and can be mated to the deck decompression chamber. This tethered pressure chamber usually has two compartments, one open to the sea, the other providing an underwater living compartment and refuge.

CHAMBER ATTENDANT   Person who attends another in a chamber.

CHARLES' LAW   *See* LAWS.

CHEMORECEPTOR   Carotic and aortic bodies that are sensitive to changes in the partial pressures of oxygen and carbon dioxide in the blood and that play an important part in the regulation of respiration.

CHOKES   Imprecise term for the pulmonary manifestations of decompression sickness.

CIRCULAR SEARCH   *See* SEARCH PATTERN, UNDERWATER.

CLOSED BELL   *See* BELL.

CLOSED-CIRCUIT GAS SYSTEM   Life-support system or breathing apparatus in which the gas is recycled, carbon dioxide removed, and oxygen periodically added. The design minimizes gas loss by recycling.

CLOSED-CIRCUIT HOT WATER SUIT   *See* SUITS, DIVING.

CLOSED-CIRCUIT SCUBA   *See* SCUBA.

COCHLEAR POTENTIALS   Electrical response generated by stimulation in the cochlea of the inner ear.

CODE-ALPHA FLAG   Blue and white swallowtail international signal flag flown by ships when divers are in the water.

COMPRESSED AIR   Air under pressure, which may be used as a breathing mixture if sufficiently pure.

COMPRESSED AIR ILLNESS   Obsolete term for decompression sickness.

COMPRESSION   That part of a dive involving an increase in pressure upon a diver, due to either the admission of compressed gas to a chamber or descent in the water.

COMPRESSION ARTHRALGIA   *See* ARTHRALGIA, COMPRESSION.

COMPRESSION CHAMBER   *See* CHAMBER, COMPRESSION.

COMPRESSOR   Machine that raises air or other gas to a pressure higher than one atmosphere.

CONSHELF   Series of three underwater habitat programs conducted by Cousteau during 1962 and 1965.

CONSTANT VOLUME DRY SUIT   *See* SUITS, DIVING.

CONTINENTAL SHELF   Shallow (200–250 m), submerged portion of a continental mass bordered by a steep slope to the oceanic deeps.

CONTROL CONSOLE   Panel of displays and controls used to manage a diving system.

COUNTERDIFFUSION   Movement of two inert gases in opposing directions through a semipermeable membrane, as in isobaric counterdiffusion.

COVERT BUBBLES   *See* BUBBLES.

CREST   High point of a wave in any given cycle.

CRISTA   "Swinging door" arrangement within the canals of the vestibular mechanism.

CURV   Cable-operated Unmanned Recovery Vehicle, used by the U.S. Navy primarily to recover test torpedoes. CURV II and III resulted from design improvements and offer greater depth capability (7000 ft of water).

CYCLE FATIGUE LIFE   Specific value of usable service for a system or component based on varied combinations of pressurizations and the number of times the material has been stressed.

DALTON'S LAW   *See* LAWS.

DARK ADAPTATION   Process by which visual receptors gradually become more sensitive to light. Rate depends on previous degree of exposure to light: cones adapt first. At very low light intensities only the rods function, giving only black and white vision, with no detailed configurations.

DEAD SPACE   Space in a diving system in which residual exhaled air remains; it adds to the normal dead space in the lung. When dead space is increased carbon dioxide buildup may occur.

DECANTING   Colloquial term used by caisson workers to mean surface decompression.

DECIBEL   Unit of measurement of perceived differences in sound. The standard sound exerts a pressure of 0.0002 dynes per square centimeter on the eardrum, the approximate average threshold value for a tone of 1000 cycles per second.

DECK DECOMPRESSION CHAMBER (DDC)   *See* CHAMBER.

DECOMPRESSION   In diving, that phase in which the individual is ascending in the water or is in a chamber when the pressure is being lowered.

DECOMPRESSION ACCIDENT   An occurrence of decompression sickness; colloquially, a "hit."

DECOMPRESSION CHAMBER   *See* CHAMBER.

DECOMPRESSION DIVE   *See* DIVE.

DECOMPRESSION METER   Device that automatically computes decompression requirements based on depth and time of exposure; more precisely, decompression computer.

DECOMPRESSION SCHEDULE   Specific decompression procedure for a given combination of depth and bottom time as listed in a DECOMPRESSION TABLE; normally indicated in feet and minutes.

DECOMPRESSION SICKNESS (DCS)   Condition caused by too rapid a reduction in pressure and having a great variety of signs and symptoms. Synonyms: bends, caisson disease, compressed air illness.

   TYPE I (MILD)   Most common symptoms are localized pain, usually in the joints, itching, skin rash, and fatigue.

   TYPE II (SERIOUS)   Common symptoms may involve neurological (central nervous system), pulmonary, or sensory systems. Obsolete term; diver's palsy.

      NEUROLOGICAL   Common symptoms are disorientation, loss of consciousness, and varying degrees of paralysis.

      PULMONARY   Common symptoms are shortness of breath and a choking sensation.

      SENSORY   Common symptoms are vertigo, ringing in the ears, nausea, and blurred vision.

DECOMPRESSION STOP   Designated depth and time at which a diver must stop and wait during ascent from a DECOMPRESSION DIVE, depth and time are specified by the DECOMPRESSION SCHEDULE used.

DECOMPRESSION TABLE   Tabulation of DECOMPRESSION SCHEDULES.

DEEP-SEA DRESS   *See* SUITS, DIVING.

DEMAND MASK   *See* MASK.

DEMAND REGULATOR   *See* REGULATOR, DEMAND.

DENSITY   Mass per unit volume, expressed mathematically as density (d) = mass/volume. Usually expressed in grams per cubic centimeter (g/cm^3) or pounds per cubic foot (lb/ft^3).

DEPTH   When used to indicate the depth of a dive, means the maximum depth attained during the dive, measured in feet of seawater.

DEPTH GAUGE   Pressure-sensitive meter used to determine depth.

DEPTH NARCOSIS   *See* INERT GAS NARCOSIS.

DIFFERENTIAL PRESSURE   Difference in absolute pressure between two locations, such as each side of a boundary between two surfaces.

DIFFUSION   Process in which particles of liquids, gases, or solids intermingle as the result of movement caused by thermal agitation and, in dissolved substances, move from a region of higher to one of lower concentration. Example: a gas in solution diffuses from a region of greater concentration to one of less concentration. *See also* PERFUSION.

DIFFUSION COEFFICIENT   Rate at which a given gas diffuses into a living tissue, expressed in square centimeters per second (cm^2/sec). There is marked variation depending on the molecular weight of the gas and the tissue type. For example, helium in water is 3.04, while oxygen in connective tissue is 0.58.

DILUENT GASES   Inert gases used in breathing mixtures to dilute oxygen to physiologically acceptable limits.

DIVE   Exposure to increased pressure either underwater or in a hyperbaric chamber.

   AIR   Dive using compressed air as a breathing mixture.

   BREATH-HOLD   Dive without breathing equipment, performed by simply holding the breath while underwater.

   DECOMPRESSION   Commonly used term to indicate a dive in which the ascent or decompression is deliberately slowed compared to no-decompression dives. This slowing of the decompression may be in stages or may be continuous, and the most time is taken at shallower depths. It is observed to allow elimination of inert gas from the body.

   EXCURSION   Movement of a diver either upward or downward from the saturation depth; permissible safe distance and time of the excursion dive depend on the saturation depth. May also refer to a trip outside a seafloor habitat with no significant change in depth.

   MIXED-GAS   Dive using a mixture of gases as a breathing medium; the ratio of diluent gas to oxygen is changed to keep the partial pressure of oxygen at or near the normal atmospheric level. Diluent gases are usually nitrogen or helium and occasionally hydrogen.

   NO-DECOMPRESSION   The commonly called *no-D* dive. Strictly it is imprecise in that any ascent or movement toward the surface from a depth in the water allows some decompression. Refers to a dive of such duration or depth that the diver can safely return to the surface without decompression stops or deliberate slowing. Synonym, no-stop dive.

   REPETITIVE   Dive whose decompression obligation is altered by a previous exposure; usually a dive performed within 12 hours of a previous dive.

   SATURATION   Exposure of sufficient duration for the diver's tissue gases to reach equilibrium with the pressure environment; once this has occurred, the decompression time required at the end of a dive for a given depth does not increase because of additional time spent at that depth. Under such conditions, the diver works out of a habitat or other pressurized chamber.

DIVE AT ALTITUDE   Dive conducted at any altitude above approximately 1000 feet. *See also* ALTITUDE CORRECTIONS.

DIVER'S PALSY   Obsolete term. *See* DECOMPRESSION SICKNESS.

DIVING BELL   *See* BELL.

DIVING GAS   *See* GAS, BREATHING.

DIVING REFLEX   Response of man and animals to the immersion of the head in water shown as a bradycardia that is a reflex phenomenon accompanied by an intense peripheral vasoconstriction and by a drastic reduction in cardiac output, only the blood circulation to the brain and the cardiac tissue being maintained.

DIVING STAGE   Suspended platform on which the diver can be lowered into or raised from the water.

DIVING SUIT   See SUITS, DIVING.

DIVING SYSTEM   Broad term used to cover equipment for diving, generally implying use of three basic components; a surface ship or PLATFORM as a support center; a DECK DECOMPRESSION CHAMBER (DDC) that is easily monitored and large and comfortable enough for several divers and is located on board the surface ship or platform; and a transfer chamber, which can be either a PERSONNEL TRANSFER CAPSULE (PTC) or a SUBMERSIBLE DECOMPRESSION CHAMBER (SDC) used to transport divers between the surface and the underwater work site and which can be mated to the DDC.

   ONE-ATMOSPHERE   Pressure-resistant one-man system with articulated arms and legs; equipped with life-support capability and designed to operate at an internal pressure of one atmosphere.

   SATURATION   Pressurized diving system that incorporates a life-support system for long-term saturation dives.

DONALD DUCK EFFECT   Changes in quality of the voice caused by breathing light gases such as helium.

DOPPLER DETECTOR   In diving medicine, a device employing the Doppler effect to detect moving bubbles in the circulation. Synonyms: Doppler flow meter, Doppler monitor.

DOPPLER EFFECT   Physical principle based on the changes in frequency of sound reflected from moving objects.

DOUBLE-LOCK CHAMBER   See CHAMBER.

DRAEGER BREATHING APPARATUS   Apparatus manufactured by the German firm of Draeger.

DRIFT DIVING   Diving while allowing the current to carry both the diver and boat along.

DRILLING PLATFORM   Structure or ship from which offshore drilling operations are conducted.

DRY SUBMERSIBLE   See SUBMERSIBLE.

DRY SUIT   See SUITS, DIVING.

DRY SUIT SQUEEZE   See SQUEEZE.

DUMP SYSTEM   Built-in chamber system that transfers exhaled gas out of the chamber to prevent oxygen buildup. Synonyms: overboard dump system.

DYNE   Unit of measurement for the force necessary to accelerate 1 gram of material 1 centimeter per second.

DYSBARIC OSTEONECROSIS   See OSTEONECROSIS.

DYSBARISM   Loosely used and vague term denoting any pathological condition caused by a change in pressure; includes but is not synonymous with decompression sickness.

696   Appendix A

EAR SQUEEZE   *See* SQUEEZE.

ED_{50} Effective dose required to produce desired effect for 50% of subjects within a large group within a specified time.

ELECTROACOUSTIC TRANSDUCERS   Generic word for hydrophones, microphones, telephone receivers, and loudspeakers; devices for changing sound or audio waves to electric impulses or vice versa.

EMBOLISM, AIR OR GAS   Gas bubbles in the arterial system caused by gas or air passing into the pulmonary veins after rupture of the alveoli.

EMBOLUS   Clot, bubble, or other plug brought by the blood from another vessel and forced into a smaller vessel in such a way as to obstruct the circulation.

EMERGENCY ASCENT   *See* ASCENT.

EMERGENCY BUOYANT ASCENT   *See* ASCENT.

EMERGENCY CONTROLLED ASCENT   *See* ASCENT.

EMPHYSEMA   Swelling or inflation due to the abnormal presence of gas in body tissues.

    ALVEOLAR   Distintention of the air sacs (alveoli) of the lung with gas, usually caused in divers by increased intrapulmonary air pressure associated with ascent.

    MEDIASTINAL   Gas trapped in the space between the lungs where the heart is located. Synonym, pneumomediastinum.

    SUBCUTANEOUS   Gas in the tissues immediately under the skin (often in the neck) caused by lung alveolar rupture. Affected tissues are swollen and crackle when touched.

ÉPAULARD   Unmanned, untethered acoustically controlled vehicle for deep ocean survey.

EQUIVALENT AIR DEPTH (EAD)   Air breathing depth that has a nitrogen partial pressure equivalent to that at the diving depth.

EQUIVALENT BOTTOM TIME   Hypothetical period of time taken to represent a decompression obligation, which is added to bottom time of a subsequent dive to determine the decompression obligation for the latter dive.

ERGOMETER   Apparatus for measuring muscular work.

EXCURSE   To make an EXCURSION.

EXCURSION   Movement of a diver either vertically (up or down) or horizontally from the work platform, bell, chamber, or habitat at the saturation depth.

EXCURSION DIVE   *See* DIVE.

EXPIRATORY RESERVE   Amount of air that can be exhaled out of the lungs after normal expiration.

EXTERNAL EAR SQUEEZE   *See* SQUEEZE.

EYE SQUEEZE   *See* SQUEEZE.

FACE MASK   *See* MASK.

FACEPLATE   That part of the diving mask or helmet through which the diver sees.

FACE SQUEEZE   *See* SQUEEZE.

FAST TISSUE   In considering tissue saturation with gas (nitrogen) while under pressure, those tissues that half-saturate quickly (blood, 5 min) compared with those tissues that saturate slowly (tendon, 75 min).

FATHOM   Obsolete term for unit of measurement of depth in the ocean for countries using the English system of units; equal to 6 feet (1.83 m).

FEEDBACK   Information returned from a source and used in regulating behavior.

FICK'S LAW   *See* LAWS.

FICK'S PRINCIPLE   Principle of conservation of matter as it relates to the transport of substances by the blood.

FINS   *See* SWIM FINS.

FIXED BOTTOM STATIONS   Underwater work sites that are maintained at one atmosphere of pressure, highly dependent on land- or sea-based support equipment; example, underwater welding chamber.

FLARE   Pyrotechnic device for light or signal.

FLOAT   Marking device that floats on the surface of the water.

FLOTATION DEVICE   Inflatable vest used to assist ascent or provide positive buoyancy; also used underwater for fine buoyancy control.

FOULING   Snarling or catching of an air line or umbilical in wreckage or underwater structures; also, organic growth on underwater surfaces.

FREE AIR SPACE   Air space trapped in an underwater structure.

FREE DIVING   Diving without tether, umbilical, or marking device.

FRENZEL MANEUVER   Maneuver to equalize pressure in the middle ear with the ambient pressure against the outer surface of the eardrum. In this maneuver the nose is compressed shut, the mouth is open, and the glottis is closed; the action is to move the back of the tongue up and backward, resulting in increased rhinopharyngeal pressure that forces air through the eustachian tube.

GAS   In diving, any respirable mixture used by the diver.

   BREATHING   Oxygen, or a mixture of oxygen and other gases, breathed through a supply system in diving, flying, or hyperbaric chambers, and in medical treatment or when the ambient medium is not respirable.

   DILUENT   *See* DILUENT GASES.

   INERT   *See* INERT GAS.

   MIXED   Breathing medium consisting of oxygen and one or more inert gases synthetically mixed.

   SEPARATED   Term describing the presence of gas in the body in sites such as joints and between muscle where the description "bubble" would not be appropriate; also used by extension to describe all unspecified collections of gas, including bubbles.

GAS CONSOLE   Station for monitoring and controlling flow of gas to the diver. Synonym, gas rack.

GAS EXCHANGE   *See* INERT GAS ELIMINATION, INERT GAS UPTAKE, PERFUSION, DIFFUSION.

GAS LAWS   Mathematical descriptions of relations of pressure, temperature, and volume under ideal conditions. *See also* LAWS.

GAS NUCLEATION   Process of forming gas nuclei.

GAS NUCLEI   Since bubbles are difficult to produce in pure liquids, it is generally assumed that "nuclei" are necessary for bubble formation; gas nuclei are defined, according to a circular argument, as that which is necessary for bubble formation; also called *microbubbles*.

GAS RACK   *See* GAS CONSOLE.

GAS SWITCHING   Changing the composition of the breathing gas.

GAS WASHOUT   *See* INERT GAS ELIMINATION.

GAUGE PRESSURE   *See* PRESSURE.

GENERAL GAS LAW   *See* LAWS.

GILL, ARTIFICIAL   Device for obtaining oxygen by diffusion from water.

GRADIENT   Degree of change of one quantity with respect to another; for example, the degree of change of temperature with ocean depth.

GRAHAM'S LAW   *See* LAWS.

HABITAT   Life-support system of limited mobility, capable of providing functional living and working space in the underwater environment; highly dependent on land- or sea-based support equipment; has an internal pressure equal to the pressure of the ambient underwater pressure. It has free access for the diver to enter and leave it through an open hatch in the bottom. An example is SEALAB. For a complete listing and classification of underwater habitats see the *NOAA Diving Manual* (2nd ed.), 1979, p. 14-4.

HALF TIME   Way of describing an exponential curve—the time required to reach 50% of the final state; in diving, the time required for a tissue to absorb or eliminate one-half the equilibrium amount of inert gas.

HAPTIC   Pertaining to the cutaneous system of senses.

HARD HAT   Common term for diving helmet. *See* HELMET.

"HARD-LINE" SYSTEMS   Communication system similar to a telephone and consisting of a microphone, cable, and receiver.

HARNESS ASSEMBLY   Combination of straps used to attach diving equipment to the diver.

HEAVY GEAR   *See* SUITS, DIVING.

HELGOLAND   German underwater habitat built in 1968 that has been used in the Baltic Sea, the North Sea, and the Western Atlantic off the coast of Massachusetts. Mission took place between 1969 and 1975.

HELIOX   Breathing mixture of helium and oxygen used at depths because it has little narcotic effect. Synonym, oxyhelium. Abbreviation, He-O_2.

HELIUM   Symbol He; atomic number 2; atomic weight 4.003. A colorless, odorless gas, used as a replacement for nitrogen in the gas mixture for deep-sea divers because it is less narcotic. Breathing helium-oxygen mixtures causes temporary speech distortion (DONALD DUCK EFFECT), which hinders communication. Helium also has a high thermal conductivity that results in rapid loss of body heat.

HELIUM SPEECH UNSCRAMBLER   Device designed to render intelligible the words spoken in a hyperbaric helium environment.

HELIUM TREMORS   *See* HIGH PRESSURE NERVOUS SYNDROME.

HELMET   Device worn over the head of a diver, designed to furnish breathing gas, allow visibility through primary viewports, be equipped with two-way communication, and be compatible with dry suits and the standard wet suit.

HENRY'S LAW   *See* LAWS.

HERTZ   Unit of frequency equal to one cycle per second. Abbreviation, Hz.

HIGH PRESSURE NERVOUS SYNDROME (HPNS)   Neurological and physiological dysfunction resulting from hyperbaric exposure, usually to helium at higher pressures; may include tremor, somnolence, EEG changes, visual disturbance, nausea, dizziness, and sometimes convulsions.

HIGH PRESSURE OXYGEN   *See* HYPERBARIC OXYGENATION.

HIT   Jargon for decompression sickness; not recommended because it provides no information about type or severity.

HOOKAH DIVING   Technique for supplying surface-supplied breathing media to a demand regulator carried by a diver.

HYDRAULIC   Moved or worked by liquid pressure.

HYDROGEN   Symbol H; atomic number 1; atomic weight 1.0080. A colorless, odorless, tasteless nontoxic gas. Although explosive when mixed with air in certain proportions, hydrogen has been used in diving. Hydrogen is less narcotic than nitrogen; it has thermal properties and distorts the voice in a manner similar to helium.

HYDROLAB   Underwater habitat 8 ft $\times$ 16 ft built by Perry Submarine Builders in 1966 and still in use in St. Croix, Virgin Islands.

HYDROPHONE   Electroacoustic transducer that responds to waterborne sound waves and delivers essentially equivalent electric waves. Conversion from sound energy to electric energy is achieved through the use of either the piezoelectric or magnetostrictive effect. The varying potential generated across a piezoelectric material when it is subjected to a varying mechanical force can be coupled to an amplifier as an electrical signal with the same frequency characteristics as those of the mechanical vibration that excited the material.

HYDROSPHERE   Aqueous vapor of the atmosphere. Commonly used to mean oceans, seas, lakes, and streams.

HYDROSTATIC   Of or relating to liquids at rest or to the pressures they exert or transmit.

HYPERBARIC   Pertaining to pressure greater than one atmosphere.

HYPERBARIC ARTHRALGIA   *See* ARTHRALGIA.

HYPERBARIC CHAMBER   *See* CHAMBER.

HYPERBARIC FACILITY   Entire group of systems and subsystems used to support a high-pressure chamber or chambers; used to simulate high pressures; may include a wet pot to simulate an actual underwater environment.

HYPERBARIC OXYGENATION (HBO)   Use of an oxygen breathing mixture that meets two conditions: the oxygen partial pressure is greater than 2/10 of an atmosphere, and the ambient pressure is greater than one atmosphere.

HYPERCAPNIA   Physiological state in which the systemic arterial carbon dioxide pressure is significantly above 40 torr. Elevated carbon dioxide levels may occur in a habitat or closed space, in a diving suit or breathing equipment, and thus in the lungs. Synonym, hypercarbia.

HYPEROXIA   Excess of oxygen in the body tissues produced by breathing a mixture in which the inspired oxygen pressure is greater than its partial pressure in air.

HYPEROXIC   Relating to raised partial pressures of oxygen, as in hyperoxic mixtures.

HYPERTHERMIA   Elevation of body temperature above normal. In diving, hyperthermia may occur in hyperbaric chambers as a result of environmental exposure to heat or failure of the body's thermoregulatory system.

HYPOCARPNIA   Physiological state in which the systemic arterial carbon dioxide pressure is significantly below 40 torr. Symptoms may include finger tingling, muscle spasm, dizziness, and loss of consciousness. Commonly caused by overbreathing.

HYPOTHERMIA   Reduction of body temperature as a result of environmental exposure to cold or failure of the body's thermoregulatory system. Some hypothermia accompanies most dives. Unless a diver is suitably protected, it may result in reduced performance; may be fatal if exposure is prolonged or extreme.

HYPOXIA   Tissue oxygen pressure below normal; may be produced by breathing mixtures that are deficient in oxygen, by disease states, or by toxic gases such as carbon dioxide.

HYPOXIC VENTILATORY DRIVE   Low oxygen physiological stimulus to breathing.

IDEAL GAS   Term denoting a gas that would obey the gas laws exactly.

IDEAL GAS LAW   *See* LAWS.

IGLOO   Pressurized space above the wet pot in some hyperbaric facilities, used either as a dry work area or preparation area before entry to the wet pot.

IMMERSION HYPOTHERMIA   Subnormal body temperature due to immersion in water.

INERT GAS   Any of a group of rare gases that include helium, neon, argon, krypton, xenon, and sometimes radon, and that exhibit great stability and extremely low reaction rate. Also called *noble gas*.

INERT GAS ELIMINATION (*also* GAS WASHOUT)   Transfer of inert gas (nitrogen, helium, etc.) under the influence of a pressure gradient from the tissues to the blood to the lungs, from which it is exhaled.

INERT GAS NARCOSIS   Degradation of performance caused by high partial pressures of krypton, argon, nitrogen, or any other of the noble gases. *See also* NARCOSIS.

INERT GAS UPTAKE   Absorption of inert gas by the tissues of the body under the influence of a pressure gradient. Rate of uptake depends on duration of exposure and partial pressure and nature of the gas.

INFLATABLE FLOTATION DEVICE   *See* FLOTATION DEVICE.

INKLE   Mild, transient, and poorly localized symptom of decompression sickness; not recommended us a useful term.

INTERFACE   Surface separating two media across which there is a discontinuity of some property; also used to mean the surface of the sea.

INTEROCEPTORS   Sensors associated with the visceral organs.

INTERVENTION DIVE   Commonly called bounce dive.

INTRAPLEURAL PRESSURE   Pressure within the space between the chest wall and the lungs (pleural space). Abbreviation, Ppl.

ISOBARIC   Relating to a process taking place without change of ambient pressure.

ISOMETRIC RELAXATION   Relaxation of a muscle without shortening.

JACKSTAY SEARCH   See SEARCH PATTERN, UNDERWATER.

JIM   Atmospheric manned diving system consisting of an armored, jointed diving suit with manipulators for hands.

J-VALVE   Spring-loaded check valve that begins to close when scuba cylinder pressure approaches a predetermined level, generally 300 or 500 pounds per square inch.

KINESTHESIS   Muscle, tendon, and joint sense that helps to yield information about the position of the body in space.

LAWS (physical laws relating to diving)

> BOYLE'S LAW   At a constant temperature the volume of an ideal gas varies inversely with the pressure.
>
> CHARLES' LAW   At a constant pressure the volume of an ideal gas varies directly with the absolute temperature.
>
> DALTON'S LAW   The pressure exerted by one gas of a mixture of gases is equal to the pressure the single gas would exert if it alone occupied the same volume (partial pressure).
>
> FICK'S LAW   Law that describes the way in which diffusion occurs in fluids. The amount of a solute that diffuses in a unit of time through a solvent depends on the following: the concentration gradient, measured over a specified time; the area over which diffusion is taking palce; the ambient temperature; the type of molecule and interaction between the molecules of solvent and solute. See also FICK'S PRINCIPLE.
>
> GENERAL GAS LAW   Boyle's and Charles' laws can be conveniently combined into what is known as the general gas law. Expressed mathematically: $P_1 V_1/T_1 = P_2 V_2/T_2$, where P_1 = initial pressure (absolute), V_1 = initial volume, T_1 = initial temperature (absolute), P_2 = final pressure (absolute), V_2 = final volume, T_2 = final temperature (absolute).
>
> GRAHAM'S LAW   Diffusivity is inversely proportional to the square root of molecular weight; the law is rather accurate in gases, but only approximately so in liquids.
>
> HENRY'S LAW   At a constant temperature the amount of a gas that dissolves in a liquid with which it is in contact is proportional to the partial pressure of that gas.
>
> IDEAL GAS LAW   Law that defines the relationships among pressure, temperature, volume, and quantities of substances (moles) of any ideal gas. The equation is $PV = NRT$, where P = absolute pressure, V = volume, N = number of moles of gas, R = universal gas constant, and T = absolute temperature.

PASCAL'S LAW   The component of the pressure in a fluid in equilibrium that is due to forces externally applied is uniform throughout the body of the fluid. Externally applied pressure is transmitted equally throughout all fluid-filled spaces.

POISEUILLE'S LAW   Law dealing with laminar flow. For practical application it states that as resistance is increased, the flow is reduced in direct proportion. Thus if the length of a hose line is doubled, the pressure must be doubled to maintain the same flow.

LD_{50} Lethal dose for 50% of subjects within a large group within a specified time.

LIFELINE   Line between the diver and his tender, used to signal and supply the diver, to assist him in normal ascent, and to retrieve him in an emergency. Usually part of the umbilical.

LIFE-SUPPORT SYSTEM   System designed to produce a controlled environment for chamber occupants. May include capability to supply metabolic oxygen, control temperature and humidity, and remove CO_2.

LIFT BAGS   Gas-containing bags of various sizes used to lift objects in the water.

LIFT LINE   Rope line attached to the lift bags and down to the object to be lifted.

LIQUID BREATHING   Experimental technique involving flushing the lungs with a highly oxygenated liquid from which the subject derives enough oxygen to sustain life; so far this technique hasn't been able to provide for adequate elimination of carbon dioxide.

LIVE BOATING   Diving from a vessel that is underway.

LOCK   Pressurizable compartment or one used to transfer personnel or supplies between two pressure levels, such as the air lock, man lock, medical lock, service lock.

LOCKING IN   Going in to an already pressurized chamber.

LOCKOUT   Relating to the release (locking out) of divers from an underwater bell, chamber, habitat, or submersible.

LOCKOUT SUBMERSIBLE   A vehicle, usually maintained at a dry one-atmosphere pressure, which has a chamber that can be pressurized to the ambient underwater pressure to allow egress of a diver or divers; if necessary, can be used to decompress the divers back to one atmosphere of pressure.

LORRAIN SMITH EFFECT   Pulmonary toxic effect of high pressure oxygen in small animals, first observed by the physiologist J. Lorrain Smith.

MASK   Diving equipment worn over the face to provide an air pocket for better vision; may also have a breathing valve.

   BAND (SURFACE-SUPPLIED)   Full-face mask affixed to the head by a network of rubber straps.

   DEMAND   Mask with a demand regulator in which the gas is activated by the negative pressure associated with inhalation. *See also* REGULATOR, DEMAND.

   FULL-FACE   Mask in which gas supply is continuous and independent of respiration; sometimes called free-flow.

   LIGHTWEIGHT DIVING   Full face cover through which surface-supplied breathing gases are delivered to a diver. Gases may flow freely through the mask or be delivered through an oronasal assembly.

ORONASAL   Breathing mask that covers and allows breathing through both nose and mouth.

MASKING   Partial or complete obscuring of one sensory process by another.

McCANN RESCUE CHAMBER   U.S. Navy rescue bell (or chamber) used to rescue men from a sunken submarine. Used successfully in the U.S.S. *Squalus* rescue.

MECHANORECEPTORS   Receptors in the body that are sensitive to mechanical energy (for touch, pressure, audition).

MEDIASTINAL EMPHYSEMA   *See* EMPHYSEMA.

MESOSCAPH   Same as a bathyscaph except for depth of operation; an example is *Ben Franklin*.

MICROPHONE   Electroacoustic transducer that responds to sound waves and delivers essentially equivalent electric waves.

MIDDLE EAR SQUEEZE   *See* SQUEEZE.

MIXED-GAS DIVING   Diving with breathing mixture composed of inert gases with oxygen, hydrogen-oxygen, or other mixtures. Often the ratio of the diluent gas to oxygen is changed to keep partial pressure of oxygen at or near normal atmospheric (normoxic) level.

MODULATED SYSTEMS   Amplitude modulation employs a carrier frequency varied by a superimposed speech signal. Systems of this type consist of a microphone, power module, amplifier, modulator, and underwater transducer.

MODULATION   Variation in value of some parameter characterizing a periodic oscillation. Best known are amplitude modulation (AM) and frequency modulation (FM). Another type uses a single-sideband suppressed carrier (SSB). AM and FM radio receivers are common radio receiver devices for detecting these modulations.

MOMSEN LUNG   Former U.S. Navy submarine escape apparatus.

MONOPLACE CHAMBER   *See* CHAMBER.

MOON POOL   Open-water center part of certain diving ships, constructed so that a bell can be raised or lowered through it.

MOUTHPIECE   Relatively watertight channel for the flow of breathing gas between the life-support system and the diver. It consists of a flange that fits between the lips and teeth, and two bits, one on either side of the mouthpiece opening; it is held in place by slight pressure of lips and teeth.

MULTIPLACE CHAMBER   *See* CHAMBER.

M-VALUE   Difference between the amount of inert gas partial pressure in the supersaturated tissues and the partial pressure of the gas in the mixture being breathed; or, the maximum value of the partial pressure of dissolved gas that can be tolerated in a specific compartment of the human body and still permit the diver to ascend safely to the next stop. Term devised by R.D. Workman.

NARCOSIS   State of stupor or unconsciousness usually caused by a drug. In diving, caused by effects of gases breathed at pressure. Gases vary in their narcotic potency and may interact with each other to produce effects that are greater than those produced individually. Symptoms may include lightheadedness, loss of judgment, and occasional euphoria.

704   Appendix A

INERT GAS   Narcosis produced by INERT GASES.

NITROGEN   Narcotic effects resulting from breathing compressed air at depths greater than about 100 feet. Synonym, compressed air narcosis.

NEAR-DROWNING   History, signs, and symptoms consistent with drowning, yet the patient has survived.

NEGATIVE-PRESSURE BREATHING   Breathing with the intrapulmonary pressure lower than the surrounding pressure. For example, breathing air at atmospheric pressure when the body is immersed to the neck in water.

NEON   Symbol Ne; atomic number 10; atomic weight 20.183. A colorless, odorless gas found in air (1 part in about 65,000 parts ordinary air). Has been used in diving because it has little narcotic effect.

NEOPRENE   Oil-resistant synthetic rubber made by polymerizing chlorophrene. Nonexpanded neoprene is used for masks, fins, and O-rings: expanded neoprene, with gas bubbles blown in, is used for wet suits.

NIGGLE   Mild, transient, and poorly localized symptoms of decompression sickness not requiring treatment. Not recommended as a useful term.

NIL-SUPERSATURATION   No or zero supersaturation. *See also* SUPERSATURATION.

NITROGEN   Symbol N; atomic number 7; atomic weight 14.008. A colorless, odorless, tasteless nontoxic inert gas. Found in great abundance in our atmosphere (78.03% nitrogen by weight). Nitrogen is commonly used as a diluent with oxygen in diving gas mixtures but has several disadvantages because of narcotic effects when breathed under pressure. *See also* NARCOSIS.

NITROGEN NARCOSIS   Intoxication caused by breathing of high partial pressures of nitrogen at hyperbaric pressures. *See also* INERT GAS NARCOSIS.

NITROX   Breathing mixture containing nitrogen and oxygen in various proportions. Used in diving when the oxygen partial pressure must be reduced because of the depth of the dive and the danger of oxygen poisoning.

NO-DECOMPRESSION DIVE   *See* DIVE.

NO-DECOMPRESSION LIMITS   Specified times at given depths from which no-decompression stops are required on return to the surface. Synonyms: no-stop curve, no-stop limits.

NO JOINT JUICE   Slang term. *See* ARTHRALGIA.

NON-RETURN VALVE   *See* VALVE, NON-RETURN.

NORMAL ASCENT RATE   60 Feet per minute.

NORMOXIA   Tissue oxygen pressure with levels of oxygen equivalent to normal partial pressures of oxygen found in air at one atmosphere.

NORMOXIC   Relating to normal partial pressures of oxygen equivalent to those found in air at one atmosphere.

NO-STOP LIMITS   *See* NO-DECOMPRESSION LIMITS.

NUCLEATION   *See* GAS NUCLEATION.

OBSERVATION BELL   *See* BELL.

OCEAN ARMS III   Atmospheric Roving Manipulator System), a two-man manipulator-equipped bell that is extremely versatile and has set a depth record for a fixed-buoyancy, manipulator-equipped bell with a dive of 2842 feet.

OCTOPUS RIG   Essentially a single-hose regulator with an extra low pressure port to which an additional second stage has been fitted. This double regulator is for emergency buddy breathing or to use in case of failure of the primary regulator.

OMITTED DECOMPRESSION   Controlled ascent in which a diver comes to the surface at a rate greater than 60 feet per minute or without one or more of his decompression stops.

ONE-ATMOSPHERE DIVING SUIT   *See* DIVING SYSTEM.

ONE-MAN CHAMBER   *See* CHAMBER, MONOPLACE.

OPEN BELL   *See* BELL, OPEN.

OPEN-CIRCUIT HOT WATER SUIT   *See* SUITS, DIVING.

ORAL NASAL MASK, ORONASAL MASK   Breathing mask covering nose and mouth; designed to reduce dead air space and thus eliminate the likelihood of CO_2 buildup.

OSTEONECROSIS

   DYSBARIC   Changes in structure of bone in which the relative density of the affected bone is increased by sclerosis. Observed changes are the result of a healing process following insult. Found in caisson workers and more recently in divers; probably due to inadequate decompression. Synonyms: aseptic bone necrosis, avascular bone necrosis.

   JUXTA-ARTICULAR   Osteonecrosis occurring near the joint articulation, usually hip or shoulder. May lead to collapse of the joint, together with pain and dysfunction.

   MEDULLARY   Osteonecrosis occurring in the shaft of the bone; usually symptomless and detected by radiography.

OTITIS   Inflammation of the ear; may be marked by pain, fever, abnormalities of hearing, tinnitus, and vertigo; a very common problem in diving.

   EXTERNA   Superficial infection of the auditory canal; a common occurrence in habitat living and wet pot and open-sea diving; usually caused by a mold or bacterium.

   MEDIA   Inflammation or infection of the middle ear; in diving, often used to describe a condition in which the middle ear fills with fluid. Compare SQUEEZE.

OTOLITHS   Small calcium deposits in the endolymph of the inner ear, which, upon movement of the head, activate neuronal endings to aid in maintaining equilibrium.

OVAL WINDOW RUPTURE   *See* PERILYMPH FISTULA.

OVERBOARD DUMP SYSTEM   *See* DUMP SYSTEM.

OXYARC BURNING   Process for cutting metals using a hollow electrode through which a stream of oxygen is delivered.

OXYGEN   Symbol O; atomic number 8, atomic weight 16.000. A colorless, odorless, tasteless, and under normal conditions, nontoxic gas. Found free in the atmosphere, 23.15% by weight in dry air and 20.98% by volume. The most abundant element in the ocean (15.8% oxygen). Oxygen is essential in cellular respiration of all animals and man but may be toxic at elevated partial pressures.

OXYGEN AT HIGH PRESSURE   *See* HYPERBARIC OXYGENATION.

OXYGEN BREATHING   Breathing of 100% oxygen; in diving, used in some closed-circuit scuba and in the treatment of decompression sickness and/or to enhance the elimination of inert gas during the final stages of decompression.

OXYGEN CLEANING   Method of cleaning an oxygen-supply system to ensure elimination of all hydrocarbons and other potentially dangerous contaminants.

OXYGEN DUMP SYSTEM   *See* DUMP SYSTEM.

OXYGEN POISONING   Deleterious effects caused by breathing high partial pressures of oxygen. Prolonged exposure can result in effects that become progressively more severe as the inspired partial pressure and/or the duration of exposure increases. Depending on level and length of exposure, may cause lung damage, enough involvement of the central nervous system to cause convulsions, or death.

OXYGEN TOXICITY   Deleterious or poisonous quality of oxygen at high partial pressure. Has come by popular usage to be interchangeable with OXYGEN POISONING.

OXYHELIUM   Mixture of helium and oxygen with the partial pressure of oxygen equivalent to air at the surface.

PARADOXICAL SHIVERING   Uncontrollable shivering under conditions of high helium partial pressures, accompanied by subjective feeling of warmth.

PARTIAL PRESSURE   *See* PRESSURE.

PASCAL'S LAW   *See* LAWS.

PAUL BERT EFFECT   Convulsions caused by oxygen at raised pressures, first observed by the French physiologist Paul Bert.

PERFUSION   Flow of blood (or lymph) through an organ or tissue, by which gases and chemical substances are disturbed and exchanged. *See also* DIFFUSION.

PERILYMPH FISTULA   Round or oval window rupture allowing the fluid (perilymph) surrounding the middle ear to escape to the inner ear. Rupture of the round or oval windows is caused by stretching them beyond capacity or by a sudden reversal in position, usually occurring during a forceful attempt to clear the ears.

PERSONNEL TRANSFER CAPSULE (PTC)   A chamber for the transfer of personnel between the surface and the work site that can be mated to the DECK DECOMPRESSION CHAMBER (DDC); can be maintained at one atmosphere or can be pressurized, depending on type of system used. *See also* BELL.

pH   Measure of alkalinity and acidity. A pH of 7 is neutral; above that is alkaline; below that, acid.

PHOTON   Measure of brightness defined as the retinal illumination that results when a surface brightness of one candle per square meter is seen through a pupillary area of one square milimeter.

PHOTOPIC VISION   Visual function performed by the cones; color vision; fine detail (high acuity); does not function below 10^{-2} millilamberts.

PINGER   *See* BEACON.

PINNIPED   Animal that has finlike feet or flippers.

PLATFORM   Any man-made structure from or on which oceanographic instruments are suspended or installed, or from which diving operations are conducted.

PLUG, BLOW-OUT   Device installed in the gas cylinder valve assembly, designed to fail under pressure before the cylinder fails.

PNEUMATIC   Moved or worked by air pressure.

PNEUMOFATHOMETER   Hollow tube connected at one end to a gauge at the surface and open under the surface at the diver's end; used to measure water pressure at the diver's end of the tube.

PNEUMOGAUGE HOSE   Durable, lightweight, flexible hose attached to a low pressure air supply source on the surface and open at the diver's end; used to monitor the diver's depth. Usually attached to the umbilical with the open end terminating at the diver's chest.

PNEUMOPERICARDIUM   Condition in which gas is present in the membranous sac that contains the heart.

PNEUMOTHORAX   Presence of gas outside the lungs and within the chest cavity. Usually the result of rupture of the visceral pleura (outer lining of the lung), allowing air to flow into the chest cavity while the lung collapses.

POISEUILLE'S LAW   *See* LAWS.

POLARIZED LIGHT   Light that has been broken up into its seven basic colors by passing through a prism or similar device.

POSITIVE BUOYANCY   *See* BUOYANCY.

PRESSURE   Force acting on a unit area; expressed mathematically Pressure = Force/Area, or P = F/A.

    ABSOLUTE   The sum of all pressures acting on an object; in diving, the sum of the atmospheric pressure and the hydrostatic pressure acting on a submerged object.

    AMBIENT   The absolute pressure surrounding an object.

    ATMOSPHERIC   Pressure exerted by the earth's atmosphere, which varies with altitude above sea level; at sea level, atmospheric pressure is equal to 760 millimeters of mercury or 1.03 kilograms per square centimeter (14.7 lb/in.^{2}).

    DESIGN   Pressure rating of a component established from physical characteristics and stress analysis.

    GAUGE   Difference between absolute pressure and atmospheric pressure; gauge pressure is converted to absolute pressure by adding 14.7 if the dial reads in pounds per square inch or 1.03 if the dial reads kilograms per square centimeter.

    HYDROSTATIC   Pressure of a column of water acting upon a body immersed in the water, equal in all directions at a specific depth; it increases at a rate of 0.445 pounds per square inch per foot of descent in fresh water.

    PARTIAL   Pressure exerted by one component in a gaseous system, described by Dalton's and Henry's laws. The partial pressure of a gas is equal to the product of the ambient pressure and the fraction of the total pressure in a mixture that can be ascribed to that gas.

WORKING Approximate pressure that must not be exceeded in normal operations.

PRESSURE EQUIVALENTS *See* Appendix C, Pressure Conversion Table.

PRESSURE HEAD Difference in pressure between two components of a system.

PRESSURE-PROOF Having the structural ability to resist ambient pressure without leakage.

PRESSURE UNITS *See* Appendix C, Pressure Conversion Table.

PRESSURIZE To increase the internal pressure of a closed vessel.

PROFILE In diving, a graphic presentation of the depth and time relationships during a dive.

PROPRIOCEPTORS Sense organs found in muscles, tendons, joints, and in the labyrinth that provide information concerning movement and position of the body in space.

PSYCHOMOTOR TESTS Tests that are based on other psychological processes (sensory, perceptual) and call for a motor reaction such as pressing a key, holding a stylus as steady as possible, manipulating controls.

PULMONARY BAROTRAUMA Damage to lung alveoli due to changes in pressure, usually as a result of increased internal pressure; may result in air embolism, pneumothorax, or emphysema, and is probably second only to drowning as a cause of death in diving.

PURGING Ventilation or flushing of a space such as a gas-filled chamber to change the composition of the gas or to remove contaminants. Electronic instruments used in hyperbaric chambers may be purged with an inert gas to reduce the fire hazard.

PUSH–PULL Breathing system used by divers that supplies gas to the diver at appropriate pressure (push) and recovers his exhaust gas for recovery and reuse (pull), for the purpose of conserving helium. Special valves are necessary to permit recovery of the exhaust gas without risk of subjecting the diver's lungs to a suction or reduced pressure. Push-pull systems may involve compressors and recovery pumps (sometimes called depressors) located within the diving bell or at the surface.

PVHO Pressure Vessel for Human Occupancy; term adopted by the American Society for Mechanical Engineers (ASME) to describe hyperbaric chambers.

RANKINE (°R) *See* TEMPERATURE.

RAPTURE OF THE DEEP Synonym for INERT GAS NARCOSIS.

REBREATHER Closed-circuit or semiclosed-circuit underwater breathing apparatus.

RECOMPRESSION A second or subsequent compression.

RECOMPRESSION CHAMBER *See* CHAMBER, HYPERBARIC.

RECOVERY In diving, to retrieve an object from the deep.

REDUCER Device to regulate the pressure in a gas system.

REFRACTIVE INDEX Ratio between the sine of the angle of incidence and the sine of the angle of refraction; can be represented as the ratio of the velocity of light in air to the velocity of light in the medium (refractive index in a vacuum = 1.00).

REGULATOR, DEMAND Apparatus in which the gas supply is activated by the negative pressure associated with inspiration.

REPETITIVE DIVE   Any dive conducted within 12 hours of a previous dive.

RESIDUAL NITROGEN   Term denoting a theoretical concept that describes amount of nitrogen remaining in a diver's tissues following a hyperbaric exposure.

RESIDUAL NITROGEN TIME   Amount of time, in minutes, that must be added to the bottom time of a repetitive dive to compensate for the nitrogen still in solution in a diver's tissues from a previous dive.

RESPIRATORY ACIDOSIS   Accumulation of acid in the blood caused by a buildup of carbon dioxide.

RESPIRATORY QUOTIENT (RQ)   Ratio between the volume of carbon dioxide expired and the volume of oxygen inspired in a given time.

REVERBERATION   Reechoing or, in the case of light, reflection.

REVERSED EARS, REVERSED SQUEEZE   External ear squeeze commonly caused by obstruction in the external auditory canal caused by wax, foreign body, mechanical ear plugs, or a tight-fitting diving hood.

SAND HOG   Popular term meaning worker in a caisson or compressed air tunnel.

SAT DIVE   Slang term for SATURATION DIVE.

SATURATION   Condition in which the partial pressure of a gas dissolved in a fluid is equal to its maximum possible partial pressure under existing ambient conditions of temperature and pressure. *See also* STEADY STATE.

SATURATION DEPTH   That depth or pressure at which a diver's tissues are saturated or reach a steady state. Synonym, storage depth.

SATURATION DIVE   Dive of such a duration that no more gas can be absorbed into the tissues of the body. The tissues and the free gas in the environment are in equilibrium.

SCHEDULE, DECOMPRESSION   *See* DECOMPRESSION SCHEDULE.

SCOTOPIC VISION   Visual functioning at low or nighttime levels of illumination; performed by the rods; characterized by poor acuity and no color vision, but extreme sensitivity to light (night vision).

SCUBA   Acronym derived from Self-Contained Underwater Breathing Apparatus. Commonly used to describe apparatus in which the inspired gas is delivered by demand regulator and exhaled into the surrounding water (open-circuit) and the gas supply is carried on the diver's back. Also called *autonomous diving* by the French.

CLOSED-CIRCUIT   Self-contained underwater breathing apparatus in which the breathing gas is recirculated through purifying and oxygen-replenishing systems. Oxygen replenishment is normally controlled by admitting air to the breathing bag or controlled by oxygen sensors. No exhaled gas is lost into the surrounding water.

SEMICLOSED CIRCUIT   Self-contained underwater breathing apparatus in which the breathing gas is recirculated through purifying and oxygen-replenishing systems. Oxygen levels are maintained by regulating the flow of the gas. A portion of the exhaled gas is lost into the surrounding water.

SEALAB   Underwater habitat in the U.S. Navy manned underwater program which had Sealab I, II, and III.

SEA-LINK   Submersible built and operated by the Link Foundation.

SEARCH PATTERN, UNDERWATER   Procedure used to locate something underwater.

    ARC   Search of an area using semicircular sweeps of increasing radius; particularly useful in waters where there is strong current.

    CIRCULAR   Search of an area using concentric circles of increasing radius around a fixed point.

    JACKSTAY   Search of an area by two or more divers using a series of overlapping rectangular patterns defined by straight pre-positioned lines on the sea floor or a ship's hull (jackstay).

    "Z"   Search of an area using a single jackstay, and moving one end at a time, forming the letter "Z". This is the most thorough method, using two divers in contact with each other, but it is the slowest of the search methods.

SEATOPIA   Japanese underwater habitat used for a two-day mission in 1972 off the coast of Yokosuka. The habitat is now at the Yokosuka shipyard and will not be used again.

SEAWATER   Seawater is known to contain at least 75 of the 92 elements that occur in nature. The four most abundant elements in seawater are oxygen, hydrogen, chlorine, and sodium. Seawater always is slightly alkaline because it contains several alkaline earth minerals, principally sodium, calcium, magnesium, and potassium. The temperature of seawater varies from $-1°C$ to $30°C$. The specific gravity of seawater is affected both by salinity and temperature, and their effects are interrelated. For example, water with a high enough salt content to sink toward the bottom will remain at the surface if the water is sufficiently warm. Conversely, water with a relatively low salt content will sink if it is sufficiently chilled. Seawater also is an excellent electrical conductor, an interaction that is the source of many corrosion problems in the ocean. The viscosity of seawater varies inversely with temperature and is nearly twice as great at $1°C$ as it is at $32°C$. This property affects the speed of sailboats in cold and warm waters.

SELF-CONTAINED DIVING   *See* SCUBA.

SEMICLOSED-CIRCUIT SCUBA   *See* SCUBA.

SENSOR   Device that responds to a physical stimulus and transmits the resulting impulse; in diving, most commonly used in connection with monitoring of oxygen, pressure, or temperature.

SHALLOW WATER BLACKOUT   American usage: unconsciousness following hyperventilation and breath hold with free diving. British usage: carbon dioxide toxicity with rebreathing equipment.

SIGNAL   Coded communication other than voice. Signals commonly used in diving are flags, line pulls, hammer taps, and hand signals.

SIGNATURE   Any characteristic pattern by which an object can be detected or identified; in diving, usually used to define the acoustic or magnetic characteristics of an object.

SINGLE DIVE   Any dive conducted 12 hours or more after any previous dive.

SINGLE-LOCK CHAMBER   *See* CHAMBER.

SINGLE REPETITIVE DIVE   Dive for which the bottom time used to select the decompression schedule is the sum of the residual nitrogen time and the actual bottom time of the dive.

SINUS SQUEEZE OR BAROTRAUMA   *See* SQUEEZE.

SKIN DIVING   *See* DIVE, BREATH-HOLD.

SLATE, DIVER'S   Piece of equipment used for writing messages or recording data underwater.

SLOW TISSUES   In considering tissue saturation with gas (nitrogen) while under pressure, those tissues that half-saturate slowly (tendon, 75 min), compared with those tissues that half-saturate fast (blood, 5 min).

SNORKEL   Tube held in the mouth with the open end above the surface of the water, allowing the swimmer or diver to breathe comfortably without turning the head.

SODA LIME   Active chemical ingredient in a carbon dioxide scrubbing system in a closed life-support system, or in a diver-carried rebreather.

SODASORB   Trade name for soda lime.

SONAR   Acronym derived from the expression Sound Navigation And Ranging; the method or equipment for determining by underwater sound techniques the presence, location, or nature of objects in the sea.

SOUND VELOCITY   Rate of travel at which sound energy moves through a medium, usually expresed in feet per second. The velocity of sound in seawater is a function of temperature, salinity, and the changes in pressure associated with changes in depth. An increase in any of these factors tends to increase the velocity. Temperature has the greatest influence, with pressure and salinity exercising less influence. At 70°F and normal salinity of 34 parts per thousand by weight, the sound velocity is 4935 feet per second at the ocean surface (speed of sound in air is 1090 ft/sec).

SPATIAL ORIENTATION   A person's ability to remain unconfused by the various alignments of objects or patterns with respect to the person.

SPECIFIC GRAVITY   Ratio of the density of a substance to the density of fresh water at 4°C. Fresh water has a specific gravity of 1.0; substances heavier than fresh water have specific gravities greater than 1.0, and substances lighter than fresh water have specific gravities less than 1.0. The human body has a specific gravity of approximately 1.0, which varies slightly from one person to another.

SPECTRUM   Band of radiant energy that can be projected after being passed through a prism.

SPEECH DISTORTION   So-called DONALD DUCK EFFECT, usually associated with breathing helium under pressure.

SPINAL CORD HIT   Type II decompression sickness involving the spinal cord; often associated with paralysis.

SPIROKINESIS   Proposition that all animals have a fundamental circling mechanism.

SPITCOCK   Auxilary exhaust valve in a diving helmet.

SPONTANEOUS PNEUMOTHORAX   Pneumothorax occurring without apparent cause.

SQUEEZE   Deformation of tissue or some portion of the body due to a difference in pressure.

DRY SUIT   Squeeze consisting of pinching of the skin in the folds of a dry suit, caused by insufficient pressure inside the suit during descent.

EXTERNAL EAR (*also* REVERSED EAR)   Squeeze caused by sealing of the space between the external ear and the eardrum during decompression. Can be caused by tightly fitting hood, bathing cap, or ear plugs.

EYE   Squeeze of the eyes caused by using goggles not compensated for pressure.

FACE   Squeeze of the face caused by failure to compensate for increased ambient pressure.

MIDDLE EAR   Squeeze caused by inability to equalize the pressure in the middle ear through the eustachian tube as the exernal pressure builds up against the eardrum.

SINUS   Squeeze caused by blockage of the opening between one of the sinuses and the nose; may be due to a common cold or sinusitis.

WHOLE-BODY   Squeeze caused by excessive external pressure when the diver is wearing a variable-volume dry suit with a rigid helmet. The two most common causes are falling through the water at a rapid rate and failure of the non-return valve in the helmet exhaust system when hose connection is broken at or near the surface.

STAGGERS   Early descriptive term to describe forms of decompression sickness that affect the inner ear or the central nervous system; associated with vestibular decompression sickness.

STANDARD SUIT   *See* SUITS, DIVING.

STANDBY DIVER   A suited or partially suited diver ready to assist the working diver should an emergency arise.

STATOMETER   Instrument for measuring standing steadiness.

STEADY STATE   Situation in which the net result of completed processes is zero. In diving, used to describe the condition in which there is no net gain or loss of gas molecules into or from the tissues, although gas molecules are constantly being exchanged with the environment.

STEINKE HOOD   Device filled with air and worn over the head for underwater submarine escape.

STOP, DECOMPRESSION   *See* DECOMPRESSION STOP.

STPD   Indication that a volume has been corrected to standard conditions of temperature (0°C), pressure (760 mmHg), and dry gas. This correction is universally used for O_2 consumption ($\dot{V}_{O_2}$) and CO_2 production ($\dot{V}_{CO_2}$).

SUBCLINICAL BUBBLES   *See* BUBBLES.

SUBMARINE   Propelled underwater vehicle used primarily for military missions, which can operate autonomously for a long period of time.

SUBMERSIBLE   Manned vehicle or ship for underwater operation.

CABLE-CONTROLLED   Unmanned submersible with the ability to move under the remote control of a surface operator and the ability to carry out specific tasks via manipulators. In additiion may carry observational and sensing equipment such as echo-sounders, magnetometers, sonar, and cameras. Generally of open-frame design and operate at low speeds. Not suitable for surveying extensive areas of the ocean bottom.

CABLELESS   Unmanned submersible designed for oceanographic data collection or bottom observation along a preprogrammed course.

DRY   Submersible in which the occupants are maintained in a dry environment at near-atmospheric conditions.

LOCK-OUT   Submersible that has a compartment maintained at one-atmosphere pressure for the pilot or observer, and a compartment that can be pressurized to ambient pressure so that the diver can enter and exit or lock out to perform underwater work.

SELF-PROPELLED   A submersible operating under its own power.

WET   A free-flooding submersible in which the occupants are exposed to the ambient environment.

SUBMERSIBLE DECOMPRESSION CHAMBER (SDC)   *See* CHAMBER.

SUITS, DIVING   Specialized protective clothing used by divers underwater.

- CLOSED-CIRCUIT HOT WATER   Dry suit and a special set of underwear through which heated water is circulated. The water is pumped from a heater, through a series of loops in the underwear, and back to the heat source. The heater may be carried by the diver or may be on the surface.

- CONSTANT-VOLUME DRY   Dry suit designed to be partially inflated to prevent squeeze and to provide insulation against cold.

- DEEP-SEA DIVING   Dry diving suit with helmet, weights, boots, and umbilical. Synonyms: hard-hat, heavy gear, deep-sea dress, Mark V (USN).

- DRY   Diving suit designed to exclude water from the surface of the body.

- HOT WATER OPEN-CIRCUIT   Wet suit modified by a system of tubes integrated into the suit, designed to allow hot water to be distributed evenly over the body. After use, the hot water is dumped into the surrounding environment.

- STANDARD   British usage for DEEP-SEA DIVING SUIT.

- VARIABLE-VOLUME DRY   Dry suit with both an inlet gas valve and an exhaust valve, so that together with the weighted belt the diver can maintain buoyancy control.

- WET   Closed-cell, synthetic rubber diving suit that provides a thermal barrier by trapping a thin layer of body-warmed water next to the diver's skin. May include boots, gloves, hood, or vest.

SUPERSATURATION   Theoretical term used in diving to mean the state in which the tension of a dissolved gas is greater than its inspired partial pressure, contrary to HENRY'S LAW; popularized by J.S. Haldane.

SUR-D TABLES   *See* SURFACE DECOMPRESSION.

SURFACE DECOMPRESSION   Procedure in which a portion of the in-water decompression is omitted and the diver is brought to the surface and recompressed in a chamber to complete the decompression; sometimes confused with DECANTING, a term that should be restricted to caisson workers.

SURFACE HABITAT   *See* CHAMBER, DECK DECOMPRESSION.

SURFACE INTERVAL   Elapsed time between surfacing from the dive and the time when the diver leaves the surface on the next dive.

SURFACE-SUPPLIED DIVING   Form of diving in which the breathing gas is supplied from a compressor or from cylinders on the surfce.

SURFACE-SUPPORTED DIVING   *See* ATTENDED DIVING.

SWIM FINS   Devices worn on the feet of the diver or swimmer to increase the propulsive force of the legs.

SWIMMER DELIVERY VEHICLE (SDV)   Type of wet submersible used for underwater transport of divers.

SWIMMER'S EAR   Otitis externa due to exposure to water.

SWIMMER VEHICLE   Any one of a number of devices used to aid the swimmer in attaining swim speeds greater than could be accomplished by using fins.

TARAVANA   Decompression sickness resulting from a series of breath-hold dives. Name used by the natives of Tuamotu Island.

TEKTITE   Underwater habitat used for two Department of Interior programs in the U.S. Virgin Islands: TEKTITE I—1969; TEKTITE II—1970.

TELEMETRY   Technique of measuring a variety of quantities in place, transmitting the value to a station and there interpreting, indicating, or recording the quantities. Transmission may be electrical, electromagnetic, or sonic.

TEMPERATURE   Degree of hotness or coldness measured on a definite scale. May be measured in degrees Celsius, centigrade, Fahrenheit, and Rankine, and in Kelvin.

CELSIUS (°C)   Named after a Swedish astronomer who invented the centigrade scale. At present the centigrade scale described below is properly called the Celsius scale.

CENTIGRADE (°C)   Thermometric scale on which the interval between the freezing point and the boiling point of water is divided into 100 degrees, 0° representing the freezing point and 100° the boiling point. Temperatures measured in centigrade may be converted into Fahrenheit by using the formula °F = (1.8 × °C) + 32.

FAHRENHEIT (°F)   Thermometric scale named after its inventor, a Dutch instrument maker, and based on the coldest temperature attainable with a mixture of water, snow, and salt, which was designated as zero. On this scale at sea level pure water freezes at 32° above zero and boils at 212° above zero. Fahrenheit may be converted to centigrade as follows: °C = (°F − 32)/1.8.

KELVIN (K)   Thermometric scale named after its inventor, Baron Kelvin (William Thomson), a British scientist. The complete absence of heat (i.e., where molecular or atomic movement ceases completely) is designated as absolute zero and is equivalent to −273.16°C. Utilizing degree units equivalent to centigrade units, the freezing and boiling points of pure water are 273.16 K and 373.16 K, respectively.

RANKINE (°R)   A thermometric scale named after its inventor, a British engineer and scientist; wherein the complete absence of heat (i.e., where molecular or atomic movement ceases completely) is designated as absolute zero and is equivalent to −459.69°F. Utilizing degree units equivalent to Fahrenheit units, the freezing and boiling points of pure water are 491.69°R and 671.69°R, respectively.

TENDER   The individual responsible for seeing that the diver receives care both while topside and underwater. Synonym, attendant; *also*, a diving support vessel (British usage).

TETHERED DIVING   *See* ATTENDED DIVING.

THERMAL BALANCE   State characterized by stable body temperature, in which heat gain equals heat loss.

THERMAL STRESS   Condition in which the body attempts to maintain normal temperature when the surrounding temperature is either higher or lower than that of the body.

THERMOCOUPLE   A pair of dissimilar electrical conductors so joined that an electromotive force is developed by the thermoelectric effects when the junctions are at different temperatures.

THERMOGENESIS   Production of heat, especially in the animal body.

TIDAL VOLUME   Amount of gas inspired and expired during each respiration cycle, measured by averaging over several breaths.

TISSUE HALF TIME   *See* HALF TIME.

TORR   Unit of pressure equal to 1/760 of an atmosphere and very nearly equal to the pressure of a column of mercury one millimeter high at 0°C and standard gravity.

TOTAL BOTTOM TIME   Total elapsed time starting when the diver leaves the surface to the time (next whole minute) that ascent begins (in minutes).

TOYNBEE   Maneuver to equalize the pressure in the middle ear with the ambient pressure against the outer surface of the eardrum. In this maneuver the nose is compressed shut, the mouth is closed, the glottis is closed, and the action is to swallow, which reduces the pressure and often opens the eustachian tube, allowing equalization; this is an easy and safe maneuver.

TRANSDUCER   Any device for converting energy from one form to another (electrical, mechanical, or acoustical).

TREATMENT DEPTH   Depth (or pressure) to which a patient is compressed for treatment.

TREATMENT MIX (GAS)   The breathing gas mixture used in the treatment of decompression sickness.

TREATMENT TABLE   A collection of decompression schedules used to treat decompression sickness or air embolism.

TRIMIX   A gas mixture involving three breathing gases, usually oxygen, helium, and nitrogen.

TROUGH   The low point of a wave in any given cycle.

TYPE I DECOMPRESSION SICKNESS (DCS)   *See* DECOMPRESSION SICKNESS.

TYPE II SICKNESS (DCS)   *See* DECOMPRESSION SICKNESS.

ULTRASONIC   Higher than audible frequency range (i.e., above 20,000 Hz).

ULTRASOUND DETECTOR   Device using high-frequency sound waves; used in diving to detect bubbles in the diver's body.

UMBILICAL   Composite of hoses and lines supplying life support to the diver.

UNITS OF PRESSURE MEASUREMENT   *See* Conversion Table, Appendix C.

UPTD   Unit Pulmonary Toxicity Dose, unit of measure devised by the Institute for Environmental Medicine at the University of Pennsylvania, and used for calculating the total oxygen exposure incurred during all phases of a dive, including decompression.

VALSALVA MANEUVER   Maneuver to equalize the pressure in the middle ear with the ambient pressure against the outer surface of the eardrum. In this maneuver the nose is compressed shut, the mouth is shut, the glottis is open, and an attempt is made to exhale through the nose, resulting in forcing air through the eustachian tube into the middle ear, but also causing increased pulmonary pressure, which has been known to cause rupture of the lung tissues.

VALVE, NON-RETURN   Valve that prevents reverse flow through the gas supply umbilical.

VARIABLE-VOLUME DRY SUIT   *See* SUITS, DIVING.

VENTILATORY CAPACITY (WORK LIMITS)   A function of maximum breathing capacity, timed vital capacity, and maximum expiratory flow rate, all of which are maximum-effort dynamic ventilatory measures and all reflect the work limits of the anatomical respiratory apparatus.

VESSEL   Hollow structure designed for carrying or transporting something on or under water.

VESTIBULAR BENDS/HIT/DECOMPRESSION SICKNESS   Decompression sickness involving the inner ear, often associated with vertigo. *See also* DECOMPRESSION SICKNESS.

VESTIBULAR KINESTHESIS   Sensitivity to movement of the skull.

VESTIBULAR SYSTEM   General term used to describe the whole neural mechanism involved in receiving the sensory data from the static sense, and providing for the making of the necessary responses for the adjustment of the equilibrium of the organism with reference to gravity or other forces affecting it.

VIEWPORT   Observation window of a bell, submersible, chamber, or habitat.

VISCOSITY   Property of a fluid or gas that resists change in the shape or arrangement of its elements during flow.

VITAL CAPACITY (VC)   Maximum volume of gas that can be exhaled from the lungs following a maximum inspiration. It is the sum of expiratory reserve volume, inspiratory reserve volume, and tidal volume (about 4600 ml).

WATER BREATHING   *See* LIQUID BREATHING.

WATER EFFECT   Term coined by H. Bowen to describe the cause of reduced human performance upon immersion in water.

WATER PRESSURE   *See* PRESSURE, HYDROSTATIC.

WAVELENGTH   Ratio of speed to frequency.

WEIGHT BELT   *See* BELT.

WET POT   One chamber of a hyperbaric facility capable of being filled with water and pressurized to simulate a given underwater depth.

WORK OF BREATHING   Amount of work the diver must exert to breathe through his equipment. The work of breathing depends on depth, type of equipment and gas mixture, and condition of the lungs. *See also* BREATHING RESISTANCE.

"Z" SEARCH   *See* SEARCH PATTERN, UNDERWATER.

B

Abbreviations and Acronyms

These commonly used abbreviations and acronyms often appear in the diving literature without identification. The list, which is by no means complete, includes abbreviations of technological and biomedical terms and of some of the national laboratories active in underwater research and technology. We have not attempted to include acronyms for specific research experiments, such as FLAR, SCORE, FAMOUS, PRUNE, and SHAD because we feared that such a list would be incomplete, and would in any case soon be obsolete.

ABLJ	**a**djustable **b**uoyancy **l**ife **j**acket (British)
ADS	**a**dvanced **d**iving **s**ystem or **a**tmospheric **d**iving **s**ystem
AEDU	**A**dmiralty **E**xperimental **D**iving **U**nit (UK)
AMTE	**A**miralty **M**arine **T**echnology **E**stablishment (UK)
AMTE (PL)	**A**dmiralty **M**arine **T**echnology **E**stablishment (**P**hysiological **L**aboratory) (UK) (formerly RNPL)
ANSI	**A**merican **N**ational **S**tandards **I**nstitute
ARMS	**a**tmospheric **r**oving or **r**emote **m**anipulator **s**ystem
ASME	**A**merican **S**ociety of **M**echanical **E**ngineers
ATA	**at**mosphere **a**bsolute
atm abs	**atm**osphere **abs**olute
ATP	**a**mbient **t**emperature and **p**ressure
BC	**b**uoyancy **c**ompensator
BIBS	**b**uilt-**i**n **b**reathing **s**ystem
BTV	**b**éance **t**ubaire **v**olontaire (France)
CDBA	**c**learance **d**iver's **b**reathing **a**pparatus (UK)
CERB	**C**entre d'**E**tudes et de **R**echerche **B**iophysiologiques Appliquees a'la Marine (France)
CFFF	**c**ritical **f**licker **f**usion **f**requency
CNS	**c**entral **n**ervous **s**ystem
COMEX	**Com**pagnie Maritime d'**Ex**pertises (French diving company)
CPAP	**c**ontinuous **p**ositive **a**irway **p**ressure
cps	**c**ycles **p**er second

CPTD	cumulative pulmonary toxicity dose
CURV	Cable-Operated Unmanned Recovery Vehicle (US)
DAWS	diver alternative work system
DCIEM	Defence and Civil Institute of Environmental Medicine (Canada)
DCS	decompression sickness
DDC	deck decompression chamber
DDS	deep diving system
DICORS	Diver Communication Research System
DSEA	Davis submarine escape apparatus
DSRV	deep submergence rescue vehicle
ΔP	pressure difference, or change in pressure
EAD	equivalent air depth
ECG (EKG)	electrocardiogram
ED_{50}	median effective dose
EDU	Experimental Diving Unit (US) *(see also* NEDU)
EEG	electroencephalogram
EMG	electromyogram
ENG	electronystagmogram
EOD	explosive ordnance disposal
fsw	feet of seawater
GERS	Groupe d'Etudes et de Recherches Sous la Mer (France)
GISMER	Groupe d'Intervention Sous la Mer (France)
HBO	hyperbaric oxygen/oxygenation (see also OHP, HPO)
HPNS	high pressure nervous syndrome
HPO	high pressure oxygen *(see also* HBO, OHP)
INM	Institute of Naval Medicine
IRV	inspiratory reserve volume
JAMSTEC	Japan Marine Science and Technology Center
LD_{50}	median lethal dose
MAST	medical antishock trousers
MDB	mobile diving barge
msw	meters of seawater
NCEL	Naval Civil Engineering Laboratory (US)
NCSL	Naval Coastal Systems Laboratory (US)
NEDU	Navy Experimental Diving Unit (US) *(see also* EDU)
NIOSH	National Institute of Occupational Safety and Health
NMRI	Naval Medical Research Institute (US)
NOAA	National Oceanic and Atmospheric Administration
NSMRL	Naval Submarine Medical Research Laboratory (US)
NUI	Norwegian Underwater Institute (now called NUTEC)
NUTEC	Norwegian Underwater Technical Institute
OHP	oxygen at high pressure *(see also* HBO, HPO)
ONR	Office of Naval Research
OSHA	Occupational Safety and Health Administration
PEEP	positive end expiratory pressure
psi	pounds per square inch

PTC	**p**ersonnel **t**ransfer **c**apsule
PVHO	**p**ressure **v**essel for **h**uman **o**ccupancy
RCV	**r**emotely **c**ontrolled **v**ehicle
RNPL	**R**oyal **N**aval **P**hysiological **L**aboratory (UK) (now AMTE (PL))
RQ	**r**espiratory **q**uotient
RUWS	**r**emote **u**nmanned **w**ork **s**ystem
SABA	**s**wimmer's **a**ir **b**reathing **a**pparatus (UK)
SCAL	**s**kin diver **c**ontact **a**ir **l**enses
SCUBA	**s**elf-**c**ontained **u**nderwater **b**reathing **a**pparatus
SDC	**s**ubmersible **d**ecompression **c**hamber
SDDE	**s**urface **d**emand **d**iving **e**quipment
SDV	**s**wimmer **d**elivery **v**ehicle
SEAL	**s**ea **a**ir **l**and (assault force) (US)
SET	**s**ingle-man **e**scape **t**ower
SLSS	**s**wimmer's **l**ife **s**upport **s**ystem
SPAR	**s**ubmersible **p**ipe **a**lignment **r**ig
SPCC	**s**trength, **p**ower, and **c**ommunication **c**able
SPL	**s**ound **p**ressure **l**evel; the intensity of a sound usually expressed in decibels
SSBA	**S**urface **S**upplied **B**reathing **A**pparatus
STPD	**s**tandard **t**emperature, **p**ressure **d**ry gas
UBA	**u**nderwater **b**reathing **a**pparatus
UDT	**u**nderwater **d**emolition **t**eam (US)
UPTD	**u**nit **p**ulmonary **t**oxicity **d**ose
UWH	**u**nderwater **w**elding **h**abitat
VC	**v**ital **c**apacity

C

Pressure Conversion Table

Given unit	Standard abbreviation	Pa	b	atm	at	psi	torr
Pascal	Pa	1	1×10^5	9.8692×10^{-6}	1.0197×10^{-5}	1.4504×10^{-4}	7.5006×10^{-3}
Bar	b	1×10^5	1	9.8692×10^{-1}	1.0197×1	1.4504×10	7.5006×10^2
Standard physical atmosphere	atm	1.0133×10^5	1.0133×1	1	1.0332×1	1.4696×10	7.6×10^2
Technical atmosphere	at	9.8067×10^4	9.8067×10^{-1}	9.6784×10^{-1}	1	1.4223×10	7.3556×10^2
Pounds/square inch	psi	6.8948×10^3	6.8948×10^{-2}	6.8046×10^{-2}	7.0307×10^{-2}	1	5.1715×10^1
Torricelli	torr	1.3332×10^2	1.3332×10^{-3}	1.3158×10^{-3}	1.3595×10^{-3}	1.9337×10^{-2}	1

Since the pressure exerted by a column of water depends on the specific gravity of the water, which varies with temperature and locality, depth equivalents should state the specific gravity (sp gr) used, e.g., 3 meters (sp gr seawater = 1.025). The preferred value is sp gr = 1.01972, which gives the equivalence 10 meters = 1 bar. The relationship is pressure exerted by 1 meter seawater (bars) = specific gravity × 9.80665×10^{-2}. Other pressure units equivalent to one standard atmosphere are:

1 atm = 1.0332 kg/cm³
 = 760 mmHg (sp gr 13.6 g/cm³)
 = 1033 cmH₂O (sp gr 1.0 g/cm³)
 = 33.07 feet of seawater (sp gr 1.025 g/cm³)
 = 10.08 meters of seawater (sp gr 1.025 g/cm³)

Author Index

Anthonisen, N. R., 71

Bachrach, A. J., 531
Bayne, C. G., 144
Behnke, A. R., Jr., 128
Bennett, P. B., 109
Bergman, W. R., 645
Biersner, R. J., 520
Bradley, M. E., 190

Edmonds, C., 406
Evans, D. E., 99

Faiman, M. D., 35
Farmer, J. C., Jr., 192, 312, 409
Fife, W. P., 136

Ginsburg, H. M., 445
Goad, R. F., 283

Hallenbeck, J. M., 316
Hamilton, R. W., 12, 328, 391, 654
Hart, G. B., 621
Hempleman, H. V., 223

Hickey, D. D., 206
Hong, S. K., 153, 178

Kindwall, E. P., 273
Kinney, J. A. S., 199
Kizer, K. W., 441

Leitch, D. R., 316
Linaweaver, P. G., Jr., 489
Lundgren, C. E. G., 86, 206

Nicodemus, H. F., 460

Påsche, A., 86
Pearson, R. R., 333
Peterson, D. H., 625

Sheffield, P. J., 601
Shilling, C. W., 1, 6, 35, 406, 421, 567
Sims, J. K., 427
Stahl, C. J., 661

Tabeling, B. B., 369

Walder, D. N., 397
Walsh, J. M., 445

Subject Index

Absolute pressure, 36
Accident, diving
  authority for investigation, 664–666
  autopsy, 666–677
  causes, 568
  chamber, 613–621
  check list, 678–681
  contributing factors, 663–664
  determining cause, 280
  investigation, 661–681
  reporting, 661–662
  stress and panic, 546–553
Acclimatization
  breath-hold diving, 216–217
  cold, 168
  tunnel workers, 255–256
Acidosis, drowning, 372
Acuity, visual, underwater, 199
Adaptability, women diving, 136
Adipose tissue, women divers, 137
Aerodontalgia, 68
Aeroembolism: *see* Decompression sickness
Age
  for diving, 570
  physical examination diving, 494
  psychological prediction, 521
Air
  breathing gas, 38
  diving, 2, 38, 645–657
  pollution, 582–583
Air embolism
  emergency diving casualty, 73, 273
  signs and symptoms, 276
  treatment, 276–277
  see also Embolism
Airway protection in anesthesia, 461
Alcohol
  and diving, 571
  and heat loss, 167
  and HPNS, 188

Alimentary system, diving physical examination, 503–504
Alternobaric vertigo, 197
Altitude and diving, 589–590
Alveolar pressure, 73–76, 333–336
Ama
  diving women, 136
  energy metabolism, 181
  heat loss immersion, 157–159
Ambient pressure, 36
Ametropia underwater, 201
Anesthesia
  anesthetic and other drugs, 479–481
  course of action, 483–485
  general, 475–476
  inhalation agents, 476
  intravenous, 476–483
  regional, 466–475
  under pressure, 460–485
Antibiotic therapy, 455
Argon narcosis, 130
Arterial gas embolism, 336–344
  causes, 349–350
  diagnosis, 352–354
  signs and symptoms, 350–352
  therapy, 354–361
  types, 350
Arthralgia
  hyperbaric, 190–192
  osmotic fluid shifts, 191
Aseptic bone necrosis: *see* Dysbaric osteonecrosis
Aspiration and drowning, 372–373
Aspirin in decompression sickness therapy, 279–280
Atelectasis, 273
Atmospheric diving systems
  anthropomorphic diving suits, 21
  observation bells, 21
  submersibles, 21
Atmospheric pressure, 36

726 Subject Index

Audiovestibular symptoms, decompression
    sickness, 290-291
Auditory function, pressure effects, 193-195
Aural barotrauma, 60-61
    see also Otologic barotrauma; Barotrauma
Aviation decompression sickness, 607-608

Barotrauma
    aural, 60-61
    blowup, 61
    breath-hold diving, 218
    cause of pulmonary, 334-336
    emergency evaluation, 273
    gastrointestinal, 66
    otologic barotrauma, 192-193, 409-416
    paranasal sinus, 418-420
    pulmonary, 66-67, 333-349
    sinus, 67, 418-420
    squeeze, 67-68
    toothache, 68
    vertigo, 68
Basal metabolic rate (BMR), 182
Behavior underwater, 531-565
Bell
    diving system, 16-20
    equipment
        life support, 16-20
        safety, 16-20
    first bell, 223-224
    open diving, 650
Bends: see Decompression sickness
Bert, Paul
    decompression sickness early work, 226, 285
BIBS: see Built-In Breathing System
Blast
    clinical aspects, 423-425
    definition, 421
    physical aspects, 422-423
    prevention, 425-426, 592
    treatment, 425
Blood
    changes in diving, 257
    volume in drowning, 374
Blood volume in drowning, 374
Blowup, 61
Bounce diving, 4
Boyle, Robert
    bubble in viper's eye, 223
    decompression sickness, 223, 283
Boyle's Law, 49-51
Bradycardia
    autonomic nervous system, 105-106
    breath-hold diving, 206-220
    gas density, 101-102
    helium and nitrogen, 104-105
    hydrostatic pressure, 102-104

Bradycardia (cont.)
    hyperbaric pressure, 100
    oxygen partial pressure, 100-101
    saturation exposures, 106
    see also Cardiovascular; Circulatory function
Brain, drowning, resuscitation, 376-377, 383
Breath-hold diving, 2-3, 72-73, 157, 206-220
    breaking point, 207-214
    depth limits, 214-216
    mammalian dive reflex, 206-207
    medical considerations, 217-220
        barotrauma, 218
        cardiological, 217
        decompression sickness, 219
        drowning, 217
        vertigo, 219
    physiology, 206-217
Breathing: see Respiration and respiratory
Bubble
    detection, 149
    and embolism, 336-339
    formation, 258-264
    migration, 337-339
    silent, 258-283
    viper's eye, 223
Built-in Breathing System (BIBS), 14
Buoyancy
    control equipment, 638-640
    immersion effects, 56-57, 97-98
Burst lung: see Pulmonary overinflation

Caisson, 12-14, 238
    contribution to diving, 602-603
    decompression, 286
    first use, 284
    St. Louis Bridge, 13, 226, 284, 602
Caisson disease: see Decompression sickness
Caloric value, 178-179
Calorimeter, energy output, 179-180
Calorimetry, heat loss measurement, 158-159
Carbon dioxide
    in breath hold, 207-214
    control of breathing, 44-45
    control of ventilation, 81-84
    description, 43-44
    in diving, 46
    effects, narcosis, 132
    food energy, 178-179
    human production, 44
    in narcosis, 132
    of pathophysiology, 45-46
    purging, 15
    retention, 45-46, 81-84
    transport, 45
    ventilation control, 81-84

Carbon monoxide
  description, 47
  in diving, 47–48
  pathophysiology, 48–49
  poisoning, treatment of, 49
  therapy, 49
  toxicity, 48–49
Cardiac
  breath-hold diving, 217
  function, 91–94
  monitoring, 146
  output (CO), 91
  see also Cardiovascular
Cardiovascular
  decompression sickness symptoms, 291
  diving physical, 502–503
  drowning response, 375
  drugs, 452
  hyperbaric exposure effects, 99–107
  monitors, 146–147
  saturation exposure, 106
  stress effects, 544–546
  see also Bradycardia; Circulatory function
Case histories
  chamber accidents, 610–619
  CNS hit, 3–4
  Dr. Jaminet, St. Louis Bridge, 284–285
  mixing equipment failure, 37
  near-drowning, 385–387
  pressure equalization, 37
  tank corrosion, 37
Casualty
  diving
    medical evaluation, 273–280
Cave diving, 8, 551–552
Central nervous system
  damage in drowning, 376–377
  drugs acting on, 449–451
  type decompression sickness, 290
Cerebral
  blood flow, 341
  gas embolism, 340–344
Chamber
  accidents, 613–621
  monoplace, 26, 621–625
  multiplace, 26, 601–621
  operators, 610
  safety codes, 609–610
Charles' law, 51
Chest wall in diving, 71–72
Chokes, decompression sickness, 291, 317
Choking, unconscious diver, 393
Cholera, polluted water, 408
Cigarettes, 571–572
  carbon monoxide toxicity, 48
Ciguatera poisoning, 435–436

Circulatory function
  immersion, 91–94
  see also Bradycardia; Cardiovascular
Closing volume, lung, 87
Cold water
  acclimatization, 168
  adaptation, 181–182
  and alcohol, 167
  diving, 10, 156–162, 370
  drowning, 370
  immersion, 157–158, 165–167
  and marijuana, 168
  metabolic adaptation, 181
  stress factor, 538–544
  wet suit protection, 159–162
Color vision underwater, 203
Comfort zone, 156
Communication, voice, 146, 651
Compressed air illness: see Decompression sickness
Compression
  effects, 128
  phase of diving, 225
  see also HPNS
Compressor, air, 24
Conduction, heat, 59
Contact lenses, underwater, 201
Contamination, breathing gas, 273, 582
Contraceptives
  and diving
    intrauterine, 138
    oral, 138
Convection, heat transfer, 60, 154, 155
Coral trauma, marine infections, 429–430
Cutaneous, symptoms decompression sickness, 288–289
Cylinders
  gas, 23–24
  scuba diving, 630–632

Dalton's Law, 52–54
Damant, decompression procedures, 233
DAN: see Divers Alert Network
Deck decompression chamber (DDC), 14–15
  purging or ventilation, 32
Decompression
  abbreviations, definitions, 234
  dive, 2
  physiological factors, 225–228
  stop, 2
  surface, 15
  table development, 296–301
  theory, 223–272
  time calculation, 234–236
  working hypothesis, 235–237
  see also Decompression sickness

Decompression sickness
  audiovestibular symptoms, 290–291
  breath-hold divers, 219
  central nervous system type, 290, 316–326
  cutaneous symptoms, 288–289
  decompression theory, 223–272
  definition, 283
  diagnosis, 287–295
  drugs, 279–280
  emergency evaluation, 273
  emergency therapy, 277–280
  history, 283–287
  inner ear, 312–316
  lymphatic symptoms, 288–289
  musculoskeletal symptoms, 289–290
  neurological forms, 290, 316–326
  peripheral nervous system, 290
  return to work after, 328–331
  signs and symptoms, 277–278, 287–291, 318–320
  spinal cord, 317
  therapy
    denitrogenation, 278
    drugs, 279–280
    hydration, 278–279
    recompression, 286–287
  treatment tables, 296–303
  tunnel workers, 13
  women divers, 137–139
Denitrogenation, decompression sickness therapy, 278
Density of gas, 55
Dermatitis, schistosome cercarial, 430
Design pressure, 36
Diet
  and diving, 178–188, 572
  saturation diving, 187–188
Diffusion, gas, 54–55
  decompression theory, 248–254
Disorientation, 219
Diuresis, effect of immersion, 94–95
Dive, diver, diving
  accident investigation, 661–684
  accidents, panic, 546–553
  acclimatization, breath-hold, 216–217
  age, 570
  air, 2, 38, 645–657
  air embolism, 73, 273, 336–344
  and alcohol, 571
  altitude, 589–590
  ama, 136, 142, 181
  argon narcosis, 130
  atmospheric systems, 21
  bell, 650
    first, 223–224
  blast, 421–426
  blowup, 61, 63

Dive, diver, diving (cont.)
  bounce, 4, 665
  bradycardia, 100–106
  breath-hold, 3–4, 72–73, 157, 206–221
  cardiovascular effects, 99–127
  casualty evaluation, 273–280
  cave, 8, 551
  circulatory effects, 91–94
  cold water, 10, 156–162, 370
  commercial physical examination, 515–516
  decompression, 2, 15, 223–272
  delay return after DCS, 328–331
  diet, 178–188, 572
  disorientation, 219
  Divers Alert Network, 274, 307
  dizziness, 196–197
  drowning hazard, 593
  emergency care, 273–280
  emotional stability, 576–577
  and energy, 57–60, 178–186
  environment, 1–6, 568
  equipment, 584, 601–660
  excursion, 6, 657–660
  and eye, 199–204
  fatigue, 572–575
  effect on fetus, 140–143
  fins, 637–638
  flying after, 590–591
  fouling hazards, 582
  gas cylinders, tanks, 23–24, 630–632
  gastrointestinal, 66, 95–97, 424
  Greek sponge, 284
  habitat, 30–31, 660
  harbor, 7–8
  hazards, 568
  heat, 58–60
  heliox, 264
  helium, 78
  high pressure nervous syndrome, 109–126
  hot water garment, 649
  hydrogen, 43
  ice, 10–11, 596–597
  infection, 406, 577
  kelp, 8–9
  lake, 7
  laws, gas, 47–54
  mammals, 73, 206–207
  masks, 636, 646
  medics (diving), 274
  menstruation, 138–139
  metabolism, 181–186
  microbes, 406
  mixed gas, 2, 651–654
  nitrogen, 42
  no-decompression (no-D), 2
  obesity, 572

Dive, diver, diving (*cont.*)
ocean, 6–7
oral contraceptives, 138
organization and planning, 578
panic, 553–560
pathophysiology, 37–47
performance, women, 136
personnel transfer capsule, 19
physical examination, 489–518
physical fitness, 506–507, 575–576
physical standards, 490–492
physics, 35–68
physiology, 71–221
polluted water, 9, 405–408, 582–583
and pregnancy, 140–143, 309–310
protective clothing, 640–643, 647–649
psychologic standards, 520–529
pulmonary effects, 71–85
radiation hazard, 587
recompression, 26, 583, 601–625
reflex, 206–207, 370
regulators, 633–636
renal effects, 94–95
rescue chambers, 28–30
respiration, 71–84
return to after DCS, 328–331
river, 7
safety, 567–600
saturation, 4–6, 20–21, 106, 266, 654–660
scuba, 3–4, 607, 625–644
selection, 520–569
signals, 584–588
sonar hazard, 581
sound, 58
squeeze, 67–68, 72
stress, 553–560
submersibles, 595–596
surface decompression, 15, 244
surface supplied, 4, 645–660
system, 16–26
table calculation, 242–248
tanks, 630–633
thermal protection, 9–11, 18, 159–162
training, 570
transfer capsule, 19
tube skid, 23
types, 1–6
under ice, 10–11
U.S. Navy tables, 242–248
ventilatory response, 80–84
vertigo, 68, 196–198
vestibular function, 68, 195–198
vital signs, monitoring, 149–152
weight loss, 183–184
welding chamber, 30–32
wet pot, 27

Dive, diver, diving (*cont.*)
wet suit, 9–11, 159–162, 640–642, 647–648
women, 136–139
wreck, 9–10
Diver's palsy: *see* Decompression sickness
Diving Accident Network: *see* Divers Alert Network
Divers Alert Network (DAN), 274, 307
Diving medic, 274
Diving reflex, 206–207, 370
Dizzy diver, 196–197
Doppler monitoring, 144, 149–152
Drowning
acidosis, 372
aspiration, 372, 373
blood volume, 374
breath-hold diving, 217
cardiovascular system, 375
case histories, 385–387
central nervous system, 376–377
definition, 369
diving hazard, 593
diving reflex, 370
electrolyte changes, 374
fresh water, 373
hematology, 376
history, 370–371
hypoxemia, 372
hypoxia, 372–373
infection, polluted water, 408
lung pathology, 373–374
physiological changes, 372–378
renal function, 376
resuscitation, 378
salt water, 373
unconscious diver, 393
water temperature, 370
Drowning therapy
brain resuscitation, 383
drugs
antibiotics, 383–384
corticosteroids, 383–384
emergency room care, 380
hyperbaric oxygen, 384
immediate first aid, 378–379
in-hospital monitoring and therapy, 382–383
respiratory care, 380–382
transportation, emergency, 379
Dynamics, gas flow lungs, 74–80
Dysbaric osteonecrosis, 14, 256, 291–292, 397–405
description, 397–398
diagnosis, radiology, 398–400
etiology, 402–403
pathology, 402
protocol radiographic examination, 513–514

Subject Index

Dysbaric osteonecrosis (*cont.*)
  therapy, 401–402
  x-ray procedures, 403–405
Dysbarism: *see* Decompression sickness

Ear
  anatomy, 4–6, 193–194
  barotrauma, 60–61, 193, 409–416
  diving physical examination, 495–497
  external ear canal, 414
  inner ear decompression sickness, 312–316
  inner ear barotrauma, 414–416
  inner ear injury stable depths, 417–418
  middle ear barotrauma, 409–414
  noise, 418
  otitis externa, 416–417
  otologic barotrauma, 409–416
  physiology, 4–7, 193–195
Elastic recoil, 71
Electrical safety, 592
Electrolyte changes in drowning, 371–374
Electrolyte metabolism in divers, 186–187
Embolism
  cause, 349–350
  cause of pulmonary, 23, 344–347
  cerebral gas, 340–344
  emergency evaluation, 276
  emergency therapy, 276–277
  gas, 67, 333–361
  intravascular gaseous, 336–344
  therapy, 354–361
  see also Arterial gas embolism; Pulmonary barotrauma; Venous gas embolism
Emergency
  care of diving casualties, 273–280
  diagnosis, 275
  diving casualty evaluation, 273–280
  therapy under pressure, 445–459
Emergency medical technicians: *see* Diving medics
Emergency telephone numbers, 306–308
Emphysema
  mediastinal, 66
  subcutaneous, 66
  pulmonary interstitial, 334
Emotional stability and diving, 576–577
Energy
  and diving, 57–60, 178–186
  of food, 178–181
Environment
  natural diving, 6–11
  man-made diving, 12–32
  diving, 568
  natural hazards, 579–580
  on-site (traffic, sonar, radioactivity), 581
  object, 581–583

Equipment
  anesthesia surgery, 362–363
  diving, 584, 601–660
  scuba, 629–644
  air supplied diving, 645–649
  mixed gas diving, 651–654
Erysipelothrix, marine infection, 429
Eupneic pressure, 89
Evaporation
  heat, 60
  heat loss, 154
Exercise, heat production, 163–165
Excursion diving, 6, 657–660
Experimental Diving Unit, 606
Expiratory reserve volume (ERV), 87–88
Explosives underwater, 422
Eye
  bubble in viper's eye, 223
  and diving, 199–204
  diving physical examination, 497–498

Facilities, hyperbaric, 12–32
Fat: *see* Adipose tissue; Obesity
Fatigue
  diving, 572–575
  stress, 537–538
Female: *see* Women
Fetus, effect of diving on, 140–143
Fins, diving, 637–638
Fire safety, 25, 592
Flying after diving, 590–591
Food, energy value, 179–181
Fouling, diving hazard, 582
Function
  circulatory, 81–84
  respiratory, 71–84
Functional residual capacity, lung (FRC), 71–87

Gas
  compression in lung, 71–73
  characteristics, 54–56
  contamination, 273, 582
  cylinders, 23–24, 630–632
  density in lung, 80, 101–102
  exchange in lung, 80
  expansion in lung, 71–73
  flow dynamics in lung, 74–80
  inert narcosis, 128–134
  intravascular gaseous emboli, 336–344
  laws, 49–54
  pathophysiology, diving, 37–49
  storage, 23–24
  toxic, unconscious diver, 393
  trapping, 333–334
Gas gangrene, 428

Gastric pressure, 95–97
Gastrointestinal
  barotrauma, 66
  blast damage, 424
  immersion effects, 95–97
Gauge pressure, 36
General gas law, 51–52
Glycerol, decompression sickness therapy, 279
Gravity, effects in water, 86
Greek sponge divers, 284

Habitat
  diving, 660
  thermal balance, 169–175
  undersea, 30–32, 595–596
Haldane, J. S.
  decompression theory, 229–237
Half time concept, 230–234
Harbor diving, 7–8
Hazards, diving, 568
Hearing measurement, 194
Heart
  breath-hold diving, 217
  cold immersion, 157–163
  immersion, 91–94
  patent foramen ovale, 337
  rate, 104–105
    monitoring, 146–147
Heat
  comfort zone, 156
  conduction, 59
  convection, 60
  in diving, 58–60
  evaporation, 60
  exchange, 153–156
  radiation, 60
  specific heat, 59
  temperature, 59
  transfer coefficient, 156–157
  see also Heat exchange; Heat loss; Heat production; Temperature; Thermal balance
Heat exchange
  air at 1 atm, 153–156
  helium-oxygen, 172–175
Heat loss
  blood flow, 162–163
  convective, 154–155
  diving, 156–164
  evaporation, 154
  exercise, 163–165
  immersion, 7–9, 157–159
  radiation, 155
  respiratory tract, 155
  skin, 155
  wet suit protection, 159–163

Heat production
  exercise, 163–165
  see also Metabolism
Heliox diving, 264
Helium
  deep dives, 78
  description, 42–43
  early work, 606
  gas density, 101–102
  heart rate, 104–105
  heliox diving, 264
  narcosis, 130
Hematology in drowning, 376
Henry's law, 54
Hepatitis, polluted water, 408
High pressure nervous syndrome (HPNS), 109–126
  adaptation, 120
  alcohol consumption, 188
  compression rate, 117–118
  excursions, 118–120
  inert gas effects, 133–134
  narcotic agents, 120–126
  susceptibility, 117
History of decompression sickness, 283–287
Hot water diving garment, 649
Humidity, 24
Hydration in decompression sickness, 278–279
Hydrogen
  diving gas, 43
  narcosis, 131
Hydrostatic pressure, 36–37
  respiratory effects, 87–91
  heart rate, 102, 104
Hyperbaric
  arthralgia, 190–192
  cardiovascular effects, 99–107
  effects on drugs, 445
  environmental, thermal balance
    dry, 169–175
    wet, 175–176
  facilities, 12–32
  oxygen therapy, chambers, 608–609
  oxygen therapy, drowning, 384
Hypercapnia: *see* Carbon dioxide
Hyperglycemia in unconscious diver, 392
Hyperthermia in unconscious diver, 394
Hyperventilation, 3, 394
  panic reaction, 558–559
Hypothermia
  immersion, cold water, 165–167
  symptoms, 165–166
  treatment, 166–167
  unconscious diver, 394
Hyperventilation, stress, 560

Hypoxia
  of ascent, 212
  drowning, 372–373
  respiratory stimulus, 81
  unconscious diver, 392
  see also Oxygen

Ice, diving under, 10–11, 596–597
Immersion
  buoyancy effects, 97
  circulatory function, 91–94
  diuresis, 94
  effects, 86–87
  gastrointestinal system effects, 95–97
  heat loss, 7–9, 157–159
  hypothermia, 166–167
  natriuresis, 94
  renal effects, 94–95
Inert gas
  narcotic effect, 128–134
  and HPNS, 133–134
Inherent unsaturation, 253–254
Infection
  diving related, 577
  marine microorganisms, 427–431
  polluted water diving, 406–409
Inner ear: see Ear
Inner ear decompression sickness, 312–316
  animal studies, 314
  human studies, 313–314
  relation to central nervous system, 313
  therapy, 314–316
Interaction of drugs with environment, 448–449
  clinical application, 448–459
  anesthetic, 479–481
  and diving, 570–571
Intrauterine devices and diving, 138
Intubation, tracheal, 464–466

Jaminet, A.
  physician St. Louis bridge, 284–285
Joint
  lubrication, 191–192
  pain, 190–192

K-value, 231, 253
Kaliuresis, 95
Kelp diving, 8–9
Kidneys, function after near-drowning, 376

Laboratory, ocean floor, 5
Lake diving, 7
Laws, gas, 47–54
Leptospirosis, 408
Light
  absorption underwater, 201–203
  distortion underwater, 190–200

Light (cont.)
  in diving, 57–58
  refraction underwater, 199
  scatter underwater, 201–203
Lock
  long, 13
  man, 13
  medical, 13
  mud, 13
  pass-through, 13
Lung
  anatomical changes, drowning, 373–374
  barotrauma, 66–67, 72–80, 333–340
  blast effect, 424
  drowning pathology, 373–374
  dynamics of gas flow, 74–80
  effects of pressure, 71–80
  function, monitoring, 71–84
  funcitonal residual capacity (FRC), 71, 87
  maximum voluntary ventilation (MVV), 78–80
  residual volume (RV), 71
  squeeze, 72
  total lung capacity (TLC), 71
  vital capacity (VC), 71, 87
  volume measurement, 71
  see also Pulmonary; Pulmonary barotrauma
Lymphatic symptoms in decompression sickness, 288–289

M-value, 247–248
Mammals
  dive reflex, 206–207
  diving, 73
Marijuana and heat loss, 168
Marine microorganisms, infection from, 427–431
Marine organisms
  algae, 431
  Dogger Bank itch, 431
  nematocyst, 432
  red tide, 431
  sponges, 432
Marine trauma, treatment, 436–437
Masks, diving, 636, 646
Maximum voluntary ventilation (MVV), 77
Mediastinal emphysema, 66, 67, 334–336
Medic: see Diving medic
Medical
  examination, commercial divers, 515–516
  hyperbaric facilities, 26
Menstruation and diving, 138–139
Metabolism
  cold adaptation, 181
  electrolyte, 186–187
  energy, ama, 181
  energy, divers, 181–186
  saturation divers, 183–186

Microbes, diver, 406
Middle ear: see Ear
Mixed gas diving, 2, 651-654
Moisture, gas, 55
Monitor
    cardiovascular, 146-147
    design requirements, 145
    Doppler, 149-152
Monitoring
    cardiovascular, 146-147
    Doppler, 149-152
    heart rate, 147
    pulmonary, 147-148
    temperature, 148-149
    vital signs, 144-152
Monoplace chambers, 26, 621-625
    application, 624
    maintenance, 624
    safety, 624
    system description, 621-624
Multiplace chambers, 26, 601-621
Musculoskeletal
    diving physical examination, 504-505
    symptoms decompression sickness, 289-290

Narcosis
    argon, 130
    clinical use, 134
    effects quantification, 131
    helium, 130
    mechanism of action, 132-133
    nitrogen, 128-130
    xenon, 130
Natriuresis
    immersion, 94
    saturation diving, 185-186
Near-drowning: see Drowning
Neon, 43
    narcosis, 131
Nervous system, autonomic
    heart rate, 104-105
Neurological, decompression sickness, 290-291, 316-326
Nitrogen
    description, 41
    in diving, 42
    heart rate, 104-105
    narcosis, 128-130
    pathophysiology, 41-42
    vision underwater, 204
No-decompression dive, 2
No-D dive, 2

Obesity, diver, 572
Ocean diving, 6-7
Octopus, 434
Octopus rig, 636
Oral contraceptives and diving, 138
Osteonecrosis: see Dysbaric osteonecrosis
Otitis externa, 416-417
Otologic barotrauma, 192-193, 409-416
    see also Barotrauma
Otorhinolaryngeal drugs, 452-455
Overinflation, pulmonary, 333-336
Oxygen
    breath-hold diving, 2-3, 206-220
    central nervous system damage, 40, 296
    decompression, 253, 254
    description, 38-39
    hyperbaric therapy, drowning, 384
    hypoxia, drowning, 372-373
    life support, 24
    metabolism, 179-181
    partial pressure, 39, 100-101
    pathophysiology, 38-41
    pulmonary toxicity, 40
    saturation diving, 658
    therapy gas embolism, 357-358
    toxicity, 39-41
    uses, 41
    vision underwater, 203-204
    window, 254
    see also Hypoxia

Panic
    behavioral reactions, 555-558
    diver, 553-560
    physiological events, 558-560
Paranasal sinus barotrauma, 418-420
Patent foramen ovale, 337
Partial pressure, 37
    of oxygen, 39, 100-101
Pathophysiology
    carbon dixoide, 43-47
    carbon monoxide, 47-49
    diving gases, 37-47
    nitrogen, 41-42
    oxygen, 41-42
Performance, women diving, 136
Perfusion, 248-254
Personnel transfer capsule (PTC), 19
Pharyngoconjunctival fever, 408
Physical examination
    age, 494
    alimentary system, 503-504
    body build, 494
    cardiovascular system, 502-503
    diving, 489-518
    ear, nose, throat, 495-497
    eyes, 497-498
    musculoskeletal system, 504-505
    nervous system, 494-495

Physical examination (*cont.*)
  respiratory system, 497-502
  sex, 494
  skin, 505-506
Physical fitness to dive, 506-507, 575-576
Physical standards
  commercial diving, 490-491
  military, diving, 490
  recreational diving, 491-492
  scientific and technical diving, 491
  semiprofessional, 491
Physics of pressure, 35-68
Physiology
  diving, 71-221
  stress, 531-565
Pneumomediastinum: *see* Mediastinal emphysema
Pneumopericardium, 334
Pneumoperitoneum, 334
Pneumothorax, 66, 73, 334-336
  spontaneous, 441-443
Poisonous marine organisms, 431-436
Polluted water diving, 9
  infection, 408-409
  hazard, 582-583
Pregnancy and diving, 140-143, 309-310
Pressure
  effects on diver, 60-68, 225
  effects on heart rate, 102-104
  hydrostatic, 102-104
  nomenclature, 36
  physics, 35-68
  pulmonary, 71-81
  transpulmonary, 73
  units, 36
  visual effects, 204
  see also Partial pressure; Inert gas
Protective clothing, 640-643, 647-649
  hot water inner garment, 649
Psychological
  age, 523
  diver social skills, 525-527
  mechanical aptitude, 520
  selection research, 520-521
  social adjustment, 524
  standards in diving, 520-529
  tests, 522-525
Puffer poisoning, 436
Pulmonary
  breath-hold diving, 72-73, 206-220
  function, 87-90
  gas exchange, 80
  interstitial emphysema, 334
  monitoring, 147-148
  overinflation, 38, 333-336
  oxygen toxicity, 39-40

Pulmonary (*cont.*)
  see also Lung; Pulmonary barotrauma;
    Respiration and respiratory
Pulmonary barotrauma, 66-67, 72-80, 333-349
  blast effect, 424
  definitions, 333-334
  diagnosis, 347-349
  etiology, 72-80, 344-347
  pneumothorax, 66, 73, 334-336
Pulse rate: *see* Heart rate

Quads, 23

Radiation
  diving hazard, 581
  heat, 60
Radiographic examination, dysbaric osteonecrosis, 513-514
Recompression
  chamber, 26, 583, 601-625
  gas embolism, 355-356
  therapy, 601-619
Refraction of light under water, 199-201
Regulators, diving equipment, 633-636
Renal
  diuresis, immersion, 94
  function in drowning, 376
  immersion effects, 94-95
  kaliuresis, 95
  natriuresis, 94
Rescue chambers, 28-30, 595
Residual volume, lung (RV), 71
Respiration and respiratory
  breath-hold diving, 206-217
  carbon dioxide, 81-84
  diving, 71-84
  diving physical, 497-502
  function, 87-90
  heat loss, 28
  immersion effects, 87-91
  inspiratory force, 93
  model, 76
  quotient (RQ), 44, 179-180
  symptoms, decompression, sickness, 291
  system, 71-84
  work, 89
Resuscitation, drowning, 378
River diving, 7
Rupture, lung, 72-73

Safety
  diver, 567-600
  precautions, 578-579
Saturation diving
  basic forms, 266

Saturation diving (cont.)
  cardiovascular effects, 106
  deep diving, 654–660
  description, 4–6
  systems, 20–21
Scombroid poisoning, 435
Scuba
  community, 626–627
  development, 625–626
  diving, 3–4, 607, 625–644
  equipment, 629–644
  procedures, 627–629
Sea snake envenomization, 434–435
Sedatives, decompression sickness therapy, 280
Selection, diving, 520, 569–578
Sex
  diving physical examination, 494
  of offspring of divers, 143
Shallow water blackout, unconsciousness, 394
Shock, decompression sickness, 291
Signals
  diver warning, 584–585
  flags, 585
  hand, 587–588
  lights, 585
  line, 586
Sinus
  barotrauma, 67, 418–420
  paranasal, 418–420
Skin
  diving physical examination, 505–506
  heat loss, 155
  infection, polluted water, 406–409, 582–583
Smoking
  carbon monoxide toxicity, 48
  cigarettes, 571–572
Snorkels, diving, 637
Snorkel swimming, 93
Sonar, diving hazard, 581
Sound in diving, 58
Specific heat, 59
Squeeze, 67–68
  lung, 72
Steroids
  decompression sickness therapy, 279
St. Louis bridge, caisson work, 13, 284–285, 602
Stress
  cardiovascular effects of, 544–546
  cold, 538–544
  concept, 531–534
  diver panic, 553–560
  diving accidents, 546–553
  fatigue, 537–538
  hazards, 549–553
  motivation, 536

Stress (cont.)
  physical factors, 557–544
  physiology, 531–565
  training to alleviate, 534–536
Subcutaneous emphysema, 67
Submarines
  escape, 594–595
  escape training
    pulmonary barotrauma, 334–335
  rescue, 595
Submarine Escape Training Tank, 605–606
Submersibles, 595–596
  decompression chamber, 19
Surface decompression, 15, 244
Surface supplied diving, 4, 645–660
Surgery, anesthesia under pressure, 460–485
System
  certification, 22
  deep diving, 5, 20
  diving, 16–25
  one atmosphere, 21
  saturation, 5, 20

Table calculation, diving, 229–248
  New York tunnel, 13–14
  U.S. Navy initiative, 242–248
Tanks, scuba diving, 630–633
Teeth, pain, 68
Taktite II, saturation selection, 527
Temperature
  critical water, 156–157
  heat, 59
  monitoring, 148–149
  water, 11
Tetanus, marine infection, 428
Therapy
  diving accidents
    emergency care, 274–275
    emergency evaluation, 273
    immediate action, 275
  drowning, 378–385
  drugs, 448–459
  gas embolism, 354–361
  hyperbaric oxygen (HBO), 41
  see also Drowning therapy
Thermal
  balance
    dry hyperbaric environment, 169–175
    water at one atmosphere, 156–169
    wet hyperbaric environment, 175–176
  considerations
    diving, 153–176
  protection
    wet suits, 9–11, 159–162
Tissue saturation rates, 230–233

Tolerance, cold water diving, 156–162
Toothache, 68
Total lung capacity (TLC), 71
Training
  diver, 570
  stress alleviation, 534–536
Transfer capsule, personnel, 19
Transpulmonic pressure, 335
Treatment: *see* Therapy
Tube skid, 23
Tunnels, 12–14, 238, 254–258
  decompression, 286
Types of diving, 1–6
Typhoid, polluted water, 408

Ultrasound, 149–152
Umbilical, 35
Unconscious diver, 391–397
  environmental factors, 392–394
  physiological factors, 394–395
  predisposing conditions, 392
  recovering, 395–396
  resuscitation, 396–397
Units of pressure, 36
Urea excretion, saturation dive, 185–186
Urine: *see* Renal
U.S. Navy diving tables, 242–248
U.S. Navy Experimental Diving Unit, 606

Venous gas embolism, 336–337
Venomous marine organisms, 431–436
Ventilation
  control, 81–84
  immersion, 87–91
  see also Respiration and respiratory
Vertigo
  breath-hold diving, 219
  diving, 68, 196–198
Vestibular function
  in diving, 68, 195–198
  vertigo, 68, 196–198
Viscosity, gas, 55–56
Visibility underwater, 199–204
  see also Vision underwater
Vision underwater
  color perception, 203

Vision underwater (*cont.*)
  correction, 201
  distance estimation, 199–200
  distortion, 200–201
  hyperbaric oxygen, 203–204
  loss of, 199
  nitrogen effects, 204
  physiological factors, 203–204
  pressure effects, 204
Vital capacity (VC), 71, 87
Vital signs monitoring, 144–152
Voice communication, 146
Vomiting underwater, 96

Water
  temperature and drowning, 370
  vapor diffusion coefficients, 171
Weight loss in saturation diving, 183–184
Weightlessness, 86
Welding chamber, 30–32
Wet pot, 27
Wet suit
  thermal protection, 9–11, 159–162, 640–642, 647–648
  see also Protective clothing
Women
  decompression sickness, 137–138
  diving, 136–139
  fat burden, 137
  intrauterine devices, 138
  menstruation, 138–139
  oral contraceptives, 138
  physical performance, 136
  pregnancy, 140–143
  specific diving, 136
  sex of offspring, 143
  shark attack, 143
  sport diving 136
  work underwater, 136
Work, return to diving after decompression sickness, 328–331
Wreck diving, 9–10

Xenon narcosis, 130
X-ray protocol, lumbosacral spine, 510–513